D1208808

Clinical
Sleep Disorders

Clinical Sleep Disorders

EDITORS

PAUL R. CARNEY, MD, DABSM

Assistant Professor of Pediatrics, Neurology, Neuroscience, and Bioengineering Chief, Division of Pediatric Neurology; Director, Comprehensive Pediatric Epilepsy and Neurophysiology Program, University of Florida College of Medicine and McKnight Brain Institute, Gainesville, Florida

RICHARD B. BERRY, MD, DABSM

Professor of Medicine, Pulmonary and Critical Care Division, University of Florida; Staff Physician and Medical Director of the Sleep Laboratory, Malcom Randall Veterans Affairs Medical Center; Medical Director, Sleep Disorders Center, Shands at AGH, Gainesville, Florida

JAMES D. GEYER, MD, DABSM

Director of Sleep Medicine and Clinical Neurophysiology, Neurology Consultants, PC, Tuscaloosa, Alabama; Director of Sleep Medicine and Epilepsy, The Alabama Neurologic Institute, Birmingham, Alabama

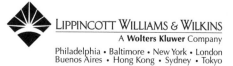

LIPPINCOTT WILLIAMS & WILKINS
A **Wolters Kluwer** Company
Philadelphia • Baltimore • New York • London
Buenos Aires • Hong Kong • Sydney • Tokyo

Acquisitions Editor: Anne M. Sydor
Developmental Editor: Scott Scheidt
Production Manager: Nicole Walz
Senior Manufacturing Manager: Ben Rivera
Marketing Manager: Adam Glazer
Design Coordinator: Holly McLaughlin
Cover Designer: Armen Kojoyian
Production Service: TechBooks
Printer: Maple Press

© 2005 by LIPPINCOTT WILLIAMS & WILKINS
530 Walnut Street
Philadelphia, PA 19106 USA
LWW.com

Library of Congress Cataloging-in-Publication Data
Clinical sleep disorders / editors, Paul R. Carney, Richard B. Berry, James D. Geyer.
 p. ; cm.
 Includes bibliographical references and index.
 ISBN 0-7817-4637-X (case)
 1. Sleep disorders. 2. Sleep—Physiological aspects. I. Carney, Paul R.
II. Berry, Richard B., 1947- III. Geyer, James D.
 [DNLM: 1. Sleep Disorders. 2. Sleep—physiology. WM 188 C6422 2005]
RC547.C565 2005
616.8′498—dc22
                                        2004021488

10 9 8 7 6 5 4 3 2 1

To my beautiful wife, Lucia, and to my daughters, Paulina and Constanza, who endured the many hours of my absence, and to my parents for their love and wisdom.

—PC

To my lovely wife, Cathy, and to my children, David and Sarah. They are my greatest joy. I also dedicate the book to the loving memory of my parents, Dr. Louie and Sarah Berry.

—RB

Dedicated to my beautiful daughters, Sydney and Emery, and to my wife, Stephenie, for her support and assistance. A special thanks to my parents. I hope that this book will honor the memory of my mentor in sleep medicine, Mike Aldrich.

—JG

CONTENTS

It has been estimated that 20 percent of adults and children have sleep disordered symptoms and signs; however, internists, pediatricians, family physicians, and house staff report considerable difficulty in managing the most common sleep conditions, and promptly refer patients to the sleep specialist. In the last decade, significant diagnostic and therapeutic advances have been made for a number of conditions such as sleep disordered breathing, insomnia, sleepiness, and associated cardiovascular and neurological disorders. Since office practice is demanding and fast-paced, practitioners must have access to current evaluations and treatment recommendations in a format that lends itself to speedy review and increases their confidence as principal care providers.

The goal of *Clinical Sleep Disorders* is to write a comprehensive and current text, and provide sleep specialists and primary care providers with succinct authoritative reviews on the evaluation and treatment of sleep disorders. The book is designed to meet the rigorous demands of a wide range of readers, including physicians from all specialties involved in sleep medicine, resident house-staff, nurses, respiratory therapists, sleep technologists, and students. Whether the patient is managed independently by the primary care physician or referred to the sleep specialist, the book is intended to improve satisfaction of both the patient, the sleep specialist, and the primary care physician.

The first section of the book, *Understanding Normal Sleep*, reviews the neurobiology of human sleep, breathing during wakefulness and sleep, dreaming, and sleep ontogeny. In the second section, *Symptomatic Sleep Problems*, we include a review of the evaluation and treatment of conditions encountered in the outpatient setting, including the approach to the sleepy patient and sleep deprivation, approach to the patient with problems initiating sleep, approach to restless legs, and approach to nocturnal spells. The third section, *Sleep Disorders*, reviews specific sleep conditions, including obstructive sleep apnea, upper airway resistance syndrome, central sleep apnea, periodic legs syndrome, parasomnias, narcolepsy, idiopathic hypersomnia, chronobiologic sleep disorders, and pediatric sleep disorders. In the fourth section, *Sleep Related Medical and Neurological Disorders*, we review the evaluation and treatment of sleep disorders and dementia and related degenerative diseases, diencephalic and brainstem sleep disorders, sleep and epilepsy, and sleep and medical disorders. In the *Appendix Section*, we review methodology and technical problems and solutions related to polysomnography, the multiple sleep latency test, CPAP/BiPAP, airway pressure methodologies, specific sleep related questionnaires, and how to develop a sleep laboratory/center. The book will have met its overall objective if practical state-of-the-art management advice is provided to a busy physician.

Carney PR, Berry R, Geyer J.

ACKNOWLEDGMENTS

The editors would like to thank the patients, their families, the nurses, and the laboratory technicians who helped make this book possible. We would also like to thank Anne Sydor and Scott Scheidt of Lippincott Williams & Wilkins for their excellent editorial support and guidance on this project, and we would like to thank Ms. Chris Grimm of the University of Florida for her excellent secretarial support.

CONTRIBUTORS

Richard P. Allen
Department of Neurology and Sleep Medicine,
Johns Hopkins University, Bayview Medical Center,
Baltimore, Maryland

W. McDowell Anderson
Division of Pulmonary and Critical Care Medicine,
University of South Florida; James A. Haley VA Hospital,
Tampa, Florida

Arthur Andrews
Division of Pulmonary and Critical Care Medicine,
University of South Florida; James A. Haley VA Hospital,
Tampa, Florida

Charles Bae
Cleveland Clinic Foundation, Department of Neurology,
Section of Sleep Medicine,
Cleveland, Ohio

M. Safwan Badr
Division of Pulmonary, Critical Care, and Sleep Medicine,
Department of Internal Medicine,
Wayne State University School of Medicine,
Detroit, Michigan

Danielle Becker
Department of Clinical and Health Psychology,
University of Florida,
Gainesville, Florida

Selim R. Benbadis
Departments of Neurology and Neurosurgery;
Comprehensive Epilepsy Program,
University of South Florida College of Medicine,
Tampa, Florida

Richard B. Berry
Professor of Medicine,
Pulmonary and Critical Care Division,
University of Florida;
Staff Physician and Medical Director of the Sleep
    Laboratory,
Malcom Randall Veterans Affairs Medical Center;
Medical Director, Sleep Disorders Center, Shands at AGH,
Gainesville, Florida

Bradley F. Boeve
Department of Neurology and Sleep Disorders Center,
Mayo Clinic College of Medicine,
Rochester, Minnesota

Susan Bongiolatti
University of Florida, Gainesville, Florida

Paul R. Carney
Assistant Professor of Pediatrics, Neurology,
    Neuroscience, and Bioengineering Chief,
Division of Pediatric Neurology;
Director, Comprehensive pediatric Epilepsy and
    Neurophysiology Program,
University of Florida College of Medicine and
    McKnight Brain Institute,
Gainesville Florida

Nancy Collop
Department of Medicine, Johns Hopkins University,
Baltimore, Maryland

David G. Davila
Sleep Disorders Center, Baptist Medical Center,
Little Rock, Arkansas

O'Neill F. D'Cruz
Department of Neurology,
University of North Carolina-Chapel Hill,
Chapel Hill, North Carolina

Stephenie Dillard
Cytopath, Pelham, Alabama

Stephan Eisenschenk
Department of Neurology, University of Florida,
Gainesville, Florida

Nancy Foldvary-Schaefer
Cleveland Clinic Foundation,
Department of Neurology,
Section of Sleep Medicine,
Cleveland, Ohio

Runi Foster
University of Florida College of Medicine,
Gainesville, Florida

James D. Geyer
Director of Sleep Medicine and
    Clinical Neurophysiology,
Neurology Consultants, PC,
Tuscaloosa, Alabama;
Director of Sleep Medicine and Epilepsy,
The Alabama Neurologic Institute,
Birmingham, Alabama

Robin Gilmore
Department of Neurology, University of Florida,
Gainesville, Florida

Susan M. Harding
Division of Pulmonary, Allergy, and Critical Care
    Medicine,
University of Alabama at Birmingham,
Birmingham, Alabama

Jeffrey W. Hawkins
Division of Pulmonary, Allergy, and Critical Care
    Medicine,
University of Alabama at Birmingham,
Birmingham, Alabama

Linda F. Hayward
University of Florida College of Veterinary Medicine and
    McKnight Brain Institute,
Gainesville, Florida

Andrew D. Krystal
Department of Psychiatry, Duke University
    Medical Center,
Durham, North Carolina

Kasey K. Li
Stanford Sleep Disorders Clinic and Facial
    Reconstructive Surgical and Medical Center,
Stanford, California

Kenneth Lichstein
Department of Psychology, University of Memphis,
Memphis, Tennessee

Atul Malhotra
Brigham and Women's Hospital,
Boston, Massachusetts

Vaughn McCall
Department of Psychiatry, Wake Forest University School
    of Medicine,
Winston Salem, North Carolina

Sidney Nau
Department of Psychology, University of Memphis,
Memphis, Tennessee

Wendy Norman
Department of Pediatrics, University of Florida,
Gainesville, Florida

Juan Ochoa
Department of Neurology, University of Florida,
Jacksonville, Florida

Lyle J. Olson
Mayo Clinic College of Medicine,
Rochester, Minnesota

Jennifer Parr
DCH Regional Medical Center Sleep Laboratory,
Tuscaloosa, Alabama

Troy A. Payne
Neurology Clinic of St. Cloud, Director of Adolescent
    Sleep Medicine and Epilepsy Monitoring Laboratory,
St. Cloud Hospital, St. Cloud, Minnesota

Barbara Phillips
Pulmonary Division, University of Kentucky
    Medical Center,
Lexington, Kentucky

Mario Pulido
Department of Neurology, University of Florida,
Jacksonville, Florida

Kathryn Reid
Northwestern University, Center for Sleep and
    Circadian Biology,
Evanston, Illinois

Deborah M. Ringdahl
Division of Pediatric Neurology
Department of Pediatrics
University of Florida College of Medicine,
Gainesville, Florida

James A. Rowley
Associate Professor of Medicine, Division of Pulmonary,
    Critical Care, and Sleep Medicine,
Department of Internal Medicine,
Wayne State University School of Medicine,
Detroit, Michigan

Mark H. Sanders
University of Pittsburgh Medical Center,
Montefiore University Hospital,
Pittsburgh, Pennsylvania

Wolfgang W. Schmidt-Nowara
Sleep Medicine Associates of Texas,
Dallas, Texas

Betty J. Seals
DCH Regional Medical Center,
Tuscaloosa, Alabama

Edward J. Stepanski
Director, Sleep Disorder Service and Research Center,
Rush University Medical Center,
Chicago, Illinois

Michael H. Silber
Department of Neurology and Sleep Disoreder Center,
Mayo Clinic College of Medicine,
Rochester, Minnesota

Christie G. Snively
Division of Pediatric Neurology
Department of Pediatrics
University of Florida College of Medicine,
Gainesville, Florida

Virend K. Somers
Division of Cardiovascular Diseases, Department of
    Internal Medicine, Mayo Clinic College of Medicine,
Rochester, Minnesota

David Surhbier
Division of Pediatric Neurology, University of Florida,
Gainesville, Florida

Anna Svatikova
Mayo Clinic College of Medicine,
Rochester, Minnesota

Mugdha Thakkur
Department of Psychiatry, Duke University
    Medical Center,
Durham, North Carolina

Bradley V. Vaughn
Department of Neurology, University of
    North Carolina-Chapel Hill,
Chapel Hill, North Carolina

David P. White
Brigham and Women's Hospital,
Boston, Massachusetts

Phyllis Zee
Northwestern University, Feinberg School of Medicine,
Chicago, Illinois

Introduction

Chapter 1

Introduction to Sleep and Sleep Monitoring—The Basics

Richard B. Berry, James D. Geyer, and Paul R. Carney

OVERVIEW OF SLEEP STAGES AND CYCLES

Sleep is not homogeneous and is characterized by sleep stages based on electroencephalographic (EEG) or electrical brain wave activity, electro-oculographic (EOG) or eye movements, and electromyographic (EMG) or muscle electrical activity (1–3). The basic terminology and methods involved with monitoring each of these types of activity will be discussed below. Sleep is composed of nonrapid eye movement (NREM) and rapid eye movement (REM) sleep. NREM sleep is further divided into stages 1, 2, 3, and 4. Stages 1 and 2 are called light sleep and stages 3 and 4 are called deep or slow-wave sleep. There are usually four or five cycles of sleep, each composed of a segment of NREM sleep followed by REM sleep. Periods of wake may also interrupt sleep during the night. As the night progresses, the length of REM sleep in each cycle usually increases. The hypnogram (Fig. 1-1) is a convenient method of graphically displaying the organization of sleep during the night. Each stage of sleep is characterized by a level on the vertical axis of the graph with time of night on the horizontal axis. REM sleep is often highlighted by a dark bar.

Sleep monitoring was traditionally by polygraph recording using ink-writing pens which produced tracings on paper. It was convenient to divide the night into epochs of time that correspond to the length of each paper page. The usual paper speed for sleep recording is 10 mm/s; a 30-cm page corresponds to 30 seconds. Each segment of time represented by one page is called an epoch; sleep is staged in epochs. Today most sleep recording is performed digitally, but the convention of scoring sleep in 30-second

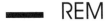

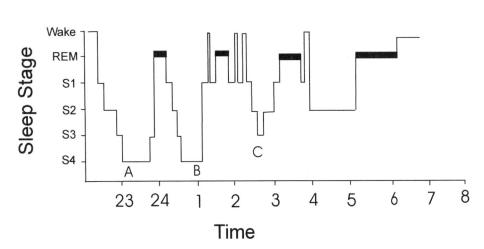

FIGURE 1-1. Normal hypnogram: The various stages of sleep are represented by levels on the vertical axis; time of night is shown on the horizontal axis. In this patient there were four sleep cycles each composed of a segment of NREM sleep followed by REM sleep. The length of REM sleep increased toward morning. Conversely, most of the stage 3 and 4 sleep was in the early portion of the night. (From Berry RB. *Sleep medicine pearls* 2nd ed. Philadelphia: Hanley and Belfus, 2003:29. With permission.)

epochs or windows is still the standard. If there is a shift in sleep stage during a given epoch, the stage present for the majority of the time names the epoch. When the tracings used to stage sleep are obscured by artifact for more than one-half of an epoch, it is scored as movement time (MT). When an epoch of what would otherwise be considered MT is surrounded by epochs of wake, the epoch is also scored as wake. Some sleep centers consider MT to be wake and do not tabulate it separately.

SLEEP ARCHITECTURE DEFINITIONS

The term sleep architecture describes the structure of sleep. Common terms used in sleep monitoring are listed in Table 1-1. The total monitoring time or total recording time (TRT) is also called total bedtime (TBT). This is the time duration from lights out (start of recording) to lights on (termination of recording). The total amount of sleep

stages 1, 2, 3, 4, REM, and MT is termed the *total sleep time* (TST). The time from the first sleep until the final awakening is called the *sleep period time* (SPT). SPT encompasses all sleep as well as periods of wake after sleep onset and before the final awakening. This wake time is termed the WASO (wake after sleep onset). Therefore, SPT = TST + WASO. The time from the start of sleep monitoring (or lights out) until the first epoch of sleep is called the *sleep latency*. The time from the first epoch of sleep until the first REM sleep is called the *REM latency*. It is useful to determine not only the total minutes of each sleep stage, but also to characterize the relative proportion of time spent in each sleep stage. One can characterize stages 1 to 4 and REM as a percentage of total sleep time (%TST). Another method is to characterize the sleep stages and WASO as a percentage of the sleep period time (%SPT). Sleep efficiency (in percent) is usually defined as either the TST × 100/SPT or TST × 100/TBT.

The normal range of the percentage of sleep spent in each sleep stage varies with age (2,3) and is impacted by sleep disorders (Table 1-2). In adults there is a decrease in stage 3 and 4 sleep with increasing age, while the amount of REM sleep remains fairly constant. The amounts of stage 1 sleep and WASO also increases with age. In patients with

▶ **TABLE 1-1. Sleep Architecture Definitions**

- Lights out—start of sleep recording
- Light on—end of sleep recording
- TBT (total bedtime time)—time from lights out to lights on
- TST (total sleep time) = minutes of stages 1, 2, 3, 4, and REM
- WASO (wake after sleep onset)—minutes of wake after first sleep but before the final awakening
- SPT (sleep period time) = TST + WASO
- Sleep latency—time from lights out until the first epoch of sleep
- REM latency—time from first epoch of sleep to the first epoch of REM sleep
- Sleep efficiency—(TST × 100)/TBT
- Stage 1, 2, 3, 4, and REM as % TST—percentage of TST occupied by each sleep stage
- Stage 1, 2, 3, 4, and REM, WASO as % SPT—percentage of SPT occupied by sleep stages and WASO

▶ **TABLE 1-2. Representative Changes in Sleep Architecture**

	20-Year-Old	60-Year-Old	Severe Sleep Apnea
WASO%SPT	5	15	20
1% SPT	5	5	10
2% SPT	50	55	60
3 and, 4%SPT	20	5	0
REM%SPT	25	20	10

severe obstructive sleep apnea there is often no stage 3 and 4 sleep and a reduced amount of REM sleep. Chronic insomnia (difficulty initiating or maintaining sleep) is characterized by a long sleep latency and increased WASO. The amount of stages 3 and 4 and REM sleep is commonly decreased as well. The REM latency is also affected by sleep disorders and medications. A short REM latency (usually <70 minutes) is noted in some cases of sleep apnea, depression, narcolepsy, prior REM sleep deprivation, and the withdrawal of REM suppressant medications. An increased REM latency can be seen with REM suppressants (ethanol and many antidepressants), an unfamiliar or uncomfortable sleep environment, sleep apnea, and any process that disturbs sleep quality.

DIFFERENTIAL AMPLIFIERS, DIGITAL POLYSOMNOGRAPHY, SENSITIVITY, AND FILTERS

EEG, EOG, and EMG activity is recorded by differential AC amplifiers that amplify the difference in voltage between two inputs (Fig. 1-2). Signals common to both inputs are not amplified (common mode rejection). This permits the recording of very small signals that are superimposed upon larger scalp-voltage changes and 60-cycle interference from nearby AC power lines. Common mode rejection depends on the impedance at input 1 and input 2, being relatively equal (4,5). A poorly conducting electrode (high impedance) will result in a large amount of 60-Hz artifact being present. By convention in EEG recording, if input 1 is negative relative to input 2, the deflection is upward (up polarity). For each tracing, one must specify the electrode to be used at inputs 1 and 2 (also called a derivation). In bipolar recording, each amplifier records the difference between two electrodes of interest (A–B and C–D). Using selector panels, it is possible to change the electrodes recorded from a given amplifier during monitoring. In modern digital sleep monitoring, one may record the activity of numerous electrodes against a common electric reference (referential recording). Any combination of

various tracings of interest can be obtained by digital subtraction (electrode A-reference) − (electrode B-reference) = electrode A − electrode B either during recording or during review (see Table 1-3) (5,6). For example, if the sleep technologist failed to observe that EMG2 went bad during the recording, the reviewer can change the chin EMG display from EMG1–EMG2 to EMG1–EMG3. In modern digital recording, it is common to have a mixture of referential (EEG, eye electrodes, EMG electrodes), true bipolar (chest, abdominal movement, airflow), and DC (oxygen saturation) recording.

Many digital recording systems still use analog amplifiers that produce a continuous signal output. An analog-to-digital conversion board converts the signal to a digital form that can be stored and manipulated by a computer. The sampling rate must be more than twice the frequencies being recorded to avoid signal distortion. In addition, signals with a frequency higher than one-half the sampling rate must be filtered out, as they can cause aliasing distortion (5). The usual paper speed for sleep recording is 10 mm/s, which produces 30-second pages (30-cm wide paper). When reviewing digital recording, one can choose various time windows. A 30-second window (equivalent to 10 mm/s) is used for sleep staging. Time windows of 60 to 240 seconds may be used to view and score respiratory events. Alternatively, viewing data in 10-second window (equivalent to 30 mm/s) is the usual window for viewing clinical EEG and displaying interictal or epileptic activity. It also can be useful for measuring the frequency of a complex of oscillations or viewing the EKG. The traditional EKG speed is 25 mm/s, which is quite close to 30 mm/s. Some systems allow split screens with different time windows in each. A summary view is often provided with all-night condensed graphs of the hypnogram, SaO_2 tracing, continuous positive airway pressure (CPAP) levels, respiratory events, and body position. This allows a useful overview of the entire recording. One can usually click on a given area of the summary and be taken to that point in the tracings.

In paper monitoring of sleep, the EEG is usually recorded at a sensitivity of 50 μV/cm in adults. In children,

Differential amplifier

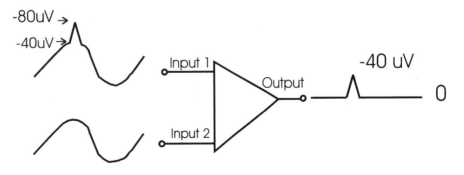

FIGURE 1-2. Schematic representation of a differential amplifier. Only differences between the inputs 1 and 2 are amplified. Signals common to both inputs are rejected (common mode rejection). By convention, a signal that causes input 1 to be negative compared with input 2 results in an upward deflection.

▶ **TABLE 1-3.** Montages for Sleep Monitoring

Bipolar		Referential	
Minimal	Typical:	Recording (each against reference electrode)	Displays[a]
C4-A1 (C3-A2)	C4-A1	C4	C4-A1
ROC-A1	C3-A2	C3	C3-A2
LOC-A2	O2-A1	O2	O1-A2
Chin EMG1-EMG2	O1-A2	O1	O2-A1
	ROC-A1	ROC	ROC-A1
	LOC-A2	LOC	LOC-A2
	Chin EMG1-EMG2	A1	Chin EMG1-EMG2
		A2	
		EMG1	
		EMG2	
		EMG3	

[a]Note: any combination of referentially recorded electrodes can be displayed.

a lower sensitivity (100 μV/cm) is used because of the very high-amplitude EEG activity. Digital recording often uses 100 μV per channel width. For simplicity, many systems amplify signals at a set gain before they are digitally recorded. The signals can be amplified or diminished by changing the digital gain to produce a satisfactory display without changing the actual recorded voltage. One can set default gains and filters so that a minimal amount of manipulation is needed to obtain a satisfactory display view of the signals.

Any signal of interest can be contaminated by unwanted low- or high-frequency signals of 50 to 60 Hz (from nearby AC power lines). Filters allow these components to be diminished. For example, a low filter (high-pass filter) attenuates the amplitude of low-frequency signals. A high filter (low-pass filter) attenuates the amplitude of high-frequency signals. A range of possible low filter settings (off, 0.01, 0.03, 0.1, 0.3, 1, 3, 10, 30) is provided with each designation, meaning that at a setting of X, the amplitude of a signal at X Hz will be attenuated by a set amount (usually 30 or 50%) depending on the amplifier

manufacturer. Lower frequencies will be attenuated even more (Fig. 1-3). It is important to realize that frequencies slightly above the low-filter setting X also will be attenuated, although to a much lesser degree. Sometimes the strength of filters is given in decibels, which is defined as 20 log (voltage-out/voltage-in), where voltage-out and voltage-in are the amplitude of the signal entering and leaving the filter, respectively. A signal reduction of 30% and 50% (voltage-out/voltage-in ratios of 0.7 and 0.5, respectively) correspond to -3 and -6 db reductions. Another terminology used for filters setting uses "1/2 amplitude." A low filter with a 1/2 amplitude low setting of 1 Hz means that a signal with a frequency of 1 Hz will be attenuated by 50%. Similarly a high filter with a setting of 1/2 amplitude high-filter setting of 30 Hz will attenuate a 30-Hz signal by 50%. Higher frequency signals will be attenuated even more. A range of high filter settings is typically provided (off, 1, 3, 15, 35, 70, 100).

Most amplifiers also provide optional notch filers to attenuate a narrow range of frequency (i.e., 50–60 Hz). Some recommend that notch filters not be used routinely,

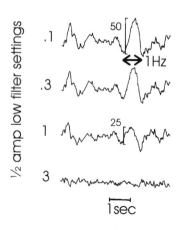

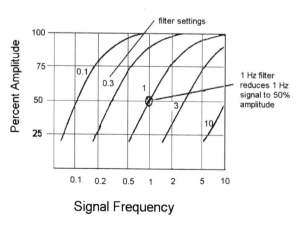

FIGURE 1-3. The effect of various low-filter settings on a typical EEG signal is shown along with the properties of a standard low-frequency filter (high pass filter). A signal at 1 Hz is reduced by 50% at a $^1/_2$ amplitude low-filter setting of 1 Hz. The larger low-filter setting of 3 Hz completely attenuates the low-frequency components of the signal. Note that even at a smaller low-filter setting of 0.3, the 1 Hz signal is attenuated slightly.

▶ **TABLE 1-4.** **Standard Sensitivity and Filter Settings**

	Sensitivity	*Low Filter*	*High Filter*
EEG	50 μV = 1 cm; 100 μV = 1 channel width	0.3	35
EOG	50 μV = 1 cm; 100 μV = 1 channel width	0.3	35
EMG	50 μv = 1 cm; 100 μV = 1 channel width	10	100
EKG		0.1	35
Airflow (thermistor)	Variable	0.1	15
Chest	Variable	0.1	15
Abdomen	Variable	0.1	15
Sao$_2$ (%)	1 Volt = 0–100 or 50–100%	DC	15
Nasal pressure machine flow	Variable	DC or AC with low filter setting of 0.01	15 100 to see snoring

as the sudden appearance of increased 60-Hz activity is a clue that one or more electrodes may have gone bad. Traditional electronic filters use resistance–capacitance circuits (RC filters). Standard filter settings for different variables monitored during sleep studies are shown in Table 1-4. Many digital polysomnography units actually record the signal over a wide frequency range (for example, DC to 100 Hz). Although signals are acquired over a wide frequency range, they are viewed after application of desired digital low and high filters. These alter the display, but not the recorded data. This allows multiple choices of filters, if desired by the technologist or reviewer.

INTRODUCTION TO ELECTROENCEPHALOGRAPHIC TERMINOLOGY AND MONITORING

EEG activity is characterized by the frequency in cycles per second or hertz (Hz), amplitude (voltage), and the direction of major deflection (polarity). The classically described frequency ranges are: delta (<4 Hz), theta (4–7 Hz), alpha (8–13 Hz), and beta (>13 Hz). Alpha waves (8–13 Hz) are commonly noted when the patient is in an awake, but relaxed, state with the eyes closed (Fig. 1-4). They are best recorded over the occiput and are attenuated when the eyes are open. Bursts of alpha waves also are seen during brief awakenings from sleep—called arousals. Alpha activity can also be seen during REM sleep. Alpha activity is prominent during drowsy eyes-closed wakefulness. This activity decreases with the onset of stage 1 sleep. Near the transition from stage 1 to stage 2 sleep, vertex *sharp waves*—high-amplitude negative waves (upward de-

flection on EEG tracings) with a short duration—occur. They are more prominent in central than in occipital EEG tracings. A sharp wave is defined as deflection of 70 to 200 milliseconds in duration.

Sleep spindles are oscillations of 12 to 14 Hz with a duration of 0.5 to 1.5 seconds. They are characteristic of stage 2 sleep. They may persist into stages 3 and 4, but usually do not occur in stage REM. The K complex is a high-amplitude, biphasic wave of at least 0.5-second duration. As classically defined, a K complex consists of an initial sharp, negative voltage (by convention an upward deflection) followed by a positive-deflection (down) slow wave. Spindles frequently are superimposed on K complexes. Sharp waves differ from K complexes in that they are narrower, not biphasic, and usually of lower amplitude.

As sleep deepens, slow (delta) waves appear. These are high-amplitude, broad waves. Whereas delta EEG activity is usually defined as <4 Hz, in human sleep scoring, the slow-wave activity used for staging is defined as EEG activity slower than 2 Hz (longer than 0.5-second duration) with a peak-to-peak amplitude of >75 μV. The amount of slow-wave activity *as measured in the central EEG tracings* is used to determine if stage 3 or 4 is present (1) (see below). Because a K complex resembles slow-wave activity, differentiating the two is sometimes difficult. However, by definition, a K complex should stand out (be distinct) from the lower-amplitude, background EEG activity. Therefore, a continuous series of high-voltage slow waves would not be considered to be a series of K complexes.

Sawtooth waves (Fig. 1-4) are notched-jagged waves of frequency in the theta range (3–7 Hz) that may be present during REM sleep. Although they are not part of the

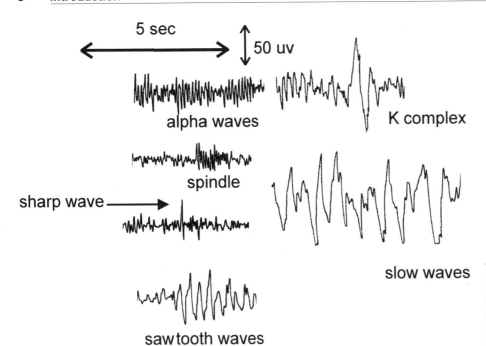

FIGURE 1-4. Several of the important EEG patterns for sleep staging are illustrated. (From Berry RB. *Sleep medicine pearls* 2nd ed. Philadelphia: Hanley and Belfus, 2003:2. With permission.)

criteria for scoring REM sleep, their presence is a clue that REM sleep is present.

Electroencephalographic Monitoring Techniques

The traditional Rechtschaffen and Kales (R&K) guidelines for human sleep staging were based on central EEG monitoring (1). However, most sleep recording today also includes occipital electrodes. Alpha activity is more prominent in occipital tracings. The terminology for the electrodes adheres to the International 10–20 nomenclature. In this nomenclature, electrodes are placed at 10% or 20% of the distance between structural landmarks on the head (Fig. 1-5). Even subscripts refer to electrodes on the right and odd to electrodes on the left side of the head. The positions of the right and left central electrodes (C4 and C3), occipital electrodes (O2 and O1), and mastoid electrodes (A2 and A1) are shown in Fig. 1-5. The usual derivations use the central or occipital electrodes referenced to the opposite mastoid electrode (C4-A1, O1-A2). The greater distance between electrodes increases the voltage difference. A minimum of one central EEG derivation must be recorded for sleep staging. In modern digital recording, typically all of the electrodes (C4, C3, O2, O1, A1, A2) are recorded. Of note, additional electrodes may be added if one suspects seizure activity. This will be discussed in detail in later chapters.

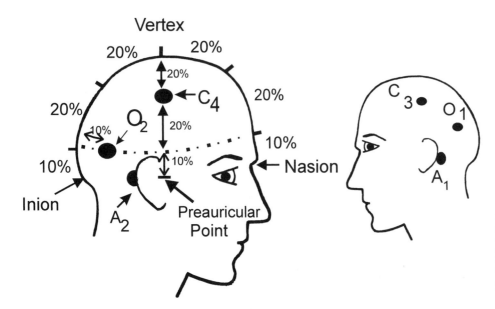

FIGURE 1-5. Locations of C4, C3, O2, O1, A1, A2, using the 10–20 system, are illustrated. (From Berry RB. *Sleep medicine pearls* 2nd ed. Philadelphia: Hanley and Belfus, 2003:8. With permission.)

EYE MOVEMENT RECORDING

The main purpose of recording eye movements is to identify REM sleep. Electro-oculographic (eye movement) electrodes typically are placed at the outer corners of the eyes—at the right outer canthus (ROC) and the left outer canthus (LOC) (Fig. 1-6). In a common approach, two eye channels are recorded and the eye electrodes are referenced to the opposite mastoid (ROC-A1 and LOC-A2). However, some sleep centers use the same mastoid electrode as a reference (ROC-A1 and LOC-A1). To detect vertical as well as horizontal eye movements, one electrode is placed slightly above and one slightly below the eyes (4,5).

Recording of eye movements is possible because a potential difference exists across the eyeball: front positive (+), back negative (−). Eye movements are detected by electro-oculographic recording of voltage changes. When the eyes move toward an electrode, a positive voltage is recorded (see Fig. 1-7). By standard convention, polygraphs are calibrated so that a negative voltage causes an upward pen deflection (negative polarity up). Thus, eye movement toward an electrode results in a downward deflection (4,7). Note that movement of the eyes is usually conjugate, with both eyes moving toward one eye electrode and away from the other. If the eye channels are calibrated with the same polarity settings, eye movements produce

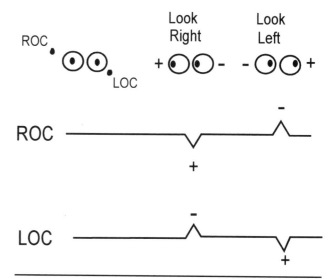

FIGURE 1-7. The effects of conjugate eye movements on deflections in tracings from ROC (right outer canthus) and LOC (left outer canthus) are illustrated. The front of the globe is positive with respect to the back. (From Berry RB. *Sleep medicine pearls* 2nd ed. Philadelphia: Hanley and Belfus, 2003:12. With permission.)

out-of-phase deflections in the two eye tracings (e.g., one up, and one down). Figure 1-7 shows the recorded results of eye movements to the right and left (assuming both amplifier channels have negative polarity up). The same approach can be used to understand the tracings resulting from vertical eye movements. Because ROC is positioned above the eyes (and LOC below), upward eye movements are toward ROC and away from LOC. Thus, upward eye movement results in a downward deflection in the ROC tracing and an upward deflection in the LOC tracing.

There are two common patterns of eye movements (Fig. 1-8). Slow eye movements (SEMs), also called slow-rolling eye movements, are pendular oscillating movements that are seen in drowsy (eyes closed) wakefulness and stage 1 sleep. By stage 2 sleep, SEMs usually have disappeared. REMs are sharper (more narrow deflections), which are typical of eyes-open wake and REM sleep.

In the two-tracing method of eye movement recording, large-amplitude EEG activity or artifact reflected in the EOG tracings usually causes *in-phase defections*. In Fig. 1-9, a K complex (A) causes an in-phase deflections in the eye tracings, while REM result in *out-of-phase* deflections.

ELECTROMYOGRAPHIC RECORDING

Usually, three EMG leads are placed in the mental and submental areas (see Fig. 1-6). The voltage between two of these three is monitored (for example, EMG1-EMG3). If either of these leads fail, the third lead can be substituted. The gain of the chin EMG is adjusted so that some activity is noted during wakefulness. The chin EMG is an essential element only for identifying stage REM sleep. In

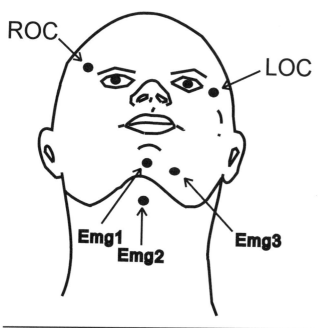

FIGURE 1-6. Positions of standard eye movement electrodes at the right outer canthus (ROC) and left outer canthus (LOC) are depicted. Typically, ROC is placed slightly above the eyes and LOC slightly below so that vertical, as well as horizontal, eye movements can be detected. Common positions used to monitor the chin EMG are also shown. While three electrodes are typically placed, the difference between only two is typically displayed at any time. (From Berry RB. *Sleep medicine pearls* 2nd ed. Philadelphia: Hanley and Belfus, 2003:18. With permission.)

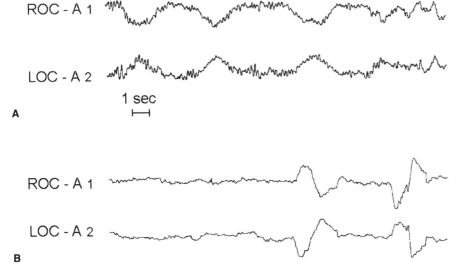

ROC - A 1

LOC - A 2

1 sec

A

ROC - A 1

LOC - A 2

B

FIGURE 1-8. Typical patterns of eye movements are illustrated. Tracing A: Slow eye movements (SEMs) are pendular and common in drowsy wake and stage 1 sleep. Tracing B: Rapid eye movements (REMs) are sharper (shorter duration) and seen in eyes open wake or REM sleep. (From Berry RB. *Sleep medicine pearls* 2nd ed. Philadelphia: Hanley and Belfus, 2003:14. With permission.)

stage REM, the chin EMG is relatively reduced—the amplitude is equal to or lower than the lowest EMG amplitude in NREM sleep. If the chin EMG gain is adjusted high enough to show some activity in NREM sleep, a drop in activity is often seen on transition to REM sleep. The chin EMG may also reach the REM level long before the onset of REMS or an EEG meeting criteria for stage REM. Depending on the gain, a reduction in the chin EMG amplitude from wakefulness to sleep and often a further reduction on transition from stage 1 to 4 may be seen. However, a reduction in the chin EMG is not required for stages 2 to 4. The reduction in the EMG amplitude during REM sleep is a reflection of the generalized skeletal-muscle hypotonia present in this sleep stage. Phasic brief EMG bursts still may be seen during REM sleep. In Fig. 1-9, there is a fall in chin EMG amplitude just before the REMs (B) occur. The combination of REMs, a relatively reduced chin EMG, and a low-voltage mixed-frequency EEG is consistent with stage REM.

SLEEP STAGE CHARACTERISTICS

The basic rules for sleep staging are summarized in Table 1-5. Note that some characteristics are required (bold) and some are helpful but not required. The typical patterns associated with each sleep stage are discussed below.

Stage Wake

During eyes-open wake, the EEG is characterized by high-frequency low-voltage activity. The EOG tracings typically show REM, and the chin EMG activity is relatively high (Fig. 1-10). During eyes-closed drowsy wake, the EEG is characterized by prominent alpha activity (>50% of the epoch). Slow-rolling eye movements are usually present. The level of muscle tone is usually relatively high (Fig. 1-11).

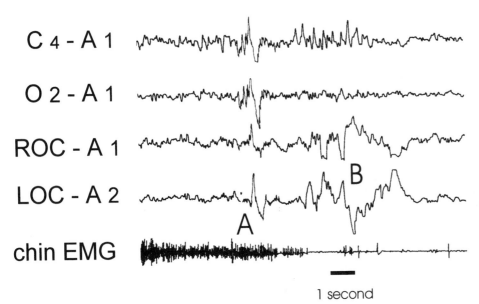

C 4 - A 1

O 2 - A 1

ROC - A 1

LOC - A 2

A

B

chin EMG

1 second

FIGURE 1-9. Transition from stage 2 sleep to stage REM. ROC and LOC are right and left outer canthus electrodes, respectively. The chin EMG fell to the REM level just prior to the onset of rapid eye movements. Note that REMs (**B**) result in out-of-phase deflections in the eye tracings, while the K complex (**A**) results in in-phase deflections. (From Berry RB. *Sleep medicine pearls* 2nd ed. Philadelphia: Hanley and Belfus, 2003:18. With permission.)

▶ **TABLE 1-5.** Summary of Sleep Stage Characteristics

	Characteristics[a,b]		
Stage	*EEG*	*EOG*	*EMG*
Wake (eyes open)	Low-voltage, high-frequency, attenuated alpha activity	Eye blinks, REMs	Relatively high
Wake (eyes closed)	Low-voltage, high-frequency >50% alpha activity	Slow-rolling eye movements	Relatively high
Stage 1	Low-amplitude mixed–frequency **<50% Alpha activity** **NO spindles, K complexes** Sharp waves near transition to stage 2	Slow-rolling eye movements	May be lower than wake
Stage 2	**At least one sleep spindle or K complex** **<20% Slow-wave activity**[b]		May be lower than wake
Stage 3	**20–50% Slow-wave activity**	[†]	Usually low
Stage 4	**>50% Slow-wave activity**	[†]	Usually low
Stage REM	**Low-voltage mixed-frequency** Sawtooth waves—may be present	**Episodic REMs**	**Relatively reduced** (equal or lower than the lowest in NREM)

[a]Required characteristics in bold.
[b]Slow wave activity, frequency <2 Hz; peak to peak amplitude >75 μV; >50% means slow wave activity present in more than 50% of the epoch; REMs, rapid eye movements.
[†]Slow waves usually seen in EOG tracings.

Stage 1

The stage 1 EEG is characterized by low-voltage, mixed-frequency activity (4–7 Hz). Stage 1 is scored when less than 50% of an epoch contains alpha waves and criteria for deeper stages of sleep are not met (Fig. 1-12). Slow-rolling eye movements often are present in the eye movement tracings, and the level of muscle tone (EMG) is equal or diminished compared to that in the awake state. Some patients do not exhibit prominent alpha activity, making detection of sleep onset difficult. The ability of a patient to produce alpha waves can be determined from biocalibrations at the start of the study. The patient is asked to lie quietly with eyes open and then with the eyes closed. Alpha activity usually appears with eye closure. When patients do not produce significant alpha activity, differentiating

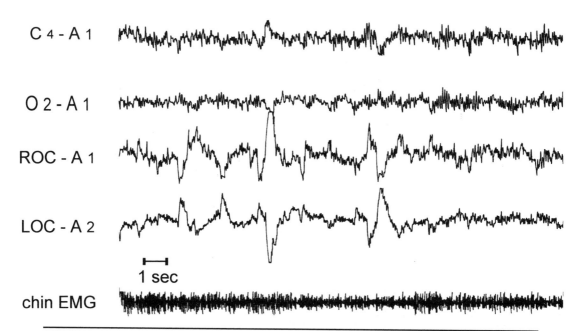

FIGURE 1-10. Stage wake-eyes open (15-second tracing). The EEG shows low-amplitude high-frequency activity. The EOG shows REMs. The chin EMG is relatively high. (From Berry RB. *Sleep medicine pearls* 2nd ed. Philadelphia: Hanley and Belfus, 2003:20. With permission.)

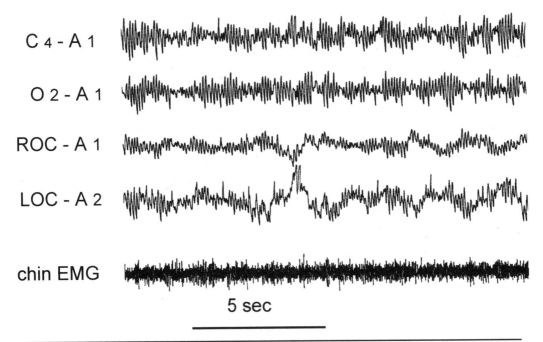

FIGURE 1-11. Stage wake-eyes closed (drowsy). The EEG shows more alpha activity for more than 50% of the epoch, and the EOG tracing may show slow eye movements. The chin EMG is relatively high in amplitude. (From Berry RB. *Sleep medicine pearls* 2nd ed. Philadelphia: Hanley and Belfus, 2003:22. With permission.)

wakefulness from stage 1 sleep can be difficult. Several points are helpful. First, the presence of REMs in the absence of a reduced chin EMG usually means the wake is present. However, SEMs can be present during drowsy wake and stage 1 sleep. In this case one must differentiate wake from stage 1 by the EEG. In wake, the EEG has considerable high-frequency activity. In stage 1, the EEG is mixed frequency with activity in the 4 to 7 Hz range. Note the slower (wider) EEG activity at point T in Fig. 1-12. This activity is in the theta range. Often the

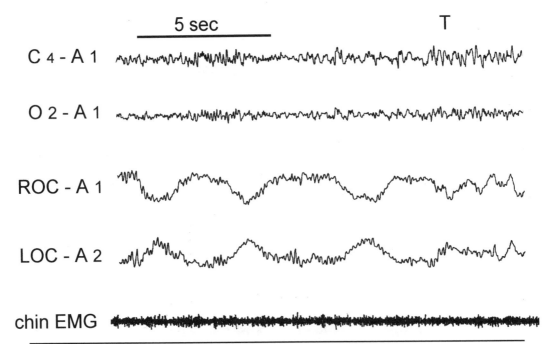

FIGURE 1-12. Stage 1 (15-second tracing). The EEG shows alpha activity for less than 50% of the epoch and has a low-voltage mixed-frequency activity. Waves in the theta range are seen at (T). Slow eye movements are usually present. (From Berry RB. *Sleep medicine pearls* 2nd ed. Philadelphia: Hanley and Belfus, 2003:24. With permission.)

easiest method to determine sleep onset in difficult cases is to find the first epoch of unequivocal sleep (usually stage 2) and work backward. The examiner can usually be confident of the point of sleep onset within one or two epochs.

Stage 2

Stage 2 sleep is characterized by the presence of one or more K complexes (Fig. 1-13) or sleep spindles (Fig. 1-14). To qualify as stage 2, an epoch also must contain less than 20% of an epoch may contain slow (delta) wave EEG activity (<6 seconds of a 30-second epoch). Slow-wave activity is defined as waves with a frequency <2 Hz and a minimum peak-to-peak amplitude of >75 μV. Stage 2 occupies the greatest proportion of the total sleep time and accounts for roughly 40% to 50% of sleep.

Stages 3 and 4

Stages 3 and 4 NREM sleep are called slow-wave, delta, or deep sleep. Stage 3 is scored when slow-wave activity (frequency <2 Hz and amplitude >75 μV peak-to-peak) is present for 20% to 50% of the epoch (Fig. 1-15). Stage 4 is scored when more than 50% of the epoch is occupied by slow-wave activity meeting the above criteria (Fig. 1-16). Spindles may be present in the EEG. Frequently, the high-voltage EEG activity is transmitted to the eye leads. The EMG often is lower than during stages 1 and 2 sleep, but this is variable. Stage 3 sleep in younger patients often is brief and represents a transition from stage 2 to stage 4 sleep. In older patients, the slow-wave amplitude is lower, and the total amount of slow-wave sleep is reduced. In these patients, the amount of stage 3 sleep may exceed the amount of stage 4 sleep. Many sleep laboratories report combined stage 3 and 4 sleep (rather than the amount of stage 3 and stage 4 separately). The amplitude of the slowwaves (and amount of slow-wave sleep) is usually highest in the first sleep cycles. Typically, stages 3 and 4 occur mostly in the early portions of the night (Fig. 1-1). Several parasomnias (disorders associated with sleep) occur in stages 3 and 4 sleep and, therefore, can be predicted to occur in the early part of the night. These include somnambulism (sleep walking) and night terrors. In contrast, parasomnias occurring in REM sleep (for example, nightmares) are more common in the early morning hours.

Stage REM

Stage REM sleep is characterized by a low-voltage, mixed-frequency EEG, the presence of episodic REMs, and a relatively low-amplitude chin EMG. Sawtooth waves (see Fig. 1-17, point A) also may occur in the EEG. There usually are three to five episodes of REM sleep during the night, which tend to increase in length as the night progresses. The number of eye movements per unit time (REM density) also increases during the night. Not all epochs of REM sleep contain REMs. Epochs of sleep otherwise meeting criteria for stage REM and contiguous with epochs of unequivocal stage REM (REMs present) are scored as stage REM (see Advanced Staging Rules). Bursts of alpha waves can occur during REM sleep, but the frequency is often 1 to 2 Hz slower than during wake.

Stage REM is associated with many unique, physiologic changes, such as widespread skeletal muscle hypotonia and sleep-related erections. Skeletal muscle hypotonia is a protective mechanism to prevent the acting out of dreams. In a pathologic state known as the REM behavior disorder, muscle tone is present, and body movements and even violent behavior can occur during REM sleep.

Arousals

Arousal from sleep denotes a transition from a state of sleep to wakefulness. Frequent arousals can cause

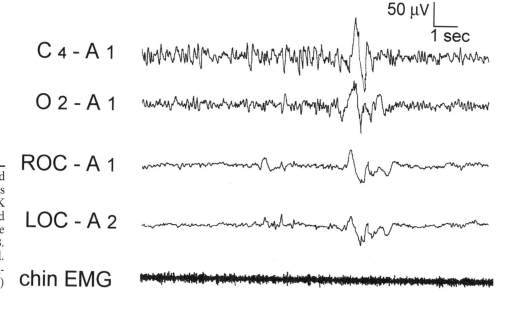

FIGURE 1-13. A 15-second tracing of stage 2 sleep is shown. The EEG shows a K complex that is transmitted to the eye channels (in-phase deflection). (From Berry RB. *Sleep medicine pearls* 2nd ed. Philadelphia: Hanley and Belfus, 2003:26. With permission.)

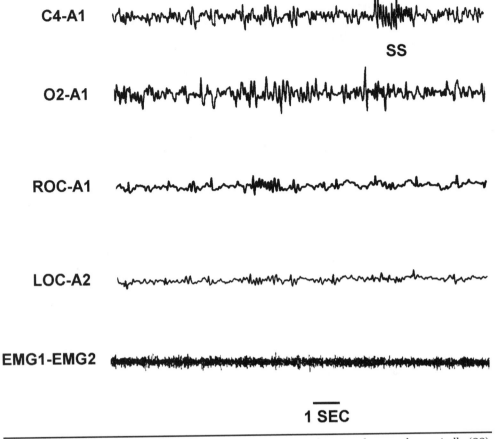

FIGURE 1-14. A 15-second tracing of stage 2 sleep is shown. The EEG shows a sleep spindle (SS), and the eye movement channels show an absence of slow eye movements.

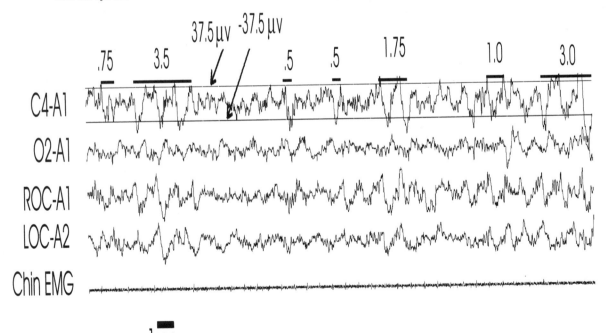

FIGURE 1-15. A 30-second tracing of stage 3 sleep. Amplitude gridlines are placed at −37.5 and +37.5 μV (difference 75 μV) to assist with sleep staging. The dark lines and numbers are the seconds of slow-wave activity with 75 μV peak-to-peak amplitude. The slow-wave activity was present for 11 s, meeting criteria for stage 3 sleep.

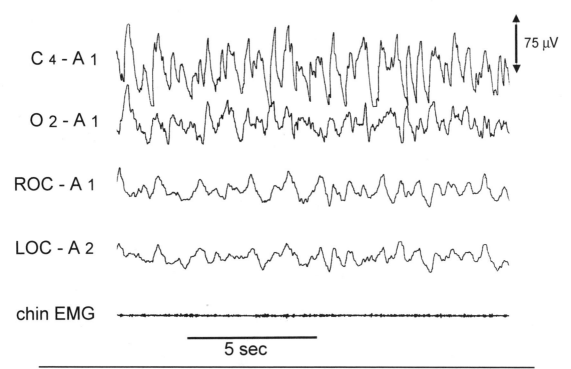

FIGURE 1-16. A 15-second tracing of stage 4 sleep is shown. There is prominent slow-wave activity meeting voltage criteria (greater than 75 μV peak-to-peak) throughout the tracing. Note that slow-wave activity is also seen in the eye channels. (From Berry RB. *Sleep medicine pearls* 2nd ed. Philadelphia: Hanley and Belfus, 2003:28. With permission.)

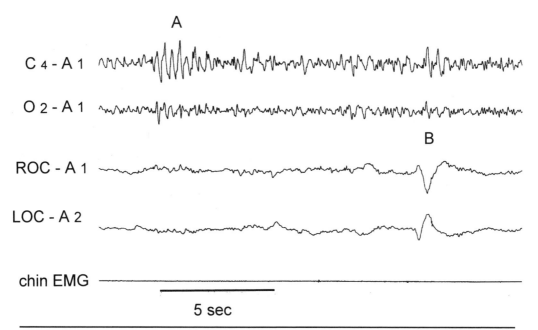

FIGURE 1-17. Stage REM. A 15-second tracing of stage REM is shown. The EEG is low-amplitude mixed-frequency. In this case, a sawtooth wave is noted at **(A)**. The eye tracings show a rapid eye movement at **B**. The chin EMG amplitude is low. (From Berry RB. *Sleep medicine pearls* 2nd ed. Philadelphia: Hanley and Belfus, 2003:30. With permission.)

daytime sleepiness by shortening the total amount of sleep. However, even if arousals are brief (1–5 seconds) with a rapid return to sleep, daytime sleepiness may result, although the total sleep time is relatively normal (8). Thus, the restorative function of sleep depends on continuity as well as duration. Many disorders that are associated with excessive daytime sleepiness also are associated with frequent, brief arousals. For example, patients with obstructive sleep apnea frequently have arousals coincident with apnea/hypopnea termination. Therefore, determination of the frequency of arousals has become a standard part of the analysis of sleep architecture during sleep testing.

Movement arousals were defined in the Rechtschaffen and Kales (R&K) scoring manual (1) as an increase in EMG that is accompanied by a change in pattern on any additional channel. For EEG channels, qualifying changes included a decrease in amplitude, paroxysmal high-voltage activity, or an increase in alpha activity. Subsequently, arousals were the object of considerable research, but the criteria used to define them was variable. A report from the Atlas Task Force of the American Academy of Sleep Medicine (formerly the American Sleep Disorders Association or ASDA) has become the standard definition (9). According to the ASDA Task Force, an arousal should be

scored in NREM sleep when there is "an abrupt shift in EEG frequency, which may include theta, alpha, and/or frequencies >16 Hz, but not spindles," of 3 seconds or longer duration. The 3-second duration was chosen for methodological reasons; shorter arousals may also have physiologic importance. To be scored as an arousal, the shift in EEG frequency must follow at least 10 continuous seconds of any stage of sleep. Arousals in NREM sleep may occur without a concurrent increase in the submental EMG amplitude. In REM sleep, however, the required EEG changes must be accompanied by a concurrent increase in EMG amplitude for an arousal to be scored. This extra requirement was added because spontaneous bursts of alpha rhythm are a fairly common occurrence in REM (but not NREM) sleep. Arousals from NREM and REM sleep are shown in Fig. 1-18. Note that according to the above recommendations, increases in the chin EMG in the absence of EEG changes are not considered evidence of arousal in either NREM or REM sleep. Similarly, sudden bursts of delta (slow-wave) activity in the absence of other changes do not qualify as evidence of arousal. Because cortical EEG changes must be present to meet the above definition, such events are also termed electrocortical arousals. Note that the above guidelines represent a consensus on events likely

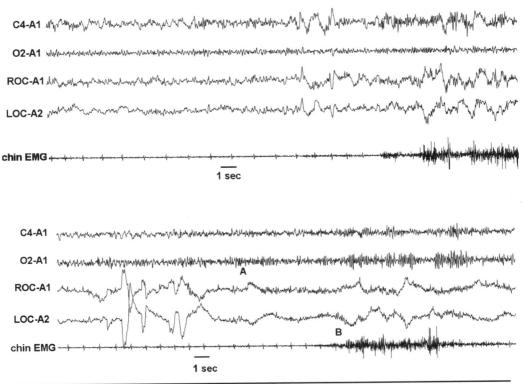

FIGURE 1-18. Examples of two tracings of 30 seconds duration showing arousals from NREM (upper tracings) and REM (lower tracings) sleep. An increase in EMG is noted in the upper tracings but this is not required to score an arousal from NREM sleep. The shift in EEG frequency is best seen in this example in the central electrodes. In the bottom tracings REM sleep is shown with a burst of alpha at (A). However, an arousal is scored only when there is an increase in the EMG associated with an EEG frequency shift (A). (See text for arousal definitions)

to be of physiologic significance. The committee recognized that other EEG phenomena, such as delta bursts, also can represent evidence of arousal in certain contexts.

The frequency of arousals usually is computed as the arousal index (number of arousals per hour of sleep). Relatively little data is available to define a normal range for the arousal index. Normal young adults studied after adaptation nights frequently have an arousal index of five per hour or less. In one study, however, normal subjects of variable ages had a mean arousal index of 21 per hour, and the arousal index was found to increase with age (10). However, a respiratory arousal index (arousals associated with respiratory events) as low as 10 per hour has been associated with daytime sleepiness in some individuals with the upper-airway resistance syndrome (11). While some have argued that patients with this disorder really represent the mild end of the obstructive sleep apnea syndrome, most would agree with the concept that respiratory arousals of sufficient frequency can cause daytime sleepiness in the absence of frank apnea and arterial oxygen desaturation.

ADVANCED SLEEP STAGING RULES

There are additional scoring rules to handle special situations. These rules are necessary because K complexes, sleep spindles, and REMs are episodic (1,3). The 3-minute rule concerns stage 2 sleep. This rule, as outlined by the classic R&K sleep staging manual, states that if the pe-riod of time between spindles or K complexes is shorter than 3 minutes and if the intervening sleep would otherwise meet criteria for stage 1 (less than 50% alpha activity) with no evidence of intervening arousal, then this period of sleep is scored as stage 2. If the period of time is 3 minutes or longer, then the intervening sleep is scored as stage 1. Figure 1-19 shows five epochs (30 seconds each) of sleep, with K complexes (K) in epochs 69 and 73. The central and occipital EEG tracings in epochs 70 to 72 are assumed not to contain sleep spindles, K complexes, or evidence of arousal. The time between the K complexes is less than 3 minutes; therefore, this intervening sleep is scored as stage 2.

Staging of REM sleep also requires special rules (REM rules) to define the beginning and end of REM sleep. This is necessary because REMs are episodic, and the three indicators of stage REM (EEG, EOG, and EMG) may not change to (or from) the REM-like pattern simultaneously. Rechtschaffen and Kales (R&K) recommend that any section of the record that is contiguous with uneqivocal stage REM and displays a relatively low-voltage, mixed-frequency EEG be scored as stage REM regardless of whether REMs are present, providing the EMG is at the stage REM level. To be REM-like, the EEG must not contain spindles, K complexes, or slow waves. In Fig. 1-20, epoch 71 is staged as REM sleep because the EMG and EEG are REM-like and the epoch is contiguous in unequivocal REM sleep (no intervening arousals). A more complete discussion of the 3-minute and REM rules are contained in the R&K guidelines (1) and other references (3,7).

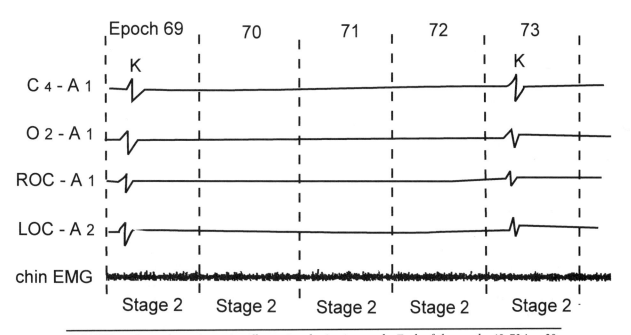

FIGURE 1-19. A schematic tracing illustrating the 3-mintue rule. Each of the epochs 69–73 is a 30-second epoch. There are K complexes in epoch 69 and 73, but no K complexes or sleep spindles in epochs 70–72. Because the time between the K complexes is less than 3 minutes, the intervening epochs are staged as stage 2. (From Berry RB. *Sleep medicine pearls* 2nd ed. Philadelphia: Hanley and Belfus, 2003:42. With permission.)

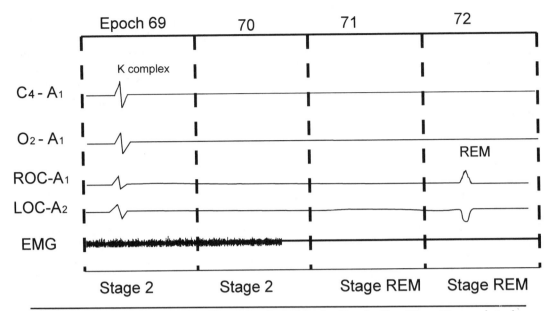

FIGURE 1-20. A schematic tracing illustrating the REM rules. Epochs 69 to 72 are 30 seconds in duration. Epoch 72 is an unequivocal epoch of REM sleep, as it contains a REM; the EMG and EEG are consistent with REM sleep. The EEG in epochs 70 and 71 is REM-like (no spindles or K complex). However, the EMG is above the REM level for most of epoch 70. As epoch 71 is contiguous with unequivocal REM and would otherwise qualify as stage REM, except for the absence of a rapid eye movement, it is scored as stage REM. (From Berry RB. *Sleep medicine pearls* 2nd ed. Philadelphia: Hanley and Belfus, 2003:23. With permission.)

Atypical Sleep Patterns

Four special cases in which sleep staging is made difficult by atypical EEG, EOG, and EMG patterns will be briefly mentioned. In alpha sleep, prominent alpha activity persists into NREM sleep. The presence of spindles, K complexes, and slow-wave activity allows sleep staging despite prominent alpha activity. Causes of the pattern include pain, psychiatric disorders, chronic pain syndromes, and any cause of nonrestorative sleep (12,13). Patients taking benzodiazepines may have very prominent "pseudo-spindle" activity (14–16 rather than the usual 12–14 Hz) (14). Slow eye movements are usually absent by the time stable stage 2 sleep is present. However, patients on some serotonin reuptake inhibitors (fluoxetine and others) may have prominent slow and rapid eye movements during NREM sleep (15). While a reduction in the chin EMG is required for staging REM sleep, patients with the REM sleep behavior disorder may have high chin activity during what otherwise appears to be REM sleep (16).

Sleep Staging in Infants and Children

Newborn term infants do not have the well-developed adult EEG patterns to allow staging according to R&K rules. The following is a brief description of terminology and sleep staging for the newborn infant according to the state determination of Anders, Emde, and Parmelee (17). Infant sleep is divided into active sleep (corresponding to REM sleep), quiet sleep (corresponding to NREM sleep), and indeterminant sleep, which is often a transitional sleep stage. Behavioral observations are critical. Wakefulness is characterized by crying, quiet eyes open, and feeding. Sleep is often defined as sustained eye closure. Newborn infants typically have periods of sleep lasting 3 to 4 hours interrupted by feeding and total sleep in 24 hours is usually 16 to 18 hours. They have cycles of sleep with a 45- to 60-minute periodicity with about 50% active sleep. In newborns, the presence of REM (active sleep) at sleep onset is the norm. In contrast, the adult sleep cycle is 90 to 100 minutes, REM occupies about 20% of sleep, and NREM sleep is noted at sleep onset.

The EEG patterns of newborn infants have been characterized as low-voltage irregular (LVI), tracé alternant (TA), high-voltage slow (HVS), and mixed (M) (Table 1-6, Fig. 1-21). Eye movement monitoring is used as in adults. An epoch is considered to have high or low EMG if over one-half of the epoch shows the pattern. The characteristics of active sleep, quiet sleep, and indeterminant sleep are listed in Table 1-7. The change from active to quiet sleep is more likely to manifest indeterminant sleep. Nonnutritive sucking commonly continues into sleep.

As children mature, more typically adult EEG patterns begin to appear. Sleep spindles begin to appear at 2 months and are usually seen after 3 to 4 months of age (18). K complexes usually begin to appear at 6 months of age and are fully developed by 2 years of age (19). The point at which sleep staging follows adult rules in not well defined, but usually is possible after age 6 months. After about 3 months, the percentage of REM sleep starts to diminish

▶ **TABLE 1-6. EEG Patterns Used in Infant Sleep Staging**

EEG Pattern	
Low-voltage irregular (LVI)	Low-voltage (14–35 μV)[a], little variation Theta (5–8 hz) predominates Slow activity (1–5 Hz) also present
Tracé alternant (TA)	Bursts of high-voltage slow waves (0.5–3 Hz) with superimposition of rapid low-voltage sharp waves 2–4 Hz In between the high-voltage bursts (alternating with them) is low-voltage mixed-frequency activity of 4 to 8 s in duration
High-voltage slow (HVS)	Continuous moderately rhythmic medium-to high-voltage (50–150 μV) slow waves (0.5–4 Hz)
Mixed (M)	High-voltage slow- and low-voltage polyrhythmic activity Voltage lower than in HVS

[a] μV, microvolts.

and the intensity of body movements during active (REM) sleep begins to decrease. The pattern of NREM at sleep onset begin to emerge. However, the sleep cycle period does not reach the adult value of 90 to 100 min until adolescence.

Note that the sleep of premature infants is somewhat different from term infants (36–40 weeks gestation). In premature infants quiet sleep usually shows a pattern of tracé discontinu (20). This differs from tracé alternant as there

is electrical quiescence (rather than a reduction in amplitude) between bursts of high-voltage activity. In addition, delta brushes (fast waves of 10–20 Hz) are superimposed on the delta waves. As the infant matures, delta brushes disappear and tracé alternant pattern replaces tracé discontinu.

RESPIRATORY MONITORING

The three major components of respiratory monitoring during sleep are airflow, respiratory effort, and arterial oxygen saturation (21,22) (Table 1-8; Fig. 1-22). Many sleep centers also find using a snore sensor to be useful. For selected cases, exhaled or transcutaneous P_{CO_2} may also be monitored.

Traditionally, airflow at the nose and mouth was monitored by thermistors or thermocouples. These devices actually detect airflow by the change in the device temperature induced by a flow of air over the sensor. It is common to use a sensor in or near the nasal inlet and over the mouth (nasal–oral sensor) to detect both nasal and mouth breathing. While temperature sensing devices may accurately detect an absence of airflow (apnea), their signal is not proportional to flow and they have a slow time response time (23). Therefore, they do not accurately detect decreases in airflow (hypopnea) or flattening of the airflow profile (airflow limitation). Exact measurement of airflow can be performed by use of a pneumotachograph. This device can be placed in a mask over the nose and mouth. Airflow is determined by measuring the pressure drop across a linear resistance (usually a wire screen). However, pneumotachographs are rarely used in clinical diagnostic

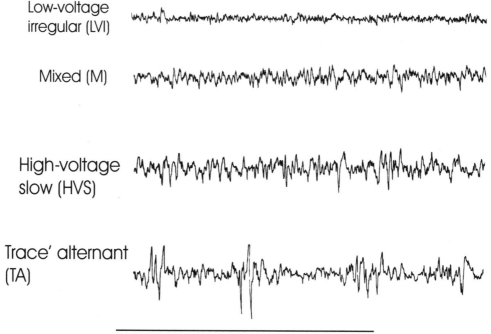

FIGURE 1-21. EEG patterns of the newborn infant.

▶ **TABLE 1-7. Characteristics of Active and Quiet Sleep**

	Active Sleep	Quiet Sleep	Indeterminant
Behavioral	Eyes closed Facial movements: smiles, grimaces, frowns Burst of sucking Body—small digit or limb movements	Eyes closed No body movements except startles and phasic jerks Sucking may occur	Not meeting criteria for active or quiet sleep
EEG	LVI, M, HVS (rarely)	HVS, TA, M	
EOG	REMs A few SEMs and a few dysconjugate movements may occur	No REMs	
EMG	Low	High	
Respiration	Irregular	Regular Post-sigh pauses may occur	

studies. Instead, monitoring of nasal pressure via a small cannula in the nose connected to a pressure transducer has gained in popularity for monitoring airflow (23,24). The nasal pressure signal is actually proportional to the square of flow across the nasal inlet (25). Thus, nasal pressure underestimates airflow at low flows and overestimates airflow at high flow rates. In the midrange of typical flow rates during sleep, the nasal pressure signal varies fairly linearly with flow. The nasal pressure versus flow relationship can be completely linearized by taking the square root of the nasal pressure signal (26). However, in clinical practice, this is rarely performed. In addition to changes in magnitude, changes in the shape of the nasal pressure signal can provide useful information. A flattened profile usually means that airflow limitation is present (constant or decreasing flow with an increasing driving pressure)

▶ **TABLE 1-8. Polysomnography**

Variables	Purpose	Methods
Central, occipital EEG Eye monitoring Chin EMG	Presence and stage of sleep arousals	Surface scalp and face electrodes
EKG	Cardiac rate and rhythm	Skin electrodes
Airflow (diagnostic)	Apnea, hypopnea	Nasal–oral thermistor Nasal pressure RIPsum (changes approximate tidal volume) Exhaled CO_2
Airflow (positive airway pressure titration)	Apnea, hypopnea	Flow signal from positive-pressure device
Respiratory effort	Classify apneas and hypopneas	Chest and abdominal bands (RIP, Piezo bands) Intercostal EMG Esophageal pressure
Pulse oximetry	Arterial oxygen saturation, Desaturations	Pulse oximetry
R, L Leg EMG	LM, PLMs	Anterior tibial EMG
Snoring	Snoring, upper-airway narrowing	Microphone or vibration transducer
End-tidal P_{CO_2}	Estimate of arterial P_{CO_2} (detect hypoventilation)	Capnography—exhaled CO_2
Transcutaneous P_{CO_2}		Transcutaneous P_{CO_2}

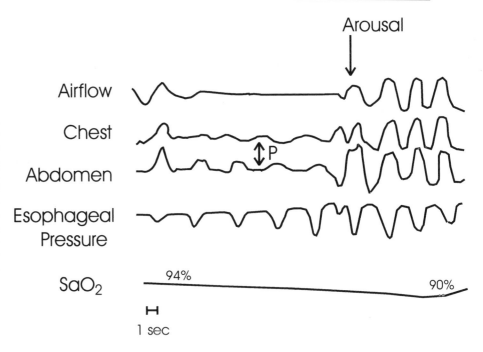

FIGURE 1-22. An obstructive apnea defined by absent airflow despite persistent respiratory effort. During the event the chest and abdominal tracings (piezo belts) show paradoxical movement (P). The esophageal pressure shows a crescendo increase in effort toward apnea termination. This is not easily appreciated from chest and abdominal movement. The nadir in arterial oxygen desaturation occurs after apnea termination. The position of the arousal that was associated with the event is also indicated.

(23,24). The unfiltered nasal pressure signal also can detect snoring if the frequency range of the amplifier is adequate. The only significant disadvantage of nasal pressure monitoring is that mouth breathing often may not be adequately detected (10%–15% of patients). This can be easily handled by monitoring with both nasal pressure and a nasal–oral thermistor. An alternative approach to measuring flow is to use respiratory inductance plethysmography. The changes in the sum of the ribcage and abdomen band signals (RIPsum) can be used to estimate changes in tidal volume (27,28). During positive-pressure titration, an airflow signal from the flow-generating device is often recorded instead of using thermistors or nasal pressure. This flow signal originates from a pneumotachograph or other flow-measuring device inside the flow generator.

In pediatric polysomnography, exhaled CO_2 is often monitored. Apnea usually causes an absence of fluctuations in this signal although small expiratory puffs rich in CO_2 can sometimes be misleading (7,22). The end-tidal P_{CO_2} (value at the end of exhalation) is an estimate of arterial P_{CO_2}. During long periods of hypoventilation that are common in children with sleep apnea, the end-tidal P_{CO_2} will be elevated (>45 mm Hg) (22).

Respiratory effort monitoring is necessary to classify respiratory events. A simple method of detecting respiratory effort is detecting movement of the chest and abdomen. This may be performed with belts attached to piezo-electric transducers, impedance monitoring, respiratory-inductance plethysmography (RIP), or monitoring of esophageal pressure (reflecting changes in pleural pressure). The surface EMG of the intercostal muscles or diaphragm can also be monitored to detect respiratory effort. Probably the most sensitive method for detecting effort is monitoring of changes in esophageal

pressure (reflecting changes in pleural pressure) associated with inspiratory effort (24). This may be performed with esophageal balloons or small fluid-filled catheters. Piezo-electric bands detect movement of the chest and abdomen as the bands are stretched and the pull on the sensors generates a signal. However, the signal does not always accurately reflect the amount of chest/abdomen expansion. In RIP, changes in the inductance of coils in bands around the rib cage (RC) and abdomen (AB) during respiratory movement are translated into voltage signals. The inductance of each coil varies with changes in the area enclosed by the bands. In general, RIP belts are more accurate in estimating the amount of chest/abdominal movement than piezo-electric belts. The sum of the two signals (RIPsum $= [a \times RC] + [b \times AB]$) can be calibrated by choosing appropriate constants: a and b. Changes in the RIPsum are estimates of changes in tidal volume (29). During upper-airway narrowing or total occlusion, the chest and abdominal bands may move paradoxically. Of note, a change in body position may alter the ability of either piezo-electric belts or RIP bands to detect chest/abdominal movement. Changes in body position may require adjusting band placement or amplifier sensitivity. In addition, very obese patients may show little chest/abdominal wall movement despite considerable inspiratory effort. Thus, one must be cautious about making the diagnosis of central apnea solely on the basis of surface detection of inspiratory effort.

Arterial oxygen saturation (Sa_{O_2}) is measured during sleep studies using pulse oximetry (finger or ear probes). This is often denoted as Sp_{O_2} to specify the method of Sa_{O_2} determination. A desaturation is defined as a decrease in Sa_{O_2} of 4% or more from baseline. Note that the nadir in Sa_{O_2} commonly follows apnea (hypopnea) termination by approximately 6 to 8 seconds (longer in severe desaturations). This delay is secondary to circulation time and instrumental delay (the oximeter averages over several cycles before producing a reading). Various measures have been applied to assess the severity of desaturation, including computing the number of desaturations, the average minimum SaO_2 of desaturations, the time below 80%, 85%, and 90%, as well as the mean SaO_2 and the minimum saturation during NREM and REM sleep. Oximeters may vary considerably in the number of desaturations they detect and their ability to discard movement artifact. Using long averaging times may dramatically impair the detection of desaturations.

ADULT RESPIRATORY DEFINITIONS

In adults, apnea is defined as absence of airflow at the mouth for 10 seconds or longer (21,22). If one measures airflow with a very sensitive device, such as a pneumotachograph, small expiratory puffs can sometimes be detected during an apparent apnea. In this case, there is "inspiratory apnea." Many sleep centers regard a severe decrease in airflow (to <10% of baseline) to be an apnea.

An obstructive apnea is cessation of airflow with persistent inspiratory effort. The cause of apnea is an obstruction in the upper airway. In Fig. 1-22, an obstructive apnea (no airflow with coexistent movement in the chest and abdomen) is followed by the corresponding nadir in the arterial oxygen saturation. In central apnea there is an absence of inspiratory effort. A mixed apnea is defined as an apnea with an initial central portion followed by an obstructive portion (Fig. 1-23). A hypopnea is a reduction in airflow for 10 seconds or longer (21). The apnea + hypopnea index (AHI) is the total number of apneas and hypopneas per hour of sleep. In adults, an AHI of <5 is considered normal.

Hypopneas can be further classified as obstructive, central, or mixed. If the upper airway narrows significantly airflow can fall (obstructive hypopnea). Alternatively, airflow can fall from a decrease in respiratory effort (central hypopnea). Finally, a combination is possible (mixed hypopnea) with both a decrease in respiratory effort and an

increase in upper airway resistance. However, unless accurate measures of airflow and esophageal or supraglottic pressure are obtained, such differentiation is usually not possible. In clinical practice, one usually identifies an obstructive hypopnea by the presence of airflow vibration (snoring), chest–abdominal paradox (increased load), or evidence of airflow flattening (airflow limitation) in the nasal pressure signal. In Fig. 1-24 two obstructive hypopneas each followed by an arterial oxygen desaturation are depicted. In both examples the nasal pressure shows a flattened profile not seen in the thermistor. In the second example there is chest-abdominal paradox during the event. Note the sudden transition from a flattened nasal pressure profile to a more rounded profile at event termination. A central hypopnea is associated with an absence of snoring, a round airflow profile (nasal pressure), and absence of chest–abdominal paradox. However, in the absence of esophageal pressure monitoring, a central hypopnea cannot always be classified with certainty. In addition, obstructive hypopnea may not always be associated with chest–abdominal paradox. Because of the limitations in exactly determining the type of hypopnea, most sleep centers usually report only the total number and frequency of hypopneas.

The exact requirements for an event to be classified as a hypopnea are a source of controversy (30,31). A task force of the AASM recommended that if an accurate measure of airflow is used, a 50% reduction in airflow for 10 s or longer would qualify as a hypopnea (28). Alternatively, any reduction in flow associated with an arousal or a 3% or greater drop in the SaO_2 (desaturation) would also meet criteria. In contrast, the Clinical Practice Review committee of the same organization defined a hypopnea as a 30% reduction in airflow of 10 seconds or longer, associated with a 4% or greater desaturation (32). The presence or absence of arousal is not a factor in their definition. The rationale for this recommendation is that there is considerable variability in scoring arousals, and studies using an associated 4% drop in the SaO_2 to define hypopnea have shown an association between an increased AHI and cardiovascular risk. The Center for Medicaid and Medicare Services (CMS) has

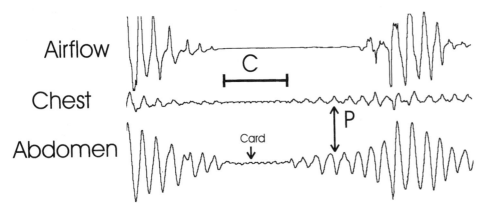

FIGURE 1-23. A mixed apnea with an initial central portion (C) during which there is no inspiratory effort followed by an obstructive portion with paradoxical chest–abdominal movement (P). The small fluctuations in the chest and abdominal tracings during the central portion are from cardiac pulsations (Card).

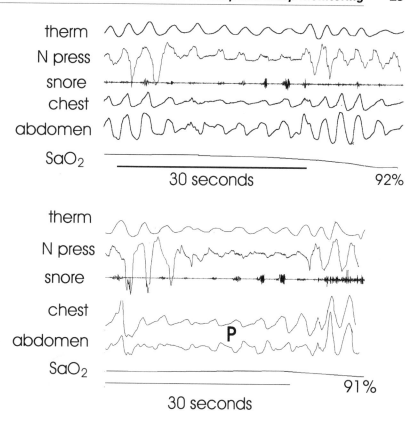

FIGURE 1-24. Two examples of obstructive hypopneas. Note that the nasal pressure tracing (N press) shows a greater decrement in flow than the thermistor (therm) signal and that the shape of the nasal pressure signal flattens. In the top hypopnea, there is a decrease in chest and abdominal movement during the hypopnea but no paradox. In the lower hypopnea, there is clear paradoxical movement (P) of the chest and abdomen.

adopted this definition of hypopnea for use in the criteria to determine if CPAP treatment will be reimbursed.

Respiratory events that do not meet criteria for either apnea or hypopnea can induce arousal from sleep. Such events have been called upper-airway resistance events (UARS), after the upper-airway resistance syndrome (11). An AASM task force recommended that such events be called respiratory effort-related arousals (RERAs). The recommended criteria for a RERA is a respiratory event of 10 seconds or longer followed by an arousal that does not meet criteria for an apnea or hypopnea, but is associated with a crescendo of inspiratory effort (esophageal monitoring) (28). Typically, following arousal, there is a sudden drop in esophageal pressure deflections. The exact definition of hypopnea that one uses will often determine whether a given event is classified as a hypopnea or a RERA.

One can also detect flow-limitation arousals (FLA) using an accurate measure of airflow, such as nasal pressure. Such events are characterized by flow limitation (flattening) over several breaths followed by an arousal and sudden, but often temporary, restoration of a normal-round airflow profile. One study suggested that the number of flow-limitation arousals per hour corresponded closely to the RERA index identified by esophageal pressure monitoring (33). Some centers compute a respiratory arousal index (RAI), determined as the arousals per hour associated with apnea, hypopnea, or RERA/FLA events. The AHI and respiratory disturbance index (RDI) are often used as equiv-

alent terms. However, in some sleep centers the RDI = AHI + RERA index, where the RERA index is the number of RERAs per hour of sleep, and RERAs are arousals associated with respiratory events not meeting criteria for apnea or hypopnea.

One can use the AHI to grade the severity of sleep apnea. Standard levels include normal (<5), mild (5 to <15), moderate (15–30), and severe (>30) per hour. Many sleep centers also give separate AHI values for NREM and REM sleep and various body positions. Some patients have a much higher AHI during REM sleep or in the supine position (REM-related or postural sleep apnea). Because the AHI does not always express the severity of desaturation, one might also grade the severity of desaturation. For example, it is possible for the overall AHI to be mild, but for the patient to have quite severe desaturation during REM sleep.

PEDIATRIC RESPIRATORY DEFINITIONS

Periodic breathing is defined as 3 or more respiratory pauses of at least 3 seconds in duration separated by less than 20 seconds of normal respiration. Periodic breathing is seen primarily in premature infants and mainly during active sleep (34). Although controversial, some feel that the presence of periodic breathing for >5% of TST or during quiet sleep in term infants is abnormal. Central apnea in infants is thought to be abnormal if

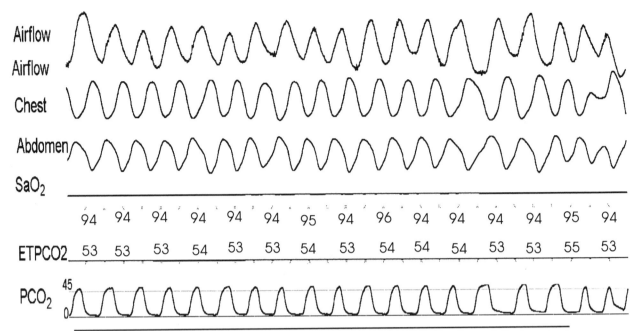

FIGURE 1-25. Obstructive hypoventilation in a 4-year-old girl with loud snoring and diaphoresis at night. The Pco_2 is a capnogram of the exhaled CO_2. The ETPCO2 tracing shows the current the end-tidal Pco_2 value. In this case the $PETCO_2$ is elevated at 53 mg Hg and the chest and abdomen show paradoxical breathing. The airflow channel (nasal oral thermistor) shows no discrete event. In this patient, the Sao_2 remained normal; however, in many cases it will be mildly to moderately reduced.

the event is >20 seconds in duration or associated with arterial oxygen desaturation or significant bradycardia (34–37).

In children, a cessation of airflow of any duration (usually two or more respiratory cycles) is considered an apnea when the event is obstructive (34–37). Of note, the respiratory rate in children (20–30/min) is greater than in adults (12–15/min). In fact, 10 seconds in an adult is usually the time required for 2 to 3 respiratory cycles. Obstructive apnea is very uncommon in normal children. Therefore, an obstructive AHI >1 is considered abnormal. In children with obstructive sleep apnea (OSA), the predominant event during NREM sleep is obstructive hypoventilation rather than a discrete apnea or hypopnea. Obstructive hypoventilation is characterized by a long period of upper-airway narrowing with a stable reduction in airflow and an increase in the end-tidal Pco_2 (Fig. 1-25). There is usually a mild decrease in the arterial oxygen desaturation. The ribcage is not completely calcified in infants and young children. Therefore, some paradoxical breathing is not necessarily abnormal. However, worsening paradox during an event would still suggest a partial airway obstruction. Nasal pressure monitoring is being used more frequently in children and periods of hypoventilation are more easily detected (reduced airflow with a flattened profile). Normative values have been published for the end-tidal Pco_2. One paper suggested that a peak end-tidal $Pco_2 > 53$ mm Hg or end-tidal $Pco_2 > 45$ mm Hg for more than 60% of TST should be considered abnormal (35).

Central apnea in infants was discussed above. The significance of central apnea in older children is less certain. Most do not consider central apneas following sighs (big breaths) to be abnormal. Some central apnea is probably normal in children, especially during REM sleep. In one study, up to 30% of normal children had some central apnea. Central apneas, when longer than 20 seconds, or those of any length associated with Sao_2 below 90%, are often considered abnormal, although a few such events have been noted in normal children (38). Therefore, most would recommend observation alone unless the events are frequent.

LEG MOVEMENT MONITORING

The EMG of the anterior tibial muscle (anterior lateral aspect of the calf) of both legs is monitored to detect leg movements (LMs) (39). Two electrodes are placed on the belly of the upper portion of the muscle of each leg about 2 to 4 cm apart (Fig. 1-26). A electrode loop is taped in place to provide strain relief. Usually each leg is displayed on a separate channel. However, if the number of recording channels is limited, one can link an electrode on each leg and display both leg EMGs on a single tracing (Fig. 1-27). Recording from both legs is required to accurately assess the number of movements. During biocalibration, the patient is asked to dorsiflex and plantarflex the great toe of the right and then the left leg to determine the adequacy of the

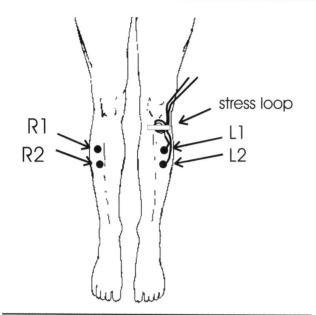

TABLE 1-9. Biocalibration Procedure

Eyes closed	EEG: Alpha EEG activity
	EOG: slow eye movements
Eyes open	EEG: attentuation of alpha rhythm
	EOG: REMs, blinks
Look right, look left, look up, look down	Integrity of eye leads, polarity, amplitude
	Eye movements should cause out-of-phase deflections
Grit teeth	Chin EMG
Breathe in, breathe out	Airflow, chest, abdomen movements adequate gain? Tracings in phase? (polarity of inspiration is usually upward).
Deep breath in, hold breath	Apnea detection
Wiggle right toe, left toe	Leg EMG, amplitude reference to evaluate LMs

FIGURE 1-26. Placement of electrodes for anterior tibial EMG recording. A two channel recording (R1-R2 and L1-L2) is recommended. If there are limited channels, the legs can then be linked on one channel (R1-L1, R2-L2, R1-L2, or R2-L1). In this case, all electrodes are placed in case one is lost during recording.

electrodes and amplifier settings. The amplitude should be 1 cm (paper recording) or at least one-half of the channel width on digital recording.

An LM is defined as an increase in the EMG signal of a least one-fourth the amplitude exhibited during biocalibration that is one-half to 5s in duration (39). Periodic LMs (PLMs) should be differentiated from bursts of spike-like phasic activity that occur during REM sleep. To be considered a PLM, the movement must occur in a group of four or more movements, each separated by more than 5 and less than 90 seconds (measured onset to onset). To be scored as a periodic leg movement in sleep, a LM must be preceded by at least 10 seconds of sleep. In most sleep centers, LMs associated with termination of respiratory events are not counted as PLMs. Some may score and tabulate this type of LM separately. The PLM index is the number of periodic leg movements divided by the hours of sleep (TST in hours). Rough guidelines for the PLM index are: >5 to <25 mild, 25 to <50 moderate, and ≥50 per hour severe (40).

A PLM arousal is an arousal that occurs simultaneously with or following (within 1–2 seconds) a PLM. The PLM arousal index is the number of PLM arousals per hour of sleep. A PLM arousal index of > 25 per hour is considered severe. LMs that occur during wake or after an arousal are either not counted or tabulated separately. For example, the PLMW (PLMwake) index is the number of PLMs per hour of wake. Of note, frequent LMs during wake, especially at sleep onset, may suggest the presence of the restless legs syndrome. The latter is a clinical diagnosis made on the basis of patient symptoms.

POLYSOMNOGRAPHY, BIOCALIBRATIONS, AND TECHNICAL ISSUES

A summary of the signals monitored in polysomnography is listed in Table 1-8. In addition, body position (using low-light video monitoring) and treatment level (CPAP, bilevel pressure) are usually added in comments by the

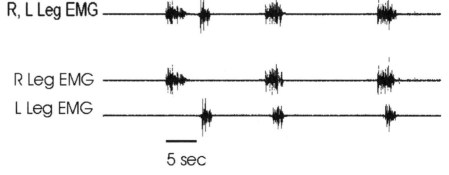

FIGURE 1-27. Sample tracing of right and left legs combined (upper tracing) and on separate channels (lower two tracings). Because the first right and leg LM onset is more than 5 seconds apart, they are considered separate movements. Therefore, the PLM count for the tracing is four.

technologists. In most centers, a video recording is also made on traditional video tape or digitally as part of the digital recording. It is standard practice to perform amplifier calibrations at the start of recording. In traditional paper recording, a calibration voltage signal (square wave voltage) was applied and the resulting pen deflections, along with the sensitivity, polarity, and filter settings on each channel, were documented on the paper. Similarly, in digital recording, a voltage is applied, although it is often a sine-wave voltage. The impedance of the head electrodes is also checked prior to recording. An ideal impedance is <5000 ohms although 10 or less is acceptable. Electrodes with higher impedances should be changed.

A biocalibration procedure is performed (Table 1-9) while signals are acquired with the patient connected to the monitoring equipment (4,5). This procedure permits checking of amplifier settings and integrity of monitoring leads/transducers. It also provides a record of the patient's EEG and eye movements during wakefulness with eyes closed and open. A summary of typical commands and their utility is listed in Table 1-9.

REFERENCES

1. Rechtschaffen A, Kales A, eds. *A manual of standardized terminology techniques and scoring system for sleep stages of human sleep.* Los Angeles: Brain Information Service/Brain Research Institute, UCLA, 1968.
2. Williams RL, Karacan I, Hursch CJ. *Electroencephalography of human sleep: Clinical applications.* New York: Wiley, 1974.
3. Caraskadon MA, Rechtschaffen A. Monitoring and staging human sleep. In: Kryger MH, Roth T, Dement WC, eds. *Principles and practice of sleep medicine.* Philadelphia: WB Saunders, 2000:1197–1215.
4. Keenan SA. Polysomnographic techniques: An overview. In: Chokroverty S, ed. *Sleep disorders medicine.* Boston: Butterworth - Heinemann, 1999:151–169.
5. Butkov N. Polysomnography. In: Lee-Chiong TL, Sateia MJ, Carskadon MA, eds. *Sleep medicine.* Philadelphia: Hanley and Belfus, 2002:605–637.
6. Geyer JD, Payne TA, Carny PR, et al. *Atlas of digital polysomnography.* Philadelphia: Lippincott Williams and Wilkins, 2000.
7. Berry RB. *Sleep medicine pearls,* 2nd ed. Philadelphia: Hanley and Belfus, 2003.
8. Bonnet MH. Performance and sleepiness as a function of frequency and placement of sleep disruption. *Psychophysiology.* 1986;23:263–271.
9. American Sleep Disorders Association—The Atlas Task Force: EEG arousals: Scoring rules and examples. *Sleep.* 1992;15:174–184.
10. Mathur R, Douglas NJ. Frequency of EEG arousals from nocturnal sleep in normal subjects. *Sleep.* 1995;18:330–333.
11. Guillemenault C, Stoohs R, Clerk A, et al. A cause of excessive daytime sleepiness: The upper airway resistance syndrome. *Chest.* 1993;104:781–787.
12. Butkov N. Atlas of clinical polysomnography, Ashland OR. *Synapse Media.* 1996;110–112.
13. Hauri P, Hawkins DR. Alpha-delta sleep. *Electroencephalogr Clin Neurophysiol.* 1973;34:233–237.
14. Johnson LC, Spinweber CL, Seidel WR, et al. Sleep spindle and delta changes during chronic use of short acting and long acting benzodiazepine hypnotic. *Electroencephalogr Clin Neurophysiol.* 1983;55:662–667.
15. Armitage R, Trivedi M, Rush AJ. Fluoxetine and oculomotor activity during sleep in depressed patients. *Neuropsychopharmacology.* 1995;12:159–165.
16. Schenck CH, Bundlie SR, Patterson AL, et al. Rapid eye movement sleep behavior disorder. *JAMA.* 1987;257:1786–1789.
17. Anders T, Emde R, Parmalee A. *A manual of standardized terminology, techniques and criteria for scoring of state of sleep and wakefulness in newborn infants.* Los Angeles: Brain Information Service, University of California Los Angeles, 1971.
18. Tanguay P, Ornitz E, Kaplan A, et al. Evolution of sleep spindles in childhood. *Electroencephalogr Clin Neurophysiol.* 1975;38:175.
19. Metcalf D, Mondale J, Butler F. Ontogenesis of spontaneous K complexes. *Psychophysiology.* 1971;26:49.
20. Sheldon SH, Riter S, Detrojan M. *Atlas of sleep medicine in infants and children.* Armonk, NY: Futura, 1999.
21. Block AJ, Boysen PG, Wynne JW, et al. Sleep apnea, hypopnea, and oxygen desaturation in normal subjects: A strong male predominance. *N Engl J Med.* 1979;330:513–517.
22. Kryger MH. Monitoring respiratory and cardiac function. In: Kryger MH, Roth T, Dement WC, eds. *Principles and practice of sleep medicine.* Philadelphia: WB Saunders, 2000:1217–1230.
23. Norman RG, Ahmed MM, Walsleben JA, et al. Detection of respiratory events during NPSG: Nasal cannula/pressure sensor versus thermistor. *Sleep.* 1997;20:1175–1184.
24. Berry RB. Nasal and esophageal pressure monitoring. In: Lee-Chiong TL, Sateia MJ, Caraskadon MA. eds. *Sleep medicine.* Philadelphia: Hanley and Belfus, 2002:661–671.
25. Monserrat JP, Farré R, Ballester E, et al. Evaluation of nasal prongs for estimating nasal flow. *Am J Respir Crit Care Med.* 1997;155:211–215.
26. Farré R, Rigau J, Montserrat JM, et al. Relevance of linearizing nasal prongs for assessing hypopneas and flow limitation during sleep. *Am J Respir Crit Care Med.* 2001;163:494–497.
27. Tobin M, Cohn MA, Sackner MA. Breathing abnormalities during sleep. *Arch Intern Med.* 1983;143:1221–1228.
28. American Academy of Sleep Medicine Task Force. Sleep-related breathing disorders in adults: Recommendation for syndrome definition and measurement techniques in clinical research. *Sleep.* 1999;22:667–689.
29. Chada TS, Watson H, Birch S, et al. Validation of respiratory inductance plethysmography using different calibration procedures. *Am Rev Respir Dis.* 1982;125:644–649.
30. Redline S, Kapur VK, Sanders MH, et al. Effects of varying approaches for identifying respiratory disturbances on sleep apnea assessment. *Am J Respir Crit Care Med.* 2000;161:369–374.
31. Redline S, Sander M. Hypopnea, a floating metric: Implications for prevalence, morbidity estimates, and case finding. *Sleep.* 1997;20:1209–1217.
32. Meoli AL, Casey KR, Clark RW. Clinical Practice Review Committee-AASM. Hypopnea in sleep disordered breathing in adults. *Sleep.* 2001;24:469–470.
33. Ayappa I, Norman RG, Krieger AC, et al. Non-invasive detection of respiratory effort related arousals (RERAs) by a nasal cannula/pressure transducer system. *Sleep.* 2000;23:763–771.
34. American Thoracic Society. Standards and indication for cardiopulmonary sleep studies in children. *Am J Respir Crit Care Med.* 1996;153:866–878.
35. Marcus CL, Omlin KJ, Basinki J, et al. Normal polysomnographic values for children and adolescents. *Am Rev Respir Dis.* 1992;146:1235–1239.
36. American Thoracic Society. Cardiorespiratory studies in children: Establishment of normative data and polysomnographic predictors of morbidity. *Am J Resp Crit Care Med.* 1999;160:1381–1387.
37. Marcus CL. Sleep-disordered breathing in children—State of the art. *Am J Resp Crit Care Med.* 2001;164:16–30.
38. Weese-Mayer DE, Morrow AS, Conway LP, et al. Assessing clinical significance of apnea exceeding fifteen seconds with event recording. *J Pediatr.* 1990;117:568–574.
39. ASDA Task Force. Recording and scoring leg movements. *Sleep.* 1993;16:749–759.
40. Diagnostic and Classification Steering Committee. Thorpy MJ. Chairman. *International classification of sleep disorders: Diagnostic and coding manual.* Rochester, MN: American Sleep Disorders Association, 1990:65–71.

Understanding Human Sleep

Chapter 2

Normal Human Sleep

Charles J. Bae and Nancy Foldvary-Schaefer

INTRODUCTION

Sleep is a universal phenomenon for human beings, defined most consistently as a temporary loss of consciousness. The meaning of sleep has been the subjects of debate since antiquity, likened to death by many over the centuries. Greek mythology described many gods for sleep and dreaming (1). Hypnos is the Greek god of sleep. His twin brother, Thanatos, is the god of death. Hypnos lived in a dark valley where the sun did not shine and the only sound heard was from the river of forgetfulness, called Lethe. Hypnos had three sons: Morpheus, Icelus, and Phantasus. Morpheus was responsible for creating dreams; he directed his brothers to produce dream content. Phantasus created images of inanimate objects and Icelus created those of men and beasts. More contemporary literature is replete with references to sleep and dreaming. For example, many of William Shakespeare's characters had sleep disorders including nightmares, somniloquoy, somnambulism, insomnia, and sleep apnea (2).

Sleep is an active physiologic state characterized by dynamic fluctuations in central nervous system, and hemodynamic, ventilatory, and metabolic parameters. The purpose of sleep has not been fully elucidated, although it is known that sleep is important in memory consolidation and healing. There is a fine balance between the homeostatic and circadian processes involved in the regulation of the sleep–wake cycle. This chapter reviews normal sleep in adult humans. The biology of sleep is discussed elsewhere.

The study of human sleep encompasses monitoring of several physiologic parameters. Loomis first described

non-rapid eye movement (NREM) sleep stages in 1937 (3). In the early 1950s, Aserinsky directly observed eye movements of sleeping infants (4). He and Kleitman recorded eye movements in humans during sleep, determining that rapid eye movements (REMs) were associated with dreaming. REM sleep was described in 1953 (5). In 1968, Rechtschaffen and Kales published standards for sleep staging using electroencephalography (EEG), electromyography (EMG), and electrooculography (EOG) (6).

NORMAL SLEEP CYCLE

Sleep is comprised of NREM and REM stages, and NREM sleep is further subdivided into stages 1 through 4 (Fig. 2-1). Stages 1 and 2 are considered light NREM sleep, while stages 3 and 4 are considered deep NREM sleep, also known as delta or slow-wave sleep (SWS). The normal sleep cycle begins in stage 1, or drowsiness. Stage 1 is followed by stage 2 sleep that, in turn, is followed by SWS. After a brief return to stage 2, REM sleep begins. Most adults have 5 to 7 sleep cycles per night, lasting approximately 90 minutes, with the first being the shortest. Slow-wave sleep predominates in the first one-third of the night, while REM sleep increases during the last few hours of sleep. The first period of REM sleep usually occurs 70 to 90 minutes after sleep onset. By the second decade of life, humans spend 2% to 5% of sleep time in stage 1 sleep, 45% to 55% in stage 2 sleep, 13% to 23% in SWS sleep, and 20% to 25% in REM sleep (3).

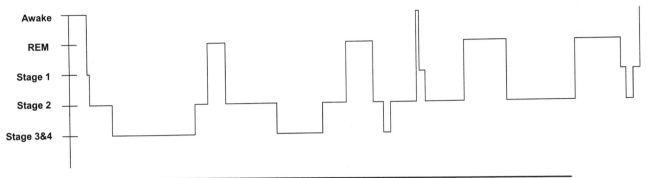

FIGURE 2-1. Normal adult histogram. Sleep onset occurs within minutes. There is a predominance of SWS during the first one-third of the sleep period. REM sleep increases as the night progresses, and the majority occurs in the last one-third of the sleep period.

Sleep patterns change across the lifespan (Table 2-1). The duration of the normal sleep cycle varies with age, as does the distribution of sleep stages. For example, the average duration of a sleep cycle is 60 minutes in newborns and 90 minutes in adolescents (4,8). The duration of the sleep period decreases with age. Newborns sleep for up to 16 hours per day; by 6 months of age, sleep time is reduced to approximately 12 hours (5). In adulthood, the normal sleep period is 7.5 to 8 hours (6).

The proportion of REM and NREM sleep changes with age. Newborns spend more time in REM sleep than do children and adults. A full-term infant spends approximately 50% of total sleep time in REM sleep, and sleep-onset REM periods (SOREMPs) are common. By 3 months of life, the amount of daytime REM sleep decreases as the sleep cycle gradually matures into that seen in older children and adults (4). Rapid eye movement sleep constitutes 20 to 25% of sleep time by 1 year of age, thereafter remaining relatively stable into adulthood (7). In contrast, the amount of SWS begins to decrease in the third decade of life, disappearing entirely in some individuals by 90 years of age (7).

Various changes in the sleep cycle are observed in subjects over the age of 60 years, as depicted in Fig. 2-2. Sleep is more fragmented in the elderly, demonstrated by an increase in arousals and awakenings throughout the night (7). Sleep fragmentation may be related to medical or psychiatric disorders as well as the increased prevalence of sleep-related breathing disorders and periodic limb movements during sleep with advancing age (7). Sleep efficiency is reduced and there is more wake time in bed (8). Slow-wave sleep percentage declines and light NREM sleep (stages 1 and 2) constitutes a larger amount of the sleep period (8).

Sleep architecture is commonly affected by environmental factors. The "first-night effect" describes various alterations in sleep quality induced by a foreign environment, such as the sleep laboratory (Fig. 2-3) (9,10). Sleep structure tends to normalize on subsequent nights as one becomes acclimated to the environment. Findings consistent with the first-night effect include reduced sleep efficiency, increased awakenings and arousals, prolonged sleep and REM latency, reduced REM and SWS, and an increase in stage 1 sleep.

SLEEP STAGES

Wakefulness

A discussion about sleep stages is not complete without first describing the electroencephalographic feature of wakefulness. First described by Hans Berger in 1929, the alpha rhythm is comprised of 8 to 13 Hz waves over the posterior head regions during relaxed wakefulness with eyes closed (Fig. 2-4) (11,12). The lower limit of 8 Hz is usually reached by 8 years of age. The frequency of the alpha rhythm lies between 9 and 11 Hz in most adults, decreasing slightly with advancing age. However, the mean is maintained at or above 8 Hz in healthy individuals in the seventh and eighth decades of life (13). A posterior dominant rhythm of less than 8 Hz during wakefulness in an adult is abnormal. The frequency of the

TABLE 2-1. Sleep Characteristics Across the Lifespan[a]

	Infants	Adults	Elderly
Total sleep time (hr)	14–15	7.5–8.5	6
Wake time after sleep onset (%)	<5	<5	15–26
Stage 1 (%)		2–5	4–15
Stage 2 (%)	50	45–55	60
Slow wave sleep (%)		13–23	5–20
REM (%)	50	20–25	18
REM:NREM	50:50	20:80	20:80
Cycle duration (min)	50–60	90–110	90–110

[a] From references 3, 4, 28, and 29.

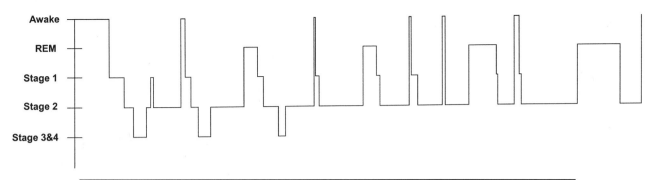

FIGURE 2-2. Sleep in the elderly. In older individuals, sleep latency is prolonged and sleep is fragmented by arousals and awakenings. The overall amount of SWS is decreased, with a relative preservation of REM sleep.

alpha rhythm should be similar over the two hemispheres. An interhemispheric asymmetry of 1 Hz or greater is abnormal.

On referential montages, the distribution of the alpha rhythm is usually maximal at the occipital electrodes (O1, O2). However, the amplitude may be highest in the parietal or posterior temporal regions and occasionally is more widespread. Using the P4 to O2 derivation, the voltage of the alpha rhythm in adult is in the range of 15 to 45 μV. Higher voltages are observed in younger individuals. The voltage decreases with age, reflecting changes in bone density and increased electrical impedance of intervening tissue. In normal individuals, mild voltage asymmetry is common, and the right hemisphere typically shows higher amplitudes. Asymmetries are considered significant when the amplitude over one hemisphere is less than 50% of that seen over the contralateral side. To be considered abnormal, voltage asymmetries should be present on both referential and bipolar montages.

Reactivity to sensory stimuli and mental activation is one feature that distinguishes the normal alpha rhythm from abnormal activity in the alpha frequency range. The alpha rhythm is best observed during relaxed wakefulness with the eyes closed. Attenuation or blocking of the alpha rhythm occurs with eye opening, concentrated mental effort, heightened levels of alertness, and auditory or tactile stimulation.

During polysomnography (PSG), it is often useful to quantify the waking background rhythm on the conventional EEG epoch length of 10 seconds. This is particularly useful in the differentiation of wakefulness and REM sleep. The alpha rhythm of wakefulness is 1 to 2 Hz faster than alpha waves occurring during REM sleep. During wakefulness, respirations are regular and EMG activity (axial and appendicular) is at the highest level of the recording.

Non-Rapid Eye Movement (NREM) Sleep

Stage 1 Sleep

Stage 1 sleep, also known as drowsiness, is a transitional state characterized by slow eye movements, gradual waning of the wake background rhythm,

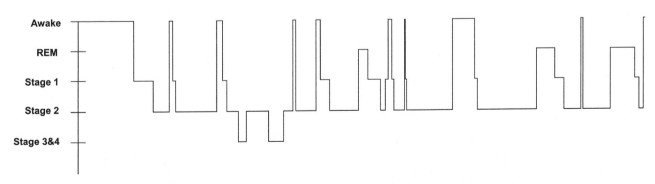

FIGURE 2-3. The first night effect. Sleeping in a foreign environment may produce alterations in sleep quality. Sleep onset and REM latency are prolonged. The total sleep time is reduced due to an increased number of arousals and awakenings. There is a decreased amount of SWS and REM sleep, with an increased amount of stage 1 sleep.

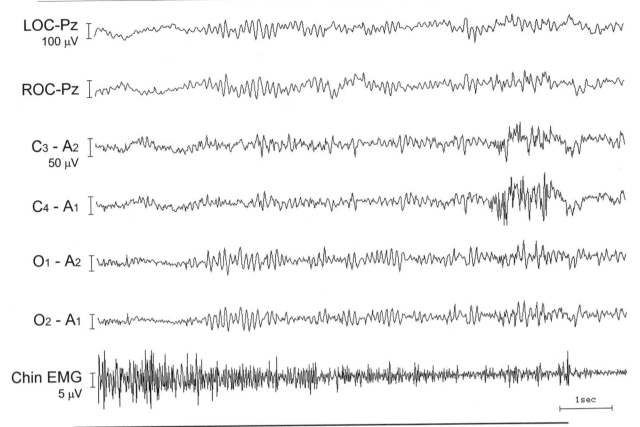

FIGURE 2-4. Normal wake rhythm. Ten-second epoch demonstrating relaxed wakefulness. The normal background rhythm in adults consists of 8 to 13 Hz sinusoidal activity maximal over the posterior head regions. Axial EMG is elevated.

frontocentral theta activity, and vertex waves (Fig. 2-5). The predominant background of the drowsy state is low- to medium-amplitude delta and theta activity intermixed with faster frequencies. Slow pendular eye movements are observed. Slow eye movements have a frequency of less than 0.5 Hz, whereas rapid eye movements are typically greater than 1 Hz (14). During stage 1 sleep, there is usually a reduction in muscle activity and movement artifact. Due to its sporadic and sometimes abrupt appearance, drowsiness may be misinterpreted as abnormal paroxysmal activity.

Vertex waves are diphasic, and surface negative sharp transients are maximally distributed in the central regions. First appearing in drowsiness, vertex waves may persist into stage 2 and SWS. In adults, vertex activity is bilaterally synchronous and symmetric. The amplitude of vertex waves may approach 200 μV in children, typically declining with age. Persistent asymmetries are abnormal, usually suggesting dysfunction on the side of lower amplitude. In children, vertex waves may appear in runs of spiky transients, making the differentiation between sleep and epileptiform activity challenging.

Positive occipital sharp transients (POSTS) are surface-positive triangular waves occasionally followed by a lower-voltage negative phase that can be seen in light sleep,

especially in children. POSTS usually appear in runs of bilaterally synchronous 4- to 5-Hz waves, but mild asymmetries are common. These waveforms first appear in drowsiness but may persist in deep stages of NREM sleep. On a 30-second epoch, POSTS may not be readily apparent.

Stage 2 Sleep

Stage 2 sleep is characterized by sleep spindles and K complexes superimposed on a background of mixed frequencies with less than 20% delta activity (Fig. 2-6). Stage 2 sleep constitutes 45% to 55% of total sleep time. Sleep spindles, or sigma activity, are rhythmic sinusoidal waves of 10 to 14 Hz seen in the central regions. Their duration ranges from 0.5 to 2 seconds. Sleep spindles are asynchronous at the time of their first appearance at 6 to 8 weeks post-term until the age of 2 years (15).

K complexes are diphasic waves having an initial negative sharp component followed immediately by a slow positive phase. A sleep spindle is often superimposed on the positive phase. K complexes are at least 0.5 seconds in duration and symmetric over the central regions. K complexes may occur singly or in trains, spontaneously or

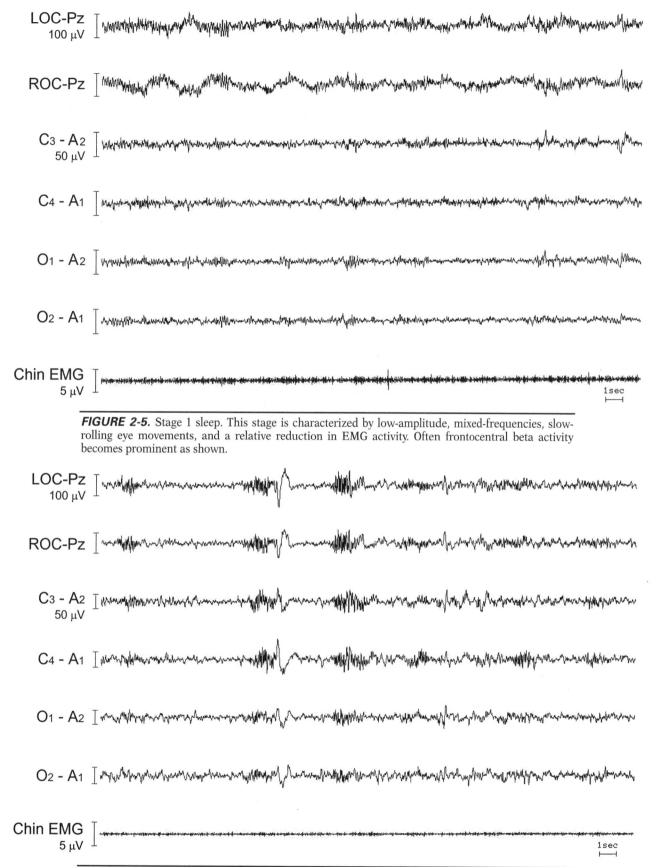

LOC-Pz
100 μV

ROC-Pz

C3 - A2
50 μV

C4 - A1

O1 - A2

O2 - A1

Chin EMG
5 μV

1sec

FIGURE 2-5. Stage 1 sleep. This stage is characterized by low-amplitude, mixed-frequencies, slow-rolling eye movements, and a relative reduction in EMG activity. Often frontocentral beta activity becomes prominent as shown.

LOC-Pz
100 μV

ROC-Pz

C3 - A2
50 μV

C4 - A1

O1 - A2

O2 - A1

Chin EMG
5 μV

1sec

FIGURE 2-6. Stage 2 sleep. The hallmarks of this stage are sleep spindles and K complexes superimposed on a mixed-frequency background.

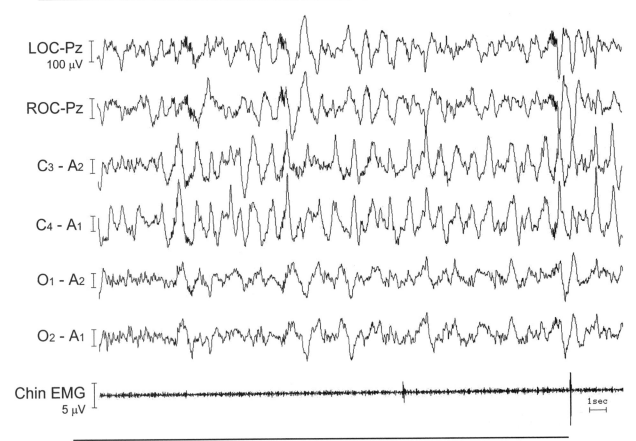

FIGURE 2-7. Slow-wave sleep. Stages 3 and 4 are collectively referred to as slow-wave sleep. High-amplitude (>75 μV), slow frequencies (<2 Hz) comprise the background activity. Sleep spindles may be observed.

following an auditory stimulus (16). They are present by 5 months of age.

Stage 3 and 4 Sleep

Stages 3 and 4 are collectively referred to as delta or SWS. Stage 3 sleep is scored when 20% to 50% of the background is comprised of delta activity of less than 2 Hz and greater than 75 μV, as shown in Fig. 2-7 (17). Spindles may be present, but are less frequent and lower in frequency than in stage 2. Stage 4 is scored when at least 50% of the background is comprised of delta activity of less than 2 Hz and amplitude greater than 75 μV (17). Most sleep laboratories do not make the distinction between stage 3 and 4 sleep. Thirteen to 25% of sleep time is spent in SWS.

Rapid Eye Movement (REM) Sleep

REM sleep is characterized by low-voltage, mixed frequencies with admixed alpha activity that is usually 1 to 2 Hz slower than the waking alpha rhythm. REM sleep is subdivided into phasic and tonic components. During tonic REM sleep, suppression of EMG activity is noted and the EEG shows low-voltage mixed-frequency background. No phasic REMs are observed and respiration is often fairly regular. During phasic REM (Fig. 2-8), twitches of EMG activity and irregularities in heart rate and respirations occur in association with REMs. Runs of 2- to 6-Hz notched waves, referred to as sawtooth waves, may be seen in the frontocentral regions, usually in association with bursts of eye movements. Muscle tone is at the lowest level of the recording. REM sleep normally occurs 60 to 90 minutes after sleep onset. The latency to REM sleep is shorter in sleep-deprived individuals, neonates, patients with narcolepsy, and subjects withdrawing from alcohol and REM suppressant medications. Features characteristic of each sleep stage are summarized in Table 2-2.

TRANSITIONAL PERIODS

In normal subjects, the transition between wakefulness and sleep and sleep and wakefulness is gradual, characterized by changes in EEG and other physiologic and behavioral parameters (10). In the transition from wakefulness to sleep, there is a waxing and waning of the alpha rhythm that is gradually replaced by frontocentral theta activity and vertex waves. Slow eye movements are commonly observed. Bursts of high-voltage (100–300 μV), monomorphic waves, in the range of 2.5 to 4.5 Hz, are often

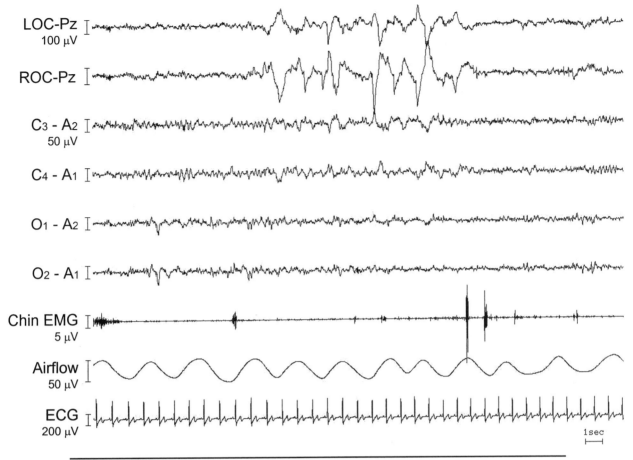

FIGURE 2-8. REM Sleep. This is a 30-second epoch demonstrating REM sleep. Rapid eye movements, twitches of EMG activity, and minor airflow irregularities are present.

▶ **TABLE 2-2. Normal Sleep Periods[a]**

Stage 1 sleep (drowsiness)	Low-voltage, mixed-frequency, slow-rolling eye movements, vertex waves
Stage 2 sleep	Sleep spindles, K complexes superimposed on mixed frequencies
Stage 3 and 4 sleep	Delta activity <2 Hz and >75 μV occupying at least 20% of the background (also referred to as slow-wave sleep or delta sleep). Stage 3 sleep—delta activity 20–50%; stage 4–delta activity >50%
REM sleep	Low-voltage, mixed frequencies with rapid eye movements, sawtooth waves, and the lowest axial EMG of the recording
Normal adult sleep cycle	5–7 per night, each lasting 90–110 min. Slow-wave sleep predominates in first one-third of sleep period; REM predominates in last one-third of sleep period.

[a]From references 3,4,28, and 29.

observed at the transition from wakefulness to sleep in infants and children. Known as hypnogogic hypersynchrony, this pattern is most common in children under the age of 10 years, and decreases during the second decade of life, only rarely observed in young adults (18,19). A similar pattern, known as hypnopompic hypersynchrony, is observed at the transition from sleep to wakefulness (Fig. 2-9) and is most common in children between the ages of 10 and 14 years (18). Due to their paroxysmal appearance, both patterns are commonly mistaken for seizure activity.

Arousals and awakenings are a normal part of sleep in most healthy adults. A number of different arousal patterns have been described (20). Arousals from stage 1 consist of low-voltage fast activity or a reversion to the waking background rhythm. Once stage 2 is achieved, arousals typically begin with a K complex followed by a brief train of alpha-range frequencies with or without intermixed high-voltage delta transients and an increase in EMG activity. Arousals from SWS are generally not observed in normal adults and their presence should raise the suspicion of a NREM parasomnia. Because bursts of alpha activity are normally seen in REM sleep, a simultaneous increase in EMG activity is required for arousals in this stage (20). The threshold to

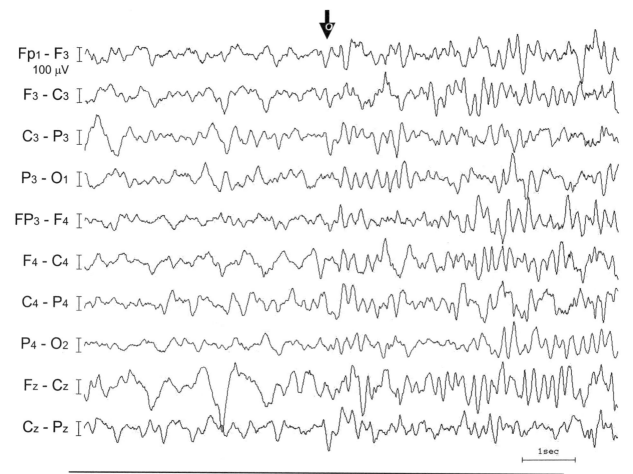

FIGURE 2-9. Hypnopompic hypersynchrony. This is a 10-second epoch of an arousal in a young child. Upon waking, there is high-voltage, monomorphic theta activity (arrow). Due to its paroxysmal nature, this pattern may be misinterpreted as epileptic in nature.

arousal increases as sleep deepens. It has been shown that auditory arousal thresholds increase to 64% of the maximum value within a minute of sleep onset (21).

Many normal adults experience unusual behavioral phenomena at the transition between sleep and wakefulness. Hypnic jerks are benign, involuntary movements involving the head, arms or legs, occurring in transitional periods, and dissipating as sleep deepens. With a prevalence of 60% to 70% in normal adults, hypnic jerks are considered benign (22). Sleep paralysis is a frightening phenomenon of muscle paralysis during wakefulness, representing an intrusion of REM sleep into the waking state. Episodes range in duration from seconds to minutes and occur when falling asleep or waking up. Isolated episodes of sleep paralysis are experienced by 40%–50% of normal individuals (22). Some adults may experience hypnogogic or hypnopompic sensory hallucinations. These are typically described as dreamlike, but can be terrifying. Hypnogogic hallucinations occur in the setting of acute recovery from REM suppression and in 15%–90% of narcoleptic patients, depending on the study (22). Sleep inertia is a state of reduced cognitive performance immediately after awak-

ening. Its expression is dependent upon the stage of sleep from which one awakens. Sudden awakening from SWS is associated with a maximum amount of sleep inertia, and sleep deprivation may increase its expression due to the potential increase in SWS (23). Symptoms typically last from 5 minutes to as long as a few hours following severe sleep deprivation (23).

NEED FOR SLEEP

Most people believe that the average normal adult requires 8 hours of sleep for good health and optimal performance. In fact, sleep needs vary from one individual to another. It is difficult to assess how much sleep is needed to function optimally. It is more practical to measure how performance is affected by sleep loss. Time spent in bed is not equivalent to time spent sleeping, but time spent in bed is a variable that can be controlled.

Two recent studies have shown that a sleep restriction of 6 hours or less produces cognitive performance deficits as measured by psychomotor vigilance tests. One study assessed the effect of 3, 5, 7, and 9 hours in bed over 7 days followed by a recovery period of 3 days (24). Performance was not affected in the group that spent 9 hours in bed. In the group that spent 5 or 7 hours in bed, performance initially declined and then stabilized. Performance declined without stabilization in the group that spent 3 hours in bed and did not return to baseline levels even after 3 days of recovery sleep. Therefore, performance becomes more impaired as the amount of sleep loss increases. Another study compared the effect of sleep restriction of 4, 6, or 8 hours over 14 days to 3 days of sustained wakefulness (25). Restricting sleep to 4 to 6 hours per night produced cognitive performance deficits similar to 1 to 2 days of total sleep deprivation.

Two recent studies highlight the importance of adequate sleep in maintaining good health. Over 1.1 million adults in the United States participated in a questionnaire study addressing the association between self-reported sleep and mortality (26). A relationship was found between total sleep time and mortality. An average sleep period of 7 hours per night was associated with the lowest mortality hazard, while those who slept for more than 8 hours or less than 6 hours had an increased mortality hazard. Another study including over 110,000 Japanese adults also found that 7 hours of sleep per night was associated with a lower mortality than 4 hours or less and 8 hours or more (27). It appears that sleeping "too much" or "too little" may be detrimental, although further research is required to explain these findings.

FUTURE DIRECTIONS

Sleep is a complex physiologic process that evolves with age. There is a delicate balance between sleep and wakefulness that can be disrupted by a multitude of factors, both internal and external. Further work is needed to identify the factors affecting sleep in different age groups and to clearly elucidate the effects of sleep deprivation on health and longevity.

REFERENCES

1. Hamilton E. *Mythology.* Boston: Little, Brown, 1969.
2. Furman Y, Wolf SM, Rosenfeld DS. Shakespeare and sleep disorders. *Neurology.* 1997;49:1171–1172.
3. Carskadon MA, Dement WC. *Normal human sleep: An overview,* 2000.
4. Anders TF, Sadeh A, Appareddy V. Normal sleep in neonates and children. In: Ferber R, Kryger MH, eds. *Principles and practice of sleep medicine in the child.* Philadelphia: W.B. Saunders, 1995: 7–18.
5. Coons S. Development of sleep and wakefulness during the first 6 months of Life. In: Guilleminault C, ed. *Sleep and its disorders in children.* New York: Raven Press, 1987:17–27.
6. Chokroverty S. An overview of sleep. In: Chokroverty S, ed. *Sleep disorders medicine: Basic science, technical considerations and clinical aspects,* 2nd ed. Boston: Butterworth-Henemann, 1999:7–20.
7. Bliwise DL. Sleep in normal aging and dementia. *Sleep.* 1993;16:40–81.
8. Redline S, Kirchner HL, Quan SF, et al. The effects of age, sex, ethnicity and sleep-disordered breathing on sleep architecture. *Arch Intern Med.* 2004;164:406–418.
9. Agnew HW, Webb WB, Williams RL. The first-night effect: An EEG study of sleep. *Psychophysiology.* 1966;2:263–266.
10. Toussaint M, Luthringer R, Schaltenbrand N, et al. First-night effect in normal subjects and psychiatric inpatients. *Sleep.* 1995;18:463–469.
11. Markand ON. Alpha rhythms. *J Clin Neurophysiol.* 1990;7:163–189.
12. Berger H. On the electroencephalogram of man. Second report. *J Psych Neurol.* 1930;40:160–179.
13. Obrist WD. Problems of aging. In: Remond A, ed. *Handbook of electroencephalography and clinical neurophysiology.* Vol. 6A. Amsterdam: Elsevier, 1976:275–292.
14. Radtke R. Sleep disorders: Laboratory evaluation. In: Ebersole JS, Pedley TA, eds. *Current practice of clinical electgroencephalography.* Philadelphia: Lippincott Williams & Wilkins, 2003:803–832.
15. Ellingtson RJ. Development of sleep spindle bursts during the first year of life. *Sleep.* 1982;5:39–46.
16. Aldrich MS. *Normal human sleep. Sleep medicine.* New York: Oxford University Press, 1999:3–26.
17. Rechtschaffen A, Kales A. *A manual of standardized terminology, techniques and scoring system for sleep stages of human subjects.* Los Angeles: UCLA Brain Information Service/Brain Research Institute, 1968.
18. Gibbs FA, Gibbs EL. *Normal controls. Atlas of electroencephalography.* Vol. 1. Cambridge: Addison-Wesley, 1950.
19. Eeg-Olofsson O, Petersen I, Sellden U. The development of the EEG in normal children from the age of 1 to 15 years: paroxysmal activity. *Neuropediatrie.* 1971;4:375–404.
20. EEG arousals: scoring rules and examples: a preliminary report from the Sleep Disorders Atlas Task Force of the American Sleep Disorders Association. *Sleep.* 1992;15:173–184.
21. Bonnet MH, Moore SE. The threshold of sleep: perception of sleep as a function of time asleep and auditory threshold. *Sleep.* 1982;5:267–276.
22. *International classification of sleep disorders, Revised: Diagnostic and coding manual.* Rochester: American Sleep Disorders Association, 2001.
23. Tassi P, Muzet A. Sleep inertia. *Sleep Med Rev.* 2000;4:341–353.
24. Belenky G, Wesensten NJ, Thorne DR, et al. Patterns of performance degradation and restoration during sleep restriction and subsequent recover: A sleep dose-response study. *J Sleep Res.* 2003;12:1–12.
25. Van Dongen HP, Maislin G, Mullington JM, et al. The cumulative cost of additional wakefulness: Dose-response effects on neurobehavioral functions and sleep physiology from chronic sleep restriction and total sleep deprivation. *Sleep.* 2003;26:117–126.
26. Kripke DF, Garfinkel L, Wingard DL, et al. Mortality associated with sleep duration and insomnia. *Arch Gen Psych.* 2002;59:131–136.
27. Tamakoshi A, Ohno Y. Self-reported sleep duration as a predictor of all-cause mortality: Results from the JACC study, Japan. *Sleep.* 2004;27:51–54.
28. Bliwise DL. Sleep and aging. In: Pressman MR, Orr WC, eds. *Understanding sleep: The evaluation and treatment of sleep disorders.* Washington, DC: American Psychological Association, 1997:441–464.
29. Bliwise DL. Normal aging. In: Kryger MH, Roth T, Dement WC, eds. *Principles and practice of sleep medicine,* 3rd ed. Philadelphia: W.B. Saunders, 2000:26–42.

The Neurobiology of Sleep

Wendy M. Norman and Linda F. Hayward

INTRODUCTION AND HISTORICAL PERSPECTIVE

Since the time of Greek philosophers and before, the function of sleep has been contemplated. In Greek mythology, sleep was considered a state similar to death and as such, the goddess of night, Nxy, was portrayed as the mother of both the god of sleep, Hypnos, and the god of death, Thanatos. Aristotle recognized that sleep was characterized by relative inattention to the environment and physical immobility and suggested that sleep reflected the time needed to replenish "power" lost from systems involved in sensory perception during wakefulness. As a result, sleep was originally considered a time of brain inactivity. It is now recognized, however, that sleep is an extremely active process as evidenced by highly predictable changes in brain electrical activity, muscle activity, and autonomic control. Yet, the biological function of sleep remains elusive.

To provide an overview of the current state of knowledge regarding the neurobiology of sleep, we have divided this chapter into five main sections (Table 3-1). First, we will briefly discuss the phylogenetic characteristics of sleep. Important information regarding the function of sleep has come from comparisons between the duration of sleep and physiologic changes during sleep across species. Second, the distinct patterns of human electroencephalogram (EEG) that are currently recognized as general descriptors of specific phases of the sleep cycle are thought to be mediated through reciprocal connections between the thalamus and cortex. Thalamocortical neuronal activation is regulated by alternating input from brainstem sites and descending inputs from the hypothalamus and suprachiasmatic nucleus (SCN). As such, we will discuss the hypothalamic circuitry currently thought to control sleep and how input from these regions interacts with different areas of the brainstem involved in the generation of rapid-eye movement (REM) sleep. Third, current mechanisms underlying changes in EEG activity will be mentioned. Fourth, we will review current information regarding the neuromodulation of sleep. Finally, we will briefly mention a current theory on how the switch from wakefulness

TABLE 3-1. Highlights of Important Neural Control Centers for Sleep and Wakefulness

Anterior hypothalamus: ventrolateral preoptic nucleus (inhibitory)—sleep promoting

Posterior hypothalamus: lateral and dorsomedial hypothalamus (orexin, excitatory)—wake promoting

Tuberomammillary nucleus: forebrain histaminergic cell group (excitatory)—wake promoting

Pedunculopontine tegmental nucleus and laterodorsal tegmental nucleus: midbrain and pontine cholinergic neurons—wake promoting and important for REM sleep production

Locus coeruleus (norepinephrine) **and dorsal raphe** (serotonin): brainstem monoaminergic cell groups—wake promoting

TABLE 3-2. Characteristics of NREM Sleep Stages

Stage 1
1. Background beta and a few alpha waves (<50% of a given segment)
2. Hippocampal theta waves
3. Involuntary slow eye rolls
4. Duration of 3 to 5 min

Stage 2
1. Background of beta waves
2. Some spindles and K complexes (high amplitude, biphasic waves)
3. No eye movements
4. Duration of 30 min

Stage 3[a]
1. Background 20 to 50% delta waves
2. Spindles and K complexes

Stage 4[a]
1. Background >50% delta waves
2. Minimal spindles
3. Duration of 20 to 30 min

[a] Together, stages 3 and 4 are referred to as slow-wave sleep.

to sleep is generated and the future directions of sleep research.

PHYLOGENY OF SLEEP

Sleep has a number of diverse, important actions, judging by the spectrum of adverse consequences of sleep deprivation: cognitive deficits, including memory loss, short attention span and poor attention, loss of speech fluency, loss of divergent (flexible) thinking, depression, and decreased growth. However, the fundamental function of sleep, the primary driving force for its development remains unclear. Studies of animals' sleep evolution through the ages and comparisons of sleep among contemporary animal species are yielding interesting insights and hypotheses about the original function of sleep.

Animal models also contribute profoundly to studies of sleep neurobiology. To interpret these data successfully, it is important to understand how animal sleep compares to human sleep.

Sleep Characteristics of Various Species

Definition

Sleep characteristics vary across species and thus, several criteria are used to qualify a behavior as sleep. Sleep is defined as a sustained quiescent period, spent in a species-specific characteristic posture or site, and during which the threshold for response to stimuli is raised, although a stimulus of sufficient strength will rapidly reverse the state (1,2). Additional criteria require that the sleep/rest rhythm follows a circadian rhythm and that there is evidence of sleep rebound after a period of deprivation (3,4).

Sleep in Humans

Sleep as we know it in humans is a complex behavioral and electrophysiologic phenomenon. In addition to the above behavioral characteristics, the EEG cycles between one of two states: non-rapid eye movement (NREM) sleep and REM sleep. NREM sleep is characterized by a high-amplitude, low-frequency EEG with delta (<4 Hz), theta (4–8 Hz), and spindle (12–14 Hz) waves. The density of slow waves reflects the intensity or depth of sleep. Four stages of NREM sleep are recognized, with a progressive increase in slow-wave density from stage 1 to 4 (Table 3-2). The EEG of stage 2 NREM sleep is characterized by the presence of either sleep spindles or K complexes (high-amplitude biphasic waves). Some high-amplitude slow-wave activity may be present. Stages 3 and 4 are defined by progressively more slow-wave activity (20–50% for stage 3 and >50% for stage 4 of each segment of sleep).

The EEG of REM sleep resembles that of wakefulness with high-frequency, low-amplitude waves. REM sleep is distinguished from wakefulness by a loss of muscle tone, especially in the antigravity muscles, intermittently broken by muscle twitching, rapid eye movements, suspended thermoregulation, and autonomic irregularities manifesting as irregular respiration and irregular heart beats (Table 3-3). PGO waves are another important component of REM sleep found in deep brain structures in animals. These waves are spiky EEG waves that arise in the pons, are transmitted to the lateral geniculate nucleus (a visual system nucleus), and to the visual occipital cortex. Hence the origin of the name of the waves is given by these structures (pons-lateral geniculate nucleus–occipital cortex). These waves have not been recorded in humans (deep brain recording needed) but are assumed to exist. The saccades of quick conjugate eye movements (REMs) that occur during REM sleep are the origin of the name of this sleep stage.

▶ **TABLE 3-3.** **Components of REM Sleep**

1. EEG Desynchronization
2. PGO waves
3. REMs
4. Muscle atonia
5. Hippocampal theta (sawtooth waves in EEG)
6. Muscle twitches
7. Suspended thermoregulation
8. Cardiovascular changes
9. Respiratory changes

Mammals

The sleep characteristics described above occur in nearly all mammals. Therefore, most mammalian species are reasonable choices as models for sleep research. However, there are some species differences among mammals worth noting. In mammalian species other than man and some primates (chimpanzee, rhesus, and squirrel monkey), NREM sleep is not differentiated into stages as it is in humans, but refers to all four stages. It is often simply referred to as slow-wave sleep, being equivalent to stages 3 and 4 in the human. Also, in other mammalian species, the duration of a sleep cycle (NREM–REM) is shorter than the 90 minutes recorded for humans (5). For example, it is about 28 minutes in cats and 10 to 12 minutes in rats (2). Humans tend to sleep during one phase in the day, whereas many mammals sleep in a "polyphasic" manner. For example, although the cat obtains a large portion of its sleep during the night, it can certainly be observed napping frequently during the daytime.

A subpopulation of aquatic mammals (cetaceans, eared seals, and manatees) exhibit unihemispheric sleep where one cortical hemisphere shows EEG signs of wakefulness while the other shows slow waves (6). Interestingly, only NREM, not REM sleep, occurs in animals with unihemispheric sleep. At the same time as unihemispheric sleep is occurring, there are behavioral signs of wakefulness, such as swimming. One eye is open and the other is closed. The study of unihemispherical sleep has led to the idea that sleep can be localized to those parts of the brain that have recently been activated. For example, dolphins were sleep deprived in a preselected hemisphere by repeatedly arousing them when that hemisphere showed signs of sleep. During recovery from the sleep deprivation, only the sleep-deprived hemisphere showed a sleep-rebound effect by compensating for lost sleep time (7).

Birds and Reptiles

Birds cycle between NREM and REM sleep as do mammals, although the percentage of time spent in REM sleep is over one-third less. In contrast to mammals, unihemispheric sleep is pervasive among birds and found in species such as domestic chickens, gulls, and pigeons (6). It comprises about 20% of sleep time in gulls.

Reptiles show periods of behavioral rest, with relaxed muscle tone and reduced response to stimuli. During these times, brain waves decrease in frequency and increase in amplitude. Spike discharges, thought to be the equivalent of slow waves, appear on the EEG. Traditionally, it is assumed that these waves are generated in a bihemispherical manner, however, specific unihemispherical recordings have not been attempted. More recently, reports of reptiles "sleeping" with one eye closed and the other open, reminiscent of unihemispheric sleep, have appeared in each of the three orders of reptiles studied: Squamata (snakes and lizards), Crocodilia (crocodiles, alligators, and caimans), and Chelonia (turtles and tortoises) (6).

Amphibians and Fish

Few studies have been done in these species. In the toad (Bufo bufo), the tectal EEG waveforms decreased in frequency from 16 to 13 Hz at sleep onset and in resting goldfish, from 16 to 25 Hz to 6 to 9 Hz (8).

Insects

By applying the criteria above, it has been determined that the fruit fly, (Drosophila melanogaster), sleeps (9). Periods of rest occur during the 12-hour dark phase of a 24-hour cycle. During rest, the flies are in a species-specific posture (prone) and have an increased arousal threshold. Sleep rebound occurs after sleep deprivation and EEG correlates of sleep have been recorded. Because so much is known about the relatively simple genome of this organism, it promises to provide fundamental information about the genetic regulation of sleep and functional consequences of disorders.

Theories on the Function of Sleep

A number of diverse explanations for the primary function of sleep have been submitted. A few of the more prominent ones are reviewed here.

Energy Conservation Theories

In 1975, Berger put forward that the goal of sleep is to reduce the metabolic rate below that obtained from resting alone (10). Attention is drawn to similarities between the slow waves of sleep and the EEG during entry into hibernation and shallow torpor. The suggestion was that these phenomena share a common purpose: to save energy. Among other detractors though, great doubt is cast on this theory by the realization that, at best, sleep has a metabolic savings of 15%, and more likely of just 5% to 10% (11,12).

A second metabolic theory to emerge from the study of mammalian sleep states is that the goal of sleep is to enforce periods of inactivity and so keep energy expenses at an affordable rate relative to energy intake. In summary, sleep quotas for different species were correlated with body mass, brain weight, food (including caloric) intake, and the type of diet. Multiple regression analyses showed that brain weight and body weight could account for up to about 30% of the variance in sleep time among various mammalian species (1,13,14). However, based on this theory alone, the need for sleep is still far from totally accounted for.

Memory Reinforcement

A currently popular belief is that sleep evolved as an adaptation to the increasing demands placed on the brain as more time became required to process complex sensory information, especially vision. Time was also needed to maintain the now vast stores of sensory and motor memories (8). By adopting sleep, neural circuits used during wakefulness to acquire new input could be temporarily turned over to processing and storing (memorizing) the information during sleep.

The slow waves of NREM sleep are thought to reinforce individual neural components of complex memory circuits and also the links between the components. Because individual components rather than the entire complex memory are reinforced, it is referred to as "uncoordinated reinforcement." This is done without fast waves and so without awareness and, therefore, avoids having to simultaneously process new sensory input. NREM sleep is thought to be the earliest form of sleep, perhaps evidenced by its presence in reptiles. It would have been associated with behaviors such as closing the eyelids and retiring to secure, dimly lit resting sites.

During further evolution toward warm-bloodedness, mechanisms continued to develop to encourage uninterrupted sleep during stronger stimuli, such as higher arousal thresholds and further reduced muscle tone to the point of atonia, especially in antigravity muscles. At this point, it was possible to allow fast waves (often associated with wakefulness) to participate in sleep. Fast waves, the principle component of REM sleep, are thought to bind the components of a particular memory together, that is, to form a so-called "coordinated reinforcement" of memory. These waves are used during REM sleep to reinforce both sensory (particularly visual) and motor circuits. Now, motor systems could be activated during sleep without waking the animal with muscle contractions because muscle contractions were inhibited. Reinforcement of the motor circuits during sleep was thought to be important for the survival of warm-blooded animals (8). With their thermoregulatory capabilities, they were able to move over a greater diversity of terrains 24 hours a day.

It is proposed, therefore, that REM sleep developed along with warm-bloodedness. In agreement, it is found only in warm-blooded animals. However, a number of avian and mammalian species do not exhibit REM— mostly those exhibiting unihemispherical sleep (8). It is suggested that because unihemispherical sleep is often accompanied by continual movement, such as swimming in the aquatic species and perhaps flying in birds, there is no need for REM sleep to further reinforce muscle movements.

In support of the memory consolidation theory is evidence that rats presented with novel stimuli show relevant spatiotemporal activity in the stimulated neuronal ensemble for up to 48 hours after the stimulus was presented (15). Reverberation of activity was strongest during slow-wave sleep, less during waking, and variable during REM sleep. It is suggested by this group that sustained neuronal reverberation during slow-wave sleep and gene-related neuronal plasticity during REM contribute to the memory consolidating role of sleep.

ESSENTIAL BRAIN REGIONS FOR SLEEP

The involvement of the hypothalamus in sleep regulation was first suggested in the 1930s. At that time, a Viennese neurologist, Baron Constantin Von Economo, identified select populations of patients with symptoms of either prolonged insomnia or excessive sleepiness associated with an endemic encephalitis. Upon autopsy it was identified that those patients with prolonged insomnia had lesions located near the anterior hypothalamus in the region of the ventrolateral preoptic nucleus (VLPO). Conversely, patients with symptoms of excessive sleepiness were identified to have lesions of the posterior hypothalamus. This led to the hypothesis that regions in the anterior and posterior hypothalamus had opposing influences on the sleep–wake cycle. We will discuss below how these hypothalamic regions interact with neurons of the brainstem reticular-activating system as well as histaminergic neurons of the tuberomammillary nucleus, and the suprachiasmatic nucleus (SCN) to promote sleep or wakefulness over a 24-hours cycle (Fig. 3-1).

Hypothalamus and Sleep

Suprachiasmatic Nucleus

Two general sleep control mechanisms are recognized: a homeostatic mechanism and a circadian mechanism. The homeostatic mechanism dictates that a given quota of sleep duration and intensity needs to be obtained over a short term and that current sleep needs depend on the individuals' immediate prior history of sleep/wakefulness. Sleep deprivation causes a "rebound" effect where, at the nearest available opportunity, an individual will sleep with an increased duration and intensity (increased cortical slow waves) to compensate for lost sleep (16–18). The circadian mechanism, located in the SCN of the

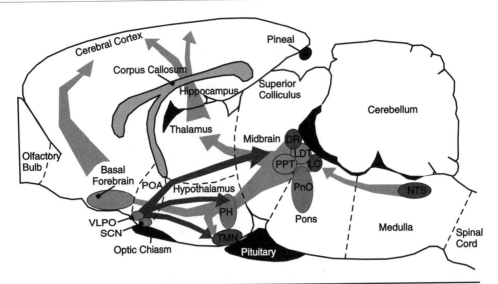

FIGURE 3-1. Schematic of location of sleep- and wake-promoting regions in the brain. Sagittal view of a rat brain redrawn from Paxinos and Watson's *Rat Brain Stereotaxic Atlas* (134) showing the location of major brain regions involved in wakefulness and sleep behavior. Monoaminergic nuclei are shown as dark shaded circles. Cholinergic nuclei include the PPT and LDT. Other important nuclei are shown as light shaded circles. Major ascending excitatory, wake-promoting projection pathways are illustrated by gray arrows, including the nucleus of the solitary tract (NTS), locus coeruleus (LC), laterodorsal tegmental nucleus (LDT), pendunculopontine tegmental nucleus (PPT), dorsal raphe (DR), oral pontine region (PnO), the posterior hypothalamus (PH), including orexigenic neurons in the lateral hypothalamus, the tuberomammillary nucleus (TMN), and the suprachiasmatic nucleus (SCN). The primary sleep promoting site is located in the ventrolateral preoptic nucleus (VLPO). The VLPO contains inhibitory neurons that project and suppress activity in wake-promoting regions.

hypothalamus, dictates that the animal should sleep during a set time frame each day. Both mechanisms are present in all species studied to date, including flies and scorpions. Yet how these two mechanisms interact to regulate an individual's sleep cycle is not completely understood.

The SCN is thought to promote arousal by generating a signal that increases in strength throughout the biological day (active period) and decreases at night. Loss of input from the SCN causes a loss of sleep consolidation (19,20). Pathways through which the circadian signal is transmitted to possible substrates of the homeostatic mechanism are being found (Fig. 3-2A). In rodents, the majority of SCN neurons project to the dorsomedial hypothalamus, which then acts as a distributor for SCN information. The dorsomedial hypothalamus sends projections to three major populations of target neurons (21). The first includes hypothalamic nuclei known to participate in sleep–wake regulation—the VLPO and the extended VLPO area. The second constitutes a group of hypothalamic neuroendocrine cells that secrete orexin, corticotrophin-releasing hormone, thyrotropin-releasing hormone, and gonadotrophin-releasing hormone (22). The third group are autonomic cells that project to brainstem and spinal cord autonomic (both sympathetic and parasympathetic) nuclei. Apart from hypothalamic connections, an indirect connection through which the SCN drives locus coeruleus neurons has been located (23). The SCN also influences

melatonin and body temperature cycles directly, independent of dorsomedial hypothalamus contributions.

Do the substrates for homeostatic control feedback information influence circadian-rhythm generators? Sleep deprivation is known to disrupt the circadian rhythm (24). Sleep deprivation studies in rats show that the slow waves of NREM sleep feed back onto the circadian-rhythm generators to slow the signal output from the generator (25). The faster waves of REM sleep increase the firing rate of SCN cells. Identities of the neural substrates, pathways, and transmitters are unknown, but evidence suggests that the SCN is able to track the amount of the different types of sleep and perhaps adjust its schedule accordingly.

Lateral Hypothalamus and Orexin

The lateral hypothalamus, located in the posterior hypothalamus, is the exclusive source of recently discovered, arousal-promoting neuropeptides, orexin 1 and 2 (also known as hypocretin 1 and 2). Genetic deficiencies occurring in knockout mice (26) and human families indicate that signs of orexin deficiency include narcolepsy, cataplexy, decreased food intake, and perhaps metabolic disturbances (27).

Studies of orexin levels in cerebrospinal fluid (CSF) have added information about its possible functions in normal individuals. Orexin levels in cerebrospinal fluid are

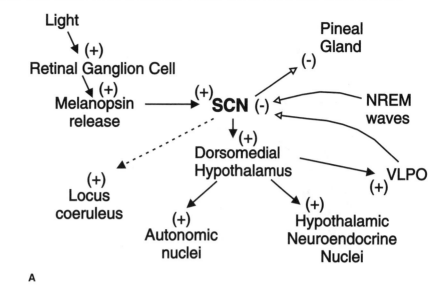

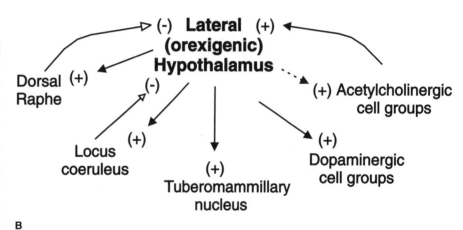

FIGURE 3-2. Interconnections of wake-promoting brain regions. **A.** Influence of suprachiasmatic nucleus (SCN) on sleep-associated centers, autonomic, and hormonal control centers. VLPO is ventrolateral preoptic nucleus. **B.** Influence of lateral hypothalamus on wake-promoting regions in the brainstem and forebrain. Solid lines indicate strong interconnections. Dashed lines indicate weak interconnections. Filled arrows and (+) represent excitatory connections. Open arrows and (–) represent inhibitory connections.

lowest during NREM sleep and highest during wakefulness (28). This, together with findings that lateral hypothalamic neurons start firing before the transition from sleep to wakefulness, suggests a role for orexins in sleep–wake transitions (29). During wakefulness, levels are higher during activity compared to quiet periods (30) causing many to believe that orexins are involved in promoting motor, especially food-seeking, activity.

Orexin-producing lateral hypothalamic neurons send abundant, strong, excitatory projections to wake-promoting noradrenergic, histaminergic, dopaminergic, and cholinergic nuclei (31) and are likely to regulate these centers (Fig. 3-2B). In turn, slice studies show inhibitory effects of noradrenaline and serotonin on orexin production, whereas acetylcholine input excites orexin-producing cells (32). This arrangement suggests the presence of self-regulating feedback loops. In addition, the SCN influences orexin production according to the individuals' circadian rhythm.

Based on information at hand, Seigel (31) has hypothesized that the role of orexins is "to facilitate motor activity in association with motivated behaviors and coordinate this with activation of attentional and sensory systems."

Ventrolateral Preoptic Nucleus

Opposing the arousing effect of posterior hypothalamic and brainstem centers is a "sleep-generating" nucleus in the anterior hypothalamus, in the preoptic area. Immunostaining with c-Fos has identified two groups of sleep-active neurons in this area (33). The first, located in the VLPO, is associated with NREM sleep (34). The second, located dorsal and medial to the first (the extended VLPO), is more closely linked to REM sleep (35). VLPO neurons are activated by sleep-inducing factors, such as adenosine and prostaglandin D_2 (36,37) (Fig. 3-3). They are also temperature (warm) sensitive (38) and so compatible with the effect of temperature on the propensity for sleep.

Neurons in the VLPO contain the inhibitory transmitters, GABA and galanin (39,40) and project to locations of "arousal" neurons, including the serotonergic dorsal raphe

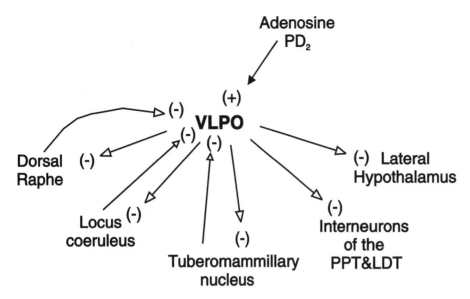

FIGURE 3-3. Interconnections of sleep-promoting brain regions. Projection sites of the inhibitory neurons in the ventrolateral preoptic nucleus (VLPO) important in promoting sleep. VLPO are activated by wake-promoting influences such as adenosine and prostaglandins (PD₂). Filled arrows and (+) represent excitatory connections. Open arrows and (–) represent inhibitory connections.

cell group, histaminergic tuberomammillary nucleus, noradrenergic locus coeruleus, and the orexigenic lateral hypothalamic nucleus (39,41,42). The VLPO also projects to cholinergic nuclei [basal forebrain and pedunculopontine tegmental nucleus (PPT) and laterodorsal tegmental nucleus (LDT)], but primarily innervates inhibitory interneurons within these regions. Projections to locus coeruleus, raphe, and PPT–LDT are derived mostly from the extended VLPO, rather than the VLPO (43). In return, VLPO neurons receive inhibitory adrenergic and serotonergic input from the locus coeruleus and raphe nuclei, respectively (44,45). GABA release into arousal areas increases during NREM sleep (46), and the VLPO has been shown to regulate the amount of delta activity, an index of sleep intensity, within NREM sleep. Because activation of VLPO neurons appears to be required for normal regulation of sleep, the VLPO is considered an essential element of the sleep–wake central circuitry.

Tuberomammillary Nucleus

It has long been recognized that antihistamines have a powerful sedative action, yet the presence of histaminergic neurons in the brain was not identified until 1984, when appropriate immunohistochemical techniques became available (47,48). To date, histaminergic neurons have been found localized to the posterior hypothalmus in the region of the tuberomammillary nucleus of the hypothalamus. Histaminergic neurons in the tuberomammillary nucleus project throughout the CNS, including the cerebral cortex, amygdala, and substantia nigra, three regions that receive the densest innervation. The tuberomammillary nucleus receives input from orexigenic neurons in the lateral hypothalamus and has descending projections to sleep-related regions of the brainstem, including locus coeruleus, dorsal raphe, the parabrachial nucleus, and nu-

cleus of the solitary tract in the dorsal medulla. Many brainstem reticular formation regions, in turn, send ascending projections back to the tuberomammillary nucleus (Fig. 3-1). The locus coeruleus and ventral tegmental regions however, send few fibers to the tuberomammillary nucleus. Tuberomammillary nucleus neurons also receive afferent input from the GABAergic neurons in the VLPO, which appear to contribute strongly to the firing rate of these histaminergic neurons in relation to behavioral state.

Histaminergic neurons in the tuberomammillary nucleus have pacemaker-like activity and fire with characteristically high rates during wakefulness, slower rates during NREM sleep, and almost completely cease discharging during REM sleep, similar to the pattern observed in the monoaminergic neurons in the brainstem reticular-activating system.

Pineal Gland

The pineal gland is positioned on the posterodorsal part of the third ventricle and, typical of all endocrine glands, it is well vascularized. The pineal gland secretes melatonin into the surrounding cerebral sinuses in response to photic information received primarily by the eyes (Fig. 3-1). Melatonin is best known for its ability to induce seasonal and circannual physiologic changes in animal species, for example, the reproductive propensity in sheep. Melatonin levels also fluctuate on a daily basis according to the individuals' light exposure, yet its influence on the circadian rhythm and sleep–wake cycle is less clear.

Retinal exposure to light, especially in the range of 460 to 470 nm (49), inhibits melatonin release. Upon exposure to light, retinal ganglion cells release a recently discovered molecule, melanopsin, into the SCN (50). The SCN response signal passes through the sympathetic intermediolateral cell column in the thoracic spinal cord and returns to the pineal gland to inhibit melatonin release. Melatonin suppression can still occur in some blind people since its secretion is independent of the integrity of rods and cones. However, if retinal ganglion cells are also damaged, melatonin fluctuations may become independent of light exposure. Because of its direct and strong link to the SCN, and because it is relatively easily measured in saliva, melatonin is often used as a marker of circadian rhythm (51).

The effects of melatonin on physiologic rhythms can be established by studying pinealectomized animals. Pinealectomy eliminates the response to changing daylight lengths in several species, and suitable melatonin replacement restores the seasonal cycles. However, the effects on the daily cycle are subtle. Rats adapt faster to light–dark phase shifts in the absence of a pineal gland (51). Reports of humans with a pinealectomy are rare, and consistent consequences of lacking the gland have been unable to be established.

Other effects can be determined by interrupting melatonin secretion during dark with a period of light and then determining which associated effects can be corrected by administering melatonin. In this way, it was found that the increase in core temperature associated with light exposure could be ameliorated by hormone replacement therapy (52). It has been suggested since that almost one-half of the nighttime decrease in body temperature associated with sleep could be attributed to secreted melatonin (53).

The effects of melatonin on sleep still remain elusive. One group described a "biological night" for humans that entailed melatonin, cortisol, body temperature, and sleep propensity fluctuations (54). The descriptors that most simultaneously and precisely correlated with the onset of dusk and dawn were melatonin, body temperature, and sleep propensity. Others lagged. This suggests that melatonin may have a role as a physiological switch for day–night activities.

Brainstem and Sleep

The brainstem was first identified to play a critical role in the control of wakefulness and sleep in the 1930s, when it was identified that transection of the brain at the level of the midbrain eliminated the low-amplitude, high-frequency cortical EEG pattern characteristic of wakefulness (55,56). Alternatively, the presence of low-frequency, high-amplitude EEG patterns typical of sleep was maintained. This suggested that the transition from wakefulness to sleep was mediated by the loss of input, possibly sensory input to the forebrain (57).

After World War II and the advent of fine-wire implantable stimulating and recording electrodes, Moruzzi and Magoun (58) subsequently documented in what is now a classic paper that activation of the brainstem reticular formation, not traditional ascending sensory pathways, produced behavioral arousal accompanied by the replacement of slow-wave EEG activity with fast-wave activity, characteristic of wakefulness. Furthermore, lesions in the brainstem reversed the effect of stimulation and resulted in a pattern of slow-wave EEG activity and behavioral immobility similar to characteristics of sleep (59). This was the first evidence to suggest that wakefulness might be maintained by activation of brainstem reticular formation neurons.

It is now established that the regions in the rostral reticular formation, referred to as the ascending reticular-activating system, send projections to the forebrain through two main pathways critical in regulating sleep–wake cycles. One pathway ascends dorsally to the thalamic nuclei and the second ascends ventrally through the lateral hypothalamus to the basal forebrain (Fig. 3-1).

The dorsal ascending pathway projects to multiple thalamic nuclei, which, in turn, have widespread projections to the cortex (60,61). Neurons localized in the LDT and PPT of the rostral pons/caudal midbrain are the primary source of ascending projections to the dorsal thalamic pathway. LDT–PPT neurons are primarily cholinergic neurons. PPT and LDT neurons are reported to fire rapidly during wakefulness, their discharge rate slows during slow-wave sleep, and then periodically increases during REM or active sleep (62). Different populations of PPT–LDT neurons may be active during wake and REM sleep ("wake-on" and "REM-on"). Accordingly, acetylcholine release in the thalamus increases during both wakefulness and REM sleep (63) and is primarily excitatory (64).

The ventral ascending pathway of the brainstem reticular-activating system projects rostrally through the lateral hypothalamus, terminating on magnocellular neurons in the substantia innominata, medial septum, and diagonal band, regions that contain cortically projecting neurons. The major brainstem cell groups involved in this ascending pathway include the locus coeruleus, one of the largest concentration of norepinephrine-containing cell groups in the brain, and serotoninergic neurons in the dorsal and median raphe nuclei. Similar to the cells in the LDT–PPT, these monoamine cell groups also demonstrate relatively high neuronal firing rates during wakefulness. Yet, as the transition from wakefulness to sleep progresses, the discharge rate of these neurons declines. During REM sleep they become inactive (65–67). The associated loss of noradrenergic and serotonergic input to brainstem and spinal motoneurons plays a significant role in loss of muscle tone throughout the body during REM sleep. The difference between locus coeruleus and raphe neuronal activity during wakefulness versus sleep, suggests that these neurons may be more critical in modulating changes in state from wakefulness to sleep, whereas LDT–PPT neurons must be critically involved in generating REM sleep.

Finally, regions caudal to the pons have also been shown to contribute to the regular cycling between sleep and wakefulness. For example, slow-wave sleep characterized by cortical synchronization has been shown to be produced in awake animals by stimulation of the dorsal reticular formation in the medulla, including the nucleus of the solitary tract (68). Conversely, lesions of the same region produce desynchronized EEG patterns in sleeping animals (68,69). Furthermore, transection between the pons and medulla revealed that the medulla has the capacity to generate regular cycles of active and quiescent period, similar to sleep versus wake cycles. Yet, unlike normal sleep, a period of atonia or the loss of muscle tone and high-frequency EEG are not observed in the medulla (70,71). The nucleus of the solitary tract is the primary central termination site of many visceral afferents. Visceral neurons in the nucleus of the solitary tract, in turn, predominately project to the parabrachial nucleus in the dorsolateral pons, which, in turn, sends projections rostrally to the hypothalamus, amygdala, and thalamus. In general, nucleus of the solitary tract neurons do not send efferent projections to the brainstem reticular-activating system, suggesting the predominant effect of the dorsal medulla on sleep regulation may be through activation of limbic structures, visceral sensory processing, and autonomic regulation.

REM Sleep

By the 1950s, it was recognized that sleep was characterized by periods of rapid eye movements (REM) (72). The observation that cholinergic neurons in the LDT and PPT reduce their discharge rate during non-REM but increase their discharge rate during REM sleep, often to levels above those obtained during wakefulness, suggests that these brainstem neurons are responsible for generating REM sleep. Although the function of REM sleep continues to be under debate, REM sleep is when we experience our most vivid dreams. Thus, over the last two decades REM sleep has been the topic of rather intense study. The characteristic components of REM sleep are listed in Table 3-3.

At present, it is generally agreed that the main network of cells responsible for generating REM sleep reside in the mesopontine junction. Electrolytic lesion of the nucleus reticularis pontis oralis, which lies just ventral to the locus coeruleus, was identified to permanently destroy REM sleep in cats (73,74). Using more selective methods that restrict the lesion to neurons and not fibers of passage, the cholinergic cells located in the lateral nucleus reticularis pontis oralis and PPT–LDT regions are now thought to be critical for the generation of REM sleep, since the loss of REM sleep (including the loss of PGO spikes and atonia) by lesions in these regions is proportional to the number of cholinergic cells removed (75).

During the sleep phase, the regular cycling between REM and non-REM sleep is thought be generated, at the simplest level, by reciprocal innervation between REM-on and REM-off cells in the pontine reticular formation (76,77). REM-off cells, discharge primarily during wakefulness and, to a lesser extent, during NREM sleep, falling

silent during REM. REM-off cells include the monoaminergic cell groups located in the locus coeruleus and raphe nuclei. During wakefulness, these tonically active neurons inhibit REM-on cells in the pontine reticular formation. The discharge rate of the REM-off cells declines during the transition from wakefulness to sleep, reducing the level of inhibition suppressing REM-on cells. Although multiple factors contribute to the decline in discharge rate of REM-off neurons during the transition into sleep, active inhibition, originating from the local release of both the inhibitory neurotransmitter GABA from interneurons, as well as an inhibitory influence of serotonin and nitric oxide, appear to play a major role (78).

As sleep sets in, disinhibition of REM-on cells involves an increase in the firing rate of both cholinergic and glutamatergic neurons in the pontine reticular formation (79). Cholinergic REM-on cells increase their discharge rate exponentially before the onset of REM, and local release of glutamate stimulates both cholinergic and noncholinergic neurons. The local activation of cholinergic neurons in the PPT–LDT triggers the manifestations of REM sleep. The various manifestations are generated by effector neurons that are activated by acetylcholine ("cholinoceptive" neurons). The neurons are not themselves cholingergic and may release transmitters such as glutamate. Different groups of effector neurons in the pontine reticular formation are the most important for the manifestations of REM sleep. For example, the pontine reticular formation is thought to contain the neural generator for the production of both rapid eye movements and PGO waves. However, neurons in the mesencephalic reticular formation and medullary reticular formation also play a role. Polysynaptic input from the mesopontine region to the medulla is critical for the generation of muscle atonia, since transection of the medulla from the pons eliminates atonia but leaves PGO spikes and rapid eye movements intact during REM sleep. The timing of the PGO spikes and rapid eye movements in these transected animals however, may be abnormal. In most mammals, PGO spikes, rapid eye movements, and muscle atonia appear simultaneously. It should be noted, however, that in some individuals the onset of atonia may precede the generation of rapid eye movements.

Cholinergic REM-on cells, in turn, innervate REM-off cells. Thus, activation of REM-on cells triggers an increase in cholinergic excitation of monoaminergic cell groups. Cholinergic activation of REM-off cells will eventually contribute to the serotergic inhibition of REM-on cells and termination of REM sleep (80).

Although neurons within the nucleus reticularis pontis oralis, LDT, and PPT are essential for the generation of REM sleep, and monoaminergic input from the reticular-activating system plays an integral role in mediating the switch from NREM to REM sleep and then back again, other neurotransmitters also play an important role in REM and NREM sleep generation. Some of these include GABA release from the periaqueductal gray matter (81);

glycine release from medullary cells onto motoneurons, which play a role in REM-associated atonia (82); galanin from the VLPO; and the withdrawal of histamine release from the tubermammillary nucleus in the posterior hypothalamus. However, the specific role of each of these neurotransmitters on direct modulation of REM-on versus REM-off cells remains to be fully defined.

NEUROMODULATION OF SLEEP AND WAKEFULNESS

Over the last 40 years, a variety of neurotransmitters or neuromodulators have been identified to be linked with regulation of the sleep–wake cycle (83). Most recently was the discovery of orexin or hypocretin, a neurotransmitter produced by cells in the lateral hypothalamus that promotes wakefulness. Other wake-promoting neurochemicals include catecholamines, acetylcholine, and histamine. Conversely, sleep-promoting neurotransmitters include serotonin, galanin, GABA, and adenosine. Overproduction or underproduction of any of these neurochemicals or alterations in the receptors to which they bind has been shown, in some instance, to have a profound influence on arousal states.

Catecholamines

With the advent of immunohistochemical techniques in the 1960s, it was soon recognized that catecholaminergic neurons of the locus coeruleus were an important part of the wake-promoting region located in the reticular-activating system of the brainstem. In line with that observation was the discovery that drugs that inhibit catabolism of catecholamines cause an intense sustained arousal (84). Conversely, inhibition of catecholamine synthesis decreases wakefulness. Noradrenergic neurons of the locus coeruleus send ascending projections to many forebrain regions through the ventral ascending pathway (Figs. 3-1 and 3-3). Single-unit recording studies have demonstrated that LC neurons are most active during arousal and stressful waking conditions. The discharge of these neurons declines progressively in sleep (85). Activation of both α- and β-adrenergic receptors in select regions of the hypothalamus and thalamus has been associated with wakefulness. Adrenoceptor activation in the same regions triggers neuronal depolarization and a transition from a bursting-like neuronal discharge, a pattern characteristic of slow–wave sleep, to a tonic discharge pattern, more similar to that observed during wakefulness (86,87).

Orexin

The discovery of orexin, also known as hypocretin, was in 1998 by two separate research groups (88,89). Preprohypocretin is a peptide produced by neurons in the dorsal and lateral hypothalamus. The peptide is cleaved to produce HCRT-1 or orexin A and HRCT-2 or orexin B. In the rat, intracerebroventricular infusion of nanomolar concentrations of hypocretin increases arousal (locomotor and grooming behavior), reduces REM sleep with no change in slow-wave sleep, and affects neuroendocrine balance (decreased plasma growth hormone, prolactin, increased corticosterone, but no change in TSH) (90). Some of these actions are localized to the basal forebrain since the influence of lateral ventricle administration on wakefulness is more pronounced than fourth ventrical administration (91). Together, these observations lead to the current thought that orexigenic neurons of the hypothalamus play an integral role in the switch from wakefulness to sleep. In the absence of the neuropeptide, this switch is unstable, and the transition to sleep can occur at inopportune moments (i.e., narcolepsy).

Orexin-containing neurons in the hypothalamus have widespread projections throughout the brain (see Fig. 3-2B) [for review (31)]. HCRT is neuroexcitatory (92) and its actions may be mediated directly by activation of postsynaptic receptors or indirectly by the stimulation of local glutamate release (93). Bath application of orexin has been shown to excite cholinergic neurons in the basal forebrain (94), suggesting a link between orexin release and cholinergic-mediated cortical activation. In the rat, local administration of HCRT-1, but not HCRT-2, in the locus coeruleus suppresses REM sleep and increases awake time, at the expense of slow-wave sleep (95). Yet HCRT-2 receptor antisense administration to the pontine reticular formation in the conscious rat has been shown to increase the amount of REM time and produce cataplexy. This suggests that much remains to be learned about the function of orexin in the brain.

Histamine

At the present time, three histaminergic receptor (HR) subtypes have been cloned, and their pattern of distribution in the brain is very distinct. The actions of histamine in the brain appear to be relatively complex based on the receptor subtype activated and the region of stimulation (96). Activation of HR-1 receptors is excitatory and mediates arousal-associated increases in histamine release and the sedative action of antihistamines (97). HR-2 receptors are metabotropic receptors and primarily act to mediate more long-term changes in neuronal discharge, such as increasing the number of action potentials discharged for a given depolarizing input. In contrast, HR-3 receptors are located on the soma of histaminergic neurons, as well as other neurons, and are considered autoreceptors, inhibiting histamine synthesis and release.

The increase in discharge rate of tuberomammillary neurons during wakefulness is dependent, in part, on input from orexinergic neurons in the lateral hypothalamus. In addition, the action of orexin on wakefulness is, in turn, dependent upon histamine release from the tuberomammillary nucleus. For example, knockout mice lacking histamine receptors (subtype 1) do not show an increase in wakefulness in response to intracerebroventricular administration of orexin. Mice lacking histamine receptors however show deficits in waking, attention, and interest in novel environments (98). The decline in discharge rate of histaminergic neurons during sleep is thought to depend on inhibitory input from the VLPO (39). In addition, the decline in excitatory input from the raphe neurons or orexinergic neurons from the lateral hypothalamus may also contribute to the state-dependent discharge rate of tuberomammillary nucleus neurons.

Acetylcholine

Cholinergic agonists, such as nicotine in tobacco, have been identified to augment vigilance and as well as induce fast cortical activity. Alternatively, systemic administration of the muscarinic receptor antagonist atropine was shown to reduce vigilance and produce a dissociation between behavior and EEG activity (slow-wave activity associated with sleep was observed in moving animals) (99). Single-unit recordings from putative cholinergic neurons in both mesopontine and basal forebrain have identified that the majority of these neurons are extremely active during waking and REM sleep and less active during slow-wave sleep (62,100). Associated with the phasic activation of these neurons is a cycle-related release of acetylcholine in the thalamus and cortex, suggesting that activation of these neurons is correlated with changes in the sleep–wake cycle (63,101). Lesion of the mesopontine neurons produces little notable change in cortical activation during waking, suggesting that activation of these neurons may not be critical to appropriate regulation of the sleep–wake cycle. Alternatively, lesion or inhibition of the cholinergic neurons in the basal forebrain has been reported to produce a reduction in vigilance and a change in cortical EEG similar to that observed following atropine administration (102,103). Similarly, increases in cortical EEG activity produced by stimulation of the mesopontine neurons has also been shown to rely, to a large extent, on the activation of the basal forebrain neurons (104). Application of acetylcholine to thalamic or cortical neurons induces a prolonged excitation that is blocked by muscarinic receptor antagonists (105).

GABA–Galanin

In 1996, Sherrin and colleagues demonstrated for the first time that sleep-active neurons in the VLPO contained the inhibitory neurotransmitters GABA and galanin (33). Inhibitory VLPO neurons increase their firing rate during the onset of drowsiness and fire maximally during NREM sleep. A correlation between the amount of spontaneous sleep and the number of VLPO galanin-GABAergic neu-

rons activated has also been found (40). VLPO, sleep-active, inhibitory neurons send projections throughout the brain, with particularly dense projection patterns to wake-promoting regions (see earlier sections and Fig. 3-3). Sleep deprivation has been shown to increase the expression of galanin in preoptic neurons (106). Consequently, it appears that VLPO GABA–galanin-positive neurons promote sleep through inhibition of neurons within wake-promoting regions (see Figs. 3-1 and 3-3). In support of this hypothesis is the observation that GABA release increases in the wake-promoting regions of the posterior hypothalamus in non-REM sleep relative to waking levels (107).

GABAergic neurons, however, are found throughout the central nervous system (CNS) and are not just localized within the VLPO. Activation of GABAergic inhibitory interneurons within the brainstem reticular-activating system and the thalamic reticular nuclei are integrally involved in regulation of sleep. For example, activation of GABAergic receptors in the pontine sleep regions (nucleus pontis oralis) promotes wakefulness in unanesthetized cats. Conversely, inhibition of GABAergic input in this region prolonged naturally occurring sleep cycles, suggesting that wakefulness is reinforced by the inhibition of local inhibitory interneurons in the brainstem. The withdrawal of this inhibitory input, in turn, then promotes sleep (78).

Serotonin

Serotonin has been linked to the sleep–wake cycle since the 1950s, when it was first identified that chemicals, that inhibit serotonin catabolism, enhance slow-wave sleep. Alternatively, chemicals that inhibit serotonin production produce insomnia (84). However, the effects of serotonin on sleep are complex and, at times, contradictory. For example, selective serotonin receptor uptake inhibitors (SSRIs) increase synaptic serotonin, but usually disturb NREM sleep and inhibit REM sleep. Serotonin is also metabolized in the pineal gland to melatonin (a sleep-promoting substance). Serotonergic neurons in the sleep-promoting regions of the brainstem have been localized to the dorsal raphe nucleus. As noted above, the firing rate of these neurons is highest during wakefulness, decreases during NREM sleep, and is nearly absent during REM sleep. The actions of serotonin in many physiologic control systems, such as sleep and wakefulness, remain relatively elusive because serotonin acts on multiple receptor subtypes (at least seven 5HT subtypes currently) that can mediate a variety of postsynaptic effects, including modulation of ion-channel activity to changes in second messenger systems. To date, cholinergic neurons in the basal forebrain have been shown to primarily express the inhibitory 5HT-1A receptor subtype. Alternatively, the excitatory serotonin receptor subtypes have been identified on GABAergic neurons in the forebrain and cortex (108).

Thus, changes in serotonergic neuronal discharge during different phases of the sleep–wake cycle could indirectly mediate disfacilitation or disinhibition of certain regions, depending upon the projection site and phase-related activity of the integrating neurons. Details on how these systems interact, however, remain to be more thoroughly investigated and defined (108–110).

Adenosine

A link between adenosine release and sleep was first proposed when it was identified that caffeine acts as a stimulant through the blockade of adenosine receptors. Subsequently, it was found that adenosine is released throughout the brain as a neurotransmitter. Adenosine is also found in relatively high concentrations in the extracellular space, probably as a by-product of the use and breakdown of ATP (111,112). Extracellular adenosine levels appear to fluctuate with the sleep–wake cycle and are highest during waking; levels increase with sleep deprivation (111). Central administration of adenosine promotes sleep and induces c-Fos expression in VLPO neurons (113,114), suggesting adenosine promotes sleep. Adenosine primarily mediates its neuromodulatory effects through A1 receptors, which act through a second messenger system to inhibit neuronal activity; the AR2 receptor may also be important. Adenosine has been shown to inhibit excitatory neurotransmitter release and inhibit cholinergic neurons in the brainstem (115). Conversely, bath application of adenosine excites VLPO neurons indirectly through a reduction in presynaptic release of inhibitory neurotransitters (36,116). Accordingly, it has been hypothesized that the increase in adenosine observed during wakefulness and the associated increase in neuronal activation may act as a negative feedback mechanism to subsequently inhibit neuronal activity in wake-related neurons while activating sleep-related neurons through disinhibition (Fig. 3-3). Yet, adenosine receptor knockout mice do not show differences from wild-type controls in either sleep–wake cycle or rebound sleep response to 6 hours of sleep deprivation (117). Thus, similar to other neurotransmitters described above, it appears that adenosine may be an important neuromodulator, but is not an essential component for full expression of the circuits involved in the homeostatic regulation of the sleep–wake cycle.

CORTICAL AND HIPPOCAMPAL WAVE PATTERNS DURING SLEEP

Cortical Patterns

Cortical electrical activity exists in one of two states during sleep: the synchronized, high-amplitude, low-frequency waveforms of NREM sleep and the fast, low-amplitude waveforms of REM sleep. Anatomical and cellular bases for these waveforms are shown in Fig. 3-4A.

Cortical EEG Waves of NREM Sleep

Three types of cortical waves are commonly identified: sleep spindles, presenting as 1- to 2-seconds bursts of waxing and waning peaks at a frequency of 12 to 14 Hz in adult humans, with the bursts occurring 3 to 5 seconds apart; delta waves, which roll over the cortex at 0.5 to 4 Hz; and slow waves, which oscillate at <1 Hz. Each arises as a result of intrinsic neuronal properties and, as well, as interactions of thalamocortical networks. As a whole, the concentration of cortical slow waves reflects the intensity of sleep. They are more prominent in the early hours of sleeping and decline in incidence as the night wears on.

Sleep spindles are perhaps the most studied and understood oscillations. Their incidence is most intense in early stages of sleep (stage 2). They are usually superimposed on other slow waves. Sleep spindles are generated in the thalamus through an interaction between thalamocortical cells and thalamic reticular neurons. Rostral (perigeniculate) reticular thalamic cells inherently generate sleep spindles due to inhibitory interconnections among themselves (118). Isolated reticular thalamic cells spike burst at a frequency of 0.1 to 0.3 Hz (119). Consequent bursts in the rostral reticular thalamic nucleus induce GABA$_A$-mediated IPSPs in thalamocortical cells. Thalamocortical cells become hyperpolarized and, subsequently, produce a rebound burst of action potentials due to special Ca^{2+} currents that are prominent in these cells (120). Detailed reviews of the role of these and other currents can be found (121). The rebound burst in thalamocortical cells reactivates inhibitory neurons in the reticular nucleus, initiating the next cycle of bursting. The time it takes for a cycle to occur represents the intraspindle frequency of 6 to 14 Hz. During the spindle wave, reticular cells progressively hyperpolarize, which increases and then decreases their participation in spindle generation.

Spike-bursting thalamocortical fibers also drive cortical targets, the pyramidal cells of layer 4, to burst in spindles. Layer 4 cells activate cortical cells in deeper layers, and these project back on to the thalamic cell of origin. In addition, their collaterals feed back onto the thalamic reticular nucleus, reinforcing its burst firing along with thalamocortical cells.

Because the thalamocortical cells are hyperpolarized for most of the sleep period, they are unreactive to incoming sensory information from prethalamic sites. Therefore, the thalamus is the first point where afferent sensory information en route to the cortex is blocked during sleep. However, thalamocortical and corticocortical interactions still occur (122).

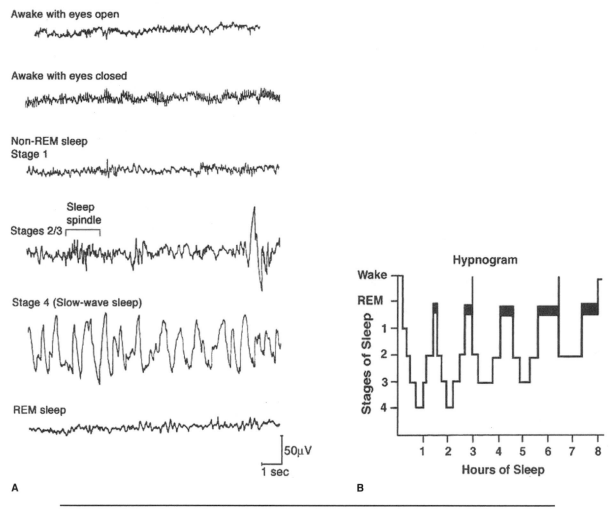

FIGURE 3-4. Waveforms and stages of sleep. (Reproduced from Siegel, JH. *The Neural Control of Sleep and Waking.* New York: Springer-Verlag, 2002. With permission.)

Delta waves appear most prominently during the later stages (3 and 4) of sleep. These waves have the highest amplitude of all EEG waveforms, up to 300 μV. They are generated by a subpopulation of thalamocortical cells that intrinsically bursts at 0.5 to 4 Hz. Rhythmic bursting results from actions of the special Ca^{2+} channels mentioned, in combination with hyperpolarization–activated Na^+/K^+ channels [see McCormick review for further details (121)]. Thalamocortical cells are more hyperpolarized when generating delta waves than when producing spindles (123). Therefore, as sleep onsets and the thalamocortical cells initially become hyperpolarized, sleep spindles appear. As sleep progresses, and the thalamocortical cells further hyperpolarize because of even less cholinergic and other activating input, the hyperpolarization-activated channels are activated and delta waves appear. Sleep spindles subside. Then, as the sleep period comes to an end, cholinergic input begins to resume, the thalamocortical cells depolarize, and sleep spindles reappear (118).

Sleep spindles and delta waves do not occur continuously but repeat in 0.7 to 0.8 Hz cycles. These slow oscillations are spontaneously generated in cortical layers 2 through 6 and are associated with a prolonged, synchronized hyperpolarization followed by a depolarization of all cortical cell types, including interneurons (123a). The long-lasting depolarization is attributed to inhibitory and excitatory postsynaptic events. Excitatory channels include NMDA and voltage-dependent Na^+ channels and inhibitory influences reflect GABA release, particularly by basket cells (123). Hyperpolarization is attributed to K^+/Ca^{2+} currents and cessation of depolarizing events (124). Corticocortical interconnections are critical and sufficient for the generation of slow waves.

Slow oscillations entrain the other forms of slow waves. For example, the depolarizing segment of the slow wave, via corticothalamic connections, can trigger thalamic reticular circuits to produce a spindle wave (124). Therefore, sleep spindles follow the patterning of slow waves.

Simultaneous hyperpolarization in many cortical cells synchronizes cortical electrical activity, and this also entrains reticular thalamic cells so that these cells also display slow waves. Rhythmic changes in the membrane potential of reticular thalamic cells and thalamocortical cells also entrain delta waves (118). The K complex, defined as a well-delineated negative sharp wave immediately followed by a positive slow-wave component, and exceeding 0.5 seconds in total duration, is formed by the combination of slow oscillations and delta waves. Slow oscillations can be seen equally well in stages 2 through 4 of human sleep (125).

Cortical Fast Waves of REM Sleep

The REM sleep cortical EEG is characterized by low-voltage, spontaneous, fast (20–50 Hz) oscillations, or gamma waves, that represent very localized synchronization in intracortical, intrathalamic, and corticothalamic networks. It occurs in conjunction with atonia in antigravity muscles and rapid eye movements.

The transition from the NREM sleep EEG to the REM sleep EEG requires depolarization of thalamocortical and thalamic reticular neurons. As the new, relatively depolarized membrane potential is approached, burst firing is inhibited and single-action potentials can be generated at a frequency of 20 to 50 Hz. Brainstem-derived neurotransmitters are implicated in the depolarization process. During REM sleep, thalamocortical cells are depolarized by acetylcholine from the pedunculopontine and laterodorasal tegmental nuclei through muscarinic acetylcholine receptors. These two brainstem nuclei recommence activity after being silenced during NREM sleep because the dorsal raphe nucleus, which inhibits these cholinergic nuclei, becomes quiet during REM sleep (126). In contrast to the awake state, norepinephrine from the locus coeruleus and serotonin from the nucleus raphe and histamine from the tuberomammillary nucleus do not contribute to the depolarization during REM sleep, since these cells are now inactive (43). As the brainstem nuclei release acetylcholine into the thalamus, burst firing from thalamic cells gradually decreases and the generation of single spikes increases.

A similar process occurs in reticular thalamic cells. In a slight twist, muscarinic acetylcholine input from the pontine nuclei hyperpolarizes the reticular cells and inhibits their firing. However, burst firing is not enabled (118).

In contrast to the awake state, medullary nuclei contribute to fast-frequency cortical oscillations during REM sleep. Medullary neurons increase their firing rate about a minute before the transition from NREM to REM sleep occurs (127).

Finally, the cholinergic basal forebrain contributes to the fast oscillatory (gamma) waves of REM sleep (128). It acts in a dual manner, first, by diffusely activating the entire cortex via muscarinic receptors, and, second, it activating thalamic circuits.

Hippocampal Patterns

Theta Waves

The hippocampus produces theta waves—high-voltage waves with a frequency of 4 to 10 Hz. More specifically, they are produced by synchronous outputs from pyramidal cells of the CA1 gyrus, dentate gyrus, and medial enterorhinal gyrus (129). They occur continuously during both REM sleep and wakefulness in an indistinguishable manner and also appear during stage 1 of NREM sleep (130). The frequency of theta waves increases in association with some phasic activities, such as PGO waves and phasic motor activities. Tonic theta waves are abolished by cholinergic antagonists, such as atropine, giving rise to the proposal that their production depends on acteylcholine input to the hippocampus (130). In contrast, the phasic component of theta waves persists after atropine administration and represents a noncholinergic–dependent component of these waves. Hippocampal synchronization is now known to result from cholinergic and GABAergic input from medial septal cells (131).

Theta waves have been linked to particular voluntary locomotor behaviors and spatial memory (132), but their significance for sleep remains unclear, except for their function as a marker for REM sleep.

Stages of Sleep

In addition to dividing sleep into REM and NREM sleep, NREM sleep in primates and humans is further subdivided into four stages, according to EEG characteristics (see Fig. 3-4B and Table 3-2). Detailed descriptions of each of these stages can be found elsewhere (133), but the general classification system is as follows.

In the awake state with focused attention, the EEG consists of high-frequency (20–40 Hz) low-voltage (5–10 μV) beta waves. As attention is lost, a more relaxed, "meditative" state onsets, with the appearance of slightly higher amplitude, lower-frequency (8–12 Hz) alpha waves, especially over the occipital cortex.

The subject then begins to drift into stage 1 sleep. Beta and a few alpha waves form the background EEG. Hippocampal theta waves appear, especially in children and adolescents. This is in association with involuntary slow eye rolls and is the transition from wakefulness to sleeping, which lasts about 3 to 5 minutes.

Stage 2 sleep is seen as a background of beta waves interspersed with sleep spindles and K complexes. Eye movements cease. Stage 2 lasts for about 30 minutes, during which the incidence of spindling increases.

In stage 3, background beta activity is largely replaced by delta waves. Spindles and K complexes are still present.

In stage 4, delta waves become more prominent and occupy more than 50% of the trace, while spindling becomes minimal. In humans, Stage 4 onsets after about 60 minutes of sleep and lasts 20 to 30 minutes. Together, stages 3 and 4 are termed slow-wave sleep.

After completing stage 4, a subject quickly (in a matter of minutes) cycles backward through stages 3, 2, and 1 and then into REM sleep, characterized by beta EEG waves, REM, and muscle atonia. The first REM sleep period lasts 5 to 10 minutes, but increases on each successive cycle as the proportion of slow waves decreases. About 90 minutes is taken to pass through a full cycle of sleep stages.

ANTERIOR-POSTERIOR HYPOTHALAMIC SLEEP–WAKE SWITCH

As the previous section outlines, the importance of select regions of the hypothalamus, forebrain, and brainstem in coordinating the elements of sleep versus wakefulness are currently being investigated and, at present, much regarding the mechanisms of sleep is unknown. Although sleep has been defined as a necessary physiologic state, the exact function of sleep remains elusive. Moreover, the mechanism(s) responsible for switching an individual from the awake state to sleep also is unknown. Yet the discovery of orexin has provided an important clue to the influence of neurotransmitter on stabilizing wakefulness (e.g., in the absence of orexin's action, a dysregulated state of sleep–wakefulness occurs, as in narcolepsy). Saper and colleagues have put forward a model to describe the transition from sleep to waking and back (43). In general, it is hypothesized that sleep-generating and arousal-promoting cell groups exhibit reciprocal activity during a sleep–wake cycle through patterns of reciprocal inhibition. This reciprocal pattern of activity is self-reinforcing, since VLPO neurons, active during sleep, inhibit monoaminergic neuron in the arousal system (primarily in the brainstem). Conversely, arousal system neurons, active during wakefulness, inhibit the sleep-generating system of the VLPO. As such, VLPO activation suppresses arousal system neurons and reciprocally excites sleep-promoting neurons through removing the arousal-mediating inhibition of VLPO neurons. This same relationship of self-promoting disinhibition then also would occur with monoaminergic neurons active during wakefulness, thus promoting extremely stable states of either wakefulness or sleep once the transition to the new state has been made. Outside or larger scale influences such as circadian inputs or the accumulation of homeostatic signals promoting the "need" for sleep would then shift the circuit from wakefulness to sleep. As these inputs change following a period of sleep and change from night to day, the transition to wakefulness would be promoted. Activation of orexin-releasing neurons in the lateral hypothalamus, in turn, promotes stability of wakefulness through direct excitation of brainstem reticular-activating

system neurons and possibly the presynaptic inhibition of sleep-promoting regions. The loss of orexin input then leads to an unstable waking state, such as observed in narcoleptics.

FUTURE DIRECTIONS

The future directions of research into the neurobiology of sleep will no doubt include a more detailed analysis of genes and proteins involved in regulating sleep, as discovered through gene array analysis and proteonomics. It is hoped that these new approaches will provide new insights into the function of sleep as evidenced by the cellular changes that occur during sleep or following sleep deprivation that can then be translated back to behavioral effects. Forthcoming will also be exciting new data on the role of specific genes in sleep–wake cycling from the rapid mutagenesis screening of the *Drosophila* genetics that have already yielded incredibly exciting information on the genes regulating chronobiology. Ongoing studies have identified *Drosophila* mutants that vary in time of sleep and lack elements of normal homeostatic sleep regulation (9). More detailed analysis of these mutants should complement gene array analysis from mammalian systems to unravel those critical cellular pathways regulating sleep and regulated by sleep.

REFERENCES

1. Zeplin H. Mammalian sleep. In: Kryger M, Roth T, Dement WC, eds. *Principle and practice of sleep medicine.* Philadelphia: WB Saunders, 2000:82–92.
2. Tobler I. Is sleep fundamentally different between mammalian species? *Behav Brain Res.* 1995;69:35–41.
3. Hendricks J, Stefanie MF, Panckeri KA, et al. Rest in Drosophila is a sleep-like state. *Neuron.* 2000;25:129–138.
4. Shaw P, Cirelli C, Greenspan RJ, et al. Correlates of sleep and waking in Drosophila melanogaster. *Science.* 2000;287:1834–1837.
5. Seigel J. Techniological developments. In: Seigel J, ed. *The neural control of sleeping and waking.* New York: Springer, 2002:9–26.
6. Rattenborg N, Amlaner CJ, Lima SL. Behavioral, neurophysiological and evolutionary perspectives on unihemispherical sleep. *Neurosci Biobehav Rev.* 2000;24:817–842.
7. Oleksenko A, Mukhametov LM, Polyakova IG, et al. Unihemispheric sleep deprivation in bottlenose dolphins. *J Sleep Res.* 1992;1:40–44.
8. Kavanau J. REM and NREM sleep as natural accompaniments of the evolution of warm-bloodedness. *Neurosci Biobehav Rev.* 2002;26:889–906.
9. Cirelli C. Searching for sleep mutants of *Drosophila melanogaster. BioEssays.* 2003;25:940–949.
10. Berger R. Bioenergetic functions of sleep and activity rhythms and their possible relevance to aging. *Fed Proc.* 1975;34:97–102.
11. Ravussin E, Lillioja S, Anderson TE, et al. Determinants of 24-hour energy expenditure in man. Methods and results using a respiratory chamber. *J Clin Invest.* 1986;78:1568–1578.
12. Shapiro C, Goll CC, Cohen GR, et al. Heat production during sleep. *J Appl Physiol.* 1984;56:671–677.
13. McNab B. The influence of food habits on the energetics of eutherin mammals. *Ecol Monogr.* 1986;56:1–19.
14. Lee A, Martin R. Life in the slow lane. *Nat Hist.* 1990;8:34–42.

15. Ribeiro S, Gervasoni D, Soares ES, et al. Long-lasting novelty-induced neuronal reverberation during slow-wave sleep in multiple forebrain areas. *PLoS Biol.* 2004;2:126–137.
16. Van Twyver H. Sleep patterns in five rodent species. *Physiol Behav.* 1969;4:901–905.
17. Hediger H. The biology of natural sleep in animals. *Experientia.* 1980;36:13–16.
18. Borbely A, Achermann P. Sleep homeostasis and models of sleep regulation. In: Kryger M, Roth T, Dement WC, eds. *Principle and practice of sleep medicine,* Philadelphia: WB Saunders, 2000;377–390.
19. Dijk D, Cajochen C. Melatonin and the circadian regulation of sleep initiation, consolidation, structure, and the sleep. *EEG J Biol Rhythms.* 1997;12:627–635.
20. Dijk D, Czeisler CA. Paradoxical timing of the circadian rhythm of sleep propensity serves to consolidate sleep and wakefulness in humans. *Neurosci Lett.* 1994;166:63–68.
21. Kalsbeek A, Buijs R. Output pathways of the mammalian suprachiasmatic nucleus: Coding circadian time by transmitter selection and specific targeting. *Cell Tissue Res.* 2002;309:109–118.
22. Chou T, Scammell TE, Gooley JJ, et al. Critical role of dorsomedial hypothalamic nucleus in a wide range of behavioral circadian rhythms. *J Neurosci.* 2003;23:10691–10702.
23. Aston-Jones G, Chen S, Zhu Y, et al. A neural circuit for circadian regulation of arousal. *Nature Neurosci.* 2001;4:732–738.
24. Antle M, Mistleberger RE. Circadian clock resetting by sleep deprivation without exercise in the Syrian hamster. *J Neurosci.* 2000;20:9326–9332.
25. Deboer T, Vansteensel MJ, Detari L, et al. Sleep states alter activity of suprachiasmatic nucleus neurons. *Nat Neurosci.* 2003;6:1086–1090.
26. Chemelli R, Willie JT, Sinton CM, et al. Narcolepsy in orexin knock-out mice: Molecular genetics of sleep regulation. *Cell.* 1999;98:437–451.
27. Taheri S, Bloom S. Orexins/hypocretins: Waking up the scientific world. *Clin Endocrinol.* 2001;54:421–429.
28. Zeitzer J, Buckmaster CL, Parker KJ, et al. Circadian and homeostatic regulation of hypocretin in a primate model: Implications for the consolidation of wakefulness. *J Neurosci.* 2003;23:3555–3560.
29. Koyama YKT, Takahashi K, Okai K, et al. Firing properties of neurons in the laterodorsal hypothalamic area during sleep and wakefulness. *Psych Clin Neurosci.* 2002;56:339–340.
30. Martins P, D'Almeida V, Pedrazzoli M, et al. Increased hypocretin-1 (orexin-a) levels in cerebrospinal fluid of rats after short-term forced activity. *Regul Peptide.* 2004;117:155–158.
31. Siegel J. Hypocretin (orexin): Role in normal behavior and neuropathology. *Annu Rev Psychol.* 2004;55:125–148.
32. Yamanaka A, Muraki Y, Tsujino N, et al. Regulation of orexin neurons by the monoaminergic and cholinergic systems. *Biochem Biophys Res Commun.* 2003;303:120–129.
33. Sherin J, Shiromani PJ, McCarley RW, et al. Activation of ventrolateral preoptic neurons during sleep. *Science.* 1996;271:216–219.
34. Lu J, Greco MA, Shiromani P, et al. Effects of lesions of the ventrolateral preoptic nucleus on NREM and REM sleep. *J Neurosci.* 2000;20:3830–3842.
35. Lu J, Bjorkam AA, Xu M, et al. Selective activation of the extended ventrolateral preoptic nucleus during rapid eye movement sleep. *J Neurosci.* 2002;22:4568–4576.
36. Morairty S, Rainnie D, McCarley R, et al. Disinhibition of ventrolateral preoptic area sleep active neurons by adenosine: A new mechanism for sleep promotion. *Neuroscience.* 2004;123:451–457.
37. Osaka T, Hayaishi O. Prostaglandin D2 modulates sleep-related and noradrenaline-induced activity of preoptic and basal forebrain neurons in the rat. *Neurosci Res.* 1995;23:257–268.
38. Guzman-Marin R, Alam MN, Szymusiak R, et al. Discharge modulation of rat dorsal raphe neurons during sleep and waking: Effects of preoptic/basal forebrain warming. *Brain Res Bull.* 2000;875:23–34.
39. Sherin J, Elmquist JK, Torrealba F, et al. Innervation of histaminergic tuberomammillary neurons by GABAergic and galaninergic neurons in the ventrolateral preoptic nucleus of the rat. *J Neurosci.* 1998;18:4705–4721.
40. Gaus S, Strecker RE, Tate BA, et al. Ventrolateral preoptic nucleus contains sleep-active, galaninergic neurons in multiple mammalian species. *Neuroscience.* 2002;115:285–294.
41. Steininger T, Gong H, McGinty D, et al. Subregional organization of preoptic area/anterior hypothalamic projections to arousal-related monoaminergic cell groups. *J Comp Neurol.* 2001;429:638–653.
42. Szymusiak R, Steininger T, Alam N, et al. Preoptic area sleep-regulating mechanisms. *Arch Ital Biol.* 2001;139:77–92.
43. Saper C, Chou TC, Scammell TE. The sleep switch: Hypothalamic control of sleep and wakefulness. *Trends Neurosci.* 2001;24:726–731.
44. Gallopin T, Fort P, Eggermann E, et al. Identification of sleep-promoting neurons in vitro. *Nature Neurosci.* 2000;404:992–995.
45. Chou T, Bjorkum AA, Gaus SE, et al. Afferents to the ventrolateral preoptic nucleus. *J Neurosci.* 2002;22:977–990.
46. McGinty D, Szymusiak R. Hypothalamic regulation of sleep and arousal. *Front Biosci.* 2003;8:s1074–1083.
47. Watanabe T, Taguchi Y, Shiosaka S, et al. Distribution of the histaminergic neuron system in the central nervous system of rats; A fluorescent immunohistochemical analysis with histidine decarboxylase as a marker. *Brain Res.* 1984;295:13–25.
48. Panula P, Yang HY, Costa E. Histamine-containing neurons in the rat hypothalamus. *Proc Natl Acad Sci USA.* 1984;81:2572–2576.
49. Brainard G, Hanifin JP, Greeson JM. Action spectrum for melatonin regulation in humans: Evidence for a novel circadian photoreceptor. *J Neurosci.* 2001;21:6405–6412.
50. Provencio I, Rollag MD, Castrucci AM. Photoreceptive net in the mammalian retina. This mesh of cells may explain how some blind mice can still tell day from night. *Nature Neurosci.* 2002;415:493.
51. Arendt J. Importance and relevance of melatonin to human biological rhythms. *J Neuroendocrinol.* 2003;15:247–431.
52. Strassman R, Qualls CR, Lisansky EJ, et al. Elevated rectal temperature produced by all-night bright light is reversed by melatonin infusion in men. *J Appl Physiol.* 1991;71:2178–2182.
53. Cagnacci A, Elliott JA, Yen SS. Melatonin: A major regulator of the circadian rhythm of core temperature in humans. *J Clin Endocrinol Metab.* 1992;75:447–452.
54. Wehr T, Aeschbach D, Duncan WC, Jr. Evidence for a biological dawn and dusk in the human circadian timing system. *J Physiol.* 2001;535:937–951.
55. Bremer F. Cerveau "isole" et physiologie du sommeil. *C R Soc Biol.* 1935;118:1235–1241.
56. Bremer F. Cerveau. Nouvelles recherches sur le mecanisme du sommeil. *C R Soc Biol.* 1936;122:460–464.
57. Kleitman N, Camille N. Studies on the physiology of sleep. VI. The behavior of decorticated dogs. *Am J Physiol.* 1932;100:474–479.
58. Moruzzi G, Magoun H. Brain stem reticular formation and activation of the EEG. *Electroenceph Clin Neurophysiol.* 1949;1:445–473.
59. Lindsley D, Schreiner LH, Knowles WB, et al. Behavioral and EEG changes following chronic brain stem lesions. *Electroenceph Clin Neurophysiol.* 1950;2:483–498.
60. Steriade M. Mechanisms underlying cortical activation: neuronal organization and properties of the midbrain reticular core and intralaminar thalamic nuclei. In: Pompeiano O, Ajmone Marsan C, eds. *Brain mechanisms and perceptual awareness.* New York: Raven Press, 1981:327–335.
61. Jasper H. Diffuse projection systems: The intergrative action of the thalamic reticular system. *Electroenceph Clin Neurophysiol.* 1949;1:405–410.
62. El Mansari M, Sakai K, Jouvet M. Unitary characteristics of presumptive cholinergic tegmental neurons during the sleep-waking cycle in freely moving cats. *Exp Brain Res.* 1989;76:519–529.
63. Williams J, Comisarow J, Day J, et al. State-dependent release of acetylcholine in rat thalamus measured by in vivo microdialysis. *J Neurosci.* 1994;14:5236–5242.
64. Steriade M. Acetylcholine systems and rhythmic activities during the waking-sleep cycle. *Prog Brain Res.* 2004;145:179–196.
65. McGinty D, Harper R. Dorsal raphe neurons: Depression of firing during sleep in cats. *Brain Res.* 1976;101:569–575.
66. Aston-Jones G, Chiang C, Alexinsky T. Discharge of noradrenergic locus coeruleus neurons in behaving rats and monkeys suggests a role in vigilance. *Prog Brain Res.* 1991;88:501–520.
67. Aston-Jones G, Bloom FE. Activity of norepinephrine-containing

locus coeruleus neurons in behaving rats anticipates fluctuations in the sleep-waking cycle. *J Neurosci.* 1981;1:876–886.

68. Magnes J, Moruzzi G, Pompeiano O. Synchronization of the EEG produced by low-frequency electrical stimulation of the region of the solitary tract. *Arch Ital Biol.* 1961;99:33–61.

69. Bonvallet M, Dell P, Hiebel G. Tonus sympathique et activite electrique corticale. *Electroenceph Clin Neurophysiol.* 1954;6:119–144.

70. Siegel J, Tomaszewski KS, Nienhuis R. Behavioral states in the chronic medullary and mid-pontine cat. *Electroenceph Clin Neurophysiol.* 1986;63:274–288.

71. Siegel J, Nienhuis R, Tomaszewski KS. Rostral brainstem contributes to medullary inhibition of muscle tone. *Brain Res.* 1983;268:344–348.

72. Aserinsky E, Kleitman N. Regularly occurring periods of eye motility, and concomitant phenomena, during sleep. *Science.* 1953;118:273–274.

73. Jouvet M. The role of monoamines and acetylcholine-containing neurons in the regulation of of the sleep-waking cycle. *Ergeb Physiol.* 1972;64:166–307.

74. Kayama Y, Koyama Y. Control of sleep and wakefulness by brainstem monoaminergic and cholinergic neurons. *Acta Neurochir Suppl.* 2003;87:3–6.

75. Webster H, Jones BE. Neurotoxic lesions of the dorsolateral pontomesencephalic tegmentum-cholinergic cell area in the cat. II. Effects upon sleep-waking states. *Brain Res.* 1988;458:285–302.

76. Hobson J, McCarley RW, Wyzinki PW. Sleep cycle oscillation: Reciprocal discharge by two brainstem neuronal groups. *Science.* 1975;189:55–58.

77. McCarley R, Hobson JA. Neuronal excitability modulation over the sleep cycle: A structural and mathematical model. *Science.* 1975;189:58–60.

78. Xi M, Morales FR. Chase MH, Evidence that wakefulness and REM sleep are controlled by a GABAergic pontine mechanism. *J Neurophysiol.* 1999;82:2015–2019.

79. Siegel J. *The neural control of sleep and waking.* New York: Springer-Verlag, 2002.

80. Pace-Schott E, Hobson JA. The neurobiology of sleep, genetics, cellular physiology, and subcortical networks. *Nature Rev Neurosci.* 2002;3:591–605.

81. Sastre J, Buda C, Kitahama K, et al. Importance of the ventrolateral region of the periaqueductal gray and adjacent tegmentum in the control of paradoxical sleep as studied by muscimol microinjections in the cat. *Neuroscience.* 1996;74:415–426.

82. Chase M, Soja PJ, Morales FR. Evidence that glycine mediates the postsynaptic potentials that inhibit lumbar motoneurons during the atonia of active sleep. *J Neurosci.* 1989;9:743–751.

83. Jones B. Basic mechanisms of sleep–wake states. In: Kryger M, Roth T, Dement WC, eds. *Principles and practice of sleep medicine,* Philadelphia: WB Saunders, 2000:134–154.

84. Jones B. The respective involvement of noradrenaline and its deaminated metabolites in waking and paradoxical sleep: A neuropharmacological model. *Brain Res.* 1972;39:121–136.

85. Jacobs B. Single unit activity of locus coeruleus neurons in behaving animals. *Prog Neurobiol.* 1986;27:183–194.

86. McCormick D. Neurotransmitter actions in the thalamus and cerebral cortex and their role in neuromodulation of thalamocortical activity. *Prog Neurobiol.* 1992;39:337–388.

87. Mohan Kumar V, Datta S, Chhina GS, et al. Alpha adrenergic system in medial preoptic area involved in sleep–wakefulness in rats. *Brain Res Bull.* 1986;16:463–468.

88. de Lecea L, Kilduff TS, Peyron C, et al. The hypocretins: hypothalamus-specific peptides with neuroexcitatory activity. *Proc Natl Acad Sci USA.* 1998;95:322–327.

89. Sakurai T, Amemiya A, Ishii M, et al. Orexins and orexin receptors: A family of hypothalamic neuropeptides and G protein-coupled receptors that regulate feeding behavior. *Cell.* 1998;92:573–585.

90. Hagan J, Leslie RA, Patel S, et al. Orexin A activates locus coeruleus cell firing and increases arousal in the rat. *Proc Natl Acad Sci USA.* 1999;96:10911–10916.

91. Espana R, Baldo BA, Kelley AE, et al. Wake-promoting and sleep-suppressing actions of hypocretin (orexin): Basal forebrain sites of action. *Neuroscience.* 2001;106:699–715.

92. Brown R, Sergeeva O, Eriksson KS, et al. Orexin A excites serotonergic neurons in the dorsal raphe nucleus of the rat. *Neuropharmacology.* 2001;40:457–459.

93. John J, Wu MF, Kodama T, et al. Intravenously administered hypocretin-1 alters brain amino acid release: An in vivo microdialysis study in rats. *J Physiol.* 2003;548:557–562.

94. Eggermann E, Serafin M, Bayer L, et al. Orexins/hypocretins excite basal forebrain cholinergic neurones. *Neuroscience.* 2001;108:177–181.

95. Bourgin P, Huitron-Resendiz S, Spier AD, et al. Hypocretin-1 modulates rapid eye movement sleep through activation of locus coeruleus neurons. *J Neurosci.* 2000;20:7760–7765.

96. Lin J, Sakai K, Vanni-Mercier, G, et al. Involvement of histaminergic neurons in arousal mechanisms demonstrated with H3-receptor ligands in the cat. *Brain Res.* 1990;523:325–330.

97. Haas H, Panula P. The role of histamine and the tuberomamillary nucleus in the nervous system. *Nat Rev.* 2003;4:121–130.

98. Huang Z, Qu WM, Li WD, et al. Arousal effect of orexin A depends on activation of the histaminergic system. *Proc Natl Acad Sci USA.* 2002;99:1098.

99. Domino E, Yamamoto K, Dren AT. Role of cholinergic mechanisms in states of wakefulness and sleep. *Prog Brain Res.* 1968;28:113–133.

100. Detari L, Juhasz G, Kukorelli T. Firing properties of cat basal forebrain neurons during sleep–wakefulness cycle. *Electroenceph Clin Neurophysiol.* 1984;58:362–368.

101. Marrosu F, Portas C, Mascia MS, et al. Microdialysis measurement of cortical and hippocampal acetylcholine release during sleep-wake cycle in freely moving cats. *Brain Res.* 1995;671:329–332.

102. Cape E, Jones BE. Differential modulation of high frequency gamma electroencephalogram activity and sleep–wake state by noradrenaline and serotonin microinjections into the region of cholinergic basalis neurons. *J Neurosci.* 1998;18:2653–2666.

103. Lo Conte G, Casamenti F, Bigl V, et al. Effect of magnocellular forebrain nuclei lesions on acetylcholine output from the cerebral cortex, electrocorticogram and behavior. *Arch Ital Biol.* 1982;120:176–188.

104. Dringenberg H, Olmstead MC. Integrated contributions of basal forebrain and thalamus to neocortical activation elicited by pedunculopontine tegmental stimulation in urethane-anesthetized rats. *J Neurosci.* 2003;119:839–853.

105. Steriade M. Acetylcholine systems and rhythmic activities during the waking–sleep cycle. *Prog Brain Res.* 2004;145:179–196.

106. Fujihara H, Serino R, Ueta Y, et al. Six-hour selective REM sleep deprivation increases the expression of the galanin gene in the hypothalamus of rats. *Brain Res Mol Brain Res.* 2003;119:152–159.

107. Nitz D, Siegel JM. GABA release in posterior hypothalamus across sleep–wake cycle. *Am J Physiol.* 1996;271:R1707–R1712.

108. Morales M, Bloom FE. The 5HT-3 receptor is present in different subpopulations of GABAergic neurons in the rat telencephalon. *J Neurosci.* 1997;17:3157–3167.

109. Sharpley A, Cowen PJ. Effect of pharmacologic treatments on the sleep of depressed patients. *Biol Psych.* 1995;37:85–98.

110. Dugovic C. Role of serotonin in sleep mechanisms. *Rev Neurol (Paris).* 2001;157:S16–S19.

111. Porkka-Heiskanen T, Strecker RE, McCarley RW. Brain site-specificity of extracellular adenosine concentration changes during sleep deprivation and spontaneous sleep: An in vivo microdialysis study. *Neuroscience.* 2000;99:507–517.

112. Porkka-Heiskanen T, Alanko L, Kalinchuk A, et al. Adenosine and sleep. *Sleep Med Rev.* 2002;6:321–332.

113. Portas CM, Thakkar M, Rainnie DG, et al. Role of adenosine in behavioral state modulation: A microdialysis study in the freely moving cat. *Neuroscience.* 1997;79:225–235.

114. Scammell TE, Gerashchenko DY, Mochizuki T, et al. An adenosine A2a agonist increases sleep and induces Fos in ventrolateral preoptic neurons. *Neuroscience.* 2001;107:653–663.

115. Rainnie D, Grunze HC, McCarley RW, et al. Adenosine inhibition of mesopontine cholinergic neurons: Implications for EEG arousal. *Science.* 1994;263:689–692.

116. Chamberlin N, Arrigoni E, Chou TC, et al. Effects of adenosine on gabaergic synaptic inputs to identified ventrolateral preoptic neurons. *Neuroscience.* 2003;119:913–918.

117. Stenberg D, Litonius E, Halldner L, et al. Sleep and its homeostatic

regulation in mice lacking the adenosine A1 receptor. *J Sleep Res.* 2003;12:283–290.

118. Steriade M. Brain electrical activity and sensory processing during waking and sleep states. In: Kryger M, Roth T, Dement WC, eds. *Principle and practice of sleep medicine.* Philadelphia: W.B. Saunders, 2000:93–111.

119. Steriade M, Domich L, Oakson G, et al. The deafferented reticular thalamic nucleus generates spindle rhythmicity. *J Neurophysiol.* 1987;57:260–273.

120. Jahnsen H, Llinas R. Ionic basis for the electro-responsiveness and oscillatory properties of guinea-pig thalamic neurones in vitro. *J Physiol.* 1984;349:227–247.

121. McCormick D, Bal T. Sleep and arousal: Thalamocortical mechanisms. *Annu Rev Neurosci.* 1997;20:185–215.

122. Timoffev I, Contreras D, Steriade M. Synaptic responsiveness of cortical and thalamic neurons during various phases of slow oscillation sleep in the cat. *J Physiol.* 1996;494:265–278.

123. Steriade M, Dossi RC, Nunez A. Network modulation of a slow intrinsic oscillation of cat thalamocortical neurons implicated in sleep delta waves: Cortically induced synchronization and brainstem cholinergic suppression. *J Neurosci.* 1991;11:3200–3217.

123a. Steriade M, Nunea A, Amzica F. A novel slow (<1 Hz) oscillation of neocortical neurons in vivo: depolarizing and hyperpolarizing components. *J Neurosci.* 1993;13:3252–3265.

124. Contreras D, Steriade M. Cellular basis of EEG slow rhythms: A study of dynamic corticothalamic relationships. *J Neurosci.* 1995;15:604–622.

125. Amzica F, Steriade M. The K-complex: Its slow (<1 Hz) rhythmicity and relation to delta waves. *Neurology.* 1997;49:952–959.

126. Amici R, Sanford LD, Kearney K, et al. A serotonergic (5-HT2) receptor mechanism in the laterodorsal tegmental nucleus participates in regulating the pattern of rapid-eye-movement sleep occurrence in the rat. *Brain Res.* 2004;996:9–18.

127. Steriade M, Sakai K, Jouvet M, et al. Bulbo-thalamic neurons related to thalamocortical activation processes during paradoxical sleep. *Exp Brain Res.* 1984;54:463–475.

128. Berntson G, Shafi R, Sarter M. Specific contributions of the basal forebrain corticopetal cholinergic system to electroencephalographic activity and sleep/waking states. *Eur J Neurosci.* 2002;16:2453–2461.

129. Seigel J. Brainstem mechanisms generating sleep. In: Kryger M, Roth T, Dement WC, eds. *Principle and practice of sleep medicine,* Philadelphia: W.B. Saunders, 2000:112–133.

130. Vanderwolf C. Robinson TE, Reticulo-cortical activity and behavior: A critique of the arousal theory and a new synthesis. *Behav Brain Sci.* 1981;4:459–514.

131. Vertes R, Kocsis B. Brainstem-diencephalo-septohippocampal systems controlling the theta rhythm of the hippocampus. *Neuroscience.* 1997;81:893–926.

132. Vanderwolf C. Hippocampal electrical activity and voluntary movement in the rat. *Electroencephalogr Clin Neurophysiol.* 1969;26:407–418.

133. Rechtschaffen A, Kales A. *A manual of standardized terminology: Techniques and scoring system for sleep stages of human subjects.* Los Angeles: UCLA Brain Information Service/Brain Research Institute, 1968.

134. Paxinos G, Watson C. *The rat brain in stereotaxic coordinates.* 4th edn. New York: Academic Press, 1998.

Chapter 4

Breathing during Sleep: Ventilation and the Upper Airway

James A. Rowley and M. Safwan Badr

INTRODUCTION

The pathogenesis of sleep apnea syndrome remains poorly understood. The occurrence of apnea during sleep and not wakefulness implicates the removal of the wakefulness stimulus to breathe as a key factor underlying apnea and upper-airway obstruction during sleep. Development of sleep apnea or hypopnea involves an interaction between "host" risk factors and changes related to sleep state per se. Host risk factors could include gender, age, body mass index, and neck circumference, all of which have been associated with an increased prevalence of obstructive sleep apnea (1–4). In this chapter, we will address the fundamental effects of sleep on ventilation, upper-airway patency, and the interaction with risk factors, such as gender and body mass index. In addition, we will discuss how sleep-related changes may conspire to induce recurrent apnea or upper-airway obstruction in susceptible individuals.

BREATHING DURING SLEEP: VENTILATION AND THE UPPER AIRWAY

Summary of Normal Breathing and Ventilation during Sleep

Non-Rapid Eye Movement Sleep (NREM Sleep)

The respiratory system changes during sleep to meet a decreased metabolic rate. Ventilatory motor output during sleep decreases from its normal levels in wakefulness, leading to decreased tidal volume and minute ventilation. The decreased ventilation is accompanied by reduced upper-airway dilator muscle activity resulting in decreased upper-airways caliber and increased airflow resistance. These biological changes may account for the observed increase in $Paco_2$ and decrease in Pao_2 during sleep, despite the diminished overall metabolism rate in the body. A decrease in chemoresponsiveness during sleep may also explain the increased $Paco_2$. Overall, breathing becomes more dependent on chemical stimuli, which is integrated in the brainstem.

Rapid Eye Movement Sleep (REM Sleep)

In contrast to NREM sleep, REM sleep is characterized by variability in ventilation. This variability consists of sudden changes in respiratory amplitude and frequency associated with the periods of phasic rapid eye movements. Because of this variability, minute ventilation in REM sleep has been shown to be the same, increased, or decreased compared with NREM sleep. Upper-airway resistance has also been reported variably as either the same or increased compared to wakefulness and NREM sleep. Finally, hypercapnic and hypoxic ventilatory chemoresponsiveness is decreased in REM sleep compared to wakefulness and possibly even NREM sleep.

Effect of Sleep on Control of Breathing

Control of Breathing

Breathing is a rhythmic and automatic activity controlled by many mechanisms. The central nervous system (CNS) tightly controls the respiratory cycle. This regulation of breathing occurs at two different levels. The first level, the brain cortex, allows humans to breathe voluntarily during wakefulness. The second level, the brainstem, regulates involuntary respiration, controlling it through many integrated responses between the peripheral and the central nervous systems. Inspiration and expiration are under neural effect through groups of neurons located in the medulla, known as the respiratory center, which is divided into two separate sites, dorsal and ventral. The dorsal group is mainly responsible for the inspiration phase and the ventral site mainly maintains the expiratory phase. The spontaneous function of the respiratory center in the medulla is usually modified by other neurons in the pons, known as the pneumotaxic center. These neurons interact directly with mechanical receptors in the airways and lung. The CNS controls breathing not only through a mechanical feedback mechanism, but also by chemical feedback coming from the blood. Ventilation is the main function of breathing and considered a target of the breathing control mechanism.

Ventilatory chemoreceptors are classified either as peripheral or central, depending on the anatomic location. These two types of receptors are highly integrated to respond to a change in partial arterial pressure of carbon dioxide ($Paco_2$), partial arterial pressure of oxygen (Pao_2), or pH, which will influence the firing rate of specific respiratory motoneurons in the brainstem. In particular, central chemoreceptors are located on the ventral surface of medulla and are distinguishable from other respiratory centers. These chemoreceptors respond to changes in arterial $Paco_2$ and the pH of the cerebrospinal fluid (CSF). Peripheral chemoreceptors are located in the carotid and aortic bodies. The peripheral chemoreceptors mainly sense the Pao_2, in addition to $Paco_2$ and pH, and send impulses to the medulla via the glossopharyngeal cranial nerve.

Ventilatory Control during Wakefulness and Sleep

Chemoresponsiveness refers to changing ventilation in response to changes in chemical stimuli. Chemosensitivity is influenced by changes in neural activity during sleep. Thus, hypoxic and hypercapnic chemoresponsiveness contributes to maintaining ventilation during sleep. Conversely, hypocapnia is a potent inhibitor of ventilation during NREM sleep and is a key mechanism of central apnea (5).

Hypercapnic Ventilatory Response (HCVR)

When arterial $Paco_2$ rises, ventilation is stimulated linearly to bring the $Paco_2$ level back to its normal range. Control of this response occurs as a central chemoresponse mainly in the ventral part of medulla. The sleep state is characterized by decreased HCVR in human adults compared to wakefulness (6–10). While the sensitivity to $Paco_2$ does not appear to differ within NREM sleep stages, the HCVR during REM stage is depressed further compared with NREM sleep (6,8).

Potential determinants of chemoresponsiveness during sleep include metabolic rate, age, gender, and the mechanics of the respiratory system. There is no empiric evidence of age effect on HCVR (11). Conversely, there are conflicting findings regarding the effect of gender on HCVR. Some have found no difference between the genders (8,9), whereas others have found a gender difference during wakefulness, but not sleep (6). One group found an increased HCVR during sleep in women compared with men (7). Thus, it is unclear if there is a gender difference in HCVR.

The use of ventilation to express chemoresponsiveness requires that chemical stimuli do not alter upper-airway or pulmonary mechanics. Therefore, increased upper-airway resistance from wakefulness to NREM sleep would dampen ventilatory reponse to chemical stimuli and be interpreted as decreased chemoresponsiveness. The variability of the effect of changes in chemical stimuli on upper-airway caliber would further confound the interpretation of changes in chemoresponsiveness. Fortunately, recent studies have demonstrated that changes in the $Paco_2$ and chemoresponsiveness occur independent of changes in upper-airway resistance (11,12). Nonetheless, the complex interaction between ventilation and upper-airway caliber mandates caution in intepreting sleep-related changes in chemoreponsiveness.

Hypoxic Ventilatory Response (HVR)

Hypoxic ventilatory response (HVR) is the increase in minute ventilation in response to hypoxia. HVR is reported to decrease during NREM sleep compared to wakefulness, with a further decrease in REM sleep (10,13–15). Previous studies investigating the gender effect on HVR have come to conflicting conclusions. During sleep, men and women had similar HVR, although there was a large decrease in HVR from wakefulness in men, indicating that men had an increased HVR during wakefulness compared with women (13,14). Two recent studies have found similar responses to sustained isocapnic hypoxia between the two genders during wakefulness (16,17). In particular, we have recently demonstrated that the ventilatory response to brief hypoxia was similar between men and women in the absence of changes in upper-airway mechanics (17). This allowed us to conclude that there is no intrinsic gender difference in HVR during NREM sleep.

Effect of Sleep on Hypocapnic Ventilatory Response and the Apneic Threshold

The loss of wakefulness stimulus to breathe renders ventilation during NREM sleep critically dependent on chemoreceptor stimuli (Pao_2 and $Paco_2$). Reduced $Paco_2$ is a powerful inhibitory factor of ventilation during sleep. Therefore, central apnea develops when $Paco_2$ is reduced below a highly reproducible hypocapnic apneic threshold, unmasked by NREM sleep (5) (Fig. 4-1). Hypocapnia is probably the most important inhibitory factor during NREM sleep. Hypocapnia, secondary to breathing instability, is key to the genesis of central sleep apnea in congestive heart failure (18), and idiopathic central sleep apnea (19,20) and could play a role in central apnea with sleep onset and aging (21,22).

Hypocapnia and unmasking of the apneic threshold may be relevant to the pathogenesis of obstructive sleep apnea (OSA) as well. First, evidence of upper-airway obstruction in the absence of ventilatory motor output (central sleep apnea) has been observed (23) (Fig. 4-2). Second, reduction in pharyngeal dilator activity has been associated with periodic breathing (24–26) and hypocapnia in subjects with evidence of inspiratory flow limitation (27). Third, it has been shown that men are more susceptible to the development of central sleep apnea and have a decreased responsiveness to carbon dioxide than women (28), a result consistent with the increased prevalence of OSA in men. In particular, the gender differences appear, at least in part, secondary to testosterone as there was no difference in apneic threshold between the follicular and luteal stages in women (28), and the administration of testosterone to premenopausal women results in an increased apneic threshold, similar to that seen in men (29).

REM sleep is a special case because peripheral atonia is accompanied by augmented inspiratory medullary neuronal activity, and the REM sleep electroencephalogram (EEG) shares many features of the awake EEG. Whether hypocapnia inhibits ventilation during REM sleep is yet to be established in humans. In dogs, central apnea following hyperventilation can be demonstrated during REM sleep, but no systematic relationship existed with the magnitude of hypocapnia (30).

Effect of Sleep on Upper-Airway Structure and Function

The sleep state is a challenge, rather than a rest period, for the ventilatory system. Consequences of loss of wakefulness include reduced activity of upper-airway dilators,

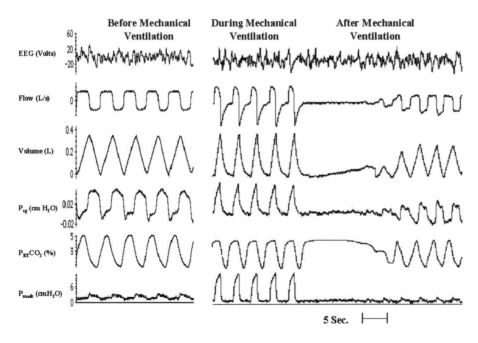

FIGURE 4-1. Induced hypocapnic central apnea during NREM sleep. Nasal mechanical ventilation was used to decrease end-tidal Pco_2 ($P_{ET}co_2$). Cessation of mechanical ventilation caused central apnea. P_{sg}, supraglottic pressure; P_{mask}, mask pressure.

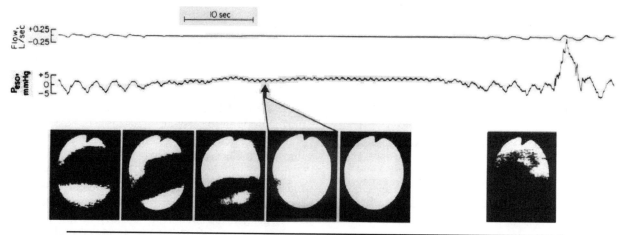

FIGURE 4-2. Complete pharyngeal obstruction during a spontaneous central apnea. Note the progressive decrease in airway caliber during the central apnea, with complete obstruction on the fourth image. The last image shows the opened airway after the arousal, during which there was again inspiratory effort. P_{eso}, esophogeal pressure.

reduced upper-airway caliber, increased upper-airway resistance, loss of load compensation, and increased pharyngeal compliance and collapsibility. Ultimately, these changes lead to reduced tidal volume and hypoventilation (Fig. 4-3).

Reduced Upper-Airway Dilating Muscle Activity

The musculature of the upper airway consists of 24 pairs of striated muscles extending from the nares to the larynx (31,32). There are at least 10 muscles that are classified as pharyngeal dilators, innervated by more than one cranial nerve motoneuron. There are two patterns of electrical discharge from these muscles: tonic (constant) activity, independent of phase of respiration, and phasic activity, occurring during one part of the respiratory cycle. It is widely accepted that upper-airway narrowing during sleep is due to a sleep-related decrease in upper-airway muscle

activity. However, data demonstrating reduced motor output to upper-airway muscles during NREM sleep remain fragmentary and based mostly on animal studies using reduced or chronically instrumented preparations. Orem et al. (33) have shown, in several studies in cats, that peak firing rate of motoneurons in the ventral respiratory group is reduced during NREM sleep. Recent work in naturally sleeping, chronically instrumented rats has shown reduced EMG activity of the genioglossus in NREM and in REM sleep (34). Overall, the available data from animal studies taken together suggest a small, but perhaps significant, reduction in the ventilatory motor output to upper airway muscles.

The effect of NREM sleep on upper airway muscle function in humans has not been conclusively studied, partly due to the difficulty in isolating the myriad influences on upper-airway muscle activity, especially changes in flow or the magnitude of negative pressure in the pharyngeal airway. However, available evidence indicates a reduction in either the tonic or phasic activity during NREM sleep for a variety of upper-airway muscles (31), including the levator palatini (35), tensor palatini (36), palatoglossus (35), and geniohyoid (37) (Fig. 4-4).

The effect of REM sleep on upper-airway muscle activity is more compelling. Activity of antigravity muscles is reduced during REM sleep. There is strong evidence that activity of phasic upper-airway dilating muscles, such as the genioglossus, is greatly attenuated during REM sleep (38,39), particularly during periods of phasic rapid eye movements (40). Reduced activity has also been shown for the alae nasi (40) and geniohyoid muscles (37).

The response of upper-airway muscle to chemical and mechanical perturbations may be more relevant physiologically than reduced baseline activity. Pharyngeal muscles display an attenuated response to negative pressure during NREM (41–43) and REM sleep (44) compared to

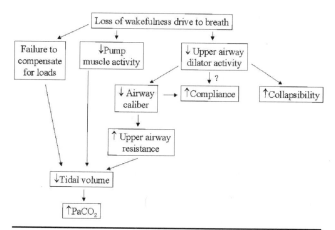

FIGURE 4-3. Effect of loss of wakefulness drive to breath on ventilation and the upper airway.

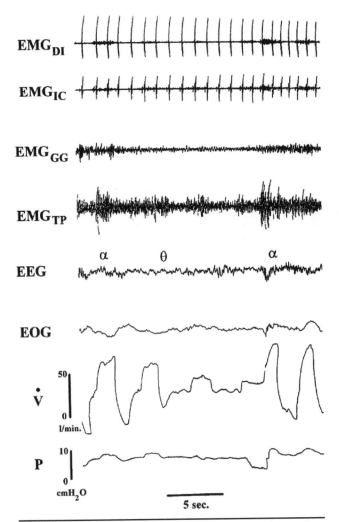

EMG_{DI}

EMG_{IC}

EMG_{GG}

EMG_{TP}

α   θ   α

EEG

EOG

$\dot{V}$

50

0

l/min.

P

10

0

cmH_2O

5 sec.

FIGURE 4-4. Raw data illustrating the decrease in electrical activity of genioglossus (EMG_{GG}) and tensor palatini (EMG_{TP}) at sleep onset in a human. EMG_{DI}, raw diaphragm EMG; EMG_{IC}, raw intercostal EMG; $\dot{V}$, airflow; P, Millar pressure. (From Worsnop C, et al., *J Appl Physiol.* 1998;85:908. With permission.)

wakefulness. Similarly, responsiveness of the genioglossus muscle to hypercapnia is also attenuated during sleep (45). Decreased responsiveness to challenges indicates that upper-airway muscles are less able to maintain upper-airway patency in the face of chemical or mechanical perturbations.

Upper-Airway Resistance

The evidence for increased upper-airway resistance during sleep is compelling, even in normal subjects (46–50). An example of increased upper-airway resistance during sleep is shown in Fig. 4-5. In particular, Kay et al. (47), studied the changes in minute ventilation and upper-airway resistance during the transition from predominant alpha electroencephalographic activity through predominant delta activity. The group found that a large decrease in minute ventilation with sleep onset was associated with a small increase

in upper-airway resistance. In subjects who achieved delta activity, there was a progressive increase in upper-airways resistance that was not associated with further decreases in minute ventilation. The large increases in resistance were not observed in subjects who remained in stage 2 sleep during the study period. The preponderance of evidence is that there are no further increases in upper-airway resistance during REM sleep (48–52).

Potential determinants of upper-airway resistance during sleep include many variables known to be associated with increased prevalence of OSA, such as gender, body mass index (BMI), and age. Two groups of investigators have found no difference in upper-airway resistance between genders (52,53) during NREM, predominantly stage 2, sleep. In contrast, Trinder et al. (54) found that while there was no difference in upper-airway resistance during the transition from wakefulness to NREM sleep, there was an increased resistance in men during slow-wave sleep. Overall, there is no conclusive gender effect on upper-airway resistance during sleep.

The effect of age on upper-airway resistance is variable across different studies. Browne et al. (55) and Thurnheer et al. (52) found no difference in upper-airway resistance between young and older subjects. The total subject groups spanned the age spectrum from 18 to older than 65 years of age. There have been contrasting results on the influence of age on upper-airway resistance during sleep. When 48 subjects were grouped broadly into two age groups (18 to 35 and 40 to 70 years), Thurnheer et al. (52) found no difference in upper-airway resistance between the two groups (136). In contrast, we performed a linear regression analysis to determine the independent predictors of upper-airway resistance in a group of 60 subjects. For this group, age was the only independent predictor of upper-airway resistance, with an increased age associated with an increased upper-airway resistance. Interestingly, BMI was not a predictor of resistance (53). The reasons for the discrepancy of studies are not clear and may be due to subtle methodologic differences or to an interaction between age and other demographic factors in our study, such as the racial composition of the population. Nevertheless, the effect of age, per se, on upper-airway resistance appears modest even in our study.

It is important to note that upper-airway resistance provides only a partial picture of the dynamic behavior of the pharyngeal airway during sleep. Specifically, upper-airway resistance is generally expressed as a single number representing the slope of pressure–flow relationship. This computation is predicated on a constant relationship between driving pressure and inspiratory flow, which is true during normal breathing in normal subjects. However, many subjects exhibit inspiratory-flow limitation, in which the pressure-flow graph (Fig. 4-4) demonstrates a changing relationship culminating in complete dissociation between pressure and flow (pressure continues to decrease with no further increase in flow). Thus, the only

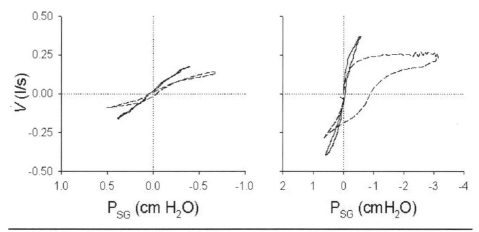

FIGURE 4-5. Left panel: Pressure-flow loops during wakefulness (solid line) and NREM sleep (dashed line). Note the increased upper airway resistance, as evidenced by a decreased slope of the pressure-flow curve, during NREM sleep. The sleep breath is nonflow limited. **Right panel:** pressure-flow loops during wakefulness (solid line) and NREM sleep (dashed line). In this example, the NREM sleep breath demonstrates inspiratory flow limitation, as evidenced by a plateau in the flow despite further decreased pressure.

physiologically meaningful measurement of resistance is the slope of the linear portion of the pressure-flow loop, which likely reflects upper-airway caliber at the narrowest point in the upper airway at the beginning of inspiration. The potential for pressure-flow dissociation mandates the use of other indices to properly characterize upper-airway structure and function during sleep.

The aforementioned discussion indicates that decreased upper-airway caliber during sleep is a physiologic phenomenon. However, a substantial decrease in upper-airway caliber may cause "fluttering" of the soft palate due to turbulent flow, producing the acoustic phenomenon known as snoring. The mechanical corollary of snoring is inspiratory flow limitation, which manifests as a plateau in flow, despite continued development of negative pressure. Figure 4-6 is an example of increased upper-airway resistance and flow limitation during sleep in a normal subject. This representative polygraphic segment depicts reduced flow with flattening of the flow profile with snoring and progressive decrease in supraglottic pressure, terminating with an arousal. Recurrent episodes of increased resistance and inspiratory flow limitation lead

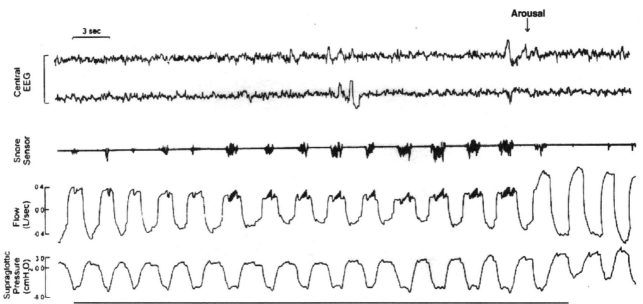

FIGURE 4-6. A representative polygraph record of progressive increase in upper-airway resistance leading to arousal. Note the progressive snoring signal and the square profile with a snoring artifact. This is terminated by an arousal (arrow) and resolution of the flow limitation and of snoring.

to increased work on breathing, hypoventilation, frequent arousals from sleep, and subsequent excessive daytime sleepiness. In fact, some authors identify this constellation of findings as a distinct clinical entity referred to as the upper-airway resistance syndrome (56), under the rubric of sleep-related breathing disorders.

It is commonly assumed that snoring and flow limitation are tightly linked to increased upper-airway resistance. However, it is plausible that resistance would be high in a stiff, but narrow, tube. To evaluate such association, we evaluated BMI and upper-airway resistance as potential determinants of the presence of inspiratory-flow limitation in >10% of breaths in a group of normal subjects (53). Using multivariate logistic regression, we determined that BMI and upper airway resistance both predicted the presence of inspiratory-flow limitation. Interestingly, increased upper-airway resistance was associated with a *decreased* likelihood of inspiratory-flow limitation, indicating that a narrow upper airway may be less susceptible to distortion by subatmospheric intrathoracic pressure. Thus, upper-airway resistance during sleep is a rather limited surrogate for susceptibility to pharyngeal closure during sleep.

Reduced Upper-Airway Caliber

Using nasopharyngoscopy during naturally occurring sleep in normal subjects, Rowley et al. have shown that pharyngeal cross-sectional area is decreased during sleep at both the retropalatal and retroglossal levels (48,49). During NREM sleep, both retropalatal cross-sectional area and retroglossal cross-sectional area decreased to ~70% of the awake baseline cross-sectional area. The decreased cross-sectional area is consistent with a decrease in upper-airway dilator activity with the onset of NREM sleep. In REM sleep, retropalatal cross-sectional area did not decrease further compared to NREM sleep (49). In contrast, retroglossal cross-sectional area did decrease further during REM compared to NREM sleep (48). The contrast between the influence of REM sleep on retropalatal and retroglossal area can be explained in two ways. First, there may not be a further decrease during REM sleep in the activity of the dilators that control the retropalatal area (including the levator and tensor palatini) in contrast to a demonstrated decrease in genioglossus activity during REM sleep. Second, it is possible that non-neuromuscular factors, such as the bony structures of the nasopharynx (including the pterygoid hamulus), could act to keep the airway open during periods of decreased neuromuscular activity.

The effect of gender on upper-airway cross-sectional area has been extensively investigated. The preponderance of studies indicates no difference in cross-sectional area between men and women during wakefulness (57–59). In contrast, using fiberoptic nasopharyngoscopy, we have shown that the retropalatal cross-sectional area was smaller in women than men during NREM sleep. However, the absolute gender difference disappeared when cross-sectional area was corrected for body surface area. In addition, sleep-related narrowing occurred to a similar degree in men and in women (approximately a 40% decrease in cross-sectional area for both genders) between wakefulness and NREM sleep (60).

Loss of Load Compensation

The ability of the ventilatory control system to compensate for changes in resistance is essential for the preservation of alveolar ventilation. Increased resistance is an example of resistive load, leading, during wakefulness, to increased effort to maintain ventilation and $Paco_2$. In contrast, hypoventilation occurs immediately upon imposing a resistive load during NREM sleep, perhaps implying that loads are not perceived during sleep (61). Therefore, resistive loading results in decreased tidal volume and minute ventilation and, hence, alveolar hypoventilation. The ensuing elevation of arterial $Paco_2$ restores ventilation toward normal levels. Teleologically, failure to respond to loads preserves sleep continuity. The cost of allowing sleep continuity is a mild elevation of $Paco_2$. In fact, elevated $Paco_2$ during sleep is one of few physiologic situations where hypercapnia is tolerated.

There has been one study comparing the ventilatory response to inspiratory resistive loading between men and women (62). In this study, there was no gender difference in the electrical activity of the genioglossus or tensor palatini during inspiratory resistive loading nor was there a difference in the ventilatory response. These data imply that there may not be a difference in the central drive or loading response between the genders. However, men were more likely to develop inspiratory flow limitation than were women, indicating that tissue factors or anatomy may be important risk factors for the increased frequency of upper-airway collapse observed in men.

Increased Pharyngeal Compliance

The walls of the pharyngeal airway consist of compliant soft tissue structures, amenable to changes in pressure during the respiratory cycle. During wakefulness, upper-airway caliber is constant during inspiration, with a decreased caliber during expiration, returning to inspiratory values at end-expiration; this finding has been observed in both normal subjects (59,63) and patients with sleep apnea (63) using either computerized tomographic (CT) scanning or nasopharyngoscopy. Using nasopharyngoscopy, NREM sleep was associated with significant dynamic within-breath changes in cross-sectional area, reaching a nadir at midinspiration (63). Interestingly, BMI was a better predictor of the magnitude of narrowing than the apnea–hypopnea index (AHI). It is not clear why sleep reversed the pattern of change in upper-airway cross-sectional area, but this may be due to sleep-related increase in upper-airway compliance, a decrease in pharyngeal caliber, and, subsequently, decreased (more negative) inspiratory intraluminal pressure.

The dynamic changes in upper-airway patency during sleep can be best investigated using compliance as a measurement. Traditionally, compliance is the change in volume for a given change in pressure. Compliance of the pharyngeal wall is an important modulator of the effect of pressure changes on upper-airway patency. The occurrence of pharyngeal narrowing and flow limitation suggests, but does not prove, increased pharyngeal compliance during sleep. However, determination of "true" compliance is not feasible with current available methodology. A "functional" compliance can be defined as the change in cross-sectional area for a given change in pressure. The minimum prerequisite measurements include cross-sectional area and luminal pressure at the same level. Traditionally, upper-airway compliance has been measured in a static fashion by measuring changes in cross-sectional area at different levels of pressure applied to the upper airway (64–66). Use of this technique has demonstrated that compliance is increased as the pharyngeal caliber decreases (64,65,67) and that the upper airway of patients with OSA is more compliant than that of normal subjects (64–66,68). However, the major limitation of this technique is that it does not allow measurement of the dynamic changes in the upper airway during eupneic breathing. Also, no direct comparisons between wakefulness and sleep have been performed using this technique.

In contrast, we have combined measurement of cross-sectional area via fiberoptic nasopharyngoscopy and measurement of intraluminal pressure at the same level during NREM and REM sleep. These studies have confirmed that retropalatal compliance is increased during NREM sleep compared to wakefulness (Fig. 4-7); in contrast,

retropalatal compliance during REM sleep is similar to that in wakefulness (49). At the retroglossal level, however, compliance was not increased during either NREM or REM sleep compared to wakefulness (48). Thus, pharyngeal compliance was not increased, despite the known absence of upper-airway muscle activity during REM sleep. The dissociation between compliance and reported muscle activity in these studies is consistent with studies in patients with OSA in which the demonstrated increased pharyngeal compliance occurs despite an increased activity of the genioglossus muscle during wakefulness (69) and sleep (70), perhaps as a compensation for anatomically reduced caliber. This finding clearly speaks for a major role for non-neuromuscular factors as determinants of pharyngeal compliance.

Using their method of measuring compliance, Rowley et al. (60) have recently shown that men have an increased retropalatal compliance compared with women during NREM sleep. Thus, increased pharyngeal compliance in men may explain the gender difference in obstructive sleep apnea. However, the finding of increased compliance in men was lost after adjusting for neck circumference, indicating that risk factors other than gender are important in explaining gender differences in upper-airway function. Specifically, men and women have different craniofacial characteristics and distribution of pharyngeal soft tissue and fat. These findings also are supportive of an important role for non-neuromuscular factors in the determination of upper-airway compliance.

Collapsibility

Collapsibility refers to the propensity of the upper airway to collapse or obstruct under certain conditions. While often used interchangeably with compliance, it differs from compliance in that it measures the changes in

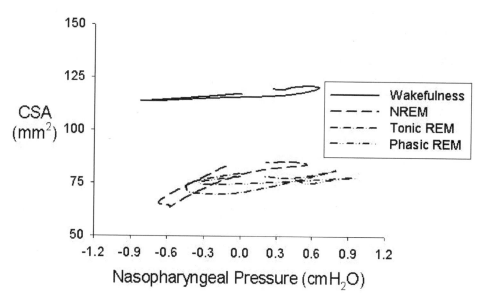

FIGURE 4-7. Group mean pharyngeal cross-sectional area (CSA) plotted against nasopharyngeal pressure for wakefulness (solid line), NREM sleep (dashed line), and tonic and phasic REM sleep (dash–dot lines). Pharyngeal compliance was defined as the slope of the relationship between CSA and nasopharyngeal pressure. Note the large changes in CSA during NREM sleep for similar changes in pressure, compared to wakefulness and REM sleep, indicating an increased airway compliance during NREM sleep.

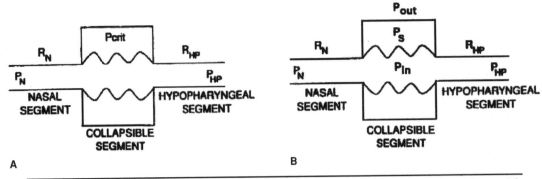

FIGURE 4-8. A: Starling resistor model of the upper airway as originally represented. In this model, P_{crit} was assumed to be equal to the pressure surrounding airway with no contribution from the airway wall itself. P_N, nasal (upstream) pressure; P_{HP}: hypopharyngeal (downstream) pressure; R_N: resistance in the nasal segment; R_{HP}: resistance in the hypopharyngeal segment. **B:** Generalized upper airway Starling resistor showing the three pressures that influence the flow-limiting site: outside pressure (P_{out}), surrounding pressure (P_s), and intraluminal pressure (P_{in}). In this model, the properties of the airway wall (as measured by the transmural pressure, P_{in}-P_{out}), contribute to collapsibility, and P_{crit} is not equated with P_s. (From Rowley, JA, et al. Effect of tracheal and tongue displacement on upper airway airflow dynamics. *J Appl Physiol*. 1996;80:2171. With permission.)

upper-airway area for given changes in pressure and not the propensity to collapse. Upper-airway collapsibility has been primarily measured using the critical closing pressure or P_{crit}.

Measurement of critical closing pressure or P_{crit} is based upon the concept of the Starling resistor (71). In a Starling resistor, maximal flow through the resistor is dependent upon the resistance of the segment upstream and the pressure surrounding the collapsible segment (Fig. 4-8). In normal subjects, the application of progressively negative nasal pressure (upstream pressure) results in inspiratory-flow limitation, followed by complete upper-airway obstruction (72). Thus, this model of upper-airway mechanics has several advantages as a method to study upper-airway collapsibility. First, it most closely approximates the inspiratory-flow limitation that characterizes the breathing of many subjects with snoring. Second, the model allows a functional approach to the upper airway, which is key, given the complicated anatomy of the upper airway.

Using this model, it has been shown that across the spectrum of sleep-disordered breathing from inspiratory-flow limitation and snoring through obstructive apneas, P_{crit} becomes progressively more positive, indicative of increased propensity for airway collapse (72–74). Upper-airway collapsibility has also shown to be increased in the supine body position (75) and after sleep fragmentation (76). P_{crit} did not change during REM sleep in a study of patients with OSA (77). Rowley et al. (53) studied the influence of gender on P_{crit} in 16 normal subjects and found no difference between the genders, in contrast to the gender difference in upper-airway compliance. These latter results indicate that compliance and collapsibility are different measurements of upper-airway function and mechanics.

The P_{crit} model has also been applied in an animal preparation. In this preparation, the upper airway is isolated from the lower respiratory system. Negative pressure to the isolated airway results in a condition of inspiratory-flow limitation, similar to that seen in humans. This model permits the further study of the physiologic basis for changes in P_{crit} by allowing manipulation of these factors in a more controlled fashion. Using this model, a series of experiments were performed to determine neuromuscular and non-neuromuscular factors that determine airway collapsibility. The most potent neuromuscular factor is hypercapnia, which decreases airway collapsibility (78–80) (Fig. 4-9). In contrast, hypoxia did not change collapsibility in this model (80). The effect of hypercapnia was modulated by both mucosal afferents, which tend to further decrease collapsibility, and vagal afferents, which tend to increase collapsibility (80). Finally, it was determined that hypercapnia is most likely acting by stimulating the palatal muscles, as the effect of hypercapnia was not diminished after cutting the hypoglossal nerve and strap muscles in this preparation (78).

The two primary non-neuromuscular factors tested using this model included tracheal traction and tongue displacement. Increased tracheal traction stiffens the upper airway and decreases airway collapsibility (81,82). On the other hand, there was no independent effect of tongue displacement on changes in airway collapsibility (81). However, there was an interactive effect between tongue displacement and caudal tracheal displacement, such that there was an effect of tongue displacement at increasing degrees of tracheal traction. These data resulted in a modification of the original Starling resistor model, which stated that collapsibility was equivalent to the pressure surrounding the airway. In the revised model, airway collapsibility, as measured by P_{crit}, is determined by both the

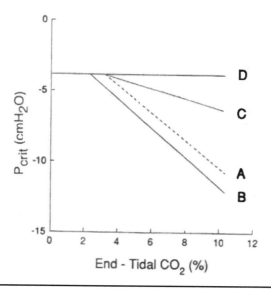

FIGURE 4-9. Schematic illustrating influence of chemoreceptor, airway mucosal receptor, and vagally mediated pulmonary reflexes on P_{crit} versus end-tidal CO_2 ($ETco_2$). **Curve A:** response of P_{crit} to increasing $ETco_2$ in absence of airway and pulmonary reflex modulation. **Curve B:** effects of airway mucosal receptor reflexes on P_{crit}–CO_2 relationship. **Curve C:** effects of pulmonary receptor reflexes on P_{crit}–CO_2 relationship. **Curve D:** P_{crit} after neuromuscular blockade. (From Seelagy, MM, et al. Reflex modulation of airflow dynamics through the upper airway. *J Appl Physiol.* 1994;76:2692. With permission.)

pressure surrounding the airway and the transmural pressure across the airway. Thus, the intrinsic properties of the airway wall, such as longitudinal tension (which is manipulated with tracheal traction), are important determinants of airway collapsibility.

Upper-Airway Patency: Neuromuscular and Non-neuromuscular Determinants

Upper-Airway "Dilating" Muscles

The muscles of the upper airway perform multiple functions pertinent to deglutition and phonation, as well as respiration. Some upper-airway muscles, such as the genioglossus, are classified as dilators by virtue of their phasic inspiratory activity. Other muscles such as the tensor palatini demonstrate activity throughout the respiratory cycle (tonic activity), and are presumed to "stiffen" the upper-airway wall and decrease pharyngeal collapsibility. It is widely accepted that upper-airway dilators play a critical role in preserving pharyngeal patency (83). There is evidence from electromyography (EMG) studies that activity of upper-airway "dilators" begins about 200 milliseconds before onset of thoracic pump activity in normal subjects (84,85). In contrast, upper-airway muscle activity may be delayed relative to thoracic pump activity in patients with sleep apnea (84).

Several studies have investigated the mechanical corollary of upper-airway muscle activation during eupneic

breathing. Kobayashi et al. (86) studied the relationship between electrical activity of the genioglossus (EMG_{GG}) and pharyngeal dimensions in laryngectomized patients breathing through a tracheal stoma with no pressure or flow changes in the upper airway. Expansion of the glossopharyngeal airway and, hence, upper-airway dilatation occurred with inspiratory-related activation of the genioglossus. Likewise, Schnall et al. (87) noted upper-airway resistance decreased with electrical stimulation of the genioglossus, but only when the upper-airway lumen was compromised by extrinsic pressure (simulating the sleep effect). Kuna and Brennick (88,89) recently demonstrated in a feline preparation with an isolated upper airway that stimulating upper-airway muscles resulted in increased pharyngeal cross-sectional area. However, this effect varied by the pharyngeal region and the pressure range.

The aforementioned studies suggest that upper airway "dilators" actually dilate the lumen of the upper airway. This would require shortening of the pharyngeal muscle fibers. However, electrical activity is not an appropriate surrogate for muscle fiber shortening. A study in awake goats (90) studied the relationship between EMG_{GG} activity and muscle fiber length during eupnea and hypercapnia. When the animals breathed through the intact upper airway, genioglossus fiber lengthening occurred during inspiration, despite elevated EMG_{GG} by hypercapnia. Thus, negative intraluminal pressure during inspiration represents an afterload, leading to passive lengthening rather than shortening of the genioglossus muscle fibers. Genioglossus muscle fiber shortening during inspiration occurred only when the animals breathed through an open tracheostomy. Accordingly, activation of upper-airway dilating muscles cannot always be translated into actual dilatation of the upper airway. Conversely, upper-airway dilatation may occur without upper-airway muscle recruitment. In one study in sleeping humans, increased end-expiratory lung volume resulted in decreased upper-airway resistance and increased retropalatal cross-sectional area in association with reduced EMG_{GG} (91).

A related question is the role of upper-airway dilating muscles in preventing upper-airway collapse. There is evidence that stimulation of the hypoglossal nerve results in decreased collapsibility (stiffer airway) in the isolated upper-airway model (92) and increased maximal airflow and decreased the AHI in patients with OSA (93,94). Conversely, there was no change in collapsibility after the hypoglossal nerve was cut during hypercapnia (78). Likewise, it is unclear whether complete atonia increases upper-airway collapsibility. For example, the pharyngeal airway becomes more collapsible in dead infants (95,96), but not in paralyzed animal preparations (97,98). Likewise, increased pharyngeal compliance in patients with sleep apnea cannot be attributed to decreased upper-airway dilating muscle activity per se since patients with OSA have increased activity of the genioglossus muscle during wakefulness (69) and sleep (70), perhaps as a compensation for anatomically reduced caliber. Finally, the pharyngeal airway is narrowed during hypocapnic central apnea (99); more pronounced narrowing (or even closure) occurred in patients with sleep apnea relative to normals despite complete inhibition of upper-airway dilating muscle activity in all subjects. Thus, non-neuromuscular factors contribute to upper-airway patency in sleeping humans.

Transmural Pressure

A collapsing transmural pressure can be generated either by a negative intraluminal pressure or a collapsing surrounding pressure. The role of negative intraluminal pressure in the pathogenesis of upper-airway obstruction is widely presumed (83). Accordingly, a subatmospheric intraluminal pressure generated by the thoracic pump muscles causes upper airway obstruction by "sucking" the hypotonic upper airway. Several pieces of evidence indicate, however, that this is not a cause of upper-airway obstruction. First, there are no data showing that subatmospheric intraluminal pressure causes upper-airway obstruction in sleeping human beings. In addition, it has been demonstrated that pharyngeal obstruction does not require negative pressure. In particular, using fiberoptic nasopharyngoscopy, it has been shown that complete upper-airway collapse occurs during central apnea in patients with sleep apnea (23). Second, in the isolated upper-airway model discussed above, the applied negative pressure, of a magnitude of -75 to -100 cm H_2O, causes inspiratory-flow limitation, and not upper-airway collapse (79,81).

The occurrence of complete upper-airway obstruction in the absence of negative intraluminal pressure supports the hypothesis that upper-airway patency is determined by the extrinsic or surrounding pressure. For example, Isono et al. (65) compared the mechanics of the pharynx in anesthetized paralyzed normals and in patients with OSA. The pharynx was patent at atmospheric intraluminal pressure in normals and required negative intraluminal pressure for closure. In contrast, patients with OSA had positive closing pressure; that is the pharynx was closed at atmospheric intraluminal pressure. Similarly, the P_{crit} in patients with predominantly apnea is positive, as opposed to the negative P_{crit} in normal subjects (72,73).

The potential components of the surrounding pressure include the tongue, tonsils, and pharyngeal fat. Enlarged tonsils are a frequent causative factor in the pathogenesis of upper-airway obstruction, with known cure of OSA after tonsillectomy (100). Disease associated with macroglossia, such as acromegaly (101,102) and hypothyroidism (103,104), are also associated with the development of sleep apnea. Using cephalometric analysis, several investigators have found a relationship between increased tongue volume and the severity of sleep apnea (105–109). However, in physiologic studies, the influence of tongue position on upper-airway collapsibility is less

clear. In older studies, passive manipulation of the tongue has been shown to alter pharyngeal patency (95,110–112). However, in more recent investigations, it was not found to be a major determinant of airway collapsibility in the isolated upper-airway model (78,81).

CT and magnetic resonance imaging (MRI) of the upper airway have clearly shown the presence of pharyngeal fat, which could theoretically predispose to airway collapse. In males, there is evidence of increased soft tissue volume and pharyngeal fat at the level of the nasopharynx (113), which, in part, could explain the larger prevalence of sleep apnea. Pharyngeal fat volume was found to correlate with the AHI in one study of 30 subjects (including 21 patients with sleep apnea), and both AHI and pharyngeal fat volume decreased with weight loss (114). However, Schwab et al. (115) in a study of 68 subjects, 26 with sleep apnea, did not find a difference in pharyngeal fat pad size between normal subjects and patients with sleep apnea. Further investigations are needed to determine the role of the pharyngeal fat pad in the pathogenesis of upper-airway obstruction.

Intrinsic Properties of the Upper Airway

The collapsing effects of the transmural pressure on upper-airway patency are modulated by the compliance of the pharyngeal wall. Using nasopharyngoscopy to measure cross-sectional area during neuromuscular paralysis, Isono et al. (65) have shown that the nasopharynx is patent at normal atmospheric pressures. In addition, in the isolated upper airway model of collapsibility, P_{crit} is negative during complete paralysis, indicating that at normal atmospheric pressures, the airway is open (80,81). These studies indicate that the pharyngeal wall has an intrinsic "stiffness" or resistance to collapse. The determinants of this intrinsic stiffness have not been fully elucidated, primarily as the pharynx is a very complex structure, consisting of muscles (which may have different properties in a passive state as compared with a stimulated state), bony structures (particularly in the nasopharynx), blood vessels, and soft tissue.

The upper airway is connected to the thoracic cage and the mediastinum by several structures. Increased lung volume during inspiration is associated with increased upper airway caliber in awake human beings, likely because of thoracic inspiratory activity providing caudal traction on the upper airway, independent of upper airway dilating muscle activity (116). Caudal traction may transmit subatmospheric pressure through the trachea and ventrolateral cervical structures to the soft tissues surrounding the upper airway, increasing transmural pressure, and, hence, dilating the pharyngeal airway. In sleeping subjects, this mechanism has been shown by reduced upper-airway resistance and increased retropalatal airway size when end-expiratory lung volume was increased by passive inflation (92). In addition, caudal tracheal traction likely increases the longitudinal tension of the pharngeal airway (117,118).

Therefore, caudal traction both dilates and stiffens the pharyngeal airway. It is likely that patients with OSA are more dependent on the effects of increased lung volume because dilatation and/or stiffening may be more prominent in the more highly compliant upper airway found in apneics (65,66,119).

Vascular perfusion of the upper airway is another potential determinant of wall stiffness (120). In the cat, pharmacologic vasoconstriction has been shown to decrease airway collapsibility (120a). Similarly, vasoconstriction and vasodilatation have been shown to cause a decrease and increase in upper-airway resistance, respectively (121,122). Finally, increased central venous pressure attenuates the changes in pharyngeal cross-sectional area between functional residual capacity and end-inspiratory volume, indicative of a decreased compliance of the pharyngeal wall (123). However, the effect of changes in vascular blood volume in the neck on upper airway patency in sleeping human beings remains unknown.

Once upper-airway closure occurs, surface mucosal forces may impede subsequent upper-airway opening and promote further narrowing and occlusion (99). Mucosal lining forces may be particularly important in patients with OSA with mucosal inflammation from repeated trauma. In awake humans, surfactant has been shown to decrease the opening and closing pressures of the upper airway (124). In sleeping humans, surfactant or other topical lubricants have been shown to decrease upper-airway resistance in normal subjects (125) and the AHI in sleep in patients with sleep apnea (125,126).

In the passive (paralyzed) nasopharynx, the relationship between pharyngeal transmural pressure and cross-sectional area is curvilinear. The implication of the curvilinear relationship is that the airway becomes more compliant as the cross-sectional area decreases. Therefore, baseline airway cross-sectional area is itself a determinant of upper-airway compliance. There is evidence that the pharyngeal airway is smaller during wakefulness in patients with OSA relative to that of normal people (59,127,128), thus supportive of the concept that a smaller airway predisposes to increased airway collapse. In addition, the pharyngeal airway in patients with sleep apnea has an anterior/posterior configuration unlike the horizontal configuration in normal subjects (59,116). However, the exact implications of the observed lateral narrowing to the pathogenesis of upper-airway obstruction during sleep are yet to be determined.

Craniofacial Structure

Craniofacial structure is an important determinant of upper-airway patency. Clinically, this is most evident in children with craniofacial abnormalities such as Pierre–Robin and Treacher–Collins syndrome, both of which are associated with an increased prevalence of sleep apnea (129). In adults, several anatomic abnormalities have been associated with sleep apnea, including retrognathia, micrognathia, and overjet (130,131). A high-arched palate has also been associated with sleep-disordered breathing, particularly in thin, young women (132).

Several investigations have utilized lateral cephalometry to analyze the contribution of craniofacial structure to the development of sleep apnea (107,108,133–139). Although these studies vary widely in methodology, sample size, gender ratios, and the presence and degree of obesity, several common craniofacial differences have been observed. Common craniofacial abnormalities that have been associated with increased severity of sleep apnea include: (a) smaller airway dimensions, particularly those involving the maxilla and mandible; (b) mandibular retrognathia; (c) decreased posterior airspace; (d) an inferiorly placed hyoid bone; and (e) increased soft palate dimensions and length. These abnormalities would decrease the dimensions of the naso- and oropharynx, increasing the risk of upper-airway collapse. In one study in 57 male patients with OSA, airway collapsibility, as measured by the P$_{crit}$ (140), correlated with soft palate length, hyoid bone distance, and an inferiorly placed hyoid bone.

Differences in craniofacial structure could theoretically explain the gender difference in the prevalence of sleep apnea (141,142). Using MRI, Malhotra et al. (143) found that gender differences in airway length, soft palate cross-sectional area, and airway volume (all increased in men), could explain the difference in airway collapsibility. Similarly, cephalometric data have been used to examine differences between races, particularly between Caucasians and African-Americans and Caucasians and Polynesians. Redline et al. found that bony and soft tissue factors and brachycephaly are associated with sleep apnea in Caucasians, while only soft tissue factors are important in African-Americans (109,144). In contrast, Polynesians with sleep apnea had more mandibular retrognathia and larger nasal aperture width, whereas neck circumference, tongue, and soft palate dimensions were associated with sleep apnea in Caucasians (106). Taken together, these data indicate that different structural factors contribute to upper airway obstruction in different races.

It should be noted that in many of these studies, abnormal craniofacial structures were found to be most important in the nonobese patients with sleep apnea. In other words, obesity remains the predominant factor in the etiology of the majority of patients with OSA. However, in a recent study in a large sample of men, obesity alone explained only 26% of the variance in the AHI, illustrating the importance of craniofacial structures (134). In addition, there was an interaction between obesity and craniofacial structures, such that in patients with unfavorable airway dimensions were susceptible to larger increases in sleep apnea severity with modest changes in BMI. Therefore, even in obese subjects, craniofacial structures may contribute to upper-airway obstruction (145).

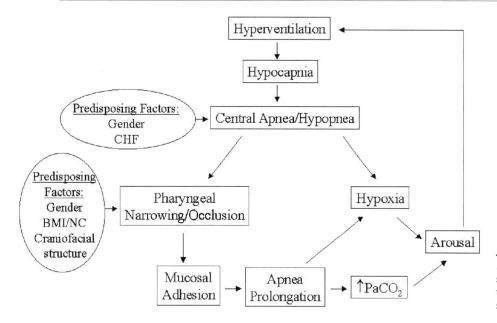

FIGURE 4-10. A proposed scheme of the pathophysiology of upper airway obstruction during sleep

Upper-Airway Obstruction: Putting the Pieces Together

Upper-airway obstruction results from an interaction between unfavorable upper-airway morphology and central breathing instability. Although precise pathogenesis is yet to be determined, common features can be assembled in plausible proposed mechanism(s) (Fig. 4-10). The underlying defect is a small pharynx susceptible to collapse. Recent evidence suggests that host risk factors such as neck circumference (3,106), body mass index (53,63), and craniofacial structure (108,134,135,139), are important determinants of an at-risk airway. Any or all of these risk factors leads to narrowing of the pharyngeal lumen, which manifests as snoring and inspiratory-flow limitation (53).

Whereas narrowing of the upper airway is a risk factor, it may not be sufficient, *ipso facto*, to induce upper-airway obstruction. We propose that central ventilatory control instability, in the form of periodic breathing, may be a key mechanism of recurrent upper-airway obstruction during sleep. This has been shown in experimentally induced periodic breathing with upper-airway obstruction occurring at the nadir of ventilatory motor output (24–26). Likewise, in some patients, periodic breathing may persist after correction of OSA with tracheostomy (146). Male gender (28), aging, and congestive heart failure (18) are possible risk factors that increase the risk of sustained breathing instability and sleep apnea.

According to this postulate, the cascade of events leading to upper-airway obstruction is initiated with reduced ventilatory motor output to upper-airway dilators. The reduction in ventilatory drive leads to reduced pharyngeal stiffness via reduction of neural output to upper-airway dilating muscles. The ensuing pharyngeal narrowing occurs because of the collapsing transmural pressure caused primarily by collapsing extraluminal forces. The narrow-

ing of the pharyngeal airway leads to an increased velocity of flow and, subsequently, to a further reduction in intraluminal pressure (the Bernoulli principle) and further pharyngeal narrowing. Eventually, complete pharyngeal obstruction occurs. Mucosal adhesive forces and gravity lead to prolongation of apnea, asphyxia, and arousal from sleep. The ensuing ventilatory overshoot leads to hyperpnea, hypocapnia, and subsequent reduction of ventilatory motor output, as sleep is resumed.

The aforementioned sequence does not explain how the cycle is initiated. In patients with severe sleep apnea, removal of the wakefulness stimulus to breathe per se may be sufficient to cause upper-airway obstruction. Sleep state instability at sleep onset may be the trigger in others.

In conclusion, our proposed scheme suggests that abnormal anatomy leads to snoring and inspiratory-flow limitation, whereas ventilatory control instability leads to periodic breathing and, hence, upper-airway obstruction.

FUTURE DIRECTIONS

The pathogenesis of sleep-related breathing disorders remains elusive. The relative contribution of upper-airway narrowing and flow limitation versus central breathing instability may reflect different pathophysiologic entities and thus may, influence treatment of the condition. The critical target is to unravel the complex mechanisms of periodic breathing on a neuronal, cellular, and molecular level and to elucidate the potential interactions of age, gender, or even race.

Most studies on the effect of sleep on ventilatory control and upper-airway fuction have focused on middle-aged adults with more studies conducted on men/women than females. Understanding the ontogeny and the gender difference in the physiology of respiration during sleep may provide great insight into the pathophysiology of sleep apnea and facilitate the development of treatment modalities targeted toward the precise pathophysiologic defect.

Evidence is emerging that sleep apnea is more prevalent and/or severe in African-Americans relative to Caucasians. Although this may be due to an interaction with environmental factors such as socioeconomic status or comorbid conditions, race-related differences in upper-airway structure or other inherited variables await systematic studies.

HIGHLIGHTS

1. Upper-airway resistance is increased during sleep relative to wakefulness.
2. Sleep is characterized by loss of immediate compensation to added loads.
3. Hypoventilation is a universal finding during sleep, attributed to increased upper-airway resistance, as well as central decrease in ventilatory motor output.
4. Ventilation during NREM sleep is critically dependent on chemical stimuli. Sleep unmasks a highly sensitive hypocapnic apneic threshold; thus, central apnea occurs if Pa_{CO_2} is reduced below the apneic threshold.
5. Gender difference in the prevalence of sleep-related breathing disorders is due to differences in central ventilatory control as well as upper-airway structure. Men are more likely to develop central apnea for a given reduction in Pa_{CO_2}. Similarly, upper airway length and neck circumference are larger in men than women. The latter finding accounts for the difference in pharyngeal compliance during sleep.

REFERENCES

1. Ancoli-Israel S, Kripke D, Klauber MR, et al. Sleep-disordered breathing in community-dwelling elderly. *Sleep.* 1991;14:486–495.
2. Redline S, Kump K, Tishler PV, et al. Gender differences in sleep-disordered breathing in a community-based sample. *Am J Respir Crit Care Med.* 1994;149:722–726.
3. Young T, Palta M, Badr MS. Sleep-disordered breathing (letter). *N Engl J Med.* 1993;329:1429–1430.
4. Young T, Palta M, Dempsey J, et al. The occurrence of sleep-disordered breathing among middle-aged adults. *N Engl J Med.* 1993;328:1230–1235.
5. Skatrud JB, Dempsey JA. Interaction of sleep state and chemical stimuli in sustaining rhythmic ventilation. *J Appl Physiol.* 1983;55:813–822.
6. Berthon-Jones M, Sullivan CE. Ventilation and arousal responses to hypercapnia in normal sleeping humans. *J Appl Physiol.* 1984;57:59–67.
7. Davis JN, Loh L, Nodal J, et al. Effects of sleep on the pattern of CO_2 stimulated breathing in males and females. *Adv Exp Med Biol.* 1978;99:79–83.
8. Douglas NJ, White DP, Weil JV, et al. Hypercapnic ventilatory response in sleeping adults. *Am Rev Respir Dis.* 1982;126:758–762.
9. Gothe B, Altose MD, Goldman MD, et al. Effect of quiet sleep on resting and CO2-stimulated breathing in humans. *J Appl Physiol.* 1981;50:724–730.
10. Hedemark LL, Kronenberg RS. Ventilatory and heart rate responses to hypoxia and hypercapnia during sleep in adults. *J Appl Physiol.* 1982;53:307–312.
11. Browne HA, Adams L, Simonds AK, et al. Aging does not influence the sleep-related decrease in the hypercapnic ventilatory response. *Eur Respir J.* 2003;21:523–529.
12. Morrell MJ, Harty HR, Adams L, et al. Changes in total pulmonary resistance and PCO2 between wakefulness and sleep in normal human subjects. *J Appl Physiol.* 1995;78:1339–1349.
13. Berthon-Jones M, Sullivan CE. Ventilatory and arousal responses to hypoxia in sleeping humans. *Am Rev Respir Dis.* 1982;125:632–639.
14. Douglas NJ, White DP, Weil JV, et al. Hypoxic ventilatory response decreases during sleep in normal men. *Am Rev Respir Dis.* 1982;125:286–289.
15. White DP, Douglas NJ, Pickett CK, et al. Hypoxic ventilatory response during sleep in normal premenopausal women. *Am Rev Respir Dis.* 1982;126:530–533.
16. Sajkov D, Neill A, Saunders NA, et al. Comparison of effects of sustained isocapnic hypoxia on ventilation in men and women. *J Appl Physiol.* 1997;83:599–607.
17. Tarbichi AGS, Rowley JA, Shkoukani MA, et al. Lack of gender difference in ventilatory chemoresponsiveness and post-hypoxic ventilatory decline. *Respir Physiol Neurobiol,* in press: 2003.
18. Xie A, Skatrud JB, Puleo DS, et al. Apnea-hypopnea threshold for CO_2 in patients with congestive heart failure. *Am J Respir Crit Care Med.* 2002;165:1245–1250.
19. Xie A, Rutherford R, Rankin F, et al. Hypocapnia and increased ventilatory responsiveness in patients with idiopathic central sleep apnea. *Am J Respir Crit Care Med.* 1995;152:1950–1955.
20. Xie A, Wong B, Phillipson EA, et al. Interaction of hyperventilation and arousal in the pathogenesis of idiopathic central sleep apnea. *Am J Respir Crit Care Med.* 1994;150:489–495.
21. Bradley TD, McNicholas WT, Rutherford R, et al. Clinical and physiologic heterogeneity of the central sleep apnea syndrome. *Am Rev Respir Dis.* 1986;134:217–221.
22. Pack AI, Cola MF, Goldszmidt A, et al. Correlation between oscillations in ventilation and frequency content of the electroencephalogram. *J Appl Physiol.* 1992;72:985–992.
23. Badr MS, Toiber F, Skatrud JB, et al. Pharyngeal narrowing/occlusion during central sleep apnea. *J Appl Physiol.* 1995;78:1806–1815.
24. Hudgel DW, Chapman KR, Faulks C, et al. Changes in inspiratory muscle electrical activity and upper-airway resistance during periodic breathing induced by hypoxia during sleep. *Am Rev Respir Dis.* 1987;135:899–906.
25. Onal E, Burrows DL, Hart RH, et al. Induction of periodic breathing during sleep causes upper airway obstruction in humans. *J Appl Physiol.* 1986;61:1438–1443.
26. Warner G, Skatrud JB, Dempsey JA. Effect of hypoxia-induced periodic breathing on upper airway obstruction during sleep. *J Appl Physiol.* 1987;62:2201–2211.
27. Badr MS, Kawak A, Skatrud JB, et al. Effect of induced hypocapnic hypopnea on upper airway patency in humans during NREM sleep. *Respir Physiol.* 1997;110:33–45.
28. Zhou XS, Shahabuddin S, Zahn BK, et al. Effect of gender on the development of hypocapnic apnea/hypopnea during NREM sleep. *J Appl Physiol.* 2000;89:192–199.
29. Zhou XS, Rowley JA, Demirovic F, et al. Effect of testosterone on the apneic threshold in women during NREM sleep. *J Appl Physiol.* 2003;94:101–107.
30. Xi L, Smith CA, Saupe KW, et al. Effects of rapid-eye-movement sleep on the apneic threshold in dogs. *J Appl Physiol.* 1993;75:1129–1139.
31. Horner RL. Motor control of the pharyngeal musculature and implications for the pathogenesis of obstructive sleep apnea. *Sleep.* 1996;19:827–853.
32. van Lunteren E, Strohl KP. The muscles of the upper airways. *Clin Chest Med.* 1986;7:171–188.
33. Orem J, Montplaisir J, Dement WC. Changes in the activity of respiratory neurons during sleep. *Brain Res.* 1974;82:309–315.
34. Horner RL, Liu X, Gill H, et al. Effects of sleep–wake state on the genioglossus vs. diaphragm muscle response to CO(2) in rats. *J Appl Physiol.* 2002;92:878–887.

35. Tangel DJ, Mezzanote WS, White DP. Influences of NREM sleep on activity of palatoglossus and levator palatini muscles in normal men. *J Appl Physiol.* 1995;78:689–695.
36. Tangel DJ, Mezzanote WS, White DP. Influence of sleep on tensor palatini EMG and upper airway resistance in normal men. *J Appl Physiol.* 1991;70:2574–2581.
37. Wiegand D, Latz B, Zwillich CW, et al. Upper-airway resistance and geniohyoid muscle activity in normal men during wakefulness and sleep. *J Appl Physiol.* 1990;69:1252–1261.
38. Sauerland EK, Harper RM. The human tongue during sleep: Electromyographic activity of the genioglossus muscle. *Exp Neurol.* 1976;51:160–170.
39. Sauerland EK, Orr WC, Hairston LE. EMG patterns of oropharyngeal muscles during respiration in wakefulness and sleep. *Electromyogr Clin Neurophysiol.* 1981;21:307–316.
40. Wiegand L, Zwillich CW, Wiegand D, et al. Changes in upper-airway muscle activation and ventilation during phasic REM sleep in normal men. *J Appl Physiol.* 1991;71:488–497.
41. Horner RL, Innes JA, Murphy K, et al. Evidence for reflex upper airway dilator muscle activation by sudden negative pressure in man. *J Physiol.* 1991;436:15–29.
42. Wheatley JR, Mezzanote WS, Tangel DJ, et al. Influence of sleep on genioglossus muscle activation by negative pressure in normal men. *Am Rev Respir Dis.* 1993;148:597–605.
43. Wheatley JR, Tangel DJ, Mezzanote WS, et al. Influence of sleep on response to negative airway pressure of tensor palatini muscle and retropalatal airway. *J Appl Physiol.* 1993;75:2117–2124.
44. Shea SA, Edwards JK, White DP. Effect of wake-sleep transitions and rapid eye movement sleep on pharyngeal muscle response to negative pressure in humans. *J Physiol.* 1999;520:897–908.
45. Stanchina ML, Malhotra A, Fogel RB, et al. Genioglossus muscle responsiveness to chemical and mechanical stimuli during non-rapid eye movement sleep. *Am J Respir Crit Care Med.* 2002;165:945–949.
46. Kay A, Trinder J, Bowes G, et al. Changes in airway resistance during sleep onset. *J Appl Physiol.* 1994;76:1600–1607.
47. Kay A, Trinder J, Kim Y. Progressive changes in airway resistance during sleep. *J Appl Physiol.* 1996;81:282–292.
48. Rowley JA, Sanders CS, Zahn BK, et al. The effect of rapid-eye movement (REM) sleep on retroglossal cross-sectional area and compliance in normal subjects. *J Appl Physiol.* 2001;91:239–248.
49. Rowley JA, Zahn BK, Babcock MA, et al. The effect of rapid eye movement (REM) sleep on upper airway mechanics in normal human subjects. *J Physiol.* 1998;510:963–976.
50. Wiegand L, Zwillich CW, White DP. Collapsibility of the human upper airway during normal sleep. *J Appl Physiol.* 1989;66:1800–1808.
51. Hudgel DW, Martin RJ, Johnson B, et al. Mechanics of the respiratory system and breathing pattern during sleep in normal humans. *J Appl Physiol: Respir Environ Exercise Physiol.* 1984;56:133–137.
52. Thurnheer R, Wraith PK, Douglas NJ. Influence of age and gender on upper airway resistance in NREM and REM sleep. *J Appl Physiol.* 2001;90:981–988.
53. Rowley JA, Zhou ZS, Vergine I, et al. The influence of gender on upper airway mechanics: upper airway resistance and Pcrit. *J Appl Physiol.* 2001;91:2248–2254.
54. Trinder J, Kay A, Kleiman J, et al. Gender differences in airway resistance during sleep. *J Appl Physiol.* 1997;83:1986–1997.
55. Browne HAK, Adams L, Simonds AK, et al. Impact of age on breathing and resistive pressure in people with and without sleep apnea. *J Appl Physiol.* 2001;90:1074–1082.
56. Guilleminault C, Stoohs R, Clerk A, et al. A cause of excessive daytime sleepiness. The upper-airway resistance syndrome. *Chest.* 1993;104:781–787.
57. Brown IG, Zamel N, Hoffstein V. Pharyngeal cross-sectional area in normal men and women. *J Appl Physiol.* 1986;61:890–895.
58. Martin SE, Mathur R, Marshall I, et al. The effect of age, sex, obesity and posture on upper-airway size. *Eur Respir J.* 1997;10:2087–2090.
59. Schwab RJ, Gefter WB, Hoffman EA, et al. Dynamic upper airway imaging during awake respiration in normal subjects and patients with sleep disordered breathing. *Am Rev Respir Dis.* 1993;148:1385–1400.
60. Rowley JA, Sanders CS, Zahn BK, et al. Gender differences in upper-airway compliance during NREM sleep: Role of neck circumference. *J Appl Physiol.* 2002;92:2535–2541.
61. Wiegand L, Zwillich CW, White DP. Sleep and the ventilatory response to resistive loading in normal men. *J Appl Physiol.* 1988;64:1186–1195.
62. Pillar G, Malhotra A, Fogel R, et al. Airway mechanics and ventilation in response to resistive loading during sleep: Influence of gender. *Am J Respir Crit Care Med.* 2000;162:1627–1632.
63. Morrell MJ, Badr MS. Effects of NREM sleep on dynamic within-breath changes in upper airway patency in humans. *J Appl Physiol.* 1998;84:190–199.
64. Isono S, Morrison DL, Launois SH, et al. Static mechanics of the velopharynx of patients with obstructive sleep apnea. *J Appl Physiol.* 1993;75:148–154.
65. Isono S, Remmers JE, Tanaka A, et al. Anatomy of pharynx in patients with obstructive sleep apnea and in normal subjects. *J Appl Physiol.* 1997;82:1319–1326.
66. Kuna ST, Bedi DG, Ryckman C. Effect of nasal airway positive pressure on upper airway size and configuration. *Am Rev Respir Dis.* 1988;138:969–975.
67. Isono S, Feroah TR, Hajduk EA, et al. Interaction of cross-sectional area, driving pressure, and airflow of passive velopharynx. *J Appl Physiol.* 1997;83:851–859.
68. Hoffstein V, Zamel N, Phillipson EA. Lung volume dependence of pharyngeal cross-sectional area in patients with obstructive sleep apnea. *Am Rev Respir Dis.* 1984;130:175–178.
69. Mezzanotte WS, Tangel DJ, White DP. Waking genioglossal electromyogram in sleep apnea patients versus normal controls (a neuromuscular compensatory mechanism). *J Clin Invest.* 1992;89:1571–1579.
70. Suratt PM, McTier RF, Wilhoit SC. Upper airway muscle activation is augmented in patients with obstructive sleep apnea compared with that in normal subjects. *Am Rev Respir Dis.* 1988;137:889–894.
71. Gold AR, Schwartz AR. The pharyngeal critical pressure. The whys and hows of using nasal continuous positive airway pressure diagnostically. *Chest.* 1996;110:1077–1088.
72. Schwartz AR, Smith PL, Gold AR, et al. Induction of upper airway occlusion in sleep individuals with subatmospheric nasal pressure. *J Appl Physiol.* 1988;64:535–542.
73. Gleadhill IC, Schwartz AR, Wise RA, et al. Upper-airway collapsibility in snorers and in patients with obstructive sleep hypopnea and apnea. *Am Rev Respir Dis.* 1991;143:1300–1303.
74. Gold AR, Marcus CL, Dipalo F, et al. Upper airway collapsibility during sleep in upper airway resistance syndrome. *Chest.* 2002;121:1531–1540.
75. Penzel T, Moller M, Becker H, et al. Effect of sleep position and sleep stage on the collapsibility of the upper airways in patients with sleep apnea. *Sleep.* 2001;24:90–95.
76. Series F, Roy N, Marc I. Effects of sleep deprivation and sleep fragmentation on upper-airway collapsibility in normal subjects. *Am J Respir Crit Care Med.* 1994;150:481–485.
77. Schwartz AR, O'Donnell CP, Baron J, et al. The hypotonic upper-airway in obstructive sleep apnea. Role of structures and neuromuscular activity. *Am J Respir Crit Care Med.* 1998;157:1051–1057.
78. Rowley JA, Williams BC, Smith PL, et al. Neuromuscular activity and upper airway collapsibility. Mechanisms of action in the decerebrate cat. *Am J Respir Crit Care Med.* 1997;156:515–521.
79. Schwartz AR, Thut DC, Brower RG, et al. Modulation of maximal inspiratory airflow by neuromuscular activity: effect of CO_2. *J Appl Physiol.* 1993;74:1597–1605.
80. Seelagy MM, Schwartz AR, Russ DB, et al. Reflex modulation of airflow dynamics through the upper airway. *J Appl Physiol.* 1994;76:2692–2700.
81. Rowley JA, Permutt S, Willey S, et al. Effect of tracheal and tongue displacement on upper airway airflow dynamics. *J Appl Physiol.* 1996;80:2171–2178.
82. Thut D, Schwartz AR, Roach D, et al. Tracheal and neck position influence upper airway airflow dynamics by altering airway length. *J Appl Physiol.* 1993;75:2084–2090.
83. Remmers JE, deGroot WJ, Sauerland EK, et al. Pathogenesis of upper airway occlusion during sleep. *J Appl Physiol.* 1978;44:931–938.
84. Hudgel DW, Harasick T. Fluctuation in timing of upper airway and chest wall inspiratory muscle activity in obstructive sleep apnea. *J Appl Physiol.* 1990;69:443–450.

85. Strohl KP, Hensley MJ, Hallett M, et al. Activation of upper airway muscles before onset of inspiration in normal humans. *J Appl Physiol.* 1980;49:638–642.

86. Kobayashi I, Perry A, Rhymer J, et al. Inspiratory coactivation of the genioglossus enlarges retroglossal space in laryngectomized humans. *J Appl Physiol.* 1996;80:1595–1604.

87. Schnall RP, Pillar G, Kelson SG, et al. Dilatory effects of upper airway muscle contraction induced by electrical stimulation in awake humans. *J Appl Physiol.* 1995;78:1950–1956.

88. Kuna ST. Effects of pharyngeal muscle activation on airway size and configuration. *Am J Respir Crit Care Med.* 2001;164:1236–1241.

89. Kuna ST, Brennick MJ. Effects of pharyngeal muscle activation on airway pressure–area relationships. *Am J Respir Critical Care Med.* 2002;166:972–977.

90. Brennick MJ, England SJ, Parisi RA. Influence of preload and afterload on genioglossus muscle action in awake goats. *FASEB J.* 1992;6:A1805.

91. Begle RL, Badr S, Skatrud JB, et al. Effect of lung inflation on pulmonary resistance during NREM sleep. *Am Rev Respir Dis.* 1990;141:854–860.

92. Schwartz AR, Thut DC, Russ B, et al. Effect of electrical stimulation of the hypoglossal nerve on airflow mechanics in the isolated upper airway. *Am Rev Respir Dis.* 1993;147:1144–1150.

93. Schwartz AR, Bennett ML, Smith PL, et al. Therapeutic electrical stimulation of the hypoglossal nerve in obstructive sleep apnea. *Arch Otolaryngol Head Neck Surg.* 2001;127:1216–1223.

94. Schwartz AR, Eisele DW, Hari A, et al. Electrical stimulation of the lingual musculature in obstructive sleep apnea. *J Appl Physiol.* 1996;81:643–652.

95. Reed WR, Roberts JL, Thach BT. Factors influencing regional patency and configuration of the human infant upper airway. *J Appl Physiol.* 1885;58:635–644.

96. Wilson SL, Thach BT, Brouillette RT, et al. Upper airway patency in the human infant: influence of airway pressure and posture. *J Appl Physiol.* 1980;48:500–504.

97. Fouke JM, Teeter JP, Strohl KP. Pressure-volume behavior of the upper-airway. *J Appl Physiol.* 1986;61:912–918.

98. Olson LG, Strohl KP. Airway secretions influence upper airway patency in the rabbit. *Am Rev Respir Dis.* 1988;137:1379–1381.

99. Badr MS, Skatrud JB, Dempsey JA, et al. Effect of mechanical loading on expiratory and inspiratory muscle activity during NREM sleep. *J Appl Physiol.* 1990;68:1195–1202.

100. Carroll JL, Loughlin GM. Obstructive sleep apnea syndrome in infants and children: diagnosis and management. In: Ferber R, Kryger M, eds. *Principles and practice of sleep medicine in the child.* Philadelphia: W.B. Saunders, 1995:193–216.

101. Grunstein RR, Ho KK, Sullivan CE. Effect of octreotide, a somatostatin analog, on sleep apnea in patients with acromegaly. *Ann Intern Med.* 1994;121:478–483.

102. Grunstein RR, Ho KY, Sullivan CE. Sleep apnea in acromegaly. *Ann Intern Med.* 1991;115:527–532.

103. Kapur VK, Koepsell TD, deMaine J, et al. Association of hypothyroidism and obstructive sleep apnea. *Am J Respir Crit Care Med.* 1998;158:1379–1383.

104. Skjodt NM, Atkar R, Easton PA. Screening for hypothyroidism in sleep apnea. *Am J Respir Crit Care Med.* 1999;160:732–735.

105. Coltman R, Taylor R, Whyte K, et al. Craniofacial form and obstructive sleep apnea in Polynesian and Caucasian men. *Sleep.* 2000;23:943–950.

106. deBerry-Borowiecki B, Kukwa A, Blanks RH. Cephalometric analysis for diagnosis and treatment of obstructive sleep apnea. *Laryngoscope.* 1988;98:226–234.

107. Lowe AA, Ozbek MM, Miyamoto K, et al. Cephalometric and demographic characteristics of obstructive sleep apnea: An evaluation with partial least squares analysis. *Angle Orthod.* 1997;67:143–153.

108. Redline S, Tishler PV, Hans MG, et al. Racial differences in sleep-disordered breathing in African-Americans and Caucasians. *Am J Respir Crit Care Med.* 1997;155:186–192.

109. Sakakibara H, Tong M, Matsushita K, et al. Cephalometric abnormalities in non-obese and obese patients with obstructive sleep apnoea. *Eur Respir J.* 1999;13:403–410.

110. Safar P. Failure of manual respiration. *J Appl Physiol.* 1959;14:84–88.

111. Safar PL, Escarraga S, Chang F. Upper airway obstruction in the unconscious patient. *J Appl Physiol.* 1959;14:760–764.

112. Shelton RL, Bosma JF. Maintenance of the pharyngeal airway. *J Appl Physiol.* 1962;17:209–214.

113. Whittle AT, Marshall I, Mortimore IL, et al. Neck soft tissue and fat distribution: Comparison between normal men and women by magnetic resonance imaging. *Thorax.* 1999;54:323–328.

114. Shelton KE, Woodson H, Gay S, et al. Pharyngeal fat in obstructive sleep apnea. *Am Rev Respir Dis.* 1993;148:462–466.

115. Schwab RJ, Gupta KP, Gefter WB, et al. Upper airway and soft tissue anatomy in normal subjects and patients with sleep-disordered breathing. Significance of the lateral pharyngeal walls. *Am J Respir Crit Care Med.* 1993;152:1673–1689.

116. Van de Graaf WB. Thoracic influence on upper airway patency. *J Appl Physiol.* 1988;65:2124–2133.

117. Roberts JL, Reed WR, Thach BT. Pharyngeal airway-stabilizing function of sternohyoid and sternothyroid muscles in the rabbit. *J Appl Physiol.* 1984;57:1790–1795.

118. Van de Graaff WB. Thoracic traction on the trachea: Mechanisms and magnitude. *J Appl Physiol.* 1991;70:1328–1336.

119. Brown IG, Bradley TD, Philllipson EA, et al. Pharyngeal compliance in snoring subjects with and without obstructive sleep apnea. *Am Rev Respir Dis.* 1985;132:211–215.

120. Olson LG, Fouke JM, Hoekje PL, et al. A biomechanical view of upper airway function. In: Mathew OP, Sant'Ambrogio G, eds. *Respiratory function of the upper airway.* New York: Marcel Dekker, 1988:359–389.

120a. Mayor AH, Schwartz AR, Rowley JA, et al. Effect of blood pressure changes in airflow dynamics in the upper airway of the decerebrate cat. *Anesthesiology.* 1996;84:128–134.

121. Wasicko MJ, Hutt DA, Parisi RA, et al. The role of vascular tone in the control of upper airway collapsibility. *Am Rev Respir Dis.* 1990;141:1569–1577.

122. Wasicko MJ, Leiter JC, Erlichman JS, et al. Nasal and pharyngeal resistance after topical mucosal vasoconstriction in normal humans. *Am Rev Respir Dis.* 1991;144:1048–1052.

123. Shepard JW, Jr., Pevernagie DA, Stanson AW, et al. Effects of changes in central venous pressure on upper airway size in patients with obstructive sleep apnea. *Am J Respir Crit Care Med.* 1996;153:250–254.

124. van der TT, Crawford AB, Wheatley JR. Effects of a synthetic lung surfactant on pharyngeal patency in awake human subjects. *J Appl Physiol.* 1997;82:78–85.

125. Morrell MJ, Arabi Y, Zahn BR, et al. Effect of surfactant on pharyngeal mechanics in sleeping humans: implications for sleep apnoea. *Eur Respir J.* 2002;20:451–457.

126. Jokic R, Klimaszewski A, Mink J, et al. Surface tension forces in sleep apnea: The role of a soft tissue lubricant; A randomized double-blind, placebo-controlled trial. *Am J Respir Crit Care Med.* 1998;157:1522–1525.

127. Bradley TD, Brown IG, Grossman RF, et al. Pharyngeal size in snorers, nonsnorers and patients with obstructive sleep apnea. *N Engl J Med.* 1986;315:1237–1331.

128. Haponik EF, Smith PL, Bohlman ME, et al. Computerized tomography in obstructive sleep apnea. Correlation of airway size with physiology during sleep and wakefulness. *Am Rev Respir Dis.* 1983;127:221–226.

129. Carroll JL, Loughlin GM. Obstructive sleep apnea syndrome in infants and children: clinical features and pathophysiology. In: Ferber R, Kryger M, eds. *Principles and practice of sleep medicine in the child.* Philadelphia: W.B. Saunders, 1995:163–191.

130. Kushida CA, Efron B, Guilleminault C. A predictive morphometric model for the obstructive sleep apnea syndrome. *Ann Intern Med.* 1997;127:581–587.

131. Schellenberg JB, Maislin G, Schwab RJ. Physical findings and the risk for obstructive sleep apnea. *Am J Respir Crit Care Med.* 2000;162:740–748.

132. Guilleminault C, Stoohs R, Kim YD, et al. Upper airway sleep-disordered breathing in women. *Ann Intern Med.* 1995;122:493–501.

133. Brander PE, Mortimore IL, Douglas NJ. Effect of obesity and erect/supine posture on lateral cephalometry: relationship to sleep-disordered breathing. *Eur Respir J.* 1999;13:398–402.

134. Dempsey JA, Skatrud JB, Jacques AJ, et al. Anatomic determinants of sleep-disordered breathing across the spectrum of clinical and nonclinical male subjects. *Chest.* 2002;122:840–851.

135. Ferguson KA, Ono T, Lowe AA, et al. The relationship between obesity and craniofacial structure in obstructive sleep apnea. *Chest.* 1995;108:375–381.

136. Hierl T, Humpfner-Hierl H, Frerich B, et al. Obstructive sleep apnoea syndrome: Results and conclusions of a principal component analysis. *J Craniomaxillofac Surg.* 1997;25:181–185.

137. Partinen M, Guilleminault C, Quera-Salva MA, et al. Obstructive sleep apnea and cephalometric roentgenograms. The role of anatomic upper airway abnormalities in the definition of abnormal breathing during sleep. *Chest.* 1988;93:1199–1205.

138. Tangugsorn V, Skatvedt O, Krogstad O, et al. Obstructive sleep apnoea: A cephalometric study. Part I. Cervico-craniofacial skeletal morphology. *Eur J Orthod.* 1995;17:45–56.

139. Tsuchiya M, Lowe AA, Pae EK, et al. Obstructive sleep apnea subtypes by cluster analysis. *Am J Orthod Dentofacial Orthop.* 1992;101:533–542.

140. Sforza E, Bacon W, Weiss T, et al. Upper airway collapsibility and cephalometric variables in patients with obstructive sleep apnea. *Am J Respir Crit Care Med.* 2000;161:347–352.

141. McNamara JA. A method of cephalometric evaluation. *Am J Orthod.* 1984;86:449–469.

142. Saksena SS. *A clinical atlas of roentgenographic measurements in norma frontalis.* New York: Alan R. Liss, 1990.

143. Malhotra A, Huang Y, Fogel RB, et al. The male predisposition to pharyngeal collapse: Importance of airway length. *Am J Respir Crit Care Med.* 2002;166:1388–1395.

144. Cakirer B, Hans MG, Graham G, et al. The relationship between craniofacial morphology and obstructive sleep apnea in whites and in African-Americans. *Am J Respir Crit Care Med.* 2001;163:947–950.

145. Fogel RB, Malhotra A, Dalagiorgou G, et al. Anatomic and physiologic predictors of apnea severity in morbidly obese subjects. *Sleep.* 2003;26:150–155.

146. Onal E, Lopata M. Periodic breathing and the pathogenesis of occlusive sleep apneas. *Am Rev Respir Dis.* 1982;126:676–680.

Sleep and Normal Human Physiology

James Geyer and Stephenie Dillard

INTRODUCTION

Although the function of sleep remains unknown, much is known about its physiologic consequences. Very few, if any, bodily systems are untouched by the drastic changes in consciousness and brain behavior. Some changes are mild and of limited clinical consequence and are secondary to changes in other systems. Others are quite dramatic and of great clinical significance. This chapter reviews the latter group and will serve as the background for understanding physiologic changes accompanying various disorders discussed in the other chapters. It provides a basic review of sleep-related physiology in the autonomic nervous system, respiratory system, cardiovascular system, immune system, gastrointestinal system, renal system, genital/reproductive system, and temperature regulation. Wherever possible, the differences between sleep-related physiologic changes and circadian effects are noted.

AUTONOMIC NERVOUS SYSTEM

Anatomy

Many of the physiologic changes occurring during sleep are related, at least in part, to alteration of autonomic nervous system activity. Basic laboratory evaluation of some of the changes in autonomic function has been challenging because, not only do the sympathetic and parasympathetic effects change from one organ system to the next, but there is great variability in those effects among various animal species. When comparing animal models, some species vary only in the degree of effect, whereas others show totally opposite responses to the same stimulus, making extrapolation to humans difficult, if not impossible.

The central autonomic nervous system is located in the brainstem, with the nucleus tractus solitarius (located in the dorsal aspect of the medulla just ventral to the dorsal vagal nucleus) serving as a central node in the system (1). The general visceral afferents arise from the gastrointestinal, cardiovascular, and respiratory systems. Multiple central autonomic efferent pathways arising from the nucleus tractus solitarius lead to the lateral hypothalamus, paraventricular hypothalamic nucleus, stria terminalis in the forebrain, central nucleus of the amygdala, midbrain central gray matter, dorsal pontine lateral parabrachial nucleus, and ventral medulla (1).

Multiple nuclei, including the ventral medullary nuclei, paraventricular hypothalamic nucleus, and pontine raphe nuclei, provide input into the interomediolateral nucleus, the sympathetic preganglionic center located in the spinal cord. The parasympathetic preganglionic neurons are located primarily in the nucleus ambiguus and the dorsal motor nucleus of the vagus. The vagus nerve is a major component of the primary common pathway for the autonomic nervous system (1).

NORMAL AUTONOMIC CHANGES IN SLEEP

Significant sleep-related changes in autonomic function affect the cardiovascular system, respiration, thermal control, musculoskeletal activity, pupillary reflex, and genital function. In general, at sleep onset there is an increase in parasympathetic tone and a concomitant decrease in sympathetic tone, which continues during non-REM (NREM) sleep (2). With the transition to tonic REM sleep, the parasympathetic activity continues to increase and the sympathetic activity is further suppressed. During phasic REM sleep, there is an increase in the sympathetic activity, which occurs in bursts (2).

The increase of parasympathetic tone in NREM sleep and tonic REM sleep results in pupillary constriction. The autonomic changes initiated with phasic REM sleep (central parasympathetic inhibition and increased sympathetic tone) result in phasic pupillary dilatation.

Musculoskeletal System

Somatic Skeletal Muscle

The somatic skeletal muscles typically have their highest muscle tone during wakefulness. The tone then decreases with sleep onset and during NREM sleep, but should achieve its lowest level during REM sleep. Anyone who has watched a family pet dream is aware of the transient bursts of myogenic activity that occur during phasic REM sleep. Failure to decrease muscular activity

during this phase of sleep results in REM sleep behavior disorder.

Projections from the nucleus reticularis pontis oralis located in the dorsal pontine tegmentum synapse in the medullary reticular formation and then project to the spinal cord. Firing of these neurons during REM sleep results in the release of the neurotransmitter glycine in the spinal cord, which generates inhibitory postsynaptic potentials (IPSPs). The IPSPs, in turn, decrease the firing of the motor neurons, thus generating relative atonia (3).

Cranial motor neurons also appear to be affected by IPSPs originating from the dorsal pontine tegmentum. These pathways are less well understood, but may be mediated by the inhibitory neurotransmitter GABA$_B$ (3).

Upper-Airway Muscles

The genioglossus muscles serve to pull the tongue down and forward. During inspiration, the activity in this muscle occurs as phasic bursts superimposed on tonic discharges. These discharges diminish during NREM sleep and are further suppressed during REM sleep, resulting in a partial atonia, which can allow the tongue to fall back toward the retropharyngeal space (4). This alteration of upper-airway anatomy is partially responsible for obstructive sleep apnea (OSA). Genioglossal activity is enhanced by tricyclic antidepressants, such as protriptyline and nortriptyline and is suppressed by alcohol, benzodiazepines, and some anesthetic agents, lending support to the theory that inhibition of this muscle is GABA-mediated.

The masseter muscles close and elevate the mandible. Phasic activity in the masseters starts at approximately the same time as the genioglossus activity.

The palatoglossus and levator palatini have phasic activity on inspiration and tonic activity during expiration. The tensor veli palatini has tonic activity during both inspiration and expiration. The palatoglossus, levator palatini, and tensor veli palatini have decreased tone during sleep, which reaches its minimal level during REM sleep (5).

The hyoid musculature contributes to the size and shape of the upper airway. The interactions of the various hyoid muscles are quite complex and beyond the scope of this discussion. Bursts of activity are present in the hyoid musculature during inspiration during both wakefulness and NREM sleep.

The posterior cricoarytenoid muscle is the primary vocal cord abductor. It has phasic burst activity during inspiration in both wakefulness and NREM sleep. With the onset of REM sleep, the expiratory burst activity becomes fragmented and less sustained (6).

Diaphragmatic Activity

The diaphragm serves as the primary bellows for respiratory function and air movement. As one would expect, the rhythmic firing of the diaphragm occurs in both wakefulness and during all phases of sleep, but the percentage of motor units firing is decreased during REM sleep (7). There may also be some variability of the decrease in diaphragmatic activity during a single breath. In addition, brief pauses in diaphragmatic activity may occur during normal phasic REM sleep.

Thermal Regulation

Body temperature typically falls by several degrees Celsius during nocturnal sleep. The body retains its thermoregulatory capability during NREM sleep, but the thermoregulatory response is attenuated during REM sleep (8). At sleep onset, the metabolic rate falls to a greater degree than can be explained by decreased motor activity and digestive function alone.

The normal 1° to 2°C drop in body temperature during nocturnal sleep is accomplished by two separate mechanisms. Approximately one-half of the decrease is related to circadian temperature variation, which is independent of sleep (9). This is superimposed on a sleep-related reduction in the body's thermal setpoint, which occurs because of a combination of increased heat dissipation and decreased heat generation (10). This effect typically peaks during the third sleep cycle, resulting in the minimum body temperature for the night (10).

The reduction in body temperature associated with NREM sleep appears to be related to a change in the thermal sensitivity of the preoptic nucleus of the hypothalamus, which contributes to both slow-wave sleep and thermoregulation. During REM sleep, there is a loss of this thermoregulatory response and body temperature tends to increase with cyclic variability. These changes are not related to motor atonia, but are determined by an alteration of central thermal regulation or, potentially, an alteration in the afferent neural input to the thermoregulatory center.

Total sleep time, slow wave, and REM sleep are maximized at thermoneutrality (approximately 29°C) (11). The wake time, sleep latency, and movement time all increase in a cold environment, and there is a decrease in total sleep time, REM sleep, and stage 2 sleep (11). Likewise, in a warm environment, wake time is increased with reductions in both REM and NREM sleep. Fragmentation of sleep occurs at higher environmental temperatures, and elevated environmental temperature causes more sleep fragmentation than does environmental noise.

An increase in waking body and brain temperature is associated with an increase in slow wave sleep (12). A warm bath, aerobic exercise, heating pads, etc., can increase the percentage of slow-wave sleep occurring approximately 4 hours after exposure. There is also evidence that fever will decrease slow-wave sleep and REM sleep, while increasing wake time and light sleep. These changes appear to be secondary to the elevated brain temperature itself and

are at least partially independent of the humoral byproducts of infection, such as cytokines (13).

Renal Function

Renal perfusion and glomerular filtration rate decrease during NREM sleep, resulting in decreased urine production, largely due to sleep-related cardiovascular function. Furthermore, water reabsorption increases during NREM sleep. Urine production decreases even further during REM sleep. There is a decrease in secretion of aldosterone during sleep, primarily due to the supine position. Only a small portion of the decrease in aldosterone secretion can be attributed to changes unique to the sleep state.

Genital Function

There are few changes in genital function during NREM sleep. In men, REM sleep is associated with penile tumescence (erection) (14). The erection typically begins at the beginning of REM sleep and continues throughout the REM sleep period. In most instances, the erection is lost at the end of the REM sleep period but, in some cases, may continue into wakefulness. Similar changes occur in the erectile tissue of women during REM sleep. Sleep-related erections occur as a result of increased blood flow to the erectile tissue, which is caused by increased parasympathetic activity resulting in local vasodilatation, decreased venous outflow, and increased bulbocavernosus muscular activity. The detumescence is a result of the increased sympathetic activity at the end of REM sleep. In addition to these autonomic changes, it is also likely that the central nervous system (CNS) may also provide input into these sleep-related erections.

Sleep-related erections are not typically affected by pre-sleep sexual activity, fantasies, or reported dream content.

Gastrointestinal Function

The effects of sleep on the gastrointestinal system are driven by a combination of increased parasympathetic activity, circadian rhythm factors, CNS activity, and the subserosal neural plexus activity. The study of the gastrointestinal system is inherently difficult and becomes even more so during sleep because of the potential for sleep disruption caused by monitoring devices; therefore, controversy remains regarding a number of aspects of digestion during sleep.

Salivation

Salivation decreases during sleep, in large part because of increased parasympathetic activity. Saliva is an important component of gastric acid neutralization, and the decrease in salivary flow can contribute to an increase in nocturnal gastroesophageal reflux. Swallowing decreases the duration of acid contact with the esophageal mucosa. The prolonged contact during sleep increases the risk of esophagitis secondary to acid reflux.

Esophageal Motility

The frequency of swallowing is markedly decreased during sleep (15). When swallowing does occur, the ensuing esophageal peristalsis appears to be normal and unchanged when compared with swallowing occurring during wakefulness (16). In a more recent study, the frequency of primary peristaltic contractions declines from wakefulness to stage 4 sleep (17).

Most episodes of nocturnal reflux appear to correspond to decreases in lower esophageal sphincter pressure (18). The relative negative pressure of the midesophagus then draws the regurgitated stomach contents even further into the esophagus.

The upper esophageal sphincter, the cricopharyngeal muscle, is a skeletal muscle which is tonically contracted to prevent aspiration. There is a minimal decrease in the upper esophageal sphincter pressure during sleep. Although the cricopharyngeal muscle is a skeletal muscle, there is minimal change in pressure throughout REM sleep.

Gastric Function

Gastric acid secretion follows a circadian rhythm, with the peak basal acid secretion occurring between 10 PM and 2 AM (19). Patients with duodenal ulcer disease have the same pattern when compared to normal controls, except that their total acid secretion is increased. This circadian pattern is mediated by the vagus nerve. There appears to be a significant night-to-night and subject-to-subject variability in acid secretion. The data regarding impact of sleep stage on acid secretion is contradictory, with one study revealing no significant change in acid secretion or serum gastrin levels across sleep stages (20).

The gastric smooth muscle generates an endogenous electrical cycle, which drives gastric motor function and occurs at a frequency of approximately three cycles per minute. There is some evidence that the power of this rhythm decreases during non-REM sleep, with some recovery toward baseline during REM sleep.

Intestinal Function

Intestinal absorption is directly related to the transit time. The motor activity, beginning in the stomach, appears to propagate along the intestinal tract. Some studies have shown variability in the frequency of migrating motor complexes during sleep (21,22). There is a circadian rhythm-associated decrease in migrating motor complex velocity during sleep. Studies have, however, shown conflicting results.

Colonic Function

There is a decrease in the colonic myoelectric activity and contractile activity, which, in turn, results in decreased colonic motility. On awakening in the morning, the colonic motility increases significantly. Sudden nocturnal awakening seems to result in segmental colonic contractions without propagation (23).

Anorectal Function

Rectal motor activity increases during sleep with *retrograde* contractions. Despite the presence of cyclic rectal contractions, the anal pressure remains above the rectal pressure. Both of these factors inhibit defecation during sleep.

Endocrine Function

Most hormones follow a predictable fluctuating pattern through a 24-hour cycle. Circadian rhythms, ultradian rhythms, and stage of sleep may all affect hormone secretion.

Growth Hormone

Plasma growth hormone concentration typically peaks approximately 90 minutes after sleep onset, usually during stages 3 and 4 sleep. However, there are several exceptions to this secretory pattern (24). Secretion of growth hormone is not related to sleep prior to 3 months of age, and growth hormone concentration peaks prior to sleep onset in 25% of young males (25). Senior adults have a less significant relationship between sleep and growth hormone concentration (26). Although sleep causes the greatest fluctuations in growth hormone levels, there is also some evidence of ultradian and circadian effects, albeit to a lesser extent. Patients with OSA or narcolepsy have a decreased correlation between sleep and growth hormone concentration (27). In acromegaly, growth hormone concentration is high and unrelated to delta sleep (28).

Adrenocorticotropic Hormone (ACTH)

ACTH and cortisol secretion follow a circadian pattern with superimposed sleep-related inhibition, which is maximal during delta sleep. Cortisol secretion peaks between 4 and 8 AM (29). Daytime naps do not perturb cortisol secretion (30). The circadian pattern of cortisol secretion is unchanged in Cushing's disease.

Prolactin

Prolactin concentration begins increasing approximately 1 hour after sleep onset and is maximal between 5 and 7 AM, but is unrelated to sleep stage (31). Prolactin concentration reaches its nadir during wakefulness. There is also a circadian component, which is independent of sleep (32). Prolactin secretion is unaffected by advancing age (33).

Gonadotropic Hormones

Hypothalamic gonadotropin-releasing hormone stimulates secretion of luteinizing hormone (LH) and follicle-stimulating hormone (FSH). During puberty, in both girls and boys, LH and FSH concentrations increase during sleep (34). A relationship to sleep has not been identified in other age groups.

Thyroid-Stimulating Hormone

Thyroid-stimulating hormone (TSH) follows a circadian pattern with low daytime levels, increasing evening levels, and peak levels at night, prior to sleep, with subsequent sleep-related inhibition (35). Bright light exposure shifts the TSH circadian pattern depending on the timing of the light exposure.

Melatonin

Melatonin is produced by the pineal gland and released into the blood and cerebrospinal fluid (CSF). Its production is regulated by the suprachiasmatic nucleus (SCN) and is inhibited by increased illumination (36). It is highest in young children and lowest in senior adults (37,38).

Cardiovascular Function

Relative autonomic stability, driven by vagal nerve function, predominates during NREM sleep. Heart rate variation during NREM sleep follows a sinusoidal pattern. A normal respiratory sinus arrhythmia is produced by the normal respiratory activity coupled with cardiorespiratory center activity. During normal inspiration, the heart rate has a brief acceleration in order to accommodate venous return and increased cardiac output (39). During expiration, there is a progressive decrease in heart rate. This normal cardiac rhythm variability is a marker for cardiac health and its absence is associated with increasing age, loss of normal vagus nerve function, and possible cardiac pathology. Small reductions in arterial blood pressure can also serve to increase the respiratory rate.

During REM sleep, the heart rate becomes increasingly variable with episodes of tachycardia and bradycardia (Fig. 5-1) (40). Respiratory patterns are also irregular and may result in oxygen desaturation (Fig. 5-2) (40). The neurons controlling the principal diaphragmatic respiratory muscles typically are not inhibited during REM sleep, but accessory airway muscles may have partial atonia. There may be a transient 35% increase in heart rate especially during phasic REM sleep. A second REM sleep-related increase in heart rate may be secondary to CNS activation. In animal models, this has been correlated to pontogeniculo-occipital activity (PGO spikes) and eye movements (41).

Beta blockers, such as atenolol, tend to reduce this phenomenon, suggesting that REM sleep-induced surges are primarily mediated by cardiac sympathetic efferent activity. Cardiac rate decelerations during REM sleep precede eye movement bursts by several seconds and may be mediated by cardiac vagus nerve efferent fiber burst activity (42).

Sleep-Related Arrhythmia

Cardiac arrhythmias have been related to several CNS structures. Stimulation of the posterior hypothalamus results in a dramatic increase in the incidence of ventricular fibrillation (43). Discontinuation of diencephalic and hypothalamic stimulation is arrhythmogenic. Some of the protective effects of beta blockade may be secondary to central beta adrenergic receptor blockade. The beta blockers, most effective for protection against cardiac arrhythmias, are also typically lipophilic and, therefore, cross the blood–brain barrier (44).

The increased vagal nerve activity during NREM sleep contributes to cardiac electrical stability, reduced rate pressure product and cardiac metabolic activity, and decreases the risk of cardiac arrhythmia. The decreased blood pressure during NREM sleep, however, can contribute to myocardial hypoperfusion.

The surges in autonomic activity and increased heart rate during REM sleep increase the risk for ventricular arrhythmias. The heightened sympathetic activity during REM sleep results in a decreased oxygen supply to oxygen demand ratio, coronary vasoconstriction, and alteration of both preload and afterload. A pharmacologic decrease in cardiac sympathetic tone (by stellate ganglion blockade) has antifibrillatory effects. The relationship between sleep state, cardiac ischemia, and myocardial infarction is incompletely understood at this time.

Circulation

Control of circulation during sleep is complicated by several factors including the metabolic requirements of a particular organ as well as the effect of the sleep state upon that organ.

Cerebral Blood Flow

During REM sleep, there is an increase in the blood flow to the entorhinal cortex, anterior cingulate gyrus, amygdala, thalamus, dorsal mesencephalic nuclei, and pontine tegmentum (45). The blood flow to these structures decreases during NREM sleep, and there is also a decrease in cerebral blood flow during postsleep wakefulness when compared with presleep wakefulness, which is most prominent in the limbic structures.

Spinal cord blood flow increases during REM sleep. Data concerning metabolic effect versus sleep state effect is inconclusive at present.

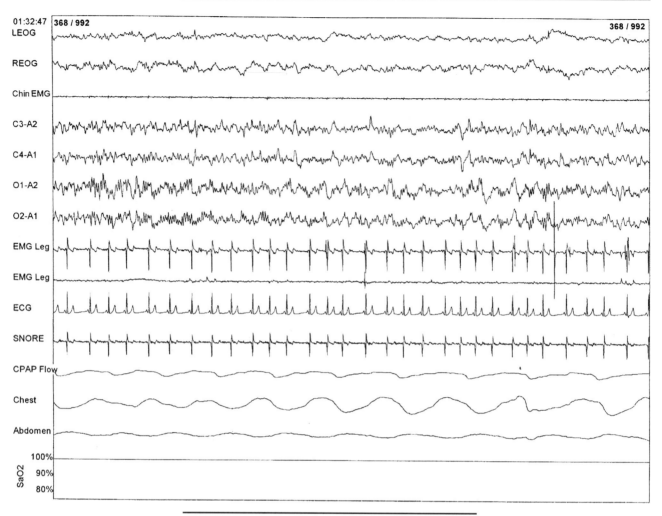

FIGURE 5-1. Cardiac rhythm variability during REM sleep.

There is an increase in oxygenated hemoglobin delivery accompanying the transition from NREM sleep to REM sleep. Cerebral metabolic rate for glucose and for oxygen both increase during REM sleep.

Mild hypercapnia develops during NREM sleep and appears to counteract the circulatory effect of the decreased cerebral metabolic rate during NREM sleep. $Paco_2$ is an important determinant of cerebral blood flow during sleep in OSA and other related disorders.

Flow-metabolism coupling controls cerebral blood flow changes during sleep (46). Both cerebral autoregulation and chemical regulation may play roles in the adjustment of cerebral blood flow under pathophysiologic conditions.

Renal Circulation

Renal blood flow is not sleep-state dependent. However, during REM sleep, the blood flow does increase because of thermoregulatory effects.

Splanchnic Circulation

No significant change in splanchnic blood flow occurs during sleep.

Cutaneous Circulation

As previously discussed, the thermoregulatory setpoint decreases in the transition from wakefulness to NREM sleep. This results in cutaneous vasodilation. In REM sleep, the cutaneous blood flow changes because of thermoregulatory inhibition. The percentage change in blood flow depends upon the neural control of the various cutaneous structures.

Muscular Circulation

There is no significant change in muscle blood flow during the transition from wakefulness to NREM sleep. During REM sleep there is a decrease in flow to red muscle fibers. The blood flow change to white fibers varies by species (47,48).

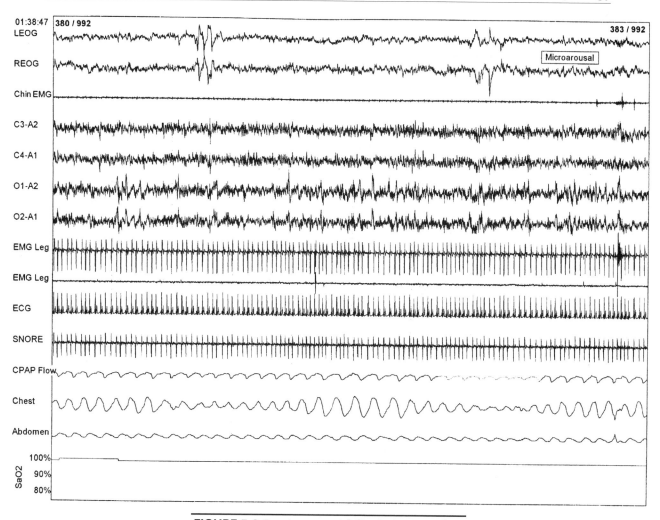

FIGURE 5-2. Respiratory variability during REM sleep.

Coronary Circulation

Changes in coronary artery blood flow are not directly related to heart rate or arterial blood pressure. Episodic increases in coronary blood flow with associated decreases in coronary vascular resistance appear to occur primarily during phasic REM sleep. The heart rate also tends to be elevated during the increases in coronary flow, possibly secondary to increased cardiac metabolism and coronary vasodilatation. With coronary artery stenosis, there are phasic decreases in blood flow during REM sleep despite increases in cardiac rate, which is secondary to a decrease in diastolic coronary perfusion time caused by the increased heart rate (49).

Power Spectral Analysis

Heart rate power spectral recordings confirms both decreased sympathetic activity during NREM sleep and increased parasympathetic activity when compared to wakefulness (50). During REM sleep, both of these components appear to move toward levels recorded during wakefulness. The shifts in heart rate power spectral analysis occur prior to the change in EEG activity, except at sleep onset when there is no preceding change prior to the alteration in EEG activity.

RESPIRATORY PHYSIOLOGY

During normal respiration, the discharge frequency of the dorsal respiratory group (ventrolateral nucleus of the tractus solitarius) increases during inspiration (51). This is governed by the pulmonary stretch receptors, which project to the dorsal respiratory group via the vagal nerve.

The ventral respiratory group consists of the nucleus ambiguus, nucleus retroambiguus, and Botzinger complex. Neurons mediating inspiration fall into several different categories: early onset and augmenting, early onset and decrementing, late inspiratory, early expiratory and decrementing. The early onset and augmenting function is mediated by either propriobulbar cells, bulbospinal cells, or vagal motoneurons. Early onset and decrementing neurons are propriobulbar with efferent activity into the contralateral ventral respiratory group. Late inspiratory neurons are propriobulbar in the dorsal respiratory group and ventral respiratory group. The early expiratory and decrementing neurons are also propriobulbar.

The ventral medullary surface has three chemosensitive zones. Experimental blockade of the ventral medullary surface suppresses respiratory response to changing pH (52). Medullary respiratory activity decreases during NREM sleep.

The pontine respiratory group (pneumotaxic center of Lumsden) contributes to inspiration, expiration, and phase-spanning activity. Although the pontine respiratory group is not obligatory for the generation of respiration, it is important for respiratory modulation and vagal afferent input.

Experimental midbrain reticular stimulation reduces the duration of expiration and increases phrenic nerve activity (53). Respiratory activation declines following stimulation of the midbrain. The respiratory after-discharge is an enhancement of respiratory activity following an excitatory stimulus.

The activity of serotonin- and norepinephrine-containing neurons in the brainstem is maximal during active wakefulness, decreases during NREM sleep, and is at its lowest during REM sleep (54). Serotonin and norepinephrine inhibit central respiratory neurons.

Chemoreceptors

Carbon dioxide levels are sensed both in the carotid body and central chemoreceptors located in the medulla. The response to rising $PaCO_2$ levels results in an increased respiratory rate. This produces a feedback mechanism to maintain the $PaCO_2$.

The carotid body senses the PaO_2, with output to the medulla. The ventilatory response to a decrease in PaO_2 is slow and occurs typically after PaO_2 falls below 60 mm Hg. Once the PaO_2 has fallen below 30 mm Hg the medullary activity is depressed, which may paradoxically contribute to further decreased ventilation.

Mechanical Receptors

Receptors in the bronchial tree and chest wall also send impulses to the medulla via the vagus nerve, which transmits information regarding stretch, irritation, deflation, etc.

Respiratory Rate

Respiratory rate decreases during the transition from wakefulness to NREM sleep, but increases during REM sleep, occasionally exceeding the waking level (55). The airflow during REM sleep is, however, lower than during either wakefulness or NREM sleep.

Ventilatory Response during Sleep

Ventilatory responses to chemical stimuli and respiratory reflexes are inhibited during REM sleep, especially phasic REM sleep. The irregular respiratory pattern during REM sleep does not depend on chemoreceptor or vagal nerve activity, but appears to be secondary to brainstem respiratory neuron activity (56).

Hypoxic ventilatory response falls during the transition from wakefulness to NREM sleep; there is a further drop during REM sleep in both men and women. The hypercapnic ventilatory response falls by approximately 50% during the transition from wakefulness to NREM sleep (57). It also falls further during REM sleep.

Supplemental Resistance and Respiration

NREM sleep blunts the respiratory response to added airflow resistance. This effect does not seem to be as prominent in patients with asthma (58). The effect during REM sleep is less well understood.

Respiratory Arousal Response

Isocapnic hypoxia is a poor stimulus for arousal. The arousal threshold in normal controls is not significantly different in NREM versus REM sleep. The arousal response appears to be further suppressed in the presence of OSA during REM sleep in animal models.

Hypercapnia typically results in an arousal once end-tidal CO_2 rises 15 mm Hg above the waking level (59). Hypoxia seems to increase the sensitivity to CO_2 increases.

Increased upper-airway resistance or airway occlusion tends to result in awakening. The arousal frequency was lowest during NREM delta sleep in normal controls, but patients with OSA tend to have longer apneas in REM sleep.

NON-RAPID EYE MOVEMENT SLEEP

NREM sleep is characterized by regularity of both respiratory frequency and amplitude. Minute ventilation decreases by 0.4 to 1.5 liters per minute during NREM sleep, with decreases occurring progressively from stage 1 to 4 (60). The thoracic and abdominal muscular contributions to breathing increase during NREM sleep.

Compared to the wakeful state, upper-airway resistance approximately doubles during NREM sleep. Palatal and hypopharyngeal components contribute to this increased resistance and result in decreased ventilation during NREM sleep.

Alveolar ventilation is decreased during NREM sleep. This results in an increase in alveolar and arterial PCO_2 of 3 to 7 mm Hg with a concomitant decrease in alveolar and arterial PO_2 during NREM sleep (61).

Sighs are deep breaths with increased tidal volumes, which serve to open alveoli and result in increased pulmonary compliance. Sighs appear to be most common during stage 1 and 2 NREM sleep.

RAPID EYE MOVEMENT SLEEP

Unlike NREM sleep, REM sleep is characterized by irregularity of both respiratory amplitude and frequency (Fig. 5-2). Central apneas and periodic breathing are also more common during REM sleep (Fig. 5-3). These irregularities occur predominantly during phasic REM sleep. The onset of phasic REM sleep is typically associated with a decrease in the amplitude of respiration (Fig. 5-4).

The contribution of the thoracic and abdominal muscles is decreased during REM sleep. The diaphragmatic activity is increased.

Upper-airway resistance during REM sleep is variable. Phasic REM sleep typically results in increasing upper-airway resistance, whereas the effects of tonic REM sleep have not been completely characterized.

Hypoventilation occurring during REM sleep may result in hypoxemia.

Sighs occur during REM sleep, but are less common than during NREM sleep or wakefulness. They may also be associated with arousals and subsequent central apneas.

Functional residual capacity decreases during REM sleep. This may contribute, in part, to hypoxia during REM sleep. Airflow resistance increases during sleep, with the peak resistance occurring during NREM sleep.

PREGNANCY

Pregnancy results in reduced functional residual capacity and residual volume, especially when in the supine position. This increases the risk of more profound hypoxemia during sleep, especially in the presence of OSA.

ALTITUDE

Periodic breathing is more prevalent at high altitude because of relative hypoxemia and hypocapnia. The lower

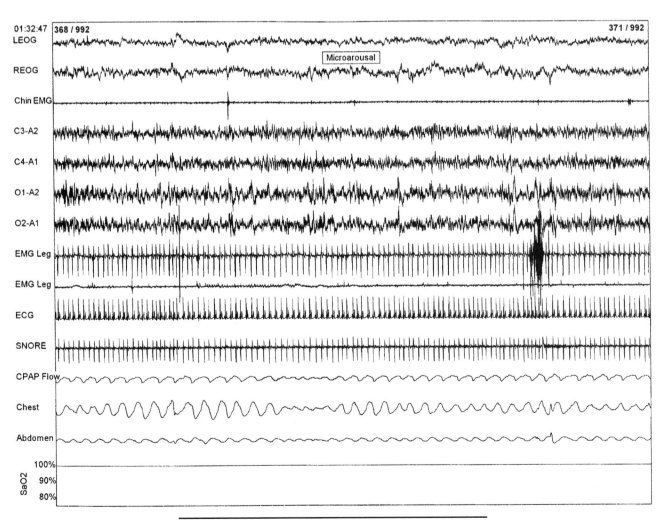

FIGURE 5-3. Periodic breathing and apnea during REM sleep.

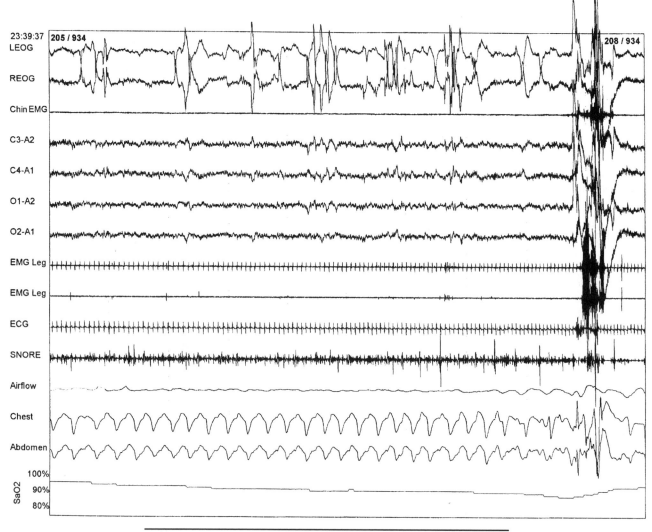

FIGURE 5-4. Decreased respiratory effort amplitude in phasic REM sleep.

oxygen levels result in relative hyperventilation, which, in turn, results in a hypocapnic alkalosis. This may cause central apnea and subsequent hypoxemia (62).

Furthermore, poor sleep quality is more common at higher altitudes related, at least in part, to periodic breathing and frequent arousals. Prophylactic treatment with a carbonic anhydrase inhibitor can reduce the alkalotic respiratory inhibition and subsequently decrease the amount and severity of periodic breathing (63). Low-dose benzodiazepine treatment can improve sleep quality by decreasing arousals without significant worsening of respiratory function.

REFERENCES

1. Chokroverty S. *Functional anatomy of the autonomic nervous system: Autonomic dysfunction and disorders of the CNS. American Academy of Neurology Course No. 144.* Boston: American Academy of Neurology, 1991;77.

2. Parmeggiani PL, Morrison AR. Alterations of autonomic functions during sleep. In: Lowey AD, Spyer KM, eds. *Central regulation of autonomic functions.* New York: Oxford University Press, 1990: 367.

3. Soja PJ, Morales FR, Chase MH. Postsynaptic control of lumbar motoneurons during the atonia of active sleep. In: Issa FG, Suratt PM, Remmers JE, eds. *Sleep and respiration.* New York: Wiley, 1990: 9.

4. Bartlett D, Jr, Leiter JC, Knuth SL. Control and actions of the genioglossus muscle. In: Issa FG, Suratt PM, Remmers JE, eds. *Sleep and respiration.* New York: Wiley, 1990:99.

5. Tangle DJ, Mezzanotte WS, Sandberg EJ, et al. Influences of sleep on tensor palatini EMG and upper airway resistance in normal men. *J Appl Physiol.* 1991;70:2574.

6. Kuna SI, Insalaco G. Respiratory-related intrinsic laryngeal muscle activity in normal adults. In: Issa FG, Suratt PM, Remmers JE, eds. *Sleep and respiration.* New York: Wiley, 1990:117.

7. Orem J. Neuronal mechanisms of respiration in REM sleep. *Sleep.* 1980;3:251.

8. Takagi K. Sweating during sleep. In: Hardy JG, Gagge AP, Stolwijk JAJ, eds. *Physiological and behavioral temperature regulation.* Springfield, IL: Thomas, 1970:669–675.

9. Aschoff J. Circadian control of body temperature. *J Therm Biol.* 1983;8:143.

10. Aschoff J. Circadian rhythm of activity and body temperature.

In: Hardy JD, Gagge AP, Stolwijk JAJ, eds. *Physiological and behavioral temperature regulation.* Springfield, IL: Thomas, 1970: 905.

11. Berger JR, Phillips NH. Comparative physiology of sleep, thermoregulation and metabolism from the perspective of energy metabolism. In: Issa FG , Suratt PM, Remmers JE, eds. *Sleep and respiration.* New York: Wiley, 1990:41.

12. Shapiro CM, Allan M, Driver H, et al. Thermal load alters sleep. *Biol Psych.* 1989;26:736–740.

13. Horne JA, Percival JE, Traynor JR. Aspirin and human sleep. *Electroencephalogr Clin Neurophysiol.* 1980;49:409–413.

14. Karacan I, Goodenough DR, Shapiro A, et al. Erection cycle during sleep in relation to dream anxiety. *Arch Gen Psych.* 1966;15:183–189.

15. Lichter J, Muir RC. The pattern of swallowing during sleep. *Electroencephalogr Clin Neurophysiol.* 1975;38:427–432.

16. Orr WC, Johnson LF, Robinson MG. The effect of sleep on swallowing, esophageal peristalsis, and acid clearance. *Gastroenterology.* 1984;86:814–819.

17. Castiglione F, Emde C, Armstrong D, et al. Nocturnal esophageal motor activity is dependent on sleep stage. *Gut.* 1993;34:1653–1659.

18. Dent J, Dodds WJ, Friedman RH, et al. Mechanism of gastroesophageal reflux in recumbent asymptomatic human subjects. *J Clin Invest.* 1980;65:256–257.

19. Moore JG, Englert E. Circadian rhythm of gastric acid secretion in man. *Nature (London).* 1970;226:1261–1262.

20. Orr WC, Hall WH, Stahl ML, et al. Sleep patterns and gastric acid secretion in duodenal ulcer disease. *Arch Intern Med.* 1976;136:655–660.

21. Thompson DG, Wingate DL. Characterisation of interdigestive and digestive motor activity in the normal human jejunum. *Gut.* 1979;20:A943.

22. Finch P, Ingram D, Henstridge J, et al. The relationship of sleep stage to the migrating gastrointestinal complex in man. In: Chistensen J, ed. *Gastrointestinal motility.* New York: Raven Press; 1980:261–265.

23. Bassotti G, Bucaneve G, Betti C, et al. Sudden awakening from sleep: Effects on proximal and distal colonic contractile activity in humans. *Eur J Gastroenterol Hepatol.* 1990;2:6.

24. Honda Y, Takahashi K, Takahashi J, et al. Growth hormone secretion during nocturnal sleep in normal subjects. *J Clin Endocrinol Metab.* 1969;29:20.

25. Gronfier C, Luthringer R, Follenius M. A quantitative evaluation of the relationship between growth hormone secretion and delta wave electroencephalographic activity during normal in sleep and after enrichment in delta waves. *Sleep.* 1996;19: 817.

26. Van Kauter E, Turek FW. Endocrine and other biological rhythms. In: DeGroot LJ, Besser M, Burger SG, et al., eds. *Endocrinology.* 3rd edn. Philadelphia: WB Saunders, 1995:2487.

27. Clark RW, Schmidt HS, Malarkey WB. Disordered growth hormone and prolactin secretion in primary disorders of sleep. *Neurology.* 1979;29:855.

28. Carlson HE, Gillin JC, Gorden P, et al. Absence of sleep related growth hormone peaks in aged normal subjects and in acromegaly. *J Clin Endocrinol Metab.* 1972;34:1102.

29. Weitzman ED, Fukushima D, Nogeri C, et al. Twenty-four hour pattern of the episodic secretion of cortisol in normal subjects. *J Clin Endocrinol Metab.* 1971;33:14.

30. Weibal L, Follienus M, Spiegel K, et al. Comparative effect of night and daytime sleep on the twenty-four hour cortisol secretory profile. *Sleep.* 1995;18:549.

31. Sassin J, Frantz A, Weitzman E, et al. Human prolactin: 24 hour patterns with increased release during sleep. *Science.* 1972;17: 1205.

32. Partsch CJ, Lerchl A, Sippel WG. Characteristics of pulsatile and circadian prolactin release and its variability in man. *Exp Clin Endocrinol Diabetes.* 1995;103:33.

33. Parker DC, Rossman LG, Kripke TF, et al. Endocrine rhythms across sleep–wake cycles in normal young men under basal state conditions. In: Orem J, Barnes CD, eds. *Physiology in sleep.* New York: Academic, 1980:145.

34. Fevre M, Segel T, Marks JF, et al. LH and Melatonin secre-

tion patterns in pubertal boys. *J Clin Endocrinol Metab.* 1978;47: 1383.

35. Lucke C, Hehermann R, von Mayersbach K, et al. Studies in circadian variations of plasma TSH, thyroxine and triiodothyronine in man. *Acta Endocrinol.* 1976;86:81.

36. Penev PD, Zee PC. Melatonin: A clinical perspective. *Ann Neurol.* 1997;42:545.

37. Kennaway DJ, Goble FC, Stamp GE. Factors influencing the development of melatonin rhythmicity in humans. *J Clin Endocrinol Metab.* 1996;81:1525.

38. Waldhauser F, Frisch H, Waldhauser M, et al. Fall in nocturnal serum melatonin during prepuberty and pubescence. *Lancet.* 1994: 362.

39. Task Force of the European Society of Cardiology and the North American Society of Pacing and Electrophysiology. Heart rate variability: Standards of measurement, physiological interpretation and clinical use. *Circulation.* 1996;93:1043–1065.

40. Dickerson LW, Huang AH, Nearing BD, et al. Primary coronary vasodilation associated with pauses in heart rhythm during sleep. *Amer J Physiol.* 1993;264:R186–196.

41. Rowe K, Moreno R, Lau RT, et al. Heart rate surges during REM sleep are associated with theta rhythm and PGO activity in the cat. *Amer J Physiol.* 1999;277:R843–849.

42. Taylor WB, Moldofsky H, Furedy JJ. Heart rate deceleration in REM sleep: An orienting reaction interpretation. *Psychophysiology.* 1985;22:110–115.

43. Verrier RL, Calvert A, Lown B. Effect of posterior hypothalamic stimulation on the ventricular fibrillation threshold. *Amer J Physiol.* 1975;228:923–927.

44. Hjalmarson A, Olsson G. Myocardial infarction. Effects of beta-blockade. *Circulation.* 1991;84(suppl 6):VI 101–107.

45. Maquet P, Peters J-M, Aerts J, et al. Functional neuroanatomy of human rapid-eye-movement sleep and dreaming. *Nature (London).* 1996;383:163–166.

46. Lenzi P, Zoccoli G, Walker AM, et al. Cerebral blood flow regulation in REM sleep: A model for flow-metabolism coupling. *Arch Ital Biol.* 1999;137:165–179.

47. Reis DJ, Moorhead D, Wooten GF. Differential regulation of blood flow to red and white muscle in sleep and defense behavior. *Amer J Physiol.* 1969;217:541–546.

48. Zoccoli G, Lalatta costerbosa G, Bach V, et al. Muscle blood flow during the sleep–wake cycle in the rat. *J Sleep Res.* 1994;2(suppl. 1):283.

49. Kirby DA, Verrier RL. Differential effects of sleep stage on coronary artery hemodynamic function during stenosis. *Physiol Behav.* 1989;45:1017–1020.

50. Bonnet MH, Arand DL. Heart rate variability: Sleep stage, time of night, arousal influences. *Electroencephalogr Clin Neurophysiol.* 1997;102:390–396.

51. de Castro D, Lipski J, Kanjhan R. Electrophysiological study of dorsal respiratory neurons in the medulla oblongata of the rat. *Brain Res.* 1994;639:49–56.

52. Cherniack NS, von Euler C, Homma I, et al. Graded changes in central chemoreceptor input by local temperature changes on the ventral surface of medulla. *J Physiol (London).* 1979;287:191–211.

53. Cohen MI, Hugelin A. Suprapontine reticular control of intrinsic respiratory mechanisms. *Arch Ital Biol.* 1965;103:317–334.

54. Trulson ME, Trulson VM. Activity of nucleus raphe pallidus neurons across the sleep-waking cycle in freely moving cats. *Brain Res.* 1982;237:232–237.

55. Orem J. Medullary respiratory neuron activity: Relationship to tonic and phasic REM sleep. *J Appl Physiol Respir Environ Exercise Physiol.* 1980;48:54–65.

56. Orem J, Montplaisir J, Dement W. Changes in the activity of respiratory neurons during sleep. *Brain Res.* 1974;82:309–315.

57. Bulow K. Respiration and wakefulness in man. *Acta Physiol Scand.* 1963;59(suppl. 209):1–110.

58. Ballard RD, Tan WC, Kelly PL, et al. Effect of sleep and sleep deprivation on ventilatory response to bronchoconstriction. *J Appl Physiol.* 1990;69:490–497.

59. Birchfield RI, Sieker HO, Heyman A. Alterations in respiratory function during natural sleep. *J Lab Clin Med*. 1959;54:216–222.

60. Krieger J, Mangin P, Kurtz D. Incidence of sleep disordered breathing in normal younger and older subjects. Correspondence analysis of related factors. *Sleep 1982: 6th Eur Congr Sleep Res*. Basel, Switzerland: Karger; 1983:308–311.

61. Ostergaard T. The excitability of the respiratory centre during sleep and during Evipan anaesthesia. *Acta Physiol Scand*. 1944;8:1–15.

62. White DP, Gleeson K, Pickett CK, et al. Altitude acclimatization: influence on periodic breathing and chemoresponsiveness during sleep. *J Appl Physiol*. 1987;63:401–412.

63. Cain SM, Dunn JD. Low doses of acetazolamide to aid accommodation of men to altitude. *J Appl Physiol*. 1966;21:1195–1200.

Chapter 6

Chronobiology and Circadian Rhythms

Arthur Andrews and Selim Benbadis

INTRODUCTION

The rotation of the Earth on its axis over a 24-hour period produces the well-known changes in the physical environment experienced by its inhabitants. The resultant light–dark cycle and the demands it imposes has produced evolutionary change in all forms of life since the beginning of time. The past several decades of investigation have demonstrated that the 24-hour nature of life is not simply a result of these external cues, but, indeed, due to an internal time-keeping system in the brain (1).

Sleep across species occurs within rigidly defined times of day and night. The 24-hour or circadian biochemical, physiologic, and behavioral rhythms are regulated by a biological clock. The regularly occurring variation in these parameters has analogs in all eukaryotic species, including single-celled algae (2). The suprachiasmatic nucleus (SCN) located in the hypothalamus has been thought to be the source of this rhythmicity (3) (Fig. 6-1). Sleep is regulated by the dual interaction of circadian and homeostatic processes. The individual's state of wakefulness or sleep at any moment in time is dependent upon the interaction between sleep debt and the circadian clock (4). Many diverse species share common genetic and molecular elements in regard to circadian systems.

Indeed, the awareness of sleep disorders as a major health concern has increased dramatically over the last decade. The number of sleep disorder centers in the United States has doubled since 1996 (4). Sleep disorders and the treatment of these disorders have significant socioeconomic consequences.

CIRCADIAN RHYTHMS VERSUS SLEEP–WAKE RHYTHMS

Circadian Rhythms

Reproducible changes of essentially all physiologic and behavioral variables occur over a 24-hour period (5). Circadian rhythms are the manifestation of an endogenous oscillatory signal with a near 24-hour period that occurs in synchrony with the 24-hour periodicities in the physical

(A)

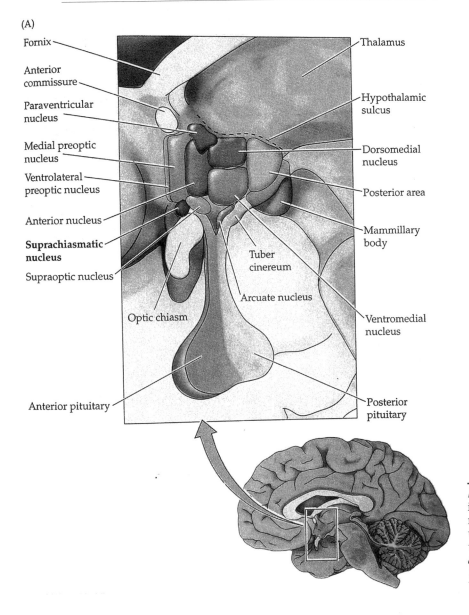

Fornix

Anterior commissure

Paraventricular nucleus

Medial preoptic nucleus

Ventrolateral preoptic nucleus

Anterior nucleus

Suprachiasmatic nucleus

Supraoptic nucleus

Anterior pituitary

Optic chiasm

Tuber cinereum

Arcuate nucleus

Thalamus

Hypothalamic sulcus

Dorsomedial nucleus

Posterior area

Mammillary body

Ventromedial nucleus

Posterior pituitary

FIGURE 6-1. The hypothalamus, showing the location of the suprachiasmatic nucleus (SCN). The name derives from the location of the nucleus just above the optic chiasm. (From Purves, D. *Sleep and wakefulness in neuroscience*, 2nd edn. Sunderland, Sinauer Associates, 2001. With permission.)

environment. The aforementioned endogenous oscillator is termed the *circadian clock*. The internal milieu of the organism is also organized so that internal changes crucial to health are coordinated. The internal clock must adjust its period each cycle to compensate for differences between its intrinsic periods and the 24-hour period of the environmental day and be synchronized in order for rhythms to occur at appropriate phases (3). This process is known as *entrainment*. Adaptation and survival mandate that the circadian clock be synchronized and entrained by environmental cues.

Sleep–Wake Rhythms

Many rhythms are dependent on the sleep–wake state of the organism and not primarily the circadian timekeeper. An animal placed in an environment where all possible 24-hour external cues are eliminated will continue to demonstrate diurnal rhythms. The period is approximately 24 hours and is called circadian (1). The sleep–wake cycle is one such rhythm. The human sleep–wake cycle is not simply driven by the circadian pacemaker, but instead is generated through interactions of circadian rhythmicity, a sleep–wake oscillatory process, circadian photoreception, as well as feedback from the sleep–wake cycle onto these processes (6). As one can infer, the interplay of influence from the sleep–wake system and the circadian system manifests as the expression of physiologic, behavioral, and biochemical processes of the organism. Both waking performance and sleep consolidation are contributed to equally by these two systems (6). The sleep–wake oscillator acts as a homeostat and regulates the level of sleep debt. As the normal day progresses, the SCN generates an arousal signal that increases in strength. This signal begins to decline by 10 PM, with nadir at 6 AM. It is the presence of this arousal signal that produces the monophasic sleep–wake cycle and maintains its timing. Sustained wakefulness leads to increased sleep need. This requirement for

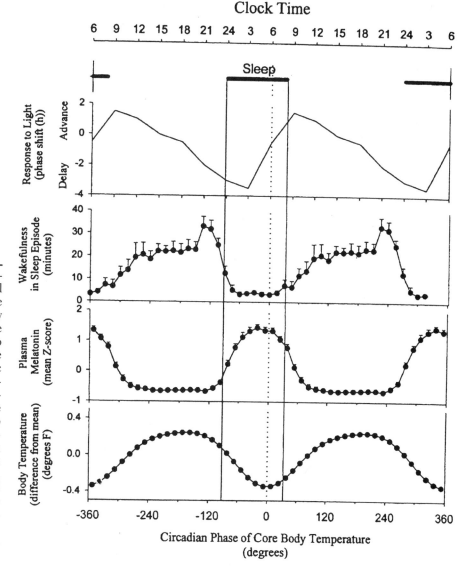

FIGURE 6-2. Schematic representation of the timing of the habitual sleep episode in young adults relative to the circadian rhythm of core body temperature, plasma melatonin, wake propensity, and the responsiveness to light. The circadian variation in the responsiveness to light is a schematic representation. Note that the maximum of the melatonin rhythm is located ~2 h before the nadir of the circadian temperature rhythm. Sleep disruption (wakefulness within scheduled sleep episodes) is maximal when sleep is scheduled just before the rise of melatonin. (From Dijk, D., Lockley, S. Functional genomics of sleep and circadian rhythm; Invited review: Integration of human sleep–wake regulation and circadian rhythmicity. *J Appl Physiol.* 2002;92:852–862. With permission.)

sleep is opposed by the circadian pacemaker. Rapid eye movement (REM) sleep is primarily under the control of circadian rhythmicity and is normally at its peak near the end of the sleep period. Slow-wave sleep timing primarily reflects sleep–wake homeostasis (7). Interestingly, there is also evidence that the SCN also promotes sleep. The SCN clock is also responsible for the endogenous regulation of moment-to-moment waking behavior as measured by fatigue, alertness, and cognitive performance (3).

Certain drug therapies that combin chronobiotic/hypnotic effects have been shown to shorten the time to adaptation of both circadian rhythmicity and sleep–wake homeostasis to a shift in dark/sleep cycle. Buxton and colleagues used the benzodiazepine triazolam to successfully facilitate adaptation to an 8-hour delay shift of sleep–wake and dark–light cycles simulating westward travel (7).

The circadian rhythms of alertness and performance efficiency run in parallel to body temperature. Alertness is the ability to maintain attention. The ability to successfully complete tasks as varied as working memory, com-

plex executive functions, and logical reasoning is termed performance (3). The controlled laboratory setting is helpful in eliminating the differences that can be obtained in peak performance as a result of level of task. The nadir of alertness and performance typically occurs early in the morning at 4 to 6 AM at the time of the low point in core body temperature (8). An individual's subjective report of an insufficient amount of energy to complete a task is considered fatigue (Fig. 6-2).

ANATOMY AND PHYSIOLOGY OF THE HUMAN (MAMMALIAN) CIRCADIAN SYSTEM

Nearly 30 years ago, the paired SCN of the anterior hypothalamus was found to be the pacemaker for mammalian circadian rhythms. Animal lesion studies were the primary means to this discovery. The metabolic activity of the SCN has been shown to peak during the subjective day for both nocturnal and diurnal animals (3). Individual SCN neurons have intrinsic 24-hour oscillatory properties in culture. *In vivo* these neurons generate a coordinated circadian signal to the remainder of the brain and the peripheral organs (1). DeCoursey and co-workers (9) demonstrated that transplantation of SCN-containing fetal neural tissue into arrhythmic hamsters restored circadian locomotor activity.

SCN neurons are very densely packed. Animal anatomic studies suggest that there is a dorsomedial and ventrolateral subdivision (10). Neurochemicals in the ventral SCN respond to photic stimuli, whereas neurochemicals synthesized in the dorsal SCN demonstrate endogenous rhythms, but do not respond to changes in light (3).

An environmental synchronizing source is required to entrain the SCN circadian clock to the 24-hour day. Indeed, the light–dark cycle serves this purpose in the majority of mammals. Pulses of light effect increases or decreases in the firing rates of specialized neurons in the SCN (11).

The retinohypothalamic tract is a direct projection from the retinal ganglion cells to the SCN. Photic input from the retinohypothalamic tract (RHT) is mediated by an excitatory amino acid, such as glutamate. Neuropeptide Y, monoamines, gamma-aminobutyrate (GABA), and acetylcholine also appear to mediate important projections to the clock; pharmacologic manipulation of those systems can impact circadian phase and amplitude (2). Additional areas of the brain also provide input to the SCN. These include the thalamus, brainstem, and certain forebrain areas.

Nonphotic entrainment on the SCN is thought to be accomplished via serotonin and geniculate–hypothalamic tract (GHT) pathways. Neuropeptide Y is the neurotransmitter of the GHT. Serotonergic (5HT) projections from the brainstem raphe nuclei project directly and indirectly. These projections are now considered to be important in the circadian effects of nonphotic stimuli. Nonphotic stimuli can induce increased arousal and therefore changes in behavior that can influence the phase and period of circadian rhythms in certain animals (11).

Studies in the rat have found several pathways from the SCN to arousal and sleep centers. Adrenergic (locus coeruleus), serotonergic (dorsal raphe), histaminergic (tuberomammillary nucleus), and orexin systems receive projections from the SCN (Fig. 6-3). Using immunohistochemical techniques and retrograde transport of fluorescent dyes, Watts et al. described four major efferent projections from the SCN (12). These projections include: (a) fibers to the optic tracts terminating in the ventral lateral geniculate nucleus; (b) a group of fibers to the anteroventral periventricular nucleus, medial preoptic area, lateral septum, bed nucleus of the stria terminalis, parataenial nucleus, and parts of the paraventricular nucleus of the thalamus; (c) ventral to the paraventricular nucleus of the hypothalamus; and (d) anterior hypothalamic area,

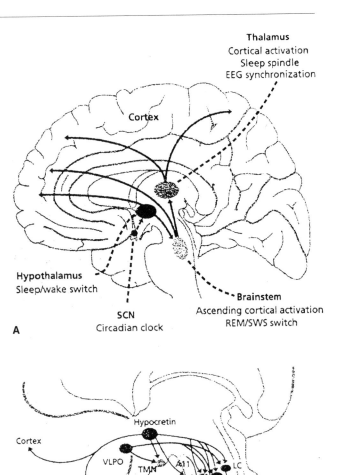

FIGURE 6-3. The suprachiasmic nucleus (SCN) projects to the major brain centers controlling alertness and sleep. These include areas in the hypothalamus, brain stem, and thalamus. For simplicity, projections of the SCN to the hypothalamus are the only ones shown. (From Mignot E, Taheri S, Nishino S. Sleeping with the hypothalamus: Emerging theraputic targets for sleep disorders. *Nature Neurosci.* 2002;5:1072–1075. With permission.)

retrochiasmatic area, lateral hypothalamus, and ventromedial hypothalamus (3).

MOLECULAR GENETICS OF CIRCADIAN RHYTHMS

The major source of the generation of the circadian rhythm is within the neurons of the SCN. A feedback cycle involving the various transcribed gene products is the driving force of the oscillatory machinery. The organism is, therefore, able to prepare itself for the regular environmental changes.

Period (*Per*), the first gene that encodes a clock component, was found in the fruit fly *Drosophila* in 1971 (3). Transgenic flies having a heat-inducible copy of *Per* demonstrate long-lasting phase shifts in locomotor activity circadian rhythm when subjected to temperature pulses (13). In addition, the lack of a *Per* gene or a missense mutation of *Per* has been shown to cause lack of locomotor activity and shortening/lengthening of the free-running period of the locomotor rhythm, respectively. Timeless (*Tim*) is an additional oscillatory component in *Drosophila*.

Tim may be important in regulating the entry of *Per* into the nucleus. In *Drosophila* lacking *Tim*, the loss of behavioral circadian rhythms is associated with loss of daily fluctuations of *Per* mRNA (14). The *Tim:Per* complex suppresses the transcription of *Tim* and *Per*.

The molecular components of the circadian *Clock* gene in *Drosophila* and the filamentous fungi *Neurospora* were identified in the 1980s (1). In 1997, the first mammalian circadian clock gene *Clock* was identified and sequenced. Mice with homozygous mutations in the *Clock* gene demonstrate progressive lengthening of circadian rhythms and eventually become arrhythmic in constant darkness (15).

The heterodimeric transcription factor *Clock-Bmal1* causes the transcription of three *Per* genes, *Tim* genes, and two cryptochrome genes (Cry), whose products act in the negative limb of this feedback loop to inactivate the *Clock:Bmal1* heterodimer (16).

Darlington and co-workers showed that in *Drosophila*, a *Clock:Bmal1* complex drives the expression of *Per* and *Tim* by binding to a site on their promoters (17). The formed heterodimers of *Per* and *Tim* inhibit *Clock:Bmal1* in a negative feedback fashion. Accumulating *Per: Tim* heterodimer and its movement to the nucleus allows the inhibition of *Per* and *Tim* transcription induced by *Clock:Bmal1* (3). A new cycle of manufacture begins as levels of *Per* and *Tim* mRNA fall.

Additional circadian clock genes have been identified in *Drosophila*, including cycle (*cyc*), double-time (*dbt*), and vrille (*vri*). *Bmal1* is the mammalian ortholog to *cyc* and *CKIe* is the ortholog to *dbt* (18; see illustration.)

The mammalian retina is an additional location of circadian oscillator as it can be entrained, free runs under constant conditions, and is temperature-compensated (19). External cues or *zeitgebers* can act to entrain this nearly 24-hour rhythmic oscillation and cause advancement or delay.

ENVIRONMENTAL CUES/INFLUENCES (ZEITGEBERS)

Zeitgebers are defined as rhythmic changes in the external environment and are essential for the entrainment of circadian rhythms. Entrainment takes place due to the required daily corrective phase shifts. Circadian rhythms can be entrained to zeitgeber periods that are longer or shorter than 24 hours (8). Light–dark cycle, social contact/social interaction, knowledge of time of day, timing of meals, ambient temperature, sleep–wake schedules, and electromagnetic fields are included in this category. In the absence of zeitgebers, desynchronization occurs, whereby circadian rhythms become "free running," with an intrinsic period of approximately 24 hours. Of note, some older studies suggested that the period was 25 hours, but new studies estimate that the period is around 24.2 hours (20). The sleep–wake cycle is the means by which social cues entrain circadian rhythms. The mechanism by which the sleep–wake cycle entrains certain circadian rhythms has not been fully established, but likely involves its control over light input to the retina and a more direct effect on the individual's endogenous oscillator. Social cues and the individual's desire to remain awake can overcome the circadian-driven sleep propensity. The administration of bright light has also been shown to accelerate re-entrainment of human circadian rhythm. This phenomenon was demonstrated by Honma and co-workers. Subjects spent 15 days without knowledge of the natural day–night alternation. The social schedule was phase advanced on day four and each subjective morning was either accompanied or not by bright light at 4,000 to 6,000 lux. The subjects treated with light demonstrated a significantly more rapid shift (21). Duffy et al. (22) inverted the schedule of rest, sedentary activity, and social contact of 32 subjects with or without exposure to bright light. Based on core temperature measurements, it was found that those exposed to bright light showed a significant phase shift with adaptation to the new schedule as compared with those who did not receive light.

Light

Bright light is emphasized as the most important zeitgeber. It is believed that sunlight can produce intensities greater than 100,000 lux as opposed to indoor light, which is typically 500 lux or less (23). A single light pulse given to an organism under constant conditions without time cues immediately resets the clock by an amount dependent upon the time of day at which it is given (24). The circadian pacemaker functions as a clock because its endogenous period is adjusted to the external 24-hour period via light–induced phase shifts that reset the pacemaker's oscillation (10). As stated earlier, light information reaches the SCN via the retinohypothalamic tract (a monosynaptic pathway from retinal ganglion cells to the SCN) and via a second pathway termed the geniculate–hypothalamic tract (11). Information is then transmitted to the pineal gland to regulate melatonin secretion. Indeed, bright light exposure may, at times, be inadequate in an uncontrolled environment and, therefore, social cues acting via the sleep–wake cycle can be very important.

Feeding

Feedings given at the same time each day will set in motion certain routine responses in the organism, such as changes in activity level and body temperature (3).

Temperature

Temperature has been shown to entrain circadian rhythms in some species and has been proved less effective in others. The effect is not thought to be a direct impact on the circadian apparatus, but is possibly an indirect effect through ambient temperature's impact on the organism's state of arousal, light exposure, and activity level.

The actual body temperature is determined by heat production and heat loss. Heat loss occurs through the skin, the largest human organ. Sleep onset latency correlates best with the amount of heat dissipation preceding sleep and is characterized by rediffusion of heat from the core to the periphery of the body (25).

Activity

Activity level has been shown to induce phase shifts in animals. The majority of this work has been done in hamsters in the frequently used wheel-running experiments.

THE HUMAN CIRCADIAN RHYTHM

Influence of Sleep and Circadian Rhythms on Physiology

Physiological rhythms occur at the appropriate phase of the light–dark cycle. This allows for the availability of metabolic energy, neurotransmitter synthesis, enzyme activity, and hormone production at critical times of the day (26). The multiple physiologic and behavioral rhythms are known to have consistent peaks and troughs in the day or night. Examples include activity level, core temperature, cognitive function, urine production, catecholamine excretion peaks in the day, and melatonin synthesis and sleep in the nighttime.

Effect of Light

Light exerts a differential effect on the circadian pacemaker over a range of lux. Animal studies have demonstrated that the photoreceptive system involved in mediating vision is not involved in this response. Phase shifts of the endogenous circadian rhythms, such as plasma or saliva melatonin, core body temperature, cortisol, and propensity to sleep can be induced by broad-spectrum light exposure even when the sleep–wake cycle is kept constant (27,28). Badia and co-workers (29) evaluated the effects of bright light compared to dim light. Each were administered in blocks of time or continuously in the nighttime

and/or daytime under sustained wakefulness. Bright light conditions were found to increase temperature under alternating conditions and to reduce the decline in temperature under continuous conditions. Sleepiness was reduced and alertness and nighttime performance were improved when compared with dim light. Campbell and Dawson studied the enhancement of nighttime alertness and performance with bright ambient light (1,000 lux) compared with dim light (</ = 100 lux) in a simulated night-shift experiment. Cognitive performance and overall alertness were significantly higher in those subjects exposed to bright ambient light (30). It is recognized that night workers experience a misalignment between the sleep–wake cycle and the output of the hypothalamic pacemaker that regulates the circadian rhythms of certain physiologic and behavioral variables. Exposure of these workers to bright light on the order of 7,000 to 12,000 lux at night and to near complete darkness during the day leads to circadian adaptation to daytime sleep and nighttime work within days (31).

Artificial light administration has been useful in the treatment of various sleep disorders including hypersomnia in association with seasonal affective disorder, advanced sleep-phase syndrome (ASPS), delayed sleep-phase syndrome (DSPS), non–24-hour sleep-phase syndrome, jet lag, and shift work. Factors such as duration, intensity, and timing of light exposure are crucially important.

Light Therapy for Specific Disorders

Delayed Sleep-Phase Syndrome

DSPS patients experience difficulty in initiating sleep prior to 1–3 AM. Sleep is maintained for a normal time period. These individuals begin their social interactions and work behaviors later in the morning and are much more active at nighttime. Shifts in core body temperature minimum and peak melatonin rhythm are shifted to later in the morning.

In DSPS, light exposure is typically scheduled immediately upon awakening (32). The patient is awakened most commonly between 6 to 9 AM in order to administer therapy. Intensity at 2,000 to 2,500 lux is suggested. In addition, patients may be asked to wear dark goggles from 4 PM to dusk.

Advanced Sleep-Phase Syndrome

Early initiation of sleep and rising early in the morning often times before 3 AM, characterize ASPS. Core body temperature minimum and peak melatonin rhythm occur earlier in the morning.

In ASPS therapy can be administered with 2,500 lux for 4 hours between 8 PM and 12 AM or 4,000 lux for 3 hours between 8 PM and 11 PM in attempts to delay sleep onset (27).

Non–24-Hour Sleep-Phase Syndrome

Non–24-hour sleep-phase syndrome is characterized by progressive phase delays of sleep onset and awakening relative to the 24-hour day (32). These patients may have hypersomnia or insomnia depending on which phase of the circadian cycle they are in when sleeping. Core body temperature cycles may be greater in length than normal. Several investigators have studied the effects of bright light in efforts to achieve phase advances or entrainment in sighted individuals but data is insufficient. In some cases, the blind may benefit from light therapy—3,300 lux for 1 hour between 6 and 8 AM.

Jet Lag

Jet lag occurs when an individual engages in transmeridian travel across multiple time zones. As the earth rotates on its axis every 24 hours, the globe is divided into 24 1-hour time zones, each with 15 meridians (26). Therefore, individuals experience a change in the light–dark cycle as well as the activity/rest rhythm in order to adjust to the new time zone. Subsequent effects include difficulty initiating or maintaining sleep, daytime sleepiness, decrements in daytime alertness and performance, gastrointestinal distress, and other psychosomatic manifestations (27). There is conflicting data regarding the benefits of light therapy in this situation, but it is thought to be safe and potentially helpful. One approach would be to administer light in the 2,000 to 5,000 lux range for 3 hours in the morning for 3 days at destination after travel east.

Shift Work

Shift work refers to working early morning, night, or on a rotating basis. The individual may experience myriad symptoms, including a decline in ability to do job–related tasks, somnolence, tiredness, and gastrointestinal disturbance. Bright light therapy has been shown to affect a shift of circadian rhythm in experimentally controlled exposure to light and darkness. In the field, one approach may be the use of 5,000 to 10,000 lux for 3 to 6 hours prior to the core body temperature minimum, combined with the use of No. 5 lens goggles upon return home to prevent natural light exposure (27).

Seasonal Affective Disorder

Seasonal affective disorder (SAD) with or without associated hypersomnolence is an atypical, recurring depression, often occurring in fall and winter and remitting fully in springtime. Light therapy has shown significant benefit in this setting. Routinely used parameters for treatment range from 30 minutes to 4 hours per day at 2,500 to 10,000 lux.

Jiuan et al. evaluated plasma melatonin levels in 42 patients with SAD after 10 to 14 days of treatment with 10,000 lux for 30 minutes. Morning light produced phase advances of the melatonin rhythm, while evening light produced delays.

Baseline and routine eye examinations are suggested and treatment in patients with progressive retinal disease is a relative contraindication. Some authors suggest routine exams for those patients concurrently taking potentially photosensitizing medications.

Patients are monitored for several weeks to allow appreciation of any deleterious responses. Noncompliance with daily light therapy generally equates to relapse. The time to relapse is, however, variable (32).

Melatonin: Circadian Rhythm Marker and Potential Therapeutic Agent

Melatonin was first isolated in 1959. The sleep-inducing characteristics were discovered soon afterward. Melatonin is synthesized in a two-step enzymatic conversion from the neurotransmitter serotonin. The molecule is lipid soluble and freely crosses most membrane barriers. The half-life of melatonin is approximately 30 to 53 minutes. The pineal gland is the primary location of this process. The retina is known to be an additional source of uncertain importance. Noradrenalin stimulates the pinealocyte to produce melatonin (33). Metabolism occurs in the liver to the hydroxylated form 6-sulfatoxymelatonin (34). Humans and rodents have been found to have melatonin receptors and binding sites in the SCN. Interestingly, melatonin is produced only during nighttime darkness (35). Sleep in normals occurs during melatonin secretion. The dim-light melatonin onset (DLMO) is a method by which the onset of melatonin production can be used as a marker for circadian phase position (Fig. 6-4). The phase of the SCN can be measured indirectly by dim-light melatonin secretion and timing of the core body temperature minimum. Melatonin serves this function because the circadian variation in sleep propensity is closely associated with the circadian rhythm of plasma melatonin (6) The effects of melatonin on the circadian phase are exactly opposite those of light. Melatonin given before the body temperature minimum phase advances while light phase delays. On the other hand, early morning light phase advances. The times when these stimuli coincide with sensitive zones of their respective phase-response curves (PRCs) are at the twilight transitions. We are entrained to the 24-hour day via this relationship. Light can serve to suppress and entrain melatonin production.

It is known that photoperiodic breeding species, which breed according to changes in daylength, use melatonin secretion to gauge appropriate timing (33). Melatonin has been used extensively in the study and treatment of sleep disorders. The ability to rapidly shift peak melatonin secretion correlates with improved performance and a faster adjustment to night-shift work (36). Exogenously administered melatonin has received much attention over the

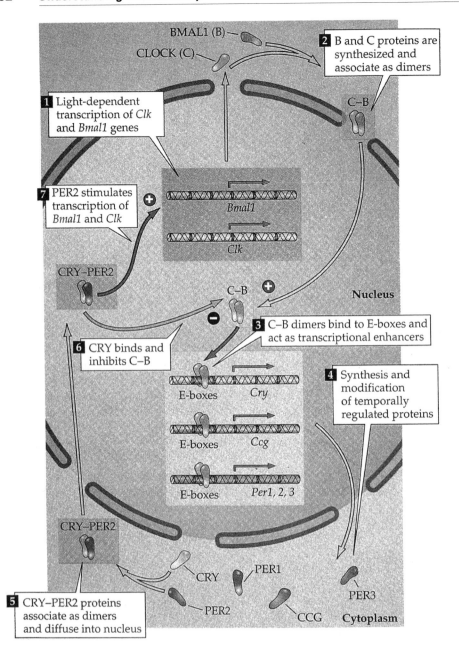

FIGURE 6-4. Diagram illustrating molecular feedback loop that governs circadian clocks. (From Purves, D. *Sleep and wakefulness in neuroscience.* 2nd edn. Sunderland, Sinauer Associates, 2001. With permission.)

recent years given its potential benefits. At low physiologic doses (0.3–0.5 mg) it shifts the circadian phase if given at appropriate times. At higher doses, it has a direct hypnotic effect. It is thought to be safe at physiologic doses of 0.3 to 0.5 mg. However, the safety of higher doses has not been systematically studied. The absorption of oral melatonin can be delayed if taken concurrently with large meals. The fast-release formulation is thought to be more appropriate for patients with difficulties in sleep initiation. Sleep maintenance is treated more appropriately with slow-release forms. Exogenously administered melatonin will produce phase shifting and, therefore, must be given at the appropriate time.

In the adult population one of the more interesting aspects of melatonin use in sleep disorders is the therapy for age-related insomnia. Irina et al. (37) performed a double-blind, placebo-controlled study on insomniacs over 50 years old. Placebo and three different doses of melatonin were used. Sleep efficiency and plasma melatonin levels were increased with the 0.3- and 3.0-mg doses (Fig. 6-5) (37).

Circadian Rhythm of Endocrine Secretion

The temporal release of certain hormones is dependent primarily on circadian rhythmicity; others depend on

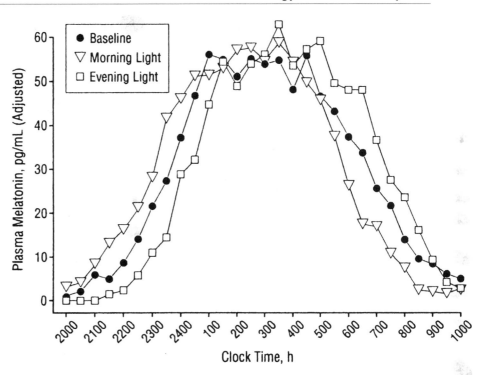

FIGURE 6-5. Mean plasma melatonin concentration measured under dim light conditions (1–5 lux, with darkness during sleep) at 30-min intervals in overnight sessions at baseline and after 10 to 14 days of treatment; morning or evening light, presented in crossovers. The three underlying curves for each of 8 subjects were normalized to compensate for varying amplitude by weighting each data point by grand mean area-under-the-curve. (From circadian time of morning light administration and therapeutic response in winter depression. *Arch General Psych.* 2001;58:69–75. With permission.)

sleep–wake homeostasis. The 24-hour profiles reflect the superposition of circadian signals on an ultradian or pulsatile release and result from the interaction of the circadian clock with sleep–wake homeostasis. Food intake, postural changes, and levels of physical activity are examples of rhythmic and nonrhythmic factors that can impact the diurnal hormonal secretory patterns (38).

Plasma cortisol levels typically rise quickly within a period of a few hours after sleep onset. The levels of cortisol peak in the early morning, at 7 to 8 AM, and decline as the day progresses. A period of consistently low cortisol levels occurs close to 12 AM.

Growth hormone demonstrates its major secretory pulse in normal young males shortly after sleep onset. In normally cycling young women, there are frequent daytime pulses accounting for the majority of the 24-hour secretion (38). Levels tend to decline as the amount of delta sleep declines with aging.

Daytime levels of thyrotropin are steadily low. Levels rise nocturnally, with peak near the time of sleep onset in a manner most consistent with a circadian effect.

The 24-hour profile of prolactin is characterized by low levels near noon, which increase in the afternoon and rise quickly soon after the initiation of sleep. The peak occurs in mid-sleep.

Indeed, older individuals may differ in regard to the amount of input they receive from social interactions, levels of physical activity, and light exposure. The changes in sleep architecture that occur during the aging process have been well described. These changes involve a decrease in overall sleep efficiency, with more frequent and prolonged

arousals, decreased delta sleep, and decreased REM stages. Both factors can have significant impact on endocrine hormonal release and function. Cortisol and growth hormone are studied examples of this phenomenon. Van Cauter et al. studied the mean profiles of cortisol and growth hormone (GH) in young and older men who were subjected to a 12-hour shift of the sleep–wake and light–dark cycles. The circadian control of cortisol secretion was evidenced by the insignificant change found after manipulation of the sleep–wake cycle. The GH secretory pulse followed the shift in the sleep–wake cycle, indicating its dependency on the timing of sleep (5). The patterns of cortisol and GH secretion also indicate that there is dampening of the temporal variation of both hormones with the aging process. There also appears to be an advance in the morning rise of cortisol in older individuals. It is suggested that the changes of amplitude reduction and phase advance may relate to age-related changes in the circadian system, but there are individual differences. The differences may relate to the amount and intensity of encountered zeitgebers (5).

CONCLUDING REMARKS

The human organism's successful adaptation to the demands placed upon it by the environment is, in large part, a function of the proper function and entrainment of the internal pacemaker. Physical environmental as well as societal demands have important effects on the individual's chronobiology. The last several years have seen the discovery of critically important genes involved in the control of the circadian rhythm. Indeed, much work remains to be done in order to continue to advance our understanding of circadian phenomena.

REFERENCES

1. Turek FW, Dugovic C, Zee PC. Current understanding of the circadian clock and the clinical implications for neurological disorders. *Arch Neurol.* 2001;58:1781–1787.
2. Richardson GS, Malin HV. Circadian rhythm sleep disorders: Pathophysiology and treatment. *J Clin Neurophysiol.* 1996;13(1):17–31.
3. Kryger MH, Roth T, Dement WC, eds. *Principles and practice of sleep medicine.* 3rd edn. Philadelphia: WB Saunders, 2000.
4. Mignot E, Taheri S, Nishino S. Sleeping with the hypothalamus: Emerging therapeutic targets for sleep disorders. *Nature Neurosci.* 2002;(5 suppl):1071–1075.
5. Van Cauter E, Plat L, Leproult R, et al. Alternations of circadian rhythmicity and sleep in aging: Endocrine consequences. *Hormone Res.* 1998;49:147–152.
6. Dijk DJ, Lockley SW. Functional genomics of sleep and circadian rhythm invited review: Integration of human sleep–wake regulation and circadian rhythmicity. *J Appl Physiol.* 2002;92:852–862.
7. Buxton OM, Copinschi G, Van Onderbergen A, et al. A benzodiazepine facilitates adaptation of circadian rhythms and sleep–wake homeostasis to an eight hour delay shift simulating westward jet lag. *Sleep.* 2000;23(7):915–927.
8. Eastman CI. Circadian rhythms and bright light: Recommendations for shift work. *Work Stress.* 1990;4(3):245–260.
9. Shearman LP, Sriram S, Weaver DR, et al. Interacting molecular loops in the mammalian circadian clock. *Science.* 2000;288:1013–1019.
10. Herzog ED, Schwartz WJ. Functional genomics of sleep and circadian rhythm invited review: A neural clockwork for encoding circadian time. *J Appl Physiol.* 2002;92:401–408.
11. Dijk DJ, Boulos Z, Eastman CI, et al. Light treatment for sleep disorders: Consensus report. II. Basic properties of circadian physiology and sleep regulation. *J Biol Rhythms.* 1995;10(2):113–125.
12. Darlington TK, Wagner-Smith K, FernandaCeriani M, et al. Closing the circadian loop CLOCK-induced transcription of its own inhibitors per and tim. *Science.* 1998;280:1599–1603.
13. Edery I, Rutila JE, Rosbash M. Phase shifting of the circadian clock by induction of the drosophila period protein. *Science.* 1994;263:237–240.
14. Lee C, Parikh V, Itsukaichi T, et al. Resetting the Drosophila clock by photic regulation of PER and a PER-TIM complex. *Science.* 1996;271:1740–1744.
15. Shearman LP, Sriram S, Weaver DR, et al. Interacting molecular loops in the mammalian circadian clock. *Science.* 2000;288:1013–1019.
16. Reick M, Garcia JA, Dudley C, et al. NPAS2: An analog of clock operative in the mammalian forebrain. *Science.* 2001;293:506–509.
17. Darlington TK, Wager-Smith K, Fernanda CM, et al. Closing the circadian loop: CLOCK-induced transcription of its own inhibitors per and tim. *Science.* 1998;280:1599–1603.
18. Albrecht U. Functional genomics of sleep and circadian rhythm invited review: Regulation of mammalian circadian clock genes. *J Appl Physiol.* 2002;92:1348–1355.
19. Tosini G, Menaker M. Circadian rhythms in cultured mammalian retina. *Science.* 1996;272:419–421.
20. Elmore SK, Betrus PA, Burr R. Light, social zeitgebers, and the sleep–wake cycle in the entrainment of human circadian rhythms. *Res Nursing Health.* 1994;17:471–478.
21. Honma KI, Honma S, Nakamura K. Differential effects of bright light and social cues on reentrainment of human circadian rhythms. *Amer J Physiol* 1995;268 *(Regulatory Integrative Comp. Physiol. 37):* R528–R535.
22. Duffy JF, Kronauer RE, Czeisler CA. Phase-shifting human circadian rhythms: Influence of sleep timing, social contact and light exposure. *J Physiol.* 1996;495:289–297.
23. Eastman CI. Squashing versus nudging circadian rhythms with artificial bright light: Solutions for shift work? *Perspect Biol Med.* 1991;34(2):181–195.
24. Minors DS, Waterhouse JM, Wirz-Justice A. A human phase-response curve to light. *Neurosci Lett.* 1991;133:36–40.
25. Van Someren EJW. More than a marker: Interaction between the circadian regulation of temperature and sleep, age-related changes, and treatment possibilities. *Chronobiol Intern.* 2000;17(3):313–354.
26. Comperatore CA, Krueger GP. Circadian rhythm desynchronosis, jet lag, shift lag, and coping strategies. *Occupational Med State of the Art Rev.* 1990;5(2):323–334.
27. Chesson AL, Littner M, Davilla D. Practice parameters for use of light therapy in the treatment of sleep disorders. Standards of practice committee, *Amer Acad Sleep Med Sleep.* 1999;22(5):641–660.
28. Drennan M, Kripke DF, Gillin JC. Bright light can delay human temperature rhythm independent of sleep. *Amer J Physiol.* 1989;257 *(Regulatory Integrative Comp. Physiol. 26):* R136–R141.
29. Badia P, Myers B, Boecker M, et al. Bright light effects on body temperature, alertness, EEG and behavior. *Physiol Behavior.* 1991;50:583–588.
30. Campbell SS, Dawson D. Enhancement of nighttime alertness and performance with bright ambient light. *Physiol Behavior.* 1990;48:317–320.
31. Czeisler CA, Johnson MP, Duffy JF, et al. Exposure to bright light and darkness to treat physiologic maladaptation to night work. *N Engl J Med.* 1990;322(18):1253–1259.
32. Terman M, Lewy AJ, Dijk DJ, et al. Light treatment for sleep disorders: Consensus report. IV. Sleep phase and duration disturbances. *J Biol Rhythms.* 1995;10(2):135–147.
33. Arendt J, Broadway J. Light and melatonin as zeitgebers in man. *Chronobiol Intern.* 1987;4(2):272–282.
34. Jan JE, Freeman RD, Fast DK. Melatonin treatment of sleep–wake cycle disorders in children and adolescents. *Develop Med Child Neurol.* 1999;41:491–500.
35. Lewy AJ, Ahmed S, Sack RL. Phase shifting the human circadian clock using melatonin. *Behavioural Brain Res.* 1996;73:131–134.
36. Quera-Salva MA, Guilleminault C, Claustrat B. Rapid shift in peak melatonin secretion associated with improved performance in short shift work schedule. *Sleep.* 1997;20(12):1145–1150.
37. Zhdanova IV, Wurtman RJ, Regan MM, et al. Melatonin treatment for age-related insomnia. *J Clin Endocrinol Metabol.* 2001;86(10):4727–4730.
38. Copinschi G, Spiegel K, Leproult R. Pathophysiology of human circadian rhythms. Mechanisms and biological significance of pulsatile hormone secretion. *Novartis Found Symp.* 227,2000;143–162.

Chapter 7

Ontogeny of Sleep

Paul R. Carney, Danielle Becker, and Susan Bongiolatti

INTRODUCTION

After the discovery of electroencephalographic waves in dogs by the English physician Caton (1) in 1875, and of the alpha waves from scalp electroencephalogram (EEG) by the German physician Hans Berger (2) in 1929, researchers began to obtain recordings of brain electrical activity from fetuses and infants. Lindsley (3) recorded fetal cardiac and cerebral electrical activity and Hughes (4) performed EEG studies in premature infants. Following the discovery of rapid eye movement (REM) sleep by Aserinsky and Kleitman (5) in 1953, it was also noted that REM and non-rapid eye movements (NREM) sleep could be differentiated by 30 weeks conceptional age (CA) (6). With improved ventilation and neonatal intensive care, healthy 23 to 30 weeks CA infants are more likely to survive without hypoxic ischemic injury, and state differentiation could be identified as early as 27 weeks CA. Sleep and wakefulness patterns develop rapidly during the prenatal and newborn period and continue to change during the first years of life. Sleep patterns then remain stable and without significant changes until late adulthood.

DIFFERENTIATION OF SLEEP AND WAKEFULNESS STATES

Newborns have a polyphasic sleep pattern and spend about two-thirds of their time sleeping during the first weeks of life. This polyphasic sleep pattern gradually changes into the monophasic adult pattern (7). Brain electrical activity, body and eye movements, and respiratory patterns are used to differentiate sleep and wake states. On falling asleep, a normal newborn enters into REM sleep, also referred to as active sleep. Random spontaneous movements of arms, legs, and facial muscles accompany active sleep. In premature infants (<37 weeks CA), it can be difficult to distinguish REM from wakefulness. Body movements and brainstem electrical activity are present at approximately 10 weeks CA, and cerebral cortical activity can be identified at 17 weeks CA. Rhythmic cycling body movements begins at 20 to 24 weeks CA (6). High-voltage slow waves and low-voltage 8 to 14 Hz activity is separated by 20- to 30-second intervals of low-voltage nearly isoelectric background. This EEG activity occurs in an asynchronous fashion over the two hemispheres and is usually accompanied by irregular respiration and irregular eye movements. The discontinuous EEG pattern is often referred to as tracé discontinu. Irregular respiration and occasional eye movements accompany tracé discontinu sleep.

Between 27 and 30 weeks CA, the EEG is usually discontinuous and background activity is asynchronous. With increasing age, the periods between bursts become increasingly shorter. Central and temporal sharp wave transients are common features during this age. Posterior predominant delta waves with superimposed 14 to 24 Hz activity called *delta brushes* appear. During quiet sleep, the EEG is discontinuous and eye movements are rare. During active sleep, continuous delta or theta–delta activity predominates. Cardiac and respiratory rhythms are more regular and apparent during quiet sleep than during active sleep. At 33 to 34 weeks CA, muscle tone decreases during active sleep relative to quiet sleep (8). The terms indeterminate sleep and transitional sleep are used to describe periods of sleep that cannot be classified as either quiet or active sleep.

Between 30 and 33 weeks CA, a low-voltage, mixed-frequency, and nearly continuous EEG pattern occurs during active sleep. However, during quiet sleep, the EEG remains discontinuous, and bursts of high-voltage delta activity followed by 10 seconds of low-voltage activity can be observed. Temporal and frontal sharp transients and delta brushes remain the prominent EEG patterns. With the emergence of distinctive active and quiet sleep patterns, transitional sleep also becomes more prominent at 32 to 33 weeks CA (9). At 34 weeks CA, NREM–REM cycle duration is approximately 45 minutes, which increases to 60 minutes at 38 weeks CA or full-term infant.

Between 33 and 37 weeks CA, features including smiling, grimaces, and body twitches are present during active sleep. By 37 weeks CA, active sleep is well differentiated. Medium-voltage and continuous EEG, rapid eye movements, irregular breathing patterns, muscle atonia, and phasic twiches of the face and extremities are present. During quiet sleep, breathing patterns are regular and body movements are rare. The EEG during quiet sleep shows an alternating pattern (tracé alternant) in which 1-to 10-second bursts of moderate- to high-amplitude delta activity alternate with 5- to 10-second intervals of low-voltage mixed-frequency theta activity. Beginning at approximately 37 weeks CA, the EEG becomes more continuous with increasing age.

DEVELOPMENT OF SLEEP–WAKE CYCLE

Infancy

The term infant spends about one-third of the time in the awake state. The remaining two-thirds (~16 hours) of time is equally divided between NREM and REM sleep. Sleep–wake states alternate in 3- to 4-hour cycles, with randomly timed phases of wakefulness, active sleep, and quiet sleep. Within the first month following birth, sleep–wake phase organization begins to adapt to the light–dark cycle and to associated social cues. The circadian rhythm of temperature appears first. Soon after birth, circadian wake rhythm then appears (~day 45 of life). Circadian sleep rhythm appears around day 56 of life (10). By 10 to 12 weeks of age, the development of neural systems produces a steady diurnal distribution of sleep and wake.

During the first 3 months of life, infants spend 50% of their sleep time in REM (active sleep) and 50% in NREM (quiet sleep). The proportion of sleep in REM and NREM changes dramatically during the first year of life. Sleep time declines to 13 hours at 1 year of life. REM sleep declines from 7 to 8 hours at birth to 6 hours by 6 months of life and then to 4 to 5 hours by 1 year of life. During the first month of life, sleep-onset REM occurs two-thirds of the time, declining to 20% by 6 months of life. At term, sleep-onset REM occurs only occasionally (9,11). With a steady decline in the proportion of REM sleep, NREM sleep becomes more predominant during the first half of sleep, and REM sleep predominates during the latter half of the sleep cycle. The latency before entering REM sleep gradually increases during the first year. The REM–NREM cycle length is between 60 to 70 minutes during the first year of life. By 4 to 5 years of age, the cycle length gradually increases to 90 minutes. By 10 years of life, total REM sleep resembles adult proportions of approximately 20% to 25% of total sleep time (TST), with the child averaging 9 hours of total sleep in a single nocturnal sleep period (12). (Fig. 7-1).

The appearances of specific wave forms in the EEG represent a significant milestone in sleep ontogeny. Sleep spindles begin to appear at 4 weeks of age, rapidly develop through 8 weeks of age, and characterize NREM sleep by 3 months (13). Sleep spindles increase in number by 6 months of age, although there is often interhemispheric asynchrony of spindles until the age of 2 years (14). K complexes are detectable on the EEG by

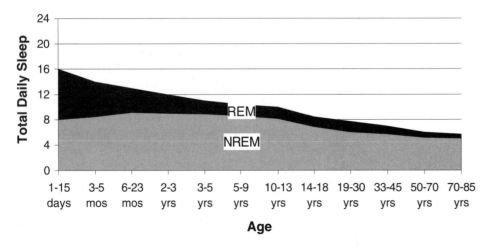

FIGURE 7-1. Changes in duration of NREM and REM sleep with age. (Adapted from Roffwarg HP, Munzio JN, Dement WC. Ontogenetic development of the human sleep–dream cycle. *Science.* 1966;152:604–619. With permission.)

3 months and are fully developed by 2 years of age (15). High-voltage, low-frequency theta (4–8 Hz) or delta (0.5–4 Hz) waves are detectable, particularly over the occipital area, at around 1 month of age. The four stages of NREM sleep are distinguishable electrophysiologically by 6 to 12 months of age. The circadian rhythm in a child's sleep patterns, detectable by 3 to 6 months, gradually comes under the control of external stimuli, including light exposure. It is common by 6 months of life to sleep throughout the night, with the appearance of a predominantly biphasic pattern, with an afternoon nap. The cycles of REM sleep develop by 3 months.

Childhood

As children progress through the first decade of life, adult patterns begin to emerge. During the first year of life, TST gradually decreases and, by 2 years of age, sleep occupies around 11 hours at night and up to 2.5 hours of sleep during one or two daytime naps. Thirty percent of a child's sleep is REM. Total daily sleep continues to decrease, but at a progressively slower rate during childhood. The afternoon nap is often retained until the age of 5 years. During childhood, sleep latency is shorter than in later life, averaging 5 to 10 minutes. Sleep efficiency is approximately 95%, and the percentage of stages 3 and 4 NREM sleep is greater than at any other age. Body movements during sleep begin to decrease in frequency, although they are more often seen in middle childhood than in adolescents or young adults (10). Between 5 and 10 years of age, sleep architecture matures to an adultlike pattern, with slow-wave sleep occurring during the first one-third to one-half of the nocturnal sleep time and REM sleep increasing in volume and intensity as the night progresses (10). Stage 4 NREM sleep decreases from 18% in 6- to 7-year-olds, to 14% in 11-year-old children. This decline in stage 4 NREM sleep is associated with an increase in stage 2 NREM sleep. Other NREM sleep stage proportions remain the same. REM latency decreases from 140 minutes in 6- to 7-year-olds to 124 minutes in 10- to 11-year-old children. The number of REM periods and amount of activity during REM also decreases with increasing age (7,16). TST decreases to around 9 hours daily, as seen in adults.

Adolescence

In adolescence, the sleep architecture assumes the pattern that will be carried into adulthood. The onset of puberty and adolescence is accompanied by the beginning of a decline in delta wave sleep, which continues steadily with age. From age 10 to 20, there is dramatic decrease in delta wave sleep of approximately 40% (17). REM latency is reduced during adolescence, and stage 1 and 2 sleep may be increased relative to preadolescent children (18). REM sleep constitutes approximately one-quarter of the total sleep in an adolescent. Although some researchers have

suggested that adolescents require more sleep (19), total daily sleep often reduces from childhood to 7 to 9 hours. Significant daytime sleepiness is found among many adolescents (20), and irregular sleep wake patterns may develop. In general, adolescents frequently go to sleep later at night and wake up later in the morning (when not restricted by early morning school schedules, for example). This change in the nightly sleep pattern may reflect a change in the circadian sleep–wake rhythm that occurs during puberty, or it may be related to increases in academic, work, and social demands (21).

Young and Middle Adulthood

The sleep pattern of adults remains relatively stable throughout young and middle adulthood with the exception of the continued decline in slow-wave sleep (stages 3 and 4) (22), which begins in adolescence and continues throughout life. In most adults, stage 3 constitutes 3% to 8% of sleep and stage 4 constitutes 10% to 15%. Stage 2 sleep predominates in adult sleep, comprising 45% to 55% of total sleep. Overall, 75% to 80% of adult sleep is NREM sleep, while 20% to 25% of total sleep time is occupied by REM sleep. NREM and REM sleep typically occurs in four to six alternating episodes throughout the night, with NREM stages initiating sleep. Typically, during the first one-third of the sleep period, NREM delta wave sleep episodes are longer, while REM sleep stages are shorter. In the last one-third of the sleep period, delta wave sleep wanes and REM stages become longer. Although there are individual differences in the optimal amount of sleep, the average adult sleeps 7 to 8 hours a day. The daily circadian sleep wake cycle becomes more stable during young and middle adulthood relative to adolescence, although the stability erodes with increasing age (7).

Older Adulthood

Older adults experience an overall decrease in sleep efficiency, changes in sleep architecture and disturbances of sleep patterns, including increased nighttime awakening, increased daytime napping, difficulty initiating sleep, and decreased total sleep time (23,24). Stage 1 sleep increases to 8% to 15% of total sleep and stage 2 sleep increases to nearly 80% (7). Meanwhile, slow-wave sleep duration and amplitude decreases and may disappear completely by age 90. Older adults also experience more frequent episodes of transient arousal, brief (3–15 second) periods of alpha wave intrusion (25). There are no major decreases in the amount of REM sleep from earlier adulthood (remaining at approximately 20%); however, REM sleep latency shortens and the first episode of REM sleep is often prolonged relative to younger adults. Sleep tends to develop a "polyphasic" quality in older adults, marked by episodes of napping for brief intervals throughout the day. Total nighttime sleep tends to be reduced.

▶ **TABLE 7-1. Changes in Sleep from Infant to Adulthood**

	Infant	Child	Adult
Sleep state percentages REM/NREM	50/50	20–25/75–80	20/80
Total sleep time (h)	16	11	7–9
Periodicity of sleep states (min)	50–60	90	90–100
Sleep onset state	REM sleep onset	NREM sleep onset	NREM sleep onset
Temporal organization of sleep states	REM–NREM cycles equally throughout sleep period	NREM stages 3–4 (SWS) predominant in first one-third of night	NREM stages 3 and 4 (SWS) predominant in first one-third of night

The previously mentioned shortened REM latencies may be related to changes in circadian rhythms that occur with increasing age (7). In older adults, there is a desynchronization of circadian rhythms associated with physiologic systems, such as sleep, hormones, and body temperature (23). The changes in circadian rhythms, including the circadian sleep–wake cycle may be associated with such factors as a decrease in nocturnal melatonin, decreased exposure to natural light cues, and reduced social and work obligations.

A summary of the maturational changes that characterize sleep state organization in infants to adults is presented in Table 7-1.

REFERENCES

1. Caton R. The electric currents of the brain. *BMJ.* 1875;2:278.
2. Berger J. Uber das Electroenkephalogramm des Menschen. *Arch Psych Nervenber.* 1929;87:527–570.
3. Lindsley DB. Heart and brain potentials of human fetuses in utero. *Amer. J Psychol.* 1942;55:412.
4. Hughes JG. Electroencephalography of the newborn infant: VI. Studies on premature infants. *Pediatrics.* 1951;7:707.
5. Aserinsky E, Kleitman N. Regularly occurring periods of eye motility and concomitant phenomena during sleep. *Science.* 1953;118:273–274.
6. Parmalee AH. Sleep states in premature infants. *Develop Med Child Neurol.* 1967;9:70.
7. Williams RL, Karacan I, Hursch CJ. *Electroencephalography (EEG) of human sleep: Clinical applications.* New York: Wiley, 1974.
8. Dreyfus-Brisac C. Ontogenesis of sleep in human premature infants after 32 weeks conceptional age. *Develop psychobiol.* 1970;3:391.
9. Curzi-Dascolova L. Sleep state organization in premature infants of less than 35 weeks gestational age. *Pediatr Res.* 1993;34:624.
10. Sheldon S. Sleep in infants and children. In: Lee-Chiong T, Sateia M, Carskadon M, eds. *Sleep medicine.* Philadelphia: Hanley & Belfus, 2002:99–103.
11. Coon S and Guilleminault C. Development of sleep–wake patterns and non-rapid eye movements sleep stages during the first six months of life in normal infants. *Pediatrics.* 1982;69:793.
12. Williams RL, Gokcebay N, Hirshkowitz M, et al. Ontogeny of sleep. In: Cooper R, ed. *Sleep.* London: Chapman & Hall Medical, 1994:60–75.
13. Tanguay P, Ornitz E, Kaplan A, et al. Evolution of sleep spindles in childhood. *Electroencephalogr Clin Neurophysiol.* 1975;38:175.
14. Parkes JD. *Sleep and its disorders.* London: Saunders, 1985.
15. Metcalf D, Mondale J, Butler F. Ontogenesis of spontaneous k-complexes. *Psychophysiology.* 1971;8:340.
16. Feinberg I. Effects of age on human sleep patterns. In: Kales A, ed. *Sleep, physiology, and pathology: A symposium.* Philadelphia: Lippincott, 1969:39–52.
17. Carskadon MA. The second decade. In: Guilleminault C, ed. *Sleeping and waking disorders: Indications and techniques.* Menlo Park, CA: Addison Wesley, 1982.
18. Dahl RE, Carskadon MA. Sleep and its disorders in adolescence. In: Ferber R, Kryger MH, eds. *Principles and practice of sleep medicine in the child,* Philadelphia: WB Saunders, 1995:19–27.
19. Carskadon MA, Harvey K, Duke P, et al. Pubertal changes in daytime sleepiness. *Sleep.* 1980;2:453–460.
20. Carskadon MA, Dement WC. Sleepiness in the normal adolescent. In: Guilleminault C, ed. *Sleep and its disorders in children.* New York: Raven Press, 1987:53–66.
21. Carskadon MA, Vierira C, Acebo C. Association between puberty and delayed hase preference. *Sleep.* 1993;16(3):258.
22. Feinberg I, Koresko RL, Heller N. EEG sleep patterns as a function of normal and pathological aging in man. *J. Psychiatr. Res.* 1967;5:107.
23. Cohen-Zion M, Gehrman PR, Ancoli-Isreal S. Sleep in the elderly. In: Lee-Chiong T, Sateia M, Carskadon M, ed. *Sleep medicine.* Philadelphia: Hanley & Belfus: 2002:115–123.
24. Foley DJ, Monjan AA, Borwn SL, et al. Sleep complaints among elderly persons: An epidemiologic study of three communities. *Sleep.* 1995;18:425–432. .
25. Carskadon MA, Van Den Hoed J, Dement WC. Insomnia and sleep disturbances in the aged: Sleep and daytime sleepiness in the elderly. *J Geriatr Psych.* 1980;13:135–51.

Clinical Presentations of Sleep Medicine

Sleepiness

Barbara Phillips

Now blessings light on him that first invented this same sleep: it covers a man all over, thoughts and all, like a cloak; Tis meat for the hungry, drink for the thirsty, heat for the cold, and cold for the hot. Tis the current coin that purchases all the pleasures of the world cheap; and the balance that sets the king and the shepherd, the fool and the wise-man even. There is only one thing that I dislike in sleep; Tis that it resembles death; there's very little difference between a man in his first sleep, and a man in his last sleep.

Miguel De Cervantes

Sleepiness is a prevalent and ill-defined symptom, experienced by almost everyone at some time. Sleepiness and fatigue have been used interchangeably in some publications, resulting in confusion and ambiguity. Sleep is to sleepiness as food is to hunger; *sleepiness* refers specifically to an increased likelihood of falling asleep. *Fatigue* refers to many different conditions, some of which do not include sleepiness; the term refers specifically to increased difficulty sustaining a high level of performance (1). Obvi-

ously, sleepiness is a normal human state and is desirable at times (e.g., bedtime). Just ask any insomniac!

Sleepiness is problematic when it disrupts daily living. Problem sleepiness is estimated to affect 0.5% to 25% of the population. Problem sleepiness has two primary causes: lifestyle factors, including sleep deprivation and medication effects, and sleep disorders, including sleep-disordered breathing, narcolepsy, and idiopathic hypersomnia.

This chapter will review a historical perspective of sleepiness, the epidemiology of problem sleepiness, and determinants of sleepiness. A discussion of tools used to measure sleepiness, the consequences of sleepiness and sleep deprivation, and a brief overview of countermeasures are also included.

HISTORICAL PERSPECTIVE

In 1989, Allan Hobson wrote, "More has been learned about sleep in the past 60 years than in the preceding

6,000" (2). Although sleep and sleep disturbance have fascinated humans since the beginning of recorded time, it was not until the 19th century that the beginning of understanding about why we sleep and what happens if we do not began to emerge. In the 1920s, Nathanial Kleitman undertook sleep deprivation experiments and began to explore the consequences of sleepiness (3). Later that same decade, Hans Berger began recording brain electrical activity and noticed striking differences between the waking and sleeping electroencephalograms (EEG) of humans (4). Understanding of the causes and consequences sleepiness itself has recently assumed center stage in "Sleep Medicine," fueled by rapid developments in the understanding of narcolepsy, improved tools to measure sleepiness, and the comprehension that sleepiness can be deadly in this era of rapidly moving vehicles.

EPIDEMIOLOGY OF PROBLEM SLEEPINESS

Several factors account for an increasing prevalence of sleepiness in the past century. Development of electricity (with reliable, inexpensive light), migration from the farm to the city (but away from the biologic tie to the rhythm of the sun), and the ability to travel across time zones have enabled us to be a 24-hour society. Up to one-third of this nation's population works in shifts. Shift work has consistently been shown to result in poorer sleep quality and reduced daytime alertness (5). Increased intensity of hospital-based medical care and increased volume of air traffic are two examples of occupational sleep loss for physicians and air traffic controllers, respectively (6,7). Adolescents are increasingly required to report to school at inappropriately early hours, with reduction in nocturnal sleep time to less than 7 hours of sleep a night, at a time when their bodies need much more than that (8,9). In addition to these societal causes of increased sleepiness, the prevalence of obstructive sleep apnea (OSA), the most common sleep disorder associated with sleepiness is clearly increasing; reasons for this include the explosion of obesity and the aging of the population (10). Taking these and other factors together, Bonnett and Arand (11) estimate that at least one-third of Americans are seriously, chronically sleep deprived and sleepy, and assert, "We must recognize the alertness function of sleep and the increasing consequences of sleepiness with the same vigor that we have come to recognize the society impact of alcohol."

In contrast to calculations of the prevalence of sleep deprivation, surveys of humans have found the endorsement of sleepiness varies from 0.5% to 36% (12). Young adults (who often have young children and multiple jobs), the elderly, and shift workers are more likely to report sleepiness and to be sleepy by objective testing. In a population-based study in Finland, 11% of women and 7% of men reported sleepiness almost every day (13); very similar findings were reported from a large study in Sweden (14).

DETERMINANTS OF SLEEPINESS

Like most things in biology and nature, the variables affecting sleepiness and alertness are multiple and vary among individuals. Our understanding of the causes of sleepiness has lagged because of confusion about how to define and measure it. However, among the determinants of sleepiness are prior sleep, time of day, genetics, individual characteristics, medications, and disease, including both intrinsic sleep disorders and many medical conditions.

Prior Sleep

Both the amount of sleep that humans need and their ability to cope with inadequate amounts of it vary among individuals. Conventional wisdom urges 8 hours of sleep a night, but adolescents clearly need more than that (8,9). Kripke reignited the debate about sleep need and its consequences with his American Cancer Society survey of more than a million individuals, demonstrating that lowest mortality rates were observed in those who slept 7 hours a night, and that those who reported sleeping 8 or more hours or 6 or less hours had increased mortality. It is likely that there are more subtle consequences of inadequate sleep time than mortality, however (see the section, "Consequences"). Although there is tremendous variability in human sleep need, all of us get sleepier the longer we are awake, and less sleepy the longer we sleep. Sleep is a biologic need like food or water and is necessary for survival. *Homeostatic pressure* is a term that has been applied to the increasing tendency to sleep with increasing time spent awake (15,16). In other words, the longer we stay awake, the sleepier we get. Although it is difficult to measure homeostatic pressure other than by measuring sleep latency (SL), characteristic EEG changes do occur with sleep deprivation: slow-wave sleep (SWS) increases, spindling decreases (17), and REM sleep is likely to occur earlier. Homeostatic pressure (or "process S") interacts with circadian rhythm (or "process C") in the "two-process" model of sleep (18,19).

Time of Day

Sleepiness varies by time of day, in a predictable, modifiable circadian rhythm. Kleitman was probably the first to report that people who stayed up all night were less sleepy the following morning than they were in the middle of their sleepless night (3). The suprachiasmatic nucleus (SCN) is the biologic clock that regulates hour-to-hour waking behavior. In forced desynchrony protocols, which theoretically eliminate or mask the homeostatic influence on sleep, subjective sleepiness and vigilance are lowest at about 6 AM, shortly after the nadir in core body temperature. There is also a midafternoon dip in core body temperature and alertness, which corresponds to the siesta time that many cultures routinely enjoy. A simplified way of understanding the two-process model is that homeostatic pressure (process S) makes us fall asleep, but circadian pressure (process C) helps us to stay asleep. SWS (deep NREM) is thought to reflect homeostatic pressure, whereas REM sleep is regulated by circadian rhythm.

Genetics

Many sleep disorders, including narcolepsy, sleep apnea, and restless legs syndrome (RLS) have a genetic component. It is increasingly clear that sleep need has a genetic basis as well. The population-based Finnish twin study of over 12,000 people yielded an estimate that about one-third of sleepiness is genetic (20). Using a rat model, Franken and colleagues have calculated that SWS need is under genetic control (21). While the gene (or genes) that govern the heritable aspect of sleepiness and sleep need have not been discovered, it is likely that orexins (hypocretins) will be implicated as significant heritable regulators of sleep in the general population. There is a wide range of evidence indicating that the orexins are involved in the regulation of the sleep–wake cycle (22).

Medications and Neuropharmacology of Sleep

Almost every medication has an effect on sleep structure or daytime alertness, and evaluation of patients with sleep complaints or problems should include a critical investigation of medication history. A comprehensive review of effects of all drugs is beyond the scope of this chapter. Instead, we will focus on a review of the pharmacology of sleep and sleepiness and a discussion of medications most pertinent to chest physicians.

Pharmacology of Sleep

At least three systems control and regulate sleep: circadian/homeostatic pressure, brain centers, and neurotransmitters. Neurotransmitters of sleep and wakefulness augment or mediate the propensity for sleeping and waking states. Table 8-1 lists some of the putative mediators of wake, NREM, and REM sleep (23).

Classic examples of effects of medications on wakefulness are that first-generation antihistamines promote sedation and drowsiness and catecholamine stimulants (e.g., isoproterenol) promote wakefulness. Examples of drug effects on NREM sleep include the fact that adenosine receptor blockers (e.g., theophylline, caffeine) promote wakefulness and GABA receptor agonists (e.g., benzodiazepines) promote sleep; serotonin reuptake antagonists (SSRIs) can cause insomnia. Examples of pharmacologic effects on REM sleep are that nicotinic drugs (e.g., nicotine patches) promotes REM sleep and dreaming. Anticholinergic drugs (e.g., tricyclic antidepressants) depress REM sleep. Most

> **TABLE 8-1. Neurotransmitters of Sleep and Wakefulness**

Neurotransmitters of Wakefulness
Dopaminergic agents, including catecholamines
Norepinephrine
Histamine
Acetylcholine
Glutamate
Serotonin
Neurotransmitters of NREM Sleep
Adenosine
GABA (gamma-aminobutyric acid)
Neurotransmitters of REM Sleep
Cholinergics
Nicotinics
Muscarinics

medications affect sleep structure or daytime alertness in some way.

Pulmonary Medications and Sleep

For individuals with hypoxemia due to chronic obstructive pulmonary disease (COPD) or sleep-disordered breathing, oxygen may improve sleep quality, but does not improve daytime alertness. Theophylline is associated with increased sleep complaints in patients with COPD, asthma, and cystic fibrosis. Although there is evidence on both sides of the issue, studies claiming theophylline improves sleep frequently lack placebo groups and have high dropout rates (24). Corticosteroid use is associated with insomnia in asthmatics, in patients with optic neuritis, and in cancer patients. Polysomnographic (PSG) data on patients taking oral steroids demonstrate decreased REM sleep and increased wake after sleep onset (WASO) (25). The effects of inhaled steroids on sleep have not been studied, but they are unlikely to disrupt sleep. Inhaled ipratropium bromide improves both sleep quality and SaO_2 in patients with COPD (26).

Antihistamines

The effects of antihistamines on sleep and alertness are incompletely studied (27). The FDA classifies antihistamines as sedating or nonsedating. Polysomnographic data on the effects of antihistamines on sleep structure are very sparce. However, the available evidence suggests that disruption of sleep architecture and increased sedation is common with first-generation antihistamines due to their high lipophilicity (28). Sedating antihistamines shorten sleep latency compared to placebo, cause measurably reduced alertness, may prolong total sleep time, impair driving, and affect performance on neuropsychologic tests. Second-generation antihistamines cause less clinically significant sedative effects, but comprehensive studies of

▶ **TABLE 8-2.** Sedating and Nonsedating Antihistamines

Nonsedating	Sedating
Astemizole	Chlorpheniramine
Fexofenadine	Terfinadine
Loratadine	Clemastine
Terfenadine	Diphenhydramine
	Promethazine
	Triprolidine
	Hydroxyzine

their effects on humans are lacking. Table 8-2 lists common sedating (first-generation) and nonsedating (second-generation) antihistamines.

With regard to administration of many medications, chronobiology is important. For example, in patients with asthma, oral corticosteroids are more effective if given at 3 PM, theophylline is more effective if given in the evening, and long-acting beta agonists at bedtime reduce nocturnal awakenings.

Nicotine

Of interest to pulmonologists are the effects of cigarette smoking on sleep. Cigarette smoking is associated with increased risk of insomnia, RLS, and both snoring and sleep apnea (29,30). Some of these effects are mediated through nicotine, but others result from direct toxicity of smoke.

Cardiac Medications

In general, antihypertensive agents may decrease the duration of REM sleep. Beta blockers, alpha agonists, and alpha antagonists can lead to sedation, which may be transient and is dose-related. Diuretics may cause sleep disruption secondary to nocturia. Compared with placebo, lipophilic beta blockers increase REM latency, reduce REM sleep, increase wakefulness, deplete endogenous melatonin stores, and may be associated with nightmares (31). HMG-CoA reductase inhibitors ("statins") are associated with insomnia. The Sleep Heart Health Study reported that the use of any medications for treatment of congestive heart failure was an independent risk factor for sleepiness (32).

Antidepressants

Most antidepressants suppress REM sleep and increase REM latency (exceptions to this are nefazodone and buproprion). In addition, antidepressants can exacerbate RLS. Rapid withdrawal may lead to nightmares and parasomnias. Both insomnia and daytime sedation are common side effects of the SSRIs.

Illness

Primary sleep disorders such as narcolepsy, idiopathic hypersomnia, and sleep apnea are associated with sleepiness. These and other primary disorders are extensively covered elsewhere in this volume. The relationship between "nonsleep" disorders and sleep is complex and bidirectional. Sleepy people perceive that their health is poorer than those who are not sleepy, and people who are sick are more likely to complain of sleepiness (33). Clearly, much of the sleepiness associated with acute and chronic illness results from medication (32) and from inadequate or low-quality sleep. Among those medical conditions that are infamous for being associated with daytime sleepiness are Parkinson's disease (PD) (34), chronic renal failure (35), and dementia (36).

Illness likely mediates at least part of its effect on daytime sleepiness by affecting quality of sleep. Clearly, duration of sleep is important, but the number of arousals from sleep and the proportion of sleep spent in more restorative stages are often adversely affected by medical illness.

Environmental Influences

Given that sleepiness is the ability or tendency to fall asleep, environmental influences need to be taken into account. Activity, bright light, noise, temperature, posture, and stress can prevent or delay sleep onset in a person who is truly sleepy (37). With regard to behavior and posture, Johns has analyzed the components of the Epworth Sleepiness Scale (ESS) (see below) and concluded that lying down to rest in the afternoon and watching TV are most sleep promoting, whereas sitting and talking with someone and in a car stopped for traffic are least "somnific" (38). Much is known about the circadian rhythm in internal temperature and its relationship to sleep (in brief, sleepiness occurs as temperature falls), but the influence of environmental temperature on sleep is less well-defined. Extremes of temperature clearly disrupt sleep, and REM sleep appears to be more vulnerable to temperature extremes than is NREM. Cold (21°C) is more disruptive than warm (34–37°C), and passive external warming, e.g., hot baths, has been shown to promote sleep in some studies (39). Historically, and for theoretical reasons, exercise just prior to sleep was discouraged; in actuality, late night exercise has not been shown to impair sleep (40) and exercise, in general, is associated with improved sleep (41).

Age and Gender

A consistent finding in the literature has been that women have a greater need for sleep than do men (42). In surveys, women report spending more time in bed than do men, but also report more sleep problems, including inadequate sleep time and insomnia. However, in older, "noncomplaining" humans, women sleep better than do men (43).

Both the quality and quantity of human sleep decline with aging (42,44). From an average total sleep time of about 16 hours in the first days of life, sleep time falls to about 12 hours by the sixth month. There is a loss of about 30 minutes of sleep a night from age 1 until age 5. At adolescence, sleep need and sleep time begin to "mismatch," as teenagers exert autonomy and schedules begin to interfere with sleeping. Probably the best sleep in a human's life span is late childhood, just before onset of puberty.

Although it is not clear whether aging adults actually obtain fewer hours of sleep than middle-aged adults, they clearly experience a deterioration in sleep quality. Seniors have more fragmentation, less SWS, and more time in bed not sleeping than they did when they were younger. They experience both a reduction in homeostatic drive for sleep and reduced amplitude of the circadian signal.

MEASURING SLEEPINESS

Our ability to measure sleepiness is imperfect. Available tools include patient report (e.g., history), subjective measurements or scales, and objective measurements.

Estimating sleepiness by patient report is unreliable. Individuals both under- and overestimate the likelihood of falling asleep in given situations. Observer history may be more accurate, if obtainable.

Subjective sleepiness is most commonly assessed in a sleep center with an ESS (45) (Table 8-3). The ESS correlates with measures of sleep-disordered breathing and is

▶ **TABLE 8-3. Epworth Sleepiness Scale**[a]

How likely are you to doze off or fall asleep in the following situations, in contrast to just feeling tired? This refers to your usual way of life in recent times. Even if you have not done some of these things recently, try to work out how they would have affected you. Use the following scale to choose the *most appropriate* number for each situation:

0 = would *never* doze
1 = *slight* chance of dozing
2 = *moderate* chance of dozing
3 = *high* chance of dozing

Situation	Chance of Dozing
Sitting and reading	————
Watching TV	————
Sitting, inactive, in a public place	————
As a passenger in a car for an hour	————
Lying down in the afternoon	————
Sitting and talking to someone	————
Sitting quietly after a lunch without alcohol	————
In a car, while stopped for a few minutes in traffic	————

[a]Adapted from Reference 42.

▶ **TABLE 8-4. Classic Scores on the ESS**[a]

Subject	ESS Mean (SD)
Normal controls	5.9 (2.2)
Primary snorers	6.5 (3.0)
OSA	11.7 (4.6)
Narcolepsy	17.5 (3.5)
Idiopathic Hypersomnia	17.9 (3.1)
Insomnia	2.2 (2.0)
Periodic Limb Movement Disorder	9.2 (4)

[a]Adapted from Reference 45.

more likely to be elevated in individuals with sleep disorders than in those with no sleep pathology. A total score below 10 points (out of 24) is typically reported as normal. Although subjective, the ESS scores do correlate with pathology (Table 8-4) and improve with the effective treatment of sleep apnea (46).

Currently, the most common tool used to objectively measure sleepiness is a Multiple Sleep Latency Test (MSLT) (47,48). In the clinical MSLT protocol, a series of naps is undertaken the day following an overnight PSG. If overnight PSG indicates significant sleep pathology (e.g., OSA), or inadequate sleep (less than 300 minutes), MSLT testing is not valid. The MSLT consists of five naps that begin 2 hours apart (typically 08:00, 10:00, 12:00, 14:00, 16:00). In a clinical MSLT, naps last 20 minutes if there is no sleep, or for 15 minutes after the first epoch of unequivocal sleep. Some labs terminate the nap after any epoch of unequivocal REM sleep. The unit of measure is minutes from lights out until sleep onset (sleep latency). The MSLT score is the sleep latency averaged for all five naps. A normal sleep latency (MSLT score) is greater than 10 minutes; between 5 and 10 minutes is a "gray zone," less than 5 minutes is pathologic sleepiness. If sleep occurs in a given nap, the test continues for 15 more minutes to give REM sleep a chance to occur. An MSLT can be terminated after the fourth nap if unequivocal REM sleep has already occurred on two or more naps or if REM sleep has not occurred on any of the four naps. In clinical practice, the MSLT is most commonly used to make a diagnosis of narcolepsy or of idiopathic hypersomnia. The MSLT shows excellent interrater reliability, and scores improve with effective treatment of the underlying cause of sleepiness.

The Maintenance of Wakefulness Test (MWT) was developed because of concern that the MSLT measures ability to fall asleep, whereas the clinically relevant issue may be whether the patient can stay awake (49). In the MWT, the patient sits in a chair with eyes closed in a dimly lit room and tries to stay awake for either 20 or 40 minutes, depending on the protocol. There are typically four "naps." The range of normal depends on whether the test lasts 20 or 40 minutes, and whether the eyes are closed, but is probably about 18 minutes, (+3.6) or greater with eyes closed (50).

Unfortunately, correlation between the ESS, MSLT, and MWT is poor, probably because they measure different things (51–53). In general, all three tests show improvement with effective treatment of sleep apnea or of narcolepsy, but the MSLT, in particular, does not usually normalize after treatment (53). The ESS is clearly affected by psychological symptoms and correlates better with subjective complaints. ESS scores have been shown to correlate with the risk of falling asleep driving and near-miss accidents (54), which is not surprising, since the questionnaire includes a question about falling asleep in a car, and because it has been much better studied than other tests (it is much easier to use). The MWT is clearly affected by motivation and might be most applicable to assess fitness to drive or to work (52).

To address some of these issues, and also to devise a test that obviates the expense and interpretation ambiguity of the MST and MWT, British investigators have recently described the OSLER (Oxford SLEep Resistance) test (55). This test involves four separate 40-minute "resistance challenges," which take place in a dark room during the day. During each session, the subjects press a switch in response to a light signal; a computer keeps track of their responses. The OSLER test discriminates normal subjects from sleep apnea patients, correlates with MWT scores, and is much less expensive and easier to perform than either the MSLT or MWT.

At this writing, the identification of sleepiness remains similar to that of pornography; its definition is highly subjective. Weaver recently published an excellent and comprehensive review of these and other measures of sleepiness (53).

CONSEQUENCES OF SLEEPINESS

Although sleep deprivation and sleepiness are not synonymous, sleepiness is the most obvious and predictable result of sleep deprivation or fragmentation. Sleepiness can also result, of course, from primary sleep disorders, such as OSA and narcolepsy. The following discussion of the effects of sleep deprivation and restriction in humans focuses on three kinds of studies: experimental, population-based, and as experienced by physicians-in-training.

Experimental Studies of Humans

Physiologic Effects of Sleep Deprivation

Sleep loss can be categorized as chronic or acute, partial or total, or selective (37). An excellent and comprehensive review was recently published by Taskar and Hirshkowitz (56). In general, total sleep loss results in changes after a single night of lost sleep, but changes are modulated by many individual factors, including age, circadian phase, gender, and environment. Partial sleep loss results in fairly rapid impairment with sleep periods of 5 hours of less. The

very persistent finding that 4 to 5 hours of sleep is necessary for minimal functioning has reinforced the notion of "core sleep," that is, that the total duration of sleep includes 4 to 5 hours of requisite sleep, and the remainder is optional (57).

Nearly every human physiologic system is affected by sleep loss (37,56). Neurologically, reflexes are impaired and seizure threshold is reduced. Pain tolerance is lowered. Sleep loss impairs glucose tolerance, increases evening cortisol levels, lowers thyrotropin concentrations, and ablates the periodicity of growth hormone and prolactin secretion. Sleep loss also impairs leptin secretion, and caloric intake increases after a night of total sleep deprivation. Short-term sleep loss probably does not affect the immune system in a critical way, but has been shown to transiently affect natural killer (NR) cell activity and increase cytokine production. Pulmonary function (FEV 1, FVC, and ventilatory responsiveness) deteriorates with a night of sleep loss. Reduction in sleep time to less than 4 hours of sleep in healthy subjects was associated with increased blood pressure and sympathetic activity compared with *ad libitum* sleep (58).

"Recovery sleep" is also affected by sleep loss and sleep deprivation. In general, total sleep time and SWS are increased above baseline the first night of *ad libitum* sleep after sleep loss. In young adults, REM latency may be increased because of increased SWS in the first part of the night. The second night, REM sleep and total sleep time are increased above baseline. By the third night of recovery sleep, sleep structure is back to baseline (37).

Behavioral Effects of Sleep Deprivation

Vigilance, mood, and mathematical calculation predictably deteriorate with increasing sleep loss in a cumulative, "dose-dependent" way (37,42). The most rigorous research in this area has been done by Dinges and colleagues (59), in which a large sample size, careful monitoring, and frequent performance assessments are employed. This work has documented that cognitive performance degrades during chronic sleep restriction, even with a sleep length of 6 hours. In these studies, performance after the fifth night of 6 hours of sleep was as poor as after a night of no sleep.

Population Studies

The leisure time of American workers has decreased in the past 20 years with a reduction of sleep length for the general population from 8 to 8.9 hours a night to 7 to 7.9 hours per night (42). Only about one-third of the populations achieve 8 or more hours of sleep a night and an equal number get 6 or fewer hours of sleep a night (60). Theoretically, this has resulted in a nationwide state of chronic partial sleep deprivation. Two large studies have investigated the relationship between sleep duration and outcomes (15,61). Kripke et al. studied over one million individuals who were surveyed 6 years apart and demonstrated a U-shaped relationship between sleep time and mortality, with increased mortality occurring both in those who slept less than 6.5 and more than 7.5 hours/night (15). In this study, they controlled for 32 other variables, and noted that most of the excess mortality that was related to sleep duration was attributable to sleep durations of more than 7.5 hours, which was more than twice as common as sleep durations of less than 6.5 hours. Ayas et al. (61) also found a U-shaped relationship between sleep duration and coronary heart disease in women. In over 71,000 female health professionals who were 45 to 65 years of age and without coronary heart disease at baseline, there were statistically significant increases in the relative risk of coronary heart disease for sleep times of 6 or fewer hours (RR 1.3, CI 1.08–1.57) or 9 or more hours (RR 1.57, CI 1.18–2.11) (Fig. 8-1). The authors chose to emphasize the increased risk associated with reduced sleep times and suggested that long sleep could be a marker of underlying heart disease risk. It should be noted, however, that the significant U-shaped relationships persisted after controlling for most potential confounders including snoring, body mass index (BMI), and smoking. In fact, multiple studies have documented increased mortality associated with both long and short sleep times, with the "optimum" amount of sleep appearing to be between 7 and 8 hours (12,62,63). Since vigilance is impaired by sleep loss and since automobile accidents are the best-proven consequence of untreated sleep apnea, the relationship between sleepiness and accidents in the general population is of interest. Bhopal and Three Mile Island are frequently cited as obvious examples of the tragic consequences of impaired vigilance related to sleep loss. Those tragedies notwithstanding, a recent review of 19 epidemiologic studies of sleepiness and automobile accidents concluded, "that the direct epidemiological evidence for a causal role of fatigue in car crashes is weak, but suggestive of an effect" (64).

The NSF's 2001 poll found that both long and short sleepers had more sleep complaints than those sleeping 7 to 8 hours (60). In sum, it appears that sleep loss and sleep "excess" can be detrimental. It is likely that sleep, like caloric intake, is necessary for human survival, but that moderation might be best.

Studies of Physicians-in-Training

A specific body of literature relates to the effects of work hours and sleep loss on physicians-in-training. This topic has recently been reviewed by Veasey et al. (65). These authors review studies of surgical residents separately from other house officers and conclude that surgical residents may be more vulnerable to degradation of skills involving fine motor tasks than they are to those requiring cognition. Possible explanations for this include that surgeons self-select for resistance to the effects of sleep loss, that they are so chronically sleep-deprived that further short-term loss does not cause much of an effect, or that vulnerable residents chose not to participate in these studies. Studies of nonsurgical residents have demonstrated impairment of psychomotor function, including such things as performance on ECG interpretation, laboratory interpretation, and comprehensiveness of history and physical examination. Most performance variables are worse at night and in more junior house officers.

Little is known about the effects of house officer sleep loss on patient safety, although a huge study is underway (*http://npsf.org/html/rescatalog/catalog.html*).

The effects of sleep loss on house officers themselves are better documented; the greatest risk appears to be motor vehicle accidents, particularly when post call. Stress, depression, somatic complaints, and complications of pregnancy appear to be increased in house officers (66).

COUNTERMEASURES

Napping

Sleep is clearly the best treatment and prevention for sleepiness. A 2- to 8-hour nap prior to 24 hours of sleep loss can improve vigilance for 24 hours (66) and even 15-minutes naps taken every 2 to 3 hours can reduce performance decrements during 24 hours of sleep loss (67). It is possible that naps longer than 2 hours might be associated with sleep inertia. Timing of naps during the circadian nadir (2 AM to 9 AM) may enhance their effectiveness. For drivers, reduced risk of crashing was associated with getting at least 9 hours of sleep in the 48 hours prior to a long drive, as well as taking rest breaks, stopping when they felt they were falling asleep, and drinking coffee (68).

Sleep Duration and CHD

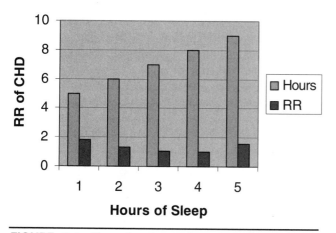

FIGURE 8-1. Sleep duration and coronary heart disease (CCHD). (Adapted from Reference 61.)

Caffeine

Caffeine is a modestly effective countermeasure; it improves alertness and MSLT scores at doses of 150 to 300 mg for up to 6 hours (37). The beneficial effect of 300 mg of caffeine is about as effective as a 3- to 4-hour prophylactic nap in anticipation of a period of sleep loss. Napping and caffeine appear to have additive effects.

Stimulants and Alerting Agents

Methylphenidate, pemoline, amphetamines, and modafinil have all shown to improve MSLT scores and limited performance tests for varying periods of time (37).

Bright Light

Limited data suggests that bright light may improve night shift performance, delay sleep onset, and increase alertness (37).

CLINICAL APPROACH TO THE SLEEPY PATIENT

The goals in evaluating sleepy patients include:

1. Distinguishing between sleepiness and fatigue
2. Distinguishing between lifestyle factors and medical illness
3. Identifying those who should be sent to a sleep center for further evaluation.

As in almost all of medicine, these goals can be accomplished by a history, physical, and some corroborative testing.

Key Historical Findings

Sleep Deprivation

- sleep schedule (obviously short times or more than an hour's difference between work and nonwork nights suggest sleep deprivation)
- work schedule (shift workers sleep less and more poorly than do nonshift workers)
- use of alarm clock (indicates inadequate time in bed)

Sleep Apnea (69)

- snoring (although about 25% of people snore, only about 5% have sleep apnea)
- witnessed apneas (the most robust historical predictor of sleep-disordered breathing)
- recent weight gain
- family history
- mood, memory, or learning changes
- headache, sore throat, or dry mouth in the morning

Narcolepsy

- history of cataplexy
- sleep paralysis, hypnogogic hallucinations (can occur in up to 50% of normals)
- first-degree relative

Medical Illness, Medication Effect

- *history of falling asleep driving*, or accidents or near-accidents when driving (this increases the risk to the patient and others and requires more urgent attention)

Key Findings on Physical Examination

Obstructive Sleep Apnea

- findings of cardiopulmonary or neurologic disease
- obesity (highly predictive of sleep apnea in Caucasians) (69)
- neck circumference >17 inches in a man or >16 inches in a woman
- hypertension (both a complication of sleep apnea and a reason to expedite diagnosis and treatment)

Corroborative Tests

- Epworth Sleepiness Scale (Table 8-3)—a score above 10 suggests pathologic sleepiness, but is neither sensitive nor specific for organic pathology
- Sleep log (Fig. 8-2)—can help identify inadequate sleep times and poor sleep hygiene
- Depression inventory (Table 8-5)—Some individuals perceive fatigue or low energy as depression. A high score on a depression inventory coupled with a low ESS score may help identify those individuals.

Sleep Center Referral

In accredited sleep centers, the entire gamut of sleep disorders can be diagnosed and treated. In actuality, the

▶ TABLE 8-5. Symptoms of Depression[a]

- Persistent sad, anxious, or "empty" mood
- Feelings of hopelessness, pessimism
- Feelings of guilt, worthlessness, helplessness
- Loss of interest or pleasure in hobbies and activities that were once enjoyed, including sex
- Decreased energy, fatigue, being "slowed down"
- Difficulty concentrating, remembering, making decisions
- Insomnia, early-morning awakening, or oversleeping
- Appetite and/or weight loss or overeating and weight gain
- Thoughts of death or suicide; suicide attempts
- Restlessness, irritability
- Persistent physical symptoms that do not respond to treatment, such as headaches, digestive disorders, and chronic pain

[a]Adapted from the National Institutes of Mental Health Website: http://www.nimh.nih.gov/publicat/depression.cfm

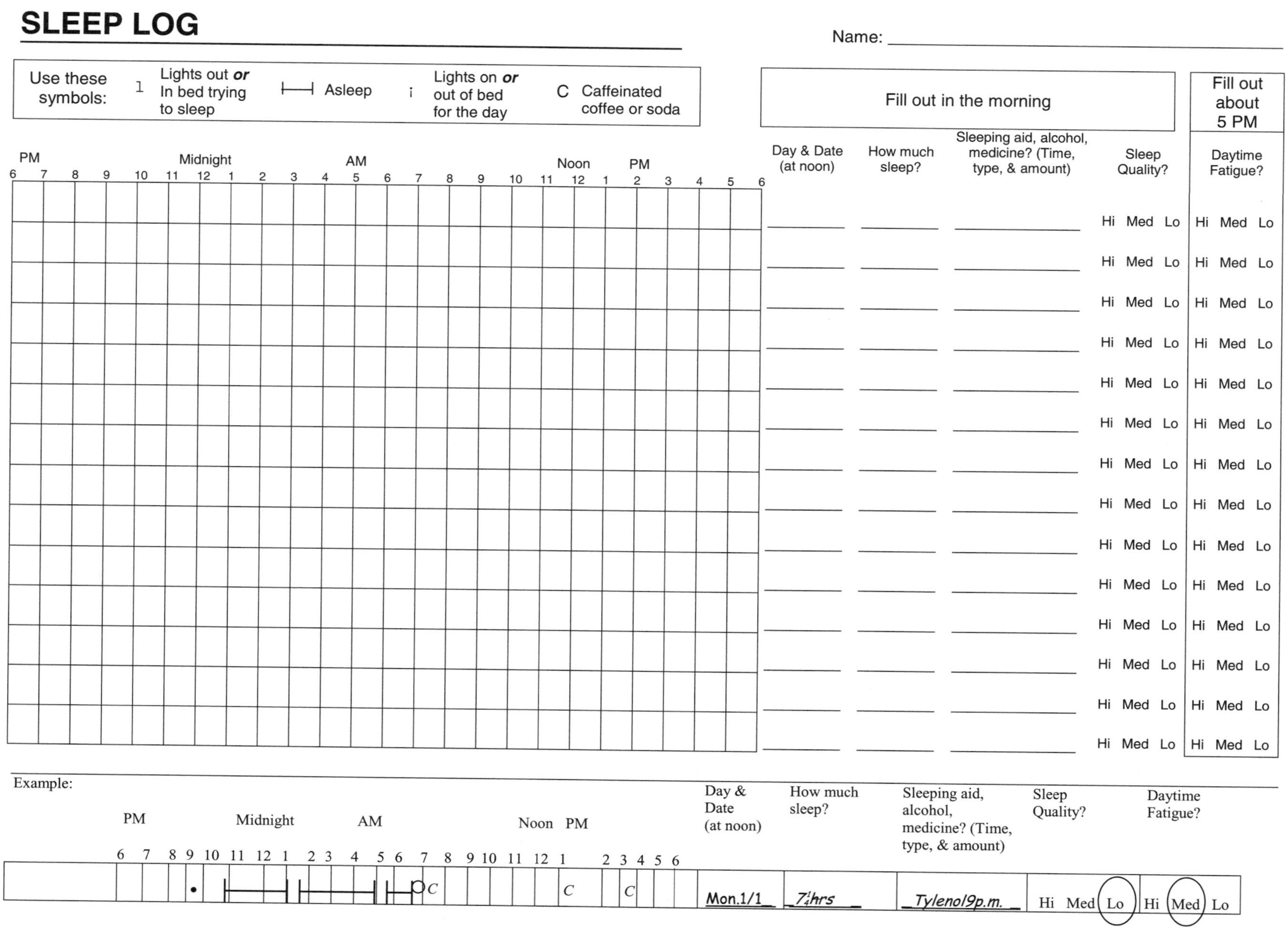

SLEEP LOG

Name: _____

Use these symbols:

⌐ Lights out **or** In bed trying to sleep | ⊢—⊣ Asleep | ¡ Lights on **or** out of bed for the day | C Caffeinated coffee or soda

	Midnight		AM		Noon		PM	
PM 6 7 8 9 10 11	12 1 2 3	4 5 6 7	8 9 10 11	12 1 2 3	4 5 6

Fill out in the morning

Day & Date (at noon)	How much sleep?	Sleeping aid, alcohol, medicine? (Time, type, & amount)	Sleep Quality?
			Hi Med Lo
			Hi Med Lo
			Hi Med Lo
			Hi Med Lo
			Hi Med Lo
			Hi Med Lo
			Hi Med Lo
			Hi Med Lo
			Hi Med Lo
			Hi Med Lo
			Hi Med Lo
			Hi Med Lo
			Hi Med Lo
			Hi Med Lo

Fill out about 5 PM

Daytime Fatigue?
Hi Med Lo
Hi Med Lo
Hi Med Lo
Hi Med Lo
Hi Med Lo
Hi Med Lo
Hi Med Lo
Hi Med Lo
Hi Med Lo
Hi Med Lo
Hi Med Lo
Hi Med Lo
Hi Med Lo
Hi Med Lo

Example:

	PM	Midnight	AM	Noon	PM
	6 7 8 9 10 11 12	1 2 3 4 5 6 7	8 9 10 11 12 1	2 3 4 5 6

Day & Date (at noon)	How much sleep?	Sleeping aid, alcohol, medicine? (Time, type, & amount)	Sleep Quality?	Daytime Fatigue?
Mon.1/1	7½ hrs	Tylenol/9 p.m.	Hi Med (Lo)	Hi (Med) Lo

FIGURE 8-2. Sleep log.

109

breakdown of patients referred to accredited sleep centers is as follows (70): Sleep apnea: 67.8, RLS: 4.9%, and narcolepsy 3.2%.

Although RLS is an important sleep disorder, it generally does not present as sleepiness. Many patients with sleepiness can and should be diagnosed by a primary care practitioner. The following groups of patients are likely to benefit from referral to a sleep center:

1. Patients in whom symptoms are suggestive of sleep apnea;
2. Patients in whom symptoms are suggestive of nar-

colepsy, who do not have symptoms suggestive of OSA (which is much more common);
3. Patients who have impaired living because of sleepiness in whom a history and physical does not disclose an explanation.

Specific Testing

In general, polysomnography is sufficient to establish the diagnosis of OSA: MSLT testing is appropriate when the diagnoses of narcolepsy or idiopathic hypersomnia are suspected. Details of MSLT testing protocol appear in Table 8-6. Occasionally, MSLT testing is helpful in a patient with sleep-disordered breathing who appears to be effectively treated and compliant with continuous positive airway pressure (CPAP). In these instances, CPAP should probably be worn during the naps.

SUMMARY

Sleepiness is a nearly universal human experience. Despite our extensive experience with this condition, we still do not have very good tools to measure or to counteract sleepiness. The effects of sleep loss range from mood impairment to possibly increased mortality. Referral to a Sleep Center for sleep testing may be helpful if OSA or narcolepsy are suspected.

▶ **TABLE 8-6. MSLT Protocol**[a]

Purpose: The MSLT can be used to objectively assess sleepiness. Patients are asked to allow themselves to fall asleep.

Protocol Background
1. Patients are tested in street clothes and not allowed into the bed between naps
2. Sleep rooms are dark and quiet
3. Drug screening is highly recommended
4. The test should follow an overnight PSG, which includes at least 300 minutes of sleep and does not reveal another cause for sleepiness (e.g., sleep apnea)
5. A sleep log for 2 weeks before testing helps to rule out chronic sleep deprivation
6. SSRIs should be stopped at least 2 weeks before. Other drugs, which affect sleep and sleepiness (BDZ, etc.), should be stopped, if possible

Performing the Test (Clinical Protocol)
1. No smoking 30 minutes before, no vigorous activity 15 minutes before, no caffeine during the test.
2. At lights out, patient is instructed "Please lie quietly, keep your eyes closed, and try to fall asleep."
3. Unit of measure: time in minutes from lights out until one epoch of unequivocal sleep or three epochs of stage 1.
4. Each nap lasts for 20 minutes or for 15 minutes after onset of sleep
5. The study is terminated after four or five naps:
   a. After four naps if NO or ≥2 SOREMs have occurred
   b. After five naps if one SOREM has occurred

Interpretation
1. Mean sleep latency (from lights out until sleep onset averaged for all naps)[b]
   a. 10–15 minutes "mild sleepiness," can be seen in normal subjects
   b. Normal is >10
   c. Gray zone is 5–10, moderate sleepiness
   d. Pathologically sleep is <5 (severe sleepiness)
2. Number SOREMs
   a. Normal is 1 or less

Diagnostic Use
Narcolepsy: Mean sleep latency <5 with 2 or more SOREMs
Idiopathic hypersomnia: Mean sleep latency less than 10 minutes, usually no SOREMs

---

[a]From reference 71.
[b]Adapted from American Sleep Disorders Association. The Clinical Use of the Multiple Sleep Latency Test. *Sleep* 1992;15:268–276.

REFERENCES

1. Pigeon WR, Sateia MJ, Ferguson RJ. Distinguishing between excessive daytime sleepiness and fatigue. Toward improved detection and treatment. *J Psychosom Res.* 2003;54:61–9.
2. Hobson J. *Sleep.* New York: Scientific American Library, 1989:P 1.
3. Kleitman N. *Sleep and wakefulness.* Chicago, IL: University of Chicago Press, 1939.
4. Berger H. Ueber das Elektroenkephalogramm des Menschen. *J Psychol Neurol.* 1930;40:160–179.
5. Monk T. Shift work. In: Kryger M, Roth T, Dement WC, eds. *Principles and practice of sleep medicine.* 3rd edn. Philadelphia: WB Saunders, 2000:600–605.
6. Luna TD. Air traffic controller shiftwork: What are the implications for aviation safety? A review. *Aviat Space Environ Med.* 1997;68:69–79.
7. Gaba DM, Howard SK. Fatigue among clinicians and the safety of patients. *N Engl J Med.* 2002;347:1249–1255.
8. Carskadon MA, Wolfson AR, Acebo C, et al. Adolescent sleep patterns, circadian timing, and sleepiness at a transition to early school days. *Sleep.* 1998;21:871–881.
9. Thorleifsdottir B, Bjornsson JK, Benediktsdottir B, et al. Sleep and sleep habits from childhood to young adulthood over a 10-year period. *J Psychosom Res.* 2002;53:529–37.
10. Young T, Shahar E, Nieto FJ, et al. Predictors of sleep-disordered breathing in community-dwelling adults: the Sleep Heart Health Study. *Arch Intern Med.* 2002;162:893–900.
11. Bonnett MH, Arand DL. We are chronically sleep-deprived. *Sleep.* 1995;18:908–911.
12. Roehrs T, Carskadon MA, Dement C, et al. Daytime Sleepiness and alertness. In: Kryger M, Roth T, Dement WC, eds. *Principles and practice of sleep medicine.* 3rd edn. Philadelphia: WB Saunders, 2000:43–52.

13. Hublin C, Karpio J, Partinen M, et al. Daytime sleepiness in an adult Finnish population. *J Intern Med.* 1996;239:417–423.

14. Broman JE, Lundh LG, Hetta J. Insufficient sleep in the general population. *Neurophysiol Clin.* 1996;26:30–39.

15. Kripke DF, Garfinkel L, Wingard DL, et al. Mortality associated with sleep duration and insomnia. *Arch Gen Psych.* 2002;59:131–136.

16. Dijk DJ, Edgar DM. Circadian and homeostatic control of wakefulness and sleep. In: Turek FW, Zee PC, eds. *Regulation of sleep and circadian rhythms.* Vol 133. New York: Marcel Dekker, 1999:111–148.

17. Knoblauch V, Krauchi K, Renz C, et al. Homeostatic control of slow-wave and spindle frequency activity during human sleep: effect of differential sleep pressure and brain topography. *Cereb Cortex.* 2002;12:1092–1100.

18. Folkard S, Totterdell P, Minors D, et al. Dissecting circadian performance rhythms: implications for shiftwork. *Ergonomics.* 1993;36:283–288.

19. Borbely AA, Achermann P. Sleep homeostasis and models of sleep regulation. In: Kryger M, Roth T, Dement WC, eds. *Principles and practice of sleep medicine.* 3rd edn. Philadelphia: WB Saunders, 2000:43–52.

20. Hublin C, Kaprio J, Partinen M, et al. Insufficient sleep—a population-based study in adults. *Sleep.* 2001;24:392–400.

21. Franken P, Chollet D, Tafti M. The homeostatic regulation of sleep need is under genetic control. *J Neurosci.* 2001;21:2610–2621.

22. Smart D, Jerman J. The physiology and pharmacology of the orexins. *Pharmacol Ther.* 2002;94:51–61.

23. Schweitzer, Paula. Drugs that disturb sleep and wakefulness. In: Kryger M, Roth T, Dement WC, eds. *Principles and practice of sleep medicine.* 3rd edn. Philadelphia: WB Saunders, 2000:441–461.

24. Salmeterol vs theophylline; Sleep and efficacy outcomes in patients with nocturnal asthma. *Chest.* 1999;115:1523–1532.

25. Moser NJ, Phillips BA, Guthrie G. Effects of dexamethasone on sleep. *Pharmacol Toxicol.* 1996;79:100–102.

26. Martin RJ, Bartelson BLB, Smith PL, et al. Effect of ipratropium bromide treatment on oxygen saturation and sleep quality in COPD. *Chest.* 1999;115:1338–1345.

27. Nolen TM. Sedative effects of antihistamines: Safety, performance, learning, and quality of life. *Clin Ther.* 1997;19:39–55.

28. DuBuske LM. Clinical comparison of histamine H-1-receptor antagonist drugs. *J Allergy Clin Immunol.* 1996;98:S307–S318.

29. Wetter DW, Young TB, Bidwell TR, et al. Smoking as a risk factor for sleep-disordered breathing. *Arch Intern Med.* 1994;154:2219–2224.

30. Phillips B, Young T, Finn L, et al. Epidemiology of restless legs symptoms in adults. *Arch Intern Med.* 2000;160:2137–2141.

31. Kostis JB, Rosen RC. Central nervous system effects of beta-adrenergic blocking drugs: the role of ancillary properties. *Circulation.* 1978;75:204–212.

32. Whitney CW, Enright PL, Newman AB, et al. Correlates of daytime sleepiness in 4578 elderly persons. The Cardiovascular Health Study. *Sleep.* 1998;21:27–36.

33. Briones B, Adams N, Strauss M, et al. Relationship between sleepiness and general health status. *Sleep.* 1996;19:583–588.

34. Gjerstad MD, Aarsland D, Larsen JP. Development of daytime somnolence over time in Parkinson's disease. *Neurology.* 2002;58:1544–1546.

35. Hui DS, Wong TY, Li TS, et al. Prevalence of sleep disturbances in Chinese patients with end-stage renal failure on maintenance hemodialysis. *Med Sci Monit.* 2002;8:CR331–CR336.

36. Ohayon MM, Vecchierini MF. Daytime sleepiness and cognitive impairment in the elderly population. *Arch Intern Med.* 2002;162:201–208.

37. Bonnet MH. Sleep Deprivation. In: Kryger M, Roth T, Dement WC, eds. *Principles and practice of sleep medicine.* 3rd edn. Philadelphia: WB Saunders, 2000:53–71.

38. Johns MW. Sleep propensity varies with behaviour and the situation in which it is measured: the concept of somnificity. *J Sleep Res.* 2002;11:61–67.

39. Bach V, Telliez F, Libert JP. The interaction between sleep and thermoregulation in adults and neonates. *Sleep Med Rev.* 2002;6:481–492.

40. Youngstedt SD, Kripke DF, Elliott JA. Is sleep disturbed by vigorous late-night exercise? *Med Sci Sports Exec.* 1999;31:864–869.

41. Naylor E, Penev PD, Orbeta L, et al. Daily social and physical activity increases slow-wave sleep and daytime neuropsychological performance in the elderly. *Sleep.* 2000;23:87–95.

42. Ferrar M, Gennaro L. How much sleep do we need? *Sleep Med Rev.* 2001;5:155–179.

43. Hume KI, Van F, Watson A. A field study of age and gender differences in habitual adults sleep. *J Sleep Res.* 1998;7:85–94.

44. Phillips BA, Ancoli-Israel S. Sleep in Aging. *Sleep Med.* 2001;2:99–114.

45. Johns MW. A new method for measuring daytime sleepiness: The Epworth sleepiness scale. *Sleep.* 1991;14:540–545.

46. Redline S, Adams N, Strauss ME, et al. Improvement of mild sleep-disordered breathing with CPAP compared with conservative therapy. *Amer J Respir Crit Care Med.* 1998;157:858–865.

47. Carskadon MA, Rechtschaffen AT. Monitoring and staging human sleep. In: Kryger M, Roth T, Dement WC, eds. *Principles and practice of sleep medicine.* 3rd edn. Philadelphia: WB Saunders, 2000:1203–1206.

48. Richardson GS, Carskadon MA, Flagg W, et al. Excessive daytime sleepiness in man: Multiple sleep latency measurement in narcoleptic and control subjects. *Electroencephalogr Clin Neurophysiol.* 1978;45:621–627.

49. Mitler MM, Guyjavarty KS, Browman CP. Maintenance of wakefulness test: a polysomnographic technique for evaluating treatment efficacy in patients with excessive somnolence. *Electroencephalogr Clin Neurophysiol.* 1982;53:658–661.

50. Doghramjii K, Mitler M, Sangal R, et al. A normative study of the maintenance of wakefulness test (MWT). *Electroencephalogr Clin Neurophysiol.* 1997;103:554–562.

51. Johns MW. Sensitivity and specificity of the multiple sleep latency test (MST), the maintenance of wakefulness test and the Epworth sleepiness scale: failure of the MSLT as a gold standard. *J Sleep Res.* 2000;9:5–11.

52. Sangal RB, Mitler MM, Sangal JM. Subjective sleepiness ratings (Epworth Sleepiness Scale) do not reflect the same parameter of sleepiness as objective sleepiness (maintenance of wakefulness test) in patients with narcolepsy. *Clin Neurophysiol.* 1999;110:2131–2135.

53. Weaver TE. Outcome measurements in sleep medicine practice and research. Part I: assessment of symptoms, subjective and objective daytime sleepiness, health-related quality of life and functional status. *Sleep Medicine Rev.* 2001;5:103–128.

54. Turkington PM, Sircar M, Allgar V, et al. Relationship between obstructive sleep apnoea, driving simulator performance, and risk of road traffic accidents. *Thorax.* 2001;56:800–805.

55. Bennett LS, Stradling JR, Davies RJ. A behavioral test to assess daytime sleepiness in obstructive sleep apnoea. *J Sleep Res.* 1997;5:142–145.

56. Taskar V, Hirshkowitz M. Health effects of sleep deprivation. *Clin Pulmon Med.* 2003;10:47–52.

57. Horne J. *Why we sleep.* New York: Oxford University Press; 1987:1–319.

58. Tochibuko O, Ikeda A, Miyajima E, et al. Effects of insufficient sleep on blood pressure monitored by a new multibiomedical recorder. *Hypertension.* 1996;27:1318–1324.

59. Dinges DF, Pack F, Williams K, et al. Cumulative sleepiness, mood disturbance, and psychomotor vigilance performance decrements during a week of sleep restricted to 4-5 hours per night. *Sleep.* 1997;20:267–277.

60. *National sleep foundation. national sleep foundation sleep survey.* Washington DC: National Sleep Foundation, 2001.

61. Ayas NT, White DP, Manson JE, et al. A prospective study of sleep duration and coronary heart disease in women. *Arch Intern Med.* 2003;163:205–209.

62. Quershi. Habitual sleep patterns and risk for stoke and coronary heart disease. *Neurology.* 1997;48:904–911.

63. Kojima M, Wakai K, Kawamura T, et al. Sleep patterns and total mortality: a 12-year follow up study. *J Epidemiol.* 2000;10:87–93.

64. Connor J, Whitlock G, Norton R, et al. The role of driver sleepiness in car crashes: A systematic review of epidemiological studies. *Accid Anal Prev.* 2001;33:31–41.

65. Veasey S, Rosen R, Barzansky B, et al. Sleep loss and fatigue in residency training. A Reappraisal. *JAMA.* 2002;288:1116–1124.

66. Bonnett MH, Arand DL. Impact of naps and caffeine on extended nocturnal performance. *Physiol Behav.* 1994;56:103–109.
67. Gillberg M, Kecklund G, Axelsson J, et al. Counteracting sleepiness with a short nap. *J Sleep Res.* 1994;3:90.
68. Cummings P, Koepsell TD, Moffat JM, et al. Drowsiness, countermeasures to drowsiness and the risk of a motor vehicle crash. *Inj Prev.* 2001;7:194–199.
69. Rowley JA, Aboussouan LS, Badr S. The use of clinical predic-

tion formulae in the evaluation of obstructive sleep apnea. *Sleep.* 2000;23:929–938.
70. Punjabi NM, Welch D, Strohl K. Sleep disorders in regional sleep centers: a national cooperative study. Coleman II Study Investigators. *Sleep.* 2000;23(4):471–480.
71. Carskadon MA, Dement WC, Mitler MM, et al. Guidelines for the Multiple Sleep Latency Test (MSLT): a standard measure of sleepiness. *Sleep.* 1986;519–524.

Chapter 9

Evaluating Sleeplessness

Edward J. Stepanski

INTRODUCTION

A presenting complaint of difficulty initiating sleep, maintaining sleep, or of inadequate sleep quality should lead to an evaluation that is distinct from that for a complaint of excessive daytime sleepiness. The differential diagnosis for a complaint of insomnia is quite different from that for excessive daytime sleepiness and, therefore, the evaluation is aimed at obtaining different information. When a patient reports both difficulty obtaining adequate quantity or quality of sleep at night, in addition to excessive sleepiness (e.g., falling asleep at work or while driving), then the complaint of sleepiness takes precedence, and the patient should be evaluated for the typical causes of this symptom. Most patients with insomnia report daytime fatigue as opposed to sleepiness. Therefore, distinguishing between fatigue and sleepiness is imperative prior to embarking on an evaluation to investigate insomnia as the primary problem. This chapter is written with the primary goal of providing practical guidelines for the evaluation of patients presenting with insomnia and will be useful to practitioners working as sleep specialists.

THEORETICAL MODEL OF CHRONIC INSOMNIA

The differential diagnosis for a complaint of insomnia is much more extensive than that for excessive sleepiness. Excessive sleepiness sufficient to cause an individual to fall asleep while driving or while at work is due to a short list of possible factors [e.g., sleep deprivation, sleep fragmentation, medication, circadian rhythm disorder, or central nervous system (CNS) pathology]. In contrast, insomnia may result from myriad behavioral, cognitive, medical, psychiatric, substance-related, or circadian factors, in addition to primary sleep disorders. An additional complication is that, in the case of chronic insomnia, several different factors may interact within a single patient to produce insomnia. Therefore, in addition to identifying

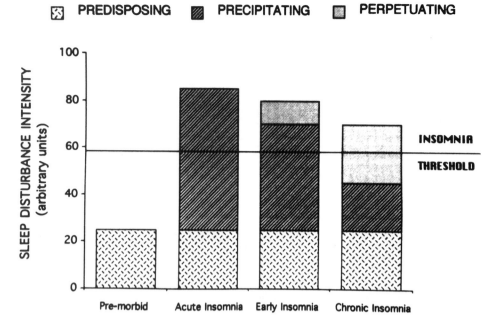

FIGURE 9-1. Theoretical model of factors contributing to chronic insomnia over time. (From Spielman AJ, Caruso L, Glovinsky P. A behavioral perspective on insomnia. *Psychiatric Clin North Amer.* 10:541–553, 1987. With permission.)

each contributory factor, it is best to determine the relative importance of these factors as contributing to the insomnia.

Understanding the role of multiple factors in a case of insomnia is simplified with use of Spielman's model of chronic insomnia (Fig. 9-1). This model classifies insomnia factors as predisposing, precipitating, or perpetuating, and shows how their relative importance changes over time (1). Predisposing factors include a tendency toward physiologic hyperarousal (2,3) or decreased homeostatic sleep drive (4). Precipitating factors can refer to a broad range of events, including pain, job stress, a noisy sleep environment, or jet lag. Perpetuating factors refer to behavioral and cognitive aspects of insomnia. Examples of these factors include spending too much time in bed, excessive worrying about the ability to sleep, a fear of being awake during the night, increased caffeine use, or eating during the night. These are phenomena that emerge once an individual is experiencing increased wakefulness at night due to predisposing and precipitating factors.

According to the Spielman model, the relative importance of these factors in producing poor sleep changes over the course of the insomnia. Prior to the start of the insomnia, each individual is hypothesized to have a certain level of predisposition to insomnia. Introduction of a precipitating factor interacts with the predisposing factors to trigger an episode of insomnia. Some individuals require only a minor precipitant (e.g., caffeinated soft drink after dinnertime) to experience significant insomnia because they have a high predisposition. Those with a low predisposition may require a heroic change before the insomnia experience. As the duration of the insomnia increases, perpetuating factors play an increasing role in maintaining the poor sleep. Although the precipitating event recedes (e.g., postoper-

ative pain is reduced), sleep remains poor due to these perpetuating factors.

Because patients with chronic insomnia often report histories with multiple potential causes of insomnia, a challenge for accurate diagnosis and treatment is to establish which causes are most important. Categorizing possible causes as predisposing, precipitating, or perpetuating helps the sleep specialist understand the contribution of these factors over the course of the insomnia. This permits the sleep specialist to establish a hierarchy of factors that need to be addressed to provide relief from the insomnia. To illustrate the use of this model in practice, consider the sample case at the end of this chapter.

CONTRIBUTING FACTORS IN CHRONIC INSOMNIA

There are many diverse factors that can contribute to poor sleep. It is helpful to organize them by general category in order to systematically evaluate possible contributing factors through the course of the evaluation.

Medical Factors

Many medical conditions are commonly associated with insomnia (5). A study of 3,445 patients being treated in a primary care setting with a diagnosis of diabetes, hypertension, congestive heart failure (CHF), postmyocardial infarction, and/or depression found that 50% of this sample had insomnia (5). Odds ratios ranged from 0.8 (diabetes mellitus) to 2.6 (depression) for mild insomnia and from 0.9 (myocardial infarction) to 8.2 (depression) for the presence of severe insomnia.

Chronic pain, CHD, chronic obstructive pulmonary disease (COPD), and Parkinson's disease (PD) are examples of other common medical conditions that have been linked to insomnia. However, the exact mechanism through which medical disorders contribute to poor sleep are not well understood. Insomnia in patients with medical disorders is probably caused through different mechanisms, depending on the nature of the illness. Patients with COPD may have increased hypercapnia when lying supine or during sleep secondary to hypoventilation, and this provides a stimulus to arousal and increased wakefulness (6). CHF can lead to periodic breathing during sleep, which is disruptive to sleep (7). Medical disorders associated with pain are presumed to disturb sleep as a consequence of arousal associated with discomfort. Autonomic dysfunction, medication effects, and depression have been proposed as possible causes of insomnia in patients with CHD (8).

It is difficult to be certain that insomnia is causally linked to a specific medical disorder in a given patient. For example, a patient with severe pain associated with osteoarthritis (OA) might only have developed poor sleep after having OA for many years. Alternatively, they might have struggled with intermittent insomnia since early adulthood, well before their symptoms of OA began. Simple coincidence of insomnia and medical illness is not sufficient to establish a causal relation between the two. Lichstein has suggested criteria that may be helpful in establishing whether insomnia is truly "secondary" to another primary disorder (9). He recommends that the contiguity between the origin of the primary disorder and the insomnia, as well as covariation between exacerbations of the primary disorder and the insomnia, be used to judge the causal relation between the two. The insomnia can absolutely be considered secondary to a primary medical disorder only when the origin and exacerbations of the insomnia are linked to the course of the medical disorder. Determining a relation between the course of the insomnia and a medical illness is more difficult when relying on a patient's attributions from historical data. A patient may perceive an illusory correlation between sleep and a medical condition or may miss a true correlation that is present. It is easier for the sleep clinician to discern a causal relation when they are following a patient over a period of months. Causes of insomnia that were not initially considered may emerge once the patient has had several cycles of insomnia while completing sleep logs (see below, *Sleep Logs*).

Psychiatric or Psychologic Factors

Psychologic factors that may contribute to insomnia encompass a wide range of phenomena. A normal variant in personality style, such as obsessive-compulsive or perfectionistic traits, may predispose an individual to insomnia. This can occur because these individuals have a high need for control and an episode of transient insomnia may trigger sufficient anxiety and concern regarding sleep that the insomnia becomes a chronic condition. In these cases, the insomnia may begin for any reason, such as a hospital stay, job stress, or travel, and then is maintained by cognitive (e.g., worry about sleep) and behavioral (eg, spending excessive time in bed) factors.

Psychiatric disorders show a strong association with insomnia, especially mood disorders (10). Depression is the most common single diagnosis for patients with insomnia presenting to sleep disorder centers (11,12). Many patients see their insomnia as the cause of their depressed mood and, therefore, seek out treatment in a sleep center instead of a psychiatry clinic. Other patients prefer somatic explanations for their symptoms, and present to sleep centers instead of psychiatry clinics for that reason. Anxiety disorders, such as posttraumatic stress disorder and panic disorder, also include insomnia among their symptoms. However, patients with anxiety disorders are more likely to see their sleep difficulty as a consequence of their anxiety, rather than the other way around. Therefore, it seems these patients are somewhat less likely to present to sleep centers than are patients with mood disorders.

The relation between mood disorders and insomnia is complex. Patients who have depression often develop insomnia as one of the symptoms of the disorder, consistent with the view that the insomnia is secondary to depression. Several theories have been proposed to explain sleep abnormalities in depressed patients. Decreased homeostatic sleep drive, circadian dysregulation, and increased rapid eye movement (REM) pressure are proposed explanations of sleep disturbance in depressed patients.

In contrast to the view that insomnia occurs secondary to depression, recent data show that an episode of insomnia is predictive of a future episode of major depression (13,14). In one study, individuals who had an episode of insomnia early in life, were twice as likely to be diagnosed with depression later in life, compared with those without an early episode of insomnia (13). These data suggest the possibility that insomnia may predispose to depression or that both share a common predisposition.

Medication Effects

Medications may cause insomnia through intended or unintended central nervous system (CNS) effects. Stimulants, selective serotonin reuptake inhibitors (SSRIs), decongestants, beta blockers, steroids, and bronchodilators are examples of classes of drugs that are associated with insomnia.

Use of hypnotic medication may also contribute to insomnia, but not because of side effects causing changes in CNS function, as described above. Instead, hypnotic medication, particularly short-acting compounds, are associated with rebound insomnia, on the first night of withdrawal (15). Although this effect is increased after multiple consecutive nights of drug administration, it can occur even after a single night of use (16). There are large individual differences in the experience of rebound insomnia, as some patients appear to be much more sensitive to this effect and have more intense rebound (16).

Cognitive–Behavioral Factors

There is a wide range of behavioral factors associated with insomnia. These are usually factors that develop once insomnia is already present to some degree, and these factors maintain the problem. Daytime behaviors, such as excessive caffeine or alcohol use, napping, or working right up to bedtime are examples. Nighttime behaviors include spending excessive time in bed, maintaining an irregular sleep–wake schedule, watching the clock at night, eating in the middle of the night, and engaging in sleep-incompatible behaviors in bed. This latter behavior can include any number of activities, such as watching TV, listening to the radio, reading books, or even surfing the Internet. Many of these behaviors are adopted in an effort to compensate for poor sleep (e.g., increased caffeine use, napping, going to bed early, and/or staying in bed late), or are attempts to improve sleep (e.g., watching TV in bed, having a snack during the night). However, although the behavior may have a short-term benefit, the long-term effect is to further contribute to a dysfunctional sleep pattern.

Behavioral factors may interfere with sleep in different ways. Large doses of coffee in the evening can interfere with sleep due to the CNS activity of caffeine. Engaging in stimulating activities in bed may lead to "conditioned" insomnia because of the association with wakefulness and the sleep environment.

Cognitive factors primarily include irrational fears about the consequences of not sleeping, as well as unreasonable expectations about sleep (17). Once an individual decides that they have a "sleep problem," their preoccupation with falling asleep quickly, or obtaining 8 hours of sleep each night, can lead to increased tension and arousal at bedtime or upon awakening during the night. Being fearful that daytime fatigue, or other insomnia-related impairment, will lead to the loss of one's job, divorce, or some other catastrophic outcome is obviously not conducive to feeling relaxed at bedtime.

Circadian Rhythm Factors

Shift-work sleep disorder can present as sleep onset or sleep maintenance insomnia, and delayed sleep-phase syndrome (DSPS) almost universally includes sleep onset insomnia as a symptom. Even when a formal circadian rhythm disorder is not diagnosed, circadian factors may play a role in insomnia and need to be evaluated. The most common example would be an individual who keeps a markedly different sleep–wake schedule on workdays versus days off. If an individual arises at 5 AM on workdays and at 9 AM on days off, we can assume that their circadian clock is set for sleep offset some time between those

two times. That is, if the "true" circadian clock sleep offset time is set about 8 AM, the individual may encounter some difficulty initiating sleep if they are going to bed at 10 PM in an attempt to obtain 7 hours in bed on a work night. This situation would be expected to be especially problematic in an individual who already struggles with insomnia for other reasons. The situation is not best understood as a case of DSPS because of the elements of conditioned insomnia. Rather, it is psychophysiologic insomnia with a circadian rhythm factor as a contributing risk factor.

Primary Sleep Disorders

Restless Legs Syndrome

Restless legs syndrome (RLS) is characterized by an unpleasant sensation in the legs, generally in the calf area, that leads to the need to move the legs in order to relieve the sensation. This usually occurs upon lying down in bed at night, but may also occur earlier in the day, especially when the individual is forced to hold his legs still, such as during a long car ride or while sitting at a movie theatre. In severe cases, patients report that they must actually arise and walk around the bedroom in order to feel relief. However, the RLS sensations often return once they lay back down in bed. Causes of RLS in the include uremia, iron-deficiency anemia (low ferritin), and peripheral neuropathy. Patients with RLS have very long sleep onset latencies and markedly decreased total sleep time, even relative to other patients with insomnia (18).

Periodic Limb Movement Disorder

Periodic limb movement disorder (PLMD) is marked by repetitive stereotyped movements of the leg muscle during sleep with a rhythmic pattern, typically with movements occurring about 30 seconds apart (19). The movements arise during NREM sleep and usually stop when the patient awakens, such that the patient is not aware of the problem. Therefore, the report of the bed partner is helpful in determining the level of suspicion for this disorder. PLMD often occurs in patients with RLS.

Sleep-Disordered Breathing

Obstructive sleep apnea (OSA), central sleep apnea, and sleep-related hypoventilation can all lead to disturbed sleep and a report of insomnia. In the case of OSA, most patients will present complaining of daytime sleepiness or snoring rather than insomnia. However, some patients with this disorder report difficulty maintaining sleep as their primary concern. Interestingly, these patients also often have poor sleep hygiene, giving them an even more insomnialike presentation (20). For example, these patients might leave the TV on in their bedroom throughout the night and watch intermittently when they awaken. They feel the TV is soothing and allows them to return to sleep more readily.

EVALUATION TECHNIQUES

Clinical Interview

A thorough clinical interview is at the center of any evaluation for a complaint of insomnia. This is in contrast to the evaluation for excessive sleepiness, where the interview will lead to hypotheses about the diagnosis, but the critical information is derived from polysomnography (PSG). Complete and accurate data from the clinical interview is essential to an appropriate diagnosis and treatment plan. Identifying a definitive diagnosis after this interview may not be possible, but the goal of this interview is to generate a list of two or three of the most important contributing factors.

Sleep History

Sleep–Wake Schedule

Obtaining a detailed sleep history is crucial in the evaluation of insomnia patients. This part of the history will include the customary bedtime, sleep onset latency, number and duration of periods of wakefulness through the night, and arising time (see Table 9-1). This information is needed for weekdays and weekends, as well as for those periods when the patient is sleeping well, compared to periods of insomnia. These data are used to characterize the severity of the insomnia and to identify possible contributing factors. For instance, some patients will extend time in bed on those nights when they have increased wake after sleep on-

▶ **TABLE 9-1. Interview Questions for the Sleep History for Insomnia**

What time do you get into bed at night?
Are you watching TV or reading at that time?
Do you fall asleep with the TV on?
If so, when do you turn it off?
How long does it take you to fall asleep once turn out the lights?
Do you sleep through the night or do you awaken?
How often do you awaken?
How long does it take you to return to sleep?
What do you do when awake at night?
Do you ever become angry or upset when awake in the middle of the night?
Do you look at the clock when you awaken during the night?
Do you ever have something to eat during the night?
What time do you get out of bed in the morning to start your day?
How long have you had this sleep pattern?
How much total sleep do you get per night?
How much sleep do you need to feel rested during the day?
What time did you go to bed and arise before you began to sleep poorly?

set and have arising times much later than usual. This may allow them more total sleep time (TST) on that night, but may then lead to greater difficulty getting back on schedule the following night. It may also give them a sleep period that is 10 to 12 hours in duration. This is how patients with insomnia who were lifelong 6- to 7-hour sleepers develop sleep periods that are much too long, and incorporate hours of wakefulness into their routine schedule.

If the insomnia occurs nightly, then the sleep schedule should be obtained for the period of time preceding the onset of the insomnia. This provides information on the discrepancies between features of the "normal" schedule and "insomnia" schedule that can provide insight into behavioral factors that may contribute to the insomnia. For example, a patient who is routinely going to bed at 10 PM because of tiredness, or in an attempt to get additional TST, may have forgotten that their bedtime prior to developing chronic insomnia (back when they were a "good sleeper") was midnight. The treatment plan will likely be aimed at re-establishing the sleep–wake schedule that was in place when the patient was sleeping well.

Sleep Period Activities

Detailed interviewing about activities before bedtime, as well as those during wakefulness at night, is also extremely important. The nature of presleep activities may explain a long sleep onset latency. Patients who do not allow a sufficient buffer zone for leisure activities between work and sleep are likely to be too tense and aroused to fall asleep quickly. Some patients may get home from work, school, or other social engagements at 10 PM, and then go to bed at 10:30 PM.

Upon awakening during the night, a patient engaging in stimulating activities may have markedly increased difficulty returning to sleep. Very specific questions must be asked about these activities because patients will often not think to volunteer this information. Patients may routinely eat upon awakening during the night, but not understand that this is relevant to their problem, and will not spontaneously report it. The same applies to having a TV, radio, or light on in the bedroom during the night, playing videogames, reading email, surfing the Internet, or any number of other activities that patients engage in when awake during the night.

Sleep Hygiene

Detailed questions about habits expected to impact sleep are needed. This includes assessing the patient's sleep environment with respect to noise (e.g., snoring spouse, street traffic) and light. Documenting the frequency and timing of napping and exercise, as well as the use of caffeinated beverages, alcohol, and tobacco is essential. A description of the variability in bedtimes and arising times from night to night should be elicited during the interview, although the most useful source of data in this regard is likely to be the sleep log (discussed below).

Daytime Consequences

Understanding the impact of poor sleep on daytime function is critical for several reasons. First, it gives another indication of the severity of the insomnia. For many patients, being awake at night is only a concern to the extent that they suffer during the day from various fatigue-related symptoms. A clear understanding of the degree of daytime impairment helps determine how aggressive the treatment should be. A patient who is having significant trouble functioning at work due to decreased attention and memory will require a different approach from one who, despite short sleep, describes no significant alteration of daytime function. Second, the patient's description of their sleep-related impairment may illuminate cognitive distortions. For example, if a patient reports that failure to obtain a promotion at work, marital conflict, or episodes of severe anxiety or depression are all consequences of insomnia, it is likely that these attributions are inaccurate. These attributions create additional pressure to obtain sleep and contribute further to insomnia.

In addition, most patients with insomnia describe tiredness or fatigue, but not sleepiness. They are able to stay awake when they choose to during the day and more likely will not be able to nap if they lie down and attempt to do so. If a patient reports falling asleep inappropriately during the day, this should suggest the possibility of sleep-disordered breathing or PLMD as a cause of sleep disturbance.

Cognitive Features

Information about the patient's fears regarding their insomnia, and their beliefs about sleep, will be needed for treatment planning. Many patients have become very fearful of insomnia, and this can cause frustration and anger. This aspect of the problem is assessed by asking the patient how often they worry about their sleep during the day and about their expectations regarding total sleep time. Once a patient decides that "I have a sleep problem that is ruining my life," there are many other changes that follow. When a patient blames insomnia for every personal failure, there is also the possibility that they receive secondary gain from the insomnia. This further complicates treatment because there is a high psychological price to be paid if they sleep well; they will no longer have an excuse for not achieving their goals.

Some patients believe that their physical integrity is being eroded due to lack of sleep. This is especially likely in older patients with medical illness who may even have been told that rest is an essential part of their treatment. They may then spend extra time in bed to get more "rest," but spend time worrying about not acquiring adequate sleep.

Medical and Psychiatric History

Careful documentation of all medical and psychiatric diagnoses, along with exacerbations of illnesses, is needed. The insomnia is considered secondary to a primary medical or psychiatric disorder when there is contiguity between the origin of the insomnia and the primary disorder (9). There should also be contiguity between exacerbations of the primary illness and episodes of insomnia. However, it can be difficult to definitively determine if insomnia is secondary to a primary medical or psychiatric illness. In cases of chronic insomnia, cognitive–behavioral factors are universally present as perpetuating factors. Therefore, medical or psychiatric causes of insomnia may act as precipitants, either chronically or intermittently, and both sets of factors will ultimately need to be addressed in the treatment plan.

Identifying psychiatric factors as early as possible is important since these factors are likely to considerably complicate treatment (Table 9-2). Patients with significant psychiatric disease will struggle and continue to have elevated distress if treatment is aimed at sleep alone. One subtype of patient with comorbid psychiatric illness and insomnia seen commonly in sleep centers is the patient who attributes all of their psychiatric/psychologic symptoms to their poor sleep and does not have insight into their psychologic problems. These patients insist that they would not be anxious, depressed, and miserable if only their sleep were improved, despite evidence to the contrary. These patients are very stressful to treat if the sleep specialist accepts these attributions and is caught up in the panic of trying to maximize sleep as the lone goal of therapy. Patients with personality disorders may be especially frustrating, since they may refuse to adhere to basic treatment recommendations, yet paradoxically insist that the sleep

▶ **TABLE 9-2. Interview Questions to Identify Psychiatric Factors in Patients with Insomnia**

Have you felt depressed lately? If yes: Tell me more about that.
Have you had difficulty with depression in the past?
If so, how was it treated? How severe did it become? Was your sleep affected?
How is your appetite? Has your weight changed recently?
How is your weight different compared to one year ago?
Have you had crying spells?
Have you had thoughts of hurting yourself or killing yourself?
Are you an anxious or nervous person? If yes: Tell me more about that.
Have you had panic attacks?
Do you have phobias?
Do you have intrusive thoughts?
Do others consider you to be perfectionistic?
Are you a person who likes everything to be very organized?
Do you need to check things many times in a row (e.g., see if the door is locked)?
Do you count things (e.g., stairs or steps to a certain location)?

specialist do something to restore normal sleep. This problem falls under treatment approaches, but is mentioned here to point out the importance of accurately diagnosing psychiatric factors prior to treatment planning.

Use of Medication

Assessing the impact of medications that are associated with insomnia is accomplished by reviewing the contiguity of the sleep disturbance and the initiation of a trial of new medication, or changes in dosages of medications. Since side effects are generally dose-dependent, it is possible that insomnia only begins when a certain medication is increased to a higher dose (e.g., fluoxetine). In some cases, it is possible to taper or discontinue medications suspected of contributing to insomnia in order to determine positively if that medication is responsible for the insomnia.

Documenting the frequency, dosage, and pattern of use of medication, especially hypnotic medication, is needed. Often these patients may be taking anxiolytic and/or hypnotic medication on a PRN schedule, and it is difficult get precise information from an interview. Use of a sleep log can be more helpful in this regard.

Past Treatment Attempts

Documenting past treatment regimens and their effectiveness will help with diagnosis and treatment planning (Table 9-3). Most patients presenting for evaluation to a sleep specialist will have already undergone pharmacologic

▶ **TABLE 9-3. Interview Questions Regarding Pharmacologic Treatment for Insomnia**

What medications have you taken for sleep?

What was the dosage?

For how long did you take it?

What time did you take it?

Did you take it every night (day)?

If no, how did you decide which nights you would take it?

Did you take the whole dosage at once, or break it into partial dosages that were taken at different times as the night progressed?

Did you ever take additional medication beyond what was prescribed?

Did you ever take additional medication in the middle of the night after awakening?

How effective was the medication at improving sleep onset? Sleep maintenance?

Was there any evidence of side effects, such as daytime sedation, motor impairment, or memory impairment?

Was daytime function improved in any way with use of medication?

Are you taking medication currently?

If not, why did you stop using sleep medication?

When you discontinued the medication, did you taper the dose or stop abruptly?

Did you experience worse sleep after discontinuing?

treatment, usually with more than one compound and perhaps at various dosages. Attention must be paid to the classes of drugs used. A patient may report having failed a clinical trial on a medication, but it is important to determine that it was a fair trial (i.e., the correct dosage for the patient or, in the case of antidepressants, for the correct duration of time). Patients may report "I took sleeping pills, but they did not work for me." This should not be accepted at face value; more detailed information is needed. If a 30-year-old patient took zolpidem, but only at a dosage of 5 mg, a therapeutic response would not be expected because the dosage is too low. Therefore, that would not be considered a treatment failure since the appropriate therapeutic dosage for that patient (i.e., 10 mg) was never used. Alternatively, a patient may report having taken antidepressants (e.g., paroxetine, 20 mg) for sleep without benefit. However, if you determine that they took the medication for only 3 days, this should not be considered a legitimate clinical trial, since benefit to sleep from remediation of an underlying depression would not be expected until after weeks of treatment.

An important dimension to assessing past hypnotic use is to determine how and when the medication was taken. If a patient reports having taken zaleplon at 8 PM and then going to bed at 10:30 PM, they have missed the therapeutic window of the medication (i.e., half-life of 1 hour) and a therapeutic response is not expected. Understanding past patterns of hypnotic use, and the impact of these trials, will be helpful in determining the future role of pharmacologic treatment in the overall management of the insomnia, and also provides information about the patient's ability to cope with their insomnia. For example, a patient who routinely takes additional medication during the night, beyond what has been prescribed, is likely to have a higher anxiety level and worse coping skills than a patient who adheres to the prescribed regimen despite a poor night of sleep. In addition, understanding which regimens were effective in the past may provide insight into the nature of the insomnia. A patient who reports having responded poorly to short-acting hypnotics, may report a positive response to a long-acting hypnotic. This scenario suggests that there may be an underlying anxiety disorder such that sedation through the day provides therapeutic benefit for both anxiety and sleep, while a short-acting compound may be insufficient to adequately reduce anxiety at night, and may also lead to rebound anxiety in the morning.

A positive response to hypnotic use does not necessarily mean this is the treatment of choice, but may offer insight into the cause of the insomnia. A patient who was placed on an appropriate dosage of sedating medication that was taken appropriately would be expected to report some degree of improvement in sleep. If this did not occur, it suggests that the accuracy of the patient's subjective report may be decreased (i.e., sleep-state misperception), or that the cause of the insomnia is not one amenable to sedation (e.g., depression, or sleep-disordered breathing).

Expectations of Treatment

Understanding what benefit patients expect from improved sleep provides insight into their attributions about their poor sleep. Patients who feel that their real or imagined failure in the workplace or at home is due to inadequate sleep is presenting with important obstacles to improvement. First, the ability to approach sleep in a rational manner is markedly reduced if one believes that their ability to be an adequate husband, father, or employee is tied to TST. The amount of tension and frustration created by lying in bed trying to fall asleep quickly in order to obtain acceptable sleep to be able to perform one's responsibilities during the day is likely to be considerable. In addition, these patients may be obtaining secondary gain from their insomnia in that they can blame any setbacks or personal shortcomings on their poor sleep, rather than take direct responsibility. In this type of case, a patient may be reluctant to give up their insomnia, despite their assertions to the contrary. A few questions about expectations from treatment are sufficient to gain insight into this area.

Sleep Logs

Information obtained from the clinical interview regarding the habitual sleep–wake schedule should be supplemented with at least 2 weeks of sleep log data. Daily charting of bedtimes and arising times, use of alcohol and caffeine, use of hypnotic medication, fatigue ratings, and napping behavior give a more precise picture of events than a self-report of habitual behavior given during the consultation. Ideally, the patient will complete the log on a daily basis, as this provides the greatest accuracy. These data may reveal patterns or variability not apparent from the patient's description of their sleep behavior. For example, use of PRN hypnotic medication may be sufficiently erratic that it is hard for a patient to describe their normative behavior in this area. For some patients, the sleep log data may deviate significantly from their description of their habitual sleep pattern. It should not be assumed that the patient has purposely misrepresented their behavior. Most individuals, normal sleepers included, have night-to-night variability in their presleep activities and bedtimes such that some "smoothing" is needed to describe a customary sleep schedule. Even though 11 PM may be the goal, this bedtime may only occur two nights per week because of family responsibilities, late games on TV, and other distractions. Given the large night-to-night variability in the sleep of patients with insomnia, providing an "average" schedule that accurately reflects their true sleep schedule is daunting. Sleep log data are much better at providing insight into the variability in sleep than are reports of habitual sleep patterns.

Psychometric Testing

Brief psychometric scales designed to quantify depression or anxiety can be helpful screening tools in the evaluation of insomnia patients. For example, the Beck Depression Inventory (BDI) consists of 20 test questions and can be completed in just a few minutes (21). Although a psychometric test is no substitute for a careful clinical interview, it can provide objective data to assist in evaluating the seriousness of mood symptoms (available at www.HarcourtAssessment.com). The test scores can confirm the clinical impression when a patient is reporting significant problems with depression or provide insight when depressive symptoms are denied during the interview. Some individuals are more candid when completing a questionnaire by themselves than when answering questions asked by a health care professional, especially concerning difficult emotional issues.

More elaborate psychometric testing might be needed when it appears that there are significant psychological issues that are difficult to diagnose with only clinical interview data.

Physical Exam

A physical exam for a patient presenting with a complaint of insomnia will be aimed at detecting evidence of medical disorders that may be contributing to poor sleep. This exam will screen for undiagnosed disorders and also evaluate the status of diagnosed disorders that might be undertreated. In particular, hyperthyroidism, lung disease, hypertension, and CHF are examples of disorders that might be suspected based on the physical exam.

Polysomnography

Abnormalities found using PSG have been shown to vary according to the insomnia subtype (18). However, PSG is not essential for many patients presenting with a complaint of insomnia and is not often used clinically. When cognitive, behavioral, or circadian rhythm factors are the primary factors contributing to poor sleep, the diagnosis and treatment plan can be decided using interview data. PSG is indicated for those patients who are suspected to have a primary sleep disorder, such as sleep-disordered breathing or PLMD, or when a patient has failed to improve following standard treatment (22). Although patients with sleep-disordered breathing usually have other presenting complaints, such as excessive daytime sleepiness or loud snoring, these patients occasionally focus on their disturbed nocturnal sleep and present as an insomnia patient. PSG is needed to definitively rule out these primary sleep disorders.

Another disorder requiring PSG to make the diagnosis is sleep-state misperception. This disorder is suspected whenever a patient reports total insomnia lasting long periods, but cannot be definitively diagnosed without objective measurement of sleep.

There is other information from a polysomnogram that may assist in making a diagnosis. Abnormal REM parameters, such as a short REM latency and long first

REM period, in conjunction with clinical data consistent with depression, would help solidify a diagnosis of depression as the primary diagnosis in a case that may otherwise be ambiguous. A diagnosis of depression should never be made based on a short REM latency alone, but it can be difficult to discriminate between a diagnosis of psychophysiologic insomnia and mood disorder in patients with features of both disorders. Objective documentation of the distribution of wakefulness at night may also help with treatment planning. For instance, patients with a long sleep onset latency or long awakenings in the middle of the night would be expected to respond better to stimulus control therapy than a patient with frequent brief awakenings during the night. Stimulus control therapy requires that a patient leave the bedroom when wide awake for about 20 minutes and return when drowsy. Although PSG would not be ordered only to obtain this ancillary information (e.g., REM latency and distribution of wakefulness), it is important to note in those instances when polysomnographic data is available (e.g., a primary sleep disorder was suspected, but ruled out). Unfortunately, many sleep specialists will interpret a polysomnogram as having ruled out sleep apnea and PLMD, but then make no use of the rest of the data to help diagnose the cause of the sleep complaint.

Actigraphy

Actigraphy measures physical activity with a portable device (usually including an accelerometer) worn on the wrist. These data can be stored for weeks and then downloaded into a computer. Sleep and wake time can be estimated by analyzing these movement data. This approach to estimating sleep and wake has been shown to correlate with polysomnographic measures in normal sleepers, with reduced agreement in patients with insomnia (23).

Actigraphy has an advantage over a sleep log in that it is an objective measure and, therefore, not subject to self-report bias or demand characteristics. It is much less expensive than PSG, although it cannot provide data on depth of sleep or other aspects of sleep architecture that require EEG measures. However, because it is inexpensive and easily tolerated by patients, it can provide data on sleep–wake function for multiple nights (Fig. 9-2). Measuring sleep across many nights is desirable given the high night-to-night variability of sleep for patients with

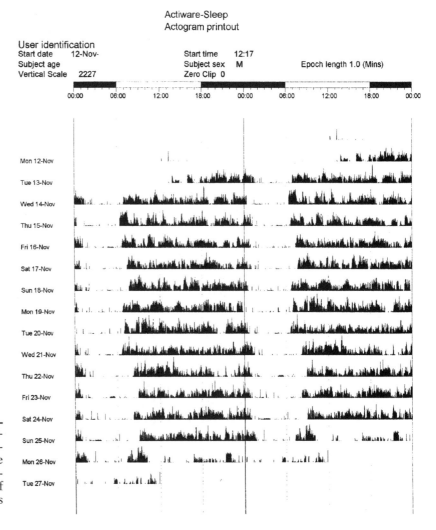

FIGURE 9-2. Printout of actigraphy data collected using an Actiwatch (Mini-Mitter Company Inc., Bend OR). This output is from the Actiware software package used with this device. The dark bars indicate various levels of activity, correlating with wakefulness. Sleep is indicated by the absence of activity.

insomnia (24). Besides estimating sleep parameters, such as TST and sleep efficiency, actigraphy can provide objective data on the temporal aspects of sleep habits; that is, the consistency of bedtimes and arising times, as well as episodes of napping, which can be determined from these data.

DIAGNOSIS: INTEGRATION OF FINDINGS

The use of the model and principles described above are illustrated through presentation and analysis of the following case example.

Sample Case

The patient is a 62-year-old man who describes persistent difficulty sleeping for the past 2 years following hip replacement surgery. He had severe postsurgical pain and, subsequently, had an episode of depression during rehabilitation. The depression was treated with 20 mg paroxetine for 6 months. He denies current problems with depression. He takes 10 mg zolpidem at 8:30 PM every night. He gets into bed about 10 or 11 PM and watches TV until he falls asleep, which may be 1 to 2 hours later. He has several awakenings during the night and usually has something to eat during one of these awakenings. He arises at 8 or 9 AM, depending on how well he slept the previous night. During the day, he reports irritability, fatigue, and trouble concentrating. He works as an attorney and feels that his daytme impairment compromises his ability to complete his work assignments. He denies ever falling asleep unintentionally during the day. Prior to this current episode of insomnia, the patient reports having occasional periods of insomnia throughout his life that he attributes to various causes: acute work stress, travel to Europe, or bereavement associated with his mother's death. These episodes of insomnia usually resolved in less than 1 month. He did use hypnotic medication on rare occasions. His usual sleep–wake schedule prior to his knee replacement surgery was 11:30 PM to 6 AM. He reports being rested in the past with 6 hours sleep, but believes he now requires more.

Analysis

This history is complex in that there are medical, psychiatric, and behavioral factors in the history. Using the Speilman model, it appears that this patient has a mild to moderate predisposition to insomnia, given his prior episodes of insomnia that occurred throughout his life. It is likely that the postsurgical pain was the initial precipitating event for the current episode of insomnia. As that event remitted, the episode of depression further precipitated poor sleep. The episode of depression was successfully treated, but, by then, there were cognitive–behavioral factors acting as perpetuating factors. Excessive time in bed, a variable sleep schedule, and chronic worry about sleep developed later, after the insomnia had been present for a few months; they now contribute to the continuation of the insomnia. This understanding helps to focus the treatment on the cognitive and behavioral factors, particularly if it is verified that the precipitating events are no longer active. Also, explaining to the patient how the factors that have caused his insomnia have changed over time can give him better insight into the problem, as well as highlight the need to make the recommended behavioral changes.

A tentative diagnosis would be psychophysiologic insomnia. Initial goals of treatment would include reducing time in bed to match his life-long average of 6 to 6.5 hours in bed. A schedule of 12 to 6:30 AM might be a place to begin, depending on the patient's enthusiasm for this schedule change. Initially, taking the zolpidem at 11:30 PM would be more appropriate, since he is currently taking the medication much too early. As treatment progresses, the medication can be tapered to 5 mg for a week or two, and then discontinued. The patient should be prohibited from eating between 12 and 6:30 AM. Cognitive therapy aimed at his fears about his insomnia may also be important at this time.

Assume that you have instituted the treatment plan above and the patient reports much improvement, but still struggles to fall asleep within 30 minutes of bedtime. During treatment, you obtain two weeks of actigraphy to help assess the patient's progress (Fig. 9-2). These data help demonstrate the effectiveness of the treatment (e.g., consolidated sleep between 1 AM and 7 to 9 AM). In addition, the patient appears to be oversleeping some mornings, and this is followed by a longer sleep onset latency the following night. It may be helpful to point this out to patients so that they can observe the relation between their sleep schedule and insomnia.

SUMMARY

Chronic insomnia requires a systematic evaluation of medical, psychiatric, cognitive, behavioral, medication-related, and circadian factors. By classifying all identified factors as predisposing, precipitating, or perpetuating, it is easier to construct a hierarchy of which factors are most important for treatment. An accurate understanding of the relevant factors consists of a thorough evaluation that minimally includes a detailed clinical interview and sleep logs. PSG is only occasionally needed, usually to rule out a primary sleep disorder.

REFERENCES

1. Spielman AJ, Caruso L, Glovinsky P. A behavioral perspective on insomnia. *Psych Clin North Amer.* 1987;10:541–553.
2. Bonnet MH, Arand D. Hyperarousal and insomnia. *Sleep Med Rev.* 1997;1:97–108.

3. Stepanski E, Zorick F, Roehrs T, et al. Daytime alertness in patients with chronic insomnia compared with asymptomatic control subjects. *Sleep.* 1988;11:54–60.

4. Besset A, Villemin E, Tafti M, et al. Homeostatic process and sleep spindles in patients with sleep-maintenance insomnia: effect of partial (21 h) sleep deprivation: *Electroenceph Clin Neurophysiol.* 1998;107:122–132.

5. Katz DA, McHorney CA. Clinical correlates of insomnia in patients with chronic illness. *Arch Internal Medi.* 1998;158:1101–1107.

6. Sandek K, Andersson T, Bratel T, et al. Sleep quality, carbon dioxide responsiveness and hypoxaemic patterns in nocturnal hypoxaemia due to chronic obstructive pulmonary disease (COPD) without daytime hypoxaemia. *Respir Med.* 1999;93:79–87.

7. Bradley TD. Sleep disturbances in respiratory and cardiovascular disease. *J Psychosom Res.* 1993;37 (suppl.1):13–17.

8. Schwartz S, McDowell Anderson W, Cole SR, et al. Insomnia and heart disease: a review of epidiemologic studies. *J Psychosom Res.* 1999;47:313–333.

9. Lichstein KL. Secondary insomnia. In: Lichstein KL, Morin CM, eds. *Treatment of late-life insomnia.* Thousand Oaks, CA: Sage, 2000.

10. Benca RM, Obermeyer WH, Thisted RA, et al. Sleep and psychiatric disorders: a meta-analysis. *Arch Gen Psychi.* 1992;49:651–668.

11. Buysse D, Reynolds C, Kupfer D, et al. Clinical diagnoses in 216 insomnia patients using the International Classification of Sleep Disorders (ICSD), DSM-IV and ICD-10 categories: a report from the APA/NIMH DSM-IV field trial. *Sleep.* 1994;17:630–637.

12. Coleman RM, Roffwarg HP, Kennedy SJ, et al. Sleep–wake disorders based on a polysomnographic diagnosis. A national cooperative study. *J Amer Med Associ.* 1982;247:997–1003.

13. Chang PP, Ford DE, Mead LA, et al. Insomnia in young men and subsequent depression. The Johns Hopkins precursors study. *Amer J Epidemiol.* 1997;146:105–114.

14. Ford DE, Kamerow DB. Epidemiologic study of sleep disturbance and psychiatric disorders: an opportunity for prevention. *JAMA.* 1989;262:1479–1484.

15. Kales A, Scharf M, Kales J. Rebound insomnia: a new clinical syndrome. *Science.* 1978;201:1039–1040.

16. Merlotti L, Roehrs T, Zorick F, et al. Rebound insomnia: duration of use and individual differences. *J Clin Psychopharmacol.* 1991;11:368–373.

17. Morin CM, Stone J, Trinkle D, et al. Dysfunctional beliefs and attitudes about sleep among older adults with and without insomnia complaints. *Psychology Aging.* 1993;8:463–467.

18. Zorick F, Roth T, Hartse K, et al. Evaluation and diagnosis of persistent insomnia. *Amer. J Psych.* 1981;138:769–773.

19. American Sleep Disorders Association. *The international classification of sleep disorders, revised: Diagnostic and coding manual.* Rochester, MN: American Sleep Disorders Association, 1997.

20. Graci GM, Stepanski EJ. The relation between sleep. hygiene behaviors and severity of sleep disordered breathing. *Sleep.* 2002;25:A348 (Abstr).

21. Beck AT. *Depression inventory.* Philadelphia: Center for Cognitive Therapy, 1978.

22. Reite M, Buysse B, Reynolds C, et al. The use of polysomnography in the evaluation of insomnia. *Sleep.* 1995;18:58–70.

23. Ancoli-Israel S, Cole R, Alessi C et al. The role of actigraphy in the study of sleep and circadian rhythms. *Amer Acad Sleep Med Rev Pap Sleep.* 2003;26:342–392.

24. Wohlgemuth W, Edinger J, Fins A, et al. How many nights are enough? The short-term stability of sleep parameters in elderly insomniacs and normal sleepers. *Psychophysiology.* 1999;36:233–244.

Nocturnal Events

Troy Payne

In the course of clinical practice many unusual nocturnal phenomena may be described by patients. The correct diagnosis can often be ascertained by distinguishing certain clinical features from the history. In other cases, the etiology of the events may only be determined by polysomnography (PSG). With modern digital equipment, additional leads can easily be applied to assist in diagnosis. Additional EEG leads should be used if a seizure disorder is suspected. Additional EMG leads can be useful in patients with movement disorders. What follows is a collection of clinical vignettes, often with a sample page from a polysomnogram. This is followed by a discussion of the differential diagnosis.

THE TWITCHER

Chief complaint: "She jerks at night in her sleep" per husband.

History of present illness: A 35-year-old woman presents with her husband. She complains that for the past 2 years she has felt tired during the day. Her family physician thought she might be depressed and put her on an antidepressant. This did not really help her sleepiness. She states she has never snored. She goes to bed regularly at 10:30 PM and falls asleep quickly. She awakens from sleep a few times in the first 2 to 3 hours. She then sleeps through the rest of the night and awakens the next morning at 6:30 AM before her alarm clock sounds at 6:45 AM. She is usually tired all day. Her husband adds that she sometimes jerks

her legs. She denies having any restless legs symptoms at night or during the day.

Medical history: Past history of anemia felt to be secondary to fibroids; hemoglobin stabilized in normal range after hysterectomy 4 years ago. Depression.

Medications: A serotonin uptake inhibitor, which she has tried for 6 months.

Family history: Her mother has insomnia and takes clonazepam at night. Her brother had febrile seizures as a child and has very rare complex partial seizures under good control with an anticonvulsant medication as an adult.

Review of systems: No headaches, vertigo, dizziness, episodes of loss of consciousness, palpitations, difficulty breathing, snoring, nausea, back pain, leg pain, incontinence, or weight change. She complains of some intermittent insomnia and daytime tiredness.

Exam: Well appearing woman who yawns a couple times and does appear tired. Sixty-eight inches tall; 155 pounds. Blood pressure 118/69 and pulse 72. Normal nasal airflow and oropharnyx by exam. Regular heart rate and rhythm. Lungs are clear to auscultation. Completely normal neurologic examination with no evidence of neuropathy. Epworth Sleepiness Scale of 14. Laboratory studies show a normal hemoglobin, ferritin, iron level, and total iron binding capacity.

Polysomnogram and Multiple Sleep Latency Test (MSLT): RDI 0.1. Minimum oxygenation 94%. There is an increase in stage 1 sleep at 32% and a decrease in the expected percentage of slow-wave sleep (SWS). Periodic leg movement

▶ **TABLE 10-1. Arousal Disorders**[a]

Confusional arousals
Sleepwalking
Sleep terrors

[a]From Reference (1).

▶ **TABLE 10-2. Sleep–Wake Transition Disorders**[a]

Rhythmic movement disorder
Sleep starts
Sleep talking
Nocturnal leg cramps

[a]From Reference (1).

▶ **TABLE 10-3. Parasomnias Usually Associated with REM Sleep**[a]

Nightmares
Sleep paralysis
Impaired sleep-related penile erections
Sleep-related painful erections
REM sleep-related sinus arrest
REM sleep-behavior disorder

[a]From Reference (1).

▶ **TABLE 10-4. Other Parasomnias**[a]

Sleep bruxism
Sleep enuresis
Sleep-related abnormal swallowing syndrome
Nocturnal paroxysmal dystonia
Sudden unexplained nocturnal death syndrome
Primary snoring
Infant sleep apnea
Congenital central hypoventilation syndrome
Sudden infant death syndrome
Benign neonatal sleep myoclonus

[a]From Reference (1).

▶ **TABLE 10-5. Twitching, Jerking, or Kicking**[a]

Periodic limb movement disorder
Rhythmic movement disorder
Restless leg syndrome
Hypnic jerks
Seizures
Obstructive sleep apnea

[a]From Reference (1).

(PLM) index 42; PLM arousal index 15.2. Mean sleep latency 4.9 minutes with no REM sleep on MSLT (Fig. 10-1).

Diagnosis and differential: Periodic limb movement disorder (PLMD) is "characterized by periodic episodes of repetitive and highly stereotyped limb movements that occur during sleep" (1). While these movements usually occur in the legs, they can also occur in the arms. There is usually extension of the toe and flexion of the ankle, knee, and hip. Most patients are not aware of the movements. The sleep disruption associated with the movements can lead to insomnia or daytime somnolence. Periodic limb movements usually start soon after onset of NREM sleep. They are usually less common in slow-wave sleep and rarer in REM sleep. There is a repetitive increase in EMG activity (most often measured over the anterior tibialis muscle) lasting 0.5 to 5 seconds. The movement can be synchronous or asynchronous with the other leg or only involve one extremity. Both legs (and even the arms) should be monitored if PLMD is suspected. The movements are between 5 and 90 seconds apart. Most of the time, the movements occur every 20 to 40 seconds. Four or more consecutive movements are needed to count them as PLMs. The PLM index is the total number of movements divided by the total hours of sleep. A PLM index over 5 is considered abnormal. Often, PLMs are associated with arousals. A PLM arousal index may also be noted on the sleep study interpretation. While many assume that the higher the PLM arousal index the more likely one is to suffer from daytime sleepiness, this has not been proven (2).

Individuals with restless leg syndrome (RLS), narcolepsy, and obstructive sleep apnea (OSA) often have PLMs on a polysomnogram. RLS is sometimes associated with anemia, uremia, and pregnancy. While all patients with PLMD and most patients with RLS have PLMs on a sleep study, only the RLS patients have the daytime annoying sensations in their limbs that improve with movement. Use of caffeine, neuroleptics, alcohol, monoamine oxidase inhibitors, or tricyclic antidepressants can cause PLMs. Withdrawal of benzodiazepines, barbiturates, and certain hypnotics can cause or aggravate PLMs. These movements are rare in children but increase in prevalence with age. PLMs may be seen in patients who are asymptomatic. Inadequate sleep habits, psychophysiologic insomnia, and other causes of daytime tiredness need to be considered and treated before placing a patient on medication for this condition.

There are a few conditions that mimic PLMs. Sleep starts or hypnic jerks are frequently mentioned by patients. These occur in drowsiness, may be associated with a feeling of falling, and do not recur repetitively throughout sleep. Seizures can cause nighttime kicking movements, but may also cause nocturnal enuresis, morning musculoskeletal soreness, or bleeding from oral laceration. An expanded additional 16-lead EEG on the polysomnogram is invaluable in identifying these individuals. Many people

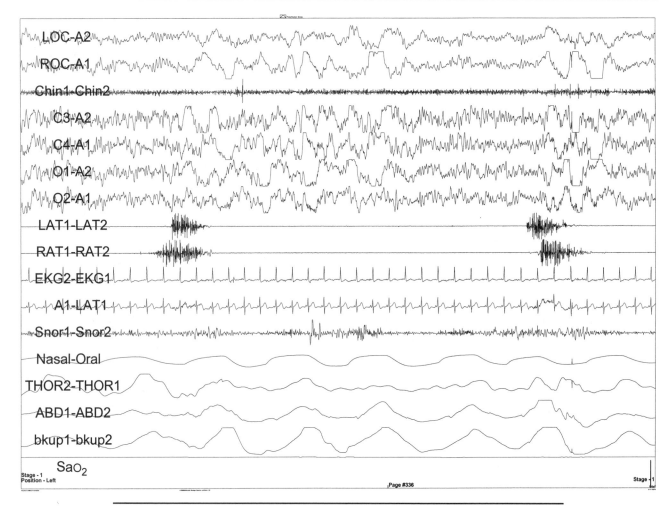

FIGURE 10-1. Periodic leg movements seen synchronously in stage 2 sleep; 30-second page.

with sleep apnea have periodic limb movements that disappear with initiation of continuous positive airway pressure (CPAP). If a patient has a high PLM index even after titrated to an appropriate CPAP pressure and continues to complain of sleepiness despite faithful use of CPAP, consider treating the PLMs.

This woman was treated with pramipexole and found her sleep much more refreshing. Her husband stated she hardly ever kicked in bed at night anymore. Similar to medical treatment for RLS, dopamine agonists, benzodiazepines, anticonvulsants, and analgesics are often helpful in the treatment of PLMs.

THE ROCKER

Chief complaint: Nocturnal movements

History of present illness: A 40-year-old patient with a static encephalopathy presents with the director of the group home into which he just moved. The patient suffered perinatal hypoxia and had developmental delays as a child. He has never had a documented seizure. His father died several years ago in a motor vehicle accident. The pa-

tient's mother recently passed away and the patient moved into the group home last month. The director states the patient usually goes to bed around 10 PM and gets up at 6:30 AM. The group home director states that a supervisor has found the patient rhythmically kicking in bed or knocking the back of his head against the bed. This almost always happens early in the night, soon after bedtime. The patient usually alerts easily from these events but has no knowledge of them. The patient has never bitten his tongue or had incontinence during these events.

Medical history: Static encephalopathy from perinatal hypoxia. Full Scale IQ (FSIQ) 61.

Medications: None.

Social history: Lived his whole life with his parents. He recently moved to group home after mother's death.

▌ **TABLE 10-6. Rocking/Repetitive Movements**[a]

Rhythmic movement disorder
Seizures
Bruxism
Periodic limb movement

[a]From Reference (1).

Family history: Father had sleep apnea and was treated with CPAP.

Review of systems: Denies restless leg symptoms, headaches, incontinence, abdominal pain, musculoskeletal pain, or nightmares.

Physical exam: Seventy inches tall; 225 pounds. His oropharynx appears normal. No maceration of tongue or buccal mucosa. No abrasions or bruising on scalp. Moderately mentally retarded. Appears to have normal tone and reflexes. No evidence of neuropathy. Has diffuse mild hypotonicity and a slightly wide-based gait.

Polysomnogram: Diffuse baseline slowing of EEG at 7 Hz. No epileptiform activity. Delayed sleep onset at 63 minutes. Rhythmic movement artifact for much of the first hour of the study. RDI 0.2. Minimum oxygenation 90%. Video showed patient bouncing legs or having rocking behaviors (Fig. 10-2).

Diagnosis and differential: Rhythmic movement disorder (RMD) "comprises a group of stereotyped, repetitive movements involving large muscles, usually of the head

and neck; the movements typically occur immediately prior to sleep onset and are sustained into light sleep" [ICSD (1), pp. 152–154]. This can manifest as repetitive head banging, leg banging, or body rolling. The movements typically start during drowsiness. Movements typically occur at a frequency of 0.5 to 2 times per second. While very common in normal infants, it is sometimes associated with a static encephalopathy, autism, or psychopathology in older children and adults. It is thought to have a self-soothing effect for some individuals. It appears to be more common in males. The noise from the movements can be disturbing to family members. My practice includes one teenager who developed a subdural hematoma from RMD. It is very important to have the technologist accurately document what was seen at the time this occurs in the sleep laboratory. Continuous video monitoring usually easily confirms the diagnosis.

The differential includes nocturnal seizures, masturbation, bruxism, and PLMD. Nocturnal seizures can usually be diagnosed by concomitant extra 16-channel EEG and

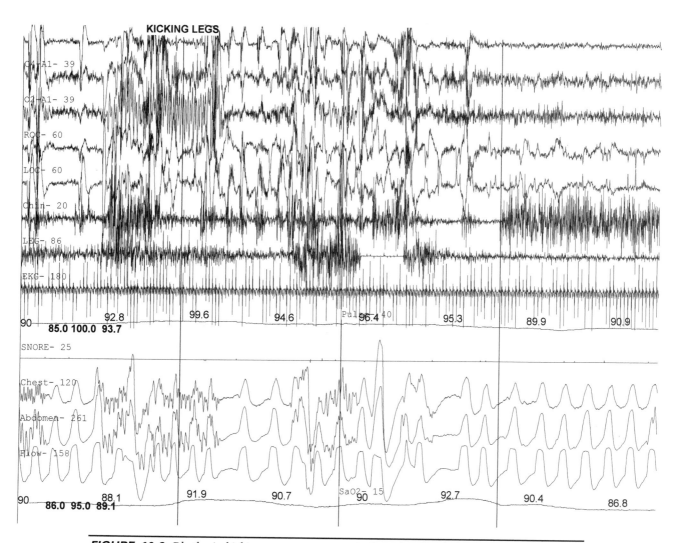

FIGURE 10-2. Rhythmic kicking movements seen during relaxed wakefulness and stage 1 sleep; 120-second page.

review of the video. Masturbation has been mistaken for RMD. Bruxism and PLMD are usually easily distinguished on the sleep study. Gasping respirations from sleep apnea can cause rhythmic movements.

This patient could have had these movements since early childhood, or they could have just started from the stress of the recent move to the group home. A counselor spent several sessions with the patient and the group home personnel to help with the transition to the new living environment. The movements improved dramatically, but worsened during times of greater stress.

THE CHEWER

Chief complaint: Headaches.

History of present illness: A 26-year-old woman presents with headaches. Patient states she has been treated by a neurologist for chronic daily headaches for the past year with only limited success. She states she often awakens with pain in her temples. Over time, a beta blocker, a calcium-channel blocker, and one anticonvulsant medication were tried, but the headaches never completely went away. When the headaches are at their worst she has trouble concentrating. She has never had scintillating scotomata, photophobia, or vomiting. She can work through the headaches. She complains of chronic fatigue and thinks she snores rarely.

Past medical history: Anxiety disorder. Chronic daily headaches.

Medications: Paxil.

Social history: Attorney. Single and lives alone. She is an intern in a prestigious law firm. She smokes half a pack of cigarettes per day. She rarely drinks alcohol.

Family history: No one in family has headaches or migraines. Sister has depression.

Review of systems: Daily headaches often worse in the morning or when in stressful situations. No recent weight change. No coughing or abdominal pain. Recently visited her family doctor and had a normal CBC and comprehensive chemistry panel.

Exam: Well groomed. Blood pressure 140/67. Pulse 86. There is mild tenderness on palpation of temporalis muscles. Moderate clicking is noticed when the mandible moved back and forth. The top surfaces of her teeth appear worn. There is normal range of motion of neck and arms. The neurologic exam is normal.

Polysomnogram: Sleep onset 42 minutes. RDI 1.1. No snoring heard. PLM index 0. Extensive muscle artifact was noted, especially early in the night. The MSLT showed a mean sleep latency of 15.2 minutes without any REM sleep (Fig. 10-3).

Diagnosis and differential: Nocturnal bruxism is "a stereotypical movement disorder characterized by grinding or clenching of the teeth during sleep" [ICSD (1), p. 182]. This often leads to abnormal destruction of the surface of teeth, which may first be noticed by a dentist. It often causes headaches or jaw and facial pain. Its prevalence has been estimated at 5%–20% or even higher (3). It is not uncommon in patients with a static encephalopathy (4). It occurs equally among males and females. Most people with bruxism are of normal intelligence. While a link has been questioned with anxiety and psychosocial stress, psychologic problems are not more common in patients with bruxism. There is a familial tendency. Temporal–mandibular joint dysfunction and malocclusion are sometimes credited as being an underlying cause or result of bruxism. There is no guarantee that correction of these abnormalities will cure bruxism in an individual. It can occur in all stages of sleep and is often disturbing to family members. Rhythmic muscle artifact is usually noted on most electrodes placed on the head.

The only significant differential diagnosis is a seizure disorder. Seizure disorders can cause masticatory movements in some individuals. Usually, there is additional history to lead to this diagnosis.

This patient was treated with gabapentin for facial pain and headaches. She was also referred to an oral surgeon. A bite block was unsuccessful. The patient decided to have surgery for her TMJ pain and had a dramatic improvement in her headaches. The patient no longer takes the gabapentin. She continues to follow her anxiety disorder with her family physician.

THE SINGER

Chief complaint: Wife states "he sings in his sleep."

History of present illness: A 62-year-old man presents with his wife. The man states he did not believe any of his wife's reports concerning his nocturnal behavior until he recently bruised his arm in the middle of the night. The man's wife states that for the last 2 years he would sing and swing his arms around in the middle of the night. He usually went to bed around 11:00 PM. About 2 hours after he went to sleep, she would awaken with him singing. She often recognized the tune. He would only sing a short phrase and then continue sleeping peacefully. Later, toward morning he would sing and swing his arms, occasionally hitting her and waking her up. Once he picked up the bedside lamp and smashed it on the floor in his sleep. The sound of the lamp breaking awakened him. The patient told his wife he was dreaming that he was a child throwing rocks in the creek. After that, the patient's wife slept in the guest

▶ **TABLE 10-7.** Chewing[a]

| Bruxism |
| Seizures |

[a]From Reference (1).

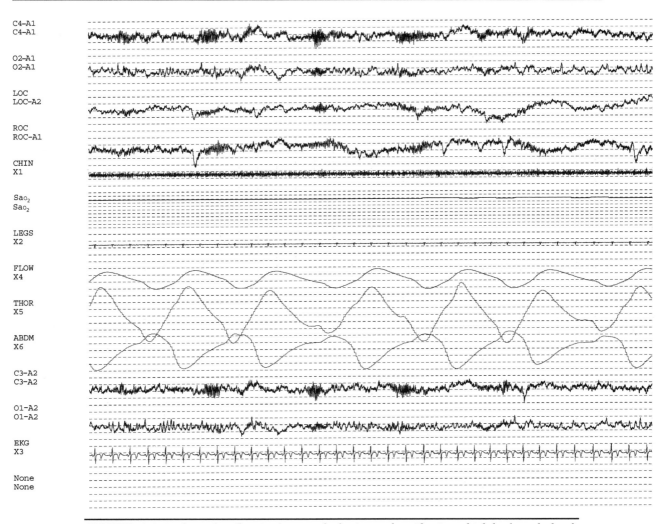

FIGURE 10-3. Teeth grinding (bruxism) causes rhythmic muscle artifact in multiple leads on the head; 30-second page.

bedroom. Last week the patient hit his arm against the wooden headboard of their bed and bruised it.

Past medical history: The patient had been diagnosed with Parkinson's disease 5 years ago.

Medications: Sinemet. Mirapex.

Social history: Retired railroad engineer. He stopped smoking 25 years ago. He drinks a couple shots of whiskey in the evening, three times a week on average.

Family history: Father had hypertension and died after having a stroke. Mother had diabetes and died of heart disease. There is no one in family with a history of seizures.

▶ **TABLE 10-8. Fighting/Acting Out**[a]

Sleep talking
REM sleep behavior disorder
Confusional arousals
Seizures
Sleep terrors

[a]From Reference (1).

Review of systems: Mild to moderate resting tremor. There has been some concern about some memory loss.

Exam: Well-dressed gentleman with a resting tremor, mostly of the right hand. Mini mental status score 23/30. Extraocular muscles intact. Cranial nerves all normal. Increased tone with mild cogwheeling in the right arm and wrist. He has only a very mildly shuffling gait. No evidence of neuropathy. There is a large bruise on the distal left forearm.

Polysomnogram: Sleep onset latency 9 minutes. Sleep efficiency 72%. Increase in slow-wave sleep and REM sleep. PLM index 8. RDI 1.2. Minimum oxygenation 87%. There was an increase in muscle tone in REM sleep. Three times during the night while in REM sleep, the patient waved his arms in the air and sang several unintelligible phrases (Fig. 10-4).

Diagnosis and differential: REM sleep-behavior disorder (RBD) is characterized "by the intermittent loss of REM sleep electromyographic atonia and by the appearance of elaborate motor activity associated with dream

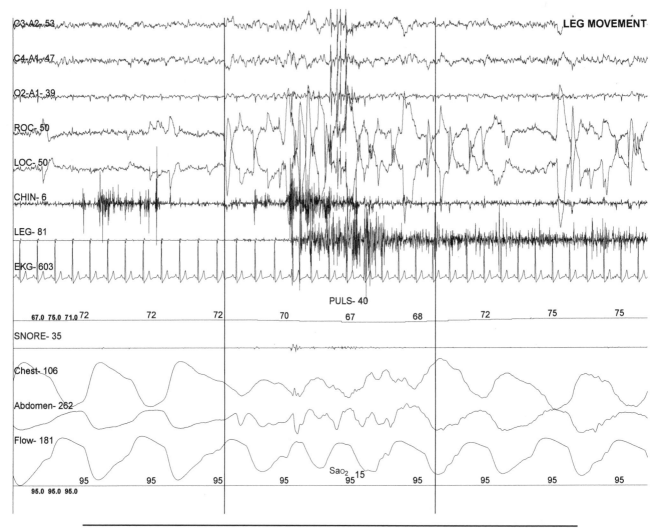

FIGURE 10-4. In REM behavior disorder (RBD) there are sections of persistent elevated muscle tone in REM sleep often accompanied by stereotyped movements that can be violent in nature; 30-second page.

mentation" [ICSD (1), p. 178]. The patient physically acts out a dream. This can lead to a variety of movements and actions. Patients can break bones, strike bedpartners, and knock items off bedside tables. Episodes can be violent. It is more common in males. It is often idiopathic but has been associated with a variety of progressive neurologic disorders including parkinsonism, dementia, and stroke. Although it can be seen at any age it is most prevalent in the 6th and 7th decades. The polysomnogram shows episodes of sustained increased muscle tone in REM sleep instead of the decreased tone normally seen at this time. The polysomnogram should be performed with continuous time-locked video. The video may show directed movements including punching and guttural utterances. If carefully awakened during an episode, the patient can often recall the content of the dream, and a reason for the movements can sometimes be ascertained. There is often an increase in NREM periodic limb movements and REM density.

A careful general medical and neurologic history is necessary. Tricyclic antidepressants and other anticholinergic medications may lead to RBD symptoms. There are also reports of transient RBD symptoms following hypnotic or alcohol withdrawal. The differential includes nocturnal seizures. Concomitant 16-channel EEG can be useful this situation. Another REM-related parasomnia, the nightmare, is sometimes confused with RBD. A nightmare is a frightening dream that often awakens the sleeper. Rarely, striking out can be part of a nightmare. RBD patients tend to be more explosive and usually do not awaken with the frightening aspect, so common in a true nightmare. The differential also includes other NREM parasomnias including sleep walking, confusional arousals, and sleep terrors.

This patient was treated with low-dose clonazepam at 0.5 mg per night with an excellent clinical result. Clonazepam has been shown to be highly beneficial in treating RBD (5).

THE SCREAMER

Chief complaint: He has had screaming spells almost every night for 3 months.

History of present illness: A 7-year-old child presents with the parents. The parents state they are exhausted. The child is well adjusted with no significant medical problems. The child sleeps alone in a room next to the parents. The mother usually has story time with the child at 8:00 PM and shortly thereafter the child is left to fall asleep. The child usually falls asleep in 15 minutes. Anytime up to 3 hours after the child goes to bed, he screams at the top of his lungs. The mother states, "he sounds like someone is stabbing him." The child is totally inconsolable. The parents stay with the child and rock him while he screams for about 10 minutes. The child then falls back asleep. This happens at least once, most nights. These episodes have occurred for 1 year. These screaming spells are affecting the parents' sleep.

Past medical history: Usual childhood viral illnesses. One case of otitis media treated with antibiotics several months ago.

Medications: None

Social history: Only child living with mother and father. Neither parents smokes cigarettes.

Family history: Father had episodes of sleep walking as a toddler.

Review of systems: No recent ear aches, abdominal pain, or diarrhea. Child does not snore.

Exam: Well-developed child with normal pediatric and neurologic examination. No tenderness on palpation of abdomen. Tympanic membranes are normal.

Polysomnogram: Sleep onset latency 4 minutes. RDI 0.1. Minimum oxygenation 97%. Episode of inconsolable screaming during slow-wave sleep (Fig. 10-5).

Diagnosis and differential: Sleep terrors are "characterized by a sudden arousal from slow-wave sleep with a piercing scream or cry, accompanied by autonomic and behavioral manifestations of intense fear" [ICSD (1), p. 148]. There are various autonomic phenomena present including tachycardia, mydriasis, diaphoresis, and flushing. Patients often sit up in bed and scream inconsolably. The facial expression is one of fear. The patient is very difficult to awaken. Once awakened, the person often seems confused. While a dream may be recalled, it is often fragmented and usually makes no sense. The patient is amnestic for the event. It is usually seen between ages 4 and 12 years of age and may persist into adulthood. It is seen in 3% of children and is much rarer in adults. Like most

▶ **TABLE 10-9. Staring**[a]

| Seizures |
| Confusional arousals |

[a]From Reference (1).

NREM parasomnias, it usually disappears in adolescence. It is seen more commonly in males. Other family members may have NREM parasomnias (6). Sleep terrors begin in slow-wave sleep, usually in the first third of the night, but can happen anytime during the night.

The differential includes nightmares, confusional arousals, and epileptic seizures. When people awaken from nightmares, they are usually clear of mind and often can remember a dream with some detail. While some children can remember an image when awakened from a sleep terror, there is no frightening story such as with a nightmare. Nightmares are more common in the last third of the night, where REM sleep is more concentrated. There is usually less autonomic phenomena in a nightmare. If there is a partial arousal during slow-wave sleep, the person often seems stuck in a confused state without the fear seen in sleep terrors. This is called a confusional arousal. These people do not have the autonomic phenomena represented in sleep terrors. Epileptic seizures can present with a cry and the patient can be confused afterward. Ictal fear can be seen in certain epileptic syndromes. Most epileptics do not have seizures solely in sleep. Focal dystonic posturing or tonic–clonic activity points to a seizure as the likely diagnosis. Sometimes, continuous video-EEG monitoring is needed to distinguish a night terror from a nocturnal seizure.

This child was treated with low-dose imipramine because the family was so disturbed and sleep deprived. After 3 months the dose was tapered and discontinued. The child continued having nocturnal events but at a lesser frequency off medication and has now outgrown the events.

THE BLANK GAZER

Chief complaint: Six months of spells of sitting up in bed in the middle of the night and staring.

History of present illness: A 5-year-old child presents with his parents and older brother. The child sleeps on the bottom of a bunk bed. His 9-year-old brother sleeps on the top mattress. The older brother states the patient will sit up in bed and mumble. He will pull the sheets off the bed and then fall back to sleep on the mattress without any sheets. He sometimes thrashes in the bed. He then wakes up later and states he is cold and accuses his older brother of pulling the sheets off the bed. On rare occasions, the patient has been caught sleep walking. Usually, the child is

▶ **TABLE 10-10. Seizures**[a]

| Epilepsy |
| REM sleep behavior disorder |
| Confusional arousals |
| Sleep walk |
| Paroxysmal dystonia |
| Rhythmic movement disorder |

[a]From Reference (1).

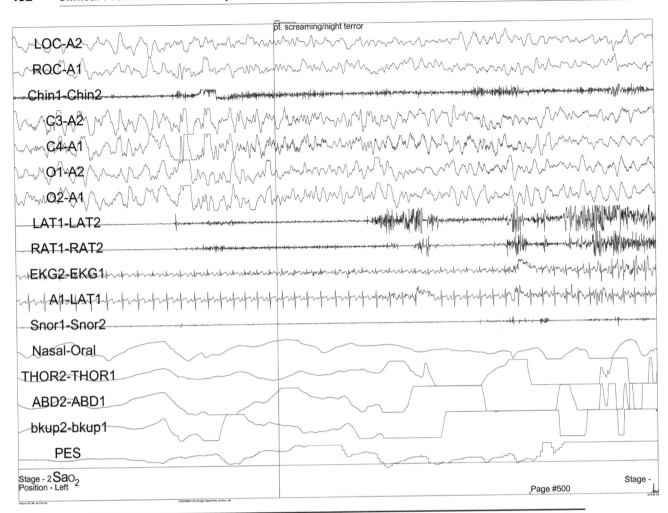

pt. screaming/night terror

LOC-A2
ROC-A1
Chin1-Chin2
C3-A2
C4-A1
O1-A2
O2-A1
LAT1-LAT2
RAT1-RAT2
EKG2-EKG1
A1-LAT1
Snor1-Snor2
Nasal-Oral
THOR2-THOR1
ABD2-ABD1
bkup2-bkup1
PES

Stage - 2 SaO_2
Position - Left

Stage -

Page #500

FIGURE 10-5. Night terrors most often occur in SWS. The patient appears frightened and often screams; 30-second page.

easily redirected back to bed. The more common episodes of confusion happen once a week. The child will most often just moan, sit up in bed, and stare without screaming or having any abnormal movements. When questioned during the event, the child seems to "stare off into space" and not recognize his own family members. The child has occasionally been incontinent with these events. The child has no recollection of any of these events the next day.

Past medical history: Normal delivery. Normal developmental milestones. He has been seen by his pediatrician and a pediatric urologist because of the incontinence that is sometimes seen with these spells. Nothing physically wrong was found with the child.

Medications: None.

Social history: Sleeps in the same room with his older brother. The parent's room is next door. He gets good grades in school.

Family history: His older brother has occasional sleep walking.

Review of systems: No bladder or abdominal pain. No rash. No headaches. Does not snore. No breathing problems.

Exam: Normal pediatric and neurologic examination. Normal sleep-deprived EEG.

Diagnosis and differential: Confusional arousals "consist of confusion during and following arousals from sleep, usually from deep sleep in the first part of the night" [ICSD (1), p. 142]. Persons may not respond or respond inappropriately. They are usually amnestic for the event. Confusional arousals usually arise in the first third of the night from slow-wave sleep (Fig. 10-6). They are sometimes associated with incontinence. Typical of many NREM parasomnias, it is common in young children, and it usually disappears with adolescence. While usually seen in children, it can be seen in adults when there is interference with awakening. Examples include sleep deprivation, metabolic encephalopathies, and use of medications that suppress the central nervous system (CNS). It is seen equally in both sexes. There is a familial predisposition to NREM parasomnias.

The differential includes sleep terrors, sleepwalking, and nocturnal seizures. Sleep terrors are associated with a frightful scream and more autonomic phenomena such as tachycardia, tachypnea, diaphoresis, and flushing.

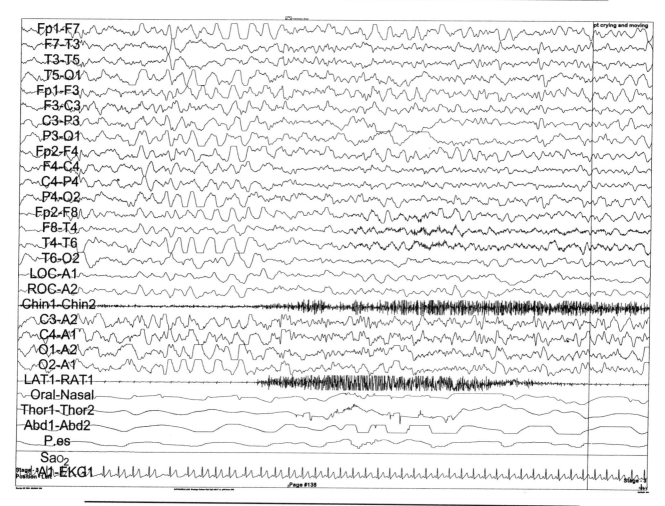

FIGURE 10-6. Confusional arousals occur in SWS. The patient is often difficult to arouse; 30-second page.

Sleepwalking is very similar to confusional arousals except that people get up and walk with sleep walking. Most epileptics with nocturnal seizures also have diurnal seizures. Sometimes video-EEG monitoring is needed to distinguish nocturnal seizures from parasomnias.

Reassurance and educational material was given to the parents and the child. It was decided not to use pharmacotherapy. It was recommended that children with confusional arousals and sleep walking may be safer not using a bunk bed.

THE CRIER

Chief complaint: I cry out in the night.

History of present illness: A 38-year-old truck driver states that she has had three episodes where she felt well when she went to bed, but awoke feeling "hung over." The patient states that the first time this happened was 6 months ago. She and her husband were taking turns driving a long distance. While her husband drove, she laid down in the back of the cab for a nap. Shortly there-

after, her husband heard her cry out a guttural sound and move around in the cab. He pulled over to check on her. The patient seemed initially confused, but quickly cleared mentally and went back to sleep. The second time this occurred, she was in a motel room as they drove cargo across the country. She woke up feeling exhausted. Her husband stated the patient cried out during the night. He thought the patient was having a nightmare. The last time it happened, the patient woke up with stiff muscles and had bitten her tongue. She does admit to some daytime tiredness.

Past medical history: The patient suffered a closed head injury 1 year ago in motor vehicle accident. The patient woke up several hours later in a hospital with a broken collarbone. A CT of the head and x-rays of the spine and chest were normal. The patient had dizziness and headaches for about 1 month after the incident. She also has a history of hypertension. An EEG showed "focal left temporal slowing and no epileptiform activity."

Medications: Atenolol.

Social history: Long-distance truck driver. Very rarely drinks alcohol. Quit smoking 2 years ago.

Family history: Brother has "passing out" spells.

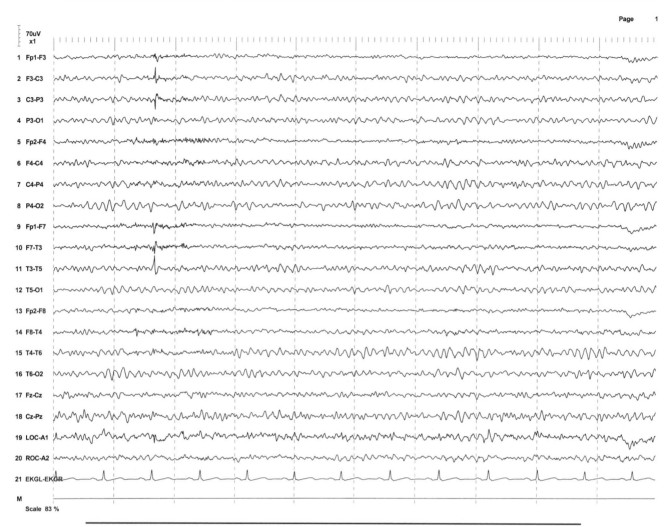

FIGURE 10-7. Focal left temporal spike discharge on an EEG performed following sleep deprivation; 10-second page. The spike is seen in F7-T3 and T3-T5 with phase reversal, tracings 10 and 11, but is also detected in the tracings 2 and 3, which are close to the region.

Review of systems: Besides these events the patient feels well. She does admit to heavy snoring. She has gained 20 pounds over last 2 years, which she feels is related to no longer smoking and her sedentary lifestyle. She does admit to being very tired some days.

Exam: She is 68 inches tall and weighs 210 pounds. She scored 30/30 on mini mental status exam. Her ESS score is 13. Her heart is regular rate and rhythm. Her lungs are clear to auscultation. The neurologic exam is normal.

Diagnosis and differential: Epilepsy is "a disorder characterized by an intermittent, sudden discharge of cerebral neuronal activity" [ICSD (1), p. 247]. There has been a growing interest in the relationship between sleep and epilepsy (7). Almost any seizure type can occur during sleep. In some epileptic syndromes seizures occur primarily during sleep (e.g., benign epilepsy with central–temporal spikes or Rolandic epilepsy). The manifestation of the seizure depends on its anatomic origin. Generalized tonic–clonic seizures are associated with loss of awareness,

tonic flexion, and then extension, a forced expiratory "cry," and then clonic rhythmic jerking of the extremities. Focal (partial) seizures may or may not be associated with alteration of consciousness, but are associated with unilateral sensory or motor phenomena. Automatisms consisting of repetitive picking movements or lip smacking may be seen. Seizures may start focal and then secondarily generalize. Sleep deprivation, noncompliance with antiseizure medication, fever, and alcohol can contribute to breakthrough seizures. Epilepsy can be idiopathic or symptomatic of an underlying discernable brain lesion. The lesions could be a tumor, stroke, brain dysgenesis, hippocampal sclerosis, or due to posttraumatic changes. The EEG may show generalized, bilateral synchronous spike and wave activity, or generalized polyspike activity in patients with generalized seizures. The EEG often shows focal, regional epileptiform activity, including spikes or sharp waves and focal slowing of background activity in patients with focal (partial) seizures. Focal epileptiform activity is more common in

NREM sleep and suppressed in REM sleep. Epileptiform activity is much more common in sleep than wakefulness in children with Rolandic epilepsy. A diurnal EEG may be all that is needed to confirm the diagnosis. An EEG after sleep deprivation or overnight continuous video-EEG may be needed in more complicated cases. Sleep deprivation from other sleep disorders, such as sleep apnea, has been shown to worsen seizures in some patients.

The differential includes nocturnal paroxysmal dystonia, sleepwalking, rhythmic movement disorder, and REM behavior disorder. Nocturnal paroxysmal dystonia occurs in a short form (15–60 seconds) and a longer form (up to 60 minutes). It is characterized by repeated stereotypical dyskinetic episodes of ballismus or choreoathetosis often associated with vocalizations in NREM sleep (8). Anticonvulsant medications are sometimes beneficial, especially in the short form. Sleepwalking, rhythmic movement disorder and RBD are not associated with epileptiform activity.

This patient had a sleep deprived EEG, which showed focal left temporal epileptiform activity (Fig. 10-7), and an MRI that was normal. She was treated with carbamazepine. The patient did well until she presented to the emergency room with a witnessed, diurnal, secondarily generalized seizure 2 months after she stopped taking the carbamazepine against a physician's advice. The patient continues to do well on carbamazepine now. The patient also had a polysomnogram, which showed an apnea-hyperapnea index (AHI) of 27 and a minimum oxygenation of 82%. She was adequately titrated on CPAP at 8 cm of water pressure. She continues to use CPAP, which, she states, makes her much more alert during the day. She decided to find a different career because her driving privileges were restricted as a result of the seizures.

REFERENCES

1. *The international classification of sleep disorders, revised.* Rochester, MN: Davies Printing, 1997.
2. Mendelson WB. Are periodic leg movements associated with clinical sleep disturbance? *Sleep.* 1996;19(3):219–223.
3. Glaros AG. Incidence of diurnal and nocturnal bruxism. *J Prosthetic Dent.* 1981;45:545–549.
4. Richmond G, Rugh JD, Dolfi R, et al. Survey of bruxism in an institutionalized mentally retarded population. *Amer J Mental Def.* 1984;88:418–421.
5. Schenk CH, Mahowald MW. A polysomnographic, neurologic, psychiatric, and clinical outcome report on 70 consecutive cases with REM sleep behavior disorder: sustained clonazepam efficacy in 89.5% of 57 treated patients. *Cleveland Clin J Med.* 1990;57(suppl):10–24.
6. Kales A, Soldatos CR, Bixler EO, et al. Hereditary factors in sleepwalking and night terrors. *Brit J Psych.* 1980;37:111–118.
7. Bazil CW, Malow BA, Sammaritano MR. *Sleep and epilepsy: The clinical spectrum.* Amsterdam: Elsevier Science, 2002.
8. Lugaresi E, Cirignotta F, Montegna R. Nocturnal paroxysmal dystonia. *J Neurol Neurosurg Psych.* 1986;49:375–380.

Pediatric and Adolescent Presentations

Danielle A. Becker and Paul R. Carney

INTRODUCTION

Pediatric and adolescent sleep-related problems are important to study given that they are frequent sources of parental concern. In addition, inadequate or disrupted sleep can have a negative impact on both the physical and mental health of a child. Insufficient sleep can play a role in a child's control of behavior, attention, and emotions.

Sleep problems occur in 20% to 30% of children (1,2). There is a wide span of sleep disorders that range from common behavioral problems to specific genetically based sleep disorders. A multitude of factors can have a negative influence on sleep, including stress, pain, eating habits, circadian phase, medical problems, and developmental transitions, to name a few. Although disrupted sleep can be caused by neurologic disorders, pulmonary abnormalities, and psychologic difficulties, they can be frequent during all ages, including infancy, toddlerhood, preschool ages,

school ages, and adolescence. However, it is important to note that the nature of specific problems is different among each age group.

Although no sleep disorder is confined to the pediatric age range, some disorders occur primarily during childhood. Other disorders may present at all ages, but have distinct presentations in children. The disorders that present in childhood may have significantly different causes and require different modes of treatment. Characteristics of some of the sleep disorders that affect infants, children, and adolescents are summarized in Table 11-1.

ROLE OF DEVELOPMENT

It is crucial to recognize that sleep is an active process that involves a cycling of physiologically diverse stages that are modified during development. These active stages of sleep

▶ **TABLE 11-1.** **Sleep Disorder Characteristics**

Sleep Disorder	*Description*	*Age*	*Prevalence*	*Diagnosis*	*Treatment*
First Three Years of Life					
Sleep-onset association disorder/problems with initiating and maintaining sleep	Inability to fall asleep or transition back to sleep alone	1–3 year olds	25–50%	Careful history, sleep logs/diaries	Responds rapidly to behavioral intervention, not begun before 6 months of age
Excessive nighttime feedings	Continued and frequent wakings, often 3–8 per night.	Infants and toddlers	Unknown	Characteristic history, multiple nighttime wakings, return to sleep only with feeding, significant fluid intake, wet diapers	Gradually decrease frequency of feedings at night
Colic	Spells of fussiness or crying continuing for more than 3 weeks predominately in the evening hours	2–4 months of age	26% of infants	Careful history and physical examination	Rhythmic rocking motions may help 18% occasionally; management strategies for parental coping
Children Ages 3–8 Years					
Confusional arousals/sleep terrors	First one-third of the night, out of stage 4 NREM sleep, vocalized distress, tachycardia, wide-eye stare, difficult to arouse, inconsolable, disoriented, morning amnesia	18 months–6 years	3% of children	Careful sleep and family history	Increase total amount of sleep, regularize sleep–wake cycle, remove any source of sleep disruption, reduce stress
Sleep-walking disorder	First one-third of the night, out of stage 4 NREM sleep, walks for 1–30 min, poor coordination, difficulty in arousing, disoriented, morning amnesia	4–12 years, rare in adolescent	15% of children have 1 attack 1–6% have 1–4 attack/week	Careful sleep and family history	Increase total amount of sleep, regularize sleep–wake cycle, remove any source of sleep disruption, reduce stress
Sleep-related breathing disorder (OSAS)	Snoring, sweating, >5 apneas or 10 apnea–hypopneas/hour	Preschool, latency age	1–2% of children have OSAS; 7–9% snore	Good sleep history, PSG, oxygen saturation	Pharmacologic, tracheostomy, adenotonsillectomy, CPAP
Adolescence					
Circadian and scheduling disorders	Late sleep onsets, difficult morning awakening, long afternoon naps, chaotic sleep schedules	Adolescence	Unknown, possibly 7% in adolescents	Sleep logs/diary, MSLT	Behavioral and supportive treatment, chronotherapy, melatonin
Narcolepsy	Excessive daytime sleepiness with irresistible sleep attacks, cataplexy, hypnogogic hallucinations, sleep paralysis	Early adolescence	0.4–0.7%	Good sleep and family history, PSG, MSLT	Structure, support, stimulant medication

require categorical shifts in awareness and responsiveness throughout the night. The specific neurologic or physiologic functions served by sleep remain unanswered. However, circumstantial evidence suggests a basic neurodevelopmental process linking sleep and the regulation of attention, arousal, affect, and social behavior (3).

The risk of specific sleep disorders appears to be related to an interaction between the biological maturation of sleep–wake states and psychological development of infants and young children (4). Examples of this can be seen starting at the first years of life, with predominance of rapid eye movement sleep (REM), associated with arousals, leading to the manifestation of dyssomnias associated with maintaining sleep. In the preschool to school-age period, non-REM (NREM) arousal parasomnias are more likely to occur at transitions between deep sleep (stages 3 and 4) and REM sleep; these are resolved by adolescence. In adolescence, the challenge of increased physiologic need for sleep and heightened academic and social demands compromise the amount of daily sleep obtained and the regularity of sleep–wake schedules, placing them at risk for circadian rhythm dyssomnias (5).

Symptomatology and significance can also present differently, depending on the age of the individual. For example, excessive daytime sleepiness in a pathologically sleepy preteen may be evidenced by their unusually long nocturnal sleep cycle, while sleepiness in younger children may be evident more by overactivity, inattentiveness, and whining, than by the appearance of sleep itself (6). Infant dyssomnias may reflect insecure attachment issues at young ages, whereas REM parasomnias (nightmares) may reflect disruptions related to stress and trauma at older ages (4).

COMPREHENSIVE EVALUATION

In order to properly assess and treat children who present with sleep problems, a comprehensive evaluation must be done on both sleep and waking behavior. An initial assessment of a child should include: (a) a detailed sleep history, (b) a general medical history, (c) a complete social history, (d) psychologic/developmental screening, and (e) a physical examination (7). It is important to obtain the age of onset, circumstances, degree of debilitation, persistence/worsening versus amelioration, and family history and practices (4). This information must be compared with age-relevant norms. Temporal descriptions of usual sleep/wake habits, napping, bedtimes, nighttime awakenings, and symptoms of daytime sleepiness or irritability are crucial as well. It is important to assess the duration, frequency, and patterns of symptoms, including timing, changes with weekends and vacations, and changes with stressors and special events. Structured sleep diaries and sleep habit questionnaires may be useful. Specific information about snoring, stopped breathing, and sleep-related behaviors, such as walking, talking, and enuresis, should

be acquired. Although sleep laboratory studies in children are required less frequently than in the adult, they are critical for the evaluation of certain complaints including: excessive sleepiness, unusual sleep-associated motor behavior, suspected sleep-associated respiratory disorders, and unexplained sleepiness (7).

New technologies have been developed to augment history taking and nighttime polysomnographic (PSG) recordings. Instruments particularly well suited for studies of young children who find it uncomfortable to sleep with electrodes in place include home-administered 24-hour ambulatory monitoring, along with alternative home-recording methodologies that do not utilize instrumentation. Body-movement detectors in mattresses that are able to track body movements and respiration, and portable, time-lapse, and infrared videosomnography are examples of noninvasive methods (1).

Once assessed, age-dependent responses to treatment must also be taken into consideration. Young children with partial arousals may respond better to schedule adjustment, assurance of sufficient sleep, and parental instruction as opposed to medication. However, adolescents and adults with somnambulism or sleep terrors may respond only to medication and perhaps psychotherapy. The occurrence of enuresis at 4 years old is difficult to treat and probably should not be. However an 8-year-old child with a similar problem is relatively easy to treat. In addition, adolescents with enuresis may respond poorly to the usual therapy for younger children. Children are more adaptive than adolescents or adults, and thus it is much easier to treat their sleep-disordered symptoms.

FIRST 3 YEARS OF LIFE

The most frequent sleep-related problem for children between ages 6 months and 3 years is difficulty going to sleep or staying asleep throughout the night (3). Multiple factors have been implicated in the occurrence of repetitive night waking and inability to fall asleep: infant temperament, nutrition, physical discomfort, mild allergy, and parental marital conflict (8,9).

Sleep-Onset Association Disorder
Clinical Features

Complaints of sleep problems in the infant and young child usually come from the parents, not the child. Nighttime wakings sometimes become worrisome to parents. However, most often the problems reflect certain established patterns of interaction between the parent and the child at time of sleep transition. Nighttime arousals are very common in all ages; however, older children and adults are usually unaware of these disruptions.

Causes

A parent may incorrectly conclude that nocturnal wakings are abnormal, becoming involved in the sleep transition process. The child may become accustomed to parental intervention and become unable to make the transition back to sleep alone, creating a sleep problem or sleep-onset association disorder. The child becomes reliant on the parent to help complete the sleep transition regardless of the time of night.

Diagnosis and Treatment

Diagnosis is usually made with a careful history. Children with this disorder often rapidly respond to simple gradual behavioral interventions, which helps the child learn a new set of sleep-associated habits (10).

Difficulties Learning to Sleep Alone

Clinical Features

Sleeping alone throughout the night without parental intervention is a learned process. All children wake up 5 to 8 times per night, at the end of each sleep cycle, but some children are able to put themselves back to sleep without parental awareness. Most infants are capable of learning this process from about 5 to 7 months of age (3).

Diagnosis and Treatment

The key is to gradually withdraw the amount of parental involvement at sleep onset. The same parental behavioral response is required for middle-of-the-night awakenings. Consistency is also of critical importance if a treatment plan is going to work, especially in conditioning the child to sleep throughout the night. If fear is affecting the progression of this process, it is important to deal with child and/or parental anxiety effectively. Fear can prevent sleep, and fear of safety for one's child can alter a planned behavioral intervention. In certain cases, it will be important to have parents problem-solve about their child's fear and how to best accommodate the behavioral treatment plan.

Excessive Nighttime Feedings

Clinical Features

Studies have shown that an increase in nighttime wakings among infants and toddlers may be related to nighttime feedings. Infants fed large quantities at night (8–32 oz) have been shown to have continued and frequent wakings, ranging up to eight per night (10–13). Repeated wakings for ingestion of fluid directly disrupt the functioning of circadian-modulated systems, which may cause further deleterious effects on sleep–wake stabilization (10,14,15).

Diagnosis and Treatment

Diagnosis can be made from a characteristic history: multiple nighttime wakings, return to sleep only with feeding, significant fluid intake during the night, and extremely wet diapers. Treatment consists of a gradual decrease in the frequency of feedings during the night (10). Frequent wakings, three or more per night in a child over 6 months of age, may cause sleep fragmentation that is harmful to the child. As feedings are decreased and associated habits are eliminated over a couple of weeks, sleep consolidation usually promptly occurs (13).

Limit Setting

Inability to set limits at bedtime can also lead to sleep deterioration. Typical bedtime struggles may consist of requests for water, stories, use of the bathroom, and adjustment of the lights (10,13). A diagnosis of this sort can be made from history. Through history taking it may become clear that the parents are unable to enforce nighttime rules with enough consistency to keep the child in bed and quiet so that he or she falls asleep. Parents may have to learn to be firm in their limit setting, enforcing a regular bedtime ritual with an endpoint. The child should also be kept in his or her bedroom with the use of a gate of some sort or closure of the door, if necessary. Positive behavior modification such as a sticker or star chart, as well as other prizes for staying in bed, may elicit a positive response (10).

Fear

Fear and nightmares are also commonly seen in early childhood, as part of normal development. A truly anxious child at night should be handled in the same manner whether the child's fears were initially expressed during waking or sleep. Mild fears often respond to supportive firmness and a stable social setting. Positive reinforcement, with rewards for staying in bed, may help motivate the child. Treatment may also consist of sleep schedule correction, progressive relaxation (16), and progressive desensitization (17).

Colic

Clinical Features

Colic is the most common medical condition that affects the sleep of young infants. It causes inconsolable fussiness and crying, typically in the late afternoon and evening. Although symptoms usually remit by 3 to 4 months of age, continuing sleep disturbances are common, secondary to altered sleep schedules and habitual patterns of parental responsiveness (13).

Diagnosis and Treatment

Colic is diagnosed when there are unexplained spells of crying in healthy infants. Treatment mainly focuses around education and management strategies for helping parents cope with the stresses of caring for the infant (18).

CHILDREN AGES 3 TO 8 YEARS

By the preschool/school-aged years, children have typically mastered the developmental hurdles of the early years and gained sufficient independence to handle sleep transitions. Disorders that appear during this stage may be related to changes in sleep patterns that coincide with the age when children first stop daytime napping.

Partial Arousal Events

Clinical Features

One of the most frequent sleep-related problems seen in children ages 3 to 8 years old is partial-arousal events from deep non-REM (NREM) sleep. NREM arousals are more likely during transitions from deep sleep (stage 4) to REM sleep, and are most prevalent in preschool and primary school years, tending to disappear by adolescence. Various forms of these partial arousals include calm sleepwalking, agitated sleepwalking, or full-blown night terrors. These disorders are similar to each other in that each of them represent a sudden partial awakening out of the deepest non-REM sleep, tending to occur 1 to 3 hours after sleep onset (3). Other shared features include: automated behavior, relative nonreactivity to external stimuli, difficulty in being aroused, fragmentary or absent dream recall, mental confusion and disorientation when awakened, and retrograde amnesia for the episode the next morning. In addition, a principal feature of partial-arousal events is that the events often cease as abruptly as they began, with a rapid return to deep sleep. The behavioral manifestation depends on the type and degree of the awakening. However, there is a developmental sequence to the manifestation of arousal disorders: sleep terrors first appear after 18 months of age, sleepwalking occurs in slightly older children of preschool and school-age years, and confusional arousals can occur at any age. Arousal disorders diminish significantly in frequency by adolescence and may even disappear.

Causes

Certain factors may influence the occurrence of partial-arousal events: age, overtiredness, inherited factors, and anxiety. The tendency to have partial arousals depends on the amount and intensity of deep stage 4 sleep, which has a developmental component. Delta sleep reaches peak levels between 3 and 5 years of age, which coincides with the period when children first stop daytime napping. Any source of tiredness, whether it be erratic sleep schedules, giving up daytime naps, sleep disruption related to apnea, stress, physical illness, or bad sleep habits, increases the likelihood of partial-arousal events (3). In addition, a positive family history for partial arousals increases the chance that a child will experience partial arousals (19). The effects of anxiety also contribute to partial arousals seen in childhood. For example, falling asleep in a tense, worried, anxious state makes the occurrence of a partial arousal more likely (20).

Treatment

Treatment of partial-arousal events includes increasing the total amount of sleep, regularizing the sleep–wake cycle, removing any source of sleep disruption, and aiding the child in falling asleep in a more relaxing, emotionally safe state (19).

Differential Diagnosis

The differential diagnoses for partial-arousal events include nightmares, nocturnal seizures, and full awakening in the night. Nightmares occur out of REM sleep, typically in the second half of the night or early morning, and resulting in a full awakening with difficulty returning back to sleep. This event is frequently remembered in the morning. Nocturnal seizures are also part of the differential, especially if events are more likely to occur at sleep onset or if there is a family history of seizures.

Confusional Arousals

Clinical Features

Confusional arousals, sometimes referred to "sleep terrors," are thought to occur in almost all young children in at least a mild form, especially before the age of 5. The arousal usually begins with a movement and moaning, progressing to crying, and perhaps calling out. Wild thrashing may be seen in an older child. The child's eyes may be open or closed, and perspiration is evident. A look of confusion, agitation, or distress is described rather than a look of "terror." Coddling does not provide reassurance and may even cause the child to become progressively more agitated. Attempts to wake the child by shaking, taking him or her into the light, yelling, or using cold water may not be successful. Theses episodes can last anywhere from 1 to 2 minutes up to 30 to 40 minutes, with 5 to 15 minutes being typical (21).

Sleep Terrors

Clinical Features

Sleep terrors are actually a variation of confusional arousals (22). These events typically begin precipitously with the child bolting upright with a "blood-curdling" scream. A child can seem aroused and appear fully awake with a racing heart rate, dilated pupils, and extremely agitated behavior. Their facial expression is one of fear. However, although appearing awake, such children may be confused, not recognize their parents, and are often inconsolable. He or she may even rise out of bed and run blindly, as if away from an unseen danger. These events are typically shorter than the confusional arousals described above, lasting only a few minutes.

Sleepwalking Disorder

Clinical Features

In calm sleepwalking, the individual may simply get up and walk about calmly, quiet, and unnoticed. The sleepwalker's body movements are poorly coordinated and their direction is purposeless. It is difficult to determine if the child is asleep or in drowsy wakefulness. Inappropriate behavior, such as urinating in the closet or next to the toilet is common. Older children usually awake fully at the end of the event and often are embarrassed to find themselves out of their bedroom and possibly at the center of attention. Nevertheless, they quickly return to bed and sleep.

Agitated sleepwalking is more often seen in older children, where the child may be upset and agitated while walking about. The presence of speech may be greater, but it is often garbled and unintelligible. Similar to calm sleepwalking, this type also may last a minute to one-half hour, resolving with the child awakening and returning to bed (21). Safety precautions (alarms that trigger when the sleepwalker rises) may need to be taken in order to keep the sleepwalker from getting into danger.

Sleep-Related Breathing Disorder

Clinical Features

The importance of sleep-disordered breathing in children has received increased awareness. Childhood obstructive sleep apnea syndrome (OSAS) is associated with significant nighttime and daytime symptoms and is characterized by episodes of partial or complete upper-airway obstruction during sleep, usually associated with a reduction in oxyhemoglobin saturation and/or hypercarbia. These problems are most often associated with large tonsils or adenoids in children. The presentation in childhood sleep apnea differs from adults in that children can have clinically significant sleep-disordered breathing with only brief obstructive events and without large drops in blood oxygen levels. Children may have frequent brief awakenings to re-establish the airway, resulting primarily in fragmented sleep (23). Nighttime symptoms include snoring, paradoxical chest–abdomen motion, retractions, observed apnea, observed difficulty breathing during sleep, cyanosis during sleep, or disturbed sleep. Daytime symptoms include

nasal obstruction, mouth breathing, and other symptoms of adenotonsillar hypertrophy, behavior problems, or excessive daytime sleepiness. The result of this disturbance may be daytime difficulties in focused attention, emotional lability, or other signs of sleep deprivation, including partial arousals during the night, or difficult awakening in the morning.

Diagnosis and Treatment

A good clinical history, eliciting information about sleep, breathing during sleep, daytime symptoms, complications, and previous airway surgery are important for diagnosis and treatment. Specific information concerning the nature and quality of the snoring and parental observations of cyanosis, apnea, inspiratory struggles, retractions, the need to shake the child to make him or her breathe, or the need to watch the child for fear he or she will stop breathing should also be collected. Laboratory studies, including a polysomnograph and a Multiple Sleep Latency Test (MSLT) are also used to classify patients. A polysomnograph provides an accurate description of the type of apnea episode (obstructive, central, mixed) and its association with REM or NREM sleep, the degree of oxygen desaturation, secondary cardiac arrhythmias, and the amount of sleep fragmentation. Treatment may include followup only, medical/pharmacologic, surgical (tracheostomy, adenotonsillectomy), and mechanical therapy [continuous positive airway pressure (CPAP), tongue retainers]. There appears to be no consensus on treatment for childhood OSAS. Current practice is based largely on what seems reasonable to practitioners.

Nocturnal Enuresis

Clinical Features

Nocturnal enuresis is considered to be one of the most prevalent and persistent sleep problems in children. Criteria for diagnosis include: (a) chronological age of at least 5 years and mental age of 4; (b) two or more incontinent events in a month between 5 and 6 years of age and one or more events after 6 years; and (c) absence of a physical disorder associated with incontinence, such as diabetes, urinary tract infection, or seizure disorder (24). Primary nocturnal enuresis is classified as continuous from infancy, with children wetting from once to twice a week to nightly, never having achieved urinary control. Secondary nocturnal enuresis indicates an enuresis relapse after a period of at least 6 months of dryness.

Treatment

Supportive therapy in combination with behavioral techniques (bell and pad method), usually result in a positive outcome.

Restless Leg Syndrome/Periodic Limb Movement Disorder

Clinical Features

Restless leg syndrome (RLS) is characterized by sensations deep in the legs produced by an irresistible urge to move. The sensation is bothersome, but usually not painful. Symptoms are worse or exclusively present when an individual is at rest and the sensations are typically lessened by voluntary movement of the affected extremity. RLS symptoms can cause difficulty in initiating and maintaining sleep along with excessive daytime sleepiness.

One variation of RLS is periodic limb movement disorder (PLMD). PLMD is characterized by leg movements or jerks, which typically occur every 20 to 40 seconds during sleep and are sustained 0.5 to 0.4 seconds in duration (25). PLMD causes disrupted sleep and excessive daytime sleepiness.

Causes

Symptoms may be caused by an underlying iron or vitamin deficiency and supplementing with iron, vitamin B_{12}, or folate (as indicated) may be sufficient to relieve symptoms (26).

Diagnosis and Treatment

RLS symptoms can begin in childhood and present as growing pains or hyperactivity because of difficulty sitting quietly. A thorough medical history is pertinent for diagnosis. Fatigue and drowsiness tend to worsen the symptoms of RLS. Thus, implementing a program of good sleep hygiene should be a first step in symptom resolution.

ADOLESCENCE

The older the child and adolescent, the more their sleep disorders resemble those of adults. During adolescence, an increased physiologic need for sleep competes with increased academic, social, and work demands that may disrupt the regularity of sleep–wake schedules (5). In addition, adolescence is a time of major developmental changes in the control of sleep and circadian systems, with emotional turmoil and stress possibly affecting the sleep system directly. Sleep deprivation may cause or exacerbate emotional difficulties experienced during this age period.

A decrease in the amount of delta sleep accompanies adolescence, with a 40% decrement observed between the ages of 10 and 20 (27). Whereas hypotheses have suggested that the age-related decline may be related to the loss of cortical synaptic density (28) that occurs during this age period, adolescents also show reduced REM latency and an increase in stages 1, 2, and awake during the night. Carskadon and associates (29) have indicated that ado-

lescents require more sleep. However despite this finding, studies have shown that adolescents frequently obtain less sleep (5), which may be attributed to their social schedules and late-night activities combined with early-morning arousals for school. Significant daytime sleepiness is often a result of this conflicting schedule (30). Delay of the circadian phase may also result as a consequence of staying up later and sleeping in later.

Insufficient Sleep

Clinical Features

Insufficient sleep is the most common cause of sleepiness in adolescents. It is defined as an insufficient number of hours in bed or available for sleep. Sleep-related problems and daytime sleepiness often occur when catch-up sleep on weekends and holidays promotes a later circadian schedule, leading to an erratic sleep–wake schedule. The erratic patterns contribute to fragmented night sleep or the inability to fall asleep early on school nights, sustaining the repeated cycle of poor and inadequate sleep. Resulting behaviors may include falling asleep in class, oversleeping in the morning, fatigue, irritability, and mood lability.

Treatment

The best treatment for insufficient sleep is to help the family understand and acknowledge the consequences resulting from inadequate sleep and its relationship to specific behaviors. Strategies to prevent poor habits may be essential. If the adolescent's daily functioning is significantly impaired by the sleep problem, a behavioral contract agreed on by the family can be a vital component of the intervention, specifying hours in bed, and targeting the specific behaviors contributing to bad sleeping habits. Choices for rewards for successes versus negative consequences for failures, as well as an accurate method of assessing compliance are important for the success of the contract.

Differential Diagnosis

A differential diagnosis for insufficient sleep is disturbed nocturnal sleep, which should be considered when symptoms of sleepiness occur despite an adequate sleep schedule. Disturbances in sleep can be difficult to assess by history alone. Significant sleep disruption may be caused by caffeine intake, as well as certain prescription medications for asthma or attention deficit and hyperactivity disorder. Another cause of disturbed nocturnal sleep with resultant excessive daytime sleepiness is obstructive sleep apnea (OSA). Nevertheless, this syndrome is uncommon in adolescents.

Circadian and Scheduling Disorders

Clinical Features

Delayed sleep-phase syndrome (DSPS) is the most common circadian problem relevant to adolescents. It usually begins with the tendency to stay up late, sleep in, or take late afternoon naps. Problems become apparent when difficulties arise around morning wakeup time and with getting to school.

Causes

The circadian system in highly susceptible adolescents can become entrained at a phase position that becomes very difficult to shift to an earlier time, resulting in long delays in falling asleep and a strenuous effort to awaken at the wrong phase of a cycle. Long afternoon naps may be taken in effort to replace missed sleep, which further retards the sleep onset at night. Occasionally an adolescent may also present with a chaotic sleep schedule, with scattered sleep across the night and day in a random fashion with no clear pattern (31).

Diagnosis and Treatment

Diagnosis is partly determined by a comprehensive assessment of all the adolescent's activities. A useful tool for the assessment of a chaotic sleep schedule is a sleep diary or sleep chart. A detailed relay of sleep habits charted on a plot may reveal a pattern not evident by history taking alone. In addition, the MSLT is useful in quantifying the amount of sleep debt that has accumulated. Treatment needs to focus on both eliminating the sleep debt and on restoring a more normal bedtime, sleep onset time, and rise time. However, the first line of treatment should be supportive: explaining the problem to the adolescent and family and encouraging motivation to make a change, having the adolescent keep a sleep–wake and daily activity log, and providing assistance with stress management and priority-setting. If supportive or behavioral management does not improve the problem, chronotherapy (resetting of the biological clock) may be necessary. A schedule should be stabilized, proceeded with a gradual realignment to the desired schedule, and then maintenance of the new alignment. After stabilization of a schedule, when the adolescent is able to fall asleep with no difficulty, small consistent advances in bedtime and wake-up time are made. It is important that naps are avoided during this time. In severe cases, successive delays in bedtime around the clock may be more favorable. The use of melatonin has also been used in the treatment of DSPS in adults (32).

Narcolepsy

The onset of narcolepsy symptoms, although most often seen between midadolescence and young adulthood, can appear from early childhood to full maturity (33). PSGs have validated the diagnosis in a number of children who had symptoms occurring before 13 years of age (34). Nevertheless, adolescence has been reported as the peak age of onset for narcolepsy. In addition, narcolepsy is suggested to be the second most prevalent cause of hypersomnolence in adolescents (35).

Clinical Features

The narcolepsy syndrome is characterized by a tetrad of symptoms including (a) excessive daytime sleepiness with irresistible sleep attacks, (b) cataplexy, characterized by sudden loss of bilateral peripheral muscle tone, often preceded by strong emotions, (c) hypnogogic hallucinations (perceptual distortions), and (d) sleep paralysis at sleep onset. It is rare for an adolescent to present with all four of these symptoms. Excessive sleepiness has been reported to be the most prominent symptom, with patients demonstrating true sleepiness following a good sleep–wake schedule with adequate hours in bed. Emotional and behavioral disturbances are also prominent features in adolescents with narcolepsy and sometimes lead to an incorrect diagnosis of a psychiatric disorder before narcolepsy has been recognized (35).

Diagnosis and Treatment

Narcolepsy is currently diagnosed by a combination of clinical findings and characteristic features on an overnight PSG. Subsequent MSLTs are used to reliably predict the severity of the individual's daytime sleepiness (35). However, a good sleep–wake schedule and good sleep hygiene are important for the accuracy of the MSLT (31). Adolescents who suffer from this disorder are vulnerable to adolescent social pressures, making education, counseling, support, and psychosocial issues equally or more important to treat than treatment with medications when working with this age group. In addition, a carefully structured sleep schedule, well judged naps during the school day, and academic courses timed to the periods of greatest alertness may be valuable. Stimulants have been the drugs of choice to treat daytime sleepiness in adult patients (36) and may aid in alleviating interference in normal activities and academic success in adolescents with this disorder (35). Tricyclic antidepressant medications have been used for the treatment of cataplexy associated with this disorder. Monamine oxidase (MAO) inhibitors have been used to manage cataplexy, sleep paralysis, and hypnagogic hallucinations.

Differential Diagnosis

Idiopathic hypersomnia is a differential diagnosis to be considered in a sleepy adolescent. In this disorder, there is often a familial history of a need for excessive sleep, with clear objective sleepiness during nap studies despite adequate nighttime sleep. Idiopathic hypersomnia is often treated with stimulant medication.

Insomnia

Clinical Features

Childhood onset insomnia or "idiopathic insomnia," can also present during adolescence. It has been suggested to be caused from an imbalance between arousal and sleep systems (37). This type of insomnia is likely to result from neurophysiologic alterations in the sleep–wake cycle, resulting in hyperarousal or hyposomnolence. An adolescent with idiopathic insomnia may complain of poor concentration, impaired vigilance and attention, low energy, bad mood, and increased fatigue. Some neurologic signs, such as dyslexia or hyperactivity, may appear. In this disorder, insomnia has been longstanding, beginning in early childhood, unceasing, and no medical or psychiatric cause can be associated with the onset of symptoms. Unless the patient is responsive to hypnotic medications, prognosis is usually poor for this disorder.

Treatment

Treatment of insomniac adolescents requires improved sleep hygiene, normalization of sleep schedules, decreased use of alcohol and other drugs, relaxation therapy, biofeedback, and psychotherapy (38–41).

Differential Diagnosis

Psychophysiologic insomnia may result from performance anxiety about getting sufficient sleep for school, leading to bedroom-associated stress and anxiety. Anxiety and depressive disorders and/or traumatic or stressful events are other common sources.

Sleep Bruxism

Clinical Features

Sleep bruxism, characterized by stereotypic movements of the mouth, leading to the grinding or clenching of the teeth during sleep, is related to stress and emotional tension. Bruxism typically appears between the ages of 10 and 20 years.

Treatment

Treatment includes interocclusal appliances, nocturnal alarms, and various behavioral regimens (42).

CONCLUSION

Regardless of the child's age, he or she may experience difficulty establishing and maintaining sleep, excessive daytime sleepiness, interruptions of sleep, things that go wrong during sleep, and variable disturbances reflecting circadian dysfunction. Differences that occur between pediatric disorders and young adult disorders pertain more to the age-related variations in presentation, significance, cause, and treatment of the problem. These differences begin to disappear as the child grows older and enters adolescence and young adulthood.

CLINICAL RELEVANCE

It has been shown that children and adolescents with behavioral, emotional, and psychiatric problems show increased rates of sleep-related symptoms and complaints (43–45). In particular, children with attention-deficit disorder hyperactivity disorder (46,47), anxiety and depression (48,49), and autism (50) have been shown to exhibit an elevated rate of sleep disturbance. Children and adolescents with sleep disorders have also been shown to display increased rates of behavioral and emotional difficulties. Studies reported that early sleep problems were predictive of later behavioral and emotional problems in later childhood (9,51,52). Inadequate sleep alone during childhood or adolescence may partially contribute to an increase in behavioral and emotional disorders. This is important for pediatricians and family practitioners to consider, given that ensuring adequate sleep is a prudent step in treatment recommendations for a variety of sleep disturbances.

FUTURE DIRECTIONS

Future directions should continue to define markers of normality and abnormality in sleep patterns among children and adolescents. The same event in a child and an adult may be considered normal in one and abnormal in the other. Obvious examples pertain to napping and enuresis, with both being normal early on but becoming relatively uncommon after 3 to 5 years of age. In addition, sleepwalking is usually considered to be a sleep disorder in adults, but it may be considered a normal developmental feature in toddlers. Adult criteria do not apply to childhood sleep disorders.

Despite the impact that disruption of sleep has on children and their psychosocial adjustment, little research has been conducted exploring sleep parameters or possible implications of sleep disturbance in children. The majority of studies on sleep disturbances focus on adult samples. As a result, it is unclear if manifestations of sleep disorders in children resemble those of adults. Clear differentiation would have important implications for treating behavioral and cognitive problems in children with excessive daytime sleepiness, given the suggested link between sleep-disordered breathing (described as a history of loud snoring, restless sleep, and/or signs of daytime sleepiness) and daytime behavioral disturbances. Behavioral disturbances reported in children with sleep-disordered breathing include sleepiness, hyperactivity, poor school performance, abnormal behavior, and aggressiveness (9,52–54). Future research should explore potential associations between the regulation of sleep and the control of attention, along with accompanying emotional, behavioral, and cognitive problems. Further exploration of these relationships may reveal information that could be beneficial in the reduction of behavioral and cognitive symptoms associated with disturbed sleep and eventually lead to an improvement of the quality of life of children who suffer from sleep disturbances.

REFERENCES

1. Anders TF, Halpern LF, Hua J. Sleeping through the night: a developmental perspective. *Pediatrics.* 1992;90:554–560.
2. Beltramini AU, Hertzig ME. Sleep and bedtime behavior in preschool-aged children. *Pediatrics.* 1983;71:153–158.
3. Dahl DE. The development and disorders of sleep. *Advan Pediat.* 1998;45:73–90.
4. Anders TF, Eiben, LA. Pediatric sleep disorders: a review of the past 10 years. *J Amer Acad Child Adolescent Psych.* 1997;36(1):9–20.
5. Carskadon MA. Patterns of sleep and sleepiness in adolescents. *Pediatrician.* 1990;17:5–12.
6. Ferber R. Introduction: pediatric sleep disorders medicine. In: Ferber R, Kryger M, eds. *Principles and practice of sleep medicine in the child.* Philadelphia: WB Saunders, 1995:1–5.
7. Ferber R. Assessment of sleep disorders in the child. In: Ferber R, Kryger M, eds. *Principles and practice of sleep medicine in the child.* Philadelphia: WB Saunders, 1995:45–53.
8. Beal VA. Termination of night feeding in infancy. *J Pediat.* 1969;75:690–692.
9. Zuckerman B, Stevenson J, Bailey V. Sleep problems in early childhood: Continuities, predictive factors, and behavioral correlates. *Pediatrics.* 1987;80:664–671.
10. Ferber R. Sleeplessness in children. In: Ferber R, Kryger M, eds. *Principles and practice of sleep medicine in the child.* Philadelphia: WB Saunders, 1995:79–89.
11. Van Tassel EB. The relative influence of child and environmental characteristics on sleep disturbances in the first and second years of life. *J Develop Behav Pediat.* 1985;6:81–86.
12. Richman N. A community survey of characteristics of one- to two-year-olds with sleep disruptions. *J Amer Acad Child Psych.* 1981;20:281–291.
13. Ferber RA. *Solve your child's sleep problems.* New York: Simon and Schuster, 1985.
14. Ferber R. Sleeplessness, night awakening, and night crying in the infant and toddler. *Pediat Rev.* 1987;9:69–82.
15. Ferber RA. The sleepless child. In: Guilleminault C, ed. *Sleep and its disorders in children.* New York: Raven Press, 1987:141–163.
16. Weil G, Goldried MR. Treatment of insomnia in an eleven-year-old child through self-relaxation. *Behav Ther.* 1973;4:282.
17. Anders TF, Keener M. Developmental course of nighttime sleep–wake patterns in full-term and premature infants during the first year of life. I. *Sleep.* 1985;8:173–192.
18. Weissbluth M. Colic. In: Ferber R, Kryger M, eds. *Principles and practice of sleep medicine in the child.* Philadelphia: WB Saunders, 1995:75–78.
19. Rosen GM, Ferber R, Mahowald MW. Evaluation of parasomnias in children. In: Dahl RE, ed. *Child and adolescent psychiatric clinics of*
North America: sleep disorder. Philadelphia: WB Saunders, 1996:601–616.
20. Dahl RE. Parasomnias. In: Ammerman RT, Last CG, Hersen M, eds. *Handbook of prescriptive treatments for children and adolescents.* Boston: Allyn & Bacon, 1994:281–299.
21. Rosen G, Mahowald MW, Ferber R. Sleepwalking, confusional arousals, and sleep terrors in the child. In: Ferber R, Kryger M, eds. *Principles and practice of sleep medicine in the child.* Philadelphia: WB Saunders, 1995:99–106.
22. Broughton RJ. Sleep disorders: disorders of arousal? *Science.* 1968;159(819):1070–1078.
23. Carroll JL. Sleep-related upper-airway obstruction in children and adolescents. In: Dahl RE, ed. *Child and adolescent psychiatric clinics of North America: sleep disorder.* Philadelphia: WB Saunders, 1996:617–647.
24. American Psychiatric Association. *Diagnostic and statistical manual of mental disorders.* 4th edn. (DSM–IV). Washington, DC: American Psychiatric Association, 1994.
25. Montpaisir J, Godbout R, Pelletier G, et al. Restless legs syndrome and periodic movements during sleep. In: Kryger MH, Roth T, Dement WC, eds. *Principles and practice of sleep medicine.* 2nd edn. Philadelphia: WB Saunders, 1994:589–597.
26. Mahowald MW. Restless leg syndrome and periodic limb movements of sleep. *Curr Treatment Options Neurol.* 2003;5:251–260.
27. Carskadon MA. The second decade. In: Guilleminault C, ed. *Sleeping and waking disorders: indications and techniques.* Menlo Park, CA: Addison-Wesley, 1982.
28. Feinberg I. Schizophrenia: caused by a fault in programmed synaptic elimination during adolescence? *J Psychi Res.* 1982;17(4):319–334.
29. Carskadon MA, Harvey K, Duke P, et al. Pubertal changes in daytime sleepiness. *Sleep.* 1980;2(4):453–460.
30. Carskadon MA, Dement WC. Sleepiness in the normal adolescent. In: Guilleminault C, ed. *Sleep and its disorders in children.* New York: Raven Press, 1987:53–66.
31. Dahl R, Carskadon MA. Sleep and its disorders in adolescence. In: Ferber R, Kryger M, eds. *Principles and practice of sleep medicine in the child.* Philadelphia: WB Saunders, 1995:19–27.
32. Dahlitz M, Alvarez B, Vignau J, et al. Delayed sleep phase syndrome response to melatonin. *Lancet.* 1991;337(8750):1121–1124.
33. Dement WC, Zarcone V, Varner V, et al. The prevalence of narcolepsy. *Sleep Res.* 1972;1:148.
34. Dahl R, Holttum J, Trubnick L. The clinical presentation of narcolepsy in children and adolescents. *J Amer Acad Child Adolescent Psychi.* 1994;33:834–841.
35. Brown LW, Billiard M. Narcolepsy, Kleine-Levin syndrome, and other causes of sleepiness in children. In: Ferber R, Kryger M, eds. *Principles and practice of sleep medicine in the child.* Philadelphia: WB Saunders, 1995:125–134.
36. Mitler MM, Shafor R, Hajdukovich R, et al. Treatment of narcolepsy: objective studies on methylphenidate, permoline, and protriptyline. *Sleep.* 1986;9:260–264.
37. Hauri P, Olmstead E. Childhood-onset insomnia. *Sleep.* 1980;3(1):59–65.
38. Anderson DR. Treatment of insomnia in a 13-year-old boy by relaxation training and reduction of parental attention. *J Behav Ther Exp Psychi.* 1979;10:263.
39. Hauri P. Biofeedback techniques in the treatment of chronic insomnia. In: Williams RL, Karacan I, eds. *Sleep disorders, diagnosis and treatment.* New York: Wiley, 1987:145–149.
40. Hauri P. Behavioral treatment of insomnia. *Med Times.* 1979;107(6):36–47.
41. Zarcone VP, Jr. Sleep hygiene. In: Kryger MH, Roth T, Dement MD, eds. *Principles and practice of sleep medicine.* 2nd edn. Philadelphia: WB Saunders, 1984:542–546.
42. Glaros A, Melamed B. Bruxism in children: etiology and treatment. *Appl and Preventative Psych.* 1992;1:191–199.
43. Kirmil-Gray K, Eagleston JR, Gibson E, et al. Sleep disturbances in adolescents: Sleep quality, sleep habits, beliefs about sleep, and daytime functioning. *J Youth Adolescence.* 1884;13:375–384.
44. Morrison DN, McGee R, Stanton WR. Sleep problems in adolescence. *J Amer Acad Child Adolescent Psych.* 1992;31:94–99.

45. Simonds JFPH. Sleep behaviors and disorders in children and adolescents evaluated at psychiatric clinics. _J Develop Behav Pediat._ 1984;5:6–10.

46. Trommer BL, Hoeppner JB, Rosenberg RS, et al. Sleep disturbance in children with attention-deficit disorder. _Ann Neurol._ 1988;24:322.

47. Kaplan BJ, McNicol J, Conte RA, et al. Sleep disturbances in preschool-aged hyperactive and nonhyperactive children. _Pediatrics._ 1987;80:839–844.

48. Ryan ND, Puig-Antich J, Ambronsini P, et al. The clinical picture of major depression in children and adolescents. _Arch General Psych._ 1987;44:854–861.

49. Dahl RE. Sleep in behavioral and emotional disorders. In: Kryger M, Roth T, Dement W, eds. _Principles and practice of sleep medicine in the child._ Philadelphia: WB Saunders, 1995:147–153.

50. Johnson CR. Sleep problems in children with mental retardation and autism. In: Dahl RE, ed. _Child and adolescent psychiatric clinics of north america: Sleep disorder._ Philadelphia: WB Saunders, 1996:673–683.

51. Pollock JI. Night-waking at five years of age: predictors and prognosis. _J Child Psychol Psych Allied Discipl._ 1994;35:699–708.

52. Minde K, Popiel K, Leos N, et al. The evaluation and treatment of sleep disturbances in young children. _J Child Psych Psych Allied Discipl._ 1993;34:521–533.

53. Lavigne JV, Arend R, Rosenbaum D, et al. Sleep and behavior problems among preschoolers. _J Develop Behav Pediat._ 1999;20:164–169.

54. Owens J, Opipari L, Nobile C, Spirito A. Sleep and daytime behavior in children with obstructive sleep apnea and behavioral sleep disorders. _Pediatrics._ 1998;102:1178–1184.

Sleep Problems of the Elderly

Stephan Eisenschenk

Sleep has become an increasingly important factor in the elderly, with the life expectancy in industrialized societies currently greater than 75 years. The 2000 United States census registered approximately 35 million citizens who were over 65 years old, and this is projected to increase to 70 million by 2030. The prevalence of sleep complaints increases with advancing age. Approximately 40% of elderly patients will present with some type of sleep complaint (1,2). However, one of the basic principals of epidemiology is that no individuals are alike. In addition, chronological age and physiological age may differ considerably. This may make it difficult to accurately determine normal and abnormal sleep physiology and behavior in the elderly.

To attempt to simplify the diagnosis of sleep disorders in the elderly, it is often easier to understand the differential diagnosis of common sleep complaints of elderly patients. Often these complaints may be subtle and relatively nondescript. Elderly patients may vary in their interpretation of sleep disturbances, having more difficulty in accurately describing their underlying sleep disturbances (3). Elderly patients also more commonly perceive sleep problems if they have difficulty falling asleep rather than maintaining sleep (4). With increased frequency of sleep disorders with advancing age, knowledge of the common sleep disorders in the elderly is imperative. This chapter will discuss the most common complaints and provide a systematic approach to the diagnosis of normal physiologic aging and sleep-related disorders in the elderly patient.

AGE-RELATED SLEEP PHYSIOLOGY IN THE ELDERLY

Although sleep can be variable in the elderly, there are common trends in sleep architecture with advancing age. Elderly patients have earlier sleep onset and morning awakening times than do persons in early adulthood. With advancing age, normal REM latency shortens with phase advancement of the sleep cycle. This is probably secondary to weakened slow-wave sleep (SWS) in the first one-third of the night. In the elderly, the amount of SWS is markedly suppressed based on reduction of slow-wave amplitude rather than a decrease in delta wave abundance (5,6). The exact age of decline of delta activity is unknown but is believed to begin as early as young adulthood (6). Despite this phase advancement, the amount of stage 1 sleep increases, while REM sleep stays approximately the same.

It is still uncertain whether elderly patients have similar sleep needs or a reduction in the need for sleep compared with younger adults. Although nocturnal sleep may be more fragmented, the need for sleep may be met by napping. Naps become more prominent in the elderly. The daytime naps taken by elderly individuals also show relatively low amounts of SWS and are more fragmented than those of younger subjects. Many normal elderly patients perceive these normal changes in sleep physiology as insomnia. If patients do not complain of excessive daytime sleepiness (EDS), then most of these patients can be reassured that their sleep patterns are normal.

Sleep architecture is also altered secondary to an increase in the number of spontaneous awakenings. Sleep lightens behaviorally, secondary to a lowered threshold for awakening stimuli. In addition, central and obstructive apneas and periodic limb movement syndrome (PLMS) increase in frequency with advancing age, which further disrupts consolidation of sleep. The higher incidence of sleep disorders in males may be part of the underlying factor for slightly poorer sleep efficiency in elderly males.

Several other factors also act as contributors to decreased sleep in older patients. These factors include inactivity, hypnotic and alcohol use, over-the-counter and prescribed medications, illness, decreased light exposure and loss of social cues, and bereavement. Neurodegenerative changes such as Alzheimer's disease also become more prominent in the elderly.

EXCESSIVE DAYTIME SLEEPINESS

It is important to differentiate fatigue from EDS in the elderly. Differentiation of EDS and fatigue is important because the causes of EDS are primarily sleep disorders, and fatigue may be induced by sleep disorders or intrinsic medical, neurologic, and psychiatric conditions (7). Prevalence rates for EDS in the elderly have been estimated to be 15% or greater (8). Psychiatric disorders including depression, bipolar disorder, drug dependency, and medical conditions including cardiopulmonary dysfunction, end-organ dysfunction, and neurodegenerative disease can all present with fatigue, but also contribute to sleep disorders. It may be difficult to differentiate the primary factor, but treatment of the underlying medical or psychiatric condition will often improve complaints of both fatigue and EDS. Even healthy elderly patients tend to have more EDS compared with middle-aged adults. The alteration of sleep physiology and higher prevalence of many sleep disorders will increase the probability of EDS with advancing age.

Although rare, there have been case reports of initial diagnosis of narcolepsy in the elderly (9). This may be related to narcolepsy being overlooked when patients present with EDS at a younger age. Many patients will continue to have symptoms even if diagnosed at an earlier age. In addition, sleep disorders, such as obstructive sleep apnea (OSA), periodic leg movements (PLM), and other parasomnias will have associated arousals. These conditions typically increase with advancing age and are discussed below based on their presentations.

Elderly patients with EDS require close scrutiny of not only their presenting symptoms but also of concurrent medications. Elderly patients will develop more frequent medical problems and will subsequently be placed on increasing numbers of medications. Both prescription and nonprescription medications may make it more difficult to differentiate between EDS and fatigue. Although many medications may cause EDS, the benefit for the patient typically will outweigh the adverse effects. Since most elderly are on multiple medications, the assessment of current medications is paramount in the determination of EDS with advancing age. Obviously, sedative hypnotics such as benzodiazepines (especially those with a long duration of action) may increase daytime sleepiness and may also exacerbate underlying sleep apnea. Even if patients are not prescribed sedative–hypnotics, many elderly patients will self-medicate with alcohol. Antidepressants may suppress REM sleep and impair daytime performance due to EDS. Although tricyclic antidepressants may improve sleep continuity, EDS is a common complaint in the elderly utilizing tricyclic antidepressants possibly secondary to suppression of REM sleep. Aspirin may have a net effect on EDS by increasing stage 2 sleep, decreasing SWS, and decreasing overall sleep efficiency. Beta-adrenergic antagonists, such as propranolol, may result in difficulty falling asleep and more frequent awakenings. Histamine-1 antagonists are frequently associated with drowsiness due to inhibition of N-methyltransferase and the blockage of central histaminergic receptors. On the contrary, histamine-2 antagonists, including cimetidine and ranitidine, usually have no significant effects on sleep. Substances that increase nocturnal wake time with resultant EDS include beta-adrenergic blockers, stimulants, caffeine, and diuretics. Other medications commonly used in the elderly that may cause EDS include antiepileptic drugs and antipsychotic agents (7,10).

In the past, medical treatment for EDS in elderly patients was more problematic due to the risk for hypertension associated with the use of stimulants. The recent approval of modafinil for narcolepsy has provided a much safer means of treating EDS in both young and older populations. In the near future, modafinil may acquire FDA approval for use in fatigue and other related disorders, potentially providing a means to improve EDS in patients without treatable underlying medical or psychiatric conditions.

DIFFICULTY FALLING ASLEEP AND MAINTAINING SLEEP

The average total sleep time (TST) increases slightly in the elderly. Nonetheless, elderly patients are more likely to be concerned with difficulty falling asleep. The prevalence of insomnia in the elderly varies between 19.0% and 38.4% with difficulty falling asleep ranging from 10% to 36.7% (11,12). Women are often more likely to have difficulties with insomnia compared with men. It has been estimated that nearly 30% of elderly patients have difficulty with maintenance of sleep (11). Current research points to both physiologic and lifestyle changes in the elderly. Patients produce less melatonin and growth hormone with advancing age. Changes in core body temperature also likely play a role. Enviromental factors including a reduction of exposure to natural light and reduction of exercise may exacerbate sleep difficulties. Frequent nocturnal arousals result in EDS. To reduce EDS, elderly patients frequently take naps. These naps often further exacerbate sleep disturbances in the elderly, secondary to difficulty with falling asleep at night, resulting in a revolving cycle.

Difficulty with maintenance of sleep is also commonly related to medical or psychiatric illness. When patients have concerns with difficulty falling asleep or maintaining sleep, it is important to assess for other possible precipitating disease processes (Table 12-1). Patients without medical and psychiatric illness have lower sleep complaints than patients with concurrent medical illness (13–16). Unfortunately, the frequency of medical and psychiatric illness increases with advancing age.

Cardiopulmonary conditions often contribute significantly to sleep disturbances in the elderly. Paroxysmal nocturnal dyspnea may produce shortness of breath with resultant insomnia. Ischemic heart disease may produce nocturnal angina in approximately 10% of cases, particularly during REM sleep. Because OSA also becomes more

prevalent, elderly patients may have increased frequency and severity of nocturnal hypoxemia (17). Cheynes–Stokes breathing is a prominent cause of arousals and is present in approximately 50% of patients with congestive heart failure (CHF). Chronic lung disease contributes to nocturnal hypoxemia secondary to increased ventilation requirements and sleep-related factors that decrease ventilatory function. Decreased accessory muscle activity during REM sleep may cause diminished ventilation and resultant hypoxemia. Management is difficult and often requires concurrent use of medications and positive airway pressure. Positive airway pressure may not only prevent hypoxemia and arousals due to apneic episodes, but also may relieve chronic respiratory muscle fatigue (17).

Other medical disease processes that produce disruption of normal sleep physiology include gastroesophageal reflux disease and rheumatologic disease, such as arthritis and fibromylagia. Chronic renal failure also increases with frequency with advancing age. Polysomnography (PSG) in chronic renal failure has demonstrated reduced SWS, poor sleep efficiency with increased arousals, increased restless legs and periodic leg movements of sleep (PLMS) due to iron-deficiency anemia, and significantly increased incidence of OSA. In chronic renal failure, increased frequency and severity of obstructive apneas may be due to fluid retention and upper-airway edema and central apneas may be more frequent secondary to metabolic acidosis (17).

Independently, sleep-related disorders also must be considered. The frequency of certain sleep-related disorders increase in frequency with advancing age and common precipitants of nocturnal arousals include nocturia, restless legs syndrome (RLS), PLMS, nocturnal leg cramps, REM behavior disorder (RBD), and sleep-related breathing disorders. Nocturia is a common precipitant of maintenance of sleep disturbances with a prevalence in the elderly of 63% to 72% (4,11). RLS occurs in approximately 5% of the population, but accounts for one-eighth of insomnia (18). It is relatively rare in younger patients, but becomes more common with advancing age. Patients with RLS will have an uncontrollable desire to move limbs secondary to associated paresthesias or dysethesias that is worse at rest and may be relieved with movement. Most patients with RLS complain of sleep disturbances, including difficulty falling asleep, frequent nocturnal awakenings, and associated EDS. RLS has been associated with several conditions that may be more prevalent with advancing age including renal insufficiency, uremia, diabetes, iron-deficiency anemia, chronic obstructive pulmonary disease (COPD), diabetes, vitamin B_{12} and folate deficiency, and peripheral neuropathy. The differential diagnosis in the elderly population includes polyneuropathy, radiculopathy, peripheral vascular disease, and vascular claudication (18,19). Approximately 80% of patients with RLS will have PLMS that may subsequently result in frequent arousals that exacerbate EDS (20).

▶ **TABLE 12-1. Medical and Psychiatric Conditions Associated with Insomnia in the Elderly**

Medical Conditions Associated with Insomnia in the Elderly
  Ischemic heart disease
  Dementia
  Cortical degenerative disorders
  Cerebrovascular disease
  Peripheral vascular disease
  Gastroesophageal reflux disease
  Incontinence
  Parkinson's disease
  Multiple systems atrophy
  Head trauma
  COPD
  Sleep-related asthma
  Fatal familial insomnia
  Arthritis
  Fibromyositis
  Hepatic encephalopathy
  Chronic renal failure
  Menopause
  Nocturnal epilepsy

Psychiatric Conditions Associated with Insomnia in the Elderly
  Depression
  Anxiety disorders
  Alcoholism
  Substance abuse

Elderly patients also tend to have more conditions associated with pain, with increased prevalence with advancing age. Approximately one-third of all pain sufferers have arthritic complaints. Nighttime pain sufferers may lose over 2 hours of sleep per night. Other pain syndromes including headaches, leg cramps, and fibromylagia may also contribute to disruption of sleep. Nocturnal leg cramps may occur in approximately 15% of the population with increased frequency with advancing age. These cramps may resolve in seconds but occasionally last a few minutes, with common precipitants including strenuous exercise, fluid and electrolyte disturbances, diabetes, caffeine, and nicotine in the elderly. Disturbance of calcium metabolism and other metabolic dysfunction is suspected (21,22).

Because many conditions increase in frequency with advancing age, medication effects must also be reviewed when patients complain of insomnia. Beta-adrenergic agonists (bronchodilators, decongestants), stimulants (amphetamines, caffeine), diuretics, and some antidepressants may increase nocturnal wake time. Elderly patients may also be at risk to develop alcohol-dependent and hypnotic-dependent sleep disorders. Other medications, including amphetamines, antipsychotics, lithium, MAO inhibitors, nicotine, selective serotonin reuptake inhibitors (SSRIs), and tricyclic antidepressants, may all suppress REM sleep and produce sleep fragmentation.

Treatment of insomnia in the elderly must include the diagnosis and treatment of underlying medical and psychiatric illness. Without adequate treatment of such underlying disease process, most patients will not have marked improvement of their symptoms. Long-standing difficulty with falling asleep or maintenance of sleep often increases the propensity for development of depression and other psychiatric conditions. The development of depression will further increase the chronic use of sedative hypnotics (23). Patients are often prescribed sedative hypnotics such as benzodiazepines for the arousals and perceived insomnia, but these agents may only exacerbate underlying sleep-related respiratory distress events. Therefore, these agents should be used with caution, and nonpharmacologic therapy should be considered either as an alternative or in conjunction with pharmacologic treatment. Common nonpharmacologic therapies include cognitive behavior therapy (24,25), sleep restriction therapy (26), light therapy (27), and exercise (28). If pharmacologic therapy is utilized, the adage of "start low and go slow" should be followed secondary to alteration of metabolism and elimination of these agents in the elderly.

UNUSUAL MOVEMENTS AND BEHAVIORS WHILE ASLEEP

Movements at night can be both normal physiologic phenomena and pathologic conditions. These activities can also be classified as sleep-related and sleep-independent conditions. With advancing age, all of these conditions may increase with both frequency and severity. Patients (or family members) may be distraught over relatively benign conditions and be less concerned over more potentially life-threatening problems. One of the most common concerns of patients in our clinics often is the hypnic jerk, which typically does not require medical intervention. Other sleep-related movements may also be benign, such as PLMS, or be more problematic including non-REM and REM-related parasomnias and also nocturnal epilepsy. Careful history taking is critical, but PSG may be necessary to differentiate conditions. Foremost, patient education of normal and abnormal movements in sleep is imperative.

Non-REM parasomnias (sleep walking, night terrors) and PLMS can often be differentiated from REM-related parasomnias based on the peak frequency of each of these conditions. In children and many younger adults sleep, walking/night terrors occur out of SWS. Hence, these behaviors tend to occur early during the night, whereas REM behavior disorder tends to occur later in the morning. However, in adults NREM parasomnias can also occur out of stage 1 and 2 sleep and therefore can occur at any time during the night. PLMS increases with advancing age, with a prevalence in the elderly of 45% compared with 5%–6% in younger adults (20). Many patients are unaware of the leg movements associated with PLMS, and more typically these are brought to the awareness of the patient and medical provider by bed partners. In situations where patients sleep alone due to medical conditions or the death of their partner, diagnosis in clinic may be difficult. Evidence of kicking off bed sheets or leg soreness upon awakening in conjunction with EDS may be the only clues. At times, it may be necessary to perform PSG to differentiate PLMS from more potentially dangerous parasomnias or sleep apnea, which can also be associated with body movements during sleep. PLMS are scored when there is a sequence of at least four muscle contractions (each lasting 0.5 to 5 seconds in duration) that recur at intervals of 5 to 90 seconds. The sleep profile of patients with PLMS include an increased light sleep (stages 1 and 2) with concurrent decreases in deep sleep (stages 3 and 4) and REM sleep, due to an increase in arousals. Because PLMS occur most commonly during stages 1 and 2 sleep, this may further exacerbate the patient's complaints of EDS due to frequent arousals. Of note, one should differentiate PLMS, a polysomnographic finding, and the periodic limb movement disorder (PLMD). The PLMD requires both PLMS and symptoms of insomnia or excessive daytime sleepiness not explained by other disorders. Because PLMS is such a common finding in older adults, one must be cautious about ascribing symptoms to them (i.e., a diagnosis of PLMD). For example, PLMS are common in patients with sleep apnea and usually do not require specific treatment. Daytime sleepiness in these patients usually resolves with effective treatment of obstructive events [nasal continuous positive airway pressure (CPAP)]. Conditions associated with PLMS include medical and neurologic conditions (dystonia, parkinsonism, motor neuron disease, myelopathy, multiple sclerosis, peripheral neuropathies, renal dysfunction, and anemia). The strongest association with other sleep-related disorders has been with RLS, but PLMS may also be seen with other sleep apnea, narcolepsy, and REM behavior disorder (29,30). The use of alcohol or tricyclic antidepressants or withdrawal from sedative-hypnotics may also produce PLMS. There may also be an increase in frequency after initiation of positive airway pressure for OSA, but this is usually a transient asymptomatic phenomenon. The treatment of PLMS is focused on reduction of movement and arousals. Dopaminergic agents are the treatment of choice because they reduce both the movements and arousals without sedation or reduction of respiratory muscle function that may be induced by sedative-hypnotic agents such as clonazepam.

REM-related parasomnias should always be considered prominently in the differential diagnosis of nocturnal seizures and other sleep-related movement while asleep. REM-related parasomnias are considered to be secondary to disturbance of normal physiologic sleep. In REM sleep, skeletal muscle atonia results from active inhibition of motor activity by pontine centers of the perilocus ceruleus region, which influences hyperpolarization of spinal motor neuron postsynaptic membranes via the ventrolateral reticulospinal tract. Normally, the atonia of REM sleep is briefly interrupted by excitatory inputs that produce REM and muscle jerks. In patients in whom there is a obscuration of non-REM and REM sleep states, patients may demonstrate oneiric behavior by acting out their dreams, also known as REM behavior disorder (RBD). This condition is most common in middle-aged to elderly males. In RBD, sudden arousals may evolve into sudden aggressive behavior resulting in injury to either the patient or others. Often RBD is preceded by other parasomnias. Approximately two-thirds of cases may be associated with medical and neurologic disease including dementia, parkinsonism, stroke, tumors, and withdrawal for sedative-hypnotics. Diagnosis is predominantly made on clinical assessment, with the peak frequency occurring in the latter one-third of the night when REM sleep is most abundant. Video–PSG can help to differentiate RBD from other conditions such as sleepwalking, psychogenic dissociative disorder, post-traumatic stress disorder, and nocturnal seizures (31). Suppression of REM sleep with clonazepam is effective for both the vivid dreams and oneiric behavior. Other treatment options include tricyclic antidepressants and carbamazepine.

By age 70, the incidence of epilepsy is nearly twice that of individuals less than 60 years old and is roughly fourfold by age 80 (32). Application of the 1980 age-specific prevalence rate of approximately 0.9% to 1.5% in the elderly reveals an estimated 300,000 to 350,000 elderly patients with epilepsy (33,34). A seizure is the clinical manifestation of abnormal excitatory discharges within the cerebral cortex that generate motor and sensory symptoms with or without alteration in consciousness. Seizures can be subdivided into: (a) primary generalized seizures, and (b) partial seizures with or without secondary generalization. Primary generalized seizures rarely manifest in the elderly. Partial seizures are more common in the elderly due to causative factors generating focal epileptogenic regions within the cortex. Although definitive etiologies of epilepsy are more readily identified in the elderly population, the causative factor remains unknown in up to 50% of cases (35,36). Structural lesions are the most common etiologies, with cortical stroke causing 33% to 50% of seizures in the elderly; the second most common cause are primary and metastatic brain tumors (6%–11%) (35–37). Other etiologies include posttraumatic epilepsy, toxic–metabolic disturbances, medications, alcohol intoxication and withdrawal, infection, subdural hematoma, and dementia. Common medications utilized in the elderly that lower seizure threshold are listed in Table 12-2 (38). If seizures are suspected, history remains the most pertinent information in most cases. It is important to remember that approximately one-third to one-half of patients will have seizures only during the awake state, one-fourth will have seizures only during sleep, and one-third will have seizures both during wake and sleep periods. Therefore, patients who present with nocturnal seizures may also have seizures while awake that may either endanger themselves or others.

The clinical manifestations of focal seizures will depend on the cortical location of the seizure focus. If a patient has a temporal lobe seizure focus, the only manifestations may be staring and nonresponsiveness, which will typically not awaken the patient's bed partner. Some of these

▶ **TABLE 12-2. Medications that May Cause Seizures**

Antidepressants	*Local Anesthetics*
Tricyclic antidepressants	Lidocaine
Bupropion	Procaine
Psychotropics	*Antibiotics*
Chlorpromazine	Penicillin
Thioridazine	Ampicillin
Trifluoperazine	Cephalosporins
Perphenazine	Pyrimethamine
Haloperidol	Isoniazid
Bronchial Agents	*Antineoplastic Drugs*
Theophylline	Vincristine
Aminophylline	Chlorambucil
Analgesics	BCNU
Fentanyl	Methotrexate
Meperidine	*Others*
Propoxyphene	Insulin
Tramadol hydrochloride	Antihistamines
Sympathomimetics	Alcohol
Phenylpropanolamine	Baclofen
Ephedrine	Cyclosporine
Terbutaline	Atenolol

patients will have automatisms with either lip smacking (oral) or repetitive hand movements (manual) that may alert others. Frontal lobe seizures may have similar presentations but may also have complex clonic or dystonic motor activity. If the focal seizure spreads throughout the cortex, the patient will manifest relatively violent tonic stiffening and/or clonic movements lasting on average from 1 to 3 minutes. These events are most likely to receive initial medical attention, but the clinician needs to be wary of the potential symptoms of focal seizures without generalization to determine the frequency and severity of the seizure disorder. Diagnostically, for isolated nocturnal events, it is recommended to perform PSG with a full array of EEG electrodes to evaluate for nocturnal interictal and ictal seizure activity. Serologic evaluation should be performed immediately for electrolyte and glucose abnormalities and for a toxicology screen. Neuroimaging with and without contrast is imperative if the initial evaluation does not delineate a possible etiology. If an initial EEG or polysomnogram are unremarkable, a sleep-deprived EEG may be necessary to enhance the possibility of detecting seizure activity.

Snoring and Gasping for Breath

Sleep-related breathing disorders are by far the most common sleep disorders. Most patients present with EDS and snoring. The prevalence of snoring and OSA increase with advancing age, with a prevalence of 70% of elderly males and 56% of elderly females (39–41). This is believed to be predominantly related to gradual weight gain with advancing age. Other age-related factors include decreased lung capacity, decreased ventilatory control, increased upper-airway collapsibility, increased muscle fatigability, decreased SWS, and reduced sleep efficiency (5). Intrinsic reduction of cardiopulmonary function will further reduce oxygenation. Furthermore, the normal aging process of reduced accessory inspiratory muscle function and obesity may produce profound episodes of apneas and hypopneas with marked desaturations.

Although the epidemiology of central sleep apnea (CSA) demonstrates no consistent epidemiologic trends, CSA may occur more commonly in middle-aged to elderly patients. During CSA, there is no EMG activity suggesting cessation of neuronal output to respiratory muscles. CSA may be idiopathic or caused by neurologic disorders or CHF, resulting in Cheyne–Stokes breathing most prominent in light NREM sleep. Other causes of CSA that may be prominent in elderly patients include multiple systems atrophy (Shy–Drager syndrome), diabetic autonomic neuropathy, medullary tumors or stroke, syringobulbia, Arnold–Chiari malformation, motor neuron disease (amyotrophic lateral sclerosis), neuromuscular junction disease (myasthenia gravis), and myopathies (42).

It is imperative that elderly patients with OSA are closely followed by their physicians. Although there are comorbidities, potential age-related outcomes with OSA include increased mortality, cardiovascular morbidity, and possible damage to other end organs (5). In patients with a marked decline in cognitive function over a few months, OSA may be a potentially reversible form of attentional dementia (43). In these cases, it is not uncommon to discover the recent initiation of sedative-hypnotics to treat perceived insomnia. The sedative–hypnotics may suppress respiratory drive and reduce the accessory muscle function that unmasks latent OSA. General treatment of patients with OSA includes review of concurrent medical disease and medications, weight loss, and sleeping in a lateral position. The treatment of choice for OSA remains CPAP. Dental devices and surgical intervention are secondary treatment options for mild and severe OSA, respectively.

SLEEP DISORDERS IN DEMENTIA AND DEGENERATIVE DISEASES

Degenerative disorders produce multifactorial sleep–wake disturbances with advancing age secondary to dysfunction of noradrenergic, serotonergic, and cholinergic systems. Compared to age-matched controls, demented patients have a greater disruption of sleep with more frequent arousals and decreased sleep efficiency, and may have increased stage 1 and decreased SWS (44–46). Patients with Alzheimer's disease often have dysregulation of their circadian rhythms, sleep excessively during the day, have nighttime awakening, and may have alteration of REM latency (44,46). In Alzheimer's disease, there may be a slight increase in prevalence of OSA but this is typically mild. Cortical degenerative processes may cause neuronal damage resulting in an increased risk of seizures (47).

Nocturnal delirium (sundowning) is agitated behavior with disorientation and confusion that typically occurs in the late evening. There are many contributors to sundowning in patients with dementia, including underlying cognitive impairment, reduced daytime light exposure, alteration of living conditions, medical illness, medications, infection, and metabolic disturbances (47). These patients tend to become less disruptive during the day due to EDS, which may further exacerbate sundowning. Resolution often depends on diagnosis and treatment of the underlying cause. Avoiding of naps and increased light exposure during the day may also be useful (48). If medical therapy is necessary for agitation, long-acting agents should be avoided since these may diminish alertness during the daytime.

In Parkinson's disease (PD), most patients have difficulty falling asleep and maintaining sleep. The resting tremor in PD typically resolves at sleep onset, but there is an increase in PLMS. In addition, there may be a prolongation of muscle tone in REM sleep resulting in RBD. In fact, RBD and other REM-related motor movement may precede the onset of clinical symptoms of PD. Medical treatment of PD with dopaminergic medications may also affect sleep. Dopaminergic agents may produce beneficial effects, including sedation at low doses with reduction of RLS and PLMS, but also may cause insomnia and dyskinesias at higher doses. Irrespective of dose, dopaminergic agents may also produce nightmares and vivid hallucinations. On the other hand, low-dose clonazepam at bedtime may be a benefit for PLMS, RBD, and insomnia in PD patients. In parkinsonlike syndromes (also known as multisystem atrophy), sleep-related disturbances similar to PD are often present and typically may be more debilitating (47).

The incidence of neuromuscular junction disease, such as myasthenia gravis, and motor neuron diseases, such as amyotrophic lateral sclerosis, also increase with frequency with advancing age. Both of these conditions may place significant stress on respiratory muscle function. This is exacerbated during REM sleep secondary to diffuse skeletal atonia. The overall effect often is severe OSA with resultant EDS. Recent studies have demonstrated the efficacy of positive airway pressure in these conditions. The positive airway pressure will improve airflow and may also relieve muscle fatigue of respiratory muscles (49).

The co-occurrence of sleep disorders with dementing illnesses has led to recognition of several syndromes. Lugaresi et al. (50) described a "fatal familial insomnia (FFI)" characterized by progressive loss of SWS with autonomic dysfunction, motor dysfunction, and dementia. Animal models have demonstrated abolition of REM atonia, resulting in dream-enacting complex movements termed oneiric behavior (51). In patients with FFI, Tinuper et al. (52) described episodes of "sleep" with vivid dreams that intruded spontaneously upon wakefulness, described as an "oneiric stuporous state." We had the opportunity to examine and study a patient who developed a progressive dementia with loss of SWS and REM atonia. The genetic deficit and postmortem findings were not consistent with FFI. We suspect that this patient had a previously unreported syndrome of progressive dementia associated with RBD and the absence of SWS, which was termed "oneiric dementia" (53).

PRESCRIBING MEDICATIONS FOR THE ELDERLY

With advancing age, the number of prescriptions an individual must take also increases. The prescribing practitioner must understand the economics of their elderly patients. Many prescription coverage programs are costly to elderly patients on a limited budget. Compliance may also be affected secondary to drug–drug interactions and significant side effects. The likelihood of dementia in the elderly exacerbates all of these factors. Simple theories to improve compliance and medical treatment in the elderly include minimizing the number of medications,

prescribing medications with once or twice daily dosing, starting at low doses and titrating slowly, and understanding the basic pharmacologic action of the patient's medications and their interactions (54). Patient and caregiver education is again paramount.

REFERENCES

1. Vitello MV. Sleep disorders and aging: understanding the causes. *J Gerontol.* 1997;52A:M189–191.
2. Schochat T, Ancoli-Israel S. Sleep and sleep disorders. In: Cassel CK, Leipzig RM, Cohen HJ, Larson EB, Meier DE, eds. *Geriatric medicine: An evidence based approach.* 4th edn. New York: Springer-Verlag, 2003:1031–1042.
3. Buysee DJ, Reynolds CF, Monk TH, et al. Quantification of subjective sleep quality in healthy elderly men and women using the Pittsburg Quality Sleep Index (PSQI). *Sleep.* 1991;14:331–338.
4. Middlekoop HAM, Smilde-van den Doel DA, Neven AK, et al. Subjective sleep characteristics of 1,485 males and females aged 50-93: effects of sex and age, and factors related to self-evaluated quality of sleep. *J Gerontol A Biol Sci Med Sci.* 1996;51:M108–M115.
5. Bliwise DL. Normal aging. In: Kryger MH, Roth T, Dement WC, eds. *Principles and practice of sleep medicine.* 3rd edn. Philadelphia: WB Saunders, 2000:26–42.
6. Feinberg I. Changes in sleep cycle patterns with age. *J Psychiatr Res.* 1974;10:283–306.
7. Aldrich MS. Approach to the patient. *Sleep medicine.* New York: Oxford University Press, 1999a:95–110.
8. Asplund R. Daytime sleepiness and napping amongst the elderly in relation to somatic health and medical treatment. *J Intern Med.* 1996;239:261–267.
9. Rye DB, Dihenia B, Weissman JD, et al. Presentations of narcolepsy after age 40. *Neurology.* 1998;50:459–465.
10. Nicholson AN, Bradley CM, Pascoe PA. Medications: Effect on sleep and wakefulness. In: Kryger MH, Roth T, Ddement WC, eds. *Principles and practice of sleep medicine.* 2nd edn. Philadelphia: WB Saunders, 1994:362–372.
11. Foley DJ, Monjan AA, Brown SL, et al. Sleep complaints amongst elderly persons: an epidemiological study of three communities. *Sleep.* 1995;18:425–432.
12. Ganglui M, Reynolds CF, Gilby JE. Prevalence and persistence of sleep complaints in rural older community sample: the MoVIES project. *J Amer. Geriatr Soc.* 1996;44:778–784.
13. Bliwise DL, King AC, Harris RB, et al. Prevalence of self-reported poor sleep in a healthy population aged 50-65. *Soc Sci Med.* 1992;34:49–55.
14. Ford DE, Kamerow DB. Epidemiologic study of sleep disturbances and psychiatric disorders. *JAMA.* 1989;262:1478–1484.
15. Morgan K, Healy DW, Healy PJ. Factors influencing persistent subjective insomnia in old age: a follow-up study of good and poor sleepers aged 65–74. *Age Ageing.* 1989;18:117–122.
16. Gislason T, Reynisdottir H, Kristbjarnarson H, et al. Sleep habits and sleep disturbances among the elderly—an epidemiological survey. *J Intern Med.* 1993;234:31–39.
17. Aldrich MS. Medical causes of disordered sleep. *Sleep medicine.* New York: Oxford University Press, 1999c:307–324.
18. Ekbom KA. Restless legs. *Acta Med Scand Suppl.* 1945;158:1–123.
19. Montplaisir J, Lapierre O, Warnes H, et al. The treatment of the restless leg syndrome with or without periodic leg movements of sleep. *Sleep.* 1992;14:496–500.
20. Ancoli-Israel S, Kripke DF, Klauber MR, et al. Sleep disordered breathing in community-dwelling elderly. *Sleep.* 1991;14:496–500.
21. Aldrich MS. Parasomnias. *Sleep medicine.* New York: Oxford University Press, 1999b:260–287.
22. Weiner IH, Weiner HL. Nocturnal leg muscle cramps. *JAMA.* 1980;244:2332–2333.
23. Dealberto MJ, Seeman T, McAvay GJ, et al. Factors related to current and subsequent psychotropic drug use in an elderly cohort. *J Clin Epidemiol.* 1997;50:357–364.
24. Edinger JD, Marsh GR, Hoelscher TJ, et al. A cognitive-behavioral

therapy for sleep maintenance insomnia in older adults. *Psychol Aging.* 1992;7:282–289.

25. Morin CM, Kowatch RA, Barry T, et al. Cognitive-behavior therapy for late life insomnia. *J Consult Clin Psychol.* 1993;61:137–146.

26. Friedman L. Bliwise DL, Yesavage JA, et al. A preliminary study comparing sleep restriction and relaxation treatments for insomnia in older adults. *J Gerontol.* 1991;46:P1–8.

27. Campbell SS, Dawson D, Anderson MW. Alleviation of sleep maintenance insomnia with timed exposure to bright light. *J Amer. Geriatr Soc.* 1993;41:829–836.

28. King AC, Oman RF, Brasington GS, et al. Moderate-intensity exercise and self-rated quality of sleep in older adults: a randomized controlled trial. *JAMA.* 1997:32–37.

29. Culpepper W, Badia P, Shaffer J. Time of night patterns in PLMS activity. *Sleep.* 1992;15(4):306–311.

30. Trenkwalder C, Walters AS, Hening W. Periodic leg movements and restless legs syndrome. In: Aldrich MS, ed. *Neurologic clinics: Sleep disorders I,* Vol. 14. Philadelphia: WB Saunders, 1996:629–650.

31. Mahowald MW, Schenk CH. REM Sleep parasomnias. In: Kryger MH, Roth T, Dement WC, eds. *Principles and practice of sleep medicine.* Philadelphia: WB Saunders, 2000:724–741.

32. Hauser WA, Annegers JF, Kurland LT. Incidence of epilepsy and unprovoked seizures in Rochester, Minnesota: 1935–1984. *Epilepsia.* 1993;34:453–468.

33. Hauser WA, Annegers JF, Kurland LT. Prevalence of epilepsy in Rochester, Minnesota: 1940–1980. *Epilepsia.* 1993b;32:429–445.

34. de la Court A, Breteler M, Meinardi H, et al. Prevalence of epilepsy in the elderly: the Rotterdam study. *Epilepsia.* 1996;37(2):141–147.

35. Hauser WA. Seizure disorders: the changes with age. *Epilepsia.* 1992;33(Suppl. 4):S6–14.

36. Luhdorf K, Jensen LK, Pleser AM. Etiology of seizures in the elderly. *Epilepsia.* 1986;27:458–463.

37. Ettinger AB, Shinnar S. New onset seizures in the elderly hospitalized population. *Neurology.* 1993;43:489–482.

38. Messing RO, Closson RG, Simon RP. Drug-induced seizures: A 10-year experience. *Neurology.* 1984;34:1582–1593.

39. Ancoli-Israel S, Kripke DF, Klauber MR, et al. Periodic limb movements in sleep in community-dwelling elderly. *Sleep.* 1991a;14:486–495.

40. Bliwise DL. Sleep in normal aging and dementia. *Sleep.* 1993;16:40–81.

41. Chervin RD, Guilleminault C. Obstructive sleep apnea and related disorders. In: Aldrich MS, ed. *Neurologic clinics: Sleep disorders I.* Vol. 14. Philadelphia: WB Saunders, 1996:583–609.

42. Guilleminault C, Robinson A. Central sleep apnea. In: Aldrich MS, ed. *Neurologic clinics: Sleep disorders I.* Vol. 14. Philadelphia: WB Saunders, 1996:611–628.

43. Bliwise DL. Is sleep apnea a cause of reversible dementia in old age? *J Amer. Geriatr Soc.* 1996;44:1407–1409.

44. McCurry SM, Logsdon RG, Teri L, et al. Characteristics of sleep disturbance in community-dwelling Alzheimer's disease patients. *J Geriatr Psychiatry Neurol.* 1999;12(2):53–59.

45. McKeith IG, Perry EK, Perry RH. Report of the second dementia with Lewy body international workshop: diagnosis and treatment. Consortium on Dementia with Lewy Bodies. *Neurology.* 1999;53:902–905.

46. Bliwise DL, Tinklenberg J, Yesavage JA, et al. REM latency in Alzheimer's disease. *Biol Psych.* 1989;25(3):320–328.

47. Aldrich MS. Sleep disorders in dementia and related degenerative diseases. *Sleep medicine.* New York: Oxford University Press, 1999d:325–337.

48. Mishima K, Okawa M, Hishikawa Y, et al. Morning bright light therapy for sleep and behavior disorder in elderly patients with dementia. *Acta Psychiatr Scand.* 1994;89:1–7.

49. Clinical indications for noninvasive positive pressure ventilation in chronic respiratory failure due to restrictive lung disease, COPD, and nocturnal hypoventilation—a consensus conference report. *Chest.* 1999;116:521–534.

50. Lugaresi E, Medori R, Montagna P, et al. Fatal familial insomnia and dysautonomia with selective degeneration of thalamic nuclei. *New Engl J Med.* 1986;315:997–1003.

51. Sastre JP, Jouvet M. Le Comportement onirique du chat. *Physiol Behav.* 1979;22:979–989.

52. Tinuper P, Monyagna P, Medori R, et al. The thalamus participates in the regulation of the sleep-waking cycle. A clinico-pathological study in fatal familial thalamic degeneration. *Electroencephalogr Clin Neurophysiol.* 1989;73:117–123.

53. Cibula JE, Eisenschenk S, Gilmore RL, et al. Progressive dementia and hypersomnolence with dream enacting behavior: oneiric dementia. *Arch Neurol.* 2002;59:630–634.

54. Beizer JL. Clinical strategies of prescribing for older adults. In: Cassel CK, Leipzig RM, Cohen HJ, Larson EB, Meier DE, eds. *Geriatric medicine: An evidence based approach.* 4th edn. New York: Springer-Verlag, 2003:83–89.

Sleep Disorders

Chapter 13

Insomnia: Causes and Treatments

Sidney D. Nau and Kenneth L. Lichstein

INSOMNIA: A COMPLEX PROBLEM AND A CHALLENGE TO TREAT

Many times insomnia is difficult to resolve, and all physicians have many patients with insomnia. This chapter aims to help the professional who is confronted with an insomniac to move from a chief complaint of insomnia to a plan for the patient's treatment, or, to a referral for treatment. We note the option to refer out for treatment due to our assumption that not all physicians will choose to treat people with persistent or severe insomnia.

Sleep is sensitive to disturbance by many internal influences, such as excessive worry, excessive anxiety, and a depressed mood. Sleep can also be disturbed by many external influences, for example, transient stress, an important life event, excessive noise, high or low room temperature, an uncomfortable bed, high altitude, jet lag, drug withdrawal, and sleeping in unfamiliar surroundings. Several types of etiologic factors can cause chronic difficulty sleeping, including circadian rhythm disorders, psychiatric disorders, pharmacologic agents, physical illnesses, sleep-related physiologic disorders, and negative conditioning effects; there are subtypes under each of these types of etiologic factor.

Subtypes of insomnia have specific therapies; it is not accurate to view insomnia as one general problem of difficulty sleeping that has only one treatment. The term insomnia has several meanings. First, it is common and appropriate to consider insomnia as a stereotype for disturbed sleep. Second, insomnia is a clinical symptom for over 30 sleep disturbance diagnostic subtypes. Finally, people with insomnia represent a large set of sleep disorders; hence, it is proper to speak of the insomnias, which are disorders that present with an insomnia complaint. The insomnias have varied causes and specific treatments with proved effectiveness for different diagnostic subtypes.

Although insomnia can be difficult to resolve, not all cases warrant referral to a specialist. As with other widespread health problems, most people with insomnia are initially seen by primary care physicians, who, of course, are not sleep specialists. A clinical assessment of limited intensity is suitable for the initial insomnia evaluation and adequate for the initial treatment selection. The cases of recent onset, and the less severe cases, can be successfully evaluated and successfully treated by physicians in general practice. The more chronic and the more severe cases may need to see an insomnia specialist.

CLINICAL EPIDEMIOLOGY AND SIGNIFICANCE

The high prevalence of insomnia is well documented; population surveys estimate one-third of all adults have one or more episodes each year (1). In one of the best U.S. surveys, 15% reported having a serious problem with insomnia during the past year (2). Insomnia increases with age. In middle-age samples, the frequency of chronic insomnia is estimated to be around 10% (3). Clinically significant insomnia prevalence in older adults is estimated at 25% and higher (1,2). Insomnia is common enough in late life to be one of the negative changes that characterize the experience of aging. In a recent U.S. poll, 67% of the adults over age 55 reported having symptoms of sleep disorders at least a few nights a week, but only 8% had been diagnosed with a sleep disorder, and fewer received treatment (4).

Clinical insomnia not only causes nights of restless, broken sleep and frustration; daytime sequelae include depressed mood, anxiety, daytime fatigue, irritability, reduced concentration, and memory complaints (5,6). Daytime functioning impairment that patients attribute to insomnia can affect the physical, emotional, cognitive, occupational, and social areas of life (7,8).

PRIMARY AND SECONDARY INSOMNIA

The majority of people with a chronic complaint of insomnia are found to have secondary insomnia (9). The frequent presence of secondary insomnia is a major reason for the importance of accurate insomnia diagnosis. When there is secondary insomnia, the difficulty sleeping is not the most pressing and dominant problem—it is not the primary problem. The course of treatment for secondary insomnia will begin by focusing on an underlying primary factor believed to have caused the patient's poor sleep. For example, the patient may have a mood disorder associated with sleep disturbance. Treatment would begin with mood disorder therapy. The patient may have sleep-related periodic limb movements (PLMs), where treatment begins with medication to suppress sleep-disturbing muscle twitches. Direct treatment for insomnia is often delayed while treatment for the other problem is initiated, but immediate treatment of secondary insomnia may also be indicated (see below). There are over 20 types of secondary insomnia.

Primary insomnia refers to two types of cases: (a) a situation where basic features of a primary insomnia have been identified, or (b) a situation where underlying causes for secondary insomnia have been ruled out, thus revealing that the insomnia is not secondary in nature. Primary insomnia is sometimes referred to as *pure* insomnia, to indicate that difficulty sleeping is at the core of the disorder. These cases are some of the most difficult insomnias to treat. When physicians refer cases on to insomnia specialists, they are often those judged to be chronic primary insomnia.

In some cases, what initially appears to be secondary insomnia is later revealed to be comorbid insomnia, where insomnia and the other disorder are independent, but co-occurring. It is difficult to discriminate primary insomnia co-occurring with another disorder (comorbid insomnia) from insomnia caused by another disorder (secondary insomnia). A recent review analyzes this diagnostic task (10). To avoid delayed treatment for persistent insomnia, we recommend that when secondary insomnia is suspected, treatment should be considered for the condition perceived to be causing the insomnia; *and* direct treatment should also be considered for insomnia. The direct treatment will prevent chronic, untreated insomnia.

TRANSIENT AND SHORT-TERM INSOMNIA (PROS AND CONS ON TREATMENT)

Most insomnia episodes last for 1 month or less (2). These are highly prevalent and are classified as transient or short-term insomnia. When an episode lasts for more than 4 weeks, it is termed chronic or persistent insomnia.

The more brief insomnias raise the questions of treatment need and timing—whether to treat an insomnia complaint, and whether to treat it right away when the patient first presents versus a decision not to treat, or at least to delay a treatment choice until the problem is shown to be more persistent. There are two common responses to these questions.

First, when the decision is "no" to treatment for short-term insomnia, limited assistance will typically be offered. General sleep management advice and a supportive manner are routinely offered. When treatment is not offered, there are implied assumptions: (a) that treatment is not necessary for symptom relief, and, (b) that treatment is not necessary to prevent the problem from persisting or worsening.

When the decision is "yes," and treatment is offered for an insomnia of recent onset, the service provider typically seeks two types of benefit: sure and possible benefits. Certainly, this early treatment can be counted on to provide symptom relief and alleviate emotional distress. A common treatment package includes a trial with sedative–hypnotic medication (11) and basic sleep hygiene advice. The second, and more speculative, type of benefit is preventive. Some physicians begin treatment early in the history of an insomnia as part of efforts to prevent chronic insomnia.

A decision to provide no treatment offers the patient only support and sleep hygiene advice. A decision not to treat short-term insomnia is reasonable, based on the statistic that, without treatment, most transient and short-term insomnias do not progress to chronic insomnia (12).

The decision to treat an insomnia of recent onset is a clinical one, based upon patient distress and professional judgment about need for intervention. Prevention of chronic insomnia is an additional treatment goal in some cases (11). There is no research to document long-term benefits from early treatment, nor data showing long-term negative consequences from early treatment.

MODEL OF CAUSES AND TREATMENTS FOR INSOMNIA

Buysse and Reynolds (13) present a conceptual framework within which to examine insomnia cases. A graphic portrayal of their ideas is presented in Fig. 13-1 and Fig. 13-2. Figure 13-1 summarizes the varied types of etiologic factors; Figure 13-2 is discussed later (see *principles for treatment planning* section). Figure 13-2 presents a multifactor model of insomnia treatment. These figures and the overview of insomnia etiologies that they portray can help a professional organize in preparation for the tasks of insomnia evaluation and treatment.

Figure 13-1 shows causes of insomnia. It begins with four general types of etiologic factors commonly noted in people with insomnia (circadian, psychiatric, pharmacologic, medical/neurologic illness). These four factors are portrayed as common precipitating factors for episodes of insomnia. In addition, the stereotypic insomnia experience includes psychophysiologic and conditioning factors that may precipitate, and that often perpetuate an insomnia.

Psychophysiologic and conditioning factors characterize single-diagnosis primary insomnia, and they

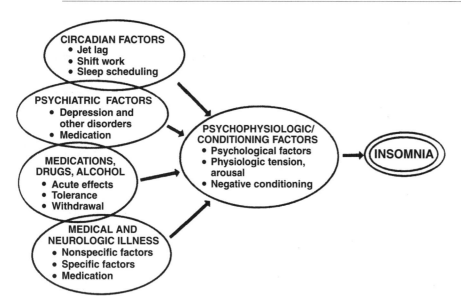

FIGURE 13-1. Several etiologic factors may contribute to the development of insomnia. Psychophysiological and behavioral factors often perpetuate an insomnia that had its origins in a medical, psychiatric, or circadian disturbance. (From Buysse and Reynolds. In: Thorpy MJ, ed. *Handbook of sleep disorders.* New York: Marcel Dekker, 1990:380. With permission.)

characterize the conditioned insomnia that is commonly overlaid on other types of persistent insomnia. Such overlay often causes multiple-diagnosis chronic insomnia (Fig. 13-1).

The psychophysiologic and conditioning factors include: (a) psychologic characteristics (such as subclinical anxiety and low mood), (b) physiologic tension/arousal, and (c) a history of negative conditioning (caused by frequent nights with excessive amounts of time spent lying awake). Negative conditioning is sometimes compounded by learning negative sleep habits (*poor sleep hygiene*), such as staying in bed late in the morning, naps, irregular bedtimes, and trying too hard to sleep. The physiologic tension/arousal of insomnia varies across individuals and may include cognitive overarousal (e.g., "mind racing,"

"thinking about all kinds of things," "thoughts jumping from topic to topic"), physiologic overarousal (e.g., tense muscles, restlessness, "feel wide awake," etc.), and arousability/sensitivity to stimuli (such as environmental sounds, temperature, light, and bedcovers).

Buysse and Reynolds emphasize that the most important components of chronic insomnia may be the psychophysiologic and behavioral/conditioning factors, since they "often perpetuate an insomnia, which had its origin in a medical, psychiatric, or circadian disturbance" (13, p. 380). The behavioral therapies for insomnia (see page 182, *Behavioral Treatments for Persistent Primary Insomnia*) are designed to reverse the behavioral/conditioning and psychophysiologic factors that can be the key perpetuating factors for a chronic insomnia.

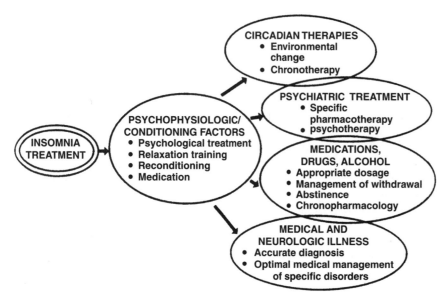

FIGURE 13-2. Treatment of insomnia must often address multiple etiologic factors. Treatment aimed at psychophysiologic-behavioral factors is often appropriate, even when medical, psychiatric, or circadian disturbance is present, since these behavioral factors may perpetuate other types of insomnia. (From Buysse and Reynolds. In: Thorpy MJ, ed. *Handbook of sleep Disorders.* New York: Marcel Dekker, 1990:408. With permission.)

Figure 13-2 (see page 179, *Principles for Treatment Planning*) outlines the types of insomnia treatment that address the varied insomnia causes shown in Fig. 13-1. Successful insomnia treatment often contains only one technique, such as pharmacotherapy, stimulus-control behavior therapy, or medical treatment for a sleep-related physiologic disorder [e.g., periodic limb movement disorder (PLMD), restless legs syndrome (RLS)]. One treatment technique is the simplest treatment plan. The complexity of factors contributing to chronically disturbed sleep often necessitates a multicomponent treatment plan. Multiple diagnoses for a person with chronic insomnia are frequently noted, which is another reason why "treatment for insomnia must often address multiple etiological factors" (13, p. 408).

CATEGORIES OF INSOMNIA SUBTYPE AND CAUSES OF INSOMNIA

The International Classification of Sleep Disorders (ICSD) presents over 30 insomnia diagnoses. As an aid to diagnosis and treatment planning, the diagnoses are grouped into nine categories. The categories are defined by the type of cause for the sleep disturbance: (a) transient or short-term factors, (b) psychophysiologic and/or conditioning factors, (c) associated with psychiatric disorders, (d) related to medications, drugs, or alcohol, (e) associated with circadian rhythm disorders, (f) secondary to sleep-related physiologic disorders, (g) related to neurologic disorders, (h) associated with other medical illness, (i) secondary to environmental factors. These groupings will also help lay the groundwork for our discussion of assessment and treatment selection.

Table 13-1 lists 29 common insomnia subtypes in the nine categories. In the following sections, the 29 subtypes are described and prevalence and typical course discussed. The subtype descriptions are based on the ICSD (12) (Table 13-1).

Transient or Short-Term Factors (The Most Frequent Cause)

Adjustment Sleep Disorder

Adjustment sleep disorder, the most common type of insomnia, is caused by a psychologic reaction to events. The sleep disturbance is correlated with a clearly identifiable stress or environmental change causing emotional arousal; the emotional reaction may be in response to normal events, such as a child preparing to begin a new school year, someone facing an important evaluation, or in relation to work or personal problems. To diagnose an adjustment sleep disorder, the insomnia must be a clear change from the patient's norm. Adjustment sleep disorder is considered a prototype for the disruptive effects of psycho-

▶ **TABLE 13-1.** Insomnia Diagnoses by Type of Etiologic Factor

1. *Transient or Short-Term Factors*
   Adjustment sleep disorder
2. *Insomnia Related to Psychophysiological and/or Conditioning Factors*
   Psychophysiologic insomnia
   Idiopathic insomnia
   Sleep-state misperception
   Inadequate sleep hygiene
3. *Sleep Disorders Associated with Psychiatric Disorders*
   Psychoses associated with sleep disturbance
   Mood disorders associated with sleep disturbance
   Anxiety disorders associated with sleep disturbance
   Panic disorder associated with sleep disturbance
   Alcoholism associated with sleep disturbance
4. *Insomnia Related to Medications, Drugs, and Alcohol*
   Hypnotic-dependent sleep disorder
   Stimulant-dependent sleep disorder
   Alcohol-dependent sleep disorder
5. *Insomnia Associated with Circadian Rhythm Disorders*
   Delayed-sleep phase syndrome (DSPS)
   Advanced sleep-phase syndrome (ASPS)
   Shift work sleep disorder
   Irregular sleep–wake pattern
6. *Insomnia Secondary to Sleep-Related Physiologic Disorders*
   Periodic limb movement disorder (PLMD)
   Restless legs syndrome (RLS)
   Central sleep apnea (CSA)
   Obstructive sleep apnea (OSA)
   Narcolepsy
7. *Insomnia Related to Neurologic Illness*
   Cerebral degenerative disorders
   Dementia
   Parkinsonism
8. *Insomnia Associated with Other Medical Illness*
   Fibrositis syndrome
   Sleep-related gastroesophageal reflux
   Chronic obstructive pulmonary disease (COPD)
9. *Insomnia Associated with Situational Factors*
   Environmental sleep disorder

logic factors on sleep. When the emotional reaction resolves, sleep returns to normal. All people are subject to having adjustment sleep disorders. Epidemiologic studies suggest that one-third of adults have at least one episode of transient insomnia each year (2).

Serious complications are usually absent. If left untreated, possible complications include negative conditioning of associations with the bedroom and decreased confidence in the ability to sleep normally, consequences which could favor the development of persistent insomnia. However, serious medical or psychologic complications are believed to be rare, unless an adjustment sleep disorder is overlaid on preexisting medical or psychiatric illness (12).

Insomnia Related to Psychophysiologic and/or Conditioning Factors

The four subtypes of insomnia in this category are referred to collectively as primary insomnia or *intrinsic insomnia*. They represent the insomnias that have been formally designated as exemplars of persistent primary insomnia, or pure insomnia (12); the first, psychophysiologic insomnia, is considered the most stereotypic primary insomnia.

Psychophysiologic Insomnia (The Classic Form of Pure Insomnia)

Psychophysiologic insomnia (14) is the most common type of persistent primary insomnia and considered the prototype for primary insomnia. Psychophysiologic insomnia is defined as a persistent, or chronic, disorder of somatized tension, maintained by learned sleep-preventing associations. Based upon repeated negative experiences with difficulty sleeping, the learned associations can be established either to internal mental contents (for example, based upon repeated associations between thoughts of bedtime and aroused anticipation of difficulty sleeping), or to external stimuli (such as many past experiences associating the bedroom environment with excess arousal during the night).

Conditioned associations to external stimuli are often caused by the frequent association of sleeplessness with situations and behaviors related to sleep, which can establish conditioned excess arousal in the prebedtime period. After many repetitions, lying awake in one's bedroom may cause conditioned excess arousal, as may behaviors that lead up to bedtime, such as brushing teeth, preparing the bedroom, or turning off the lights. Occasionally, a person with insomnia will temporarily escape this conditioned arousal and sleep well when sleeping in unfamiliar surroundings that have not been previously associated with insomnia (e.g., when visiting the home of a friend or relative).

Learned associations to internal mental contents are mainly conditioned overconcern about the inability to sleep. This overconcern can cause a circular pattern wherein difficulty sleeping leads to more effort to obtain sleep, which causes an increase in arousal, and less ability to sleep. This pattern is often referred to as *trying too hard to sleep*, and it is associated with a complementary ability to fall asleep more easily when *not trying*. For example, a person who frequently stays awake at night when *trying* to sleep, may become drowsy when listening to a lecture or watching television, despite an intent to stay awake. The drowsiness may represent an escape from the anxiety and arousal often associated with trying to sleep.

As a complication of psychophysiologic insomnia, excessive use of hypnotics or use of alcohol as a sleep aid are often noted. Tranquilizers may be used in the daytime to decrease somatized tension, and caffeine or stimulants may be used to combat fatigue.

Among patients referred to sleep disorders centers, about 15% of people with insomnia complaints receive a diagnosis of psychophysiologic insomnia (15). Among all individuals who experience a transient sleep disorder, it is not known how many go on to develop psychophysiologic insomnia. Also, the prevalence of psychophysiologic insomnia in the general population is unknown.

The widespread occurrence of learned sleep-preventing associations represents, over the course of persistent insomnia episodes, a component that is added to the initial pattern of sleep disturbance for most chronic insomnias. Learned sleep-preventing associations, while the key defining feature of psychophysiologic insomnia, also play an important role in the other forms of insomnia, based upon the common experience of negative conditioning.

Psychophysiologic insomnia and the other primary insomnias are typically diagnosed by exclusion, after all the causes of secondary insomnia have been ruled out. In addition to single-diagnosis psychophysiologic insomnia, this type of insomnia is often present in multiple-diagnosis cases of chronic insomnia, due to the overlay of conditioned sleep-preventing associations developed over time.

When trying to determine the most basic factor contributing to a possible psychophysiologic insomnia, a common differential concerns psychiatric disorders that include sleep disturbance. When an affective disorder, generalized anxiety disorder, or other psychiatric disorder is present, psychiatric treatment will usually take precedence over treatment for psychophysiologic insomnia. A recent study challenges the precedence for psychiatric treatment that causes delay in insomnia treatment. The results of Lichstein, Wilson, Johnson (16) suggest that simultaneous treatment for psychiatric disorder and behavioral treatment for insomnia can be successful.

Idiopathic Insomnia

Idiopathic insomnia (17) is a rare, lifelong inability to obtain adequate sleep. It typically begins at birth, or by early adolescence at the latest. It is presumably due to an abnormality in the neurologic regulation of sleep (the sleep–wake system). The insomnia cannot be explained by childhood psychological trauma or by medical problems that chronically disturb the sleep–wake system, such as pain or allergies.

Chronically poor sleep leads to a general decrease in sense of well-being; there can be low mood, decreased motivation, decreased vigilance and concentration, low energy, and fatigue. However, as long as sleep disturbance remains mild to moderate, psychologic adjustment remains in the normal range. If idiopathic insomnia is severe, daytime functioning may be severely disrupted and depressive features may be prominent.

Prevalence is unknown. Idiopathic insomnia is rarely observed in a pure form. The lifelong difficulty almost always causes complications that compound the problem, such as conditioned sleep-preventing associations and sleep-disruptive psychiatric symptoms. Hypnotics are often used excessively and, often, there is excessive alcohol intake in an effort to promote sleep.

Sleep State Misperception

Sleep state misperception (18) is a disorder in which a subjective complaint of insomnia occurs, but objective sleep laboratory results do not show significant difficulty falling asleep or staying asleep. In the morning after polysomnography (PSG, the term for physiologic sleep recordings), the patient will report the insomnia problem occurred during the night. The prevalence of this disorder is not known, because most insomnia patients are not referred for sleep laboratory testing.

The apparent conflict between the subjective and objective findings has not been explained. The most common explanation is that these patients experience a type of objective problem that is not measured by standard PSG measures; for example, perhaps experiential awareness that persists during sleep, which is not measurable by standard sleep recordings, contributes to a perception of being awake. This hypothetical unmeasured cognitive activity perhaps could resemble the cognitive awareness of one's own dreaming that occasionally occurs during REM sleep, during what is known as a lucid dream—but the sleep state misperception patient does not have the unusual mental activity that cues a lucid dreamer to the presence of sleep (as well as being a cue for the lucid dreamer to the presence of dreaming). Perhaps sleep state misperception patients have other physiologic abnormalities during sleep that are not detected by recording methods currently in use.

Some research has shown similar subjective results from behavioral treatment for psychophysiologic insomnia and behavioral treatment for sleep state misperception patients (19). The psychological evaluation results with sleep state misperception do not reveal evidence of psychopathology. Before treating for sleep state misperception, special care should be taken to rule out insomnia related to mental disorders.

Inadequate Sleep Hygiene

Inadequate sleep hygiene is a sleep disorder resulting from habits and activities of daily living that are inconsistent with obtaining good quality sleep and that work against maintaining full daytime alertness.

Sleep hygiene habits are important health knowledge; they include positive and negative sleep management behaviors that are under an individual's control. Negative sleep hygiene behaviors can be classified in two general categories: (a) practices that increase general level of

▶ **TABLE 13-2. Daily Living Activities That Are Inconsistent with the Maintenance of Good Quality Sleep**

1. Frequent napping
2. Variable bedtimes or variable morning risetimes
3. Frequently spending an excessive length of time in bed
4. Regular use of sleep-disruptive substances near bedtime (e.g., alcohol, tobacco, caffeine)
5. Exercise too near bedtime
6. Stimulating activities too close to bedtime
7. Use of the bed for non-sleep-related activities (such as watching television, reading, snacking)
8. Using an uncomfortable bed
9. Poor control of the bedroom environment (e.g., too much light, heat, cold, or noise)
10. Performing activities that demand strong concentration near bedtime
11. Allowing oneself to persist in sleep-preventing mental activities while in bed, such as, thinking, planning, reminiscing, etc. (When these mental activities persist, it is best to get out of bed for a while and do something relaxing until sleepy.)

arousal during nocturnal sleep times (for example, regular daytime naps), and (b) practices that disrupt the sleep pattern within an individual night (such as alcohol) or influence the pattern across nights (such as a frequently changing sleep schedule).

Table 13.2 presents a representative list of negative sleep hygiene practices. This list is based upon material from the ICSD (12).

When sleep hygiene is grossly inadequate, it can easily be revealed during a clinical evaluation. For example, a grossly excessive length of time spent in bed, frequent naps, or high variability in the time of arising will be obvious. Mild deficiencies that cause sleep disturbance may be missed during an initial interview. Daily sleep logs, when filled out for 2 weeks, can greatly help in the thorough assessment of the scheduling aspects of sleep hygiene.

Inadequate sleep hygiene behaviors may precipitate an episode of insomnia, and they may help perpetuate insomnias with varied etiologies. It is important to assess sleep hygiene in all insomnia patients because some negative sleep habits start after a sleep problem begins, in response to an episode of insomnia (such as napping and trying to sleep late in the morning—both habits that can develop due to seeking more sleep). These efforts to cope with the problem can help perpetuate the insomnia.

The prevalence of inadequate sleep hygiene disorder is not known, although it is believed to be a fairly common precipitant of insomnia episodes and a frequent contributing factor in persistent insomnia. In many cases, multiple factors have a cumulative effect that causes clinically significant insomnia, and inadequate sleep hygiene is commonly among the causal factors.

Sleep Disorders Associated with Mental Disorders

Most psychiatric disorders can have associated sleep disturbance. Five categories of psychiatric disorder are commonly seen in patients presenting with sleep complaints and need to be considered in differential diagnosis. These categories are included in the ICSD: psychoses, mood disorders, anxiety disorders, panic disorder, and alcoholism (12).

Psychoses Associated with Sleep Disturbance

Insomnia is a common feature of schizophrenia, schizophreniform disorder, and other functional psychoses. A significant decrease in total sleep time per night may precede psychotic decompensation and accompany the acute exacerbation of psychotic symptoms. Severe sleep disruption can be a significant complication with schizophrenia and lead to suicidal ideation. Acutely ill psychotic patients are more likely to experience severe sleep disturbance, while some chronic patients can show almost normal sleep during sleep laboratory testing.

Mood Disorders Associated with Sleep Disturbance

Major depression and dysthymia, mania, and hypomania, as well as other mood disorders, typically are associated with insomnia (20). In rare cases, excessive daytime sleepiness is associated with a mood disorder.

The difficulty sleeping associated with mood disorders includes two general patterns of insomnia that can help indicate the presence of depression and mania. In the depression pattern, there is difficulty falling asleep, sleep maintenance disturbance, and early morning awakening that prematurely ends the night's sleep (also termed *early final awakening* or *terminal insomnia*). The mania pattern shows sleep-onset insomnia and short sleep duration [sometimes with severely reduced total sleep time (TST)].

Frequent awakenings and early morning awakening are the most characteristic sleep features of major depression. Waking up well before the planned time of arising, followed by inability to return to sleep is the cardinal sleep complaint for major depression. Most depressed patients complain of nocturnal restlessness and daytime tiredness. In contrast, mania and hypomania patients, despite low TST, do not complain about the lack of sleep and report feeling rested and alert during the daytime. Despite their severe insomnia and daytime tiredness, most depressed patients are not objectively sleepy during daytime sleepiness testing with the Multiple Sleep Latency Test (MSLT) (21).

Among depressives, in general, younger patients are more likely to experience difficulty falling asleep at bedtime, relative to more elderly patients who experience greater difficulty with during-the-night awakenings. The characteristic pattern of insomnia associated with depression is frequently a very early sign of mood disorder, often appearing before clinical depression has become clearly established. With initiation of antidepressant medication, the insomnia complaint tends to improve more rapidly than the mood disturbance. Clinical experience indicates that at least 90% of patients with mood disorders have sleep disturbances at some time.

PSG recordings of depressed patients show abnormalities on several features of REM. The night's first period of REM sleep begins early (i.e., there is a short REM latency). Early onset of REM is the most characteristic feature of sleep laboratory results for depressed patients. Increased density of rapid eye movements during REM sleep is another abnormality associated with depression. Particularly because of REM abnormalities, PSG can be useful in confirming a mood disorder diagnosis. The PSG data can provide evidence of a biological component to the disorder, in support of somatic therapies for depression.

Anxiety Disorders Associated with Sleep Disturbance

The anxiety disorders (including, generalized anxiety disorder, simple phobias, obsessive–compulsive disorder, and posttraumatic stress disorder) are characterized by chronic anxiety and avoidance behaviors. The associated sleep disturbance is characteristically a sleep-onset or a sleep-maintenance insomnia, resulting from excessive anxiety or apprehensive expectation about life events. Typical sleep symptoms include frequent awakenings (some with anxious dreams), ruminative thinking, and anxiety attacks while awake during the night.

When the sleep disturbance has become chronic, conditioned arousal to the sleep environment may also be present. This conditioned sleep-preventing response is in addition to the excessive arousal of an anxiety disorder. This negative conditioning is not the most basic sleep-disturbing factor.

Anxiety disorders are chronic conditions. The associated sleep complaints follow a parallel temporal course. Sleep disturbance associated with anxiety disorders appears to be very common (22). Some patients develop sedative or hypnotic abuse secondary to anxiety disorder insomnia, which can lead to drug-dependency insomnia and complicate the primary disorder.

Panic Disorder Associated with Sleep Disturbance

Panic disorder is characterized by discrete episodes of intense fear or physical discomfort, which can occur unexpectedly. Panic episodes can be associated with sudden awakenings from sleep, followed by persistent arousal and difficulty returning to sleep (23).

Panic disorder is a chronic condition lasting for many years. The associated sleep complaints follow a parallel temporal course. Some patients develop sedative or hypnotic abuse, which can lead to hypnotic-dependent insomnia.

Some types of sleep-related fear episode need to be differentiated from awakenings related to panic disorder. Sleep terror episodes begin with a loud scream or yell during deep, nondreaming sleep. Sleep terror patients do not have daytime panic symptoms. Panic attacks are also not REM-related nightmares. Panic attacks tend to occur in non-REM stage 2 or 3 sleep and do not include dreamlike mental content.

Alcoholism Associated with Sleep Disturbance

Insomnia is a common consequence of chronic excessive alcohol intake (24). The long-term effects of alcohol upon sleep and daytime functioning are complex and change over time. The distribution of nocturnal sleep stages varies from person to person, and distribution can vary over the course of an individual's alcoholism disorder.

Of course, the immediate effects from a dose of alcohol include sedation. Sleep laboratory recordings show alcohol consumed near bedtime will promote sleep during the first 4 hours in bed, but will subsequently lead to increased wakefulness during the last 2 to 3 hours of an 8-hour sleep period. In addition to promoting sleep onset at bedtime, the sedative effects of alcohol can also increase snoring and obstructive sleep apnea (OSA). During the daytime, even a small dose of alcohol ingested by a sleepy individual can increase the risk for automobile accidents.

Insomnia Related to Medications, Drugs, and Alcohol

Hypnotic-dependent Sleep Disorder

Hypnotic-dependent insomnia (25) occurs in association with tolerance to or withdrawal from sedative–hypnotic medications. Several patterns of hypnotic use have been associated with insomnia due to use of sleeping pills. In the first pattern, brief use of a hypnotic, for several consecutive nights, may lead to difficulty sleeping when the drug is stopped (termed rebound insomnia), which may result in resuming use of the hypnotic. In the second pattern, sustained use of hypnotics frequently causes tolerance associated with a decrease in the drug's hypnotic effects and a return of symptoms. This often leads to an increase in the patient's dosage. In a third pattern, partial withdrawal may occur when persistent drug tolerance occurs, despite dosage increases, and causes either a generally diminished hypnotic effect or causes the hypnotic effect to dissipate well before the end of the night. Partial withdrawal can cause a secondary, drug-related sleep disturbance to occur despite continued hypnotic use. Finally, whenever there is abrupt termination of lengthy hypnotic use, severe sleeplessness can occur.

There is a hypothesized pattern of escalating dependence with long-term hypnotic use, as follows. Many patients are hesitant about the use of sleeping pills. They lose confidence and become apprehensive when the initial therapeutic benefits start to decrease. When dosages are increased to offset tolerance, daytime carryover side effects also increase, which may include excessive sleepiness. The daytime symptoms are attributed to the decreased ability to sleep at night. The patient will be distressed and may become focused on the perceived need for more effective medication. The patient may consult new physicians and try varied sedative–hypnotic compounds.

Finally, if the hypnotic therapy is stopped, sleep will return to the predrug pattern. After stopping hypnotics, the subjective quality of sleep is often judged to be worse than before starting the medication. The patient may fear the ability to sleep normally has been permanently lost. There may be central nervous system withdrawal symptoms, which can include nausea, aches, irritability, and restlessness. The experience of withdrawal symptoms can predispose the patient toward resumption of chronic hypnotic use, in search of more normal sleep and improved daytime functioning. As an important complication, anxiety, nervousness, or depression may result from a hypnotic-dependent sleep disorder, especially during withdrawal.

After hypnotic withdrawal, sleep may gradually normalize. More often, sleep disturbance will persist, and it will be important to seek to determine etiology. There could be a chronic psychophysiologic insomnia or insomnia secondary to psychiatric disorder. PSG may be indicated to assess for apnea, PLMD, and other physiologic sleep disorders.

Stimulant-dependent Sleep Disorder

The stimulant-dependent sleep disturbance is characterized by reduction of sleepiness or suppression of sleep by central nervous system (CNS) stimulants. When the drugs are withdrawn, sleepiness and sleep increase. Stimulant-dependent sleep disorder generally applies to the abuse of stimulants.

When a stimulant is prescribed for medical treatment (e.g., for asthma or attention-deficit disorder) difficulty falling asleep may occur when treatment is begun, when the dosage is increased, or the administration times are moved closer to bedtime. The difficulty usually ends after treatment changes become established. Stopping use of a prescribed stimulant may also cause transient withdrawal symptoms, such as daytime sleepiness.

When stimulants are used to suppress sleep or to maintain a drug-mediated sense of well-being, sleep problems occur. Drug tolerance develops, and this causes dosages to escalate. Inevitably, periods of high-dosage use will lead to exhaustion and periods of somnolence.

Psychiatric symptoms are prominent in association with chronic stimulant abuse. During drug administration, the symptoms may mimic paranoid schizophrenia. Because intravenous stimulant administration is common, infectious diseases may be a complication.

A mild case of stimulant abuse could be misdiagnosed as anxiety-related sleep onset insomnia. When stimulant abuse is chronic, the differential includes schizophrenia or mania.

Alcohol-dependent Sleep Disorder

The alcohol-dependent sleep disorder is characterized by regular ingestion of ethanol in the evening as a hypnotic. There may be an underlying disorder that causes sleep-onset insomnia, which the patient chooses to self-medicate with alcohol. In a representative case, alcohol ingestion begins in the evening 3 to 4 hours before bedtime. The patient may regularly consume 6 to 8 drinks. This condition is generally not associated with alcoholism nor the general adjustment problems of alcoholism. Some patients assert that they sleep well as long as they continue nightly alcohol use.

This disorder is rare. It is more frequent after age 40. In suspected cases, there may be an underlying sleep disorder in a person who drinks alcohol in the evening. This would not be diagnosed as alcohol-dependent sleep disorder.

To diagnose an alcohol-dependent sleep disorder, the patient must have taken alcohol as a sleep aid daily for 30 or more nights. The insomnia complaint must have been temporally associated with one or more attempts to discontinue use of alcohol as a hypnotic. The presence of chronic alcoholism must be ruled out.

Insomnia Associated with Circadian Rhythm Disorders

The major feature of circadian rhythm disorders is misalignment between the patient's sleep pattern and the desired time of day for sleeping. The patient is unable to sleep when sleep is desired and needed. As a consequence, periods of wakefulness may also occur at undesired times.

Delayed Sleep-phase Syndrome

The delayed sleep-phase syndrome (DSPS) (26) has the daily major sleep episode delayed, or shifted to a later time period, in relation to the desired clock time. This shift of the sleep period causes symptoms of sleep-onset insomnia and, in the morning, difficulty awakening and difficulty arising at the desired time. When not compelled to sleep on a strict schedule, such as on weekends, the patient experiences normal sleep quantity and quality, but at a delayed clock time relative to the patient's usual earlier sleep schedule.

Several additional features are basic characteristics of DSPS: (a) sleep-onset and wake-up times seem intractably later than desired and unresponsive to enforcement of a strict sleep schedule, (b) patient reports normal ability to stay asleep once sleep has begun, and (c) severe difficulty awakening at the patient's desired time for arising in the morning.

In relatively pure cases of DSPS, a carefully completed daily sleep log shows the pattern. In cases complicated by alcohol, sleeping pills, or major psychiatric disorders, the sleep logs may also show frequent awakenings during the delayed sleep periods, which reflect the additional factors. When delayed phase syndrome occurs in the context of severe psychopathology, sedative abuse, or alcohol abuse, it is often unresponsive to standard treatment with behavior therapy techniques until those factors are dealt with.

This disorder is estimated to affect 5% to 10% of patients with insomnia complaints who are seen at sleep disorders centers.

Advanced Sleep-phase Syndrome

In this disorder (27), the daily major sleep episode is advanced (shifted to an earlier time period), in relation to the desired clock times for retiring and arising. The advanced phase results in strong early evening sleepiness, falling asleep early, and a final awakening that is correspondingly earlier than desired.

There is intractable and chronic inability to delay the beginning of early evening sleep and inability to continue sleep past an early morning final awakening. There are negative social consequences because evening activities are often missed.

This disorder is not often diagnosed and it is apparently rare. Many research studies have shown a mild advance in sleep phase among elderly individuals. Theoretically, this could make elderly individuals at increased risk for advanced sleep phase syndrome (ASPS).

The early morning awakenings of depression must be differentiated from ASPS. Depression is usually accompanied by other sleep symptoms (e.g., frequent awakenings and unique abnormalities of REM sleep). PSG can help differentiate the patient's sleep pattern from the depression pattern.

Shift-work Sleep Disorder

A shift-work sleep disorder (28) consists of transient symptoms of insomnia and excessive sleepiness that recur in relation to work schedule.

A shift-work sleep complaint typically affects a third shift (night shift) employee with inability to sleep for a normal length of time, when the major sleep period is begun in the morning (e.g., at 6–8 AM). TST during the daytime sleep period is often reduced by 1 to 4 hours. Early morning shift workers and evening shift individuals can also have shift work–related difficulty sleeping. The disorder also includes excessive sleepiness during work shifts (mainly on the night shift).

The course of this disorder follows the work schedule. Full adaptation to the night shift rarely occurs. Major portions of free time may be used for recovery of sleep. The disorder affects night-shift workers in varying degrees.

Among all workers, 5% to 8% are night shift. Shift-work sleep disorder may contribute to serious physical illnesses (e.g., gastrointestinal disturbances) and drug or alcohol dependency (related to sleep management efforts). Common consequences to shift-work sleep disorder include disruption of social and family life.

It is usually possible to diagnose shift-work sleep disorder based on history information that details the sleep symptom pattern and work schedule.

Irregular Sleep–Wake Pattern

This disorder consists of circadian disorganization with variable timing of sleep and wake episodes. Sleep is broken into three or more short periods in each 24 hours.

Although average total sleep time per 24 hours is within normal limits for the patient's age, no single sleep period is of normal length, and the times when sleep will occur are hard to predict. It has been noted that the unpredictability resembles a newborn infant's disorganized sleep pattern.

Diffuse brain dysfunction is a risk factor for irregular sleep–wake pattern. An environment with a regular and unvarying daily routine can help prevent the disorder. Irregular sleep–wake pattern occasionally occurs in association with chronic depression.

This disorder is rare in the general population. It is estimated to be fairly common among severely impaired institutionalized patients.

Insomnia Secondary to Sleep-related Physiologic Disorders

Primary sleep disorders that involve sleep-related physical illness sometimes present with an insomnia complaint. The sleep-related physiologic disorders that frequently include insomnia complaints are RLS, PLMD, CSA, OSA, and narcolepsy.

Periodic Limb Movement Disorder

This movement disorder is characterized by frequent, rhythmic limb twitches or movements during sleep (29). Leg movements are most typical, but some patients have arm movements; some have both arm and leg movements. A key distinguishing feature is the timing of movements; they usually occur 20 to 40 seconds apart. Legs are still between movements. The patient is not directly aware of the movements because they are initiated during sleep; a bedpartner may notice them, but often they occur when both parties are asleep, and go unobserved.

It is not possible to confirm the presence of a clinically significant PLMD without PSG. Physiologic monitoring in a sleep laboratory reliably records all leg movements (and/or arm movements) and the degree of sleep fragmentation and restlessness caused by them.

The periodic movements can cause frequent, brief *arousals* leading to frequent *awakenings*, and/or, unrefreshing sleep and excessive daytime sleepiness. The clinical significance of PLMs must be assessed on an individual basis by how much the sleep is disrupted and by the degree of daytime sleepiness. PLMs may occur as an incidental finding.

An arousal is defined as a brief disturbance of sleep lasting a few seconds (30). An awakening is defined as an interruption of sleep lasting 30 seconds or longer (31). The disruption associated with brief arousals may be the key sleep disturbance, as periodic limb movement patients can experience unrefreshing sleep and excessive daytime sleepiness when they have frequent movement-related arousals *without* the occurrence of frequent awakenings.

PLMs occur in association with a variety of medical conditions. Patients with narcolepsy and OSA often show PLMs in sleep. Most, if not all, RLS patients have PLMs during sleep. Other causes of PLMs include chronic uremia, tricyclic antidepressants, monoamine oxidase inhibitors, and withdrawal from some medications (including, anticonvulsants, barbiturates, benzodiazepines, and other hypnotics).

The general prevalence of PLMD is unknown. It shows increased incidence with age. Studies of older adults reveal PLMs in up to 45% of individuals over age 60 (32).

Restless Legs Syndrome

This syndrome (33) is characterized by uncomfortable leg sensations and the ability of voluntary leg movement to temporarily relieve the discomfort. The leg symptoms usually occur in the evening prior to sleep onset and cause almost irresistible urges to move the legs. The temporary relief provided by leg movement and the return of symptoms upon stopping movement are the most characteristic aspects of the syndrome.

Patients typically have difficulty labeling the uncomfortable sensations and use a variety of words: ache, discomfort, tingling, restless (plus comments such as, "have to move"), uncomfortable, creeping, crawling, pulling, or itching. The discomfort is usually in the lower leg muscles, but can be from the feet and thighs, and rarely, in the arms. The symptoms are typically present only at rest just prior to the sleep period, but can occur at other times, especially when sitting for long periods (e.g., in a movie or during a long car ride).

RLS is a pattern of subjective symptoms. In order to diagnose this syndrome, it is not necessary to perform sleep laboratory testing.

This condition can be associated with pregnancy, anemia, uremia, and heavy caffeine intake. Most restless legs patients show PLMs in sleep. Predisposing factors also include rheumatoid arthritis. Differential diagnosis should routinely consider caffeinism, uremia, and anemia as causes of the leg discomfort.

RLS can cause severe insomnia, can be severely distressing, and is sometimes associated with significant psychologic disturbance. It may lead to depression.

Symptoms of RLS have been identified in 5% to 15% of normal adults. In uremia, 15% to 20% report restless legs symptoms; in rheumatoid arthritis (RA) up to 30% report them. The most common time of onset is middle age.

Central Sleep Apnea

In central apnea (34), sleep-related respiration shows intervals with marked decrease or cessation of ventilatory effort. This breathing disorder is usually associated with insomnia complaints of difficulty maintaining sleep. The apnea-related awakenings sometimes begin with a gasp for air and a sensation of choking. There can also be occasional obstructive apneas or periods of hypoventilation associated with central sleep apnea (CSA), but the dominant respiratory abnormality consists of central apnea episodes. Medical complications associated with central apnea include, systemic hypertension, congestive heart failure (CHF), and depression.

Polysomnographic monitoring documents central apnea events and the frequency of arousals associated with apneas, as well as oxygen desaturations and arrhythmias. The differential diagnosis between CSA and OSA is generally important, and PSG is necessary to document central apnea and obstructive apnea events.

CSA can be asymptomatic. Therefore, the exact prevalence is unknown. The prevalence of this condition increases with age.

Obstructive Sleep Apnea

The OSA syndrome (35) is characterized by repetitive episodes of upper-airway obstruction during sleep, usually associated with brief oxygen desaturations. There is a characteristic snoring pattern with obstructive apneas, in which loud snores or gasping breaths alternate with pauses in breathing sounds.

Each apnea ends with an arousal and resumption of breathing. The arousals to breathe have been termed protective arousals. Most individuals are unaware of the apneas or the frequent arousals. Some patients, often the elderly, are aware of the sleep disturbance caused by obstructive apneas (although unaware that apneas are occurring), and present with complaints of insomnia and unrefreshing sleep.

The complications associated with OSA include unrefreshing sleep and excessive daytime sleepiness (EDS), cardiac arrhythmia, hypoxemia during sleep, and mild hypertension.

The prevalence of OSA in the general population is estimated between 1% and 4%. It is more common among men, overweight individuals, and among the middle-aged, and older. PSG is necessary to document OSA and rule out other sleep-related breathing abnormalities.

Narcolepsy

Narcolepsy (36) is a disorder of severe excessive daytime sleepiness, typically associated with three unusual phenomena that represent fragmentary aspects of REM sleep. The three REM-related symptoms are cataplexy, hypnagogic hallucinations, and sleep paralysis. In addition to problems with severe daytime sleepiness, narcolepsy patients also experience difficulty sleeping and may complain of frequent awakenings during the night.

PSG is necessary to document excessive daytime sleepiness and to rule out other causes of sleepiness (e.g., OSA). The primary problem for a narcoleptic is excessive sleepiness, although insomnia may require treatment. Prescription stimulant medication is typically necessary for the management of daytime sleepiness associated with narcolepsy, which must be handled carefully to prevent increasing the patient's insomnia.

Insomnia Related to Neurologic Illness

Cerebral degenerative disorders, dementia, and parkinsonism are common neurologic conditions that are associated with insomnia.

Cerebral Degenerative Disorders

The cerebral degenerative disorders are slowly progressive conditions characterized by abnormal behaviors or involuntary movements, such as Huntington's disease, spastic torticollis, and blepharospasm. These disorders can produce insomnia. Sleep symptoms include, insomnia, EDS, and abnormal motor activity. The circadian sleep–wake cycle may also be disturbed. Sleep disturbance increases with the progression of the disease.

PSG may be indicated if there is a clinical need to rule out other movement disorders that are not associated with cerebral degeneration, such as PLMD and RBD.

Dementia

Dementia refers to a deterioration of intellectual capacity due to a chronic, progressive degenerative disease of the CNS. The sleep disturbance in dementia is characterized by delirium, agitation, combativeness, and wandering (37). Sleep is fragmented, with frequent awakenings; often there is difficulty falling asleep at bedtime and early final awakening.

Sleep and nocturnal cognitive abilities may be particularly disturbed in demented patients; often the nighttime hours present the most difficult management challenge for caregivers. Sleep disturbance that is characterized by wandering and confusion is often summarized as the sundowner syndrome, and the syndrome is exacerbated by physical illness or hospitalization. The sleep disturbance follows the course of the dementia. Nocturnal symptoms and sleep disturbance are often the cause for institutionalization.

The prevalence of sleep disturbance among all patients with dementia is not known, but it is common. The prevalence of severe dementia is estimated to be 5% to 15% of institutionalized patients over age 65.

Parkinsonism

Parkinsonism refers to a group of neurologic disorders with hypokinesia, tremor, and muscular rigidity. Insomnia is the most common sleep-related complaint in patients with parkinsonism, although a variety of sleep-related symptoms are common.

There is no typical sleep pattern revealed by PSG. The following features are commonly observed: (a) long sleep latency, sleep fragmentation, and reduced REM sleep, (b) tremor usually stops during sound sleep, but may reappear with arousals, (c) bradykinesia and rigidity that are associated with decreased ability to get out of bed and reduced ability to change position, (d) abnormal movements, including PLMs and isolated twitches, and (e) respiratory abnormalities (including apneas and hypoventilation).

Medications for parkinsonism can improve sleep disturbance by decreasing rigidity, but conversely may exacerbate sleep disturbance and can cause new sleep complaints. Sleep complaints generally worsen as the disorder progresses and the duration of treatment lengthens.

Parkinson's disease affects approximately 0.2% of the general population. The prevalence increases with age. Onset is commonly between ages 50 and 60. Among people who seek treatment for parkinsonism, 60% to 90% have sleep complaints.

Insomnia Associated with Other Medical Illness

There are a variety of other medical disorders that cause sleep disturbance. The more common disorders include the fibrositis syndrome, sleep-related gastroesophageal reflux, and chronic obstructive pulmonary disease (COPD).

Fibrositis Syndrome/Fibromyalgia

This syndrome (38) is characterized by diffuse musculoskeletal pain, chronic fatigue, unrefreshing sleep, and localized areas of increased tenderness in the muscles (tender points). The muscle discomfort complaints generally become stronger during the nighttime.

Fibrositis patients typically complain that their sleep is light, associated with muscle pain and joint stiffness, and they awaken feeling unrefreshed. Tiredness and fatigue persist throughout the day.

This disorder has a chronic relapsing course that can last years. The muscle discomfort and sleep disturbance often lead to anxiety and depression. Sleep complaints may improve with specific treatment, but muscle discomfort may persist. Sleep laboratory testing can help differentiate fibrositis from other causes of unrefreshing sleep. PSG with fibrositis reveals a fairly unique presence of EEG alpha wave activity (8–11 cycles per second) during non-REM sleep. This is especially common during stages 3 and 4, slow-wave sleep (SWS), where the combination of alpha and slow waves is referred to as alpha–delta sleep.

The prevalence of the fibrositis syndrome is not known, but apparently is not rare.

Sleep-related Gastroesophageal Reflux

This disorder (39) is characterized by movement of the stomach contents into the esophagus during sleep. When reflux occurs, the patient can awaken with a sour taste, burning sensations, or heartburn-type chest discomfort. The chest pain is usually substernal and is somewhat similar to the pain due to angina. Awakenings associated with this discomfort can lead to an insomnia complaint.

Daily heartburn prevalence is estimated at 7% to 10%. Sleep-related gastroesophageal reflux is a chronic disease that is difficult to cure. It warrants early treatment and preventive measures. Monitoring esophageal pH during sleep can document sleep-related gastroesophageal reflux episodes. The differential diagnosis for sleep-related gastroesophageal reflux includes peptic ulcer and angina.

Chronic Obstructive Pulmonary Disease

Chronic obstructive pulmonary disease (COPD) is described by a chronic impairment of airflow through the respiratory tract. Sleep disturbance commonly occurs due to COPD and includes difficulty falling asleep, awakenings with respiratory distress, and a feeling of being unrefreshed upon arising from sleep (40). The sleep disturbance is temporally related to the presence of COPD.

The sleep disturbance generally appears correlated with the progression of the underlying pulmonary disorder. As the COPD increases in severity, the sleep disturbance also progresses.

The majority of COPD patients will develop some associated disturbance of sleep quality.

Insomnia Associated with Situational Factors

This insomnia category represents cases of sleep disturbance due to the physiologic response to external environmental factors. Example subtypes include environmental sleep disorder and altitude-related insomnia.

Environmental Sleep Disorder

Environmental sleep disorder refers to a mix of disorders caused by the types of environmental conditions that frequently result in insomnia or excessive sleepiness. In order to warrant this diagnosis, the onset, course, and termination of the sleep complaint are tied to the causative environmental condition. Common examples of such environmental factors include excessive heat, excessive cold, noise (e.g., airport or highway), danger in the environment, excess light, snoring and movements of a bedpartner, and the need to remain alert related to caregiver responsibilities for an infant or invalid.

In contrast to the definition of an adjustment sleep disorder, the physiologic rather than psychologic aspects of the environmental factors are critical for causing environmental sleep disorder. Removal of the causative environmental factors results in an immediate or gradual return to a normal sleep pattern.

When duration is 1 to 3 months, the patient may experience mild depression, decreased concentration, fatigue, and irritability. When environmental sleep disorder becomes chronic, symptoms may include depression, decreased work performance, and chronic daytime sleepiness.

When tested in the sleep laboratory, the environmental sleep disorder patient should show greater TST than reported for the home bedroom. The sleep pattern should also be normal. Similarly, the patient may report having relatively normal ability to sleep when sleeping away from home in more favorable environmental conditions.

THE PROMISE OF INSOMNIA ASSESSMENT (AND THE TIME COMMITMENT)

The numerous subtypes of insomnia provide an opportunity to make specific diagnoses and guide patients toward optimal treatment. Progress in our understanding of the causes of insomnia presents an opportunity for more effective treatment of insomnia, but success is dependent, primarily on adequate assessment.

Studies of clinical practice, however, suggest that insomnia most often goes unrecognized by the patient's personal physician and in most instances it may not be assessed and treated. Surveys of general practice have found that physicians are often unaware of severe insomnia in their patients. Two studies found 60% to 64% of cases went unrecognized (41,42). Even when physicians identify insomnia and medication is prescribed for sleep, there is usually no documented evaluation of sleep. In one study, 88% of the medical charts for patients receiving hypnotic medication contained no progress note reference to sleep (43).

The large number of insomnia subtypes provides an opportunity for specificity in diagnosis and treatment; it also presents a potentially time-consuming assessment task. The following sections describe a structured assessment approach; the last section presents a diagnosis algorithm (Figure 13-3); the structured approach is intended to facilitate time-efficient insomnia assessment.

INSOMNIA ASSESSMENT TOOLS

Sleep History (Begin with Reason for Referral)

Insomnia evaluation begins with history taking. The information collection starts with *reason for referral*, specifically, history that focuses on (a) presenting complaints, (b) nocturnal symptoms, (c) bedpartner reports, and (d) previous treatment for sleep problems.

It is also important to promptly elicit information about *daytime consequences*. The type of consequences can be an important indicator for etiology; for example, a history of excessive daytime sleepiness would suggest the patient's most primary problem is not insomnia. Patients with a primary insomnia disorder generally do not experience severe daytime sleepiness or fall asleep unintentionally during the daytime, because their basic problem is difficulty sleeping.

Chief Complaint

History taking begins with the patient's description of sleep complaints. The chief complaint generally falls into one or more of the following categories: difficulty falling asleep, difficulty staying asleep, early morning awakenings, decreased TST, poor quality sleep, or daytime fatigue.

Nocturnal Symptoms and Events

Some common symptoms of primary and secondary insomnia disorders can be documented with patient report. These include increased arousal in the prebedtime period (suggesting conditioned arousal), restless legs symptoms, PLMs (although this usually requires the observations of a bedpartner), respiratory distress (including dyspnea, choking, and gasping), nocturnal panic attacks, pain, gastroesophageal reflux, and environmental noise. The report of

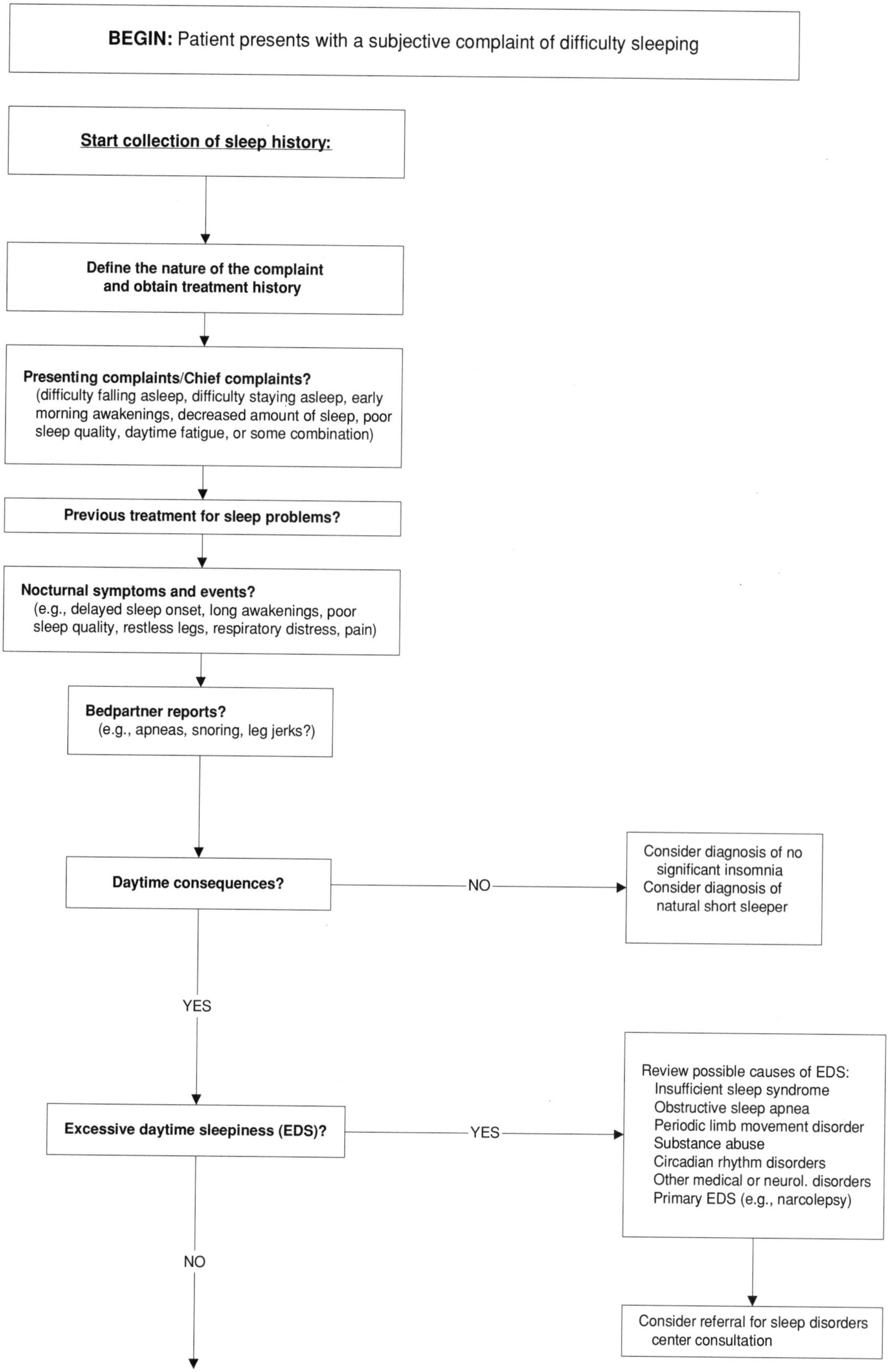

BEGIN: Patient presents with a subjective complaint of difficulty sleeping

Start collection of sleep history:

Define the nature of the complaint and obtain treatment history

Presenting complaints/Chief complaints?
(difficulty falling asleep, difficulty staying asleep, early morning awakenings, decreased amount of sleep, poor sleep quality, daytime fatigue, or some combination)

Previous treatment for sleep problems?

Nocturnal symptoms and events?
(e.g., delayed sleep onset, long awakenings, poor sleep quality, restless legs, respiratory distress, pain)

Bedpartner reports?
(e.g., apneas, snoring, leg jerks?)

Daytime consequences? ——NO——▶ Consider diagnosis of no significant insomnia
Consider diagnosis of natural short sleeper

YES

Excessive daytime sleepiness (EDS)? ——YES——▶ Review possible causes of EDS:
Insufficient sleep syndrome
Obstructive sleep apnea
Periodic limb movement disorder
Substance abuse
Circadian rhythm disorders
Other medical or neurol. disorders
Primary EDS (e.g., narcolepsy)

NO

Consider referral for sleep disorders center consultation

FIGURE 13-3. Algorithm for insomnia diagnosis and treatment selection. (*Continued*)

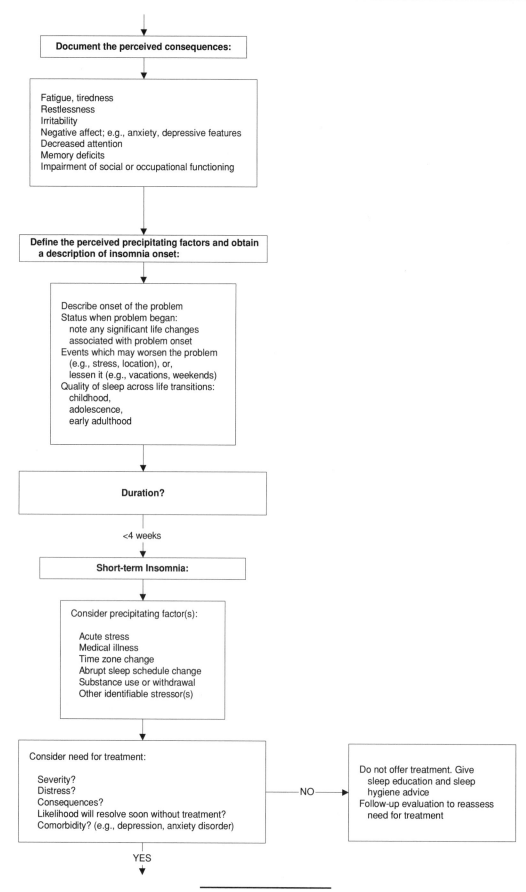

Document the perceived consequences:

Fatigue, tiredness
Restlessness
Irritability
Negative affect; e.g., anxiety, depressive features
Decreased attention
Memory deficits
Impairment of social or occupational functioning

Define the perceived precipitating factors and obtain a description of insomnia onset:

Describe onset of the problem
Status when problem began:
  note any significant life changes
  associated with problem onset
Events which may worsen the problem
  (e.g., stress, location), or,
  lessen it (e.g., vacations, weekends)
Quality of sleep across life transitions:
  childhood,
  adolescence,
  early adulthood

Duration?

<4 weeks

Short-term Insomnia:

Consider precipitating factor(s):

  Acute stress
  Medical illness
  Time zone change
  Abrupt sleep schedule change
  Substance use or withdrawal
  Other identifiable stressor(s)

Consider need for treatment:

  Severity?
  Distress?
  Consequences?
  Likelihood will resolve soon without treatment?
  Comorbidity? (e.g., depression, anxiety disorder)

—NO—

Do not offer treatment. Give
  sleep education and sleep
  hygiene advice
Follow-up evaluation to reassess
  need for treatment

YES

FIGURE 13-3. (*Continued*)

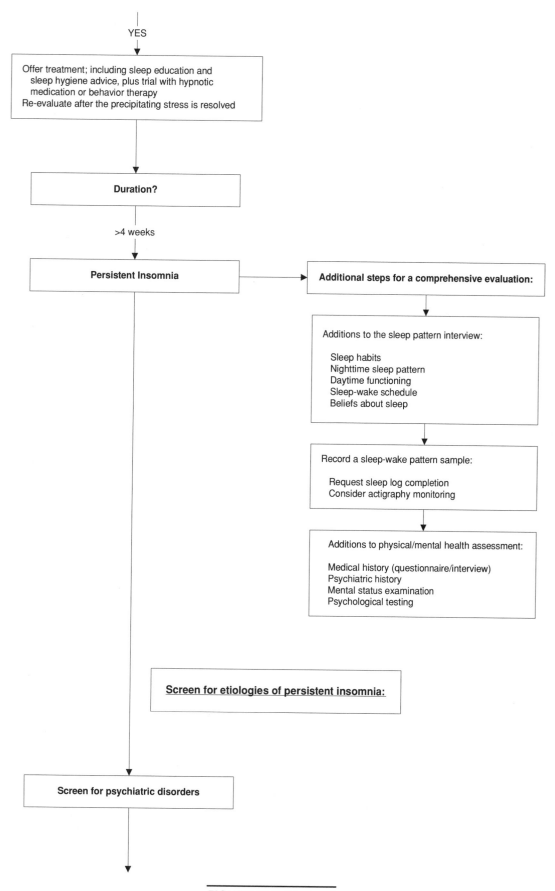

FIGURE 13-3. (*Continued*)

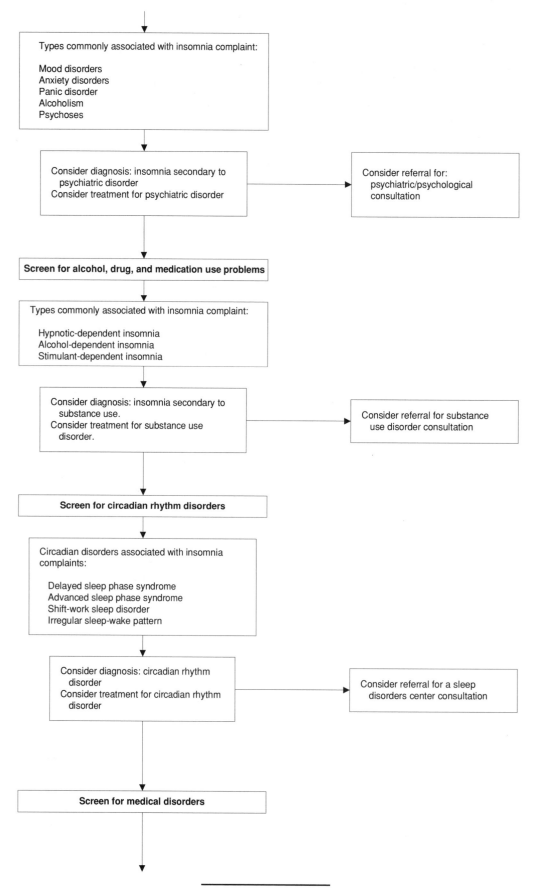

Types commonly associated with insomnia complaint:

Mood disorders
Anxiety disorders
Panic disorder
Alcoholism
Psychoses

Consider diagnosis: insomnia secondary to
  psychiatric disorder
Consider treatment for psychiatric disorder

Consider referral for:
  psychiatric/psychological
  consultation

Screen for alcohol, drug, and medication use problems

Types commonly associated with insomnia complaint:

Hypnotic-dependent insomnia
Alcohol-dependent insomnia
Stimulant-dependent insomnia

Consider diagnosis: insomnia secondary to
  substance use.
Consider treatment for substance use
  disorder.

Consider referral for substance
use disorder consultation

Screen for circadian rhythm disorders

Circadian disorders associated with insomnia
complaints:

Delayed sleep phase syndrome
Advanced sleep phase syndrome
Shift-work sleep disorder
Irregular sleep-wake pattern

Consider diagnosis: circadian rhythm
  disorder
Consider treatment for circadian rhythm
  disorder

Consider referral for a sleep
disorders center consultation

Screen for medical disorders

FIGURE 13-3. (*Continued*)

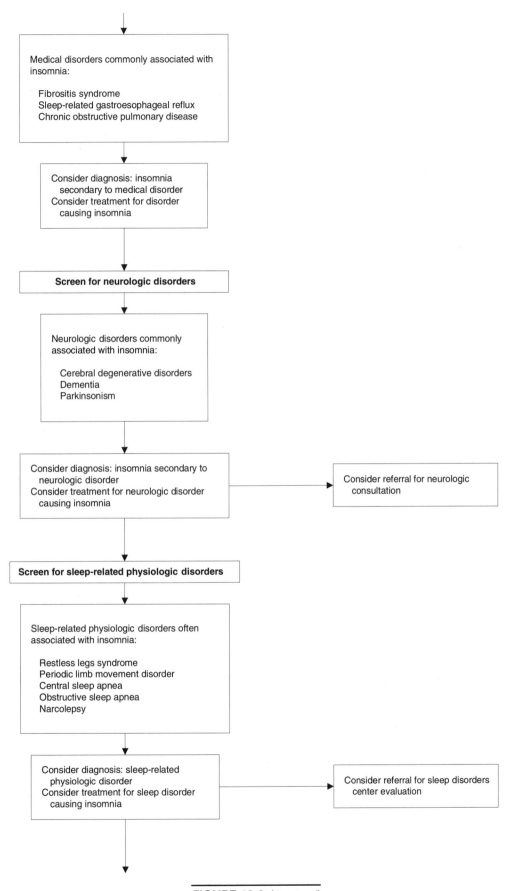

FIGURE 13-3. (*Continued*)

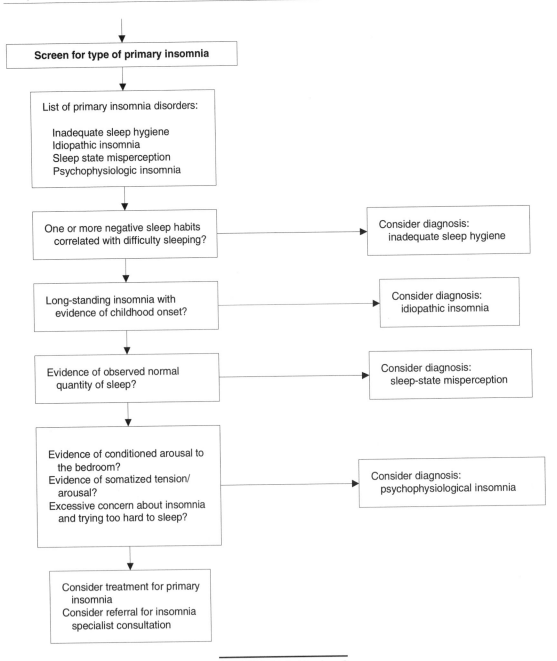

FIGURE 13-3. (*Continued*)

these symptoms and events can help guide the initial sleep interview.

Bedpartner Reports

Bedpartners (and anyone else who has observed the patient sleeping) are a potential source of information about nocturnal symptoms and the daytime consequences of insomnia. However, the validity of bedpartner observations is limited by several factors. During the night, the bedpartner will be sleeping and may have low awareness of the patient's behavior. The bedpartner can have subjective biases, e.g., the loudness of snoring and the frequency of pauses in breathing or leg jerks during sleep may be exaggerated. Despite the inherent limitations, bedpartners are sometimes the only good source of details about important nocturnal events including, limb movements during the patient's sleep, snoring, and pauses in breathing during sleep.

Previous Treatment

Questions about previous treatment outcome can reveal important information for planning future treatment. The type, duration, and judged effectiveness of past treatment should be determined. The adequacy of delivery should be assessed for previous treatment. An effort should be made to account for any previous treatments that were not effective (e.g., side effects, poor compliance).

The questions about previous treatment conclude the first stage of information collection, termed reason for referral.

Daytime Consequences

Judgments concerning the clinical significance of an insomnia complaint are heavily influenced by the reported extent to which insomnia impairs daytime functioning. A complaint of difficulty sleeping, in the absence of negative daytime effects or daytime distress, does not indicate significant insomnia. The perceived consequences of insomnia generally concern adverse effects on psychosocial, occupational, and physical functioning. The perceived adverse effects are typically described in terms of fatigue, negative affect, cognitive inefficiency, impaired motor skills, social discomfort, and nonspecific physical symptoms.

Reports of increased fatigue are common among people with insomnia and have been documented in several studies (44).

The status of subjective daytime sleepiness as a consequence of insomnia is not fully resolved, but clinically, it is believed that people with insomnia do not exhibit severe daytime sleepiness. Some studies have reported increased subjective sleepiness in people with insomnia (45), but physiological assessment with the MSLT in research studies does not show evidence of increased daytime sleepiness (46).

Other Insomnia Assessment Tools (Elements of a Comprehensive Evaluation)

When a new insomnia patient is scheduled by a sleep disorders center for evaluation by a sleep medicine specialist, the time available for a sleep history interview and, subsequently, a medical history interview (including a psychiatric history) is greater than the time available for initial evaluation activities in a private practitioner's office. A physical examination would also be a common component of a sleep disorders center insomnia evaluation. In addition, the sleep medicine specialist often decides that the patient should complete a daily sleep log (usually for 2 weeks). A mental status examination typically is performed during the psychiatric history. Psychological testing may also be indicated. The time commitment is considerable for a comprehensive insomnia evaluation; it is unlikely that an evaluation this extensive will be performed by a primary healthcare provider.

▶ **TABLE 13-3. Standard Sections of a Sleep History Interview**

The primary sleep problem; including frequency, severity, duration, and perceived consequences
Previous treatment for sleep problems
Review of nighttime sleep: presleep and sleep onset, sleep during the night, mornings.
Daytime functioning
Sleep–wake rhythms
Sleeping environment
Beliefs about sleep
Development of the sleep problem, e.g., onset of the problem, course, sleep across the life-span

Sleep History Interview

A sleep history interview may occur right after collection of reason for referral information. The typical contents of a sleep history interview are listed in Table 13-3.

A model outline for the sleep history interview is available at the American Academy of Sleep Medicine (AASM) website (aasmnet.org), which is contained in the published AASM report on insomnia evaluation, which is posted on the site (47; Table 3 of the publication).

In the office practice of a primary service provider, the amount of time available for a sleep history evaluation is limited. The basic questions about presenting complaints, nocturnal symptoms, bedpartner reports, daytime consequences, and previous treatment for sleep problems may use up a substantial portion of the total time available. Time pressure may force the interviewer to proceed to questions intended to rapidly reveal the etiology of the chief complaint.

As noted above, insomnia etiologies are quite varied and the full range of possible etiologies should be considered during the assessment of each case. The process of reviewing possible causes is discussed in *Diagnostic Evaluation Steps* and is presented in the evaluation algorithm (Fig. 13-3).

Medical History

A medical history assessment is a basic part of comprehensive care. Data from epidemiology studies suggest that there is a correlation between poor physical health and insomnia (2). A questionnaire may be used to obtain basic information about medical history, psychiatric history, and review of systems. The questions should be tailored to address medical disorders that are often associated with insomnia (e.g., anxiety disorders, depression, COPD, asthma, gastroesophageal reflux, fibrositis).

Physical Examination

In view of the varied medical disorders that are frequently associated with insomnia, a physical examination could be useful in the diagnosis of some cases. If the patient is referred to the sleep disorders center, physical examination results could be requested from the referring physician.

Psychiatric History and Mental Status Examination

Psychiatric diagnoses define the largest subgroup among sleep disorders center patients with insomnia. Insomnia attributed to psychiatric disorder accounts for an estimated 30% to 40% of patients seen in sleep disorders centers with a chief complaint of insomnia (15,48). However, only a minority of sleep disorders center patients receive a formal psychiatric evaluation pursuant to diagnosis receipt. Numerous epidemiologic studies have also shown a statistical association for insomnia with complaints of depression, tension, or anxiety. Psychiatric examination of the insomnia patient customarily includes a psychiatric history and a mental status examination.

The Sleep Log

Brief daily sleep logs are used to efficiently describe the patient's sleep pattern before treatment and to monitor for changes in the pattern during treatment. These usually contain about ten questions to be answered each morning—questions about sleeping and waking during the previous 24 hours. The logs typically include questions about bedtime, sleep latency, number and duration of awakenings, risetime, ratings of sleep quality and daytime alertness, and use of sleep aids. A daily log takes about 2 to 3 minutes to complete.

Sleep log data is particularly helpful for assessing sleep hygiene and for sampling the circadian sleep–wake pattern. A period of 2 weeks is a common interval for completion of daily sleep logs prior to starting treatment.

Psychological Testing

The Minnesota Multiphasic Personality Inventory (MMPI), the Profile of Mood States (POMS), and brief, self-administered scales that target specific psychologic state or trait features (such as anxiety or depression) have frequently been employed in insomnia research.

The shorter questionnaires that assess single psychologic features are becoming more popular because they have greater ease of use and lower labor costs. However, they are face valid and more fakable than subtle instruments (e.g., the MMPI). The short, face-valid questionnaires should only be used as a supplement to clinical interviewing.

Polysomnography

Insomnia is often significantly affected by the location where the patient sleeps. Insomnia patients can be vulnerable to increased difficulty sleeping when in a sleep laboratory, although some people with insomnia sleep better than usual during their first night in the unfamiliar laboratory surroundings (the unusual reverse first night effect, with good sleep during night one in a new location; 49). Many insomnias do not have unique physiologic manifestations that can be reliably sampled during a single night of PSG.

For these reasons, there has been long-standing controversy about the appropriateness of polysomnographic evaluation for insomnia. The American Academy of Sleep Medicine (AASM) report on the indications for use of PSG (50) offers guidelines that can be summarized by four statements: (a) PSG is indicated when sleep-related breathing disorder or narcolepsy is suspected, or unusual parasomnias or violent behavior have been witnessed, (b) PSG may be indicated when PLMs are strongly suspected or sleep-related features of certain neurologic disorders have been observed, (c) PSG is not routinely indicated for diagnosis of circadian sleep disorders, RLS, diagnosis of most psychiatric conditions (an exception is the diagnosis of a major depression, which is sometimes aided by PSG), uncomplicated parasomnias, or seizures without sleep complaints, and (d) PSG is not routinely indicated in the evaluation of transient or chronic insomnia, with the possible exceptions of prior treatment failure or cases where there is diagnostic uncertainty.

Actigraphy

Actigraphy uses a small, wearable device (usually worn on the wrist) to measure body movements continuously for long time periods, movement being an accepted indicator of sleep and wakefulness. Recent research (reviewed elsewhere; 51) suggests that actigraphy data quality has improved in recent years, and it is now appropriate for recording night-to-night variability in the sleep patterns of people with insomnia, although there is a tendency for actigraphy to overscore the presence of sleep in people with insomnia. This pattern information can be used to evaluate pre- to posttreatment therapy results, and the information is useful for clinical diagnosis of circadian rhythm disorders.

DIAGNOSTIC EVALUATION STEPS

The bulk of insomnia complaints that receive evaluation and treatment are seen by primary care physicians. A method for evaluation of insomnia complaints should present at least two levels of intensity for the evaluation process, one tailored to a primary care physician and one designed with the sleep disorders center environment in mind.

There are two complementary goals for the insomnia algorithm that follows: (a) provide a basic evaluation path that is intended for use by all professionals, and, (b) provide branches from the basic path that describe additional evaluation steps. The additional steps are intended to serve those professionals who choose to complete a more comprehensive initial evaluation of an insomnia complaint.

Insomnia Evaluation Algorithm

The insomnia evaluation algorithm (Figure 13-3, above) moves from presenting complaint to insomnia diagnosis and then to treatment recommendations. Optional branches present ways to intensify the evaluation process. This algorithm was patterned after one in the AASM report on evaluation of chronic insomnia (47).

When an algorithm branch leads to a diagnosis, it concludes with a treatment recommendation and also offers referral suggestions (for cases with which a consultation is desired). For example, when a case is diagnosed as insomnia secondary to psychiatric disorder, treatment for the psychiatric disorder is recommended and a possible referral for psychiatric/psychologic consultation is also suggested.

The following comments concern an optional track in the algorithm. When the algorithm steps move past the relative simplicity of assessment for short-term insomnia and reach the beginning of the section on evaluation of persistent insomnia, there is an outline of additional steps for completion of a comprehensive insomnia evaluation. The additional steps portray an evaluation similar to one that would be provided by an insomnia specialist.

The algorithm is presented in Figure 13-3.

Epilogue for Algorithm

The algorithm concludes the discussion of evaluation steps. The goal has been an organized review of the insomnia evaluation process, with commentary on each step. We now turn to treatment options for primary insomnia.

PRINCIPLES FOR TREATMENT PLANNING

Two previously published efforts to aid treatment planning for primary insomnia are included in this section. The intent is to provide conceptual views of insomnia that many sleep specialists find useful.

Graphic Model of Insomnia Treatment Factors

The model of etiologic factors for insomnia presented in Fig. 13-1 has a complement. The authors of the multifactor model of insomnia causes (13) present a multifactor model of treatment that portrays the same complexity of influences found in Fig. 13-1 (Figure 13-2). The array of treatment factors is intended to portray the mixture of

five components that may be included in treatment planning for insomnia (psychophysiologic/conditioning, circadian, psychiatric, substance use, and medical/neurologic illness).

In cases of primary insomnia, the focus of treatment is generally on psychophysiologic and conditioning factors, but the presence of other identified factors is common, which places additional demands on the therapist's attention (such as an irregular sleep–wake schedule, hypnotic dependence, anxiety, and depressive features). In addition, other initially undiscovered types of etiological factor may be present and later warrant treatment attention. As noted in the caption for the graphic model (Fig. 13-2), insomnia treatment must often address multiple factors. This issue will be covered in the discussion of follow-up treatment for secondary insomnia (below).

Conceptual Model of Contributing Factors in Insomnia

A widely accepted insomnia model offers a scheme of three categories for etiologic factors and describes how the status of specific factors can change during the development of an insomnia disorder (52). For example, a stressful event that precedes the onset of a persistent insomnia may be judged the *precipitating event* for the insomnia episode. Over time, the impact of the precipitating stressor will typically lessen and may become insignificant as a factor contributing to the persistence of difficulty sleeping.

When insomnia symptoms persist for weeks and months, new influences can develop and function as *maintaining factors* for the insomnia disorder. The long-term repetition of difficulty sleeping can cause conditioned sleep-preventing associations that function as the maintaining factors for a psychophysiologic insomnia disorder. This type of conditioning can occur with any persistent insomnia, primary or secondary. Other examples of common maintaining factors include the worry about sleep and excessive effort to sleep that characterize psychophysiologic insomnia and negative sleep habits that can develop after the onset of an insomnia episode. Maintaining factors are the ones most actively affecting a patient's sleep at the time of seeking help.

Predisposing factors are the third type articulated by Spielman and Glovinsky. These are individual differences that may increase a person's risk of developing persistent insomnia. A tendency for depression symptoms and a tendency for anxiety are generally considered predisposing factors for insomnia. Negative sleep habits can predispose a person for insomnia episodes that could be triggered by a period of stress-related excess arousal. The hypothesized sensitivity to subtle abnormalities of sleep that may afflict sleep state misperception patients is a possible predisposition. The presumed sleep–wake regulation weakness of idiopathic insomnia could be a uniquely dominating and possible genetic predisposition for sleep disturbance.

The analysis articulated by Spielman and Glovinsky provides a valuable tool for setting treatment priorities. In general, predisposing factors predate the patient's insomnia, so logically are neither the cause of it nor the best target for treatment. Precipitating events may be the cause for onset of an insomnia episode, but their influence tends to wane with the passage of time. The maintaining factors remain as the most active influence when patients present for treatment. Based upon the Spielman and Glovinsky analysis, identification of maintaining factors and planning their resolution is a promising strategy for beginning a primary insomnia treatment plan.

TREATMENT PACKAGE OUTLINE FOR PRIMARY INSOMNIA

Three components are recommended for a model treatment package with persistent primary insomnia: (a) promote improved self-management of sleep by offering basic information about sleep and recommending sleep hygiene improvements, (b) consider a trial with sedative–hypnotic medication, and (c) consider behavioral treatment.

Before detailing the components of the treatment package outline, the treatment of short-term insomnia needs to receive additional review. Short-term insomnia occurs at the beginning of chronic insomnia, and the management of short-term insomnia raises issues that carry over to chronic insomnia.

Treatment for Short-term Insomnia

The majority of all insomnias are short-term. The treatment of short-term insomnia is considered under the heading of treatment for persistent primary insomnia because prevention of persistent insomnia is a common argument in favor of offering treatment for short-term insomnia. One or more of the following factors typically influence the clinical decision on whether to treat a short-term insomnia: severity, patient distress, insomnia consequences, likelihood the insomnia will soon resolve without treatment, and comorbidity (e.g., depression and anxiety disorder).

If the service provider decides not to treat, then sleep education and sleep hygiene advice should be offered immediately and a follow-up evaluation to reassess need for treatment should be scheduled for 1 to 4 weeks later. If instead the decision is to treat, sleep education and sleep hygiene advice should be provided. A trial with hypnotic medication should be considered that would last 1 to 4 weeks, followed by supervised gradual withdrawal. A trial with behavioral treatment should also be considered, such as stimulus control treatment or brief relaxation training. Also, reevaluation should be planned to be performed after the precipitating stress has abated.

TREATMENT STEPS FOR PERSISTENT PRIMARY INSOMNIA

The treatment for a patient who presents with persistent insomnia will address some of the same issues that arise with short-term insomnia: education about normal sleep, sleep hygiene, consideration of hypnotic medication, and behavioral treatment.

Education about Normal Sleep and Sleep Hygiene

Education about normal sleep helps provide a foundation for teaching individuals how to sleep better. This knowledge helps shape realistic expectations. Sleep hygiene education provides research-based advice on the management of sleep. Treatment for insomnia should routinely include these two types of education. They can serve as part of the foundation for successful treatment of insomnia.

Most people receive no formal education about sleep (e.g., not covered in secondary school health classes) and remain naïve about what is normal and abnormal. Their expectations for sleep remain imprecise and dependent upon teaching received from parents. This presents an opportunity for providers to fill a void with useful facts about sleep. The single expectation that is widespread among adults concerns perceived need for sleep. The common knowledge rule that 8 hours of sleep are needed per day is actually an adult average for self-reported total sleep per night, but is used as the prescribed expectation for all adults. Based upon a normal distribution of need for sleep, an average is certain to be too little to meet some individuals' need for sleep and too much for many others. Reference studies of polysomnographically recorded sleep (53) show a range of values for all measures of sleep pattern at each age level tested (e.g., sleep latency, wakefulness during the night, percentage deep sleep, and percentage REM sleep). Patients can benefit from the knowledge that sleep needs and sleep pattern vary from person to person and vary from night to night. The standard clinical guidelines that a sleep latency of less than 30 minutes is within normal limits and that total wakefulness during the night of less than 30 minutes is also within normal limits can also be helpful to share. This basic sleep knowledge can foster some objectivity and flexibility of expectations for each night's sleep.

Incorrect beliefs and overly optimistic expectations can increase concern about sleep disturbance, which can contribute to a negative circular pattern, with worry about not getting the right amount of sleep. This causes greater effort to sleep, which increases the likelihood of further difficulty obtaining sleep and more worry about sleep.

The concept of positive sleep hygiene exemplifies the goal of self-management of health. Sleep hygiene principles are based upon research into which behaviors promote more reliable and better quality sleep and which behaviors make the occurrence of sleep more difficult to predict and undermine its quality (12,54,55). The inadequate sleep hygiene diagnosis subtype speaks to the importance of adequate sleep hygiene. Negative sleep habits can undermine the positive effects of pharmacologic and behavioral treatments for insomnia. For example, if a patient maintains a pattern of irregular morning risetimes and irregular bedtimes, the ability of hypnotic medication to consistently promote a short sleep latency can be decreased due to the inconsistent schedule. Table 13-2 summarizes a list of negative sleep habits found in the inadequate sleep hygiene section of the ICSD (12).

Representative lists of sleep management recommendations can be found at the National Sleep Foundation website (http://www.sleepfoundation.org) and the AASM website (http://aasmnet.org).

Pharmacologic Treatment of Persistent Primary Insomnia

A variety of approaches to the use of sedative–hypnotic medication should be considered, from not at all to nightly use. The varied needs and goals of patients dictate flexibility in the prescription of hypnotics.

The use of hypnotic medication is a controversial core issue and belongs in the forefront when discussing treatment for primary insomnia. Decisions about hypnotic prescription are believed to influence the likelihood that short-term insomnia will persist and develop into a chronic primary insomnia (56,57). The popularity of hypnotic medications is considerable and well documented (58). Patients desire relief from insomnia symptoms and often seek a prescription for sleeping pills. Responsibility for evaluating the pros and cons of medication therapy for each insomniac rests with each patient's personal physician.

Before giving a prescription for sleeping pills, treatment recommendations must be formulated that take into account individual differences. For some patients, hypnotic use will function as a distraction from the task of resolving an insomnia problem (e.g., disrupting concentration by causing daytime sedation effects during hypnotic treatment and withdrawal symptoms during abstinence). When a patient is motivated to attack the cause of insomnia, the use of hypnotic medication could impede progress toward that goal. Hypnotics pose a relatively high risk of sedative dependency for some patients, e.g., a person with an addiction history.

When behavioral treatment fails, hypnotics provide a potent alternative treatment that may be considered for long-term use, although standard practice recommends regular use only for up to 1 month. Of course, when a diagnosis is made and the recommended treatment fails, review of the diagnosis and further evaluation into the nature of the disorder, including PSG, should be considered. The appropriateness of long-term hypnotic use is a subject of long-standing debate. Prolonged use is associated with increased risks for tolerance problems, chronic dependency, and hypnotic-dependent insomnia.

The role of hypnotic medication in the treatment of chronic insomnia is similar to the role of analgesic medication in the treatment of chronic pain. Like hypnotics, pain medications are interventions that reliably provide symptom relief, but they do not correct the underlying pathophysiology. Also, similar to the normal practice of prescribing analgesics on an as-needed basis for chronic pain sufferers, access to hypnotics should be considered for all chronic insomnia patients. However, if the patient desires to avoid or minimize hypnotic use, that preference should be honored. The strict preconditions for when it is appropriate to consider long-term prescription of sedative–hypnotic medication are presented in the section *Pharmacological Therapy Management*.

Restoration of an acceptable sleep pattern without use of sedative–hypnotic medication is a desirable goal for all patients. The incidence of hypnotic avoidance is unknown, although many patients prefer to manage sleep without medication (59). In a recent study of hypnotic-dependent insomnia, 25% of 3,000 chronic insomnia patients who volunteered for participation were not using prescription sleep medication when they contacted the research recruiters (60). Many stated that a desire to avoid hypnotics prompted them to volunteer, although they did not meet a basic qualification for the study.

The potential benefits and risks associated with hypnotic use for chronic primary insomnia are similar to the benefits and risks when used for short-term insomnia symptom relief. Some of the risks increase with a long period of hypnotic use.

On the positive side, hypnotic medication can prevent persistent unchecked symptoms, reduce fear associated with loss of control over sleep, and promote emotional stability in patients prone to anxiety or depressive symptoms. The risks of hypnotic use include dependency. This physical and psychologic dependency may occur in cases where the patient is an adaptive and resourceful person, originally capable of reestablishing a normal sleep pattern without using hypnotic medication. Another risk is reduced motivation to identify and resolve the factors responsible for the continuation of an insomnia (e.g., stress, negative sleep hygiene, anxiety, depression, fear that the ability to sleep without medication has been lost, failure to adapt to normal changes in sleep that occur with aging, and failure to deal with developmental challenges that can provoke insomnia). In other words, the hypnotic can shift the patient's focus onto symptom relief and away from what can be done to prevent symptoms. Also, hypnotics carry risk for anterograde amnesia (61). There are increased risks for falls (62), automobile accidents, and hospitalization that are mainly associated with long half-life benzodiazepines. All three risks are highest in the elderly.

Opinions vary about the recommended duration for treatment with hypnotic medication. Recommended patterns of hypnotic use have been published by the National Institutes of Health (NIH) (63). The 1984 NIH report recommended short-term use of hypnotic medication for a period of up to 4 weeks. Behavioral treatment was favored for long-term treatment of primary insomnia. Published proposals for hypnotic use with persistent insomnia range from (a) avoidance of hypnotics when starting behavioral treatment (64), to (b) starting off unstable new primary insomnia patients with a month of nightly hypnotic use in an effort to stabilize the sleep pattern (65).

It is ideal, in some respects, to avoid initiating hypnotic therapy when starting behavioral treatment for primary insomnia; however, there are numerous exceptions. Often the need arises for consideration of a trial with sleeping pills. Many long-term insomniacs will be using hypnotics at the time of initiating alternative therapy.

If sedative–hypnotic medications are being withdrawn in conjunction with behavioral treatment, it should be done very gradually under close supervision, to minimize the amount of withdrawal symptoms and associated anxiety about recurrence of insomnia. Some experts recommend withdrawing the hypnotic before initiating behavioral treatment (64). Espie and associates studied hypnotic withdrawal before and after behavioral treatment and the early withdrawal group showed better treatment outcome (66).

When considering hypnotic therapy, or withdrawal of a hypnotic, weigh the costs and benefits carefully. Discuss them with the patient, and encourage the patient to state (and/or formulate) a preference. Some patients will be hesitant and uncomfortable with the responsibility of choosing for or against use of sleeping pills and prefer to depend on their physician's advice. It is desirable for the patient to accept some responsibility for the decision and thus take a more active role.

BEHAVIORAL TREATMENTS FOR PERSISTENT PRIMARY INSOMNIA

Behavioral treatments for insomnia developed from efforts to apply learning principles and teaching strategies to the challenge of helping insomniacs establish better sleep patterns. These are psychologic treatments originally launched by clinical researchers who practiced a behavior therapy approach to helping people solve problems. Many types of behavior therapy can be suitable for inclusion in the behavioral approach to insomnia, as long as each can pass the empirical test of demonstrated efficacy in controlled research.

There are several general principles that guide the application of all behavior therapy techniques. First, behavior therapists are trained to practice the continuous assessment of patient status and treatment results; for people with insomnia this is usually achieved through monitoring with daily home sleep logs through actigraphy which

provides a more expensive, objective alternative. Second, a related principle says to perform continuous adjustment of the treatment plan, based upon the adequacy of results. These are two therapy principles that characterize the behavioral approach. A third guideline for behavior therapy states that early in treatment, assessment of the patient needs to identify hypothesized active maintaining factors. Treatment components are then chosen to address those suspected maintaining conditions. If treatment recommendations are not successful or counterproductive, they will be promptly modified or replaced. (These assessment and treatment activities are in addition to the provision of sleep education, sleep hygiene recommendations, and decision-making about hypnotic therapy, all of which are done early in treatment.)

A trial with behavior therapy for insomnia typically consists of 6 to 8 treatment visits during 2 to 3 months. Visits usually occur at 1- to 2-week intervals, which allows time for learning insomnia management skills, time for the new behaviors to gradually become established, and time for the sleep pattern to gradually improve. It generally takes at least 1 to 2 months to gradually replace insomniac sleep patterns that have developed over a period of months or years.

The behavioral approach to insomnia treatment builds treatment plans with techniques from a set of approximately 10 to 15 published techniques. The most standard techniques are often packaged in a multicomponent treatment plan. In recent years, this type of treatment package has come to be called *Cognitive Behavior Therapy* for insomnia.

The most widely used behavioral techniques for treatment of persistent insomnia are: relaxation, stimulus control treatment, sleep restriction therapy, cognitive restructuring techniques, and cognitive behavior therapy treatment packages. Treatments with demonstrated efficacy, but less widely used, include, paradoxical intention and biofeedback. A typical cognitive behavior therapy package includes relaxation training, stimulus control and/or sleep restriction/sleep compression, plus cognitive restructuring.

After six to eight treatment sessions, if behavior therapy for insomnia is judged unsuccessful, a sleep disorders center evaluation is recommended. The sleep laboratory testing can assess for additional undiagnosed factors.

Stimulus Control

Stimulus-control therapy is built on the hypothesis that persistent insomnia is a conditioned response to *time-of-day cues* (e.g., evening routine, feelings of sleepiness, and bedtime), and *environmental cues* (the bed and bedroom), that are usually associated with sleep. Instead, bedtime and the bedroom have become associated with sleep-incompatible behaviors, e.g., worrying, tossing and turning, reading, watching TV, fretting. The noninsomniac sleeper associates bedtime and bedroom with rapid sleep onset, but the evening routine and bedroom may elicit a wakefulness response in people with insomnia. The goals of stimulus control are to help the insomniac learn to fall asleep quickly at bedtime and to maintain sleep. These goals are reached by strengthening the bed and bedroom as cues for sleep, weakening them as cues for activities that might interfere with sleep, and helping the insomniac to acquire a consistent sleep rhythm. The basic stimulus control principle is to associate the bed with sleep and avoid associating the bed with wakefulness. This principle is summarized for patients with the concise instruction, "the bed is for sleep." Patients are given this phrase as a mnemonic and as a description of what a normal night of sleep is about.

Stimulus-control treatment consists of implementing six basic instructions. The instructions are given to each patient in writing (Table 13-4). They can be found on the internet (at *http://counselling.massey.ac.nz/articles/sleep.htm*) and in therapy guides (67).

Although the stimulus-control instructions are simple and clear, experience has shown that compliance is better if they are discussed one at a time and a logical explanation is presented for each rule (67). The initial patient response to practicing stimulus-control procedures is a temporary increase in difficulty sleeping. Patients need to be counseled on the expectation of gradual changes that will progress to a new sleep pattern. Support and encouragement are typically needed to coach the patient through implementation of the stimulus-control instructions.

Treatment benefits from stimulus control have been demonstrated for both sleep onset and maintenance insomnia. Two meta-analyses (68,69) have reviewed the evidence of stimulus-control treatment effects and found an average 48% decrease in sleep latency and 48% decrease in the time spent awake during the night. The 1999 review of behavioral treatments for insomnia (70) rated stimulus control as a "generally accepted patient-care strategy that reflects a high degree of clinical certainty (pp. 1131–1132)."

Relaxation

Relaxation is a commonly recommended treatment for insomnia. The goal is to teach the patient how to be relaxed at bedtime and during awakenings. The variety of techniques includes progressive muscle relaxation, passive relaxation, biofeedback, meditation, imagery training, autogenic training, and diaphragmatic breathing. Review of research on relaxation treatments reveals variations in the strength of evidence (70), although in clinical practice these techniques are often used as if they were equivalent in effectiveness (71). We will discuss them separately.

Progressive Muscle Relaxation

Progressive relaxation (72) involves a sequence of exercises to tense and release each of the body's major muscle groups, while focusing attention on the contrasting sensations of tension and relaxation. The goal is to learn how to rapidly relax the muscles and achieve a general state of relaxation. Relaxation is considered to be a skill that improves with practice. Patients are counseled to practice regularly and to expect that the ability to relax will gradually improve with practice. Alternative relaxation techniques omit muscle tensing (e.g., passive relaxation; 73), which may be better tolerated by older patients.

The 1999 research review of behavioral insomnia treatment (70) recommended progressive relaxation as a patient care strategy, which reflects a moderate degree of clinical certainty. The text of the recommendation states this therapy "has been observed to be useful in insomnia patients who often display high levels of arousal both at night and during the daytime" (p. 1131).

Biofeedback

Biofeedback applies the technology of physiological recordings and principles of learning to the goal of promoting sleep. During biofeedback, the patient utilizes physiologic arousal information to increase the ability to reach a lower general level of arousal. Several measures related to relaxation and sleep have been monitored to provide biologic feedback for insomnia patients: (a) frontalis electromyographic activity, (b) theta frequency (4 to 7 cycles per second) EEG activity, and, (c) sleep spindle or sensorimotor rhythm frequency EEG (12 to 14 cycles per second; 74). The insomniac receives either an auditory or visual signal to show the level of activity in the target physiological measure. After repeated practice sessions, patients are

▶ **TABLE 13-4. Stimulus-Control Instructions**[a]

1. Lie down intending to go to sleep only when you are sleepy.
2. Do not use your bed for anything except sleep; that is, do not read, watch television, eat, or worry in bed. Sexual activity is the only exception to this rule. On such occasions, the instructions are to be followed afterward when you intend to go to sleep.
3. If you find yourself unable to fall asleep, get up and go to another room. Stay up as long as you wish and then return to the bedroom to sleep. Although we do not want you to watch the clock, we want you to get out of bed if you do not fall asleep immediately. Remember that the goal is to associate your bed with falling asleep quickly! If you are in bed more than about 15 to 20 minutes without falling asleep and have not gotten up, you are not following this instruction.
4. If you still cannot fall asleep, repeat rule 3. Do this as often as is necessary throughout the night.
5. Set your alarm and get up at the same time every morning, irrespective of how much sleep you got during the night. This will help your body to acquire a consistent sleep rhythm.
6. Do not nap during the day.

[a] Adapted from Reference 67.

able to shift physioslogic activity toward a more relaxed state.

Biofeedback training continues until the individual can reliably demonstrate the desired change in the target physiologic measure. The number of training sessions needed can be as high as 20 or 30; the length of training has been an obstacle to widespread use of biofeedback.

The 1999 review of behavioral treatments for insomnia (70) concluded that biofeedback is effective therapy to help patients control physiologic parameters (e.g., muscle tension) in order to attain reduction in somatic arousal.

Meditation

Meditation utilizes the passive focusing of attention upon limited internal sensations to promote relaxation (such as breathing movements or breathing sounds, muscle sensations, and stimuli from spontaneously occurring mental contents), while repeating a special word or phrase (*mantra*). Patients can quickly learn the basic procedure of a meditation technique (75) and begin practicing to build skill. Because meditation can be introduced quickly and requires little therapist time, it is sometimes chosen over progressive relaxation or biofeedback as the first type of relaxation training.

Meditation and several additional relaxation techniques (autogenic training, abdominal/diaphragmatic breathing, and hypnosis) did not receive any recommendation in the 1999 AASM review of behavioral insomnia treatments (70). The research evidence was judged too limited to officially sanction their use in the treatment of insomnia.

Imagery Training

Imagery training involves 15 to 20 minute periods of repetitive focusing on a set of pleasant or neutral images (76). Training and practice are important for positive results. Because the patient's thought processes are focused on relatively simple mental content, this technique is often perceived to be similar to meditation. The 1999 review of behavioral treatments (70) concluded there was no sufficient evidence to recommend imagery training as a stand-alone treatment. The reviewers also could not determine if this treatment would be effective when added to other interventions in a package of therapies.

Sleep Restriction and Sleep Compression

The goals of sleep restriction (77) and sleep compression (78) are a decrease in awake time during the night and an increase in the restorative benefits of sleep. The treatments are based on the observation that many people with insomnia spend too much time awake in bed trying to sleep, which causes a low percentage of time asleep during the night (low sleep efficiency). The treatments aim to consolidate sleep by restricting the amount of time the patient is allowed to be in bed. Sleep logs are used to determine

how many hours a night the patient sleeps before treatment. The patient is then restricted to no more than that number of hours in bed each night. Sleep compression gradually reduces the time allowed in bed, while sleep restriction abruptly reduces the time. This time-in-bed restriction causes some additional sleep deprivation, the effects of which are cumulative and increase the likelihood that sleep will occur when the patient is in bed. Increased daytime sleepiness often occurs early in sleep restriction treatment and the patient needs to be informed of this possibility. Daytime sleepiness is less likely to occur with sleep compression. When the patient's sleep becomes more consolidated (i.e., more efficient), the therapist will prescribe increments in the scheduled amount of time in bed.

At the beginning of treatment, the minimum time allowed in bed each night is 4.5 hours. Patients are monitored for daytime sleepiness, especially for episodes of inappropriately falling asleep. If a patient has too much difficulty staying awake, the restricted number of hours to spend in bed can be increased.

Sleep restriction has been included as a basic component of treatment packages for sleep maintenance insomnia. Patients who try too hard to sleep and spend too much time in bed trying to sleep are suitable for sleep restriction and sleep compression. The 1999 review of behavioral treatments (70) reported that sleep restriction is an effective therapy in the treatment of insomnia. The recommendation's strength was moderate.

Cognitive Therapy

The therapeutic goal of cognitive therapy is to interrupt the vicious circle of distress over poor sleep provoking dysfunctional cognitions, thus leading to more distress and more sleep disturbance. Cognitive therapy seeks to replace faulty beliefs and attitudes about sleep (79). For example, insomniacs often adhere to unrealistic expectations about sleep (such as, "I must sleep eight hours every night"), and often magnify the consequences of difficulty sleeping ("I cannot function at all after a bad night"). During cognitive therapy, treatment begins with learning the patient's dysfunctional sleep cognitions, challenging their validity, and then resolving them by replacing them with more adaptive alternatives. The treatment process is called *cognitive restructuring*.

The 1999 review of treatments (70) concluded there was insufficient evidence available for cognitive therapy to be recommended as a stand-alone treatment. The review noted that cognitive therapy is increasingly being used as one of the treatments in multicomponent behavioral therapy for chronic insomnia.

Paradoxical Intention

Paradoxical-intention treatment (80) aims to decrease the behavior of trying too hard to sleep and decrease hypothesized performance anxiety about the ability to sleep. Many people with insomnia add to their problem by worrying excessively about difficulty sleeping. They experience anticipatory anxiety associated with trying to control when sleep will occur. When the paradoxical-intention therapist instructs the patient to retire for the night and "try to stay awake," the goal is to prevent the anxiety associated with trying to sleep and thus promote relaxation and sleep. This instruction is the basic element of the treatment.

The therapist's description of paradoxical intention may be crucial to its success. A review of paradoxical-intention treatments (81) found that results were better when the treatment rationale emphasized the positive benefits of paradoxical intention or the positive qualities of the patient. The 1999 review of behavioral treatments concluded that paradoxical intention is an effective therapy in the treatment of chronic insomnia.

Multicomponent Behavioral Therapy

Clinicians and researchers have combined behavioral treatments in cognitive behavior therapy (CBT) treatment packages. The procedures of the individual behavior therapies for insomnia are compatible with each other and the goal is to increment the benefits by adding interventions. A typical package will include sleep education, relaxation training, stimulus control, and/or sleep restriction. An increasingly popular combination includes cognitive therapy plus sleep education, stimulus control, and/or sleep restriction.

The 1999 review of behavioral treatments (70) concluded that multicomponent CBT is effective for chronic insomnia, and it was recommended as a treatment option. Research indicates that a multicomponent treatment package is not always more effective than treatment with stimulus control or sleep restriction, when either is used as a single therapy (68,69). Consequently, it is important to recognize that the use of stimulus control or sleep restriction alone can provide significant benefit and is an empirically supported approach to treatment of chronic insomnia.

Benefits of Psychologic Treatment

Psychologic/behavioral treatments for insomnia offer a high expectancy for relief. These treatments decrease the time it takes to fall asleep, increase TST, and improve sleep efficiency (per meta-analyses: 68,69) although often sleep is still not completely normalized. They reduce the frequency and duration of nightly awakenings. Psychologic treatments present no physical tolerance and dependency risks, and adults rate psychologic interventions as more appropriate and acceptable than pharmacotherapy (59).

Recommendations for Initiating Behavioral Treatment

The use of stimulus control or sleep restriction treatment alone, or the use of a CBT treatment package is recommended for initiating a trial with behavior therapy for primary insomnia. The techniques included in a CBT package may be individualized to match the patient's history and the therapist's experience.

Follow-up Treatment for Secondary Insomnia

If a problem that is judged to be a secondary insomnia persists after successful resolution of the primary disorder, direct treatment for insomnia is indicated, if direct treatment has not previously been initiated. Treatment for secondary insomnia (e.g., mood disorder associated with sleep disturbance, anxiety disorder associated with sleep disturbance, PLMD, and, RLS) traditionally begins with treatment for the primary disorder. In this traditional approach to secondary insomnia, direct treatment for insomnia is delayed.

When the disorder causing secondary insomnia is treated first, it is anticipated that the insomnia will also decrease. Secondary insomnia should resolve when the disorder causing it has been resolved, *if* the two problems are fully linked as cause and effect *and* the maintaining factors issue from the primary disorder. Secondary insomnia, however, does not consistently resolve after treatment for the disorder judged to be primary, which causes prolonged delay in treatment for insomnia. It is desirable to consider direct treatment for insomnia early in the course of a secondary insomnia; this will prevent excess delay in treating the insomnia. Also, if the putative primary disorder is judged to be weakly linked with insomnia, direct treatment for insomnia is indicated in tandem with treatment for the primary disorder.

Of course, with chronic insomnia, conditioned sleep-preventing associations can develop, and a psychophysiologic insomnia can become established in addition to the initial sleep disturbance. The precipitating cause of a chronic insomnia may have been the medical disorder designated as primary, but over time conditioned associations can become dominant as maintaining factors and become the most appropriate focus of treatment.

Pharmacologic Therapy Management

The management of medication for insomnia can be extremely challenging. In addition to benzodiazepines, a number of medications from various classes have a potential place in the treatment of insomnia. Benzodiazepine and the newer non-benzodiazepine hypnotics are prescribed frequently and, not infrequently, inappropriately. For example, mistakenly prescribing a hypnotic for an undiagnosed and untreated OSA patient who presents with an insomnia complaint, rather than ordering a sleep laboratory study.

As both benzodiazepines and the new non-benzodiazepine medications both act at the benzodiazepine receptor (BZ-R) on the gamma-aminobutyric acid type-A ($GABA_A$) receptor, they are both referred to as BZ-R

▶ **TABLE 13-5. Medications Used in the Treatment of Insomnia**

Class	Medication	Half-life	Onset	Dosing (mg)
Benzodiazepine	Alprazolam	Medium	Medium	0.25–2.0
	Chlordiazepoxide	Long	Medium	10–25
	Clonazepam	Long	Medium	0.25–2.0
	Clorazepate	Long	Rapid	7.5–15
	Diazepam	Long	Rapid	2–10
	Estazolam	Medium	Rapid	1–2
	Flurazepam	Long	Medium	15–30
	Midazolam	Short	Medium	7.5–15
	Lorazepam	Medium	Medium	0.5–2
	Oxazepam	Medium	Slow	15–30
	Temazepam	Medium	Medium	15–30
	Triazolam	Short	Rapid	0.125–0.25
NBBRA[a]	Zaleplon	Short	Rapid	10–20
	Zolpidem	Short	Rapid	5–10
TCA[b]	Amitriptyline	Long	Medium	10–100
	Doxepin	Short	Rapid	10–100
	Imipramine	Medium	Rapid	10–100
	Nortriptyline	Long	Medium	10–100
Triazolopyridine	Trazodone	Medium	Rapid	25–100
Antiepileptic	Gabapentin	Short-medium	Medium	100–600
	Tiagabine	Medium	Medium	4–32
Dopamine antagonist	Quetiapine	Long	Medium	25–100

[a]NBBRA, non-benzodiazepine benzodiazepine receptor agonist.
[b]TCA, tricyclic antidepressant.

agonists (82). When these drugs bind to the BZ receptor they potentiate the effect of GABA binding to the receptor complex. When GABA binds the receptor complex, it causes an opening of the chloride ionophore moiety of the complex. The resulting influx of negative chloride ions hyperpolarizes the neuron, thus inhibiting its ability to create an action potential. BZ-R agonists enhance the ability of GABA to induce chloride influx. GABA$_A$ receptor complexes have five subunits (most have two alpha, two beta, and one gamma subunits). The alpha subunit has six subtypes (alpha$_1$–alpha$_6$). The BZ-R is near an alpha subunit. The composition of the five GABA$_A$ subunits differs at various locations. The newer BZ-R agonists (zolpidem and zaleplon) preferentially bind where the BZ-R is associated with the alpha$_1$ subunit—so called BZ-R1 agonists. The effect of BZ-R binding depends on the associated type of alpha subunit. When BZ-R agonists bind a BZ receptor associated with an alpha$_1$ subunit they have hypnotic, amnestic, and some anticonvulsant effects, but not muscle relaxant or antianxiety effects. Thus, the selective BZ-R1 agonists have less muscle relaxant and antianxiety effects than nonselective BZ-R agonists (the benzodiazepines). When anxiety is a prominent comorbid condition, benzodiazepines may be more effective than the selective BZ-R1 agonists.

PSG has shown that benzodiapzepines reduce sleep latency, increase TST, decrease stage 3 and 4 sleep, and, to a lesser extent, may decrease REM sleep. There may also be an increase in sleep spindle activity. The selective BZ-R drugs tend to reduce the amplitude of slow-wave activity less than nonselective benzodiazepines and, therefore, often do not reduce the amount of stage 3 and 4 sleep. Of note, the BZ-R1 agonists are not absolutely selective, and at higher doses the selectivity is lost (82).

The traditional benzodiazepines differ mainly in their duration of action (Table 13-5). In general, longer acting medications are more likely to have carry over effects into the waking hours. On the other hand, some of the shorter-acting medications may be associated with more rebound insomnia. Of note, despite some potential advantages of the selective BZ-R drugs, individual patients may respond to traditional BZs when they no longer respond to the selective BZ-Rs.

Although both zolpidem and zaleplon have a short half life, neither medication causes prominent rebound insomnia (83). Zaleplon has an especially short half-life and potentially could be useful as a middle of the night medication when a patient awakens but cannot return to sleep. A recent study by Walsh et al. (84) found a lack of sedation following middle-of-the-night zaleplon administration (testing 5 hours after drug administration) in sleep maintenance insomnia. Of note, for a rise time of 7:00 AM, this would suggest this medication could be taken at 2 AM with minimal daytime sedation.

While there is often concern regarding the possibility of physical addiction to BZ-R agonists, this is atypical in insomniacs unless there is a prior history of drug dependence. Physical tolerance to the drug and eventual ineffectiveness does occur in an unknown proportion of patients. Hypnotic-dependent insomnia is a significant problem, which includes drug dependency and a history of withdrawal symptoms. In general, all hypnotics should be tapered slowly to reduce rebound effects. A behavioral sleep program may also be helpful with hypnotic withdrawal (60). Other concerns include falls or other accidents from sedation or confusion from hypnotic use, especially in the elderly. It is always prudent to start with the lowest dose, especially in older patients. For example, 5 mg should be used instead of 10 mg of zolpidem. However, even at the lowest dose of hypnotics, confusion and sedation can occur in elderly patients.

The issue of tolerance is controversial because there are very few long-term studies of BZ-Rs. Certainly some patients complain the medications no longer work well but report a worsening of insomia when the drugs are stopped. A study by Scharf et al. (83) demonstrated effectiveness of zolpidem over a 5-week period (no tolerance). The investigation was placebo-controlled with sleep quality determined by PSG. In this study, there was no evidence of a reduction in stage 3 and 4 sleep, which is typical of nonselective BZ-Rs. Sustained efficacy over 6 months was also reported for the non-BZ drug eszopiclone in a large double-blind placebo controlled study. Here sleep quality was determined by patient report (85). In any case, some have challenged the conventional wisdom that long-term treatment with BZ-Rs frequently results in tolerance (86). However, until more information proves otherwise, the recommendation to use hypnotics for as short a time as possible still seems prudent.

The other group of medications that are frequently used for treatment of insomnia are the sedating antidepressants. Surveys have shown that there has been a dramatic shift from BZ-R hypnotics to the use of antidepressants to treat insomnia (87). In a recent survey, the use of trazodone exceeded zolpidem as the most commonly used medication (86).

Of note, unlike the BZ-R agonist hypnotics, none of the sedating antidepressants are FDA approved for treatment of insomnia (treatment of insomnia is "off-label"). In addition, the efficacy and safety of the sedating antidepressants as hypnotics has not been well studied. Some of the tricyclic antidepressants (amitriptyline, doxepin) that are commonly used as hypnotics have anticholinergic and cardiotoxic side effects. The antidepressant trazodone is not a tricyclic and is frequently used in low doses (50 to 100 mg) as a hypnotic. Trazodone is a serotonin type-2 receptor antagonist and a weak serotonin reuptake inhibitor. While the drug does not have anticholinergic side effects, it can cause priapism, postural hypotension (alpha blockade), and morning sedation. Despite the frequent use of this medication as a hypnotic, the evidence of efficacy is scanty at best. Yamadera et al. (88) studied the effects of trazodone on normal subjects with PSG and found an increase in stage 3 and 4 sleep, but no decrease in sleep latency or increase in TST. Walsh and co-workers (89) studied patients with primary insomnia and found a decrease in sleep latency and an increase in TST with 50 mg of trazodone compared to placebo at week 1, but not week 2 of treatment. Sleep was quantified by self-report not PSG. The incidence of adverse side effects of trazodone at antidepressant doses is known, but has never been studied at lower hypnotic doses. Nefazodone is less sedating than trazodone, but is less commonly used after reports of the rare but severe side effect of hepatic failure from the medication. Mirtazapine is another antidepressant that can be used in low doses as a hypnotic. The most worrisome side effect of this medication is weight gain. Other classes of drugs used as hypnotic include antiepileptics (neurontin) and antipsychotics (quetiapine). These medications have not been systematically studied as hypnotics and can have significant side effects. Despite the widespread off label use of sedating antidepressants as hypnotics, they would seem to be the agents of choice for the treatment of insomnia only where (a) BZ-Rs have failed, (b) drug-dependence is a major concern, (c) sleep apnea is present, or (d) depression is causing the insomnia.

As previously addressed, patients with depression frequently have insomnia complaints. Certain effective antidepressants [selective serotonin reuptake inhibitors (SSRIs), venlafaxine, bupropion] can also disturb sleep. If sleep complaints do not improve or worsen with treatment with these antidepressants it is common practice to (a) switch to a sedating antidepressant, (b) add a low dose of a sedating antidepressant at bedtime, or (c) add a BZ-R agonist at bedtime. A recent double-blind placebo-controlled cross-over study found that 100 mg of trazodone did improve sleep quality documented by PSG in a small group of patients on SSRIs (89). Another study found zolpidem to be effective for persistent insomnia (>2 weeks) on SSRI therapy for depression using a placebo-controlled patient questionnaire study. The drug was effective over the 4 weeks of the study (90).

In summary, chronic sedative/hypnotic prescribing can be a reasonable treatment option, when a set of four preconditions have been met: (a) the patient's problem is primary insomnia and it is chronic, (b) behavioral treatments have been attempted and were unsuccessful, (c) sleep laboratory studies have ruled out the presence of untreated sleep apnea or PLMD (if there is clinical suspicion of these disorders) or if treatment fails, and (d) the medication is prescribed by a single provider. When used, hypnotics should be prescribed in the lowest effective dose for as short an interval as possible.

FUTURE DIRECTIONS

1. Psychologic treatments for insomnia offer a high expectancy for relief. These treatments decrease the time it takes to fall asleep, increase TST, and improve sleep

efficiency. They reduce the frequency and duration of awakenings. Although generally successful, behavioral treatment often does not normalize sleep. New research is needed to develop behavioral treatments that more frequently normalize the sleep pattern of people with insomnia. For example, new relaxation techniques, new worry-management procedures, new types of stress-management training, and more sophisticated sleep hygiene programs may help produce better treatment outcomes.

2. For the problem of insomnia to be more fully addressed by the healthcare system, insomnia needs to be checked for more often by primary physicians, and insomnia needs to be reported more freely by patients. There appear to be barriers to doctor–patient communication about insomnia, because insomnia usually goes unrecognized. Treatment can be most effective if insomnia is identified before it progresses to a severe state. Yet, even severe insomnia is frequently not recognized by the patient's personal physician. Patient attitudes about seeking treatment for insomnia and physician attitudes about offering treatment for insomnia should be studied to provide the basis for educational efforts. For example, better education about the causes of insomnia, health risks associated with insomnia, and treatments for insomnia should facilitate more frequent identification of insomnia disorders.

3. The clinical measurement of insomnia generally depends on patient interview comments about sleep pattern. The use of more reliable and more valid measures of insomnia sleep patterns could improve treatment. Personal computers or hand-held computers could be used to collect sleep questionnaires as often as once a day, for processing by computer software in the physician's office. Objective recordings could also be performed in the home, such as wrist actigraphy measurement of sleep.

4. The sleep disorders nosology is relatively new; the current classification system has been in use since 1990. Research to document the reliability and validity of insomnia diagnoses is needed to promote progress toward high levels of diagnostic accuracy. Accuracy of diagnosis is a necessary step toward greater knowledge of how to treat the various insomnia subtypes. The applicability of insomnia diagnosis algorithms for use by primary care physicians needs to be tested. In designing and implementing such instruments, issues of usability, reliability, and, ultimately, effect on treatment outcome need to be addressed.

PEARLS

1. There is heterogeneity in the causes for persistent insomnia. Avoid blanket treatments, such as sedative

medication for symptom management. Insomnia complaints warrant assessment and differential diagnosis work-up before prescribing treatment; this will serve the accurate matching of specific therapy to specific diagnosis.

2. When treating primary insomnia, consider offering a trial with behavioral treatment. This type of psychologic treatment can help the patient learn a more healthy sleep pattern and reduce the risk of insomnia recurrence.

3. Evaluate the pros and cons of sedative–hypnotic medication for each patient with insomnia before prescribing any sleep medication.

4. Insomnia often goes unrecognized by the patient's personal physician. Physicians should routinely ask new patients about sleep.

REFERENCES

1. Bixler EO, Kales A, Soldatos CR, et al. Prevalence of sleep disorders in the Los Angeles metropolitan area. *Amer J Psychi*. 1979;136:1257–1262.
2. Mellinger GD, Balter MB, Uhlenhuth EL. Insomnia and its treatment. *Arch Gen Psych*. 1985;42:225–232.
3. Partinen M, Hublin C. Epidemiology of sleep disorders. In: Kryger MH, Roth T, Dement WC, eds. *Principles and practice of sleep medicine*, 3rd edn. Philadelphia: WB Saunders, 2000:558–579.
4. WB&A. *Sleep in America: 2003*. Annapolis, MD: WB&A Market Research, 2003.
5. Espie CA. *The psychological treatment of insomnia*. Chichester, England: Wiley, 1991.
6. Kales JD, Kales A, Bixler EO, et al. Biopsychobehavioral correlates of insomnia, V: clinical characteristics and behavioral correlates. *Amer J Psychi*. 1984;141:1371–1376.
7. Morin CM, Gramling SE. Sleep patterns and aging: comparison of older adults with and without insomnia complaints. *Psychol Aging*. 1989;4:290–294.
8. Morin CM. *Insomnia: Psychological assessment and management*. New York: Guilford, 1993.
9. Ohayon MM. Prevalence of DSM-IV diagnostic criteria of insomnia: distinguishing insomnia related to mental disorders from sleep disorders. *J Psych Res*. 1997;31:333–346.
10. Lichstein KL, McCrae CS, Wilson NM. Secondary insomnia: diagnostic issues, cognitive-behavioral treatment, and future directions. In: Perlis ML, Lichstein KL, eds. *Treating sleep disorders: Principles and practice of behavioral sleep medicine*. Hoboken, NJ: Wiley, 2003:286–304.
11. Roehrs T, Roth T. Hypnotics: efficacy and adverse effects. In: Kryger MH, Roth T, Dement WC, eds. *Principles and practice of sleep medicine*. 3rd edn. Philadelphia: WB Saunders, 2000:414–418.
12. American Sleep Disorders Association. *International classification of sleep disorders, revised: Diagnostic and coding manual*. Rochester, MN: American Sleep Disorders Association, 1997.
13. Buysse DJ, Reynolds CF. Insomnia. In: Thorpy MJ, ed. *Handbook of sleep disorders*. New York: Marcel Dekker, 1990:375–433.
14. Hauri PJ, Fischer J. Persistent psychophysiologic (learned) insomnia. *Sleep*. 1986;9:38–53.
15. Coleman RM. Diagnosis, treatment and follow-up of about 8,000 sleep/wake disorder patients. In: Guilleminault C, Lugaresi E, eds. *Sleep/wake disorders: Natural history, epidemiology, and long-term evolution*. New York: Raven Press, 1983:87–97.
16. Lichstein KL, Wilson, NM, Johnson CT. Psychological treatment of secondary insomnia. *Psychol Aging*. 2000;15:232–240.
17. Hauri PJ, Olmstead EM. Childhood onset insomnia. *Sleep*. 1980;3:59–65.

18. Carskadon MA, Dement WC, Mitler MM, et al. Self-reports versus sleep laboratory findings in 122 drug-free subjects with complaints of chronic insomnia. *Amer J Psych.* 1976;133:1382–1388.

19. Borkovec TD, Grayson JB, O'Brien GT, et al. Relaxation treatment of pseudoinsomnia and idiopathic insomnia: an electroencephalographic evaluation. *J Appl Behav Anal.* 1979;12:37–54.

20. Reynolds CF, Kupfer DJ. Sleep research in affective illness: state of the art circa 1987. *Sleep.* 1987;10:199–215.

21. Carskadon MA, Dement WC, Mitler MM, et al. Guidelines for the Multiple Sleep latency Test (MSLT): a standard measure of sleepiness. *Sleep.* 1986;9:519–524.

22. Reynolds CF, Shaw DM, Newton TF, et al. EEG sleep in outpatients with generalized anxiety: a preliminary comparison with depressed outpatients. *Psych Res.* 1983;8:81–89.

23. Hauri PJ, Friedman M, Ravaris CL. Sleep in patients with spontaneous panic attacks. *Sleep.* 1989;12:323–337.

24. Zarcone VP. Sleep and alcoholism. In Weitzman ED, ed. *Sleep disorders: Intersections of basic and clinical research. Vol. 8. Advances in sleep research.* New York: Spectrum Press, 1982:125–135.

25. Kales A, Bixler EO, Tan TL, et al. Chronic hypnotic-drug use: ineffectiveness, drug-withdrawal insomnia, and dependence. *JAMA.* 1974;227:513–517.

26. Czeisler CA, Richardson GS, Coleman RM, et al. Chronotherapy: resetting the circadian clock of patients with delayed sleep phase insomnia. *Sleep.* 1981;4:1–21.

27. Kamei R, Hughes L, Miles L, et al. Advanced-sleep-phase syndrome studied in a time isolation facility. *Chronobiologia.* 1979;6:115.

28. Walsh JK, Tepas DI, Moss PD. The EEG sleep of night and rotating shift workers. In: Johnson LC, Tepas DI, Colquhoun WP, et al., eds. *Biological rhythms, sleep and shift work.* New York: SP Medical & Scientific Books, 1981:347–356.

29. Coleman RM. Periodic movements in sleep (nocturnal myoclonus) and restless legs syndrome. In Guilleminault C, ed. *Sleeping and waking disorders: Indications and techniques.* Menlo Park, CA: Addison-Wesley, 1982:265–295.

30. American Sleep Disorders Association. EEG arousals: scoring rules and examples. A preliminary report from the sleep disorders atlas task force. *Sleep.* 1992;15:173–184.

31. Rechtschaffen A, Kales A (eds.). *A manual of standardized terminology, techniques and scoring system for sleep stages of human subjects.* Los Angeles: UCLA Brain Information Service/Brain Research Institute, 1968.

32. Ancoli-Israel A, Kripke DF, Klauber MR, et al. Periodic limb movements in sleep in community-dwelling elderly. *Sleep.* 1991;14:496–500.

33. Lugaresi E, Cirignotta F, Coccagna G, et al. Nocturnal myoclonus and restless legs syndrome. *Advan Neurol.* 1986;43:295–307.

34. Bradley TD, McNicholas WT, Rutherford R, et al. Clinical and physiologic heterogeneity of the central sleep apnea syndrome. *Amer Rev Respir Dis.* 1986;134:217–221.

35. Guilleminault C, Bassiri AG. Clinical features and evaluation of obstructive sleep apnea. In: Kryger MH, Roth T, Dement WC, eds. *Principles and practice of sleep medicine.* 3rd edn. Philadelphia: WB Saunders, 2000:869–878.

36. Guilleminault C, Anagnos A. Narcolepsy syndrome. In: Kryger MH, Roth T, Dement WC, eds. *Principles and practice of sleep medicine.* 3rd edn. Philadelphia: WB Saunders, 2000:676–686.

37. Bliwise DL. Sleep in dementing illness. In: Oldham JM, Riba MB, eds. *Review of psychiatry.* Vol. 13. Washington, DC: American Psychiatric Press, 1994:757–776.

38. Moldofsky H, Saskin P, Lue FA. Sleep and symptoms in fibrositis syndrome after a febrile illness. *J Rheumatol.* 1988;15:1701–1704.

39. Orr WC. Gastrointestinal disorders. In: Kryger MH, Roth T, Dement WC, eds. *Principles and practice of sleep medicine.* 3rd edn. Philadelphia: WB Saunders, 2000:1113–1122.

40. Douglas NJ. Chronic obstructive pulmonary desease. In: Kryger MH, Roth T, Dement WC, eds. *Principles and practice of sleep medicine.* 3rd edn. Philadelphia: WB Saunders, 2000:965–975.

41. Hohagen F, Rink K, Kappler C, et al. Prevalence and treatment of insomnia in general practice: a longitudinal study. *Eur Arch Psych Clin Neurosci.* 1993;242:329–336.

42. Schramm E, Hohagen F, Kappler, et al. Mental comorbidity of chronic insomnia in general practice attenders using DSM-III-R. *Acta Psych Scand.* 1995;91:10–17.

43. Shorr R, Bauwens S. Diagnosis and treatment of outpatient insomnia by psychiatric and non-psychiatric physicians. *Amer J Med.* 1992;93:78–82.

44. Lichstein KL, Means MK, Noe SL, et al. Fatigue and sleep disorders. *Behav Res Ther.* 1997;35:733–740.

45. Lichstein KL, Johnson RS. Pupillometric discrimination of insomniacs. *Behav Res Ther.* 1994;32:123–129.

46. Stepanski E, Zorick F, Roehrs T, et al. Daytime alertness in patients with chronic insomnia compared with asymptomatic control subjects. *Sleep.* 1988;11:54–60.

47. Sateia MJ, Doghramji K, Hauri PJ, et al. Evaluation of chronic insomnia: an American Academy of Sleep Medicine review. *Sleep.* 2000;23:243–308.

48. Buysse DJ, Reynolds CF, Kupfer DJ, et al. Clinical diagnoses in 216 insomnia patients using the International Classification of Sleep Disorders (ICSD), DSM-IV and ICD-10 categories: a report from the APA/NIMH DSM-IV field trial. *Sleep.* 1994;17:630–637.

49. Hauri PJ, Olmstead EM. Reverse first night effect in insomnia. *Sleep.* 1989;12:97–105.

50. American Academy of Sleep Medicine. Practice parameters for using polysomnography to evaluate insomnia: an update. *Sleep.* 2003;26:754–757.

51. Ancoli-Israel S, Cole R, Alessi C, et al. The role of actigraphy in the study of sleep and circadian rhythms: American Academy of Sleep Medicine review paper. *Sleep.* 2003;26:342–358.

52. Spielman AJ, Glovinsky PB. The varied nature of insomnia. In: Hauri PJ, ed. *Case studies in insomnia.* New York: Plenum Press, 1991:1–15.

53. Williams RL, Karacan I, Hursch CJ. *Electroencephalography (EEG) of human sleep.* New York: Wiley, 1974.

54. Hauri PJ. Sleep hygiene, relaxation therapy, and cognitive interventions. In Hauri PJ, ed. *Case studies in insomnia.* New York: Plenum Press, 1991:65–84.

55. Stepanski EJ, Wyatt JK. Use of sleep hygiene in the treatment of insomnia. *Sleep Med Rev.* 2003;7:215–225.

56. Zorick FJ, Walsh JK. Evaluation and management of insomnia. In: Kryger MH, Roth T, Dement WC, eds. *Principles and practice of sleep medicine,* 3rd edn. Philadelphia: WB Saunders, 2000:615–623.

57. Roehrs T, Zorick FJ, Roth T. Transient and short-term insomnias. In: Kryger MH, Roth T, Dement WC, eds. *Principles and practice of sleep medicine,* 3rd edn. Philadelphia: WB Saunders, 2000:624–632.

58. Ohayon MM, Caulet M, Arbus L, et al. Are the prescribed medications effective in the treatment of insomnia complaints? *J Psychosom Res.* 1999;47:359–368.

59. Morin CM, Gaulier B, Barry T, et al. Patients' acceptance of psychological and pharmacological therapies for insomnia. *Sleep.* 1992;15:302–305.

60. Lichstein, KL, McCrae CS, Wilson NM, et al. Treatment of hypnotic dependence in older adults. *Sleep.* 2003;26:A290.

61. Roehrs T, Merlotti L, Zorick F, et al. Sedative, memory, and performance effects of hypnotics. *Psychopharmacology.* 1994;116:130–134.

62. Ray WA, Griffin MR, Downey W. Benzodiazepines of long and short elimination half-life and the risk of hip fracture. *JAMA.* 1989;262:3303–3307.

63. National Institutes of Health. Drugs and insomnia: The use of medication to promote sleep. *JAMA.* 1984;18:2410–2414.

64. Hauri PJ. Can we mix behavioral therapy with hypnotics when treating insomniacs? *Sleep.* 1997;20:1111–1118.

65. Stepanski EJ, Zorick FJ, Roth T. Pharmacotherapy of insomnia. In Hauri PJ, ed. *Case studies in insomnia.* New York: Plenum Press, 1991:115–129.

66. Espie CA, Lindsay WR, Brooks DN. Substituting behavioural treatment for drugs in the treatment of insomnia: an exploratory study. *J Behav Ther Exp Psych.* 1988;19:51–56.

67. Bootzin RR, Epstein DR. Stimulus control. In: Lichstein KL, Morin CM, eds. *Treatment of late-life insomnia.* Thousand Oaks, CA: Sage, 2000:167–184.

68. Morin CM, Culbert JP, Schwartz SM. Nonpharmacological interventions for insomnia: a meta-analysis of treatment efficacy. *Amer J Psych.* 1994;151:1172–1180.

69. Murtagh DRR, Greenwood KM. Identifying effective psychological treatments for insomnia: a meta-analysis. *J Consult Clin Psychol.* 1995;63:79–89.

70. American Academy of Sleep Medicine. Practice parameters for

the nonpharmacologic treatment of chronic insomnia. *Sleep.* 1999;22:1128–1133.

71. Bootzin RR, Rider SP. Behavioral techniques and biofeedback for insomnia. In: Pressman MR, Orr WC, eds. *Understanding sleep: the evaluation and treatment of sleep disorders.* Washington, DC: American Psychological Association, 1997:315–338.

72. Bernstein DA, Borkovec TD. *Progressive relaxation training: a manual for the helping professions.* Champaign, IL: Research Press, 1973.

73. Lichstein KL, Johnson RS. Relaxation for insomnia and hypnotic medication use in older women. *Psychol Aging.* 1993;8:103–111.

74. Hauri PJ, Percy L, Hellekson C, et al. The treatment of psychophysiologic insomnia with biofeedback: a replication study. *Biofeedback Self-Regulation.* 1982;7:223–235.

75. Benson H. *The relaxation response.* New York: Morrow, 1975.

76. Morin CM, Azrin NH. Stimulus control and imagery training in treating sleep-maintenance insomna. *J Consult Clin Psychol.* 1987;55:260–262.

77. Spielman AJ, Saskin P, Thorpy MJ. Treatment of chronic insomnia by restriction of time in bed. *Sleep.* 1987;10:45–56.

78. Lichstein KL, Riedel BW, Wilson NM, et al. Relaxation and sleep compression for late-life insomnia: a placebo-controlled trial. *J Consult Clin Psychol.* 2001;69:227–239.

79. Morin CM, Savard J, Blais FC. Cognitive Therapy. In: Lichstein KL, Morin CM, eds. *Treatment of late-life insomnia.* Thousand Oaks, CA: Sage, 2000:207–230.

80. Turner RM, Ascher LM. A controlled comparison of progressive relaxation, stimulus control and paradoxical intention therapies for insomnia. *J Consult Clin Psychol.* 1979;47:500–508.

81. Shoham-Salomon V, Rosenthal R. Paradoxical interventions: a meta-analysis. *J Consult Clin Psychol.* 1987;55:22–28.

82. Mohler H, Fritschy JM, Rudolph U. A new benzodiazepine pharmacology. *J Pharmacol Exp Ther.* 2002;300:2–8.

83. Scharf MB, Roth T, Vogel GW, Walsh JK. A mulicenter, placebo-controlled study: evaluation zolpidem in the treatment of chronic insomnia. *J Clin Psych.* 1994;55:192–199.

84. Walsh JK, Pollak CP, Scharf MB, et al. Lack of residual sedation following middle-of-the-night Zaleplon administration in sleep maintenance insomnia. *Clin Neuropharmacol.* 2000;23:17–21.

85. Krystal AD, Walsh JK, Laska E, et al. Sustained Efficacy of Eszopiclone over 6 months of nightly treatment: results of a randomized, double-blind, placebo-controlled study in adults with chronic insomnia. *Sleep.* 2003;26:793–799.

86. Mendelson WB, Roth T, Cassella J, et al. The treatment of chronic insomnia: drug indications, chronic use and abuse liability. *Sleep Med Rev.* 2004;8:1–17.

87. Walsh JK, Schwitzer PK. Ten-year trends in the pharmacological treatment of insomnia. *Sleep.* 1999;22:371–375.

88. Yamadera H, Nakamur S, Suzuki H, et al. Effects of trazodone hydrochloride and imipramine on polysomography in healthy subjects. *Psych Clin Neurosci.* 1998;52:439–443.

89. Kaynak H, Kaynak D, Gozukirmizi E, et al. The effects of trazodone on sleep in patients treated with stimulant antidepressants. *Sleep Med.* 2004;5:15–20.

90. Asnis GM, Chakraburtty A, DuBoff EA, et al. Zolpidem for persistent insomnia in SSRI-treated depressed patients. *J Clin Psych.* 1999;60:668–676.

Narcolepsy and Idiopathic Hypersomnia

Richard B. Berry and Robin L. Gilmore

INTRODUCTION AND HISTORY

Narcolepsy is a chronic disabling disorder that affects the control of wakefulness and sleep. It may be conceptualized as a "state boundary disorder" (1) that results in an intrusion of rapid eye movement (REM) sleep features into the waking state. Willis first described the disorder in 1672. The term narcolepsy was first used to describe the syndrome by Gelineau in 1880, combining the Greek words for "somnolence" and "to seize." He described a disorder characterized by irresistible sleepiness and episodes of falling. Adie first used the term "cataplexy" in 1926 to describe brief episodes of muscle weakness triggered by emotions. In 1957, Yoss and Daly described the classic narcolepsy symptom tetrad of daytime sleepiness, cataplexy, hypnogogic hallucinations, and sleep paralysis (Table 14-1) (2). Sleep paralysis is a partial or complete paralysis of the skeletal muscles that occurs at sleep onset or sleep offset. The hallucinations of narcolepsy are vivid dreamlike images that occur upon falling asleep (hypnogogic) or waking up (hypnopompic). In 1960, Vogel reported that sleep onset REM periods (REM latency <20 minutes) are associated with narcolepsy (3).

While the etiology of narcolepsy remains uncertain, major advances in understanding the pathophysiology of the disorder have recently occurred. This is due to the discovery of the orexin (hypocretin) neuropeptide system (4,5) and demonstration that defects in this system result in impaired control of wakefulness and sleep (6–11).

An abnormality in the gene coding for the hypocretin receptor 2 was found to be responsible for familial canine narcolepsy (9). Narcolepsylike behavior was noted in orexin knockout mice (no orexin ligand) (10) and in mice developing an ablation of oxrein neurons (11).

▶ **TABLE 14-1.** Features of the Classic Narcolepsy Tetrad

Features of the Tetrad	Duration	Age at Onset	Occur (%)	Specific for Narcolepsy?
Excessive daytime sleepiness (EDS)	Continuously, with exacerbations	Typically teens–30s	100	No
Cataplexy	Seconds–minutes	Typically 3 to 5 years after EDS,[a] but may be years later	60–70	Yes
Hypnagogic/ hypnapompic hallucinations	Minutes	Teens	30–60	No
Sleep paralysis	Minutes (usually longer than cataplexy)	Teens	25–50	No

[a] Excessive daytime sleepiness. Frequency listed is for patients with narcolepsy (both with and without cataplexy; proportions will vary with the percentage of patients with cataplexy). See Table 14-3.

Subsequently, it was determined that most cases of human narcolepsy with cataplexy are associated with low or absent CSF levels of hypocretin 1 (12–14). Current information suggests this is due to a loss of hypocretin-secreting cells in the hypothalamus (15,16).

CLINICAL SYMPTOMATOLOGY

The manifestations of narcolepsy (Table 14-2) generally begin between the ages of 15 and 30 (17). However, narcolepsy can present in the pediatric age group or in patients over 60 years of age. The development, number, and severity of symptoms vary widely among individuals with the disorder. The classic symptom tetrad (Table 14-1) includes excessive daytime sleepiness (EDS), cataplexy, sleep paralysis, and hypnagogic or hypnopompic hallucinations. These symptoms will be discussed in detail in separate sections. Of note, only 10% to 15% of patients have the complete symptom tetrad (2). EDS alone or in combination with hypnagogic hallucinations and/or sleep paralysis is the presenting symptom in approximately 90% of patients (17–23). Approximately 60% to 70% of patients have cataplexy (2,17–22). Cataplexy may develop several years after the initial presentation (Table 14-1). However, most patients with cataplexy develop the symptom within 3 to 5 years of the onset of daytime sleepiness (17). Rarely, cataplexy can precede daytime sleepiness.

Cataplexy is the only symptom specific to narcolepsy (18–23). Isolated cataplexy or cataplexy with sleepiness can occur in a few rare neurologic disorders associated with mental retardation and obvious neurologic deficits. These will be discussed in a following section. In a patient with daytime sleepiness and a normal neurologic examination, cataplexy is virtually diagnostic of narcolepsy. Hypnogogic hallucinations and sleep paralysis can occur

in other sleep disorders. Sleep paralysis (SP) is reported in patients with sleep apnea or idiopathic hypersomnolence and occasionally in normal subjects, especially after periods of sleep deprivation. The symptom of hypnogogic hallucinations (HH) also is not specific for narcolepsy and

▶ **TABLE 14-2.** Manifestations of Narcolepsy

Symptoms
Excessive daytime sleepiness (EDS) (sleep attacks)
Cataplexy
Hynogogic/hypnopompic hallucinations
Sleep paralysis
Automatic behavior

Polysomnographic finding
Short sleep latency (<10 min)
Short nocturnal REM latency (<20 min)
Increased arousals
Decreased sleep efficiency
Increased stage 1 sleep
Decreased stage 3 and 4 sleep may occur
Periodic leg movements (PLMs) in sleep

MSLT
Mean sleep latency <5 min
Two or more REM onset periods in 5 naps

HLA typing
DQB1*0602 in 90–100% of narcolepsy with cataplexy patients
DQB1*0602 in 40–60% of narcolepsy without cataplexy patients

CSF hypocretin 1 level
Absent/very decreased in 90–95% of narcolepsy with cataplexy patients
Normal in patients with narcolepsy without cataplexy

Concurrent sleep disorders
Periodic leg movements (PLMs) in sleep
OSA
REM sleep-behavior disorder (RBD)

▶ **TABLE 14-3.** Features of Narcolepsy Syndromes versus Idiopathic Hypersomnia[a]

	Narcolepsy with Cataplexy	*Narcolepsy without Cataplexy*	*Idiopathic Hypersomnia*
Symptoms			
Daytime sleepiness	Yes	Yes	Yes
Hypnogogic hallucinations (%)	70–86	15–60	40
Sleep paralysis (%)	50–70	25–60	40–50
***Polysomnography* (PSG)**			
Sleep latency	Short	Short	Normal
REM latency <20 minutes	40–50%	40–50%	Normal
Disturbed nightime sleep	Yes	Yes	No
Stage 1 sleep	Increased	Mildly increased	Normal
24-Hour total sleep time	Normal to slight increase	Normal to slight increase	Very increased in some patients
MSLT			
Mean sleep latency (min)	<5	<5	<10
Sleep-onset REM periods(SOREM) (*n*)	3–3.7	2–3.3	0.2 (None)
DQB1*0602 (% positive)	90–100%	40–60%	52
CSF hypocretin 1	Undetectable in 90–95%	Normal	Normal
Neuropathology	Marked reduction in hypocretin neurons	Possibly a partial loss of hypocretin neurons or injury to critical hypocretin pathways?	Unknown
Body mass index (BMI)	Increased in 5–15%	Normal	Normal

[a]Adapted from Scammel TE, The neurobiology, diagnosis, and treatment of narcolepsy. *Ann Neurol*. 2003:53:154–166.

can occur in the same settings as SP. Aldrich (19,20) and others have suggested that SP and HH are not very useful in separating patients with narcolepsy without cataplexy from idiopathic hypersomnia or sleep apnea. In the absence of cataplexy, a diagnosis of narcolepsy depends on demonstration of sleep-onset REM (SOREM) (very short REM latency) and an absence of other disorders to explain this finding. There are group differences in the characteristics of narcolepsy patients with and without cataplexy, although overlap does exist (Table 14-3) (23,24).

Excessive Daytime Sleepiness

The excessive daytime sleepiness (EDS) of narcolepsy can occur as discrete "sleep attacks" or as constant sleepiness with intermittent worsening. Unrelenting EDS is usually the first and most prominent symptom of narcolepsy. Sleepiness may occur throughout the day, regardless of the amount or quality of prior nighttime sleep. Sleep episodes may occur at work and social events, while eating, talking, and driving, and in other similarly inappropriate situations. Only temporary relief is gained with napping. It has been said that falling asleep while standing or eating is especially suggestive of narcolepsy. Although patients may sleep at every hour of the day, the total sleep time (TST)

over a 24-hour period is normal or only slightly increased (23,25,26). As mentioned previously, EDS is usually the first symptom of narcolepsy.

Cataplexy

Cataplexy is characterized by the sudden, temporary loss of bilateral muscle tone with preserved consciousness triggered by strong emotions, such as laugher, anger, or surprise (17,21,22,27). When loss of muscle strength is severe, almost all the voluntary muscles in the body are affected, leading to complete collapse. The muscles of the eyes are not affected during cataplexy; individuals can move their eyes during a cataplectic episode. Diaphragmatic activity is also not impaired. In mild cases of cataplexy, the loss in muscle strength can be quite subtle, partially involving only a few muscle groups. For example, partial neck muscle weakness may cause the patient to have difficult keeping the head erect (head nodding), ptosis, or difficulty speaking. In some patients, partial attacks are more frequently than complete attacks. Loss of muscle function may not be evident, and the patient may experience only a vague feeling of weakness. In one study, the legs and knees were most frequently affected (27). Patients may fall to the ground, and injuries do occur. However, most people are able to find support at the onset of an attack. The attacks start abruptly and usually take several seconds to reach their maximum intensity. Episodes of cataplexy usually last from seconds to minutes; rarely does an attack last any longer than 2 minutes. Clinical signs during an attack are the loss of muscle tone and abolished tendon reflexes. The phenomenon of virtually continuous attacks of cataplexy (status catapleticus) can occur after sudden withdrawal of medications that suppress cataplexy.

Cataplexy occurs during times of intense emotional states. Unfortunately, up to 30% of patients with all causes of daytime sleepiness may report some sensation of weakness during emotion (27). A systematic survey of symptoms of muscle weakness associated with emotion in a large group of patients with daytime sleepiness found that weakness during joking (telling or hearing a joke), laughter, and anger were the most specific for cataplexy associated with narcolepsy (27). Involvement of the legs also seemed to be more specific for narcolepsy.

During the attack, the patient is completely awake and later will have total recall of the entire event. If episodes last longer than a few minutes, the patient may transition into REM sleep and experience hypnogogic hallucinations. During an attack of cataplexy, there are cardiovascular changes consisting of increased blood pressure and decreased heart rate. The decreased heart rate is secondary to the increased blood pressure (28).

Isolated cataplexy can rarely occur with syndromes other than idiopathic narcolepsy. It has been reported in Coffin–Lowry syndrome (29,30), the Prader–Willi syndrome (31), Nieman–Pick Disease type C (32–34), Moebius syndrome (35), and Norrie disease (36,37). These patients have mental retardation and/or obvious neurologic deficits in contrast to the patient with "idiopathic" narcolepsy. The Coffin–Lowry syndrome is a rare X-linked disorder in which affected males demonstrate severe mental retardation with prominent dysmorphic features usually affecting the face and hands. Typical facial features include a prominent forehead, hypertelorism, a flat nasal bridge, downward sloping palpebral fissures, and a wide mouth with full lips. Cataplexy may be seen in up to 10% of children with Niemann–Pick type C disease (32–34). This is a rare autosomal recessive disorder characterized by lysosomal accumulation of unesterfied cholesterol in many tissues as well as lysosomal storage of sphingolipids in the brain and liver. The clinical manifestations and severity are variable. Classic findings include hepatosplenomegaly, vertical supranuclear gaze palsy, ataxia, dystonia, and dementia. In one recently reported case, the CSF hypocretin was reduced, but not into the narcolepsy range (34). Cataplexy has been reported in children with Moebius syndrome (35). The Moebius syndrome consists of congenital paresis of the 7th cranial nerve, orofacial and limb malformations, and mental retardation. Norrie disease is a rare genetic condition that has also been associated with cataplexy. It is an X-linked recessive disorder causing ocular atrophy, mental retardation, deafness, and dysmor-

phic features (36). Monoamine oxidase (MAO) defects occur in some patients (37). Based on a questionnaire study one group of investigators has found cataplectic attacks among patients with Wilson's disease (38). However, before this becomes generally accepted, further studies will be needed.

Hypnogogic Hallucinations

The hallucinations of narcolepsy that occur at nocturnal sleep onset are called hypnogogic and those on awakening are termed hypnopompic. The hallucinations are typically bizarre and may be frightening. Patients sometimes have a fair degree of insight that they are hallucinatory in nature, but often consider them no less frightening. The duration is usually less than 10 minutes, and the frequency is quite variable. Visual imagery is the predominant feature for many patients. Colored forms that may be changing are sometimes of intense hues and dramatically described. A commonly described vision is that of an animal or stranger in the room. Auditory or vestibular hallucinations (sensation of falling) may also occur. Early series reported about 30% of patients with narcolepsy reported sleep-related hallucinations (2). However, later series have reported proportions up to 70% in groups of narcolepsy with cataplexy (20). Aldrich studied the results of questionnaires in groups with narcolepsy–cataplexy (NwithC), narcolepsy without cataplexy (NwithoutC), and idiopathic hypersomnia (IH). The proportion of NwithC patients reporting sleep-related hallucinations was higher than in the NwithoutC or IH groups. The proportion reporting hallucinations in the IH group was slightly higher than in the NwithoutC group (20).

Sleep Paralysis

Sleep paralysis is partial or complete paralysis during the onset of sleep or upon awakening. Patients are awake and conscious during the attack. There is no emotional precipitant. The episodes may last longer than a typical cataplectic attack. People who experience sleep paralysis sometimes experience hallucinations simultaneously. Early series reported about 25% of patients with narcolepsy having sleep paralysis (2,23). Later series have found that up to 50% to 80% of patients with NwithC report sleep paralysis (17,20). Aldrich found that more patients with NwithC reported sleep paralysis than in groups of NwithoutC patients with and IH (20). The proportion of patients reporting sleep paralysis was similar in the NwithoutC and IH groups.

Adequate ventilation is maintained during sleep paralysis as diaphragmatic function is spared. However, some patients have a sensation of dyspnea. Sleep paralysis is often very frightening, due to the inability to move, speak, or communicate during the episode. Sleep paralysis may also occur in the general population, but usually is a fairly uncommon event. In normal subjects, sleep paralysis often follows periods of sleep deprivation/reduced sleep.

Disturbed Nocturnal Sleep and Other Symptoms

Patients with narcolepsy often experience disturbed nighttime sleep with tossing and turning in bed, leg jerks, nightmares, and frequent awakenings. In general, NwithC patients have more disturbed sleep than NwithoutC patients (20). Automatic behaviors occur for which there may be partial amnesia. For example, patients report driving a car and not remembering the trip. They may find themselves doing activities that make no sense, like putting salt in iced tea. These episodes typically involve activities that are habitual or not demanding of skill. Inattentiveness related to drowsiness may occur. Aldrich reported that the proportions of patients reporting automatic behavior were similar in groups of NwithC, NwithoutC, and IH (20). Patients with narcolepsy may also have the REM behavior disorder (RBD) (39). In this disorder, skeletal muscle atonia is absent during REM sleep and dreams may be acted out. As the hypocretin system has affects on appetite, perhaps it is not surprising that some patients with NwithC have an increased body mass index (BMI) (24,40). Obstructive sleep apnea is also not uncommon (41). If cataplexy is not present, narcolepsy may be suspected only if daytime sleepiness persists after adequate treatment of the sleep apnea.

EPIDEMIOLOGY AND GENETICS

The estimated prevalence of narcolepsy is around 1 in 2,000 individuals (20,42–44). Although narcolepsy is not a rare disorder, it is often misdiagnosed or diagnosed only years after symptoms first appear. Early diagnosis and treatment, however, are important for the well-being of the affected individual. Narcolepsy is distributed equally between men and women. Approximately 125,000 people in the United States suffer from this disorder.

It is probable that there is a genetic component to the disorder. Familial canine narcolepsy is transmitted as a single autosomal recessive gene (canarc-1) with complete penetrance (44). However, the human form of the narcolepsy is not a simple genetic disease. A familial tendency for human narcolepsy has long been recognized since the disease's first description in the late 19th century (45). While the majority of cases of human narcolepsy are sporadic, there have been numerous reports of familial narcolepsy in the literature (44). Recent studies revealed that the risk of a first-degree relative of a narcoleptic developing NwithC is 1% to 2%, a 10 to 40 times higher risk than in the general population (44,46). However, studies of identical twins show a high degree of discordance for narcolepsy with cataplexy. That is, if one twin has narcolepsy, only 25% to 31% of the time will the other twin also have narcolepsy (44). Thus, factors other than genetics are important for the development of human narcolepsy.

Narcolepsy with cataplexy is strongly linked to specific human-leukocyte antigens. About 90% to 100% of patients with NwithC have the DQB1*0602 allele regardless of race (47). This allele is present in about 12% of Japanese, 25% of Caucasians, and 38% of African Americans without the syndrome. The percentage of patients with narcolepsy without cataplexy that are DQB1*0602 positive is lower (40% to 60%). In general, patients with narcolepsy who are DQB1*602 positive, have more severe symptoms (17).

PATHOPHYSIOLOGY

Before the discovery of the hypocretin system, cholinergic hypersensitivity or monoaminergic (serotonin, norepinephrine) deficiency had been hypothesized to be the cause of the daytime sleepiness and REM-associated manifestations of narcolepsy (23,48,49). Of note, narcoleptics have a normal amount of REM sleep and normal or slightly increased total sleep time (TST) over 24 hours (25,26). Therefore, the basic abnormalities are the inappropriate switches between wake and sleep, and wake and REM sleep phenomenon.

Recent advances provide compelling evidence that human narcolepsy with cataplexy may be a neurodegenerative or autoimmune disorder resulting in a loss of hypothalamic neurons containing the neuropeptide hypocretin (orexin) (15,16). The hypocretin system has been hypothesized to stabilize the wakefulness and sleep states and prevent inappropriate transitions between the states (6,7,8,23,24). Other abnormalities in the hypocretin system may be the cause of narcolepsy without cataplexy. To understand the importance of the hypocretin system, basic elements of the control of wake and sleep are presented below.

Neurologic Processes and Sleep

A number of areas in the brain are thought to be important for wakefulness and project to the cortex either directly or via the thalamus (6,50,51) (Fig. 14-1; Table 14-3). Cholinergic neurons in the lateral dorsal tegmental (LDT) and pedunculopontine tegmental (PPT) nuclei located in the dorsal pons release acetylcholine and project to the thalamus, producing thalmocortical activation. A population of these neurons is active only during wakefulness ("wake on") while another population is active during both wakefulness and REM sleep (wake on–REM on). Noradrenergic neurons releasing norepinephrine (NE) are located in the locus coeruleus (LC) situated in the caudal pons/rostral medulla. Serotononergic neurons of the dorsal raphe nuclei (DRN) in the pons release serotonin (5HT). These noradrenergic and serotonergic neurons project to the cortex and other brainstem nuclei and are most active during wakefulness, less active during NREM sleep, and minimally active during REM sleep (52,53). The ascending pathways from the LDT/PPT, LC, and DRN are

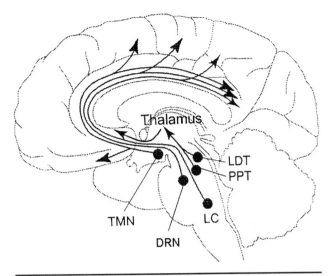

FIGURE 14-1. Major locations in the brain responsible for wakefulness. These include the noradrenergic locus coeruleus (LC), the serotonergic dorsal raphe nucleus (DRN), the cholinergic pedunculo-pontine tegmental (PPT)/lateral dorsal tegmental (LDT) nuclei, and the histaminergic tuberomammillary nucleus (TMN). (From Saper CB, et al. *Trends Neurosci.* 2001;24:726–731. With permission.)

sometimes referred to as the ascending reticular-activating system (ARAS). Histaminergic neurons in the tuberomammillary nucleus (TMN) in the ventral posterior hypothalamus also contribute to pathways maintaining wakefulness. These neurons are active during wake and inactive during NREM and REM sleep (54). Dopaminergic transmission also appears to be important for promoting wakefulness, but the site(s) of action is (are) not known with certainty. Amphetamines are believed to promote wakefulness by increasing extracellular concentrations of dopamine (55,56). The dopaminergic area in the ventral tegmental area (VTA) of the midbrain is believed to have important projections

to the LC (57,58). By altering LC activity, dopaminergic neurons or dopaminergic agonists/antagonists may have an important effect on wakefulness and sleep (59,60). The activity of dopaminergic neurons does not vary with sleep state (61). The activity of selected brain areas during wake and sleep is summarized in Table 14-4.

Non-REM sleep is produced by neurons in the preoptic area and brainstem. The ventrolateral preoptic area (VLPO) is the best-characterized non-REM sleep-producing area (62). The gamma-aminobutyric acid (GABA) containing neurons of the VLPO inhibit the wake-producing areas of the brain, including the LC, DRN, and TMN (54,62) (Fig. 14-2). The latter also send inhibitory projections to the VLPO, which has inhibitory projections to the LDT/PPT, and cholinergic activity of these areas is low during NREM sleep (Table 14-3).

Distinct LDT/PPT neurons are active during REM sleep (but not wake) and are called REM-on neurons (50,51). These cholinergic cells stimulate cholinoceptive effector cells in the pontine reticular formation (pRF). The effector neurons have ascending and descending projections that result in the manifestations of REM sleep. Some ascending projections activate the thalamus, causing cortical activation [low-voltage electroencephalogram (EEG)]. Descending pathways from the pRF (Fig. 14-3) innervate areas of the medullary reticular formation (mRF). The medullary neurons project onto spinal glycinergic interneurons. These spinal interneurons innervate spinal alpha motoneurons. The inhibitory neurotransmitter glycine decreases spinal alpha motoneuron excitability and, consequently, decreases muscle tone. The area of the reticular formation in the pons, thought critical for REM atonia, is ventral and lateral to the LC and sometimes called the peri-locus coureleus alpha area or reticularis pontis oralis (RPO) area (49,51). Areas in the medial medullary reticular formation are also part of the atonia system (63).

▶ TABLE 14-4. Neurotransmitters and Sleep

Brain Location	Neurotransmitter	Wake	NREM	REM
LDT/PPT REM On	Acetylcholine (Ach)	Off	Off	Active
LDT/PPT REM on/wake On	Acetylcholine (Ach)	Active	Off	Very active
Dorsal raphe Nucleus (DRN)	Serotonin (5HT)	Active	Reduced	Off
Locus coeruleus (LC)	Norepinephrine (NE)	Active	Reduced	Off
Tuberomammillary nucleus (TMN)	Histamine	Active	Off	Off
Ventral lateral preoptic (VLPO)	GABA	Off	Active	Reduced
Hypocretin neurons	Hypocretin	Active	Off?	Subpopulation may be active?

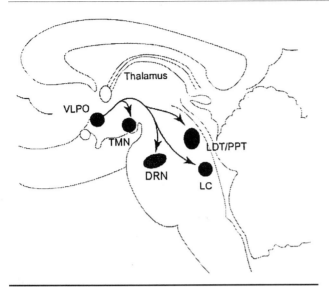

FIGURE 14-2. Neurons in the ventrolateral preoptic area (VLPO) have inhibitory projections to the locus coeruleus (LC), dorsal raphe nucleus (DRN), tubermammillary neurons (TMN), and lateral dorsal tegmental (LDT), and pedunculopontine nuclei (PPT). The inhibitory neurotransmitters of the VLPO is believed to be GABA (gamma-aminobutyric acid) and galanine. The VLPO neurons are active during NREM sleep while the LC, DRN, TMN, and LDT/PPT have reduced activity. (From Saper CB, et al. *Trends Neurosci.* 2001;24:726–731. With permission.)

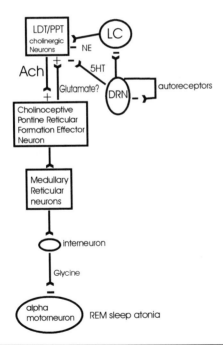

FIGURE 14-3. Schematic drawing the interactions between brain areas that generate REM sleep. The REM-on cells of the lateral dorsal tegmentum/pedunculopontine tegmentum (LDT/PPT) are active and released from inhibition by decreased activity of the locus coeruleus and dorsal raphe nucleus (DRN). Cholinoceptive effector cells of the pontine reticular formation are stimulated and generate the characteristics of REM sleep. Descending pathways stimulate cells in the medullary reticular formation. These cells activate glycinergic interneurons in the spinal cord that hyperpolarize and inhibit alpha motor neurons (atonia).

The LDT/PPT REM-on cells are inhibited by NE and 5HT from the LC and DRN, respectively. The activity of the LC and DRN is lowest during REM sleep, highest during wake, and intermediate during NREM sleep. Thus, they inhibit REM-on cells during wake and disinhibit them during REM sleep. Medications increasing serotonin or norepinephrine tend to decrease REM sleep. The REM-on LDT/PPT cells also receive reciprocal excitation from the effector pontine reticular neurons during REM sleep.

The release from inhibition of the LC and DRN and the excitation from the pontine effector neurons allows the REM-on cells of the LDT/PPT to remain active during REM sleep (Fig. 14-3).

Hypocretin System—Effects on Wake and Sleep

The hypocretins, also known as orexins, were discovered by two separate groups (4,5) almost simultaneously; hence, the two names. One group (4) called them "hypocretin 1 and 2" since the neurons synthesizing the two peptides are found only in the hypothalamus and the peptides have structural similarities with secretin. The other group (5) named the peptides "orexin A and B" based on the knowledge that the region of the hypothalamus in which the peptide-secreting cells were located was important in the regulation of feeding behaviors. *Orexis* derives from Greek and means appetite.

The hypocretin-producing cells are found in the lateral hypothalamus. The peptides hypocretin 1 and 2 (orexin A and B) are produced by cleavage of a single precursor, preprohypocretin. The hypocretin neurons have widespread axonal projections to the cortex as well as brainstem regions, important for the control of wakefulness and REM sleep (Fig. 14-4) (64). The hypocretin neuronal projections are excitatory for the TMN (65,66), DRN (67), LC (68), LDT/PPT (69), and ventral tegmental area (70). There are two hypocretin receptors (Hctr 1 and 2). Hypocretin 1 is active at both receptors. Hypocretin 2 has much higher activity at the hypocretin receptor 2 (5,71). The type of receptor present in different brain areas varies (72). For example, the LC expresses only the hypocretin receptor 1; the TMN, basal forebrain, and mesopontine dopaminergic areas express only the hypocretin receptor 2. The DRN region expresses both hypocretin receptors 1 and 2 receptors. Studies have shown that hypocretin levels in several brain centers is high during wake and low during NREM sleep (73,74). Thus, hypocretin neurons appear to be active during wake and inactive during NREM sleep. The activity of the hypocretin neurons excites wake-promoting brain centers, which allows maintenance of prolonged wakefulness. The effects of the hypocretin system on REM sleep are more complicated. Some studies have shown brain levels of hypocretin to also be high during REM sleep. This does not seem consistent with the idea that the hypocretin system suppresses REM sleep. However, various

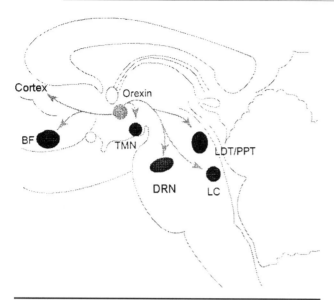

FIGURE 14-4. Projections from the hypocretin (orexin)-secreting cells of the hypothalamus are excitatory for a number of brain areas including the LDT/PPT, locus coeruleus (LC), tuberomammillary nucleus (TMN), and dorsal raphe nucleus (DRN). Other projections go to the cortex and basal forebrain (BF).). (From Saper CB, et al. *Trends Neurosci.* 2001;24:726–731. With permission.)

subpopulations of the hypocretin cells may be active during either wake or REM sleep (7). Thus, a model where certain hypocretin cells stimulate REM inhibiting sites (LC, DRN) during wake and other hypocretin cells stimulate the REM-on cells of the LDT/PPT has been proposed. Alternatively, as hypocretin promotes the REM-inhibiting activity of the DRN and LC, the net effect of the hypocretin system is to stabilize the balance between REM promoting and inhibiting areas. In summary, it has been hypothesized that the hypocretin system prevents inappropriate transitions between wakefulness and sleep, and wakefulness and REM sleep (6,7,24,71,75,76).

Hypocretins and Narcolepsy

Interest in the hypocretin system as related to narcolepsy was greatly increased after the discovery by Lin et al. that canine narcolepsy is caused by a mutation in the hypocretin receptor 2 gene (9). A very short time later, Chemelli and co-workers reported that orexin knockout mice (no ligand) had behaviors that were similar to patients with narcolepsy (10). Sporadic cases of canine narcolepsy that are hypocretin deficient have also been described. Hara et al. (11) developed a transgenic mouse that selectively loses its hypocretin neurons during development. That is, the mouse is born with functional hypocretin neurons and then loses them over time. This model may be especially relevant for human narcolepsy. Hypocretin system dysfunction could theoretically occur for several reasons including (a) destruction of hypocretin cells

(degeneration or autoimmune destruction) or their axonal pathways, (b) an inability to make functional hypocretin (abnormal gene), or (c) absent or dysfunctional hypocretin receptors (abnormal gene or antibodies against the receptor).

In humans, most cases of NwithC are hypocretin deficient. Brains of patients with narcolepsy have reduced staining for hypocretin in the hypothalamus (15,16,77). About 90% to 95% of patients with NwithC have absent CSF levels of hypocretin 1 (12,13). Mutations in hypocretin genes do not appear to be the cause of most human narcolepsy (78). To date, most evidence in humans with NwithC points to a loss of hypocretin-secreting neurons. Of note, up to 10% of patients with NwithC have normal CSF hypocretin 1 levels (12,13). Thus, other abnormalities of the hypocretin system or other mechanisms must be the cause of the syndrome in these patients.

The involvement of the hypocretin system in patients with NwithoutC is less clear. In general CSF hypocretin levels in patients with narcolepsy without cataplexy are normal (14). Some narcolepsy patients that are cataplexy negative but are positive for DQB1*0602 also have low levels. A few cases with familial narcolepsy have high CSF hypocretin levels. Therefore, other mechanisms beside hypocretin deficiency must result in the symptoms of narcolepsy. It is possible that damage to hypocretin pathways or partial loss of specific hypocretin neurons may be the etiology (24). As patients with narcolepsy but no cataplexy have sleep-onset REM sleep, it is hypothesized that hypocretin deficiency is associated with cataplexy but is not necessary for the early appearance of REM sleep. Some actually consider narcolepsy with and without cataplexy to be separate disorders. There are clinical differences (Table 14-4), although overlap certainly exists.

If loss of hypocretin neurons is the etiology of NwithC, why does this occur? Two possibilities include degeneration of these cells or destruction of the cells by autoimmune or infectious processes. The association of narcolepsy with specific HLA antigens has suggested the possibility of autoimmune mechanisms in narcolepsy. However, to date, no one has demonstrated evidence of autoimmune antibodies or abnormalities in immune function in patients with narcolepsy. However, it is possible that very localized autoimmune mechanisms may not be detected by current techniques. One study of narcoleptic brains found evidence of gliosis (77). If neurodegenerative processes cause narcolepsy, the etiology of the processes is currently unknown.

Mechanisms of Cataplexy

It is too simplistic to regard cataplexy as simply the atonia of REM sleep. While both phenomena likely have some mechanisms and pathways in common, a number of differences between REM atonia and cataplexy have been noted. While the LC neurons have nearly absent activity during both REM sleep and cataplexy, the serotonergic neurons of the DRN are active during cataplexy but are inactive during REM sleep (79,80). In addition, cataplexy, unlike REM sleep, has an emotional trigger. The pathways responsible for the effect of emotion are unknown but probably involve the limbic system. During REM sleep, many effector neurons of the pontine reticular formation are active while, during cataplexy, most are inactive. In addition, specific cells in the medial medulla that are active during cataplexy have been identified (79). Further evidence of complexity of motor control in patients with narcolepsy is the fact that some narcoleptics also have the REM behavior syndrome during which time REM atonia is absent (39).

The pharmacology of medications suppressing REM sleep and cataplexy also suggests that there are differences between the phenomena. In canine narcolepsy, medications increasing NE are more potent in preventing cataplexy than those increasing serotonin (48). Nishino suggested that selective serotonin reuptake inhibitors (SSRIs) (fluoxetine and clomipramine) may suppress cataplexy mainly via their metabolites, which are more potent blockers of NE uptake (81). However, medications increasing serotonin are potent REM sleep inhibitors. Some have suggested that cataplexy is associated with hypocretin deficiency, while the other REM-associated manifestations of narcolepsy including REM onset sleep, sleep paralysis, and hypnogogic hallucinations do not require hypocretin deficiency. Evidence for this hypothesis is the fact that most patients with NwithC have absent CSF levels of hypocretin, while NwithoutC patients have normal levels.

The mechanism by which hypocretin deficiency causes cataplexy is still controversial. Presumably, loss of facilitation of the LC and other REM-inhibiting centers is the mechanism (76). However, while reduced LC activity is thought to be an essential part of cataplexy, these neurons express only hypocretin 1 receptors. Why do hypocretin 2 receptor-deficient dogs have cataplexy (hypocretin levels and hypocretin receptor 1 are normal)? One possibility is that other brain areas, such as the dopaminergic cells of the ventral tegmental area that express hypocretin 2 receptors are excited by hypocretin and provide important excitation to the LC (59,60,82). Why does daytime sleepiness develop prior to cataplexy in most patients? One explanation might be that, as progressive hypocretin deficiency develops, earlier partial deficiency results in sleepiness followed later by severe deficiency and cataplexy.

The only neurophysiologic test that is known to be altered during cataplexy is the H reflex (18,22,28,49). This reflex relies on calf muscle (soleus) contraction monosynaptically activated following excitation of tibial sensory nerve fibers. The H reflex amplitude reflects interneuron inhibition of alpha-motoneuron excitability. Accordingly, H reflexes disappear during a cataplectic attack. Based on the knowledge that the H reflex disappears during an at-

tack, Lammers and co-workers (83) investigated the notion that the assessment of the H reflex during cataplexy-provoking situations might allow subclinical manifestations of cataplexy to be detected. However, they found that both patients and controls had similar changes in the H reflex during laughter, giving new meaning to the phrase "weak with laughter" (84). Therefore, cataplexy may simply represent an excessive activation of normal mechanisms.

DIAGNOSTIC TESTING FOR NARCOLEPSY

History

In patients with EDS, unequivocal cataplexy, and a normal neurologic examination, a clinical diagnosis of narcolepsy can be made with some certainty. In the absence of cataplexy, a nocturnal sleep study [polysomnography (PSG)] followed by a multiple sleep latency test (MSLT) is needed. Even if cataplexy is present, most physicians would still seek objective confirmation with sleep testing. Obtaining a history of unequivocal cataplexy is often difficult. This is especially true for patients with infrequent episodes. Cataplexy is difficult to induce in the clinic or in the laboratory setting (18). The diagnosis of cataplexy is based on history in the vast majority of cases.

Polysomnography

The nocturnal sleep study is used to rule out other significant sleep disorders [sleep apnea and periodic leg movements (PLMs) in sleep]. Nocturnal PSG often reveals a short sleep latency and impaired sleep quality with increased stage 1 sleep and decreased stage 3 and 4 sleep. Total sleep time may be reduced, but the amount of REM sleep is usually normal (19,20,81). NwithC patients, on average, have lower sleep efficiency, lower amounts of stage 3 and 4 sleep, more stage 1 sleep, and more awakenings than those with NwithoutC (20). PLMs in sleep are not uncommon in patients with narcolepsy (85). SOREM is defined as a REM latency <15 to 20 minutes and is present in about 40% to 50% of patients on a nocturnal sleep study (85–89). Billard and co-workers (90) found no correlation between the amount of nighttime and daytime sleep. In another study comparing narcoleptics and normal subjects using 24-hour ambulatory monitoring, Broughton and co-workers found no increase in the total amount of sleep in 24 hours, but narcoleptics had more daytime and less nighttime sleep compared to normal persons (25,26).

Multiple Sleep Latency Test and Maintenance of Wakefulness Test

The MSLT is currently the standard objective test for the assessment of sleepiness and the diagnosis of narcolepsy

(86–89). The MSLT measures the sleep latency and determines if SOREM is present in each of four or five naps spaced over the day, during which subjects are asked to lie down every 2 hours on a bed in a dark, quiet room to try to sleep. Subjects are given 20 minutes to fall asleep and are studied for 15 minutes after sleep onset to determine if REM sleep will occur. The sleep latency is defined as the time from lights out to the first epoch of any stage of sleep. Attention is paid to mean sleep latency and the occurrence of REM sleep. The standard criteria for the diagnosis of narcolepsy is a mean sleep latency of less than 5 minutes and at least two sleep-onset REM periods during five naps (87–89,91). Aldrich and co-workers (89) found that the MSLT had improved sensitivity when a sleep latency of 8 rather than 5 minutes was used as a criterion for sleep latency (89). The MSLT is usually performed following an overnight PSG that has excluded other causes of EDS, such as obstructive sleep apnea (OSA) and periodic limb movement disorder (PLMD). Ideally the night of sleep will have been deemed sufficient to exclude sleep deprivation as a cause of an abnormal MSLT. A sleep diary should document a normal amount of sleep for the preceding 1 to 2 weeks. REM-suppressing medications can alter the ability to detect REM sleep. However, acute withdrawal of REM-suppressing agents can cause a false positive test. Medications that can alter sleepiness (stimulants) or REM sleep (antidepressants) should be withdrawn at least 2 weeks before testing, if possible.

Unfortunately, the MSLT is not very sensitive or completely specific for the diagnosis of narcolepsy. Aldrich and co-workers reviewed MSLT findings in patients evaluated for daytime sleepiness (89) (Table 14-5). In some cases, a diagnosis of NwithoutC patients required a repeat MSLT. In NwithC patients a single MSLT was positive only 67% of the time. Hence, a negative MSLT does not rule out the diagnosis of narcolepsy. In patients ultimately believed to have only sleep-related breathing disorder, about 4% had a positive MSLT (89,93) (Table 14-5). It is usually recommended that sleep apnea be treated adequately before an MSLT is performed to evaluate for narcolepsy. For example, after successful treatment with continuous positive airway pressure (CPAP) for several weeks, the patient undergoes a repeat PSG and MSLT while using this therapy. If good control of sleep apnea is demonstrated during the night study, but the MSLT meets criteria for narcolepsy, one can make a diagnosis of this condition. This assumes adequate adherence to CPAP has been documented.

The maintenance of wakefulness test (MWT) was designed to test the patient's ability to stay awake. The patient is seated upright in bed in a dimly lighted room and asked to remain awake for either 20 or 40 minutes (94). The usual electroencephalography (EEG), electrooculargraphy (EOG), and electromyography (EMG) monitoring is performed to detect sleep. The test is terminated if sleep is noted or after 20/40 minutes if the patient maintains wakefulness. The test is repeated four to five times across the day and the mean sleep latency determined (20 or 40 minutes if no sleep is recorded). The MWT is frequently used to test the effect of stimulants or other treatments on daytime sleepiness. For the 40-minute test, a sleep latency of ≥ 19 minutes is considered normal. Studies of patients with narcolepsy have found the mean MWT latency is 30% to 50% of normal (6 to 9.5 minutes) (95) with many patients falling asleep in 6 minutes or less.

HLA Typing

As previously mentioned, about 90% to 100% of NwithC patients have the DQB1*0602 allele regardless of race (47). This allele is present in 25% of white Americans and 38% of African Americans without the syndrome. The percentage of NwithoutC patients that are DQB1*0602 positive is lower (40% to 60%). Because many more persons are positive for the antigen than have narcolepsy, the test is not very useful for ruling in narcolepsy. In a group of patients with possible NwithoutC, it is also not very useful in ruling out the disorder.

Cerebrospinal Fluid Hypocretin Levels

Hypocretin 1 levels of the CSF can be assayed at a few centers. At the present time, such testing is not routinely indicated but might be helpful in difficult cases. In NwithC patients, over 90% have very low or undetectable hypocretin 1 levels. In a study of patients with many neurologic diseases, only NwithC patients and a few patients with Guillain–Barré had undetectable hypocretin levels (12,13,96,97). Patients with a number of neurologic

▶ **TABLE 14-5.** Multiple Sleep Latency Test Findings in Patients Evaluated for Daytime Sleepiness[a]

	Narcolepsy with Cataplexy	Narcolepsy without Cataplexy	Sleep-Related Breathing (SDB) Disorders
$\geq$2 SOREMP (%)[b]	74	91	7
Mean sleep latency <5 min (%)	87	81	39
Both (%)	67	75	4

[a] Data from Aldrich MS. et al. *Sleep* 1997;20:620–629.
[b] SOREMP, sleep-onset REM period.
Note: In narcolepsy without cataplexy and a negative initial MSLT, a repeat MSLT established the diagnosis.

diseases had levels that were lower than normal but still detectable (97). As noted above, NwithoutC patients usually have normal levels of hypocretin (14).

Differential Diagnosis of Narcolepsy

In the presence of unequivocal cataplexy, a diagnosis of narcolepsy can be made with confidence even if other sleep disorders are present. However, if cataplexy is absent, one must consider the other disorders that can cause EDS. These include the sleep apnea syndromes, the insufficient sleep syndrome, RLS/PLMD in sleep, posttraumatic hypersomnia, inadequate sleep secondary to medical disorders or medications, depression, and idiopathic hypersomnia, and the DSPS. Idiopathic hypersomnia (IH) will be discussed at the end of the chapter.

SECONDARY NARCOLEPSY

Patients with idiopathic narcolepsy usually have a normal neurologic examination and no definite pathology on brain imaging. Secondary narcolepsy or "symptomatic narcolepsy" is defined as manifestations of the narcolepsy syndrome associated with specific brain pathology (98,99). This is usually secondary to tumors in the hypothalamic area (100), but can rarely occur from arteriovenous malformations or following cerebrovascular accidents. Hypothalamic sarcoidoses have also been reported to cause narcolepsy. Other reported associations of cerebral disease and narcolepsy include multiple sclerosis and Niemann–Pick disease type C. Daytime sleepiness following closed head injury is a well-known syndrome (101). However, most patients do not have narcolepsy. Postencephalitic narcolepsy was common in the 1920s, but no similar epidemic has been recently described.

TREATMENT OF NARCOLEPSY

Treatment of Excessive Daytime Sleepiness

The treatment of daytime sleepiness includes conservative measures (adequate sleep time, good sleep hygiene, scheduled daily naps) (102) and stimulant or alerting medications. Adequate control of daytime sleepiness can be attained in about 60% to 80% of patients. A number of medications are available to treat the daytime sleepiness of narcolepsy (95,103), including the indirect

▶ **TABLE 14-6. Medications Used to Treat Excessive Daytime Sleepiness**

Drug	Dose (Preparation)	Maximum Dose (Daily)(mg)	Half-Life (h)	Selected Side Effects
Pemoline (Cylert)	18.75–37.5 mg qd (18.75 and 37.5 mg tabs)	150	12 (adults)	Hepatitis, liver failure
Methylphenidate[a] (Ritalin)	10–30 mg bid or tid (5, 10, and 20 mg tabs)	100	2–4	Nervousness, tremulousness, headache, palpitations
Methylphenidate (SR)[b]				
Concerta	18 mg SR qam + 10–20 mg of intermediate release in afternoon (18, 27, 36, 54 mg SR tabs)	54 mg (Concerta)	8–12	Same
Medidate ER	20 mg SR qam + 10–20 mg of immediate release in afternoon (10, 20 mg SR tabs)	60 mg (Metadate)		
Dextroamphetamine[a] (Dexedrine; Dextrostat; and others)	5–30 mg qd to bid (5 and 10 mg tabs)	60	10–30	Nervousness, tremulousness, headache, palpitations
Dextroamphetamine[a] (SR preparation)	10 mg SR + 10–20 mg of immediate release in afternoon (5,10, and 15 mg SR)	60		Palpitations
Methamphetamine[a] (Desoxyn)	5–20 mg qd to bid (5 and 10 mg tabs)	60	12–34	Nervousness, tremulousness, headache, palpitations
Selegiline (Eldepryl)	20–40 mg	40	9–14	Nausea, dizziness, confusion, dry mouth[c]
Modafinil[c] (Provigil)	200–400 mg qd (100 and 200 mg tabs)	400	10–12	Headache, drug interactions, nervousness

[a]Schedule II medication.
[b]SR, slow release.
[c]Low tyramine diet required (MAOI); FDA approved for treatment of narcolepsy.

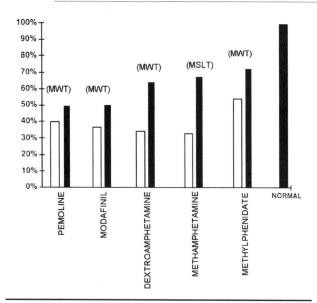

FIGURE 14-5. The relative improvements in objective sleepiness are displayed by normalizing the pre-(white bars) and post-(black bars) treatment values of the sleep latency on maintenance of MWT or MSLT as a percentage of the published normal values for the MSLT (13.4 minutes) or MWT (18.9 minutes). Note that the predrug values are not equal between the studies. The dose of drugs used was 112.5 mg for pemoline, 300 mg for modafinil, 60 mg for dextroamphetamine, 60 mg for methylphenidate, and 40–60 mg for methamphetamine. The largest changes were for methamphetamine and dextroamphetamine, whereas the highest post drug values was for methylphenidate (although baseline values were the highest for this medication). No medication came close to normalizing objective sleepiness. (From Mitler M, Aldrich MS, Koob GF, et al. ASDA standards of practice: Narcolepsy and its treatment with stimulants. *Sleep.* 1994; 17:352–371. With permission.)

sympathomimetic stimulants (which increase the synaptic availability of norepinephrine and dopamine) and a new nonstimulant, but alerting, medication, modafinil (104,105) (see Table 14-6). There are few studies directly comparing the efficacy of these medications. However, the relative objective improvement in the sleep latency after medication on the MSLT or maintenance of MWT has been compared by using the pre- and postdrug, sleep latency values as a percentage of normal for the test (95) (Fig. 14-5). Methamphetamine, dextroamphetamine, and methylphenidate appear to be the more efficacious medications. The first two may be the more potent, although methylphenidate is probably the most widely used of the three. Modafinil is moderately effective and pemoline less effective.

The wake-promoting effects of the stimulants are proportionate to their ability to inhibit the reuptake of amines (serotonin, norepinephrine, dopamine) by the dopamine transporter (DAT) (55,56). This action increases release and inhibits reuptake, with the result that synaptic levels of the neurotransmitters increase. The increase in dopamine transmission is believed to be the most important effect. The peak action of dextroamphetamine, metham-

phetamine, and methylphenidate is 1 to 3 hours from ingestion, so the medications should be taken at least 1 hour before the time of desired effectiveness. If a sleep attack has begun before medication is taken, then a nap may be the best treatment in some patients. Also note that methylphenidate has a much shorter half-life than the amphetamines and must be taken several times a day (bid to tid). Sustained action forms of the amphetamines and methylphenidate are available (Table 14-6). The side effects of these stimulants include nervousness, headache, loss of appetite, and palpitations. However, methylphenidate appears less likely to produce side effects than the amphetamine drugs. All these medications are schedule II drugs. One treatment approach is to use sustained-action forms of the medicines in the morning with short-acting forms in the afternoon or evening. Milder cases of narcolepsy often can be treated with pemoline, which has the advantage of not being a schedule II medication. However, pemoline is no longer a first-line agent because it has been associated with severe liver damage. However, some patients may tolerate pemoline better than the other stimulants. It has a long half life, and the once-a-day dosing may also increase compliance.

There are several potential problems with the use of stimulant medications. First, tolerance may develop, requiring escalating doses and leading to ineffectiveness at the highest dose. In some patients, effectiveness can be restored by a "drug holiday"—no medications for several days. Unfortunately, severe sleepiness may occur during that time. Second, the medications can increase blood pressure, although this effect is not usual in normotensive patients. Third, insomnia is a common side effect of stimulants. Thus, they should not be taken near bedtime, especially methamphetamine and dextroamphetamine, both of which have a relatively long half-life. Fourth, attacks of paranoia or hallucinations have been reported with amphetamines, but major psychiatric side effects are rare in the absence of underlying psychiatric disorders.

Modafinil is a wake-enhancing nonstimulant medication that is not a schedule II drug and can be given once daily in the morning (104–106). The mechanism of action is not known (107). The alerting effect of modafinil is not specific to patients with narcolepsy. Modafinil does not bind the receptors or uptake sites of norepinephrine, GABA, adenosine, or benzodiazepines. It binds weakly to dopamine transporter (108). Modafinil enhances the activity of many brain sites associated with wakefulness, including the tuberomammillary nucleus and hypocretin cells of the perifornical area (109). However, modafinil does not require the hypocretin system to be effective. Modafinil can reduce the extracellular GABA concentrations (110). As GABA is an inhibitory neurotransmitter, this could disinhibit a number of wake-promoting sites, such as the tuberomammillary neurons (TMN). Another possibility is that modafinil may increase dopaminergic signaling. All the brain regions activated by modafinil receive dopaminergic innervation (109). In mice lacking the DAT, modafinil does not improve wakefulness (56). At noted above, modafinil binds weakly to DAT. Newer derivatives of modafinil that do not bind DAT may help determine the importance of dopamine for the altering effects of modafinil. Enhanced dopaminergic stimulation of the LC from neurons in the ventral tegmental area has been hypothesized to be one possible mechanism of modafinil's wake-enhancing activity (59). A recent study by Gallopin and co-workers (111) found that modafinil blocks reuptake of norepinephrine (NE) by noradrenergic terminals that interface with sleep-promoting neurons of the VLPO. Higher NE at the VLPO would be wake promoting, as NE inhibits the activity of the VLPO. The mechanism by which modafinil blocks reuptake is unclear, as modafinil does not bind to NE receptors. In summary, modafinil may promote NE and dopaminergic transmission of wake-promoting centers. Continued research in this area will likely help design more effective treatments for narcolepsy.

Modafinil has been shown to be effective at decreasing subjective and objective measures of sleepiness in narcolepsy in double-blind placebo-controlled studies (104–106). There is no evidence that tolerance develops or that the drug impairs sleep quality. It has a number of advantages, including once daily dosing, low abuse potential, and the fact that it is not a schedule II medication. While generally felt to have less side effects than methylphenidate and other stimulants, this has never been proved in a randomized comparison. The general impression of most clinicians is that it may be less effective than methylphenidate (95). The major side effects of modafinil include headache, nausea, and nervousness. Headache can be minimized by a slow increase in dose. Modafinil is metabolized in the liver by the P450 system. Hence, a number of drug interactions are possible. The main interaction of significance is that certain oral contraceptives may be less effective after modafinil is started. The drug is fairly expensive (thirty 200-mg tablets are about $150). Unlike the indirect sympathomimetics, withdrawal of modafinil does not result in a rebound of REM and slow-wave sleep (SWS). Patients can be switched from stimulants to modafinil without a washout period (112). However, as stimulant medications have some anticataplectic action, patients changed from methylphenidate to modafinil may require the addition of specific medications for cataplexy (113).

Another treatment alternative that can be tried in patients not tolerating stimulants is the irreversible MAO type-B inhibitor selegiline. At doses of 10 to 40 mg/day, this drug has been shown to improve narcoleptic symptoms (114). Unfortunately, at doses over 20 mg/day, it loses its MAO B inhibitor selectivity, and a low tyramine diet is indicated to avoid the risk of hypertensive reactions. The drug also has anticataplectic activity in addition to its alerting ability. Patients who experience intolerable side effects with other agents may benefit from this medication as long as they are willing to adhere to a low tyramine diet.

Improving nocturnal sleep and treatment of concurrent sleep disorders is also important for improving daytime sleepiness. Benzodiazepine receptor agonists may improve sleep quality in some patients. If the RLS/PLMs are significantly impairing sleep, specific treatment for these problems may be helpful. The combination of narcolepsy and OSA is also not uncommon. Adequate treatment of OSA with nasal CPAP or other therapies is essential. Good sleep hygiene with a regular sleep schedule and adequate sleep is essential for narcolepsy patients. Some find short, scheduled naps to also be beneficial.

There is now evidence that the chronic use of sodium oxybate may improve daytime sleepiness by consolidating nocturnal sleep. This is discussed in the next section.

Treatment of Cataplexy

In some patients with NwithC, episodes are so uncommon or mild that treatment is not needed. In others, they constitute an important problem for patients. The medications that are useful for the treatment of cataplexy also suppress the other associated symptoms of narcolepsy, including sleep paralysis and hypnogogic hallucinations (Table 14-7).

The classic medications useful in treating cataplexy have a common property of suppressing REM sleep. In the canine form of narcolepsy, drugs increasing norepinephrine are the most efficacious (48). The tricyclic antidepressants that have been used include protriptyline, desipramine, clomipramine, and imipramine. They are commonly effective in doses less than those used for antidepressant action. Protriptyline, desipramine, and imipramine block reuptake of norepinephrine, while clomipramine is a more potent blocker of serotonin reuptake. The major problem with these medications is their anticholinergic side effects. Recently, SSRIs (fluoxetine) have also been found useful in treating cataplexy (115). They are used in typical antidepressant doses, and their effect may be more delayed than the tricyclic medications. However, as they generally are better tolerated and safer in overdose, they are widely used. Venlafaxine (Effexor), a medication that blocks the reuptake of both serotonin and norepinephrine, appears to be particularly useful in treating cataplexy and is well tolerated (113). Carbamazepine has also been reported to decrease cataplexy, although it is rarely used (116). It should be pointed out that none of the above medications are FDA approved for cataplexy treatment. Abrupt cessation of anticataplectic medications can markedly worsen cataplexy and result in nearly continuous attacks (status cataplecticus). There have also been reports of exacerbation of cataplexy by the alpha$_1$ blocker prazosin (117).

Unfortunately, a portion of patients with narcolepsy and symptomatic cataplexy do not respond well to the traditional medications or are unable to tolerate the side effects. Sodium oxybate (gamma-hydroxybutyrate) has

▶ **TABLE 14-7. Medication Used to Treat Cataplexy**[a]

Drug (Brand Name)	Dose (range)	Maximum Dose (daily)	Half Life (h)	Selected Side Effects
Tricyclic antidepressants				
Protriptyline (Vivactil)	5–10 mg bid or tid (5, 10 and 20 mg tabs)	30 mg	67–89	Dry mouth, urinary hesitancy, constipation
Clomipramine (Anafranil)	Start 50 mg qhs (75–125 mg)	250 mg	32	Dry mouth, sweating drowsiness
Imipramine (Tofranil)	Start 50 mg qhs (75–125 mg)	300 mg	6–20	Dry mouth, constipation drowsiness
Selective SRIs				
Fluoxetine (Prozac)	Start 20 mg qam (20–60 mg)	80 mg	48–216	Headache, dry mouth, sexual dysfunction
Nonselective SRIs[b]				
Venlafaxine (Effexor)	Start 37.5 mg bid 75–100 mg bid for XR[d] form start 37.5 mg qam (75–150 mg qam)	375 mg 225 mg–XR	3–7	Nausea, dry mouth, headache, blood pressure elevation, insomnia, nervousness
Other medications				
Selegiline (Eldepryl)	20–40 mg	40 mg	9–14	Nausea, dizziness, confusion, dry mouth
Sodium[c] oxybate (Xyrem)	Starting dose 2.25 mg qhs repeated in 2.5–4 h (see text)	9 gm daily in divided doses	0.5–1	Nausea, headache, confusion, enuresis sleepwalking

[a] Also effective for sleep paralysis and hypnogogic hallucinations.
[b] SRI, serotonin reuptake inhibitor.
[c] FDA approved for treatment of cataplexy.
[d] XR, extended release.

been recently approved for the treatment of cataplexy in the United States (118). The drug has been used in Europe for some time. Gamma-hydroxybutyrate (GHB) is a naturally occurring metabolite of GABA and binds strongly to GHB-specific receptors and weakly to GABA-$_B$ receptors. The method by which the medication decreases cataplexy is unknown. It may decrease daytime sleepiness by improving nocturnal sleep quality. Unfortunately, the illicit use of GHB (the date-rape drug) has complicated its use as a treatment for cataplexy. GHB is tasteless and can cause rapid sedation and amnesia. In sufficient doses, respiratory depression and death can occur (119,120). Chronic abusers of the medication can also experience a withdrawal syndrome (insomnia, anxiety, and delirium). However, a recent large double-blind placebo-controlled study showed that sodium oxybate is effective and reasonably safe as a treatment for cataplexy (118). In this study, the Epworth Sleepiness Scale (ESS) (subjective) and nocturnal awakenings were also decreased on treatment. Thus, sodium oxybate may have other long-term benefits in narcolepsy patients, such as improved nocturnal sleep quality and reduced daytime sleepiness. No rebound syndrome was noted in clinical trials. Other studies have suggested that GHB may increase the amount of SWS (121).

Sodium oxybate (Xyrem) is currently available from a single central pharmacy and is the only medication approved by the FDA for the treatment of cataplexy. The medication is a liquid (500 mg/ml) and, because of a short half-life, must be taken at bedtime and repeated 2.5 to 4 hours later (the patient typically sets an alarm clock). The recommended starting daily dose is 4.5 gm (two equal 2.25 grams doses). The effect of the drug is so rapid that after ingesting each dose of the medication, patients should lie down and remain in bed. Each dose of medication is diluted with 60 ml of water in the child-resistant dosing cups. Both doses should be prepared before going to bed. The dose in the middle of the night should be taken while sitting in bed. Food can reduce the bioavailability of sodium oxybate. Patients should eat well several hours before bedtime and then not eat for several hours before taking the medication. The starting dose can be increased to a maximum of 9 gm per day with increments of 1.5 gm per day (0.75 gm per dose) every 2 weeks. This time between dose increments is recommended to assess clinical response (a higher dose may not be needed) and to minimize side effects. The usual effective dose is 6 to 9 gm daily. The most frequent reasons for discontinuance are nausea and headache. Dizziness, confusion, sleep walking, urinary incontinence, and vomiting may occur. Problems with enuresis may be approached by a temporary reduction in dose.

Psychosocial Issues

While narcolepsy is a life-long condition, the majority of patients with the disorder can enjoy a near-normal lifestyle with adequate medication and psychosocial support systems. If not properly diagnosed and treated, narcolepsy has a devastating impact on the life of the affected individual, causing social, educational, vocational, marital, psychological, and financial difficulties.

IDIOPATHIC HYPERSOMNIA

IH remains a diagnosis of exclusion (19), with most series consisting of a heterogeneous group of patients. The disorder, if strictly defined, is rare and less common than narcolepsy. Bassetti and Aldrich estimated less than 1% of 4,000 patients seen at a university sleep center had IH (122). The prevalence has ranged anywhere from 77% to 11% of that of narcolepsy (123). The lower percentage is more typical of recent studies. Some patients historically given a diagnosis of IH were later found to have the upper-airway resistance syndrome/mild OSA when more sophisticated monitoring techniques, such as esophageal pressure monitoring, were applied. Atypical depression (hypersomnia instead of depression), the insufficient sleep syndrome, medication side effects, narcolepsy (with delayed cataplexy), and medical and neurologic disease must be excluded. IH usually presents in adolescence or early adulthood. As originally described by Roth and co-workers (124), IH consisted of hypersomnia with sleep drunkenness (difficulty waking up) and deep and prolonged sleep. Later, IH was divided into a monosymptomatic form (excessive sleepiness) similar to narcolepsy or a polysymptomatic form consisting of daytime sleepiness, a long nocturnal sleep period, sleep drunkenness (confused and slow awakening), and typically long unrefreshing naps. The polysymptomatic form may also have "neurovegetative" symptoms of orthostatic hypotension, syncope, Raynaud's phenomenon, or frequent headaches. Sleep paralysis and hypnogogic hallucinations are common in both forms of IH, but cataplexy is absent. A considerable amount of symptom overlap exists between IH, NwithC, and NwithoutC (20) (Table 14-3). Bassetti and Aldrich (122) divided a group of 42 patients with IH into three groups: classic IH (sleep attacks not irresistible, long nocturnal sleep, sleep drunkeneness, unrefreshing naps, duration of involuntary naps >1 hr, neurovegetative symptoms), narcolpetic IH (like narcolepsy without cataplexy or REM onsets), and mixed form (a few classic symptoms). The International Classification of Sleep Disorders (ICSD) (125) defines IH as "a disorder of presumed central nervous system cause that is associated with a normal or prolonged major sleep episode and excessive daytime sleepiness consisting of prolonged (1–2 hours) sleep episodes (naps) of NREM sleep." The etiology of IH is unknown and may well consist of several causes. The CSF hypocretin levels are normal (13).

PSG in IH usually shows a short sleep latency with total sleep time that is either normal or increased (12 hours or more). The nocturnal REM latency is not shortened and the amount of REM sleep is usually normal (122,125,126). Some have suggested that 24-hour sleep monitoring is useful to document the prolonged nocturnal sleep episode and increased sleep per 24 hours. The MSLT shows excessive sleepiness (mean sleep latency <10 minutes), but, in most series, the mean is longer than in narcolepsy. Less than 2 REM periods are found in five naps (19,125,126). The daytime sleepiness does not respond to an increase in nocturnal sleep time (if previously normal or slightly short). A sleep diary or clinical history should eliminate the possibility of the insufficient sleep syndrome.

When initially described, the sleepiness of IH was said to respond poorly to stimulants. However, later series have shown that about 75% of patients will improve on traditional stimulants (122) and modafinil (127).

FUTURE DIRECTIONS IN THE TREATMENT OF NARCOLEPSY AND RELATED DISORDERS

Future research will hopefully address the reason(s) for the loss of hypocretin cells in patients with NwithC and the etiology of the syndrome in NwithoutC patients (normal CSF hypocretin). More information about the involvement of the dopaminergic system in the etiology and treatment of narcolepsy will assist in understanding why hypocretin receptor 2 deficiency causes canine narcolepsy despite normal hypocretin levels and an intact hypocretin receptor 1. Recently, there have been conflicting results from two groups studying the systemic administration of hypocretin 1 to treat sleepiness and cataplexy in canine narcolepsy (128,129). One group showed a benefit, whereas the other failed to confirm the earlier results. The different findings could be related to experimental techniques or the biologic activity of the hypocretin 1 peptide utilized. Hopefully, understanding the basic mechanisms of narcolepsy will result in improved diagnostic techniques and more effective treatments.

REFERENCES

1. Broughton R, Mullington J. Chronobiological aspects of narcolepsy. *Sleep.* 1994;17(8 Suppl.):S35–44.
2. Yoss RE, Daly DD. Criteria for the diagnosis of the narcoleptic syndrome. *Proc Staff Meet Mayo Clin.* 1957;32:320–328.
3. Vogel G. Studies in the psychophysiology of dreams, III: the dream of narcolepsy. *Arch Gen Psych.* 1960;3:421–428.
4. deLecea L. The hypocretins: hypothalamus-specific peptides with neuroexcitatory activity. *Proc. Natl. Acad Sci USA.* 1998;95:322–327.
5. Sakurai T. Orexins and orexin receptors: a family of hypothalamic neuropeptides and G protein coupled receptors that regulate feeding behavior. *Cell.* 1998;92:573–585.
6. Saper CB, Chou TC, Scammell TE. The sleep switch: hypothalamic control of sleep and wakefulness. *Trends Neurosci.* 2001;24:726–731.

7. Overeem S, Scammell TE, Lammers GJ. Hypocretin/orexin and sleep: implications for the pathophysiology and diagnosis of narcolepsy. *Curr Opin Neurol.* 2002;15:739–745.
8. Nishino S. The hypocretin/orexin system in health and disease. *Biol Psych.* 2003;54:87–95.
9. Lin L, Kadotan H, Rogers W, et al. The sleep disorder canine narcolepsy is caused by a mutation in the hypocretin (orexin) receptor 2 gene. *Cell.* 1999;98:365–376.
10. Chemelli RM, Willie JT, Sinton C, et al. Narcolepsy in orexin knockout mice: molecular genetics and sleep regulation. *Cell.* 1999;98:437–451.
11. Hara J, Beuckman CT, Nambu T, et al. Genetic ablation of orexin neurons in mice results in narcolepsy, hypophasia, and obesity. *Neuron.* 2001;30:345–354.
12. Ripley BN, Overeem S, Fujiki N, et al. CSF hypocretin/orexin levels in narcolepsy and other neurological conditions. *Neurology.* 2001;57:2253–2258.
13. Mignot E, Lammers GJ, Ripley MS, et al. The role of cerebrospinal fluid hypocretin measurement in the diagnosis of narcolepsy and other hypersomnias. *Arch Neurol.* 2002;59:1553–1562.
14. Krahn Le, Pankratz S, Oliver L, et al. Hypocretin (orexin) levels in cerebrospinal fluid of patents with narcolepsy: relationship to cataplexy and HLADQB1*0602 status. *Sleep.* 2003;25:733–736.
15. Peyron C, Faraco J, Rogers W, et al. A mutation in a case of early onset narcolepsy and a generalized absense of hypocretin peptides in human narcoleptic brains. *Natur Med.* 2000;6:991–997.
16. Thannickal T, Moore RY, Nienbus R, et al. Reduced number of hypocretin neurons in human narcolepsy. *Neuron.* 2000;27:469–474.
17. Okun ML, Lin L, Pelin Z, et al. Clinical aspects of narcolepsy-cataplexy across ethnic groups. *Sleep.* 2002;25:27–35.
18. Guilleminault C. Cataplexy. In: Guilleminault C, Dement WC, Passouant P, eds. *Narcolepsy.* New York: Spectrum, 1976:125–144.
19. Aldrich MS. Narcolepsy. *Neurology.* 1992;42(Suppl. 6):34–43.
20. Aldrich MS. The clinical spectrum of narcolepsy and idiopathic hypersomnia. *Neurology.* 1996;46:393–401.
21. Guilleminault C, Wilson RA, Dement WC. A study on cataplexy. *Arch Neurol.* 1974;31:255–261.
22. Guilleminault C, Gelb M. Clinical aspects and features of cataplexy. *Advan Neurol.* 1995;67:65–77.
23. Overeem S, Mignot E, van Dijk JG, et al. Narcolepsy: clinical features, new pathophysiologic insights, and future perspectives. *J Clin Neurophysiol.* 2001;18:78–105.
24. Scammel TE. The Neurobiology, diagnosis, and treatment of narcolepsy. *Ann Neurol.* 2003;53:154–166.
25. Broughton R, Dunham W, Newman J, et al. Ambulatory 24 hour sleep–wake monitoring in narcolepsy-cataplexy compared to matched controls. *Electroencephalogr Clin Neurophysiol.* 1988;70:473–481.
26. Broughton R, Krupa S, Boucher B, Rivers M, Mullington J. Impaired circadian waking arousal in narcolepsy-cataplexy. *Sleep Res. Online.* 1998;1:159–165.
27. Anic-Labat S, Guilleminault C, Kraemer HC, et al. Validation of a cataplexy questionnaire in 983 sleep-disorders patients. *Sleep.* 1999;22:77–87.
28. Guilleminault C, Heinzer R, Mignot E, et al. Investigations into the neurologic basis of narcolepsy. *Neurology.* 1998;50(Suppl. 1):S8–S15.
29. Nelson GB, Hahn JS. Stimulus-induced drop episodes in Coffin–Lowry syndrome. *Pediatrics.* 2003;111:197–202.
30. Fryssira H, Kountoupi S, Delaunoy JP, et al. A female with Coffin–Lowry syndrome and "cataplexy." *Genet Counsel.* 2002;13:405–409.
31. Manni R, Politini L, Nobili L, et al. Hypersomnia in the Prader Willi syndrome: clinical–electrophysiological features and underlying factors. *Clin Neurophys.* 2001;112:800–805.
32. Kanbayashi T, Abe M, Fujimoto S, et al. Hypocretin deficiency in Niemann-Pick type C with cataplexy. *Neuropediatrics.* 2003;34:52–53.
33. Vanier MT, Suzuki K. Recent advances in elucidating Niemann-Pick C disease. *Brain Pathol.* 1998;8:163–174.
34. Vankova J, Stepanov I, Jech R, et al. Sleep disturbancees and hypocretin deficiency in Niemann-Pick disease type C. *Sleep.* 2003;26:427–430.
35. Tyagi A, Harrington H. Cataplexy in association with Moebius syndrome. *J Neurol.* 2003;250:110–111.
36. Vossler DG, Wyler AR, Wilkus RJ, et al. Cataplexy and monoamine oxidase deficiency in Norrie disease. *Neurology.* 1996;46:1258–1261.
37. Chen ZY, Denney RM, Breakfield XO. Norrie disease and MAO genes: Nearest neighbours. *Hum Mol Genet.* 1995;4:1729–1737.
38. Portala K, Westermark K, Ekselius L, et al. Sleep in patients with treated Wilson's disease. A questionnaire study. *Nord J Psych.* 2002;56:291–297.
39. Schenck CH, Mahowald MW. Motor dyscontrol in narcolepsy: rapid-eye-movement (REM) sleep without atonia and REM sleep behavior disorder. *Ann Neurols.* 1992;9:63–67.
40. Schuld A, Hebebrand J, Geller F, et al. Increased body mass index in patients with narcolepsy. *Lancet.* 200;355:1274–1275.
41. Chokroverty S. Sleep apnea in narcolepsy. *Sleep.* 1986;9:250–253.
42. Hublin C, Partinen M, Kaprio J, et al. Epidemiology of narcolepsy. *Sleep.* 1994;17(Suppl.):S7–12.
43. Silber MH, Krahn LE, Olson EJ, et al. The epidemiology of narcolepsy in Olmstead County, Minnesota: a population based study. *Sleep.* 2002;25:197–202.
44. Mignot E. Genetic and familial aspects of narcolepsy. *Neurology.* 1998;50(Suppl. 1):S16–22.
45. Westphal C. Eigenthü mliche mit Einschlä fen verbundene Anfä lle. *Arch Psych.* 1877;7:631–635.
46. Billiard M, Pasquie-Magnetto V, Heckman M, et al. Family studies in narcolepsy. *Sleep.* 1994;17 (Suppl.):S54–S59.
47. Mignot E, Hayduk R, Black J, et al. HLA DQB1*0602 is associated with cataplexy in 509 narcoleptic patients. *Sleep.* 1997;20:1012–1020.
48. Nishino S, Mignot E. Pharmacological aspects of human and canine narcolepsy. *Prog. Neurobiol.* 1997;52:27–78.
49. Hishikawa Y, Shimizu T. Physiology of REM sleep, cataplexy, and sleep paralysis. In: Fahn S, Hallett M, Luders HO, Marsden CD, eds. *Negative motor phenomena.* Philadelphia: Lippincott-Raven, 1995:245–271.
50. McCarley RW. Sleep Neurophysiology: basic mechanisms underlying control of wakefulness and sleep. In Chokroverty S. *Sleep disorders medicine.* 2nd ed. Boston: Butterworth Heinemann, 1999: 21–50.
51. Siegel JM. Brainstem mechanisms generating REM sleep. In Kryger M, Roth T, Dement WC, ed. *Principles and practice of sleep medicine.* 3rd ed. Philadelphiia: WB Saunders, 2000;112–133.
52. Aston-Jones G, Chiang C, Alexinsky T. Discharge of noradrenergic locus coeruleus. Neurons in behaving rats and monkeys suggests a role in vigilance. *Progr Brain Res.* 1991;88:501–520.
53. McGinty D, Harper R. Dorsal. Dorsal raphe neurons: depression of firing rate during sleep in cats. *Brain Res.* 1976;101:569–575.
54. Sherin JE, Elmquist JK, Torrealba F, et al. Innervation of histaminergic tuberomammillary neurons by GABAergic and galaniergic neurons in the ventrolateral preoptic nucleus of the rat. *J Neurosci.* 1998;18:4705–4721.
55. Nishino S, Mao J, Sampathkmaran R, et al. Increased dopaminergic transmission mediates the wake-promoting effects of CNS stimulants. *Sleep Res Online.* 1998;1:49–61.
56. Wisor JP, Nishino S, Sora I, et al. Dopaminergic role in stimulant-induced wakefulness. *J Neurosci.* 2001;21:1787–1794.
57. Ornstein K, et al. Biochemical and radioautographic evidence for dopaminergic afferents of the locus coeruleus originating in the ventral tegmental area. *J Neural Transmission.* 1987;70:183–191.
58. Maeda T, Kitahama K, Geffard M. Dopaminergic innervation of the rat locus coeruleus: a light and electron microscopic immunohistochemical study. *Microsc Res Techn.* 1994;29:211–218.
59. Keating GL, Rye DB. Where you least expect it: dopamine in the pons and modulation of sleep and REM sleep. *Sleep.* 2003;26:788–789.
60. Crochet S, Sakai K. Dopaminergic modulation of behavioral states in mesopontine tegmentum: a reverse microdialysis study in freely moving cats. *Sleep.* 2003;26:801–806.
61. Shouse MN, et al. Monamines and sleep: microdialysis findings in the pons and amygdala. *Brain Res.* 2000;860:181–189.
62. Szymusiak R, Alam N, Steininger TL, et al. Sleep-waking discharge patterns of venterolateral preoptic/anterior hypothalamic neurons in rats. *Brain Res.* 1998:803:178–188.

63. Lai YY, Siegel JM. Medullary regions mediating atonia. *J Neurosci.* 1988;8:4790–4796.
64. Peyron C, Tighe DK, van den Pol AN, et al. Neurons containing hypocretin (orexin) project to multiple neuronal systems. *J Neurosci.* 1998;18:9996–10015.
65. Erikson KS, Sergeeva O, Brown RE, et al. Orexin/hypocretin-1 excites the histaminergic neurons of the tuberomammillary nucleus. *J Neurosci.* 2001;21:9273–9279.
66. Bayer L, Eggermann E, Serafin M, et al. Orexins (hypocretins) directly excite tuberomammillary neurons. *Eur J Neurosci.* 2001;14:1571–1575.
67. Brown RE, Sergeeva O, Eriksson KS, et al. Orexin A excites serotonergic neurons in the dorsal raphe nucleus of the rat. *Neuropharmacology.* 2001;40:457–459.
68. Hagan J. Orexin A activates locus coeruleus cell firing and increases arousal in the rat. *Proc Natl. Acad Sci USA.* 1999;96:10911–10916.
69. Burlet S, Tyler CJ, Leonard CS. Direct and indirect excitation of laterodorsal tegmental neurons by hypocretin/orexin peptides. Implications for wakefulness and narcolepsy. *J Neurosci.* 2002;22:2862–2872.
70. Korokova T, Sergeeva OA, Eriksson KS, et al. Excitation of ventral tegmental domaminergic and non-dopaminergic neurons by orexin/hypocretins. *J Neurosci.* 2003;23:7–11.
71. Taheri S, Zeitzer JM, Mignot EM. The role of hypocretins (orexins) in sleep regulation and narcolepsy. *Annu Rev Neurosci.* 2002;25:283–313.
72. Marcus JN, Aschkenasi CJ, Lee CE, et al. Differential expression of orexin receptors 1 and 2 in the rat brain. *J Comp Neurol.* 2001;435:6–25.
73. Kiyaashchenko LI, Mileykoveskiy BY, Maidment N, et al. Release of hypocretin (orexin) during waking and sleep states. *J Neurosci.* 2002;22:5282–5286.
74. Alam MN, Gong H, Alam T. et al. Sleep-waking discharge pattern of neurons recorded in the rat periformical lateral hypothalamic area. *J Physiol.* 2002;538:19–631.
75. Krahn LE, Black JL, Silber MH. Narcolepsy: new understanding of irresistible sleep. *Mayo Clin Proc.* 2001;76:185–194.
76. Kilduff TS, Peyron C. The hypocretin/orexin ligand-receptor system: implications for sleep and sleep disorders. *Trends Neurosci.* 2000;23:359–365.
77. Thannickal TC, Siegel JM, Nienhuis R, et al. Pattern of hypocretin (orexin) soma and axon loss, and gliosis, in human narcolepsy. *Brain Pathol.* 2003;13:340–351.
78. Hungs M, Lin L, Okun M, et al. Polymorphisms in the vicinity of hypocretin/orexin are not associated with human narcolepsy. *Neurology.* 2001;57:1893–1895.
79. Siegel JM, Nienhuis R, Fahringer HM, et al. Neuronal activity in narcolepsy: identification of cataplexy related cells in the medial medulla. *Science.* 1991;252:1315–1318.
80. Wu MF, Gulyani SA, Yau E, et al. Locus coeruleus neurons: cessation of activity during cataplexy. *Neuroscience.* 1999;91:1389–1399.
81. Nishino S, Arrigoni J, Shelton J, et al. Desmethyl metabolites of serotonergic uptake inhibitors are more potent for suppressing canine cataplexy than their parent compounds. *Sleep.* 1993;16:707–712.
82. Reid MS, Tafti M, Nishino S, et al. Local administration of dopaminergic drugs into the ventral tegmental area modulates cataplexy in the narcoleptic canine. *Brain Res.* 1996;133:83–100.
83. Lammers GJ, Overeem S, Tijssen MA, et al. Effects of startle and laughter in cataplectic subjects: a neurophysiological study between attacks. *Clin Neurophysiol.* 2000;111:1276–1281.
84. Overeem S, Lammers GJ, van Dijk JG. Weak with laughter. *Lancet.* 1999;4;354(9181):838.
85. Mosko SS, Shampain DS, Sassin JF. Nocturnal REM latency and sleep disturbance in narcolepsy. *Sleep.* 1984;7:115–125.
86. Richardson GS, Carskadon MA, Flagg W. Excessive daytime sleepiness in man: multiple sleep latency measurements in narcoleptic and control subjects. *Electroencephalogr Clin Neurophysiol.* 1978;45:621–627.
87. Mitler MM, Van den Hoed J, Carskadon MA, et al. REM sleep episodes during the multiple sleep latency test in narcoleptic patients. *Electroencephalogr Clin Neurophysiol.* 1979;46:479–481.
88. American Sleep Disorders Association. *International classification of sleep disorders: Diagnostic and coding manual.* Lawrence, KS: Allen Press, 1990:65–71.
89. Aldrich MS, Chervin RD, Malow BA. Value of the multiple sleep latency test for the diagnosis of narcolepsy. *Sleep.* 1997;20:620–629.
90. Billard M, Quero-Salva M, De Koninck J, et al. Daytime sleep characteristics and their relationships with night sleep in the narcoleptic patient. *Sleep.* 1986;9:167–174.
91. Carskadon MA. Guidelines for the multiple sleep latency test. *Sleep.* 1986;9:519–524.
92. Standards of Practice Committee, American Sleep Disorders Association. The clinical use of the multiple sleep latency test. *Sleep.* 1992;15:268–276.
93. Chervin RD, Aldrich MS. Sleep onset REM periods during multiple sleep latency tests in patients evaluated for sleep apnea. *Amer J Respir Crit Care Med.* 2000;161:426.
94. Sangal RB, Thomas L, Mitler MM. Maintenance of wakefulness test and multiple sleep latency test: measurements of different abilities in patients with sleep disorders. *Chest.* 1992;101:898–902.
95. Mitler M, Aldrich MS, Koob GF, et al. ASDA standards of practice: narcolepsy and its treatment with stimulants. *Sleep.* 1994;17:352–371.
96. Mignot E, Chen W, Black J. On the value of measuring CSF hypocretin-1 in diagnosing narcolepsy. *Sleep.* 2003;26:646–649.
97. Nishino S, Kanbayashi T, Fujiki N, et al. CSF hypocretin levels in Guillain-Barré syndrome and other inflammatory neuropathies. *Neurology.* 2003;61:823–825.
98. Malik S, Boeve BF, Krahn LE, et al. Narcolepsy associated with other central nervous system disorders. *Neurology.* 2001;57:539–541.
99. Autret A, Lucas B, Henry-Lebras F, de Toffol B. Symptomatic narcolepsies. *Sleep.* 1996;17:S21–S24.
100. Aldrich MS, Naylor MW. Narcolepsy associated with lesions of the diecephalon. *Neurology.* 1989;39:1505–1508.
101. Guilleminault C, Van den Hoed J, Miles L. Posttraumatic excessive daytime sleepiness. *Neurology.* 1983;33:1584–1589.
102. Mullington J, Broughton R. Scheduled naps in the management of daytime sleepiness in narcolepsy-cataplexy. *Sleep.* 1993:16:444–456.
103. Littner M, Johnson SF, McCall MV, et al. Standard of Practice Committee of the AASM. Practice Parameters for the treatment of narcolepsy: an update 2000. *Sleep.* 2001;24:451–466.
104. U.S. Modafinil in Narcolepsy Study Group. Randomized trial of modafinil for the treatment of pathological somnolence in narcolepsy. *Ann Neurol.* 1998;43:88–97.
105. U.S. Modafinil in Narcolepsy Study Group. Randomized trial of modafinil as a treatment for the excessive daytime somnolence of narcolepsy. *Neurology.* 2000;53:1166–1175.
106. Mitler M, Harsch J, Hirshkowitz M, et al. Long-term efficacy and safety of modafinil for the treatment of excessive daytime sleepiness associated with narcolepsy. *Sleep.* 1994;17:352–371.
107. Saper CB, Scammell TE. Modafinil: a drug in search of a mechanism. *Sleep.* 2004;27:11–12.
108. Mignot E, Nishino S, Guilleminault C, et al. Modafinil binds to the dopamine uptake carrier site with low affinity. *Sleep.* 1994;17:436–437.
109. Scammell TE, Estabrooke IV, McCarthy MT, et al. Hypothalamic arousal regions are activated during modafinil-induced wakefulness. *J Neurosci.* 2000;20:8620–8628.
110. Ferraro L, Tanganellis S, O'Connor WT, et al. The vigilance promoting drug modafinil decreases GABA release in the medial preoptic area and in the posterior hypothalamus of the awake rat: possible involvement of the serotonergic 5-HT3 receptor. *Neurosci Lett.* 1996;220:5–8.
111. Gallopin T, Luppi PH, Rambert FA, et al. Effect of wake-promoting agent modafinil on sleep-promoting neurons from the ventrolateral preoptic nucleus: an in vitro pharmacologic study. *Sleep.* 2004;27:19–25.
112. Thorpy MJ, Schwartz JR, Kovacevi-Ristanovic R, et al. Initiating treatment with modafinil for control of excessive daytime sleepiness in patients switching from methylphenidate: an open label study assessing three strategies. *Psychopharmacology.* 2003;167:380–385.
113. Guilleminault C, Aftab FA, Karadeniz D, et al. Problems associated with switch to modafinil—A novel alerting agent in narcolepsy. *Eur J Neurol.* 2000;7:381–384.
114. Mayer G, Ewert-Meier K, Hephata K. Selegiline hydrochloride treatment in narcolepsy: a double-blind, placebo-controlled study. *Clin Neupharmcol.* 1995;18:306–319.

115. Frey J, Darbonne C: Fluoxetine suppresses human cataplexy. *Neurology.* 1994;44:707–709.

116. Vaughn BV, D'Cruz OF: Carbamazepine as a treatment for cataplexy. *Sleep.* 1996;19:101–103.

117. Aldrich M, Rogers AE. Exacerbation of human cataplexy by prazosin. *Sleep.* 1989;12:254–256.

118. The U.S. Xyrem Multicenter Study Group. A randomized, double-blind, placebo-controlled multicenter trial comparing the effects of three doses of orally administered sodium oxybate with placebo for the treatment of narcolepsy (cataplexy). *Sleep.* 2003;25:42–49.

119. Zvosec DL, Smith SW, McCutcheon JR, et al. Adverse events including death, associated with the use of 1,4-butanediol. *N Engl J Med.* 2001;344:87–94.

120. Li J, Stokes SA, Woeckener A. A tale of novel intoxication: severe cases of gamma-hydroxybutyric acid overdose. *Ann Emerg Med.* 1998;723–728.

121. Lammers GJ, Arends J, Declerck AC, et al. Gamma-hydroxybutyrate and narcolepsy: a double-blind study. *Sleep.* 1993;16:216–220.

122. Bassetti C, Aldrich MS. Idiopathic hypersomnia. *Brain.* 1997;120:1423–1435.

123. Billiard M. Idiopathic hypersomnia. *Neurol Clin.* 1996;14:573–582.

124. Roth B, Nevsimalova S, Rechtschaffen A. Hypersomnia with sleep "drunkenness." *Arch Gen Psych.* 1972:26:456–462.

125. American Sleep Disorders Association. *International classification of sleep disorders: diagnostic and coding manual.* Rochester, Minnesota: American Sleep Disorders Association, 1997:46–49.

126. Baker TL, Guilleminault G, Nino-Murcia G, et al. Comparative polysomnographic study of narcolepsy and idiopathic central nervous system hypersomnia. *Sleep.* 1986;9:232–242.

127. Bastujii H, Jouvet M. Successful treatment of idiopathic hypersomnia and narcolepsy with modafinil. *Prog Neuropsychopharmacol Biol Psych.* 1988;12:695–700.

128. John J, Wu MF, Siegel JM. Systemic administration of hypocretin-1 reduces cataplexy and normalizes sleep and waking durations in narcoleptic dogs. *Sleep Res Online.* 2000;3:23–28.

129. Fujiki N, Yoshida Y, Ripley B, et al. Effects of IV and ICV hypocretin-1 (orexin A) in hypocretin receptor–2 gene mutated narcoleptic dogs and IV hypocretin-1 replacement therapy in a hypocreting-ligand-deficient narcoleptic dog. *Sleep.* 2003;26:953–959.

Chapter 15

Restless Legs Syndrome (RLS) and Periodic Limb Movement Disorder (PLMD)

Richard P. Allen

INTRODUCTION

The development of the polysomnogram (PSG) and sleep latency tests as methods for evaluating sleep and waking nurtured the birth of sleep medicine. The PSG generally served the field well, with one notable exception. The fascination of the striking and unexpectedly common periodic limb movements occurring in sleep (PLMS) led to the assumption that these represented a significant disorder of sleep, referred to as the periodic limb movement disorder (PLMD). Considerable attention focused on PLMS with frequent diagnoses of PLMD, while an associated disorder, the restless legs syndrome (RLS), remained neglected and rarely, if ever, diagnosed in the early development of clinical sleep medicine. Now we know better. RLS represents the major movement disorder of sleep–wake medicine and PLMD a rather minor disorder of uncertain clinical status. RLS, like other sleep-related disorders, now impacts both our understanding of sleep–wake regulation and the methods used in our sleep laboratory evaluations. The emphasis had been on only the sleep parts of objective tests, but now it shifts to measure the PLM during wake as well as sleep, and a new laboratory test evaluating waking movements when resting has been developed.

This chapter reflects this change in the significance of these disorders. The primary emphasis upon RLS delays the discussion of the PLMs until later in the chapter. Some readers unfamiliar with the definitions and characteristics of PLM may prefer to first read the definitions given in the last section of the chapter and then return to reading about RLS. However, understanding the more significant clinical and scientific issues presented in the first part of the chapter does not require this specific knowledge.

RESTLESS LEGS SYNDROME (RLS)

History

RLS was probably first described in the medical literature late in the 17th century by Willis, in an original publication in Latin (1) from Oxford University that was later included in the posthumous English language compilation of his work (2). The case he describes generally sounds like RLS with inability to resist leg movements, apparently engendered by rest, that disrupted sleep and responded to treatment with an opiate. Not much is written about this disorder for the next three centuries until Ekbom's seminal work describing this condition as a commonly occurring neurologic disorder—naming it the restless legs syndrome (3). After Ekbom, RLS again was largely ignored and sometimes considered to be primarily a psychologic disorder involving anxiety or response to financial worries. The development of sleep medicine led to renewed interest in this disorder, particularly when it was discovered that PLMs occur during large parts of sleep (4). Diagnostic criteria for the disorder were included in the first published nosology of sleep disorders (5). Finally, in 1995, a newly formed international RLS study group advanced a new set of diagnostic criteria, which were then updated and supported by a consensus of experts at a workshop at the National Institutes of Health in 2002 (6). Thus, the diagnostic criteria for RLS evolved through stages from a predominately motor phenomenon described by Willis to abnormal sensory phenomena detailed by Ekbom to our current understanding of the disturbance as a strong, sometimes irresistible urge to move the legs, sometimes referred as an akathisia focused on the legs (Table 15-1).

As better diagnostic criteria developed, so did treatment. The major advance was the serendipitous finding by Akpinar that levo-dopa (*L*-dopa) produces dramatic relief from all the RLS symptoms (7). At about the same time, Montplaisir independently made the same discovery. Now RLS was both well defined and, for the first time, had available a dramatically effective treatment. This was capped by the realizations that, when severe, RLS produces the most profound chronic sleep loss of any nonpsychiatric sleep disorder other than fatal familial insomnia and that it also commonly occurs in at least European and European descendents. Thus RLS is now recognized as perhaps the third most common specific sleep disorder after sleep apnea and psychophysiologic insomnia and one seen in all sleep medicine practices. As Ekbom (3) said "The disease is so common that every practicing physician meets it."

Diagnosis

Essential Features

The RLS diagnosis depends entirely on clinical symptoms matching the four essential criteria defined by the NIH workshop (Table 15-1). The first criterion that defines the primary symptom of RLS is a strong urge to move the legs can be termed a focal akathisia. This akathisia is often, but not always, accompanied by other disagreeable sensations or paresthesias usually involving a dynamic sensation located deep in the leg, not on the surface or in the skin. Any observable physical abnormality in the leg or changes in its appearance rarely if ever occur with these paresthesias. Subjects commonly report they are unable to describe the sensory disturbance but recognize it as unpleasant and, in a minority of cases, actually painful. The remaining three essential criteria indicate the conditions in which the RLS symptoms occur. Rest involving both decreased motor and mental activity engenders or worsens the symptoms. This quiescegenic feature depends upon both the duration and degree of rest for promoting symptom onset. Obversely, activity reduces the RLS symptoms. Walking or moving the legs produces an almost immediate relief from symptoms as long as the movement continues. Sometimes intense mental activity, such as arguing or playing an involving computer game, also significantly relieves the symptoms. The symptom relief lasts for variable amounts of time once the patient returns to resting, and there is no clear indication that the intensity or duration of the activity affects the subsequent duration of rest before symptoms recur. Finally, the symptoms have a strong circadian pattern, with symptoms occurring most prominently on the descending limb of the daily temperature curve during the late afternoon, evening, and night (9). Symptoms decrease or disappear in the midmorning about 6 to 10 AM, only to reoccur the next evening or night. The quiescegenic and circadian features interact. The duration of time the patient can sit or lie still decreases as the day progresses. In mild cases, it may take as much as an hour or more of rest to engender the symptoms, which may not be severe enough to awaken the patient. Thus, if the patients falls asleep in less than 30 minutes, the symptoms will be experienced only during protracted periods of enforced rest in the afternoon or evening, such as when traveling or attending a performance or meeting. More severely affected

---

▶ **TABLE 15-1. Diagnostic Criteria for RLS for Adults and Children over 13[a]**

Essential criteria

1. An urge to move the legs, usually accompanied or caused by uncomfortable and unpleasant sensations in the legs.
2. The urge to move or unpleasant sensations begin or worsen during periods of rest or inactivity, such as lying down or sitting
3. The urge to move or unpleasant sensations are partially or totally relieved by movement, such as walking or stretching, at least as long as the activity continues
4. The urge to move or unpleasant sensations are worse or only occur in the evening or night

Features supportive of an RLS diagnosis

1. Family history
2. Symptoms responded to dopaminergic therapy
3. Periodic limb movements (during wakefulness or sleep)

[a]From the NIH RLS diagnosis workshop.

patients, however, have trouble lying still long enough to fall asleep at night and, once asleep, may even wake up with the symptoms compelling them to get out of bed and walk for a while.

Features Supportive of the Diagnosis

Three features supportive of the diagnosis may guide clinical judgment in situations of diagnostic uncertainty (Table 15-1). RLS, particularly when it starts early in life, frequently occurs in more than one member of a family. RLS in the family supports the diagnosis. Nearly all patients report reduced symptoms at least initially when treated with L-dopa or a dopamine agonist. When there is no such response, the diagnosis should be reconsidered. PLMS occur for about 80% to 90% of all RLS patients (10) and, similarly, most RLS patients have periodic limb movements while lying resting awake, either during the sleep period or during a special suggested immobilization test (SIT) (11). These movements represent the motor expression of the disorder and provide the only sign for the disorder. Their presence supports the diagnosis when other causes for the movements can be excluded; their absence makes the diagnosis unlikely.

Differential Diagnoses

Some conditions produce symptoms that mimic RLS and are commonly misdiagnosed as RLS. The most common is positional discomfort occurring from sitting or lying in a fixed position too long. This puts pressure on veins, nerves, or simply on the skin itself, producing a discomfort and a need to move to relieve the discomfort. The characteristic difference is that relief occurs with a simple change in body position without any persisting activity. RLS requires some degree of activity to reduce the symptoms after return to resting. Positional discomfort usually occurs only when sitting whereas RLS, in contrast, usually occurs whenever the patients is resting and thus should at least occasionally occur when lying down. The same considerations apply to the urge to move occurring with orthostatic hypotension (12).

Pain from arthritis or other conditions can be circadian, worse at night, and, in some cases, brought on by rest and relieved by activity. Usually, unlike the RLS situation, the relief by activity does not occur almost immediately nor persist as long as the movement continues. The urge to move is usually more clearly secondary to the desire to relieve the pain; RLS patients desire to move to relieve a focused urge to move the leg, more than to relieve some other sensation associated with the leg.

Nocturnal leg cramps are sometimes confused with RLS. For these, a specific activity of stretching the affected muscle is usually required to produce relief; RLS patients may also stretch or tense muscles to reduce symptoms, but they find that almost any other leg activity also reduces symptoms.

Habitual or unconscious movements, such as foot tapping and sleep starts, can sometimes be confused with RLS, but these are automatic behaviors occurring without awareness of any urge to move. Inferring an urge to move the leg, based on an observation of movement occurring, differs from the clear awareness of the urge to move occurring with RLS. RLS patients may also have involuntary leg movements but, independent of the involuntary or unconscious movements, must have a conscious awareness of the akathisia focused on, and even appearing to stem from, the leg.

Neuroleptic-induced akathisia appears to be similar to RLS, and the differential diagnosis depends upon the history of medication use and response to discontinuing or changing the neuroleptic.

Neuropathies, anxiety, and moving toes and painful legs can at times be misdiagnosed as RLS. These generally do not involve a primary urge to move and are either not quiescegenic or circadian.

Objective Diagnostic Tests

RLS diagnosis relies on the clinical symptoms, but the occurrence of PLMS as a motor sign for the disorder provides strong support for the diagnosis. These periodics leg movements occur during sleep (PLMS) and also when awake lying down resting (PLMW). They are measured using electromyographic (EMG) recordings from the anterior tibialis or using activity meters placed on the ankle. They occur every 5 to 90 seconds and may persist for several minutes. Each movement during sleep lasts 0.5 to 5.0 seconds, but during waking tends to be longer, lasting 0.5 to 10 seconds. More details for scoring these are provided in the last section of this chapter. In one study, PLMS >7 per hour support the diagnosis of RLS with an accuracy of 84%, but PLMW >15 per hour during the nocturnal polysomnogram provides much better support for the diagnosis, with an accuracy of 91% (11). PLMW should always be scored when doing a polysomnogram as a sign of RLS.

A specific test, the suggested immobilization test (SIT), has been developed to evaluate the sensory and motor symptoms of RLS during a period of rest. The patient sits reclining in bed at about a 45-degree angle, with legs outstretched, without any cognitive or motor stimulation for 60 minutes. The patient is told to remain awake and to lie still without moving the legs unless the movement is needed to relieve RLS symptoms. The standard PSG recording is obtained without respiratory measures and, if sleep occurs, the patient is awakened. The patient provides a rating of the sensory discomfort in the legs on a 100-mm vertical bar using an electronic device placed conveniently at the bedside to minimize disturbance of the resting aspect of the SIT once every 5 minutes. The SIT is usually done in the hour before sleep onset. In one study, the diagnostic accuracy for PLM per hour >12 was 75%; the

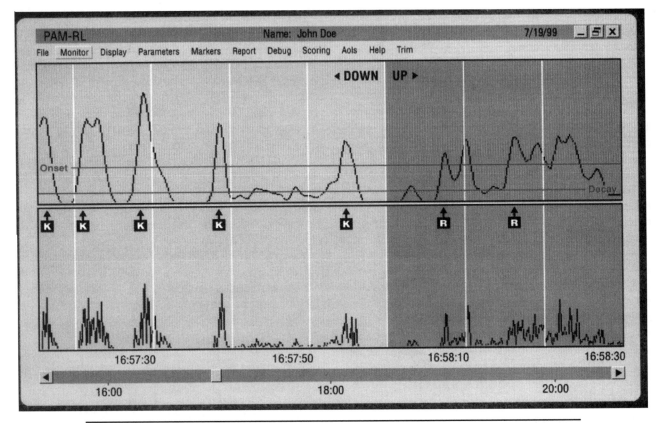

FIGURE 15-1. A 75-second leg activity recording for an RLS patient lying down awake and then getting up and walking. Actual activity data in the bottom panel and smoothed envelope of the activity in the upper panel. K indicates leg movements accepted as periodic; R indicates those rejected. Onset is the threshold for an adequate size movement and decay is the point of return to resting baseline.

sensory score >11 mm was 88% (11). It should be noted that the sensory score for leg discomfort on the SIT provides the only systematized assessment of the expression of the primary RLS symptom when provoked. While this makes it an interesting measure, it also makes it somewhat more prone to environmental and subject variation. It also may provide breaks in the SIT, thereby reducing the provocative nature of the boredom with this test. It remains to be seen whether or not the sensory score provides any advantage over the motor measurement of PLMW during the SIT.

The best laboratory objective test was the PLMW during the nocturnal PSG; the second best was the sensory score during the SIT, but the PLMW during the SIT was a close third.

Activity measure presumably could also be used to measure PLMW and PLMS together over several nights and presumably, given the repeated nights, would have at least the same degree of accuracy as the PLMS and PLMW from the PSG on a single night. Recent advances in activity measures include a device made by IM Systems in Baltimore that uses a three-dimensional sensor sampling the activity at 40 Hz and recording it at 10 Hz for up to 5 consecutive days. It also includes a position sensor that separates

the movements into those occurring when the leg is in the lying position versus standing or sitting. Its software identifies the PLM and provides a summary of the PLM per hour, adjusted for the amount of time in each body position. Validation studies comparing this activity meter to the PLMS and PLMW in a mixture of RLS and insomnia patients showed that the measurement of PLM per hour was accurate within ± 2 (correlation seconds >0.90) (13). (See Fig. 15-1 for an example of the activity recording of leg movements for an RLS patient while awake resting.) For RLS, this device also measures the amount of lying the patient is able to do during the night. There is obvious appeal to an objective test that could be obtained in the home using a device that could be mailed to the patient. The diagnostic benefits of repeated nights of activity recording have, however, not been evaluated.

Secondary Restless Legs Syndrome

RLS commonly occurs with end-stage renal disease, pregnancy, and iron deficiency and, for each of these conditions, RLS commonly starts and ends with the condition. RLS occurs in 20% to 70% of patients on dialysis, depending on the population (14,15), and has been associated with increased risk of mortality (14). RLS symptoms disappeared in 1 to 21 days after a successful kidney transplant (16). RLS occurs in about 20% to 30% of women during pregnancy, mostly in the third trimester (17–20), and resolves for most, but not all, within a few days after delivery (18, 20). The fact that RLS persisted after delivery raises the possibility that pregnancy may be a risk factor for its development. It occurs commonly in patients with iron deficiency and, for these patients, correction of the iron deficiency generally leads to remission or at least a significant reduction in the severity of the RLS symptoms.

The relationship between RLS and neuropathy remains unclear. While neuropathies have been reported to be surprisingly common among RLS patients (21,22), the best survey to date did not find a high prevalence of RLS among patients with neuropathy (23). One comparison of types of neuropathy found RLS commonly occurred for patients with Charcot–Marie–Tooth disease (CMT) type 1, but not CMT type 2, suggesting that RLS was associated or possibly secondary to neuropathy-disrupting sensory processing (24).

Several conditions that compromise iron status have also been advanced as causing RLS, such as very frequent blood donations (25), low-density lipoprotein apheresis (26), rheumatoid arthritis (27), and gastric surgery (28). It seems likely that RLS results from the iron deficiency more than other aspects of these conditions.

Diagnosis in Children

The NIH workshop that set forth the currently accepted standards for RLS diagnosis also established diagnostic criteria for children ages 2–12 (6). Adult criteria apply to children over age 13. Given the difficulties in diagnosing a primarily sensory disorder in young children, the criteria were divided into definite and probable RLS (Table 15-2). The criteria for definite RLS were made even more strict for young children than adults to decrease the risk of diagnostic error. Definite RLS requires all of the adult criteria plus an indication of some significant leg discomfort associated with the urge to move or the presence of two or three features supportive of RLS diagnosis: PLMS >5 per hour, complaint of sleep disturbance, and a biological parent or sibling with RLS. A diagnosis of probable RLS for children can be made when the child meets all of the adult criteria except the worsening of symptoms at night and has a biological parent or sibling with RLS. For very young children with limited language, describing the urge to move may be difficult and thus an alternate diagnostic criterion was established. For very young children probable RLS can be diagnosed if the child is observed to have behaviors suggesting leg discomfort associated with leg movement and occurring when sitting or lying down. The child must also have a biological parent or sibling with RLS.

Limited studies of RLS in children have suggested an association of uncertain significance with attention deficit-

▶ **TABLE 15-2. Diagnostic Criteria for RLS, Children 2–12 Years Old**[a]

Definite RLS diagnostic criteria

1. The child meets all four essential adult criteria for RLS and either
2. The child describes in his or her own words that a leg discomfort occurs, with the urge to move or
3. Two of three following supportive criteria are present
   a. Sleep disturbance for age
   b. A biologic parent or sibling has definite RLS
   c. The child has a PSG documenting PLMS/h ≥5

Probable RLS diagnostic criteria I

1. The child meets all essential adult criteria for RLS, except criterion No. 4 (the urge to move or sensations are worse in the evening or at night than during the day); and
2. The child has a biologic parent or sibling with definite RLS

Alternative probable diagnosis (particularly for younger children)

1. The child is observed to have behavior manifestations of lower extremity discomfort when sitting or lying and the discomfort presentation follows the diagnostic pattern for adults: worse during rest, relieved by movement, and worse during the evening and at night; and
2. The child has a biologic parent or sibling with RLS

[a]From the NIH RLS diagnosis workshop.

hyperactivity disorder (ADHD) (29) and growing pains (30,31).

Phenotypes

RLS appears to differ depending, to some extent, on the age of onset of symptoms. Two studies have demonstrated that an earlier age for onset of symptoms is associated with increasing occurrence of RLS among family members (32,33). Patients with RLS onset before age 45 were found to have a strong familial occurrence of RLS (33), a gradual progressive worsening of symptoms with age (34), and to be more commonly in women than men (35). In contrast, RLS patients whose symptoms started after age 45 had been found to have few family members with RLS, a rapid progression of symptoms, which then remained stable, and to be somewhat more likely to be male than female. Similar results were reported in a study using a cut-off age of 40 for defining early and late age of onset of RLS symptoms, except that this study did not report on the gender differences (19).

Epidemiology

Initial attempts to determine the prevalence of RLS relied mostly upon one or two questions describing RLS symptoms added to a large population-based survey. These rarely covered the full diagnostic criteria for RLS and had no adequate independent determination of their sensitivity or specificity for RLS diagnosis. There have been four more recent general population-based surveys using questions covering the full range of the diagnostic criteria for RLS. Two of these, conducted in Sweden, showed the RLS prevalence for adults age 18 to 64 was 11% for females (36) and 6% for males (37). The sensitivity and specificity of the diagnostic questions was not determined. Another study, using standardized questions in face-to-face interviews of senior citizens (age 65 to 83) in a survey in Augsburg, Germany, reported a slightly higher prevalence of 14% for women and 6% for men (38). The higher prevalence in Germany may reflect the age difference between the populations. Finally, a large population-based survey of adults over 21 covering five European countries and the United States provided an estimate of the overall prevalence of 7.2% (39). Since RLS occurs with a wide range of severity and, in its milder forms, can usually be managed without medical treatment, this survey also collected data on the severity of the RLS symptoms when present. It defined RLS symptoms occurring at least twice a week and reported to be subjectively distressing as moderately severe RLS that is likely to warrant medical treatment. The prevalence of the moderately severe RLS was 2.7% overall (3.7% for women and 1.7% for men). The prevalence of moderately severe RLS generally increased with age. However, 36% of these patients were less than 50 years old.

Some limited studies indicate a lower prevalence of about 3% in Japan (40) and less than 1% in both Singapore (41) and India (42). These studies have some sampling bias and need to be repeated, but, at this point, it appears RLS is less common in Asian than European populations.

The Swedish studies also examined some possible comorbid conditions and reported significant increased risk for headache and depressed mood for both males and females; for males there was increased risk for hypertension and cardiac problems.

Pathophysiology

Neural Substrate

A consideration of the possible site of RLS pathology guides much of the following considerations of RLS pathophysiology. The profound exacerbation of RLS by all centrally active dopamine antagonists but not the primarily peripherally active domperidone indicates a primary CNS pathology. The RLS abnormalities from transcranial magnetic stimulation suggest a pathology involving supraspinal, subcortical areas (43–45). The increased excitability of spinal cord regulation of a flexor reflex also indicate less a spinal abnormality than a disruption of subcortical inhibition of these reflexes (46,47). Given the response to dopaminergic medications, subcortical dopamine systems seem likely candidates for the pathology. These could be the nigrostriatal system, with its well-recognized sensory–motor regulation functions, and pos-

sible involvement of the nucleus accumbens, well recognized for its effects on motivation for behaviors. The spinal dopamine system, with its cell bodies in the A11 system, also seems a likely candidate for a role in RLS pathology, although the very diffuse nature of this system makes it hard to evaluate. One functional magnetic resonance imaging (fMRI) study showed that the primary sensory symptoms of RLS, when not accompanied by leg movement, produced increased activation in the thalamus and, surprisingly, the cerebellum. When symptoms occurred with leg movements, there was added activation of the red nucleus and brainstem areas close to the reticular formation but not of the motor cortex (48). This provides further support for a subcortical pathology. The role of the thalamus for inhibiting sensory phenomena during the transition to sleep makes it a likely candidate for involvement with a quiescegenic sensory disorder, but interpreting the cerebellar involvement remains more difficult.

Genetics and Family History

RLS commonly occurs within the same family and, in the published pedigrees from several large families, occurs with a pattern suggestive of an autosominal dominant trait. One family history study, however, reported the risk of RLS occurring among first-degree relatives of an RLS patient compared to controls was strongly affected by age of onset of RLS symptoms. The risk of RLS among other family members was 6.7 times greater than controls for RLS patients with an age of onset before 45, but only 2.9 times greater for those with a later age of symptom onset. A segregation analysis of the first-degree relatives of a sample of RLS patients similarly found a strong effect for age of onset of symptoms. The analyses favored a single autosomonal active gene for those families with an average age of onset of 30 or less but no consistent genetic pattern could be found for families with a later average age of symptom onset.

Recently, two studies using genomewide screens on large families with a high density of RLS reported significant linkages, one for some French Candadian families on chromsome12 q (in a 14.71-cM region between D12S1044 and D12S78) (49) and another in an Italian family on 14q13-21 (in a 9.1 cM, between markers D14S70 and D14S1068) (50). These linkages have not been reported to occur in other RLS families. Evaluation for occurrence of specific genotypic or allelic distributions related to the dopamine system failed to find any significant pattern for RLS patients (51), except for one study showing that females with a high activity MAOA allele had a greater risk of having RLS. This contributed to a phenotypic expression of longer sleep latency and more periodic movements on the evening SIT, suggesting an overall greater severity of RLS symptoms (52).

At this point the balance between genetic and environmental factors contributing to RLS remains uncertain.

A   B   R2* (sec⁻¹)

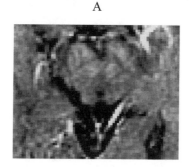
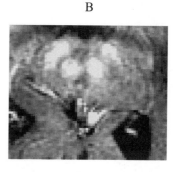
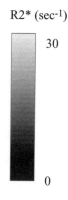

FIGURE 15-2. R2* images in **(A)** a 70-year-old RLS patient; **(B)** a 71-year-old control subject. Much lower R2* relaxation rates are apparent in the RLS case in both red nucleus and substantia nigra. (From Allen RP, et al *Neurology.* 2001;56:263–265. With permission.)

None of the standard blinded family or twin studies have been done. The genetic linkage and association studies have not been very informative and the few positive findings appear to be unique to special families and may not be directly related to any primary pathology of RLS.

Dopamine

The remarkable effectiveness of dopaminergic medications for treating RLS has naturally led to the hypothesis that RLS involves an abnormality of the central dopaminergic system. Imaging studies of the striatum, however, have failed to show any consistent dopaminergic abnormalities. One proton emission tomography (PET) study showed decreased D2 receptor binding in the putamen and caudate (53). Two subsequent SPECT studies failed to find any similar abnormality (54), but another reported reduced striatal D2 receptor binding (55). Two SPECT studies failed to find any abnormality involving the dopamine transporter (54,55). Somewhat more consistent findings have been reported for FDOPA PET, wherein two studies have reported small decreases in striatal uptake for RLS patients compared to controls (53,56). Cerebrospinal fluid (CSF) studies failed to find any abnormalities related to the dopaminergic system (57). Overall, these data do not provide a clear picture of a specific dopamine abnormality in RLS.

Iron

Given the strong clinical link between iron deficiency and RLS, it has been proposed that a primary pathology for RLS may be abnormalities producing brain iron insufficiency. CSF studies have reported decreased ferritin and increased transferrin (58), both indicating abnormally reduced CNS iron status. The regional regulation of brain iron leads to well known development, with age, of iron-rich areas in the brain. Thus an iron-deficit brain may be regional and may be, to some extent, age dependent. Specialized MRI studies evaluating regional brain iron have found for the substantia nigra (SN) a consistent decrease in iron held in ferritin that correlates with RLS severity

(59) (Fig. 15-2). Other iron or dopaminergic areas of the brain did not show this pattern of consistent decreases for RLS patients. Since the substantia nigra contains the cell bodies for the dopaminergic nigrostriatal system, an iron deficiency in this area could significantly impair the functioning of that system. Further autopsy studies comparing brain tissue from RLS patients to that from controls have confirmed this deceased iron content in the SN. In addition, the autopsy studies of the SN found decreased H-ferritin, decreased iron transporter proteins (divalent metal transporter 1 and ferroportin), and increased ferritin, all consistent with an iron insufficiency. As shown in Fig. 15-3, transferrin receptor (Tfr), however, was found to be decreased, which is contrary to the expected cellular response to iron insufficiency (60). This unexpected finding could indicate a deficiency in the posttranscriptional regulation of Tfr in RLS. There are two iron-regulatory proteins (IRP-1 and IRP-2) that serve a primary role in the cellular response to iron status, both normally increasing with decreasing iron in the cell. Another autopsy study using laser-capture microdissection to obtain neuromelanin cells of the SN found for RLS compared to controls the expected increase for IRP-2 appropriate for the iron deficiency but also an unexpected marked decrease in IRP-1 (61). Decreased IRP-1 would lead to a failure to stabilize the Tfr, resulting in a decrease in Tfr. This, in turn, could compromise the cell's ability to obtain an adequate iron status. It seems somewhat unlikely that this type of deficit would occur only in the SN neuromelanin cells, but, at this point, these studies have been limited to the SN. The degree of regional significance or specificity of this deficit remains to be determined. It should also be noted that the autopsy studies were conducted on brains from patients with an early age of onset of symptoms (before 45) and almost exclusively from females.

Medical Evaluation

Clinical Presentation and Evaluation

The diagnosis of RLS relies upon a good clinical interview and medical history documenting the four essential features of the disorder and a careful differential

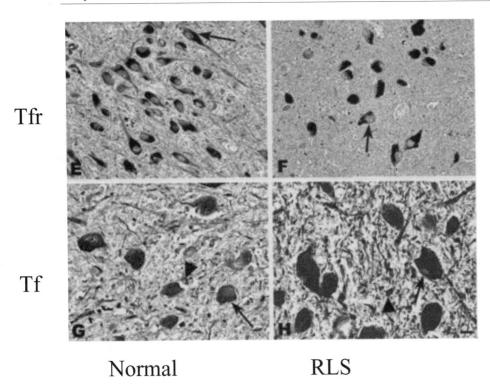

Tfr

Tf

Normal   RLS

FIGURE 15-3. Substantia nigra, transferrin receptor (Tfr), and transferrin Tf immunoreactive product is blue. Tfr reaction in neuromelanin cells and process (arrow) is less for RLS patient. Tf staining in the neuromelanin cells (arrow) and oligodendrocytes is more abundant for RLS. (From Connor, JR, et al, *Neurology.* 2003;61:304–309. With permission.)

diagnosis to exclude possible RLS mimics, as described above. A routine physical and brief neurologic examination, particularly checking for signs of neuropathy is recommended both as a potential differential diagnosis and because, when present, may complicate treatment.

Determining RLS severity aids in confirming the diagnosis and planning treatment. Mild RLS rarely occurs daily and may present only as discomfort when sitting for protracted periods, particularly in the evening. These patients complain of difficulty sitting still more than of sleep disturbance. Moderate to severe RLS generally occurs daily or at least twice a week, and the patient usually has a primary complaint of sleep disturbance. Moderate to severe RLS patients are more likely to seek treatment at a sleep medicine clinic. Rarely do the patients complain of frank daytime sleepiness, rather, they report fatigue and difficulty concentrating. Structured diagnostic interviews are available and a telephone version of one of these has been validated against standard clinical interviews (62). During the clinical interview, the symptoms specific to RLS should be defined and clearly separated from those of other disorders, such as neuropathy or psychophysiologic insomnia.

Laboratory Tests

Since iron deficiency can cause RLS and may present with no symptoms other than RLS, all patients should have a morning fasting iron evaluation, including a serum ferritin and percentage saturated test.

While other laboratory tests are not required for management of RLS, a PSG preceded by a 1-hour SIT often helps resolve uncertain diagnoses. The critical measures are the PLMW during the PSG and the SIT and the sensory scored during the SIT. If the patient complains of significant excessive sleepiness, these tests should be performed both to confirm the diagnosis and to exclude other causes of the disorder, particularly, sleep-disordered breathing (SDB). Sleepiness with severe RLS may require first treating the RLS before evaluation with a PSG for other causes of sleepiness.

An alternative to the PSG and SIT would be the multiple nights of leg activity monitoring, described earlier.

Evaluation of Severity

There are two well-validated severity scales that can be used to assist treatment planning. The Johns Hopkins Severity Scale (63) was developed for ease of use in the clinic and also for possible retrospective evaluation of the patients, based on recall of symptoms in the past. This scale is meant for clinic use with patients with nearly daily symptoms and should not be used for patients with intermittent or very mild symptoms. The scale assesses severity by the time of day for usual onset of RLS symptoms. The scores are 0 for no symptoms, 1 for onset during bedtime or the night, 2 for onset after 6 PM but before bedtime, and 3 for onset before 6 PM.

The International Restless Legs Scale (IRLS) developed and validated by the IRLSG (64) has ten items, each scored from 0 to 4, with higher scores indicating more severe RLS. In the validation study, all RLS patients scored 11 or better. The form of this questionnaire currently in use is presented in the journal *Sleep Medicine* (65) and available in English and other languages from MAPI Research Institute Lyon, France (http://www.mapi-research-inst.com). Subsequent work with this scale has found that it has two subscales: one for RLS symptoms and the other for symptom impact (66).

Objective measures from the PSG or SIT or from leg activity measures also provide useful severity assessments when available.

Treatment

Evidenced-based standards of practice for treatment of RLS have been developed by the American Academy of Sleep Medicine (67) and they have been followed by an update on the dopaminergic treatment of RLS. At this time, no medication has been approved by the United States Food and Drug Administration (FDA) for use with RLS, and only one medication, the dopamine agonist ropinirole, has been evaluated with large double-blinded, placebo-controlled clinical trials. This may change in the very near future, but, until then, clinical experience and the mostly limited clinical studies guide the treatment recommendations presented below. The ongoing large-scale evaluations of other dopaminergic treatments of RLS may alter this situation.

Pharmacological Treatment

Four major classes of medication have been reported to provide effective treatment of RLS: dopaminergics (mostly L-dopa and dopamine agonists), opioids, some anticonvulsants (mainly those also useful for treating neuropathic pain), and gabanergic hypnotics. Some examples of these medications are given below and in Table 15-3.

Among the dopaminergics, L-dopa with benserazide was the first to be evaluated (7, 8, 68). Since then, placebo-controlled double-blind studies have found that L-dopa either with carbidopa or benserazide (69–71) and the dopamine agonists bromocriptine (72), pergolide (73–75), pramipexole (76,77), rotigotine (78), and ropinirole (79–83) all provide effective treatment for all RLS symptoms at remarkably small doses compared to those customarily used for treatment of Parkinson's disease. Ropinirole and pergolide have been evaluated in clinical samples large enough to clearly establish efficacy for treatment of RLS. The striking aspects of dopaminergic treatment are both its immediate benefits shortly after being taken at an effective dose and that almost all RLS patients show at least some benefit to initial treatment.

Although opiates were the first medications used to treat RLS, only the opioid oxycodone has been evaluated for

▶ **TABLE 15-3.** Pharmacotherapy for RLS

Drugs used to treat RLS
  Dopaminergic agents (DA)
    L-dopa (with carbidopa or benserazide)
    Agonists: pergolide, pramipexole, ropinirole
  Sedative–hypnotics
    Clonazepam; estazolam; oxazepam; temazepam; triazolam;
    Zaleplon; Zolpidem
  Anticonvulsants
    Gabapentin; carbamazepine
  Opiates/opioids
    Propoxyphene; hydrocodone; codeine; tramadol; oxycodone;
    Methadone, Morphine sulfate-X
Drugs to avoid or use cautiously with RLS
  Avoid: Dopaminergic antagonists
    Antipsychotics (e.g., haloperidol),
      antinausea (e.g., metaclopramide)
  Use cautiously
    Antidepressants other than buproprion
    Sedating antihistamines

treatment of RLS in a standard placebo-controlled, double-blind trial (84). Oxycodone provided effective treatment for most of a small sample of RLS patients in that study. Clinical experience indicates that all of the opioids provide effective treatment, and it has been suggested that the more potent opioids, such as methadone, provide the best treatment for very severe RLS not adequately treated with other medications. The effective dose of opioids for treating RLS is in the same range as the usual analgesic dose.

Two anticonvulsants have been found effective for treating RLS in double-blind, placebo-controlled trials: carbamazepine (85,86) and gabapentin (87,88). Although carbamazepine was evaluated in a much larger clinical trial, its use has been limited partly by problems with adverse effects. Gabapentin has become accepted as a treatment alternative for RLS.

Among the gabanergic medications, only clonazepam has been evaluated for treatment of RLS using double-blind, placebo-controlled trials. In one older study with uncertain diagnoses, it was found to effectively reduce leg dysesthesias, but, in both of two recent studies, it failed to be any better than placebo (89,90) and, in one of these studies, it failed to significantly reduce the PLM of RLS patients, but did increase total sleep time (TST) (89). Thus the gabanergic sedative hypnotics appear not to provide effective treatment for RLS symptoms, but since they promote sleep may help a patient go to sleep and not be awakened, despite the presence of mild RLS symptoms.

Medications listed in Table 15.4 may exacerbate or even engender RLS. Centrally active dopamine antagonists, including antiemetics and antipsychotics, exacerbate and may even engender RLS (91). Several antidepressants,

▶ **TABLE 15-4.** Pharmacological and Behavioral Treatment of RLS

Sx	Sequence of Treatment Use		
	First Choice	*Second Choice*	*Third Choice*
Mild			
Intermittent	Behavioral treatment PRN sedative–hypnotic PRN lowest dose DA (if tolerated)	PRN carbidopa/L-dopa 25/100	PRN opiates
Most days	Behavioral treatment	Daily low-dose DA Daily sedative–hypnotics	Daily opiates
Moderate or severe			
Intermittent	PRN carbidopa/L-dopa PRN or daily DA	PRN or daily opiates	Daily gabapentin
Most days	Daily DA	Daily opiates	Daily gabapentin
Special considerations			
Mostly painful and daily	Daily gabapentin or opiates	Daily DA	Daily sedative–hypnotic

Break-through Sx	If on DA
	  add PRN lowest DA dose
	If not on DA
	  then PRN carbidopa/L-dopa 25/100
	  or lowest-dose DA if tolerated
		***	Nonpharmacologic
			  treatment

*a*DA, dopamine agonist; intermittent, averages no more than 2 times a week.

particularly the SSRIs, have been reported to sometimes exacerbate RLS symptoms. The adverse effects of antidepressants have, however, not been well documented. The dopamine-active antidepressant bupropion is considered not to have any adverse effect on RLS symptoms. Patients have reported that sedating antihistamines often exacerbate their RLS.

Nonpharmacological Treatment

Several nonpharmacological treatments for RLS have been advocated, but none have proved effective in adequately controlled studies or gained general clinical acceptance. Based on the diagnostic criteria for RLS, the behavioral treatment of increased physical and mental activity provides effective temporary relief from symptoms. Unfortunately, this treatment is hard to implement and maintain and is counterproductive for sleep.

Iron Treatment

Whenever iron deficiency is found in an RLS patient (morning fasting serum ferritin <18 μg/L or %SAT <16%) the standard treatment with oral iron is indicated. O'Keffe and colleagues also showed that oral iron treatment can reduce RLS symptoms for patients with serum ferritin levels less than 45 μg/L (92). Iron can be given as ferrous sulfate 325 mg TID with 200 mg vitamin C to increase absorption of the iron. Fasting morning %SAT should be considered, since a value >45% is one of the better indicators of possible hemochromatosis, a not un-

common genetic condition prone to peripheral iron overload.

Augmentation and Other Complications of Pharmacological Treatment

In addition to the usual adverse effects from the medications used to treat RLS, there are a few adverse effects that appear to be somewhat specific to RLS. The dopaminergic treatments, in particular, were found to cause a significant problem for some patients, with augmentation of the RLS symptoms so that they would start occurring earlier in the day and persist longer. Augmentation also involves a reduction of the time that the patient can remain at rest before symptoms started; an increased severity of the symptoms, with decreased duration of symptom relief from the medication and; in a small number of cases, spreading of the symptoms to involve body parts other than the legs. Augmentation has been reported to occur in about 80% of the patients treated with carbidopa/L-dopa (93), but only about 30% of the patients treated with the dopamine agonists pergolide (94) or pramipexole. The risk of augmentation on carbidopa/L-dopa increases with the dose of the medication and is particularly pronounced for doses over 50/200 (93). Augmentation with the dopamine agonists appears to be less aggressive and has been reported to be adequately managed in many cases by giving a dose earlier in the day, either as an additional or extra dose. Augmentation appears to develop within the first 6 to 18 months of treatment. It can be severe, requiring discontinuing the dopaminergic medication. The mechanism for this augmentation is not understood but raises some concerns that the dopaminergic treatments may be exacerbating the underlying pathology of RLS. Limiting L-dopa treatment to intermittent use no more than two or three times a week significantly reduces the risk of severe augmentation.

The major problem noted with long-term treatment of RLS using opioids has been the possible development or exacerbation of sleep-disordered breathing (95). Patients should be followed for any indications that this has occurred.

Summary of Clinical Treatment

Clinical management of RLS requires defining treatment goals both in terms of frequency with which symptoms occur (daily or nearly daily versus intermittent) and the time of day that symptoms occur. Table 15-4 presents one approach to treatment that has been modified somewhat from the recommendations suggested by Earley (96).

PERIODIC LIMB MOVEMENTS

History

Periodic leg movements (PLM) observed to occur persistently during sleep were referred to by Symonds as "nocturnal myoclonus" (97). Further studies indicated that these movements were neither myoclonic nor limited to the night, but rather were more appropriately described as periodic leg movements in sleep (PLMS). Since they may also occur in the arms, they are often referred to as limb rather than only leg movements (98). However, the predominant presentation, and the only one with recording and diagnostic standards involve the legs. They were initially considered to be primarily physiologic flexor movements and were, therefore, recorded from surface electromyography (EMG) electrodes placed on the belly of the anterior tibialis muscle (99). Subsequently, more detailed analyses has found these movements to be multifocal with no consistent pattern of EMG activation, but still most involve the anterior tibialis (100,101).

Standards for scoring the PSG were advanced by Coleman and then updated by a task force of the American Sleep Disorders Association (now known as the American Academy of Sleep Medicine) (99). When present in patients complaining of a sleep–wake disorder, the PLMS were seen as defining a sleep disorder referred to as periodic limb movement disorder (PLMD) (98). The finding of PLM occurring in both sleep and waking and the recognition that PLMS occurs in conjunction with many disorders has led to a conceptualization of these events as a nonspecific sign very sensitive for RLS but less so for other disorders.

Definition

PLMs are defined for PSG recordings based on essentially uncalibrated anterior tibialis surface EMG recordings. Limited calibration is provided by having the patient perform a physiologic flexor of the foot (with extension of the big toe) and requiring that the maximum amplitude of any EMG event considered to be a candidate PLM be at least 25% of this calibration amplitude. These conventions are rather loosely followed during actual scoring, and it is rare that the nature or extent of the calibration movement by the patient is described in the notes accompanying a PSG. The candidate PLM must also last 0.5 to 5.0 seconds and reoccur at least four times, with an interval between onset of movements of 5 to 90 seconds (99). If the patient is awake, the PLM criteria have been modified to permit a longer duration of 0.5 to 10 seconds (102). For sleep recordings, the PLMS are often associated with arousals, and an index of the PLMS with arousal is calculated. By convention, the number of events divided by the hours of total observation time determine the major indexes as events per hour.

For activity recordings from the ankle, the same duration and periodicity criteria apply, but here the amplitude of the movements is actually measured in acceleration units, so the minimal criterion can be consistent across different studies. This has been set for one monitor, based on matching expert scoring of PSGs, as movements with a maximum acceleration amplitude exceeding μG (103).

Major Factors Affecting Periodic Limb Movements (Sleep–Wake State, Age, and Gender)

PLMs appear to be strongly influenced by the sleep–wake state. When lying down during drowsy waking, the PLMs occur for patients with RLS with somewhat longer durations and are far less periodic than during sleep. They appear to be more common and the intermovement interval shorter as the patient becomes more sleepy. The onset of stage 1 sleep stabilizes the PLM periodicity somewhat, the duration of the movements become shorter, and the intermovement interval somewhat lengthens. With the progression to deeper stages of non-REM sleep, the intermovement interval continues to lengthen. The intermovement interval in REM sleep is similar to that in stage 1 (104). In general, then, the PLM are most common in the states of transition between sleep and waking and are less common during either deeper sleep and more alert states while resting.

PLMS increase with age and have been reported to occur at a rate >5 per hour for 45% of community-dwelling elderly >65 years old (105). What would be considered a normal value for PLMS must, therefore, be age adjusted; and at this time no standards have been established. The PLMS index was also, on average, greater for elderly (over 65) men than women. Occurrence of PLMW without RLS appears to be relatively uncommon, but until recently these have not been measured in non-RLS patients. The rates of PLMW occurrence in normal or clinical populations are unknown, as are the effects of age on PLMW.

Autonomic Arousal and Periodic Limb Movement in Sleep

Heart rates after each PLMS leg movement, when averaged over several movements, show increases of about 15% over 7 beats followed by transient decreases (3 to 5 beats) to slightly below the baseline levels before the movement (106,107). Blood pressure may also transiently increase after PLMS (108). The heart rate changes occur even when there is no EEG evidence for arousal with the PLM. The amount of heart rate change after a PLMS decreases with age (109) and appears to be much less for the PLMS associated with REM behavior disorder (RBD) (110), presumably because of the autonomic dysfunction. Thus, for most situations, PLMS result in a significant transient autonomic arousal. It has been conjectured that these repetitive and sometimes frequent autonomic arousals during sleep produce clinically significant adverse consequences but this has not been demonstrated.

Secondary Periodic Limb Movement in Sleep

PLMS has been found to be secondary to a large number of conditions other than RLS. These include multiple sclerosis (111), central sleep apneas (CSA) (111), SDB events (112), spinal cord injury (113), juvenile fibromyalgia (114), RBD (110), Parkinson's disease (PD) (115), and narcoplesy (116). It has been suggested that any disorder involving the dopaminergic motor systems will likely produce PLMS. Similarly, the experience with PLMS occurring with the termination of SDB events, even without any EEG arousal, may indicate that PLMS provide a sensitive indicator of autonomic arousal events during sleep.

Primary Periodic Limb Movement in Sleep and Periodic Limb Movement Disorder

A sleep–wake disturbance resulting from PLMS occurring in excess for age and without any of the secondary causes, such as those noted above, defines the periodic limb movement disorder (PLMD). Studies failing to find any relation between PLMS rates and sleep–wake complaints (117) raise serious doubts about the significance or even existence of PLMD. However, PLMD could be a relatively uncommon disorder easily overlooked in the studies on PLMS and clinical symptoms. While clearly not as common as once thought, PLMD may still exist as a significant sleep disorder.

SUMMARY

As in other fields of sleep medicine, remarkable advances have occurred in the study of sleep-related movement disorders. The striking PLMS are now understood to be a primary sign of RLS. PLMD is a relatively uncommon disorder, while RLS is common. The rapid growth in studies of RLS has increased our understanding of the pathology, diagnosis, and treatment. Sleep medicine clinics are expected to provide effective treatment for this disorder and hopefully the growing knowledge about RLS will guide development of future new treatments.

The clinician interested in obtaining more information will find the website of the Restless Legs Syndrome Foundation (www.RLS.org) helpful. The RLSF also publishes a regular newsletter for RLS patients.

REFERENCES

1. Willis T. *De Animae brutorum*. London: Wells and Scott, 1672.
2. Willis T. *The London practice of physick*. London: Bassett and Crooke, 1685.
3. Ekbom KA. Restless legs: a clinical study. *Acta Med Scand.* (Suppl.) 1945;158:1–122.
4. Lugaresi E, Cirignotta F, Coccagna G, et al. Nocturnal myoclonus and restless legs syndrome. In: Fahn S, Marsden CD, Van Woert MH, eds. *Myoclonus.* New York: Raven Press, 1986;295–307.
5. Thorpy M, chairman. Diagnostic Classification Steering Committee. Periodic leg movements and restless legs syndrome. In: *The international classification of sleep disorders: diagnostic and coding manual.* Rochester, New York: American Sleep Disorders Association, 1990.
6. Allen R, Hening W, Montplaisir J, et al. Restless legs syndrome: diagnostic criteria, special considerations, and epidemiology. A report from the restless legs syndrome diagnosis and epidemiology workshop at the National Institute of Health. *Sleep Med.* 2003;4(2):101–119.
7. Akpinar S. Treatment of restless legs syndrome with levodopa plus benserazide [letter]. *Arch Neurol.* 1982;39(11):739.
8. Montplaisir J, Godbout R, Poirier G, et al. Restless legs syndrome and periodic movements in sleep: physiopathology and treatment with L-dopa. *Clin Neuropharmacol.* 1986;9(5):456–463.
9. Hening WA, Walters AS, Wagner M, et al. Circadian rhythm of motor restlessness and sensory symptoms in the idiopathic restless legs syndrome. *Sleep.* 1999;22(7):901–912.
10. Montplaisir J, Boucher S, Poirier G, et al. Clinical, polysomnographic, and genetic characteristics of restless legs syndrome: a study of 133 patients diagnosed with new standard criteria. *Move Disorders.* 1997;12(1):61–65.
11. Michaud M, Paquet J, Lavigne G, et al. Sleep laboratory diagnosis of restless legs syndrome. *Eur Neurol.* 2002;48(2):108–113.
12. Heinze E, Frame B, Fline G. Restless legs and orthostatic hypotension in primary amyloidosis. *Arch Neurol.* 1967;16:497–500.
13. Gorny S, Allen R, Krausman D, et al. Evaluation of the PAM-RL system for the detection of periodic leg movements during sleep in the lab and home environments. *Sleep.* 1998;21(suppl.):183.
14. Winkelman JW, Chertow GM, Lazarus JM. Restless legs syndrome in end-stage renal disease. *Amer J Kidney Dis.* 1996;28(3):372–378.
15. Hui D, Wong T, Li T, et al. Prevalence of sleep disturbances in Chinese patients with end stage renal failure on maintenance hemodialysis. *Med Sci Monitoring.* 2002;8(5):CR331–336.
16. Winkelmann J, Stautner A, Samtleben W, et al. Long-term course of restless legs syndrome in dialysis patients after kidney transplantation. *Move Disorders.* 2002;17(5):1072–1076.
17. Suzuki K, Ohida T, Sone T, et al. The prevalence of restless legs syndrome among pregnant women in Japan and the relationship between restless legs syndrome and sleep problems. *Sleep.* 2003;26(6):673–677.
18. Lee KA, Zaffke ME, Baratte-Beebe K. Restless legs syndrome and sleep disturbance during pregnancy: the role of folate and iron. *J Womens Health Gender Based Med.* 2001;10(4):335–341.

19. Kurella B, Kraemer S, Winkler P. Restless legs syndrome and pregnancy. Results of a questionnaire-study. *German Neurol Soc.* 2002, *Göttingen* Sept. 26–29.

20. Manconi M, Govoni V, Cesnik E, et al. Epidemiology of restless legs syndrome in a population of 606 pregnant women. *Sleep.* 2003;26:A330–331.

21. Polydefkis M, Allen RP, Hauer P, et al. Subclinical sensory neuropathy in late-onset restless legs syndrome. *Neurology.* 2000;55(8):1115–1121.

22. Iannaccone S, Zucconi M, Marchettini P, et al. Evidence of peripheral axonal neuropathy in primary restless legs syndrome. *Move Disorders.* 1995;10(1):2–9.

23. Rutkove S, Matheson J, Logigian E. Restless legs syndrome in patients with polyneuropathy. *Muscle Nerve.* 1996;19:670–672.

24. Gemignani F, Marbini A, Di Giovanni G, et al. Charcot-Marie-Tooth disease type 2 with restless legs syndrome. *Neurology.* 1999;52(5):1064–1066.

25. Silber MH, Richardson JW. Multiple blood donations associated with iron deficiency in patients with restless legs syndrome. *Mayo Clin Proc.* 2003;78(1):52–54.

26. Happe S, Tings T, Schettler V, et al. Low-density lipoprotein apheresis and restless legs syndrome. *Sleep.* 2003;26:A335–336.

27. Györfi M, Szakács Z, Koumlves P. Restless legs syndrome and serum transferrin receptor and ferritin levels in patients with rheumatoid arthritis. *Sleep.* 2003;26:A334.

28. Ekbom KA. Restless legs syndrome after partial gastrectomy. *Acute Neurol Scand.* 1966;42:79–89.

29. Chervin RD, Archbold KH, Dillon JE, et al. Associations between symptoms of inattention, hyperactivity, restless legs, and periodic leg movements. *Sleep.* 2002;25(2):213–218.

30. Picchietti D. *Growing pains: RLS in children.* Orange Park, Florida: Galaxy Books, 1996.

31. Walters A. Is there a subpopulation of children with growing pains who really have restless legs syndrome? A review of the literature. *Sleep Med.* 2002;3(2):93–98.

32. Winkelmann J, Wetter TC, Collado-Seidel V, et al. Clinical characteristics and frequency of the hereditary restless legs syndrome in a population of 300 patients. *Sleep.* 2000;23(5):597–602.

33. Allen RP, La Buda MC, Becker P, et al. Family history study of the restless legs syndrome. *Sleep Med.* 2002;3 Suppl:S3–7.

34. Allen RP, Earley CJ. Defining the phenotype of the restless legs syndrome (RLS) using age-of-symptom-onset. *Sleep Med.* 2000;1:11–19.

35. Nichols DA, Allen RP, Grauke JH, et al. Restless legs syndrome symptoms in primary care: a prevalence study. *Arch Intern Med.* 2003;163(19):2323–2329.

36. Ulfberg J, Nystrom B, Carter N, et al. Restless legs syndrome among working-aged women. *Eur Neurol.* 2001;46(1):17–19.

37. Ulfberg J, Nystrom B, Carter N, et al. Prevalence of restless legs syndrome among men aged 18 to 64 years: an association with somatic disease and neuropsychiatric symptoms. *Move Disorders.* 2001;16(6):1159–1163.

38. Rothdach AJ, Trenkwalder C, Haberstock J, et al. Prevalence and risk factors of RLS in an elderly population: the MEMO study. Memory and morbidity in Augsburg elderly. *Neurology.* 2000;54(5):1064–1068.

39. Allen RP, Montplaisi J, Myers A. Profile of RLS in a large multinational population and characterization of a group likely warranting treatment: the REST (RLS Epidemiology, Symptoms and Treatment) General Population Study (Abstr). *Neurology.* 2004; in press.

40. Inoue Y, Ishizuka T, Arai H. Surveillance on epidemiology and treatment of restless legs syndrome in Japan. *J New Rem Clin.* 2000;49(3):244–254.

41. Tan EK, Seah A, See SJ, et al. Restless legs syndrome in an Asian population: a study in Singapore. *Move Disorders.* 2001;16(3):577–579.

42. Krishnan PR, Bhatia M, Behari M. Restless legs syndrome in Parkinson's disease: a case-controlled study. *Move Disorders.* 2003;18(2):181–185.

43. Tergau F, Wischer S, Paulus W. Motor system excitability in patients with restless legs syndrome. *Neurology.* 1999;52(5):1060–1063.

44. Entezari-Taher M, Singleton JR, Jones CR, et al. Changes in excitability of motor cortical circuitry in primary restless legs syndrome. *Neurology.* 1999;53(6):1201–1205.

45. Quatrale R, Manconi M, Gastaldo E, et al. Neurophysiological study of corticomotor pathways in restless legs syndrome. *Clin Neurophysiol.* 2003;114(9):1638–1645.

46. Bara-Jimenez W, Aksu M, Graham B, et al. Periodic limb movements in sleep: state-dependent excitability of the spinal flexor reflex. *Neurology.* 2000;54(8):1609–1616.

47. Aksu M, Bara-Jimenez W. State dependent excitability changes of spinal flexor reflex in patients with restless legs syndrome secondary to chronic renal failure. *Sleep Med.* 2002;3(5):427–430.

48. Bucher S, Seelos K, Oertel W, et al. Cerebral generators involved in the pathogenesis of the restless legs syndrome. *Ann Neurol.* 1997;41(5):639–645.

49. Desautels A, Turecki G, Montplaisir J, et al. Identification of a major susceptibility locus for restless legs syndrome on chromosome 12q. *Amer J Hum Genet.* 2001;69(6):1266–1270.

50. Bonati MT, Ferini-Strambi L, Aridon P, et al. Autosomal dominant restless legs syndrome maps on chromosome 14q. *Brain.* 2003;126(Pt 6):1485–1492.

51. Desautels A, Turecki G, Montplaisir J, et al. Dopaminergic neurotransmission and restless legs syndrome: a genetic association analysis. *Neurology.* 2001;57(7):1304–1306.

52. Desautels A, Turecki G, Montplaisir J, et al. Evidence for a genetic association between monoamine oxidase A and restless legs syndrome. *Neurology.* 2002;59(2):215–219.

53. Turjanski N, Lees AJ, Brooks DJ. Striatal dopaminergic function in restless legs syndrome: 18F-dopa and 11C-raclopride PET studies. *Neurology.* 1999;52(5):932–937.

54. Eisensehr I, Wetter TC, Linke R, et al. Normal IPT and IBZM SPECT in drug-naive and levodopa-treated idiopathic restless legs syndrome. *Neurology.* 2001;57(7):1307–1309.

55. Michaud M, Soucy JP, Chabli A, et al. SPECT imaging of striatal pre- and postsynaptic dopaminergic status in restless legs syndrome with periodic leg movements in sleep. *J Neurol.* 2002;249(2):164–170.

56. Ruottinen HM, Partinen M, Hublin C, et al. An FDOPA PET study in patients with periodic limb movement disorder and restless legs syndrome. *Neurology.* 2000;54(2):502–504.

57. Earley CJ, Hyland K, Allen RP. CSF dopamine, serotonin, and biopterin metabolites in patients with restless legs syndrome. *Move Disorders.* 2001;16(1):144–149.

58. Earley CJ, Connor JR, Beard JL, et al. Abnormalities in CSF concentrations of ferritin and transferrin in restless legs syndrome. *Neurology.* 2000;54(8):1698–1700.

59. Allen RP, Barker PB, Wehrl F, et al. MRI measurement of brain iron in patients with restless legs syndrome. *Neurology.* 2001;56(2):263–265.

60. Connor JR, Boyer PJ, Menzies SL, et al. Neuropathological examination suggests impaired brain iron acquisition in restless legs syndrome. *Neurology.* 2003;61:304–309.

61. Connor JR, Wang X, Patton S, et al. Decreased transferrin receptor expression in restless legs syndrome: a putative mechanism. *Neurology.* 2004;62(9):1563–1567.

62. Hening W, Allen RP, Thanner S, et al. The Johns Hopkins telephone diagnostic interview for the restless legs syndrome: preliminary investigation for validation in a multi-center patient and control population. *Sleep Med.* 2003;4(2):137–141.

63. Allen RP, Earley CJ. Validation of the Johns Hopkins Restless Legs Severity Scale (JHRLSS). *Sleep Med.* 2001;2:239–242.

64. The International Restless Legs Syndrome Study Group. Validation of the International Restless Legs Syndrome Study Group rating scale for restless legs syndrome. *Sleep Med.* 2003;4(2):121–132.

65. Hening WA, Allen RP. Restless legs syndrome (RLS): the continuing development of diagnostic standards and severity measures. *Sleep Med.* 2003;4(2):95–97.

66. Allen RP, Kushida CA, Atkinson MJ. Factor analysis of the International Restless Legs Syndrome Study Group's scale for restless legs severity. *Sleep Med.* 2003;4(2):133–135.

67. Chesson AL, Jr., Wise M, Davila D, et al. Practice parameters for the treatment of restless legs syndrome and periodic limb movement

disorder: an American Academy of Sleep Medicine report. Standards of Practice Committee of the American Academy of Sleep Medicine. *Sleep.* 1999;22(7):961–968.

68. Akpinar S. Restless legs syndrome treatment with dopaminergic drugs. *Clin Neuropharmacol.* 1987;10(1):69–79.
69. Benes H, Kurella B, Kummer J, et al. Rapid onset of action of levodopa in restless legs syndrome: a double-blind, randomized, multicenter, crossover trial. *Sleep.* 1999;22(8):1073–1081.
70. Brodeur C, Montplaisir J, Godbout R, et al. Treatment of restless legs syndrome and periodic movements during sleep with L-dopa: a double-blind, controlled study. *Neurology.* 1988;38(12):1845–1848.
71. Saletu M, Anderer P, Hogl B, et al. Acute double-blind, placebo-controlled sleep laboratory and clinical follow-up studies with a combination treatment of rr-L-dopa and sr-L-dopa in restless legs syndrome. *J Neural Trans.* 2003;110(6):611–626.
72. Walters AS, Hening WA, Kavey N, et al. A double-blind randomized crossover trial of bromocriptine and placebo in restless legs syndrome. *Ann Neurol.* 1988;24(3):455–458.
73. Trenkwalder C, Brandenburg U, Hundemer H, et al. A randomized long-term placebo-controlled multicenter trial of pergolide in the treatment of restless legs syndrome with central evaluation of polysomnographic data. *Neurology.* 2001;56(8 suppl 3):A5.
74. Wetter TC, Stiasny K, Winkelmann J, et al. A randomized controlled study of pergolide in patients with restless legs syndrome. *Neurology.* 1999;52(5):944–950.
75. Earley CJ, Yaffee JB, Allen RP. Randomized, double-blind, placebo-controlled trial of pergolide in restless legs syndrome. *Neurology.* 1998;51(6):1599–1602.
76. Saletu M, Anderer P, Saletu-Zyhlarz G, et al. Acute placebo-controlled sleep laboratory studies and clinical follow-up with pramipexole in restless legs syndrome. *Eur Arch Psych. Clin Neurosci.* 2002;252(4):185–194.
77. Montplaisir J, Nicolas A, Denesle R, et al. Restless legs syndrome improved by pramipexole: a double-blind randomized trial. *Neurology.* 1999;52(5):938–943.
78. Moller JC, Stiasny K, Benes H, et al. Rotigotine CDS (constant delivery system) in the treatment of moderate to advanced stages of restless legs syndrome—A double-blind placebo-controlled pilot study. *Sleep.* 2003;26:A340.
79. Saletu B, Gruber G, Saletu M, et al. Sleep laboratory studies in restless legs syndrome patients as compared with normals and acute effects of ropinirole. 1. Findings on objective and subjective sleep and awakening quality. *Neuropsychobiology.* 2000;41(4):181–189.
80. Freeman A, Rye D, Bliwise DL, et al. Ropinirole forrestless legs syndrome (RLS): an open-label and double-blind placebo-controlled study. *Neurology.* 2001;56(8 suppl. 3):A5.
81. Allen RP, Becker P, Bogan R, et al. Restless legs syndrome: the efficacy of ropinirole in the treatment of RLS patients suffering from periodic leg movements of sleep. *Sleep.* 2003;26:A341.
82. Walters A, Ondo W, Sethi K, et al. Ropinirole versus placebo in the treatment of restless legs syndrome (RLS): A 12-week multicenter double-blind placebo-controlled study conducted in 6 countries. *Sleep.* 2003;26:A344.
83. Garcia-Borreguero D, Montagna P, Trenkwalder C, et al. Ropinirole is effective in the treatment of restless legs syndrome (RLS): a double-blind placebo-controlled 12-week study conducted in 10 countries. *Neurology.* 2003;60(suppl. 1):A11–12.
84. Walters AS, Wagner ML, Hening WA, et al. Successful treatment of the idiopathic restless legs syndrome in a randomized double-blind trial of oxycodone versus placebo. *Sleep.* 1993;16(4):327–332.
85. Lundvall O, Abom PE, Holm R. Carbamazepine in restless legs. A controlled pilot study. *Eur J Clin Pharmacol.* 1983;25(3):323–324.
86. Telstad W, Sorensen O, Larsen S, et al. Treatment of the restless legs syndrome with carbamazepine: a double blind study. *BMJ.* 1984;288(6415):444–446.
87. Burchell BJ. Treatment of restless legs syndrome with gabapentin: A double-blind, crossover study. *Neurology.* 2003;60(9):1558.
88. Garcia-Borreguero D, Larrosa O, de la Llave Y, et al. Treatment of restless legs syndrome with gabapentin: a double-blind, cross-over study. *Neurology.* 2002;59(10):1573–1579.

89. Saletu M, Anderer P, Saletu-Zyhlarz G, et al. Restless legs syndrome (RLS) and periodic limb movement disorder (PLMD): acute placebo-controlled sleep laboratory studies with clonazepam. *Eur Neuropsychopharmacol.* 2001;11(2):153–161.
90. Boghen D, Lamothe L, Elie R, et al. The treatment of the restless legs syndrome with clonazepam: a prospective controlled study. *Can J Neurol Sci.* 1986;13(3):245–247.
91. Wetter TC, Brunner J, Bronisch T. Restless legs syndrome probably induced by risperidone treatment. *Pharmacopsychiatry.* 2002;35(3):109–111.
92. O'Keeffe ST, Gavin K, Lavan JN. Iron status and restless legs syndrome in the elderly. *Age Ageing.* 1994;23(3):200–203.
93. Allen RP, Earley CJ. Augmentation of the restless legs syndrome with carbidopa/levodopa. *Sleep.* 1996;19(3):205–213.
94. Silber MH, Shepard JW, Jr., Wisbey JA. Pergolide in the management of restless legs syndrome: an extended study. *Sleep.* 1997;20(10):878–882.
95. Walters AS, Winkelmann J, Trenkwalder C, et al. Long-term follow-up on restless legs syndrome patients treated with opioids. *Move Disorders.* 2001;16(6):1105–1109.
96. Earley CJ. Restless legs syndrome. *N Engl J Med.* 2003;348:2103–2109.
97. Symonds CP. Nocturnal myiclonus. *J Neurol Neurosurg Psychiatr.* 1953(16):166–171.
98. Diagnostic Classification Steering Committee of ASDA. *The international classification of sleep disorders.* Revised edn. Rochester: American Sleep Disorders Association, 1997.
99. Atlas Task Force of the American Sleep Disorders Association. Recording and scoring leg movements. *Sleep.* 1993;16(8):748–759.
100. Plazzi G, Vetrugno R, Meletti S, et al. Motor pattern of periodic limb movements in sleep in idiopathic RLS patients. *Sleep Med.* 2002;(3 Suppl):S31–S34.
101. Provini F, Vetrugno R, Meletti S, et al. Motor pattern of periodic limb movements during sleep. *Neurology.* 2001;57(2):300–304.
102. Michaud M, Poirier G, Lavigne G, et al. Restless legs syndrome: scoring criteria for leg movements recorded during the suggested immobilization test. *Sleep Med.* 2001;2(4):317–321.
103. IM Systems. PAM-RL Manual. Baltimore, Maryland: IM Systems, 2003.
104. Nicolas A, Michaud M, Lavigne G, et al. The influence of sex, age and sleep/wake state on characteristics of periodic leg movements in restless legs syndrome patients. *Clin Neurophysiol.* 1999;110(7):1168–1174.
105. Ancoli-Israel S, Kripke DF, Klauber MR, et al. Periodic limb movements in sleep in community dwelling elderly. *Sleep.* 1991;14:496–500.
106. Sforza E, Juony C, Ibanez V. Time-dependent variation in cerebral and autonomic activity during periodic leg movements in sleep: implications for arousal mechanisms. *Clin Neurophysiol.* 2002;113(6):883–891.
107. Sforza E, Nicolas A, Lavigne G, et al. EEG and cardiac activation during periodic leg movements in sleep: Support for a hierarchy of arousal responses. *Neurology.* 1999;52(4):786–791.
108. Ali NJ, Davies RJ, Fleetham JA, et al. Periodic movements of the legs during sleep associated with rises in systemic blood pressure. *Sleep.* 1991;14(2):163–165.
109. Gosselin N, Lanfranchi P, Michaud M, et al. Age and gender effects on heart rate activation associated with periodic leg movements in patients with restless legs syndrome. *Clin Neurophysiol.* 2003;114(11):2188–2195.
110. Fantini ML, Michaud M, Gosselin N, et al. Periodic leg movements in REM sleep behavior disorder and related autonomic and EEG activation. *Neurology.* 2002;59(12):1889–1894.
111. Gupta P, Hening W, Rahman K, et al. Periodic limb movements (PLMs) in a patient with multiple sclerosis and central sleep apnea: independent right and left leg movement periods suggest lateralized PLM oscillators. *Sleep Res.* 1996;25:417.
112. Fry JM, DiPhillipo MA, Pressman MR. Periodic leg movements in sleep following treatment of obstructive sleep apnea with nasal continuous positive airway pressure. *Chest.* 1989;96(1):89–91.
113. Dickel MJ, Renfrow SD, Moore PT, et al. Rapid eye movement sleep

periodic leg movements in patients with spinal cord injury. *Sleep.* 1994;17(8):733–738.

114. Tayag-Kier CE, Keenan GF, Scalzi LV, et al. Sleep and periodic limb movement in sleep in juvenile fibromyalgia. *Pediatrics.* 2000;106(5):E70.

115. Wetter TC, Collado-Seidel V, Pollmacher T, et al. Sleep and periodic leg movement patterns in drug-free patients with Parkinson's disease and multiple system atrophy. *Sleep.* 2000;23(3):361–367.

116. Hartman PG, Scrima L. Muscle activity in the legs (MAL) associated with frequent arousals in narcoleptics, nocturnal myoclonus and obstructive sleep apnea (OSA) patients. *Clin Electroencephalogr.* 1986;17(4):181–186.

117. Montplaisir J, Michaud M, Denesle R, et al. Periodic leg movements are not more prevalent in insomnia or hypersomnia but are specifically associated with sleep disorders involving a dopaminergic impairment. *Sleep Med.* 2000;1(2):163–167.

Chapter 16

Parasomnias

Juan G. Ochoa and Mario Pulido

INTRODUCTION

Parasomnias are one of the most intriguing sleep disorders to be depicted in famous literary publications. Shakespeare used many sleep disorders in his characters including somnambulism, sleep apnea, insomnia, and nightmares (1). Parasomnias are abnormal events occurring in association with sleep, specific stages of sleep, or sleep–awake transition phases. They may be characterized by violent or subtle motor activity, autonomic or behavioral phenomena that may cause partial or full awakening, or disturbances of sleep–stage transition (2).

Behaviors arising from sleep may result in violent or even fatal consequences; sometimes these accidental deaths may be confused with suicide (3). Although they cause disruption of normal sleep pattern, parasomnias are not associated with an intrinsic abnormality of the sleep cycle.

Parasomnias were originally considered a form of epilepsy because of the sudden activation of behavior and amnesia of the episode. It was not until 1965 that Broughton and Gastaut differentiated parasomnias as nonepileptic events. Nocturnal frontal lobe epilepsy (NFLE) is particularly similar to parasomnia, and the differential diagnosis may sometimes be difficult. In general, in parasomnias onset is in early childhood, with rare episodes of long duration, absence of stereotypy, and general disappearance after puberty. In NFLE, onset is between the age of 10 and 20, with frequently complex and stereotyped behaviors of short duration, nocturnal agitation, daytime fatigue or sleepiness, and persistence into adulthood (Table 16-1). Paroxysmal arousals, nocturnal paroxysmal dystonia, and nocturnal wandering has been considered as a manifestation of nocturnal frontal lobe epilepsy. Some cases have been reported to have a possible temporal lobe origin (4,5).

The pathophysiology of parasomnias is unknown. It has been presumed to be a disturbance of the mechanisms that regulate the transition and maintenance of the different states,—wakefulness, REM, and NREM sleep—causing a

▶ **TABLE 16-1.** Differential Diagnosis between Parasomnias and Nocturnal Frontal Lobe Epilepsy

	Parasomnia	*NFLE*
Onset (years)	3–6	10–20
Frequency (per month)	1–4	>20
Clinical semeiology	Polymorphic	Stereotyped
Course	Disappear with age	Increase or stable
Sleep relationship	First third of the night	Anytime
Sleep state	2 and NREM	3,4, NREM, and REM
Interictal EEG	Normal	50% Abnormal
Duration	Minutes	<Than a minute

dissociation of the wake and sleep neuronal network activity. The pathophysiology of the parasomnias varies significantly according to the wake–sleep state of occurrence; for example, occurrence of REM sleep during wakefulness results in cataplexy, whereas NREM sleep activity during the awake state produces microsleeps; arousal disorders typically occur during slow-wave sleep (SWS).

Some parasomnias involve violent muscle activity, while others are characterized by significant autonomic events. There is a significant variability of events and a wide degree of severity, some of which may be considered as normal because of a very rare recurrence and frequent incidence in an otherwise normal population (6). They may overlap in the same patient and may be associated with other conditions, such as Parkinson's disease (PD), cerebrovascular disease, and psychiatric disorders. Children with parasomnia frequently (more than one-half) have a diagnosis of an additional sleep disorder, partic-

ularly sleep-disordered breathing (SDB) and restless legs syndrome (RLS).

According to DSM-IV, parasomnias are classified in four groups: (1) nightmare disorder, (2) sleep terror disorder, (3) sleepwalking disorder, and (4) parasomnias not otherwise specified.

However, for better understanding of the pathophysiology, we will refer to a classification of parasomnias according to the association of the occurrence in relation to the wake–sleep cycle as presented in The International Classification of Sleep Disorders: (1) sleep–wake transition disorders, (2) arousal disorders, (3) parasomnias associated with REM, and (4) other parasomnias (Table 16-2).

SLEEP–WAKE TRANSITION DISORDERS

The sleep–wake transition disorders are benign, very common events that occur during the transition from wake to sleep state or vice versa; they may be regarded as normal phenomena and are usually present in otherwise healthy populations. Occasionally, these events may occur frequently enough to cause disruption of the normal sleep cycle and may create discomfort or be associated with injuries or anxiety. Mild cases are usually untreated, however, severe cases may warrant treatment. They are more common in young children (6 months to 4 years), and males (about four times), and usually resolve spontaneously.

There are four different sleep–wake transition disorders: rhythmic movement disorder, sleep start, sleep talking, and nocturnal leg cramps.

Rhythmic Movement Disorder

Also called stereotypic movement disorder, this a disorder typically found in children. It is characterized by rhythmic

▶ **TABLE 16-2.** Classification of Parasomnias and ICD Code

Sleep–Wake Transition Disorder	*Arousal Disorders*	*REM Parasomnias*	*Other*
Rhythmic movement disorder (307.3)	Confusional arousals (307.46-2)	REM sleep behavior disorder (780.59-0)	Sleep bruxism (306.8)
Nocturnal leg cramps (729.82)	Sleep terrors (307.46-1)	REM sleep-related sinus arrest (780.56-8)	Sleep enuresis (788.36-0)
Sleep talking (307.47-3)	Sleepwalking (307.46-0)	Nightmares (307.47-0)	Sleep-related abnormal swallowing (780.56-6)
Sleep starts (307.47-2)		Sleep paralysis (780.56-2)	Nocturnal paroxysmal dystonia (780.59-1)
		Impaired sleep-related erections (780.56-3)	Sudden nocturnal death syndrome (780.59-3)
		Sleep-related painful erections (780.56-4)	Sudden infant death syndrome (798.0)
			Primary snoring (786.09)
			Infant sleep apnea (770.80)
			Benign neonatal myoclonus (780.59)

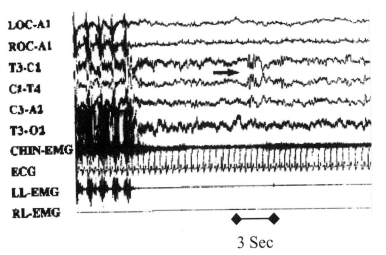

HEAD BANGING

3 Sec

FIGURE 16-1. Polysomnogram of head banging episodes represented by rhythmic EMG artifacts at the beginning of the figure. Note the presence of normal sleep stage 2, characterized by K complex and spindles (arrow) after the event.

movements in the head and neck or large muscle groups, occurring with a frequency of 0.5 to 2 Hz, which can persist for a few minutes to many hours and may occur almost nightly. They may appear in all sleep stages, but tend to be more common during sleep stage 1 and 2 (see Fig. 16-1). Head banging (jactacio capitis nocturna) typically occurs with the patient in supine position and is characterized by anteroposterior head movements.

This disorder is called head banging because frequently the child bangs his head against the pillow or the headboard. Body rocking movements are associated with anteroposterior body movements occurring in different body positions. Other movement includes rocking on hands and knees. These movements may result in soft tissue injury and, rarely, eye trauma, hemoglobinuria, internal carotid artery dissection, and subdural hemorrhage. Rhythmic activity during sleep is seen in up to 67% of normal infants and decreases to 6% by the age of 5 years. The average onset is 9 months and commonly subsides before 10 years of age. Patients with mental retardation or autism persist longer, but up to 20% of normal children persist with rhythmic movements after 10 years of age.

The pathophysiology is unknown. It has been hypothesized that the rocking movements help development of the vestibulo-ocular and vestibulospinal reflexes to improve overall motor development. Diagnosis of rhythmic movement disorder by history alone is difficult since the clinical description is similar to other sleep disorders, seizures, or psychogenic events. Even with video electroencephographic (EEG) monitoring, frontal lobe seizures may be hard to differentiate since they frequently have multiple movement artifacts that obscure the EEG. A combination of clinical features and video EEG monitoring or polysomnography (PSG) offers the best diagnostic yield (see Fig. 16-1). Differential diagnosis includes seizures, tantrums, and night terrors (7,8).

Often there is no need for treatment other than reassurance. Frequently, there is spontaneous resolution as children get older. Benzodiazepines and tricyclic antidepressants have been used with variable success. Behavior modification has had little success. Protection of the sleep environment is essential to prevent injuries.

Nocturnal Leg Cramps

Nocturnal leg cramps occur spontaneously during sleep, typically in the calf. No particular sleep state has been associated this disorder. The pathophysiology is unknown and last up to 30 minutes. Cramps may be precipitated by changes in water and electrolyte homoeostasis or by drugs, such as diuretics, laxatives, beta2 agonists, cimetidine, and phenothiazines. The cramp frequency varies from sporadic to daily occurrences. Sleep is disrupted by this sudden painful cramp (9).

Treatment is recommended according to frequency and severity of events. Multiple treatments are available (Table 16-3). Quinine can effectively prevent nocturnal leg cramps, however, it is also associated with significant side

▶ **TABLE 16-3. Treatment of Nocturnal Leg Cramps**

Treatment	Efficacy	Comment
Quinine	Good data supporting efficacy	Significant side effects
Verapamil	Effective in small well-designed studies	Well tolerated
Diltiazem	Better than placebo, probably as effective as verapamil	Well tolerated
Vitamins B and E	Limited controlled data	Safe and well tolerated
Magnesium	Good data in pregnancy	Besides diarrhea, is well tolerated
Gabapentin	Anecdotal	Safe

effects. Calcium-channel blockers have been effective, particularly verapamil and diltiazem. Interestingly, nifedipine has been found to worsen the cramps. Although verapamil, diltiazem, and nifedipine block the L-type calcium channel, nifedipine appears to elicit stronger reflex adrenergic stimulation, activating T-type calcium channels and neutralizing the calcium channel blockade. Magnesium has been used for years to treat cramps in pregnancy and appears to be effective in nonpregnant patients as well. Vitamins B and E have been reported to be effective in reducing the frequency and severity of leg cramps. The author has seen anecdotal improvement of the cramps with gabapentin. All these treatments are much better tolerated than quinine and have less serious potential side effects. Therefore, they are recommended first. There is an increasing number of reports of side effects including pancytopenia, cinchonism, and visual toxicity with the use of quinine. A combination of quinine and aminophylline has showed significant benefit for difficult-to-control patients (9–12).

Sleep Talking

Sleep talking (somniloquy) is characterized by verbal output during sleep. One the most famous literary examples of sleep talking is the episode of Lady Macbeth by Shakespeare (1). The talking is sometimes brief or incoherent but occasionally could be long and associated with anger. Sometimes the sleep talking occurs spontaneously, or it could be elicited by talking with the sleeper. It is frequently associated with other parasomnias, such as sleepwalking and confusional arousals. In fact, both in children and adults, sleeptalking is the parasomnia that has been found to co-occur most frequently with other parasomnias. Emotional stress, concomitant illness, sleep apnea, or sleep terrors can precipitate this phenomenon. Sleep talk is usually harmless and does not require treatment. However, bedpartners or family members can be disturbed.

Sleep Starts

Sleep starts or hypnic jerks are common phenomena that occur when the person is just falling asleep; these are characterized by sudden, brief contractions of muscles in the extremities or head lasting from 75 to 250 milliseconds. Also called hypnagogic jerks, they are considered normal physiologic events, although they are poorly understood. Sleep starts mainly involve lower extremities but may also involve the arms and head, with asymmetric single jerks, or asynchronous or massive body movements. Movements may be associated with vivid dreams or hallucinations.

Motor starts are the most common, but visual or auditory sleep start may also occur (a sensation of blinding light coming from inside the eyes or a loud snapping noise that seems to come from inside the head). These sensory phenomena may occur without motor jerk or may precede the body jerk. Although the sensation from sleep starts can be frightening, these occurrences are harmless. Sleep starts can be exacerbated by sensory stimuli, excessive exercise, stress, sleep deprivation, and use of stimulants.

The presumed mechanism involved with this activity is a sudden activation of the mesencephalic reticular-activating system, which is supported by the presence of a brief arousal or wakefulness after the movement. A dissociation between REM and motor inhibition is also postulated. Sometimes it is triggered when the individual is sleeping in a different position than usual, for example, a back sleeper who has fallen asleep on his stomach. They vary in intensity, but when they are strong or very frequent, disrupt wake–sleep transition and lead to insomnia. Flurazepam has been reported to improve sleep starts (13).

Arousal Disorders

The arousal disorders are very frequent parasomnias. It has been reported that up to 50% of children have experienced one of these events during childhood (14). There are three types of arousal disorders according to the International Classification of Sleep Disorders, confusional arousals, sleep terrors, and sleepwalking. They are characterized by behavioral events that occur during SWS. They occur mainly during childhood and some of them, particularly sleep terror and sleepwalking episodes, are disturbing to parents. They tend to improve with age and typically disappear after puberty or in young adulthood.

Sleepwalking may lead to accidents and self-injury. It has been hypothesized that these disorders occur because of incomplete arousal due to disturbed physiologic mechanisms of arousal. SWS fragmentation is the most common finding on polysomnographic (PSG) studies; PSG has also shown that these parasomnias occur more frequently in the first sleep cycle during SWS. There is a hypersynchronous high voltage slow-wave (1 $\pm$ 3 Hz) activity lasting up to 30 s, preceding the behavior activation (Jacobson et al., 1965). Frequent SWS interruptions by stage 0 have been found in these patients, demonstrating a chronic inability to sustain deep sleep (15,16).

The patients may experience a variety of behaviors associated with mental confusion and disorientation. Most of these patients have no memory of the events, but they may remember fragments or vague impressions of the behavior. They are relatively nonreactive to external stimuli and usually are not stereotypic, thus facilitating differential diagnosis from epileptic seizures.

Confusional Arousal

Confusional arousals occur following an attempt to awaken the patient from deep sleep, typically during the first part of the night. Sometimes this disorder is called excessive sleep inertia or sleep drunkenness. These patients react slowly to commands, may have difficulty understanding what they are asked and often they have problems with short-term memory. Patients with this disorder have very exaggerated slowness, which typically occurs when the individual is awakened from a deep sleep.

These events are very predictable, occurring frequently about 1 hour after going to bed, and are present most commonly when a child is overtired. Other conditions that may trigger these events include stuffy nose, sleep apnea, fever, sore throat, or ear infection. Complete awakenings commonly occur (child goes to the parents' room at 2:00 AM every night) and may trigger incomplete arousals early in the night that may lead either to confusional arousal or sleepwalking. Behavioral management preventing the late awakening may prevent development of early night arousal disorders. If the child has multiple events in one night, he may have events close to the morning; however, those events tend to be milder than early night ones. The behavior may resemble a temper tantrum.

Confusional arousals start slowly with gradual worsening of the behavior progressing to crying, sitting, and thrashing, which lasts from 5 to 15 minutes and, only rarely, may last up to 45 minutes. Attempting to awaken the child is typically unsuccessful. Confusional arousals are commonly seen in patients with other types of arousal disorders. Night terrors can be differentiated from confusional arousals by their abrupt onset instead of the typical gradual occurrence seen in the latter. In school-aged children, confusional arousal behavior may be related to high stress situations in a rather quiet and well-behaved child, probably as repressed feelings. Worsening of daytime behavior and control of emotions have been observed to reduce the occurrence of arousal events (17).

Treatment is very seldom needed. In severe cases, clonazepam given for a short term is very effective, and rarely is long-term therapy necessary.

Night Terrors and Sleepwalking

Sleep terrors are characterized by sudden, terrified screaming associated with an intense autonomic component (tachycardia, tachypnea, diaphoresis, and mydriasis) occurring mainly during childhood. There is disorientation and confusion upon awakening, usually without memory of the event. Often the affected individual sits upright with eyes open, not responding to other people. They may mumble or scream and parents typically describe terrified facial expressions and inability to be consoled. Children typically do not have memory of the event, but adults may partially remember the behavior and have a dreamlike feeling that usually involves a threat by imminent danger, running away from snakes, spider, monsters, etc.

Sleep terrors may be more common in males, and occur in about 3% of children and 1% of adults. Investigation of twin cohorts and families with sleep terror and sleepwalking has suggested a genetic factor (14). PSG is an excellent diagnostic test for this disorder. An abnormally low delta wave electroencephalogram (EEG) and frequent,

brief, EEG-defined arousals not associated with clinical wakefulness have been reported.

The sleepwalking events are characterized by sudden automatic behaviors including wandering around the house, sitting in bed, moving objects around, eating, urinating in closets, or going outdoors. A complex activity, such as driving an automobile, is possible, but rare. Patients are easily stopped by adding a new lock or leaving the keys in a different location. Sleepwalkers are not conscious and, therefore, do not communicate well with others during the event; they usually mumble.

Although sleepwalkers rarely fall down familiar stairs, they need to be kept clear of obstacles; walking at dangerous heights or near sharp objects may result in serious injury. Awakening sleepwalkers should be avoided, since it may cause them to be very confused; in fact, confusional arousals are very frequent in these patients. Sleepwalkers typically go back to bed by themselves. Episodes of sleepwalking usually occur 15 minutes to 2 hours after sleep onset. The prevalence of sleepwalking has been estimated to be about 15% in children and 4% to 10% in adults (14). There is no sex preference for sleepwalking not associated with injuries, but injurious sleepwalking is more predominant in males.

Functional studies with single proton emission tomography (PET) during sleepwalking have shown activation of the cerebellum and the posterior cingulate cortex and deactivation of the parietal and frontal association cortex, including the dorsolateral prefrontal cortex, mesial frontal cortex, and left angular gyrus, typically seen in normal awake walking individuals (Fig. 16-2) (18).

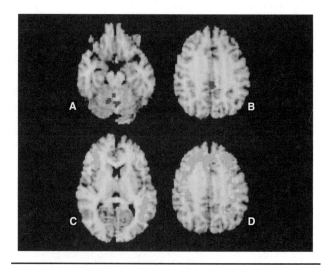

FIGURE 16-2. SPECT findings during sleepwalking after magnetic resonance imaging (MRI) correlation. (A) Anterior cerebellum activation. (B) Posterior cingulate cortex. (C) and (D) Dorsolateral prefrontal cortex, mesial frontal cortex, and parietal cortex. (From Guilleminault C. Sleepwalking and sleep terrors in prepubertal children: What triggers them? *Pediatrics.* 2003:111(1). With permission.)

▶ **TABLE 16-4.** Differential Diagnosis of Night Terrors and Nightmares

	Sleep Terrors	*Nightmares*
Age	3–8 years	Any age
Sleep cycle	NREM	REM
Gender predominance	Male	None
Memory for event	None	Yes
Aroused	No	Yes
Exacerbated by stress	Yes	Yes

Although sleepwalking and sleep terrors are two different clinical events, they may sometimes be hard to differentiate in adults because screaming can be confused with angry shouting and seeking safety with walking during the episode. Children affected by sleepwalking and sleep terrors usually have complete amnesia about such events. There are several risk factors associated with this disorder, including those associated with drugs, such as lithium carbonate, olanzapine, bupropion, zolpidem, and anticholinergics. Stress and trauma have been implicated as well (19–23).

Other sleep disorders, such as SDB and restless legs syndrome (RSL) have been associated with an increased incidence of these parasomnias. Furthermore, the improvement of the underlying sleep disorder was found to correlate with improvement of the parasomnias as well. Psychiatric disorders, including psychologic trauma, are not a common cause. Nightmares are sometimes confused with sleep terrors, but in the later there is usually complete memory of the dream (Table 16-4).

Occasionally, frontal lobe epilepsy may present clinically as nocturnal terrors, differentiated by stereotyped events, daytime events, response to antiepileptic drugs, and abnormal EEG. PSG or video EEG monitoring are excellent tools to differentiate these disorders. Proper and prompt diagnosis is essential for better management and assessment of prognosis (17,24). The indications for obtaining polysomnographic studies are summarized in Table 16-5.

▶ **TABLE 16-5.** Indications for Polysomnography in Patients with Parasomnias

Indications for Polysomnography	*Reason*
Semeiology	Stereotyped, seizurelike event
Severity	Violent, potentially injurious
Time of occurrence	Toward morning
Duration and frequency	Long lasting, frequent
Therapy	If needed or not responding to therapy
Legal	Forensic evaluation requested

Treatment

Sleepwalking and sleep terrors, especially in children, usually do not require pharmacologic treatment. However, identifying and controlling factors for potential risk of injury is warranted. Scheduled awakenings have been used as an intervention for parasomnias and appear to be effective, according to some reports, but there is insufficient data to support effectiveness; parents are instructed to wake the child 15–30 minutes prior to an expected partial arousal event.

Adult patients and children with high-risk sleep-related injury may require pharmacotherapy. Chronic treatment with benzodiazepines has been found to be very effective in adults with sleepwalking, sleep terrors, and other parasomnias. Benzodiazepines are usually well tolerated, with a low incidence of side effects and risk of abuse. Clonazepam, 0.25 to 1.5 mg taken 1 hour before sleep onset, is usually effective. Other drugs used include alprazolam, diazepam, imipramine hydrochloride, and paroxetine hydrochloride. Use of self-hypnosis techniques can be effective in milder cases in both adults and children (25).

PARASOMNIAS DURING RAPID EYE MOVEMENT SLEEP

Nightmares

Nightmares are vivid dreams occurring during REM sleep usually resulting in the individual awaking from the dream. They usually occur during the second half of the night to early morning, when REM is more common. Characteristically, the imagery and concomitant emotions are very frightening and often threaten an individual's sense of security while resting and/or awakening. Nightmares should be differentiated from other non-REM (NREM) sleep disorders, such as sleep terrors and sleep panic attacks.

Sleep terrors, also called pavor nocturnes, generally occur during the first half of the sleeping period and present with the child awakening and screaming; this is accompanied by autonomic symptoms, such as profuse sweating and an elevated heart and respiratory rate. Following these features, the individual is usually difficult to arouse and has a difficult time recollecting the event by the next morning. Traditionally, when an individual initially awakens from experiencing a nightmare, he or she has a clear recollection of the details surrounding the unpleasant features of the dream, thus differentiating it from the above-mentioned NREM sleep disorders.

The onset of nightmares is commonly around ages 4 to 6 years old. A peak in frequency and intensity until approximately age 10 to 12 years typically follows, leading some authors to believe this is a natural component of REM sleep development. It is difficult to assess the severity of an individual's nightmares since there is subjective interpretation of their significance, as well as variability in the individual personalities that may play a role in the susceptibility to stimuli, including specific fears, concerns, or stressful triggers. For example, an individual who is naturally anxious would describe his or her nightmares as being more often and/or of worse intensity. By the same token, an individual without a predisposition to anxiety might not subjectively complain of the frequency or nature of their nightmares (26,27).

The diagnostic criteria for nightmare disorder according to the DSM-IV are as follows:

1. Repeated awakening from the major sleep periods or naps with detailed recall of extended and extremely frightening dreams, usually involving threats to survival, security, or self-esteem; the awakening generally occurs during the second half of the sleep period.
2. On awakening from the frightening dreams, the person rapidly becomes oriented and alert.
3. The dream experience or sleep disturbance resulting from the awakening causes clinically significant distress or impairment in social, occupational, or other important areas of functioning.
4. The disorder does not occur exclusively in the course of another mental disorder and is not due to the direct physiologic effects of a substance or a general medical population.

The epidemiology surrounding the incidence of nightmares in adults varies depending on the clinical trials. It is believed that, in the adult population, nightmares are more common in women than in men. There is also a direct correlation between nightmares and psychiatric or psychosocial disorders.

Dissociative disorders, acute stress disorder, and post-traumatic stress disorder (PTSD) are frequently portrayed by continuous and repetitive nightmares following the acute event. In fact, nightmares are oftentimes the chief complaint of victims with PTSD and are the mainstay of management and intervention. These nightmares may subject an individual to have vivid memories of the traumatic event on a nightly, weekly, or monthly basis and may persist for years. For obvious reasons, this commonly causes significant distress for the individual. The relationship between nightmares and elevated levels of distress and anxiety has been proposed and followed closely in clinical trials since the 1970s.

Nightmares also have played a role in major depressive disorder. Reports by these patients show an increase in the frequency of their nightmares during exacerbations of their illness, while appropriate management of the depression with pharmacotherapy and proper counseling results in a decrease in the incidence of nightmares. Social problems, such as alcohol or substance abuse, also have a strong correlation with nightmares. Similar to psychologic and psychiatric conditions, these patients also report a decrease in their symptoms with appropriate therapy (28).

The treatment of nightmares has centered on cognitive–behavior therapy. Although commonly challenging for the individual, imagery rehearsal and desensitization are very effective in managing the patient's concerns. Effective interventions such as these assist in decreasing the anxiety that accompanies repetitive nightmares and subsequent sleep loss and contribute to an overall improvement in the patient's health (29).

Rapid Eye Movement Sleep Behavior Disorders

REM sleep in humans is characterized by increased electrical activity measured by EEG readings, rapid eye movement, and generalized muscle atonia. The latter is due to a suppression of muscle tone despite the elevated level of brain activity, thereby typifying this pattern as paradoxic sleep.

The mechanism by which authors have described this phenomenon is by an intrinsic regulation on behalf of the pontine nuclei near the locus ceruleus; this occurs by hyperpolarization of the alpha-motoneurons, resulting in subsequent muscle atonia. This mechanism was initially described in animal models after demonstrating that in cats with specific pontine lesions, there was a reproducible loss of REM sleep-induced atonia. This model has since been extrapolated to humans and manifests as a variety of abnormal sleep behaviors.

REM sleep-behavior disorder (RBD) is the loss of sub-cortical regulation of REM sleep atonia and generally involves skeletal muscle activity. In essence, the loss of normal REM activity allows one to "act out" their dreams. The normal hyperpolarized state of the neurons is lost and behaviors such as punching, yelling, swearing, kicking, screaming, grabbing, talking, running, crawling, and jumping out of bed are commonly described. This is clinically significant, as one might hurt themselves and/or their partner during sleep. This phenomenon may only occur while the individual is in REM sleep, making this behavior more common in the latter one-half of the night.

RBD is more common in men than in women and generally has a later onset in life, with the majority of the cases presenting after the age of 50. In recent years, studies have demonstrated a significant correlation between idiopathic RBD and neurodegenerative disorders, such as Parkinson's disease, Lewy body dementia, and multiple-system atrophy. These conditions are also termed *synucleinopathies*, since they all contain intracellular inclusion bodies containing alpha-synuclein. The association between these clinical entities and RBD lies in the decreased amount of neurotransmitters that accompanies these disorders. It has been suggested that dopaminergic striatal dysfunction may play a role in RBD.

Another association between RBD and preceding events, such as a history of prior neurologic disease, including stroke, dementia, subarachnoid hemorrhage,

▶ **TABLE 16-6.** **Clinical and Epidemiological Features Associated with REM Sleep Behavior Disorder**

Characteristic	Findings
Sex	More common in males than in females
Age	Increased prevalence >50 years old
Preceding event	Stroke Dementia Subarachnoid hemorrhage Guillian-Barré
Associated conditions	Parkinson's disease Lewy body dementia Multiple-system atrophy

and Guillain-Barré syndrome, has been noted (Table 16-6). In fact, REM sleep disorders are often the initial presenting complaint of patients who subsequently develop these conditions.

A clinical diagnosis of RBD can often be made by history alone if an individual has a classic description that is often reported by the spouse. In these cases, PSG may not be necessary; however, this type of data would help corroborate suspicions and rule out other potential differential diagnoses of RBD (30,31).

The treatment of RBD includes the use of clonazepam as the medication of choice. The only caveat to using this long-acting benzodiazepine for the treatment of RBD is that the majority of these patients are older individuals and, as previously suggested, may have other concomitant neurologic issues. The long-term use of benzodiazepines in this population may predispose these elderly patients to having an increased risk of altered cognitive function. Ideally, the lowest therapeutic dose of benzodiazepines resulting in appropriate regulation of nocturnal events without any daytime sequelae would be best suited for patient management. Medium- and short-acting benzodiazepines might be considered as an alternative treatment if any such undesired effects of sedation or impaired cognitive function should occur (32). Other treatment options include carbamazepine, L-dopa, and dopamine agonists, which are typically effective to a lesser extent than is clonazepam.

Sleep Paralysis

Sleep paralysis is a condition that is reported by individuals as a form of transient paralysis, either while falling asleep or when awakening. It is classified as a REM sleep disorder, although recently it has been postulated that this may, in fact, occur as an interruption of normal REM sleep architecture. Sleep paralysis was initially described in association with narcolepsy. It actually constitutes one of the components of the narcolepsy tetrad, along with the following: cataplexy, sleep attack, and hypnagogic hallucinations.

Sleep paralysis is defined as a transient state in which the individual is conscious of his environment, however, he or she is unable to perform any movement or action (involuntary immobility). Although individuals are unable to perform gross body movements, they are able to open their eyes and subsequently recall the events of their sleep paralysis and their environments. This phenomenon can be explained by an interruption in REM sleep, wherein the brain activity still renders a hyperpolarized state leading to muscle atonia, yet the same disruption of sleep leads to an abnormal state of awakefullness in which individuals can open their eyes and interpret the details of their surroundings. It is important to distinguish sleep paralysis from other neurologic events such as transient ischemic attacks (TIA), seizures, and strokes (Table 16-7).

Sleep paralysis may occur with sleep onset rapid eye movement (SOREM) or during normal circadian REM sleep that occurs during the latter half of the night and early morning, generally while the patient is awakening. Sleep paralysis is not limited to merely when the patient is going to bed or early in the morning while awakening. As some reports describe, similar events may also occur in the middle of the night during sporadic episodes of awakening while in REM sleep.

Individuals manifest a variety of different sensations while the described sleep paralysis is occurring. Some of

▶ **TABLE 16-7.** **Differential Diagnosis and Clinical Findings of Sleep Paralysis Compared to TIAs, Seizure Disorders, and Strokes**

Feature	Sleep Paralysis	TIA	Seizure	Stroke
Time of onset	During REM sleep	Any time	Any time	Any time
Duration of symptoms	Seconds to minutes	Generally 10 to 30 minutes	Seconds to minutes	Days to indefinite amount
Characterization of symptoms	Wakefulness with muscle atonia, hallucinations, incubus, and intruder experiences	Transient focal neurological deficit	Variable seizure presentation with postictal state	Permanent focal neurologic deficit

the more common complaints include a feeling of pressure in the chest area that may be associated with difficulty breathing, or a sensation of fear and auditory and visual hallucinations. The latter two hallucinoid experiences may also be described as hypnagogic and hypnopompic experiences.

These features have been reviewed and interpreted by multiple experimental and review studies that have classified these experiences into separate categories and have even proposed their association with primitive, instinctual responses at the level of the midbrain to situations of fear and distress. The first of these is the intruder experience, which is described, just as the name suggests, as a sensation that simulates the presence of a threatening entity and is associated with distinct vivid hallucinations that could be visual, auditory, and/or tactile in nature. The incubus experiences encompass the aforementioned sensations of respiratory distress. These patients also describe a feeling as if they were being choked or asphyxiated and complain of shortness of breath and chest pressure that may or may not be accompanied by chest pain.

The last experience described involves perceptions of changes in body positioning, time and date, and orientation toward the environment. These experiences are often described as if the patient were floating or flying. Often, these feelings may be interpreted as out-of-body experiences by the individual.

The neuroanatomic structures involved in these vivid hallucinations appear to involve the amygdaloid complex and the prefrontal gyrus and adjacent cortical structures, namely the anterior cingulate. This theory has been supported by studies that demonstrate an increase in blood flow to these structures during the subject's complaints of hallucinoid experiences.

It is interesting to note that the experiences described above have undergone different introspective interpretation by various societies and cultures on a worldwide level. Often these experiences form the foundation for supernatural reports of visits by ghosts and deceased loved ones. Other phenomena, such as evil spirits and alien abductions, may also be falsely interpreted by these different sensations experienced during episodes of sleep paralysis.

Sleep paralysis has been traditionally described as occurring more often in adolescents and young adults. Some recent studies, however, have proposed a bimodal presentation occurring in young people, mostly in the twenties, as well as in the elderly. These new data revealing the incidence of sleep paralysis in patients older than 65 years reaffirms that the greater number of cases still remains within the younger population. One explanation is that there are many social and religious beliefs surrounding these experiences that may influence the subjective data reported by these subgroups. The elderly patients may also have a more difficult time recalling the incidence of these events because of natural degenerative memory loss.

In the overall population, sleep paralysis occurs with an incidence that ranges from 4% to as high as 40% to 60%.

Again this large variation is likely secondary to variation among different groups. It is more common in women, who not only report a higher incidence, but also report a higher level of fear than do men. Sleep patterns are an important risk factor if the individual performs shift work, such as nurses or nighttime clerks (33,34).

The position in which an individual sleeps has been examined in several trials and results conclude that the supine position is strongly correlated with the incidence of sleep paralysis. Mechanics affecting the airway and related soft-tissue structures, similar to those predisposing a patient to obstructive sleep apnea (OSA), can explain this finding. In fact, there has been an association between patients who have been diagnosed with OSA and sleep paralysis. This is attributed to periods of arousal caused by a SBD. Therefore, recommendations for patients susceptible to sleep paralysis include not positioning themselves in the supine position while resting. The caveat to this recommendation, however, is that often, despite patients' efforts to lie in prone position while resting, they are often found to be supine as the night progresses, ultimately leading to episodes of sleep paralysis.

Healthy individuals undergoing PSG have been noticed to undergo changes in body position just prior to entering into REM sleep, thereby nullifying attempts to recommend avoidance of this body posture. One consideration for these patients is to recommend attaching a tennis ball to the lower back with a belt device, a technique previously used in patients with snoring complaints and OSA, as a method to hinder the patient from rolling over onto his back (35).

Rapid Eye Movement Sleep Sinus Arrest

REM sleep sinus arrest syndrome is characterized by the occurrence of prolonged asystole during REM sleep, typically up to 9 seconds. The clinical symptomatology is vague and often asymptomatic. Common symptoms include chest pain or discomfort, palpitations, fatigue, lightheadedness, presyncope, or syncope.

Autonomic changes were observed during sleep as early as 1923. Over the years, multiple observations on Holter monitoring in a diverse population have shown frequent conduction disturbances during sleep, so that asystolic periods up to 2.5 seconds in duration have been considered normal. It has been estimated that 38,000 sudden deaths occur at night and 40% of episodes of atrial fibrillation are precipitated at night.

Different types of arrhythmias have been found related to particular sleep stages. Slow-wave sleep (SWS) is associated with a relatively stable reduced heart rate, with normal variability associated with respiration and respiratory sinus arrhythmia. REM sleep results in abrupt fluctuations in heart rate. An increase in sympathetic tone during REM produces tachycardia, followed by a compensatory baroreflex-mediated deceleration in rate in response to the initial tachycardia. Therefore, there are two different types of arrhythmias influenced by sleep. The first type is affected by a phasic increase in sympathetic nervous tone during REM sleep. The second type is related to an increase in vagal tone during the night (36).

Dickerson et al. found that heart rate pauses are accompanied by increases in coronary blood flow and were concentrated during transition from SWS to desynchronized sleep and in REM sleep during the phasic stage. They found that the heart rhythm pause was almost invariably preceded by tachycardia and elevations in arterial blood pressure, presumably secondary to baroreceptor stimulation. In contrast, Verrier et al. found heart decelerations not preceded by tachycardia during tonic REM sleep, suggesting a primary central vagal response.

The proposed mechanism for the abrupt deceleration in heart rate during tonic REM sleep is a change in the centrally induced pattern of autonomic tone to the heart, manifested as a decrease in sympathetic activity or an enhancement of vagal tone or both. Respiratory modulation of the autonomic activity does not appear to be related to this deceleration because it often occurs in the absence of significant inspiratory effort. Nonetheless, long asystolic periods during REM sleep have been associated with OSA syndrome. Treatment of symptomatic or significantly prolonged asystole is recommended with a pacemaker (36,37).

Sleep-related Penile Tumescence

Sleep-related penile erections are natural events that occur during REM sleep. This phenomenon should naturally occur in all healthy men of reproductive age. Stimulation of the corpora cavernosa and spongiosum, resulting in vascular congestion with subsequent penile erection, requires involvement of autonomic nervous, neurohumoral, and peripheral vascular systems. The initial engorgement of the penile vasculature is initiated by parasympathetic stimulation while the sympathetic pathways regulate ejaculation.

The sacral plexus gives origin to the preganglionic fibers that run into the hypogastric plexus, subsequently synapsing at the postganglionic neurons. The postganglionic fibers then run alongside the internal pudendal arteries and their respective branches, rendering a network of autonomic regulation of the contractile state of these vessels. When parasympathetic stimulation occurs, as is the case with REM sleep penile tumescence, there is an increase in arterial inflow toward the corpora cavernosa followed by a decrease in outflow of the same (Fig. 16-3). There is also a possible role on behalf of the perineal muscle, which assists in pumping blood into the cavernous bodies and may serve as an auxiliary method for increasing blood flow, ultimately allowing more blood flow for penile tumescence.

The level of activity of the autonomic nervous system during REM sleep is perpetually changing. Overall, there is a predominance of the parasympathetic system with intermittent bursts of sympathetic activity. These bursts, although they may occur during REM sleep, are characteristic of stages 3 and 4 (slow-wave phase) of normal sleep architecture. The incidence of penile tumescence is inversely related to that of sympathetic bursts.

The contribution of the central and peripheral nervous systems in penile erection is supported by reports of

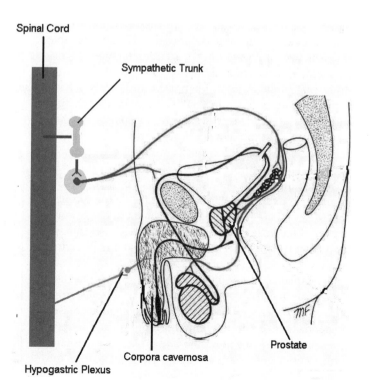

FIGURE 16-3. Anatomical display of the autonomic innervations of the male reproductive system.

Spinal Cord

Sympathetic Trunk

Prostate

Corpora cavernosa

Hypogastric Plexus

patients with complete transection of the spinal cord, where there is an inability to generate REM sleep-related penile erection. These patients do conserve the ability to respond to tactile stimuli directly to the penis, resulting in a reflex-type response. Conversely, a significant percentage of patients who have undergone incomplete lesions (such as Brown–Sequard type lesions) maintain the relationship between REM sleep and penile erections.

The central nervous system (CNS) areas reported to be involved in penile erection are the cortex and limbic structures. In early studies, subjective data suggested that nocturnal penile erections while sleeping were due to erotic dreams. Clearly there is a bias in the recollection of these dreams versus other nonerotic dreams. This theory was later absolved after documentation of the incidence of REM sleep-related erections was noted to have an incidence of six to eight episodes per night. This was not concurrent with the amount of erotic dreams experienced during the same period.

Laboratory testing and conventional methods can be utilized to determine whether an individual is capable of experiencing penile erections while sleeping. The initial test used was the *stamp test* in which a strip of postage stamps was fastened around the shaft of the penis while flaccid. The individual would then proceed to sleep under normal conditions, and the strip of stamps would be examined in the morning. The results of the test were positive for erections if the strip of stamps was separated due to an increase in penile diameter. This early identification of an organically intact penile erection mechanism was very useful in diagnosing organic versus psychogenic causes of erectile dysfunction.

Another more sophisticated technique involves measuring penis change in size using a mercury-filled strain gauge. The results of this test are displayed on a polygraphic tracing. This test has proved to be more reliable and sensitive for changes in penis circumference. If a patient should have abnormal findings on any of the different testing methods, his or her physician should still have a threshold for nonorganic causes of erectile dysfunction and perform a detailed medical, social, and psychiatric history as well as a thorough physical exam. Other reversible or nonreversible conditions may account for the patient's ailment (Table 16-8).

We mentioned earlier the participation of the neurohumoral system in regulating normal penile tumescence. Testosterone plays a key role in the endocrinologic component of the male reproductive tract. Direct associations have been made between insufficient amounts of androgens and decreased nocturnal penile tumescence. Patients may complain of a diminished libido, which is often corrected with the exogenous administration of testosterone replacement therapy. Inversely, patients with an increased concentration of the feminine hormones, such as progesterone, luteinizing hormone, and prolactin, experience similar complaints of erectile dysfunction. An array of dif-

▶ **TABLE 16-8. Reversible Causes of Impaired REM Sleep Penile Tumescence**

Etiology	Type
Trauma	Head Trauma
Iatrogenic/Drugs	Antihypertensives
	α-Adrenergic receptor agonists
	β-Receptor antagonists
	Tricyclic antidepressants
	Antipsychotics
	Cancer chemotherapeutic agents
	Cimetadine
	Disulfuram
	Digoxin
	Atropine
Behavioral	REM sleep deprivation

ferent medical conditions may account for reduced sexual drive and performance (Table 16-9).

Impaired Sleep-related Penile Erections

Impaired sleep-related penile erection is defined as the incapability to maintain an adequate penile erection during REM sleep. The criteria for determining whether the erection is adequate or not is characterized as an erection that can sustain approximately 750 g of rigidity in order to perform sexual intercourse. Many factors influence the individual's ability to sustain an adequate erection. It is empirically essential to rule out these potential causes of erectile dysfunction.

Cigarette smoking is commonly associated with its cardiopulmonary effects on the body, however, cigarette smoking also serves as a risk factor for impotence. There is a significant inverse correlation between nocturnal penile tumescence qualities and number of cigarettes smoked per day. Specifically, in patients who smoke two packs or more a day, there is a lower quality of penile rigidity when compared with individuals who smoke one pack or less per

▶ **TABLE 16-9. Factors That May Impair Sexual Function**

Type	Condition
Social	Alcohol abuse
	Tobacco abuse
Medical	Diabetes mellitus
	COPD
	Hypertension
	Narcolepsy
	Spinal cord injury
	End-stage renal disease
Psychological	Depression

day. This observation was accompanied by a shorter period of penile tumescence along with an increased rate of detumescence. Two-pack-a-day smokers also have fewer REM periods, although the average period of REM was similar in both groups.

In the setting of major depression, studies have suggested that nocturnal penile tumescence is altered in a temporal fashion, in which by overall time of tumescence is decreased. Of note, patients with major depression may produce false positive nocturnal penile tumescence test results. This has important clinical application in that these men should be evaluated and, if indicated, treated for depression before considering any surgical intervention to correct their erectile dysfunction. The caveat to this is that the same antidepressant medications may aggregate to the patient's impaired ability of erection; therefore, appropriate nocturnal penile erection studies should be performed while the patient is not taking medications.

When obtaining the clinical history with regards to impaired REM penile tumescence individuals, it is important to consider the possibility of other sleep disorders, including sleep apneas, hypopneas, and periodic leg movements (PLMs) as causes of sleep interruption. This may result in decreased time of penile tumescence, thus making it more difficult to maintain proper nocturnal penile erection. Even in cases where REM sleep is interrupted, nocturnal penile tumescence may still be affected, since this has been described to occur outside of REM sleep, especially by elderly patients. Consequently, it is imperative to screen for various sleep disorders in order to accurately determine independent factors that may account for abnormal nocturnal penile tumescence.

Sleep-related Painful Erections

Sleep-related painful erections generally transpire throughout the course of the evening, when natural REM sleep penile erections occur. These episodes differ in that the individual affected describes painful sensations associated with the events. This may lead to perpetual loss of sleep as long as this complaint proceeds. Middle-aged and elderly men often report these complaints. The cumulative effects of this condition may lead to increased levels of anxiety and distress (38).

OTHER PARASOMNIAS

The other parasomnias are a group of disorders that have characteristics different from the previous three types of parasomnias. The semeiology and severity varies significantly among them. They are classified in a different group because of their diverse clinical symptomatology and lack of uniform presentation. They may be very subtle and not require any intervention or could be life threatening.

Sleep Bruxism

Bruxism or tooth grinding is a rhythmic masticatory muscle activity characterized by repetitive three or more muscle contractions of the jaw at frequency of 1. The etiology is not clear, but it has been postulated that it may be related to abnormal orofacial sensory inputs from periodontium mucosa. Bruxism has been associated with sleep arousal, when the contact of the teeth surface is more likely to happen. The presence of sequential changes in autonomic activity observed before bruxism suggest active involvement of central and autonomic system as the main responsible mechanism, perhaps influenced by the sensory inputs.

Multiple neurochemicals including serotonin, dopamine, GABA, and noradrenaline have been involved in both the genesis and the modulation of the jaw muscle tone during sleep. It is unclear why rhythmic masticatory muscle activity during sleep is characterized by coactivation of both jaw opening and closing muscles instead of the alternating jaw opening and closing muscle activity pattern that it is typically seen during chewing function. The incidence is about 8% of the adult population, although rhythmic masticatory muscle activity without grinding occurs during the sleep of most normal subjects, up to 60% (39,40).

The consequences of bruxism may include tooth destruction, jaw pain, headaches, temporomandibular joint problems, as well as sounds that disrupt bedpartners. Patients with significant oral damage should be evaluated with formal sleep study to determine the pathophysiology and exclude seizures.

Occlusal adjustment therapy has been advocated as a treatment modality for temporomandibular disorders, but there is no clear evidence–based data to support the effect of occlusal therapy as a general method for treating a nonacute temporomandibular disorder, bruxism, or headache. The response to occlusal adjustment therapy is variable and appears to be a more subjective response. Alternative treatments such as biofeedback, counseling, avoidance conditioning, hypnosis, relaxation techniques, physical therapy, and life-style changes have been commonly used, but there is no data to assess efficacy.

Various drugs have been used to suppress bruxism in humans but the literature is still controversial and based mostly on anecdotal case reports. Benzodiazepines, nonsteroidal antiinflammatory agents, betablockers, or anticholinergic agents are among the treatments used for this condition. The more we know about bruxism, the more treatment options become available. Bruxism associated with orofacial dystonia and dyskinesia can be treated with botulinum toxin, whereas common bruxism may respond to electrical stimulation of the lip (40).

Sleep Enuresis

Nocturnal primary enuresis is a heterogeneous disorder that is not due to intrinsic neurologic or urologic

▶ **TABLE 16-10.** Treatment Options for Enuresis

Reassurance
Bell-and-pad device
Tricyclic antidepressant agents (imipramine, desipramine)
Desmopressin
Combination therapy

dysfunction. Enuresis was classified as an arousal disorder, but sleep studies found that it can occur both in REM and NREM sleep. Local urologic abnormalities account for only 2% of the pediatric cases. The underlying pathophysiologic mechanisms include a mismatch between the bladder capacity and the amount of urine produced during sleep at night and a high arousal threshold that prevents a proper response to the bladder fullness sensation. Autonomic and brainstem dysfunction have been implicated to affect micturition, which is controlled by a network of neurons involving a center in the mesopontine tegmentum of the brainstem (Barrington's nucleus) (Table 16-10) (41).

Physiologic bedwetting disappears before the child is 5 years old. The incidence of bedwetting at age 4 years is 40%, 10% in 6 year olds, 5% in 10 year olds, and 3% in 12 year olds. Nocturnal enuresis is inherited via an autosomal dominant mode in transmission with high penetrance (90%), but up to one-third of all cases are sporadic (42).

The polysomnogram is characterized by a high arousal threshold but is otherwise normal. Enuretic children who respond to desmopressin treatment have more rapid eye movement sleep than therapy-resistant children, but the significance of this finding is not clear. A large study from Scandinavia showed that enuretic children have no statistical difference in behavioral or psychological problems compared to nonenuretic children. The enuretic children were harder to arouse than controls, have lower vasopressin levels, and a normal bladder capacity.

Treatment includes supportive therapy, conditioning with a urine alarm, or medications—imipramine or desmopressin acetate. Extensive urologic evaluation is generally not indicated (43).

Children with increased nocturnal urine production usually have a good response to desmopressin therapy. Patients with urologic abnormalities, such as small bladder, generally have a poor response to desmopressin treatment, but would benefit more from combination therapy with urine alarm and antimuscarinic agents, in addition to desmopressin. Desmopressin has no major effects on sleep physiology but does delay bladder emptying (44).

Nocturnal Paroxysmal Dystonia

This entity was first described in 1981, under the term "hypnogenic paroxysmal dystonia," with a case report of five patients with seizures during sleep involving dystonic, ballistic or choreoathetoid movements. Subsequently, more cases were described and two different groups were identified, one characterized by short-lasting episodes, suddenly arousing from sleep with a fearful or astonished expression followed by dystonic posturing of the head and body, and choreoathetoid movements of the limbs. The other group is rarer and it is reported that long-lasting attacks of motor agitation with dyskinetic, dystonic, and ballistic movements occur.

The clinical features of nocturnal paroxysmal dystonia are characterized by repeated, stereotyped dystonic, ballistic, or choreoathetoid nocturnal episodes involving a single or all extremities or paroxysmal arousals occurring during NREM sleep, often involving vocalizations, mumbling, or crying. The patients typically go back to sleep and they have poor recollection of the details of the behavior, but often are aware of some occurring. Short-lasting attacks have a duration less than 2 minutes, while long-lasting attacks occur from 2 to 50 minutes. The long-lasting attacks have been observed during light sleep, sporadic recurrence, and normal EEG.

Nocturnal paroxysmal dystonia is considered to be a sleep-related subtype of nocturnal frontal lobe epilepsy and is associated with seizures in 50% of cases. The diagnosis is sometimes difficult since patients frequently have normal interictal EEG. Several studies have found interictal epileptic abnormalities using sphenoidal electrodes and others have reported electrographic seizure activity during a typical attack of nocturnal paroxysmal dystonia. Seizures involving the motor supplementary area and temporal lobe areas typically show dystonic posturing and deep frontal lobe seizures. These are characterized by semipurposeful, bilateral limb movements, with pelvic torsion or thrusting movements, that frequently are confused with pseudoseizures.

The frequent involvement of short-lasting complex bilateral movements and dystonic posturing of arms and legs suggests involvement of the excitatory neuronal network projecting from the anterior cingulate gyrus to the basal ganglia, as captured using ictal SPECT in a reported case (Fig. 16-4) (45). Short-acting nocturnal paroxysmal dystonia responds to carbamazepine therapy, whereas the long-lasting dystonias are unresponsive to anticonvulsants.

A group of disorders described to be characterized by complex motor attacks that arise suddenly from sleep and that are closely related to epileptic activity include paroxysmal arousals, nocturnal paroxysmal dystonia, and episodic nocturnal wanderings. Paroxysmal arousals are described by sudden start and a cry, frightened or confused expression, and dystonic or athetoid posture lasting few seconds, followed by falling asleep again. Autonomic activity occurred during the attacks and the electroencephalographs (EEG) sometimes showed a K complex at the onset of the episode without epileptic activity. The episodes responded to carbamazepine therapy (5,8).

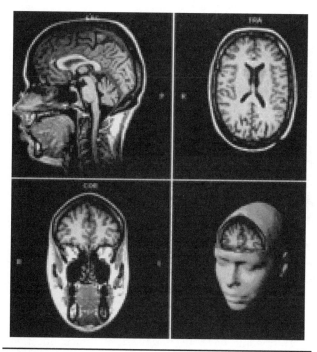

FIGURE 16-4. Subtraction SPECT with MR coregistration showing bilateral hyperperfusion of the anterior part of the cingulate gyrus during an episode of nocturnal paroxysmal dystonia. (From Espa F. Sleep architecture, slow-wave activity, and sleep spindles in adult patients with sleepwalking and sleep terrors. *Clin Neurophysiol.* 2000;111:929–939. With permission.)

Nocturnal paroxysmal wandering is described as sudden arousal followed by violent ambulation, kicking, head banging, and screaming with unintelligible speech. During these events they are unaware of the surroundings and are subject to injuries. The attacks present in clusters, more commonly during NREM during the second half of the night and in early morning. Focal epileptiform activity has been found in these patients, who responded to antiepileptic drugs. These events differed from somnambulism by the clinical characteristics and the association with epileptic activity. The evidence of these paroxysmal arousal disorders suggests an epileptic etiology, probably originating from the orbitomesial frontal lobe. The role of this brain region in regulating the sleep–wake cycle explains the nocturnal occurrences during sleep (Table 16-11).

Sudden Unexplained Nocturnal Death Syndrome (SUNDS)

This is the sudden unexplained death of a young adult during sleep. This disorder is found mainly in South-

▌ **TABLE 16-11.** **Paroxysmal Arousal Disorders**

Paroxysmal arousals
Nocturnal paroxysmal dystonia
Episodic nocturnal wanderings

east Asia and is the most common cause of "natural" death in the young, healthy Asian population. The clinical features of SUNDS are recognized as ST-segment elevation in the right precordial leads (V1–V3), inconsistently associated with right bundle branch block, and ventricular tachycardia and fibrillation on surface electrocardiogram (ECG). Autopsy and clinical findings are both unable to determine the cause of death. Genetic studies have demonstrated that Brugada syndrome (sudden death and ECG right bundle-branch block with ST-segment elevation in leads V1-V3 and normal QT interval in the absence of any structural heart disease) has been reported in individuals of European descent. SUNDS represents the same autosomal dominant familial disorder that causes sudden cardiac death (usually in males) during sleep. The data also reported that the patients were difficult to arouse and had labored breathing. From these reports it is likely that the instability of the physiologic systems, especially respiration, in particular during the REM phase, may play a role in precipitating the sudden death (Fig. 16-5).

Mutations in sodium channel 5A (SCN5A) have also been found to cause progressive conduction system disease (Lev–Lenegre syndrome), isolated conduction system disease, and sudden infant death syndrome (SIDS). Patients with features of both long QT syndrome and Brugada syndrome suggest variable clinical presentations with mutations in the same gene (46,47).

Infant Sleep Apnea

Apnea is the interruption of airflow at the nostrils and mouth lasting at least 10 seconds. Infant sleep apnea can be of central origin, due to obstruction, or it can be combined. The diagnosis of infant sleep apnea is reserved for infants who are older than 37 weeks at the onset of the apnea, without a specific cause of acute life-threatening event (ALTE) or apnea.

The clinical symptomatology includes a pale or bluish color change, hypotonia, observed cessation of breathing during sleep, or associated noisy breathing during sleep. Family history is often positive for sleep apnea or sudden infant death syndrome. Asthma or bronchitis is also commonly found in the family history.

The patency of the upper airway is dependent on the structural integrity of the rigid airway and the effective and coordinated contractions of the upper respiratory muscles. Structural or functional narrowing of the upper airway produces obstructive apnea. Structural narrowing may occur because of deformation of the upper airways or a mass lesion. Weak upper-airway muscle contractions or lack of coordination between the diaphragmatic and upper-airway muscle contractions creates a functional narrowing. Infants born before 31 weeks have a 50% to 80% chance of developing a sleep apnea whereas full-term infants have a 7% chance of having this problem.

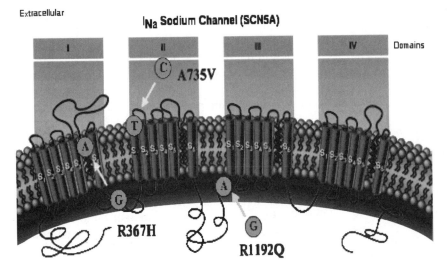

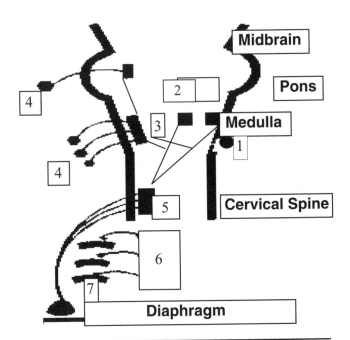

FIGURE 16-5. Illustration of the SUNDS mutations within the cardiac sodium channel SCN5A, as well as the locations of mutations previously identified in Brugada syndrome and LQTS patients. (From Diener HC. Effectiveness of quinine in treating muscle cramps: a double-blind, placebo-controlled, parallel-group, multicentre trial. *Interm J Clin Pract.* 2002;56(4): 243–246. With permission.)

In full-term newborns, REM sleep occupies more than 50% of TST and this percentage is even greater in preterm newborns (Table 16-12). During REM sleep, the irregular phasic inhibitory–excitatory respiratory pattern is co-ordinated with other brainstem phasic activity, such as rapid eye movements. Inhibition of the upper-airway muscles predisposes to further narrowing of the upper airway during REM.

Normal breathing occurs because of a well-orchestrated interplay among brainstem structures, nerves, and respiratory muscles (Fig. 16-6).

A strong diaphragmatic contraction depends on the integrity of the phrenic, diaphragm, chest wall, and the effective and coordinated contraction of the intercostal muscles. The upper airway maintains its patency and is kept patent by the integrity of the upper airway and the effective and coordinated contractions of the upper respiratory muscles. A failure of any of these conditions to occur can lead to apnea.

These structures are perfectly coordinated by the nervous system. The breathing apparatus generates and coordinates the contractions of the diaphragm, upper-airway respiratory muscles, and intercostal muscles. The dorsal respiratory groups are in the medulla and are connected with the tractus solitarius. The neurons of the ventral respiratory group in the medulla are related to the nucleus ambiguus and retroambigualis.

The medulla has both efferent and afferent connections. The efferent neurons of the respiratory groups connect with the phrenic center, alpha-motoneurons of the intercostal muscles, and the cranial nerve motor neurons of the upper-airway muscles. The dorsal and ventral respiratory

FIGURE 16-6. Physiology of breathing: Afferent fibers are from a chemoreceptor (1) in the lower medulla that monitors cerebrospinal fluid pH according to blood P_{CO_2}; respiratory group at the nucleus of the tractus solitarius, ambiguus, and nucleus retroambigualis (2) react to the signals from this sensor by modifying their discharge frequency, intensity, and coordination between upper-airway motor neurons (3), upper-airway motor muscle (4), phrenic center (5), intercostal muscle anterior horn cells (6), intercostal muscles, and diaphragm (7).

▶ **TABLE 16-12. Proportion of REM Sleep in Infants**

Age	REM Sleep
Preterm infant	>50%
Full-term newborn	50%
6-Month old	25%

groups react to the signals from the chemoreceptors (mediated by CO_2 content), which modify the electrical discharge frequency and intensity. The discharge frequency and intensity of the dorsal and ventral respiratory groups dictate the respiratory rate and tidal volume. This electric stimulation induces the contractions of upper-airway muscles and the intercostal muscles about 100 milliseconds before the onset of diaphragmatic contractions, which prevents collapse of the upper airway or the chest wall due to the negative pressure created by the diaphragm.

A structural or functional narrowing of the upper airway, or ineffective diaphragmatic contractions that fails to create negative intrapulmonary pressure, produces an obstructive apnea. Mass lesions or a deformation of the upper-airways produce a structural narrowing. Functional narrowing results from weak upper-airway muscle contractions or poor coordination between the diaphragmatic and upper-airway muscle contractions. Functional narrowing occurs with nervous system dysfunction and with loss of adhesion between the pleura (Fig. 16-7)

The dorsal and ventral respiratory groups also receive and integrate information regarding lung volume and airflow through the fifth and tenth cranial nerve. These medullary centers are regulated by structures in the pons (the apneustic and the pneumotaxic centers) and higher central nervous system that modulate the firing of the dorsal and ventral respiratory groups during sleep. The apneustic center produces a stimulus to the medulla to induce an inspiratory drive, followed by a pneumotaxic stimulus to inhibit the apneustic center, and regulates transition from inspiration to expiration. During active sleep, respiration is less dependent on chemoreceptors than quiet sleep and wake state.

Brainstem lesions produce apnea by disrupting the normal coordination of the respiratory function described above. Any brainstem lesions in neonates can cause obstructive, central, or mixed apnea during any behavioral state. Neonates with idiopathic hypoventilation syndrome have central apnea, usually during quiet sleep. The diagnosis of brainstem lesions in a neonate with apnea is based on clinical and neurologic findings, polysomnogram, imaging findings, and brainstem auditory and somatosensory-evoked responses (SSERs) (48–50).

Neonates with sleep apnea can be revived and typically have recurrent episodes until they outgrow the syndrome, which differs significantly from the sudden infant death syndrome.

Sudden Infant Death Syndrome

SIDS refers to a child who dies during sleep from no apparent cause. It was the leading cause of postneonatal mortality in the United States in 1999. Its cause is unknown. Prematurity and low birth weight appear to be the major risk factors. Many other factors are related, such as deprivation, young maternal age, three or more previous live births, maternal smoking and drinking, urinary tract infection in pregnancy, reduced birth weight, infant illness, regurgitation, history of crying or colic in the interval from birth to the week before death.

Cosleeping has been associated with increase SIDS, but other studies have reported a protective effect based on several physiologic and behavioral observations. For example, bed-sharing infants had less stage 3 and 4 sleep and more stage 1 and 2 sleep with more frequent arousals than when they slept alone. Prone infant positioning was minimized during bed sharing, and mother-infant pairs typically sleep face to face. In addition, breast feeding is significantly increased, as well as maternal vigilance (51).

The major difference is that a child with sleep apnea can usually be revived. In fact, the baby may suffer several episodes of apnea before he outgrows the syndrome.

AREAS OF
OBSTRUCTIVE APNEA

1. Soft palate
2. Larynx
3. Vocal cords
4. Tongue
5. Pleural space

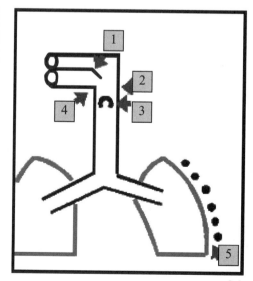

FIGURE 16-7. Areas of structural and functional narrowing.

IA

▶ **TABLE 16-13. Recommendations for Apnea Monitoring**

History of previously life-threatening episodes of unclear etiology
Siblings of babies who died from SIDS
Babies on respiratory stimulants
Babies with a tracheostomy
Premature babies with apnea episodes
Babies on oxygen for lung disease
Babies with gastroesophageal reflux treated with medications

The use of apnea monitors decreases mortality in high-risk infants, but there is no clear consensus to determine which baby requires a monitor. There are some recommended factors that can help to identify high-risk babies and prevent fatal consequences (Table 16-13). Some neurologists advocate use of apnea monitoring in all premature babies, whereas the consensus from the National Institutes of Health states that that if no apnea occurs for 1 week prior to discharge they should go home without a monitor.

The recommended time of monitoring is also controvertial but, in general, the recommendations are that neonates with an apparent or confirmed life-threatening episode should be monitored until they are free of events for at least 3 months and are at least 6 months of age. Siblings of infants who died of SIDS should be monitored until 1 month after the age at which the sibling died—at least 6 months. Premature neonates with apnea episodes should be monitored until they have not had apnea for at least 1 month, at least until their conceptional age is at least 52 weeks. Babies with respiratory stimulants and gastroesophageal reflux medications should be monitored until those medications have been stopped.

The settings of the monitor for low heart rate depends on the conceptional age (Table 16-14), but the high heart rate alarm is set at 230 beats per minute and the apnea time alarm is set to 20 seconds, which is the case for all ages. The setting of the low heart rate alarm will change according to conceptional age.

Environmental preventive techniques for the preterm infant includes supine positioning.

▶ **TABLE 16-14. Apnea Monitor Settings for Low Heart Rate According to Conceptual Age**

Conceptual Age	Low Heart Rate Alarm Settings (beats/min)
Less than 40 weeks	80
40–48 weeks	70
Older than 48 weeks	60

Congenital Central Hypoventilation

Congenital central hypoventilation syndrome (CCHS) is a relatively rare disorder characterized by autonomic nervous system dysfunction producing impairment of ventilatory homeostasis during sleep. The estimated incidence is approximately 1 in 50,000 live births. Neonates with idiopathic hypoventilation syndrome have central apnea, usually during quiet sleep. CCHS appears to have a genetic link, but no gene has been clearly implicated.

Other conditions and symptoms have been observed in these patients, such as gastroesophageal reflux, need for gastrostomy tube feedings during infancy, constipation, diarrhea, premature birth, fainting episodes, seizures, cardiac arrhythmias, cor pulmonale, episodes of profuse sweating and cool extremities, absence of fever with infections, asthma, recurrent pneumonia, hypotonia, and ophthalmologic problems. The children with this disorder frequently have learning disabilities. The treatment involves ventilatory support and management of concomitant problems (52).

Primary Snoring

Primary snoring is simply loud airway breathing sounds without any indications of reduced airflow, or other signs of sleep apnea. Snoring affects up to 10% of children. Primary snoring has been regarded as relatively benign, because it does not progress to OSA. In the majority of children, treatment is not warranted. Parents should be reassured about the low incidence of OSA and educated about the symptomatology and presentation of that condition.

Benign Neonatal Sleep Myoclonus

Benign neonatal sleep myoclonus is characterized by rhythmic myoclonic jerks involving limbs and trunk, occurring during drowsiness or quiet sleep. The myoclonus stops with awakening, and normal encephalograms are observed during or after the episodes. Benign neonatal sleep myoclonus can only be diagnosed in neurologically normal full-term infants and usually presents within a few days of birth. Sleep myoclonus usually disappears after a period of weeks and is resolved, in most cases, by 3 months of age. However, it has been reported to last up to 3 years of age. Typically there is no family history. The myoclonic activity may last from several seconds to 90 minutes. Benign neonatal sleep myoclonus is not associated with electroencephalographic seizures during the events. Myoclonus may increase heart rate during the episodes. Benign neonatal sleep myoclonus may be triggered and exacerbated by noise or rocking movements. Rocking is especially effective in triggering the events and has been used to trigger typical events at the doctor's office. The mechanism of benign neonatal sleep myoclonus is unknown but the disappearance coincides, in most cases, with the period of maturation in sleep patterns seen during the first 3 months of life and establishment of the diurnal–nocturnal pattern. It may occur during any sleep stage, but occurs more frequently during quiet sleep. During the first 12 weeks, sleep changes from REM to NREM sleep, and the total REM sleep periods continue to decrease significantly during the first 6 months of life. Immaturity of the serotonergic system has been postulated as a cause. There is no clear genetic predisposition.

The use of benzodiazepines may induce myoclonus and occasionally sustained myoclonus, which can be misdiagnosed as status epilepticus. Benign neonatal sleep myoclonus usually disappears before 6 months of age. It does not requires treatment and is not associated with subsequent neurologic deficit (53–55).

Sleep-Related Abnormal Swallowing

Swallowing is episodic during sleep, with long periods without swallow activity. Swallows occur in association with movement arousals that occur most frequently during stages REM, 1 and 2 of sleep and during rhythmic masticatory muscle activity. This syndrome is characterized by choking or coughing while sleeping due to accumulation of saliva caused by impairment of swallowing during sleep. This is a rare and benign disorder with limited clinical published data (56).

REFERENCES

1. Furman Y. Shakespeare and sleep disorders. *Neurology*. 1997; 49(4):1171–1172.
2. Krahn LE. Sleep Disorders. *Semin Neurol*. 2003;23(3):307–314.
3. Mahowald MW, Parasomnia pseudo-suicide. *J Forensic Sci*. 2003; 48(5):1158–1162.
4. Lombroso CT. Pavor nocturnus of proven epileptic origin. *Epilepsia*. 2003;41(9):1221–1226.
5. Zucconi M. NREM parasomnias: arousal disorders and differentiation from nocturnal frontal lobe epilepsy. *Clinical Neurophysiol*. 2000;(Suppl. 2):129–135.
6. Malow BA. Paroxysmal events in sleep. *J Clin Neurophysiol*. 2002;11:552–534.
7. Dyken M. Diagnosing rhythmic movement disorder with videopolysomnography. *Pediat Neurol*. 0000;16(1):8–16.
8. Malow BA. Paroxysmal events in sleep. *J Clin Neurophysiol*. 2002; 11:552–534.
9. Roffe C. Randomised, cross-over, placebo controlled trial of magnesium citrate in the treatment of chronic persistent leg cramps. *Med Sci Monitoring*. 2004;8(5):326–330.
10. Diener HC. Effectiveness of quinine in treating muscle cramps: a double-blind, placebo-controlled, parallel-group, multicentre trial. *Intern. J Clin Pract*. 2002;56(4):243–246.
11. Chan P. Randomized, double-blind, placebo-controlled study of the safety and efficacy of vitamin B complex in the treatment of nocturnal leg cramps in elderly patients with hypertension. *J Clin Pharmacol*. 1998;38(12):1151–1154.
12. Man-Son-Hing M. Meta-analysis of efficacy of quinine for treatment of nocturnal leg cramps in elderly people. *BMJ*. 1995;310:313–317.
13. Reimao R. Evaluation of flurazepam and placebo on sleep disorders in childhood. *Arq Neuropsiquiatr*. 1982;40(1):1–13.
14. Hublin C. Genetic aspects and genetic epidemiology of parasomnias. *Sleep Med Rev*. 2003;7(5):413–421.
15. Espa F. Sleep architecture, slow wave activity, and sleep spindles in adult patients with sleepwalking and sleep terrors. *Clinical Neurophysiol*. 2000;111:929–939.
16. Hartman D. Is there a dissociative process in sleepwalking and night terrors? *Postgrad Med J*. 2001;77(906):244–249.
17. Ohayon MM. Night terrors, sleepwalking, and confusional arousals in the general population: their frequency and relationship to other sleep and mental disorders. *J Clin Psych*. 1999;60(4):268–276.
18. Bassetti C, Vella S, Donati F, et al. SPECT during sleepwalking. *Lancet*. 2000 Aug 5;356(9228):484–485.
19. Landry P. Lithium-induced somnambulism. *Can J Psych*. 1998:957–958.
20. Khazaal Y. Bupropion-induced somnambulism. *Addict Biol*. 2003; 8(3):359–362.
21. Kolivakis TT. Olanzapine-induced somnambulism. *Amer. J Psych*. 2001;158:1158.   .
22. Milliet N. Somnambulism and trauma: Case report and short review of the literature. *J Trauma*. 1999;47(2):420–422.
23. Harazin J. Zolpidem tartrate and somnambulism. *Milestones Med*. 1999;164(9):669–670.
24. Guilleminault C. Sleepwalking and sleep terrors in prepubertal children: what triggers them? *Pediatrics*. 2003:111(1).
25. Schenck C. Long-term, nightly benzodiazepine treatment of injurious parasomnias and other disorders of disrupted nocturnal sleep in 170 adults. *Amer J Med*. 1996;100:333–337.
26. Nguyen T. Nightmare frequency, nightmare distress, and anxiety. *Percept Motor Skills*. 2002;95:219–225.
27. Schredl M. Effects of state and trait factors on nightmare frequency. *Eur Arch Psych Clin Neurosci*. 2003;253:241–247.
28. Raskind MA, et al. Reduction of nightmare and other PTSD symptoms in combat veterans by prazosin: a placebo-controlled study. *Amer J Psych*. 2003;160:371–373.
29. Krakow B, et al. An open-label trial of evidence-based cognitive behavior therapy for nightmares and insomnia in crime victims with PTSD. *Amer J Psych*. 2001;158:2043–2047.
30. Olson E. Rapid eye movement sleep behavior disorder: demographic, clinical and laboratory findings in 93 cases. *Brain*. 2000;123:331–339.
31. Shirakawa S, et al. Study of image findings in rapid eye movement sleep behavioral disorder. *Psych Clin Neurosci*. 2004;56:291–292.
32. Schenck CH. Managing bizarre sleep-related behavior disorders. *Parasomnias*. 2000;107(3):145–156.
33. Wing Y-K. Sleep paralysis in the elderly. *J. Sleep Res*. 1999;8:151–155.
34. Ohayon MM, et al. Prevalence and pathologic associations of sleep paralysis in the general population. *Neurology*. 1999;52(6):1194.
35. Synder S. Serotoninergic agents in the treatment of isolated sleep paralysis. *Amer J Psych*. 1982;139(9).
36. Verrier RL. Primary vagally mediated decelerations in heart rate during tonic rapid eye movement sleep in cats. *Amer J Physiol*. 1998;274(4):1136–1141.
37. Guilleminault C. Sinus arrest during REM sleep in young adults. *N Engl J Med*. 1984;311(16):1006–1010.
38. Lavie PSA. Cardiac autonomic function during sleep in psychogenic and organic erectile dysfunction. *J Sleep Res*. 1999;8:135–143.
39. Lavigne GJ. Neurobiological mechanisms involved in sleep bruxism. *Crit Rev Oral Biol Med*. 2003;14(1):30–46.
40. Kato T. Topical review: sleep bruxism and the role of peripheral sensory influences. *J Orofac Pain*. 2003;17(3):191–213.
41. Tanaka Y. Firing of micturition center neurons in the rat mesopontine tegmentum during urinary bladder contraction. *Brain Res*. 2003;965:146–154.
42. Von Gontard A. The genetics of enuresis: a review. *J Urol*. 2001; 166(6):2438–2443.
43. Kuhn B. Treatment efficacy in behavioral pediatric sleep medicine. *J Psychosom Res*. 2003;54:587–597.
44. Neveus T. The role of sleep and arousal in nocturnal enuresis. *Acta Pediatr*. 2003;92(10):1118–1123.
45. Schindler K. Hyperperfusion of anterior cingulate gyrus in a case of paroxysmal nocturnal dystonia. *Neurology*. 2001;57:917–920.

46. Vatta M. Genetic and biophysical basis of sudden unexplained nocturnal death syndrome (SUNDS): a disease allelic to Brugada syndrome. *Human Mol Genet.* 2002;11:337–345.
47. Malloy M. Sudden infant death syndrome among extremely preterm infants: United States 1997–1999. *J Perinatol Advance Online Publ.* 2004;2:9.
48. Gaultier C. Sleep apnea in infants. *Sleep Med Rev.* 1999;3(4):303–312.
49. Richard C. Apnea and periodic breathing in bed-sharing and solitary sleeping infants. *J Appl Physiol.* 1998;84:1374–1380.
50. Gaultier C. Sleep apnea in infants. *Sleep Med Rev.* 1999;3(4):303–312.
51. Ponsonby A. Sleeping position, infant apnea, and cyanosis: a population-based study. *Pediatrics.* 1997;99(1):3.
52. Vanderlaan M. Epidemiologic survey of 196 patients with congenital central hypoventilation syndrome. *Pediatr Pulmonol.* 2004;37(3):217–229.
53. Dravet C. Benign myoclonus of early infancy or benign nonepileptic infantile spasms. *Neuropediatrics.* 1986:33–38.
54. Egger J. Benign sleep myoclonus in infancy mistaken for epilepsy. *BMJ.* 2003;326:5.
55. Di Capua M. Benign neonatal sleep myoclonus: clinical features and video-polygraphic recordings. *Mov. Disorders.* 1993;8(2):191–194.
56. Lichter I. The pattern of swallowing during sleep. *Electroencephalogr Clin Neurophysiol.* 1975;38(4):427–432.

Chapter 17

Circadian Rhythm Sleep Disorders

Phyllis C. Zee and Kathryn J. Reid

INTRODUCTION

Circadian rhythms in physiology and behavior are ubiquitous in all living organisms from single cells to humans. These self-sustaining endogenous circadian rhythms are genetically regulated and persist in the absence of external time cues, with a period of approximately 24 hours (1). In mammals, the suprachiasmatic nuclei (SCN), a paired structure located in the hypothalamus, is the site of a master circadian clock (2–5). The SCN not only generates circadian rhythms, but also maintains the temporal organization of circadian rhythms to the external physical, social, and work schedules. The nadir of the circadian core body temperature and the rise in melatonin rhythm are commonly used as estimates of the phase of the circadian clock in humans.

In humans, light is the strongest synchronizing agent for the circadian clock (6), and its ability to advance or delay circadian rhythms is dependent on the time of exposure. Exposure to light in the first half of the night delays circadian rhythms, whereas, light late in the second half of the night or early morning advances circadian rhythms. In humans, the transition point between the delay and advance regions occurs near the temperature minimum (4:00 to 6:00 AM) in young adults and somewhat earlier in older adults (7–10). In addition to light, nonphotic agents such as melatonin, and physical and social activity also play a role in entrainment of human circadian rhythms (11,12). The phase shifting responses to melatonin (13–15) are generally in the opposite direction of light. Early evening administration of melatonin will advance and early morning melatonin will delay circadian rhythms.

The sleep–wake cycle is the most apparent circadian rhythm in humans. During the past decade, there has been tremendous progress in our understanding of the neural regulation of sleep and wakefulness. Our current understanding of the regulation of the human sleep–wake cycle indicates that sleep and wake behaviors are generated by a complex interaction of endogenous circadian and sleep homeostatic processes, as well as social and environmental factors. The drive toward sleep and the tendency to sleep longer and more deeply after sleep loss is referred to as "sleep homeostasis" (process S). This homeostatic drive for sleep is a function of the amount of prior wakefulness. Physiological sleepiness and alertness not only varies with prior waking duration, but also exhibits circadian variation. In humans, daily variation in physiologic sleep tendency reveals a biphasic circadian rhythm of wake and sleep propensity (16,17), with a mid-day increase in sleep tendency occurring around 2–4 PM, followed by a robust decrease in sleep tendency and increase in alertness that lasts through the early to mid-evening hours. The primary role of the circadian pacemaker is to promote wakefulness during the day and thus facilitate the consolidation of sleep during the nighttime hours (16, 18–20). The interaction between circadian and homeostatic processes typically allows for approximately 16 hours of wakefulness and 8 hours of sleep.

CIRCADIAN RHYTHM SLEEP DISORDERS

For optimal sleep and alertness, desired sleep and wake times should be synchronized with the timing of the endogenous alertness-promoting circadian rhythm. Misalignment between the circadian timing system and the 24-hour physical environment or work and social schedules can result in symptoms of insomnia and excessive daytime sleepiness (EDS). Circadian rhythm sleep disorders arise when the physical environment is altered relative to the internal circadian timing system, such as in jet lag and shift work, or when the timing of endogenous circadian rhythms are altered, such as in circadian rhythm sleep phase disorders. The latter is thought to occur predominantly because of chronic alterations in the circadian clock or its entrainment mechanisms. This chapter focuses on this second group of disorders.

The essential feature of a circadian rhythm sleep disorder (CRSD) is that the pattern of sleep disturbance is due primarily to alterations of the circadian time-keeping system or a misalignment between the endogenous circadian rhythm and exogenous factors that affect the timing or duration of sleep. The circadian-related sleep disruption leads to insomnia or EDS, which causes functional impairment or distress. The diagnosis of CRSD is primarily based on published criteria using either the International Classification of Sleep Disorders or the DSM IV-TR. In addition to physiologic and environmental factors, maladaptive behaviors often influence the presentation and clinical course of circadian rhythm sleep disorders.

CIRCADIAN RHYTHM SLEEP-PHASE DISORDERS (DELAYED SLEEP-PHASE SYNDROME AND ADVANCED SLEEP-PHASE SYNDROME)

The circadian rhythm sleep-phase disorders delayed sleep-phase syndrome (DSPS) and advanced sleep-phase syndrome (ASPS) occur when the timing of the major sleep period is delayed or advanced in relation to 24-hour clock time. A diagnosis of DSPS or ASPS requires a complaint of inability to fall asleep or maintain sleep at the desired or conventional time. Diagnostic criteria should also include a stable advanced or delayed sleep and wake pattern for a minimum period of at least 1 month—preferably

3 months. This is to differentiate these conditions from circadian rhythm misalignment caused by transient responses to changing work schedules or traveling across time zones.

Delayed Sleep-Phase Syndrome (Delayed Sleep-Phase Type, Delayed Sleep Pattern)

DSPS was first described in 1981 by Weitzman and colleagues (21). It is characterized by bedtimes and wake times that are usually delayed 3 to 6 hours relative to desired or socially acceptable sleep–wake times. The patient typically cannot fall asleep before 2–6 AM and has difficulty waking up earlier than 10 AM to 1 PM (9, 22). Attempts to advance sleep times are usually unsuccessful. When allowed to follow a preferred schedule, circadian phase of sleep is delayed, but relatively stable and sleep quality is reported to be normal. When the individual has no obligations, such as on weekends and vacations, sleep often is extended into the late morning. Patients with DSPS often report feeling most alert in the evening and most sleepy in the early morning. They typically score as definite "evening" types on the Horne and Ostberg questionnaire of diurnal preference and often are described as "night" people, or "owls" (23). In general, individuals with DSPS seek treatment because enforced socially acceptable bed times and wake up times result in insomnia, excessive sleepiness, and functional impairments, particularly during the morning hours (9).

Clinical Epidemiology

DSPS is probably the most common of the primary CRSDs (24). Although the actual prevalence of DSPS in the general population is unknown, it has been reported that among adolescents and young adults, the prevalence is 7% to 16% (9,25). It has been estimated that 5% to 10% of patients presenting with chronic insomnia to sleep clinics have DSPS (22).

Differential Diagnosis

DSPS must be distinguished from "normal" sleep patterns, particularly in adolescents and young adults, who exhibit delayed schedules without impaired functioning. Social and behavioral factors play an important role in the development and maintenance of the delayed sleep patterns. Behaviors, such as attempts to fall asleep earlier, result in prolonged sleep latency and may promote as well as perpetuate features of conditioned insomnia; activities and exposure to bright light into the late evening may promote the inability to sleep and exacerbate the delayed circadian phase. In adolescents, the role of school avoidance, social maladjustment, and family dysfunction must be considered as precipitating and contributing factors. Individuals may use alcohol and excessive caffeine to cope with symptoms of insomnia and excessive sleepiness, which, in turn, may exacerbate the underlying CRSD.

Etiology

Although the exact mechanisms responsible for DSPS are unknown, several explanations, such as a longer than usual endogenous circadian period or alterations in the entrainment of the circadian system, could account for a persistently delayed-phase relationship between the endogenous circadian rhythm and the desired or conventional times for sleep and wake (9). It has been suggested that the advance portion of the phase response curve to light may be unusually small (22) or lack of early morning light exposure (due to prolonged sleep in the morning) may promote the delayed-sleep phase under normal light–dark cycles. Furthermore, individuals with DSPS may have an altered responsiveness to light (26). Therefore, there is evidence that changes in oscillation of the circadian clock and/or the response to synchronizing agents, such as light, contribute to the alteration in the timing of sleep in DSPS.

Although circadian mechanisms are fundamental in the pathophysiology of DSPS, there is increasing evidence that alterations in the homeostatic regulation of sleep may also play an important role (27). It is commonly accepted that sleep architecture is essentially normal in patients with DSPS. Polysomnographic recordings of sleep in DSPS patients showed that sleep architecture was not disrupted when subjects were allowed to sleep at their desired sleep and wake times (28–31). However, following sleep deprivation, DSPS patients showed a decreased ability to compensate for sleep loss during the day and first hours of the night (32,33). These results suggest that changes in sleep homeostatic regulation may contribute to daytime sleepiness in individuals with DSPS.

A family history may be present in approximately 40% of individuals with DSPS, and the DSPS phenotype has been shown to segregate as an autosomal dominant trait (34). Further evidence of a genetic basis for DSPS comes from recent reports of polymorphisms in the circadian clock genes, *hPer3* and *Clock* in DSPS (35–38).

Diagnostic Evaluation

The diagnosis of DSPS relies largely on the clinical history. However, diagnostic studies such as actigraphy and sleep diaries can be very useful to confirm the delayed sleep-phase pattern. Recordings of sleep diaries and actigraphy over a period of at least 2 weeks demonstrate delayed-sleep onset and offset (Fig.17-1), with sleep onsets typically delayed until 2–6 AM and wake up times in the late morning or early afternoon. Daily work or school schedules may result in earlier than desired wake time during weekdays, but a delay in bedtime and wake up time is almost always seen during weekends and while on vacation. Polysomnographic (PSG) parameters of sleep architecture, when performed at the natural delayed sleep times, are essentially normal for age (28–31). However, if a conventional bedtime and wake up time is scheduled, PSG recording will show prolonged sleep latency and decreased total sleep time (TST).

Measurements of circadian phase can be performed by assessment of core body temperature or dim-light melatonin onset (DLMO) in plasma or saliva. These circadian measures show the expected phase delay in the timing of these circadian rhythms. In addition to physiological measures, the Horne–Ostberg questionnaire is a useful tool to assess the "circadian type" of "eveningness" and "morningness" (39, 40). Individuals with DSPS score as definite evening types.

Clinical Management

Approaches aimed at resetting circadian rhythms, such as chronotherapy, timed bright light, and melatonin have been employed for the treatment of DSPS. Chronotherapy is a treatment in which sleep times are progressively delayed by approximately 3 hours per day until the desired earlier bedtime schedule is achieved (31). Although effective, the length and repeated nature of treatment and need for adherence to restrictive social and professional schedules limit practicality in the clinical setting. However, in adolescents, in which behavioral factors often contribute to the delayed-sleep phase, chronotherapy in conjunction with enforcement of regular sleep and wake times are important components of the clinical management.

Exposure to bright light for 1–2 hours in the morning results in an advance of the phase of circadian rhythms, whereas evening light exposure causes phase delays. Therefore, bright light exposure during the early morning hours and avoidance of bright light in the evening have been shown to be effective treatments for DSPS (41, 42) (Fig. 17-2). Following 2 weeks of exposure to 2 hours of bright light of 2500 lux each morning and restricted evening light, individuals with DSPS showed earlier sleep times and reported improved morning alertness level (42). However, many patients, particularly those who are severely delayed, find it difficult to awaken earlier for the 1 to 2 hours of bright-light therapy. Despite the potential utility of bright-light therapy, the timing, intensity, and duration of treatment remain to be defined. Exposure to broad-spectrum light of 2,000 to 10,000 lux for approximately 1 to 2 hours is generally recommended for use in clinical practice.

Due to the practical limitations of chronotherapy and phototherapy, melatonin, taken orally in the evening, has been increasingly investigated as a treatment for DSPS. Several studies have demonstrated the potential benefits of melatonin administered in the evening (43–46). However, because the timing of administration and dose varied among studies, and there is a relative lack of large-scale controlled clinical trials, guidelines for the use of

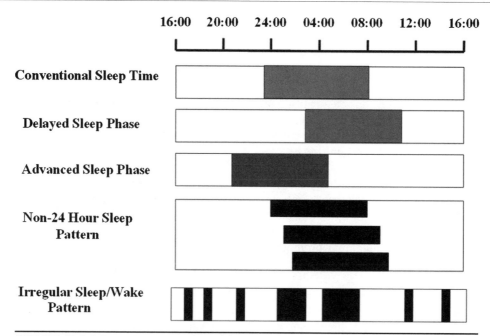

FIGURE 17-1. Schematic representation of the CRSD due primarily to alterations of the circadian timing system.

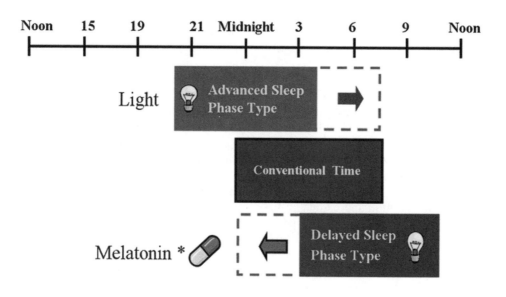

* Indicates non-FDA approved use

FIGURE 17-2. Schematic representation of treatment strategies for ASPS and DSPS. Exposure to light in the first half of the night delays circadian rhythms, whereas light late in the second half of the night or early morning advances circadian rhythms. In humans, the transition point between the delay and advance regions occurs near the temperature minimum (4:00 to 6:00 AM) in young adults and somewhat earlier in older adults. Therefore, bright-light exposure in the evening, usually between 7 and 9 PM, delays circadian rhythms and sleep–wake time in patients with ASPS, whereas light in the early morning, usually between 6 and 8 AM, will advance circadian rhythms in patients with DSPS. In severe cases, in which an estimate of circadian phase cannot be made based on habitual sleep and wake times, monitoring of circadian rhythms to determine the phase may be performed to determine the timing of light exposure. Melatonin in the evening, approximately 5 hours before habitual sleep time, has also been used to advance sleep time and circadian rhythms in DSPS.

melatonin in the treatment of DSPS is not available. The treatment of DSPS with melatonin is an unapproved use and remains empirical. Treatment success depends on many variables, including severity of the delayed-sleep phase, comorbid psychopathology, ability and willingness of the patient to comply with the treatment, school schedule, work obligations, and social pressures (9, 29, 47). A summary of treatment approaches of DSPS is shown in Fig. 17-2.

Advanced Sleep-Phase Syndrome (Advanced Sleep-Phase Type, Advanced Sleep-Phase Pattern)

ASPS is a sleep disorder in which there is a stable advance of the major sleep period, characterized by habitual and involuntary sleep onset and wake-up times that are several hours earlier relative to conventional and desired times (Fig 17-1). Individuals with ASPS usually report sleep onset of 6 to 9 PM and wake time of 2 to 5 AM (48, 49). ASPS complaints include early-morning awakenings, sleep maintenance insomnia, and also of sleepiness in the late afternoon or early evening. Individuals with ASPS typically consider themselves "larks" and score as morning types on the Horne–Ostberg questionnaire (23).

Clinical Epidemiology

The actual prevalence of ASPS is estimated at much lower than DSPS (50–53). ASPS not associated with aging is probably rare, with only a few reported cases (48, 54, 55). This condition is more common among middle-age and older adults, with an estimated prevalence of 1% of middle-age adults (51). However, it is not known whether the more commonly seen age-associated advance in sleep and wake times is the same entity as ASPS in younger individuals.

Differential Diagnosis

ASPS should be distinguished from "normal" sleep patterns, particularly in the elderly, who maintain advanced schedules without distress or impaired functioning (morning types or larks). Because depression may also present with early morning awakening, it is important to distinguish ASPS with depression and other types of mood disorders.

Etiology

Although the precise mechanisms underlying the pathophysiology of ASPS are unknown, several circadian-based mechanisms, such as an unusually short endogenous circadian period that is less than 24 hours (54), and decreased exposure or weakened response to entraining agents, such as light and physical activity (56–58), may impair phase delays and promote an advanced sleep phase. In addition to an earlier circadian phase, there is evidence that homeostatic regulation of sleep is also altered in older adults with advanced sleep phase (59).

Genetic factors have been shown to also play an important role in the pathogenesis of ASPS. Familial cases indicate an autosomal dominant mode of inheritance (54, 55). A mutation in the circadian clock gene *hPer2* was localized in a large family with this syndrome (60).

Diagnostic Evaluation

In addition to the history, actigraphy and sleep diaries can be very useful to confirm the advanced sleep-phase pattern. Recordings of sleep diaries and actigraphy over a period of at least 2 weeks demonstrate advanced sleep onset and offset (Fig.17-1), with typical sleep onsets of 6 to 9 PM and wake times of 2 to 5 AM. The Horne–Ostberg questionnaire is a practical and useful tool to assess the chronotype of "eveningness" and "morningness." Individuals with ASPS score as definite morning types (55).

When the diagnosis is unclear, or when another sleep disorder may be in the differential diagnosis, PSG is indicated. When performed at the preferred (advanced) sleep times, PSG findings are essentially normal for age. However, if conventional later bedtime and wake times are enforced, the PSG recording may show decreased sleep latency, decreased TST, and shortened REM sleep latency. Although not required, laboratory physiologic measures of circadian phase, such as core body temperature and DLMO, are useful to document the advanced circadian phase, particularly when a definite diagnosis is in question.

Clinical Management

Treatment approaches for ASPS may include chronotherapy, exposure to light in the evening, and pharmacotherapy with sedative–hypnotics or melatonin. Chronotherapy was one of the earliest treatment approaches proposed for ASPS (48), in which attempts to delay the sleep times of the ASPS patients were largely unsuccessful, but a 3-hour advance in sleep time every 2 days allowed the individual to shift to the desired later sleep schedule. Because of the behavioral restrictions, this treatment has had limited success in the clinical setting.

As with DSPS, the most commonly used treatment is timed bright-light therapy in the evening, usually between 7 to 9 PM (61–63). In these studies, bright-light exposure improved sleep efficiency and delayed the phase of circadian rhythms, but patients had difficulty maintaining the treatment regimen (64). Based on the phase-response curve to melatonin, in order to delay circadian rhythms in ASPS, melatonin should be taken during the early morning hours. Theoretically, melatonin can be useful in delaying the phase of circadian rhythms and sleep in ASPS. However, there is very little data of its usefulness in the treatment of ASPS in the clinical setting and the sedative effects of melatonin administered in the morning could be a potential limiting factor. A summary of the treatment approaches for ASPS is shown in Fig. 17-2.

Nonentrained Sleep–Wake Disorder (Non-24-Hour Sleep and Wake Disorder, Free-Running, Hypernychthermal Syndrome)

Nonentrained sleep–wake disorder is characterized by a steady daily delay drift of the major sleep period in which the intrinsic circadian pacemaker is not entrained to the physical and social 24-hour cycle (Fig. 17-1). When the timing of endogenous circadian rhythms is in phase with the desired and conventional sleep times, sleep is typically normal, and when allowed, some individuals maintain a sleep pattern in which their sleep and wake times are delayed daily by 1 to 2 hours. However, when the nonentrained circadian clock is out of phase with the timing of the desired sleep and wake times, individuals complain of insomnia and EDS.

Prevalence

This circadian rhythm sleep disorder is rare and mostly observed in blind people (65). It has been rarely reported in sighted individuals living in normal society (66). It has been estimated that about 50% of the totally blind have free-running circadian rhythms (67) and that approximately 70% have complaints of chronic sleep disturbances (68, 69).

Diagnostic Evaluation

The diagnosis of a nonentrained circadian sleep–wake cycle requires that the periodic sleep disturbances are due to the lack of a stable entrainment of circadian rhythms to the 24-hour physical environment and that this alteration is accompanied by distress or impairment in social, occupational, or other areas of functioning. Depending on the time, patients with nonentrained sleep–wake disorder may have varied complaints, from insomnia or early morning awakenings to EDS (DSM IV-TR). As with the circadian sleep-phase disorders, actigraphy and sleep diaries are useful diagnostic tools for evaluation of non–24-hour sleep–wake disorder. When recorded over 2 to 4 weeks, these measures typically show a progressive daily delay drift in the timing of sleep and wake. If available, serial measurements of physiologic or hormonal circadian rhythms, such as DLMO or core body temperature, may also be used to confirm the diagnosis by demonstrating nonentrained circadian rhythms (70).

Etiology

The average endogenous period of oscillation of the human circadian clock is slightly longer than 24 hours and synchronizing agents, such as light and social or physical activity, maintain alignment between the non–24-hour circadian rhythms with the 24-hour physical environment (71). Therefore, the high prevalence of nonentrained circadian rhythms in blind people is most likely due to the lack of photic entrainment. However, not all blind people have nonentrained circadian rhythms. In these individuals, scheduled social or physical activity may serve as synchronizing agents to maintain entrainment of circadian rhythms. In addition, despite their lack of visual light perception, there is evidence that the circadian clock of some blind individuals responds to bright light (72). This finding can be explained by recent observation that retinal ganglion cells, rather than the rods and cones, are predominantly responsible for the circadian phase shifting effects of light (73,74).

It has been postulated that in sighted individuals with non–24-hour sleep–wake sleep disorder, the etiology may be an extremely prolonged endogenous circadian period that is no longer within the range of entrainment to the 24-hour day–night cycle (75). In fact, it has been postulated that free-running circadian sleep disorder in sighted persons may be a severe form of DSPS (9). Supporting this hypothesis are case reports of DSPS patients who developed a free-running pattern after chronotherapy (76). Other possibilities include a decreased sensitivity of the circadian clock to light or alteration in the entrainment pathways, resulting in weakened entrainment or lack of entrainment of the endogenous circadian rhythm (77).

Differential Diagnosis

In sighted people, social and behavioral factors may also play an important role in the development and maintenance of the disorder. Behavioral factors predisposing to irregular schedules, medical, neurologic, and psychiatric disorders should be considered, as there is an increased incidence of psychiatric and personality disorders in patients with non–24-hour sleep–wake sleep disorder (77). In patients with cognitive disorders, lack of exposure to regular social and light–dark schedules may result in what appears to be a nonentrained sleep–wake cycle (78,79).

Clinical Management

In blind people, several approaches using nonphotic circadian synchronizing agents, such as regular schedules of sleep and social–work activities and melatonin have been successful in the management of non–24-hour sleep–wake disorder. Melatonin (10 mg), typically taken 1 hour before bedtime, has been shown to entrain the timing of sleep in blind people (80). Furthermore, in some individuals, entrainment could be maintained with a gradual reduction to just 0.5 mg at night (81).

In sighted individuals, increasing the strength of the light–dark cycle with bright light exposure and/or melatonin to entrain circadian rhythms may be useful (77). There has been also been a case report of the successful treatment of free-running sleep and wake rhythms with flurazepam and vitamin B_{12} (82). However, very little is known regarding the actual effectiveness of these treatment approaches.

Irregular Sleep–Wake Disorder (No Circadian Rhythm, Grossly Disturbed Sleep–Wake Rhythm, Low-Amplitude Circadian Rhythm)

Irregular sleep–wake disorder is characterized by lack of a clearly defined circadian sleep and wake cycle. Sleep and wake behaviors are variable, so that a major sleep or wake period is not seen within the usual 24-hour period. Diagnosis of this condition requires a complaint of insomnia and/or excessive sleepiness associated with multiple irregular sleep bouts or naps during a 24-hour period. Total sleep time (TST) per 24-hour period is essentially normal for age.

In addition to the clinical history, continuous monitoring of sleep and wake activity with actigraphy for a minimum of 2 weeks is the most useful diagnostic tool. Actigraphic recordings show disturbed or low-amplitude circadian rhythm with loss of the normal diurnal sleep–wake pattern. Irregular sleep–wake disorder should be distinguished from poor sleep hygiene and voluntary maintenance of irregular sleep schedules, as seen with shift work and frequent transmeridian travel.

The prevalence of irregular sleep–wake pattern in the general population is unknown, but estimated to be rare (24). It is most frequently seen in association with neurologic dysfunction, such as brain injury and dementia, and in children with psychomotor retardation, where a low-amplitude or irregular rhythm of sleep and wake patterns may be due to dysfunction of the central processes responsible for the generation of circadian rhythms (83–85).

In certain populations, like the institutionalized elderly and those with dementia, lack of regular exposure to bright light and social schedules has been postulated to influence the development and maintenance of irregular sleep–wake patterns (86, 87). Therefore, both dysfunction of circadian regulation and weakened exposure to environmental signals are likely involved in the etiology of irregular or arrhythmic sleep and wake patterns.

Clinical management approaches have been aimed at enhancing the amplitude of circadian rhythms and their alignment to the external physical environment. Exposure to synchronizing agents, such as bright light and structuring of social and physical activities, has been used to consolidate sleep and wake cycles in these individuals (34,58,88). In the elderly with dementia, programs of structured activities and increased social interaction to maintain wakefulness during the day and increased light exposure have been shown to consolidate sleep and wake (88–

90). A combination of bright light, chronotherapy, vitamin B_{12}, and hypnotics showed that 45% of patients with irregular sleep cycles responded to treatment (24). In children with psychomotor retardation, evening administration of melatonin may improve sleep and wake patterns (91). Despite the potential utility of the various pharmacologic and behavioral interventions, treatment is often difficult and results have been variable.

Circadian Rhythm Sleep Disorder: Shift Work Type

Shift work-associated sleep disorder is characterized by complaints of insomnia or excessive sleepiness that occur in relation to work hours that are scheduled during the usual sleep period. There are several types of shift work schedules, including rotating shifts, staggered rotating shifts, seven on–seven off night and day shifts, with a superimposed night call schedule. Sleep disturbance is most commonly reported in association with night and early-morning shifts. TST is typically curtailed by 1 to 4 hours in night and early-morning shift workers, and sleep quality is perceived as unsatisfactory (92–94). In addition to impairment of performance at work, reduced alertness may also be associated with consequences for safety.

Clinical Epidemiology

It has been estimated that 20% of the workforce in industrialized countries is employed in a job that requires shift work (95). Although, the actual prevalence of clinically significant sleep disturbance and excessive daytime sleepiness due to work schedules is unknown, based on the number of night-shift workers, an estimate of 2% to 5% is reasonable (96).

Differential Diagnosis

Symptoms of insomnia or excessive sleepiness should be differentiated from that due to other primary sleep disorders, such as other CRSD, obstructive sleep apnea (OSA) syndrome, narcolepsy, or insufficient sleep related to inadequate opportunity for sleep. The relation between the occurrence of disturbed sleep and work hour distribution should provide sufficient information to indicate the correct diagnosis. Use of sedative–hypnotics and stimulants, as well as substance dependency, should be considered as contributing factors, and may exacerbate the symptoms of shift work sleep disorder.

Etiology

Disturbance of sleep and alertness is due to a misalignment between the circadian alerting process with the time that the worker needs to sleep. The excessive sleepiness is most likely the result of both cumulative sleep loss and decreased circadian alertness during night and early morning work shifts. Individual tolerance to shift work varies considerably and may involve differences in the degree of circadian adaptation, sleep homeostatic influences, age, type of shift schedule, and family/social support.

Diagnostic Evaluation

Shift work-associated sleep disorder can usually be diagnosed by history. In addition to the history, sleep diaries and actigraphy are very useful in demonstrating a disrupted sleep–wake pattern consistent with shift work sleep disorder. Polysomnographic recordings may be useful if the nature of the sleep disturbance is unclear, or to evaluate for comorbid conditions, such as sleep-disordered breathing (SDB). Under specific conditions, when objective evaluation of sleepiness is indicated, the multiple sleep latency test (MSLT) or maintenance of wakefulness test (MWT) is useful in demonstrating excessive sleepiness during the time of the work shift.

Clinical Management

Clinical management of shift work-related sleep disorder should be aimed at realigning circadian rhythms with the sleep–wake–work schedules, as well improving the sleep and work environments to enhance sleep quality and alertness. Most of the strategies developed for adjustment to shift work have focused on the night-shift worker. In shift workers, the use of bright light and melatonin have been shown to improve the adaptation of circadian rhythms by aligning the circadian rhythm of sleep propensity with the desired sleep time (97–99). Most studies used light intensities that varied between 1,200 and 10,000 lux for a period of 3 to 6 hours of exposure during the night shift (100). More recently, intermittent bright-light exposure (~20 minutes per hour blocks) has also being shown to accelerate circadian adaptation to night shift work (101,102). Either continuous or intermittent bright-light treatment should be initiated early during the night shift and stopped approximately 2 hours prior to the end of the shift. For the night-shift worker, exposure to early morning light may prevent the phase delay that is required for alignment of the circadian rhythm of sleep propensity with the desired daytime sleep. Therefore, just as important as bright-light exposure at the correct time is avoidance of light exposure at the wrong circadian time. Several studies (101–103) have indicated that avoiding light in the early morning on the way home from work (by wearing dark glasses) can improve phase adjustment even without bright-light treatment (103). In addition to the phase-shifting properties, bright light has acute alerting effects that have been shown to improve cognitive performance during work hours (104). Because of the potential circadian-phase shifting and mild hypnotic effects of melatonin, it has also been used to improve adjustment to shift work. A recent review of the role of melatonin indicates that when taken at bedtime after the night shift, it can improve daytime sleep duration, but had limited effects on alertness (100).

Pharmacological agents such as sedative–hypnotics may be used for the management of insomnia. Although sedative–hypnotic medications may improve the quality and quantity of sleep, they do not address the issue of circadian phase alignment, and, therefore, are insufficient alone. Stimulants such as caffeine and, more recently, modafinil can be useful as short-term strategies to combat excessive sleepiness, particularly when safety is at risk and where additional strategies for improving alertness and performance in the shift work setting are required (105,106).

Family and social factors are also extremely important in determining coping ability. Family responsibilities, such as childcare and household chores, decrease the amount of time allotted for sleep. The sleep environment needs to be optimized to include decrease daytime noise, a darkened room, and an adherence to healthy sleep habits. Family dynamics surrounding shift work can place a tremendous strain on a marriage. Therefore, education for the patient, family, and employer is vital for effective management of shift work.

In summary, management of shift work sleep disorder requires multimodal strategies that address circadian alignment, sleep hygiene, improving sleep and alertness, and, very importantly, psychosocial factors. Other factors to consider are individual differences in tolerance to shift work, motivation of the patient, social/family support, and an increasingly diverse number of shift work schedules, type of work, and safety issues at risk. Therefore, for maximum success, the treatment plan needs to be individualized to address the multiple factors involved.

Jet Lag

Jet lag occurs with rapid travel across time zones, resulting in a misalignment between the timing of circadian rhythms with that of the external physical environment. Symptoms of jet lag typically consist of general malaise, daytime sleepiness, difficulty sleeping, impaired performance, and gastrointestinal upset (107). These symptoms usually last for several days, with resolution occurring as the traveler adapts to the new time zone. The severity of jet lag symptoms and the ability to adapt to the new time zone is influenced by three major factors: the direction of travel, the number of time zones crossed, and individual susceptibility. Eastward travel (requiring advancing circadian rhythms and sleep–wake hours) is usually more difficult to adjust than westward travel. Eastward travel generally results in difficulty falling asleep and westward travel in difficulty maintaining sleep (107). In addition, other factors such as the air quality, diminished physical activity level, and discomfort likely contribute to the severity of symptoms.

Treatment of jet lag symptoms should address the sleep loss associated with the time zone change, as well as circadian reentrainment. A number of general counter-measures can be employed to ameliorate the symptoms of jet lag. Maintaining good sleep hygiene is important during travel. Wearing loose clothing during the flight and ear plugs and eyeshades may be helpful (even after arrival) to promote sleep. Upon arrival, eating meals according to local time, exercise, and light exposure at appropriate clock times can be useful(108,109).

Treatments aimed at accelerating reentrainment of circadian rhythms to a new time zone include bright light, avoidance of bright light (107,110), and/or melatonin (111). The avoidance of natural bright light may be the most important practical strategy. The timing of light exposure depends on the direction of travel and the number of times zones crossed. For example, on an eastward flight, when arriving in the morning, one should remain awake, avoid bright light early in the morning, but get as much light as possible in the afternoon (112). Some studies have also shown that melatonin can help alleviate jet lag (112). It is important to note that melatonin has not been approved by the FDA for the treatment of CRSD. Furthermore, potential adverse effects such as headaches, nausea, and exacerbation of cardiovascular disease should be considered.

Given that insomnia is a major complaint of travelers with jet lag, short-term use of short-acting hypnotic medications (111,113) is also useful. A study using zolpidem (10 mg) given for three consecutive nights starting with the first night's sleep after travel was shown to improve sleep in some seasoned travelers (113). If behavioral strategies, such as bright-light exposure and good sleep hygiene, are not sufficient to alleviate jet lag, use of a short-acting hypnotic during the flight and for the first few days after arrival is a reasonable approach.

SUMMARY AND FUTURE DIRECTION

Disorders of the sleep–wake cycle due to disruptions of circadian timing or misalignment are characterized by an unconventional temporal distribution of the major sleep and wake periods within the 24-hour day. The impact of these disorders in the differential diagnosis of insomnia in clinical practice remains underappreciated. Most clinical practices do not have the tools to assess circadian rhythm profiles; coupled with a relative lack of standardized clinical treatment guidelines, this presents a barrier to effective diagnosis and treatment of these disorders. Rapid advances in the understanding of the physiologic and genetic basis of circadian rhythm and sleep regulation, as well as the recent discovery that the circadian clock is most responsive to short wavelength light in the blue range, should lead to improved and practical management strategies for CRSD.

Although there is strong evidence that a common etiology of these disorders is an alteration in the circadian timing system, behavioral and environmental factors play an important role in the presentation and maintenance of the CRSD. Therefore, in addition to physiological approaches aimed at realignment and entrainment of circadian rhythms, treatment interventions need to also address behavioral and environmental influences.

REFERENCES

1. Dunlap JC. Molecular bases for circadian clocks. *Cell.* 1999;96(2):271–90.
2. Moore RY, Eichler VB. Loss of a circadian adrenal corticosterone rhythm following suprachiasmatic lesions in the rat. *Brain Res.* 1972;42(1):201–206.
3. Stephan FK, Zucker I. Circadian rhythms in drinking behavior and locomotor activity of rats are eliminated by hypothalamic lesions. *Proc Natl Acad Sci USA.* 1972;69(6):1583–1586.
4. Ralph M, Foster RG, Davis FC, et al. Transplanted suprachiasmatic nucleus determines circadian period. *Science.* 1990;247:975–978.
5. Moore RY. Circadian rhythms: basic neurobiology and clinical applications. *Annu Rev Med.* 1997;48:253–266.
6. Czeisler CA, Allan JS, Strogatz SH, et al. Bright light resets the human circadian pacemaker independent of the timing of the sleep–wake cycle. *Science.* 1986;233(4764):667–671.
7. Boivin DB, Duffy JF, Kronauer RE, et al. Sensitivity of the human circadian pacemaker to moderately bright light. *J Bio Rhythms.* 1994;9(3–4):315–331.
8. Minors DS, Waterhouse JM, Wirz-Justice A. A human phase-response curve to light. *Neurosci Lett.* 1991;13:36–40.
9. Regestein QR, Monk TH. Delayed sleep phase syndrome: a review of its clinical aspects. *Amer J Psych.* 1995;152(4):602–608.
10. Czeisler CA, Kronauer RE, Allan JS. Assessment and modification of a subject's endogenous circadian cycle. U.S. Patent No. 5,163,426. Washington, DC: US Patent Office, 1992.
11. Aschoff J, Fatranska M, Giedke H, et al. Human circadian rhythms in continuous darkness: entrainment by social cues. *Science.* 1971;171(967):213–215.
12. Turek FW. Effects of stimulated physical activity on the circadian pacemaker of vertebrates. *J Biol Rhythms.* 1989;4(2):135–147.
13. Smith R, Turek FW, Takahashi JS. Two families of phase response curves characterize the resetting of the hamster circadian clock. *Amer J Physiol.* 1992;262:R1149–R1153.
14. Dubocovich ML, Benloucif S, Masana MI. Melatonin receptors in the mammalian suprachiasmatic nucleus. *Behav Brain Res.* 1996;73:141–147.
15. Lewy AJ, Bauer VK, Ahmed S, et al. The human phase response curve (PRC) to melatonin is about 12 hours out of phase with the PRC to light. *Chronobiol Intern.* 1998;15(1):71–83.
16. Dijk D, Czeisler C. Paradoxical timing of the circadian rhythm of sleep propensity serves to consolidate sleep and wakefulness in humans. *Neurosci Lett.* 1994;166:63–68.
17. Borbely A. Sleep: circadian rhythm vs. recovery process. In Koukkou M, Lehmann D, Angst J, ed. *Functional states of the brain: Their determinants.* Amsterdam: Elsevier/North-Holland, 1980;151–161.
18. Wever R. *The circadian system of man. Results of experiments under temporal isolation.* New York: Springer Verlag, 1979.
19. Czeisler C, Weitzman E, Moore-Ede M, et al. Human sleep: its duration and organisation depend on it circadian phase. *Science.* 1980;210:1264–1267.
20. Zulley J, Wever R. Aschoff J. The dependence of onset and duration of sleep on the circadian rhythm of rectal temperature. *Pflugers Arch.* 1981;391(4):314–318.
21. Czeisler CA, Richardson GS, Coleman RM, et al. Chronotherapy: resetting the circadian clock of patients with delayed sleep phase insomnia. *Sleep.* 1981;4:1–21.
22. Czeisler CA, Richardson GS, Zimmerman JC, et al. Entrainment of human circadian rhythms by light-dark cycles: a reassessment. *Photochem Photobiol.* 1981;34(2):239–247.

23. Horne JA, Ostberg O. A self-assessment questionnaire to determine morningness-eveningness in human circadian rhythms. *Interm J Chronobiol.* 1976;4(2):97–110.

24. Yamadera H, Takahashi K, Okawa M. A multicenter study of sleep–wake rhythm disorders: clinical features of sleep–wake rhythm disorders. *Psych Clin Neurosci.* 1996;50(4):195–201.

25. Pelayo R, Thorpy MJ, Govinski P. Prevalence of delayed sleep phase syndrome among adolescents. *Sleep Res.* 1988;17:392.

26. Rufiange M, Dumont M, Lachapelle P. Correlating retinal function with melatonin secretion in subjects with an early or late circadian phase. *Invest Ophthalmol Vis Sci.* 2002;42(7):2491–2499.

27. Shibui K, Uchiyama M, Okawa M. Melatonin rhythms in delayed sleep phase syndrome. *J Biol Rhythms.* 1999;14(1):72–76.

28. Alvarez B, Dahlitz M, Vignau J. The delayed sleep phase syndrome: clinical and investigative findings in 14 subjects. *J Neurol Neurosurg Psych.* 1992;55:665–670.

29. Thorpy MJ, Korman E, Spielman AJ, et al. Delayed sleep phase syndrome in adolescents. *J Adoles Health Care.* 1988;9(1):22–27.

30. Uchiyama M, Okawa M, Shirakawa S, et al. A polysomnographic study on patients with delayed sleep phase syndrome (DSPS). *Jpn J Psych Neurol.* 1992;46(1):219–221.

31. Weitzman ED, Czeisler CA, Coleman RM, et al. Delayed sleep phase syndrome. A chronobiological disorder with sleep- onset insomnia. *Arch Gen Psych.* 1981;38(7):737–746.

32. Uchiyama M, Okawa M, Shibui K, et al. Poor recovery sleep after sleep deprivation in delayed sleep phase syndrome. *Psych Clin Neurosci.* 1999;53(2):195–197.

33. Uchiyama M, Okawa M, Shibui K, et al. Poor compensatory function for sleep loss as a pathogenic factor in patients with delayed sleep phase syndrome. *Sleep.* 2000;23(4):553–558.

34. Ancoli-Israel S, Schnierow B, Kelsoe J, et al. A pedigree of one family with delayed sleep phase syndrome. *Chronobiol Interm.* 2001;18(5):831–840.

35. Iwase T, Kajimura N, Uchiyama M, et al. Mutation screening of the human Clock gene in circadian rhythm sleep disorders. *Psych Res.* 2002;109(2):121–128.

36. Ebisawa T, Uchiyama M, Kajimura N, et al. Association of structural polymorphisms in the human period3 gene with delayed sleep phase syndrome. *EMBO Rept.* 2001;2(4):342–346.

37. Archer SN, Robilliard DL, Skene DJ, et al. A length polymorphism in the circadian clock gene Per3 is linked to delayed sleep phase syndrome and extreme diurnal preference. *Sleep.* 2003;26(4):413–415.

38. Hohjoh H, Takasu M, Shishikura K, et al. Significant association of the arylalkylamine N-acetyltransferase (AA-NAT) gene with delayed sleep phase syndrome. *Neurogenetics.* 2003;4(3):151–153.

39. Horne JA, Ostberg O. Individual differences in human circadian rhythms. *Biol Psychol.* 1977;5(3):179–190.

40. Kerkhof GA. Inter-individual differences in the human circadian system: a review. *Biol Psychol.* 1985;20:83–112.

41. Chesson AL, Jr. Littner M, Davila D, et al. Practice parameters for the use of light therapy in the treatment of sleep disorders. Standards of Practice Committee, American Academy of Sleep Medicine. *Sleep.* 1999;22(5):641–660.

42. Rosenthal NE, Joseph-Vanderpool JR, Levendosky AA, et al. Phase-shifting effects of bright morning light as treatment for delayed sleep phase syndrome. *Sleep.* 1990;13(4):354–361.

43. James SP, Sack DA, Rosenthal NE, et al. Melatonin administration in insomnia. *Neuropsychopharmacology.* 1990;3(1):19–23.

44. Dahlitz M, Alvarez B, Vignau J, et al. Delayed sleep phase syndrome response to melatonin. *Lancet.* 1991;337(8750):1121–1124.

45. Oldani A, Ferini-Strambi L, Zucconi M, et al. Melatonin and delayed sleep phase syndrome: ambulatory polygraphic evaluation. *Neuroreport.* 1994;6(1):132–134.

46. Nagtegaal JE, Kerkhof GA, Smits MG, et al. Delayed sleep phase syndrome: a placebo-controlled cross-over study on the effects of melatonin administered five hours before the individual dim light melatonin onset. *J Sleep Res.* 1998;7(2):135–143.

47. Ohta T, Iwata T, Kayukawa Y, et al. Daily activity and persistent sleep–wake schedule disorders. *Prog-Neuropsychopharmacol Biol Psych.* 1992;16(4):529–537.

48. Moldofsky H, Musisi S, Phillipson EA. Treatment of a case of advanced sleep phase syndrome by phase advance chronotherapy. *Sleep.* 1986;9(1):61–65.

49. Kamei Y, Urata J, Uchiyaya M, et al. Clinical characteristics of circadian rhythm sleep disorders. *Psych Clin Neurosci.* 1998;52(2):234–235.

50. Schrader H, Bovim G, Sand T. The prevalence of delayed and advanced sleep phase syndromes. *J Sleep Res.* 1993;2(1):51–55.

51. Ando K, Kripke DF, Ancoli-Israel S. Estimated prevalence of delayed and advanced sleep phase syndromes. *Sleep Res.* 1995;24:509.

52. Baker SK, Zee PC. Circadian disorders of the sleep–wake cycle. In: Kryger MH, Roth T, Dement W, eds. *Principles and practice of sleep medicine,* Philadelphia: WB Saunders, 2000:606–614.

53. Burns ER, Sateia MJ, Lee-Chiong TL. Basic principles of chronobiology and disorders of circadian sleep–wake rhythm. In: Chiong TL, Sateia MJ, Carskadon MA, eds. *Sleep medicine,* Philadelphia: Hanley & Belfus, Inc, 2002:245–254.

54. Jones CR, Campbell SS, Zone SE, et al. Familial advanced sleep-phase syndrome: a short-period circadian rhythm variant in humans. *Nat Med.* 1999;5(9):1062–1065.

55. Reid KJ, Chang AM, Dubocovich ML, et al. Familial advanced sleep phase syndrome. *Arch Neurol.* 2001;58(7):1089–1094.

56. Ancoli-Israel S, Kripke DF. Prevalent sleep problems in the aged. *Biofeedback Self Regul.* 1991;16(4):349–359.

57. Moore RY. A clock for the ages. *Science.* 1999;284(5423):2102–2103.

58. Naylor E, Penev PD, Orbeta L, et al. Daily social and physical activity increases slow-wave sleep and daytime neuropsychological performance in the elderly. *Sleep.* 2000;23(1):87–95.

59. Duffy JF, Czeisler CA. Age-related change in the relationship between circadian period, circadian phase, and diurnal preference in humans. *Neurosci Lett.* 2002;318:117–120.

60. Toh KL, Jones CR, He Y, et al. An hPer2 phosphorylation site mutation in familial advanced sleep phase syndrome. *Science.* 2001;291(5506):1040–1043.

61. Campbell SS, Dawson D, Anderson MW. Alleviation of sleep maintenance insomnia with timed exposure to bright light. *J Amer Geriatr Soc.* 1993;41(8):829–836.

62. Lack L, Wright H. The effect of evening bright light in delaying the circadian rhythms and lengthening the sleep of early morning awakening insomniacs. *Sleep.* 1993;16(5):436–443.

63. Lack L, Schumacher K. Evening light treatment of early morning insomnia. *Sleep Res.* 1993;22:225.

64. Campbell SS. Intrinsic disruption of normal sleep and circadian patterns. In: Turek FW, Zee PC eds. *Regulation of sleep and circadian rhythms.* Marcel New York: Marcel Dekker, 1999:465–486.

65. Elliott AL, Mills JN, Waterhouse JM. A man with too long a day. *J Physiol.* 1971;212(2):30P–31P.

66. Weber AL, Cary MS, Connor N, et al. Human non-24-hour sleep–wake cycles in an everyday environment. *Sleep.* 1980;2(3):347–354.

67. Sack RL, Lewy AJ, Blood ML, et al. Circadian rhythm abnormalities in totally blind people: incidence and clinical significance. *J Clin Endocrinol Metab.* 1992;75(1):127–134.

68. Miles LE, Raynal DM, Wilson MA. Blind man living in normal society has circadian rhythms of 24.9 hours. *Science.* 1977;198(4315):421–423.

69. Martens H, Endlich H, Hildebrandt G. Sleep/wake distribution in blind subjects with and without sleep complaints. *Sleep Res.* 1990;9:398.

70. Klein T, Martens H, Dijk DJ, et al. Circadian sleep regulation in the absence of light perception: Chronic non-24-hour circadian rhythm sleep disorder in a blind man with a regular 24-hour sleep–wake schedule. *Sleep.* 1993;16(4):333–343.

71. Czeisler CA, Duffy JF, Shanahan TL, et al. Stability, precision, and near-24-hour period of the human circadian pacemaker. *Science.* 1999;284(5423):2177–2181.

72. Czeisler CA, Shanahan TL, Klerman FB, et al. Suppression of melatonin secretion in some blind patients by exposure to bright light. *N Engl J Med.* 1995;332(1):6–11.

73. Menaker M. Circadian rhythms. Circadian photoreception. *Science.* 2003;299(5604):213–214.

74. Guido ME, Carpentieri AR, Garbarino-Pico E. Circadian phototransduction and the regulation of biological rhythms. *Neurochem Res.* 2002;27(11):1473–1489.

75. Uchiyama M, Shibui K, Hayakawa T, et al. Larger phase angle between sleep propensity and melatonin rhythms in sighted humans with non-24-hour sleep–wake syndrome. *Sleep.* 2002;25(1):83–88.

76. Oren DA, Wehr TA. Hypernyctohemeral syndrome after chronotherapy for delayed sleep phase syndrome. *N Engl J Med.* 1992; 327(24):1762.

77. McArthur AJ, Lewy AJ, Sack RL. Non-24-hour sleep–wake syndrome in a sighted man: circadian rhythm studies and efficacy of melatonin treatment. *Sleep.* 1996;19(7):544–553.

78. Palm L, Blennow G, Wetterberg L. Correction of non-24-hour sleep/wake cycle by melatonin in a blind retarded boy. *Ann Neurol.* 1991;29(3):336–339.

79. Palm L, Blennow G, Wetterberg L. Long-term melatonin treatment in blind children and young adults with circadian sleep–wake disturbances. *Develop Med Child Neurol.* 1997;39(5):319–325.

80. Sack RL, Brandes RW, Kendall AR, et al. Entrainment of free-running circadian rhythms by melatonin in blind people. *N Engl. J Med.* 2000;343(15):1070–1077.

81. Lewy AJ, Bauer VK, Hasler BP, et al. Capturing the circadian rhythms of free-running blind people with 0.5 mg melatonin. *Brain Res.* 2001;918(1-2):96–100.

82. Kamgar-Parsi B, Wehr TA, Gillin JC. Successful treatment of human non-24-hour sleep–wake syndrome. *Sleep.* 1983;6(3):257–264.

83. Witting W, Kwa IH, Eikelenboom P, et al. Alterations in the circadian rest-activity rhythm in aging and Alzheimer's disease. *Biol Psych.* 1990;27(6):563–572.

84. Hoogendijk WJ, van Someren EJ, Mirmiran M, et al. Circadian rhythm-related behavioral disturbances and structural hypothalamic changes in Alzheimer's disease. *Intern Psychogeriatr.* 1996;8 (Supp.3):245-252, 269–272.

85. Edgar DM, Dement WC, Fuller CA. Effect of SCN lesions on sleep in squirrel monkeys: evidence for opponent processes in sleep–wake regulation. *J Neurosci.* 1993;13(3):1065–1079.

86. Pollak CP, Stokes PE. Circadian rest-activity rhythms in demented and nondemented older community residents and their caregivers. *J Amer Geriatr Soc.* 1997;45(4):446–452.

87. van Someren EJ, Hagebeuk EE, Lijzenga C, et al. Circadian rest-activity rhythm disturbances in Alzheimer's disease. *Biol Psych.* 1996;40(4):259–270.

88. Van Someren EJ, Swaab DF, Colenda CC, et al. Bright light therapy:Improved sensitivity to its effects on rest-activity rhythms in Alzheimer patients by application of nonparametric methods. *Chronobiol Intern.* 1999;16(4):505–518.

89. Okawa M, Mishima K, Hishikawa Y, et al. Circadian rhythm disorders in sleep-waking and body temperature in elderly patients with dementia and their treatment. *Sleep.* 1991;14(6):478–485.

90. Ancoli-Israel S, Martin JL, Kripke DF, et al. Effect of light treatment on sleep and circadian rhythms in demented nursing home patients. *J Amer Geriatr Soc.* 2002;50(2):282–289.

91. Pillar G, Shahar E, Peled N, et al. Melatonin improves sleep–wake patterns in psychomotor retarded children. *Pediatr Neurol.* 2000;23(3):225–228.

92. Åkerstedt T. Work hours, sleepiness and the underlying mechanisms. *J Sleep Res.* 1995;4(2 Suppl.):15–22.

93. Knauth P, Landau K, Droge C, et al. Duration of sleep depending on the type of shiftwork. *Intern Arch Occup Environ Health.* 1980;46:167–177.

94. Knauth P, Rutenfranz J. Duration of sleep related to the type of shiftwork. In: Reinberg A, Vieux N, Andlauer P, eds. *Advances in the biosciences. Vol. 30. Night and shiftwork biological and social aspects,* Oxford, New York: Pergamon Press, 1981;161–168.

95. Presser H. Towards a 24-hour economy. *Science.* 1999;284:1778–1779.

96. Akerstedt T. Shift work and disturbed sleep/wakefulness. *Occup Med (London).* 2003;53(2):89–94.

97. Dawson D, Campbell SS. Timed exposure to bright light improves sleep and alertness during simulated night shifts. *Sleep.* 1991;14(6):511–516.

98. Dawson D, Encel N, Lushington K. Improving adaptation to simulated night shift: timed exposure to bright light versus daytime melatonin administration. *Sleep.* 1995;18(1):11–21.

99. Sharkey KM, Fogg LF, Eastman CI. Effects of melatonin administration on daytime sleep after simulated night shift work. *J Sleep Res.* 2001;10(3):181–192.

100. Burgess HJ, Sharkey KM, Eastman CI. Bright light, dark and melatonin can promote circadian adaptation in night shift workers. *Sleep Med Rev.* 2002;6(5):407–420.

101. Boivin DB, James FO. Circadian adaptation to night-shift work by judicious light and darkness exposure. *J Biol Rhythms.* 2002;17(6):556–567.

102. Crowley SJ, Lee C, Tseng CY, et al. Combinations of bright light, scheduled dark, sunglasses, and melatonin to facilitate circadian entrainment to night shift work. *J Biol Rhythms.* 2003;18(6):513–523.

103. Eastman CI, Stewart KT, Mahoney MP, et al. Dark goggles and bright light improve circadian rhythm adaptation to night-shift work. *Sleep.* 1994;17(6):535–543.

104. Campbell SS, Dijk DJ, Boulos Z, et al. Light treatment for sleep disorders: consensus report. III. Alerting and activating effects. *J Biol Rhythms.* 1995;10(2):129–132.

105. Akerstedt T, Ficca G. Alertness-enhancing drugs as a countermeasure to fatigue in irregular work hours. *Chronobiol Intern.* 1997;14(2):145–158.

106. Babkoff H, French J, Whitmore J, et al. Single-dose bright light and/or caffeine effect on nocturnal performance. *Aviat Space Environ Med.* 2002;73(4):341–350.

107. Boulos Z, Campbell SS, Lewy AJ, et al. Light treatment for sleep disorders: consensus report. VII. Jet lag. *J Biol Rhythms.* 1995;10(2):167–176.

108. Waterhouse J, Reilly T, Atkinson G. Jet-lag. *Lancet.* 1997;350(9091):1611–1616.

109. Daan S, Lewy AJ. Scheduled exposure to daylight: a potential strategy to reduce "jet lag" following transmeridian flight. *Psychopharmacol Bull.* 1984;20(3):566–568.

110. Burgess HJ, Crowley SJ, Gazda CJ, et al. Preflight adjustment to eastward travel: 3 days of advancing sleep with and without morning bright light. *J Biol Rhythms.* 2003;18(4):318–328.

111. Beaumont M, Batejat D, Pierard C, et al. Caffeine or melatonin effects on sleep and sleepiness after rapid eastward transmeridian travel. *J Appl Physiol.* 2004;96(1):50–58.

112. Herxheimer A, Waterhouse J. The prevention and treatment of jet lag. *BMJ.* 2003;326(7384):296–297.

113. Jamieson AO, Zammit GK, Rosenberg RS, et al. Zolpidem reduces the sleep disturbance of jet lag. *Sleep Med.* 2001;2(5):423–430.

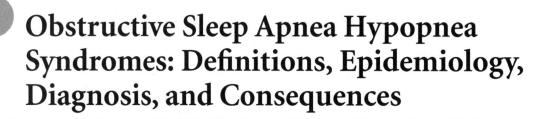

Chapter 18

Obstructive Sleep Apnea Hypopnea Syndromes: Definitions, Epidemiology, Diagnosis, and Consequences

Richard B. Berry and Runi Foster

FIGURE 18-1. An obstructive apnea is characterized by absent airflow and persistent respiratory effort (movement of chest and abdominal bands). An arterial oxygen desaturation to 82% follows this 28-second apnea. The drop in the arterial oxygen saturation (SaO_2) to 90% is from a preceding apnea. In this case, the chest and abdominal tracing deflections progressively increase during the event. This is not always seen.

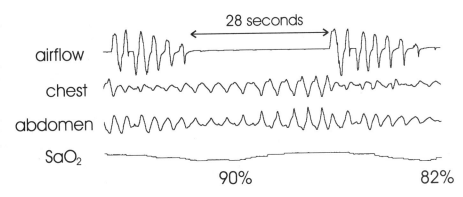

HISTORY AND DEFINITIONS

The obstructive sleep apnea hypopnea syndrome (OSAHS) was first recognized as a significant health problem only over the last three decades of the 20th century. In 1956, Burwell used the term Pickwickian syndrome to describe individuals with obesity, hypersomnolence, hypercapnia, cor pulmonale, and erythrocytosis (1). We now know that Pickwickian patients represent the "tip of the iceberg" of the larger group of patients with sleep-disordered breathing. Subsequently, the connection between nocturnal respiratory events and daytime sleepiness was recognized. Guilleminault and co-workers (2) described the obstructive sleep apnea (OSAS) syndrome defined as patients with daytime sleepiness and obstructive apneas on polysomnography (PSG). By convention, in adults, an ap-

nea is a cessation of airflow at the nose and mouth for 10 seconds or longer. An obstructive apnea is characterized by absent airflow despite persistent respiratory effort (Fig. 18-1). An apnea index of ≥ 5 was considered abnormal (3). Obstructive apneas are secondary to airway closure at a supraglottic location that reverses at apnea termination often associated with a brief awakening (arousal) (4). A fall in arterial oxygen saturation (SaO_2) of varying severity follows the event. An arterial oxygen desaturation is usually defined as a fall in the SaO_2 of 4% or more. Central apneas are defined as absent airflow for 10 seconds or longer associated with an absence of respiratory effort. Mixed apneas are those apneas consisting of an initial central apnea portion followed by an obstructive portion (Fig. 18-2). Respiratory effort is commonly detected by the movement of bands around the chest and abdomen in

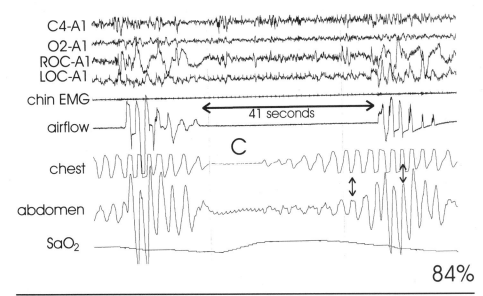

FIGURE 18-2. This tracing shows a 41-second mixed apnea. The initial portion (C) is a central apnea characterized by absent ventilatory effort. The small deflections in the abdomen tracing are from cardiac pulsations. After the central portion, an obstructive portion is noted. In this case, there is a progressive increase in chest and abdominal movement prior to apnea termination. In addition, there is paradoxical motion of the chest and abdomen tracings (small arrow) that vanishes after apnea termination. The apnea is followed by an arterial oxygen desaturation to 84%. In this case, an arousal is not seen in the central (C4-A1) or occipital (O2-A1) EEG tracings, although there is sudden movement in the eye tracings (ROC-A1 and LOC-A1). Here ROC and LOC are the right and left outer canthus electrodes, and A1 is the left mastoid electrode.

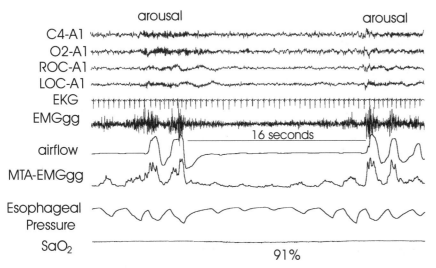

FIGURE 18-3. This tracing shows the end of one obstructive apnea followed by a 16-second obstructive apnea during NREM sleep. Arousal is noted at the termination of both events. The esophageal pressure swings increase toward the end of the event, consistent with a progressive increase in inspiratory effort. The moving time average MTA–EMGgg of the genioglossus EMG (EMGgg) was measured using a mouthpiece electrode. At the start of the apnea the genioglossus activity falls; at apnea termination there is a large increase in the EMGgg coincident with arousal and opening of the airway.

response to breathing efforts. Esophageal pressure monitoring detects changes in pleural pressure during inspiration and is a more sensitive method to detect inspiratory effort. The nadir in negative pressure swings or the size of the deflections can be used to quantify the amount of effort (5). The deflections in chest and abdominal bands during obstructive apnea may or may not increase prior to apnea termination. In NREM sleep, the esophageal pressure deflections routinely increase during the terminal portion of obstructive apnea, reflecting an increase in inspiratory effort during the apnea (Fig. 18-3).

It was soon realized that the episodes of severe airway narrowing (partial obstruction) resulting in reduction of airflow or tidal volume (hypopneas) are also important (Fig. 18-4) (6). Patients with primarily hypopneas had the same symptoms, arousals, and arterial oxygen desaturation as patients with obstructive apneas (7). Hence the

term obstructive sleep apnea hypopnea syndrome has been used to be more inclusive. However, many clinicians still use the term obstructive sleep apnea (OSA) to refer to the apnea and hypopnea syndrome. Of note, patients with the OSAHS will have variable proportions of obstructive apneas and hypopneas. For example, they may have apneas during REM sleep or in the supine position and hypopneas during NREM sleep or in the lateral position. Variable amounts of mixed and central apneas may also be present.

The apnea + hypopnea index (AHI) is the number of apneas and hypopneas per hour of sleep. The AHI has been used to quantify the severity of sleep-disordered breathing. An AHI ≥ 5 per hr in the presence of symptoms is said to define OSAHS. However, there has been considerable controversy about the definition of hypopnea and the frequency of events that is considered abnormal. As will be discussed below, the AHI value for a given patient can

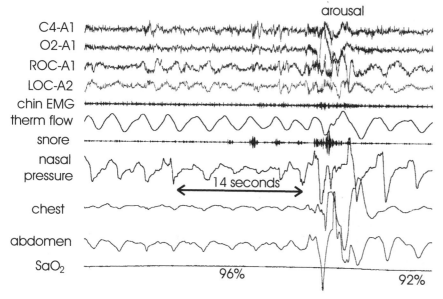

FIGURE 18-4. Obstructive hypopnea with arousal at event termination. Notice that the decrease in airflow by nasal pressure is greater than by thermistor (therm flow). Also note the flattening of the nasal pressure signal during the event. Obstructive hypopnea may be associated with paradoxical motion of the chest and abdomen band tracings, but this is not seen in this tracing. The reduction in airflow is associated with a 4% arterial oxygen desaturation and would therefore meet the hypopnea criteria based on oxygen desaturation. After arousal, the flattening in the nasal pressure signals resolves and the negative pressure swings decrease.

very tremendously depending on the definition of hypopnea and the technology used to monitor airflow (8,9). It has also been recognized that the correlation between the AHI and measures of impairment, such as subjective or objective sleepiness, although significant, is low (correlation coefficient in the range of 0.4 to 0.5) (10). However, to date, efforts to find better indexes of impairment based on polysomnographic findings, such as the arousal index, have not substantially improved the correlation with symptoms. The wide variability in symptoms is likely due, in part, to different individual susceptibility to sleep fragmentation or other factors contributing to symptoms of daytime sleepiness, such as medications or reduced sleep time. Two patients with the same AHI can have vastly different degrees of arterial oxygen desaturation. This could be relevant for many of the cardiovascular consequences of sleep apnea.

The Hypopnea Controversy

It is not possible to discuss the hypopnea controversy without briefly discussing methods of airflow monitoring. Many early sleep studies used thermal-sensitive devices (thermocouples, thermistors) to detect airflow. These are fairly accurate in detecting apnea, but the signal is not proportional to the flow rate (5,11). Thus, they tend to be less sensitive at detecting hypopneas than systems that accurately measure airflow, such as pneumotachograph–mask systems (5,11). The latter are somewhat uncomfortable and confined to research studies. Early definitions of hypopnea required a reduction in airflow coupled with a 4% or greater drop in the SaO_2 (6). This certainly meant that the reduction in airflow had physiologic significance for the patient. However, subsequently it became clear that it is possible for patients to have episodes of increased inspiratory effort sufficient to induce arousal from sleep without a drop in the SaO_2 (12,13). Guilleminault and co-workers described a group of patients who were sleepy, but traditional airflow monitoring with a thermal-sensing devices showed an AHI <5 per hour and most had minimal arterial oxygen desaturation (12). Monitoring of esophageal pressure in these patients demonstrated increased respiratory effort and subsequent arousal. In the original description, a respiratory arousal index of >10 per hour was required to diagnose these patients as having the "upper-airway resistance syndrome." Respiratory arousals were defined as arousals following a period of abnormally negative esophageal pressure. The upper-airway resistance events were associated with minimal changes in flow detected by thermal devices, but mildly reduced airflow and flattening (airflow limitation) by pneumotachograph monitoring. Thus, esophageal pressure was needed to demonstrate the events in the absence of an accurate measurement of airflow. Studies of experimental sleep disturbance in normal subjects also demonstrated that repetitive brief awakenings (arousals) could induce daytime sleepiness

in the absence of arterial oxygen desaturation (14–16). These developments suggested that the sleep-disturbing consequences of respiratory events were as clinically important as the respiratory event-associated arterial oxygen desaturation.

Despite the ability of esophageal pressure monitoring to detect subtle episodes of increased respiratory effort, the technique was never widely used in clinical sleep medicine. Instead, nasal pressure monitoring has gained popularity, being both well tolerated and more accurate at detecting changes in airflow during sleep than thermal devices (5,17). In addition, nasal pressure monitoring can often detect many of the subtle respiratory arousal events detected by esophageal pressure monitoring. A sensitive pressure transducer is connected to a nasal cannula inserted in the nose. The pressure drop across the nasal inlet is measured and is proportional to the square of the nasal flow (5,17,18). During obstructive hypopnea, the nasal pressure signal demonstrates a reduction in magnitude and the shape of the inspiratory portion shows flattening (flow plateau) during flow limitation (airway narrowing/increased upper-airway resistance) (Fig. 18-4). Patients monitored with nasal pressure will often have many more events, defined as a reduction in flow, than detected by a thermal device (17). Arousal associated with minimal changes in thermistor flow will often be seen to follow a more obvious reduction in the nasal pressure signal with flattening (Fig. 18-4).

Respiratory inductance plethysmography (RIP) provides another alternative to thermal devices for detecting respiratory events. The signal from bands around the chest and abdomen is added to give a RIPsum signal. The fluctuations in the RIPsum give an estimate of tidal volume when the device is calibrated (19–21). The individual chest and abdomen signals give an estimate of the surface area they encircle (inductance of a coil is proportional to the area it encloses). During hypopnea, the chest and abdominal band fluctuations decrease and RIPsum decrease (Fig. 18-5). Either nasal pressure or RIP will detect many instances of obvious reductions in airflow (tidal volume) in the absence of a 4% arterial oxygen desaturation. Should such events be classified as hypopneas?

A taskforce of the American Academy of Sleep Medicine (AASM) published guidelines for monitoring respiration during sleep and graded the accuracy of monitoring technology based on the literature. The task force defined a hypopnea ("Chicago criteria") based on a 50% reduction in airflow or any discernable reduction in flow associated with either an arousal or a 3% arterial oxygen desaturation (22) (Table 18-1). While this definition of hypopnea is inclusive, there are no large population studies using these definitions to determine a frequency of events associated with cardiovascular risk or to define normal limits. The AASM Taskforce also published criteria for estimation of severity of OSAHS based on the AHI. Values of 5 to <15, 15 to 30, and >30 per hour were termed mild,

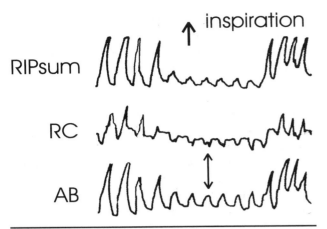

TABLE 18-1. Hypopnea Definitions[a]

	Airflow	*Other Criteria*
AASM task force "Chicago criteria"	50% Reduction Discernable but less than 50% reduction	None Arousal or ≥3% desaturation required
AASM Clinical Practice Review Committee	30% or greater reduction	4% or greater drop in the Sao[2]

[a]Airflow reduction must be 10 seconds or greater in duration.

FIGURE 18-5. This tracing shows an obstructive hypopnea detected by respiratory inductance plethysmography (RIP). Fluctuations in the RIPsum are estimates of tidal volume. The rib cage (RC) and abdominal (AB) band tracing are decreased during the hyponea and also show paradoxical motion.

moderate, and severe. These are somewhat arbitrary, but widely used.

The task force also defined a respiratory effort-related arousal (RERA) as an event lasting 10 seconds or longer with a "pattern of progressively more negative esophageal pressure, terminated by a sudden change in pressure to a less negative level and an arousal." The event may be associated with a drop in airflow, but does not qualify as a hypopnea (Fig. 18-6). In actual clinical practice, most sleep centers detect RERAs based on the nasal pressure signal rather than esophageal pressure. A flow-limitation RERA would be one associated with flattening in the airflow signal greater than 10 seconds followed by an arousal and an abrupt reversal in flow to a round shape (that does not qualify as a hypopnea). Although one may have airflow limitation without an increase in respiratory effort

and vice versa, most episodes of airflow limitation (increased upper airway resistance) during sleep are associated with increased esophageal pressure deflections. One study showed that the RERA indexes determined by nasal pressure and esophageal pressure monitoring were similar (23).

A consensus statement for the indications for continuous positive airway pressure (CPAP) treatment from another group suggested that a respiratory-disturbance index (RDI) be defined as the AHI + the RERA index. The RERA index is defined as the number of RERAs per hour of sleep. The RDI could then be used to assess the severity of sleep-disordered breathing (SDB) (24). The respiratory-arousal index can be defined as the number of arousals per hour of sleep associated with apnea, hypopnea, or a RERA.

Subsequent to publication of the above definitions, the Clinical Practice Review Committee (CPRC) of the AASM advocated another definition of hypopnea, based on a 30% reduction in airflow of 10 seconds or longer and a 4% or greater desaturation (drop in the Sao$_2$) (25). The presence or absence of arousal was not considered. The CPRC provided several reasons for their choice of hypopnea

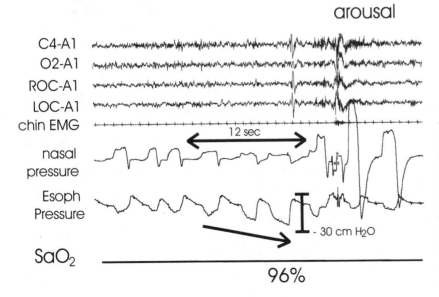

FIGURE 18-6. A respiratory effort related arousal (RERA). The esophageal pressure shows a progressive increase in negative pressure followed by an arousal and reduction in the pressure swings. No desaturation was noted. There is also a reduction in flow by nasal pressure with a flattening in the inspiratory shape. After arousal, the flattening is abruptly reversed. Of note, this event would qualify as a hypopnea if an associated desaturation was not required (reduction in flow + arousal).

definition. First, the scoring of hypopnea based on airflow and desaturation has good intra- and interscoring reliability, while the scoring of arousals does not (26,27). Second, the Sleep Heart Health study, using this definition of hypopnea, was able to show that even mild elevations of the AHI ($\geq$5 per hour) are associated with an increased risk of cardiovascular disease (28). Of note, the Centers for Medicare and Medicaid Services (CMS) has adopted the CPRC definition for hypopnea to determine qualification for CPAP reimbursement. However, the CPRC hypopnea definition does not recognize the sleep-disturbing effects of reductions in airflow associated with arousal but less than a 4% desaturation. For example, the event in Fig. 18-6 would not be considered a hypopnea if a 4% or greater arterial oxygen desaturation is required. It would qualify as a RERA (or flow-limitation RERA if esophageal pressure was not monitored). Some sleep centers report an AHI based on a hypopnea definition requiring a 4% desaturation and an RDI = AHI + RERA index. In summary, a reduction in airflow (nasal pressure) with flattening that is followed by an arousal, but less than a 4% arterial oxygen desaturation, could be classified as either a hypopnea or a flow-limitation RERA, depending on the definition of hypopnea that is used. Clearly, the hypopnea controversy is not over. However, if one reads a sleep study report or a published sleep medicine investigation, it is important to know both the definition of hypopnea and the technology used to detect airflow.

VARIANTS OF THE OBSTRUCTIVE SLEEP APNEA HYPOPNEA SYNDROME

Upper-Airway Resistance Syndrome

As noted above, Guilleminault and co-workers identified a group of patients who exhibited subjective and objective [Multiple Sleep Latency Test (MSLT)] daytime sleepiness but did not have an AHI >5 per hour (thermal devices measured airflow). The group was defined by having a respiratory-arousal index >10 per hour using esophageal pressure monitoring (12). The events were not associated with desaturation or a change in thermal device detected airflow. The symptom of sleepiness responded to CPAP treatment. The mean arousal index of the group was 33 per hour (range 16 to 52), and the mean maximally negative esophageal pressure nadir was −37 cm H_2O. There has been controversy as to whether the upper-airway resistance syndrome is a distinct entity or simply a milder form of OSAHS (29,30). Individual persons without daytime sleepiness may have a RERA index >10 per hour although the mean RERA for a group of persons without symptoms is usually lower than 10 per hour (31). Of note, the mean total arousal index in a group of normal persons using AASM criteria was 21 per hour in one study (32). The 95% confidence limit of normal for the arousal

index was very wide due to high arousal rates in older patients. It is possible that respiratory arousals cause more potent sleep disruption than "spontaneous arousals." However, this has never been experimentally addressed. In any case, there is some overlap in the arousal index between groups of normal subjects and patients with upper-airway resistance syndrome/mild OSAHS. If one uses nasal pressure monitoring for airflow and a definition of hypopnea that utilizes arousal, as well as a drop in the Sao_2, most "upper-airway resistance" patients will have an AHI >5 per hour and, hence, be classified as having the OSAHS. Alternatively, an RDI = AHI + RERA index will be greater than 5 per hour if hypopneas are required to be associated with a 4% or greater desaturation.

Obesity Hypoventilation Syndrome (OHS)

Most patients with the OSAHS do not have daytime hypoventilation. Those obese patients with daytime hypoventilation, not secondary to lung disease, are said to have the obesity hypoventilation syndrome (OHS). These patients were previously referred to as "Pickwickian" (1). Patients with the OHS are a heterogeneous group. The etiology includes upper-airway obstruction, decreased respiratory system compliance from obesity, and intrinsic or acquired abnormalities in ventilatory drive. Most OHS patients will have a high AHI and severe arterial oxygen desaturation (33–35). A few will exhibit worsening hypoventilation and severe arterial oxygen desaturation during sleep, without many discrete apneas or hypopneas. A recent study characterized the patients on the basis of their response to treatment (35). Some OHS patients could be adequately treated with CPAP alone. Opening the upper airway with CPAP during sleep restored adequate oxygenation. Others still had hypoventilation despite the absence of apnea or hypopnea. Some with persistent airflow limitation responded to higher levels of CPAP (decreasing the upper-airway resistance). Presumably they could not compensate for a high upper-airway resistance even if apnea and hypopnea were not present. Another group of patients required either nasal bilevel pressure-support ventilation or mechanical ventilation with or without oxygen. This group was felt likely to have abnormal ventilatory drive or very decreased respiratory compliance due to massive obesity. Despite the fact that the term OHS describes a very diverse group, a better terminology for the group of patients is not currently available. The sleep hypoventilation syndrome (SHVS) is an alternate term used by a Task Force of the American Academy of Sleep Medicine to include all forms of abnormal sleep-induced hypoventilation (22).

OHS patients may present with acute respiratory failure (36,37). The treatment of choice is positive airway pressure (usually bilevel positive airway pressure and oxygen). Very severe patients may require temporary endotracheal intubation and mechanical ventilation. For stable chronic OHS patients, treatment with positive airway pressure may reduce the daytime P_{CO_2}, as well as reducing apnea and hypopnea and nocturnal desaturation (33–35). Berthon-Jones and Sullivan (38) showed chronic CPAP treatment of OSA patients with daytime hypoventilation resulted in a leftward shift in the ventilatory response to carbon dioxide (ventilation plotted versus P_{CO_2}) during the day without a change in slope. The P_{CO_2} set point is lowered and there is higher ventilation at any given P_{CO_2}. Medroxyprogesterone, a respiratory stimulant, may improve the daytime P_{CO_2}, but does not reduce the AHI (39).

Overlap Syndrome

Patients with the OSAHS and chronic obstructive pulmonary disease (COPD) may have daytime hypopventilation and severe nocturnal oxygen desaturation. Of note, patients with COPD alone rarely retain CO_2 until the forced expiratory volume in 1 second (FEV1.0) is below 1.0 liter or 40% of predicted values. However, patients with the OSAHS and mild to moderate COPD may retain CO_2 (40,41). Patients with the overlap syndrome tend to have particularly severe arterial oxygen desaturation at night. They are often assumed to simply have COPD and are treated with nocturnal oxygen alone. This may incompletely reverse the nocturnal hypoxemia and worsen the CO_2 retention during sleep (42). The long-term outcome of patients with overlap syndrome may worsen if upper-airway obstruction is not addressed (43). Proper treatment usually requires CPAP or bilevel positive airway pressure and supplemental oxygen, if needed (44). The daytime P_{CO_2} may improve in some patients with adequate treatment of upper-airway obstruction during sleep.

Pathogenesis of Upper-Airway Obstruction

A detailed discussion of the pathogenesis of upper-airway obstruction is beyond the scope of this chapter. The reader is referred to several excellent reviews of this topic (45, 46). Multiple factors determine upper-airway patency during sleep (Table 18-2). Different factors may be more or less important in a given individual. Patients with the OSAHS tend to have small upper airways either secondary to bony or soft tissue alterations (47). In general, a short and posteriorly placed mandible, a long dependent palate, a large tongue, nasal obstruction, and thick lateral pharyngeal walls all predispose to upper-airway collapse during sleep. Patients with OSAHS tend to have a different shape of the upper airway with the narrowest dimension laterally versus anterior–posterior in normal persons (47,48). Dynamic imaging of the upper airway during wakefulness shows the smallest diameter at end expiration. Studies of the upper airway during general anesthesia (passive properties) have shown the upper airway of OSAHS patients to be narrower and more collapsible (49). When the Starling resistor model is applied to the upper airway, one can define a critical closing pressure (P_{crit}) during sleep such

TABLE 18-2. Factors Determining Upper-Airway Patency

Open Upper Airway	Closed Upper Airway
Active upper airway muscle activity	Decreased upper airway muscle activity
Active negative pressure reflexes	Decreased pressure reflexes (sleep)
Increased lung volume	Decreased lung volume
Less negative intraluminal pressure	More negative intraluminal pressure
Less positive extraluminal pressure	More positive extraluminal pressure
Stable ventilatory drive	Fluctuating ventilatory drive
Larger, stiffer upper airway	Smaller, more compliant upper airway
Lateral decubitus posture	Supine posture

that lower intraluminal pressures are associated with airway closure (50). In normal persons, P_{crit} is negative whereas in OSAHS patients it is positive. That is, a positive intraluminal pressure is required to keep the airway open during sleep.

During wakefulness, upper-airway muscle activity maintains an open upper airway even if the airway is anatomically narrow. Some upper airway muscles, such as the genioglossus (tongue protruder) and palatoglossus show increases of activity with inspiration (phasic activity), while others such as the tensor veli palatini (a muscle of the palate) show tonic (constant) activity (51). At the onset of NREM sleep, the activity of upper-airway muscles decreases (51–53) and upper-airway resistance increases (54) (Fig. 18-7). With stable sleep, the activity of the genioglossus may actually return to waking or higher than wakefulness levels. While chemostimulation from hypoxia and hypercapnia stimulates respiratory muscle activity during sleep, simultaneous increases in genioglossus activity appears to be related, in large part, to stimulation of upper-airway mechanoreceptors by negative pressure. (55,56). Upper-airway reflexes triggered by negative pressure also help maintain upper-airway patency during wakefulness. The sudden application of negative pressure elicits a reflex increase in the genioglossus (57) and palatal muscle activity (58). This reflex is diminished during sleep (58–60).

Patients with OSAHS tend to have higher than normal basal genioglossus activity (61, 62) and a greater genioglossus response to negative airway pressure (63). The higher activity and response to negative pressure are believed to be a compensation for an intrinsically narrowed airway. In contrast, the response of the palate muscles to negative pressure may be impaired in OSAHS patients (64). Despite evidence for higher upper-airway muscle activity during wakefulness, the upper airways of OSAHS patients are still more collapsible than those of normal persons (65).

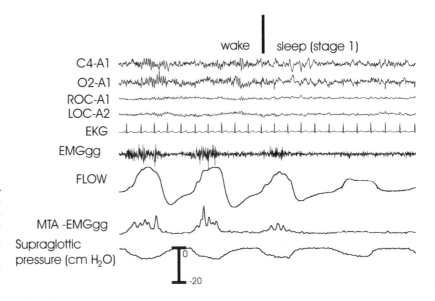

FIGURE 18-7. This tracing shows the onset of sleep with the coincident fall in genioglossus muscle activity and a fall in airflow with evidence of flow-limitation flattening. As the supraglottic pressure is similar but flow is lower, this means that upper-airway resistance has increased.

At sleep onset, some studies have suggested that OSAHS patients have a greater than normal fall in upper-airway muscle activity (66). In any case, the upper-airway activity is not sufficient to maintain an open upper airway. In Fig. 18-3, a fall in genioglossus activity as the patient returns to sleep is associated with an obstructive apnea. Posture also has important effects on airway patency (67,68) and some patients with OSAHS have apnea or hypopnea only in the supine position (postural OSAHS).

During upper-airway obstruction, phasic genioglossus muscle activity increases proportionally to esophageal pressure deflections (ventilatory drive) (Fig. 18-3) (4,69). At apnea termination, both genioglossus and palatal muscle activities are preferentially augmented (4,69,70) and the upper airway opens. While it was once assumed that increasing genioglossus activity during obstructive apnea or hypopnea was driven by hypoxia and hypercapnia, a study of the effect of upper airway local anesthesia suggests that mechanoreceptor stimulation (from increasingly negative pressure below the site of airway closure) is responsible for a large proportion of the augmentation (69).

Traditionally, a concept of a balance between negative inspiratory pressure tending to collapse the airway and upper-airway muscle dilating forces was assumed to determine the state of the airway. However, more recently, the concept of passive collapse at sleep onset has gained favor. In fact, at sleep onset, the ventilatory drive decreases and supraglottic pressure actually may initially decrease (less negative) in some patients (although resistance increases). Upper-airway closure has also been documented during central apnea where there is no inspiration or negative collapsing forces (71). Therefore, suction pressure during obstruction may help keep the airway closed, but is not necessary for the onset of airway occlusion.

Upper-airway volume also has a dependence on lung volume, with decreasing airway size as lung volume decreases (72,73). The lung volume dependence may be greater in patients with OSAHS (72). The lung volume dependence of the upper airway may be mediated via passive distending forces due to a downward tension on upper-airway structures during inspiration ("tracheal tug") (74). Another way of thinking of the tracheal tug is a decrease in extramural pressure surrounding the airway (46). Any fall in end-expiratory volume or tidal volume would then reduce upper-airway size. Functional residual capacity is known to decrease during sleep (75) and this would tend to predispose to airway closure. Morrell and co-workers (76) demonstrated a progressive fall in end-expiratory retropalatal cross-sectional area as well as end-expiratory lung volume in the breaths leading up to obstructive apnea.

Ventilatory instability generated by arousal and hyperventilation postapnea may also predispose to subsequent upper-airway closure and help perpetuate repetitive cycles of respiration and apnea. If the patient falls asleep rapidly after arousal, the arterial P_{CO_2} may be near or below the apneic threshold, the level of P_{CO_2} below which ventilation is no longer triggered during sleep (77). If the P_{CO_2} falls below the apneic threshold, a central apnea may occur, followed by an obstructive apnea when ventilatory drive returns (mixed apnea) (78). Alternatively, a hypopnea or obstructive apnea may occur as ventilatory drive and upper-airway muscle activity fall (79). Of note, obstructive apnea may occur before the nadir in inspiratory effort is reached. If one monitors esophageal pressure in patients with OSAHS, the nadir in deflections in some patients can occur two or three breaths into the apnea (Fig. 18-8) (5,13).

During REM sleep, ventilation is irregular, even in normal persons with the greatest irregularity during periods of phasic eye movements (80). As periods of REM sleep are longest and the REM density (number of eye movements per time) is the highest during the early morning hours, it is not surprising that this is the time of the greatest changes in ventilation during sleep. Although the diaphragm is

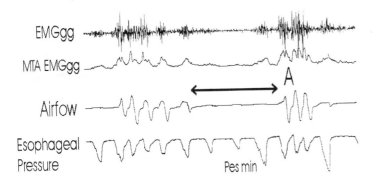

FIGURE 18-8. An obstructive apnea is shown with the raw genioglossus EMG (EMGgg) and the moving time average of the genioglossus EMG (MTA–EMGgg) as well as airflow and esophageal pressure. Note that the genioglossus EMG fall at airflow limitation (flattening) is noted on the last breath before apnea. At arousal (A) there is a large increase in genioglossus EMG. Note also that both EMGgg and the esophageal pressure deflections fall at apnea onset. In this case the nadir in esophageal deflections (Pes min) occurs on the second breath of apnea.

not affected by the generalized muscle hypotonia of REM sleep, periodic decrements in diaphragmatic activity are associated with periods of reduced tidal volume. Upper-airway muscles are also affected during REM sleep. In normal persons, during REM sleep, genioglossus tonic activity is reduced but phasic activity can still be detected if intramuscular EMG electrodes are used (Fig. 18-9). During bursts of eye movements, both diaphragmatic and genioglossus phasic activity is often decreased (81). REM sleep without phasic eye movements is called "tonic REM" and with eye movements "phasic REM." The latter is associated with more breathing irregularity. Many patients with OSAHS have a much higher AHI during REM sleep or have events only during REM (REM-related OSAHS). However, two studies have found no greater collapsibility of the upper airway during REM than NREM sleep (67,68). This variance with clinical experience could be due to the nonhomogeneous nature of REM or to the fact that drops in diaphragm activity are also important for inducing apnea and hypopnea.

Mechanisms of Apnea Termination and Arousal

Obstructive apnea or hypopnea termination is believed to depend on arousal mechanisms. During obstructive apnea in NREM sleep, upper-airway muscle activity increases, as does inspiratory effort. Airway opening does not occur until there is a preferential increase in upper-airway muscle activity (4). This is often associated with signs of cortical arousal, although the EEG changes may not meet AASM criteria (16), for example, the sudden onset of delta activity. A recent study suggested that arousal can be detected at the termination of the majority of respiratory events if frontal electroencephalographs (EEG), as well as central EEG, is monitored (82). If cortical arousal does not occur, there is still believed to be a "state" change in the brainstem—so called subcortical or autonomic arousals. The term autonomic arousal is used because an abrupt change in heart rate or blood pressure can be detected at apnea termination, even if cortical arousal is absent. While hypercapnia and hypoxia drive the increase in respiratory effort, the level of effort, rather than individual values of hypoxia or hypercapnia seems to trigger arousal (13,83). Thus the level of effort is an index of the combined arousal stimulus. Studies have suggested that information from upper-airway mechanoreceptors may contribute to the arousal stimulus (84,85). In NREM sleep, arousal appears to occur when inspiratory effort reaches an "arousal threshold." Normal subjects tend to arouse during mask occlusion when suction pressure reaches 20 to 40 cm H_2O. In contrast, many patients with OSAHS arouse only after

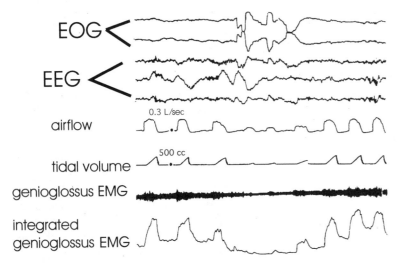

FIGURE 18-9. This tracing shows the fall in integrated genioglossus EMG activity and tidal volume during a burst of eye movements during REM sleep in a normal individual. The tracing illustrates that REM sleep is not homogeneous with respect to the effects on ventilation or upper airway muscle control. (From Wiegand L, Zwillich CW, Wiegand D, et al. Changes in upper airway muscle activation and ventilation during phasic REM sleep in normal men. *J Appl Physiol.* 1991;71:488–497. With permission.)

pressure reaches −60 to −80 cm H_2O (13). The increased arousal threshold in OSAHS patients is probably due, in part, to chronic sleep deprivation or hypoxemia. Withdrawal of CPAP for even three nights has been shown to increase the arousal threshold in OSAHS. However, chronic CPAP treatment does not restore the arousal threshold to normal (86). Patients with OSAHS could have an intrinsically increased respiratory arousal threshold. Alternatively there could be damage to mechanoreceptors from years of snoring or to chemoreceptors from repetitive nightly stimulation. A study of respiratory-related evoked potentials (RREP) in patients with mild OSAHS, suggested that there is a sleep-specific blunted cortical response to inspiratory occlusion (87). At least in these milder patients, there was no evidence of impaired mechanoreceptor function, as the RREP was normal during wakefulness. One study found that the prolongation in event duration that occurs overnight in patients with OSAHS is secondary to a blunting of the cortical response as the level of inspiratory effort at apnea termination increased during the night (88). Another study found that the within-night variation in the arousal threshold followed the cycles of NREM sleep (89) with a higher arousal threshold associated with higher EEG delta power (deeper sleep).

In REM sleep, the arousal mechanisms are less well understood. Esophageal pressure deflections do not show a steady increase. Of note, in normal subjects the arousal to mask occlusion is quicker during REM than in NREM sleep (13). In contrast, patients with OSAHS have the longest apneas and most severe desaturation during REM sleep. The reasons for the delayed arousal during REM sleep in OSAHS patients are not known.

Arterial Oxygen Desaturation

Patients with a similar AHI of events may have vastly different degrees of arterial oxygen desaturation. Studies of breath holding in normal subjects suggest that the rate of fall in the SaO_2 is inversely proportional to the baseline SaO_2 and to the lung volume (oxygen stores) at the start of breath hold (90). The rate of fall is disproportionately higher at low lung volumes, secondary to increases in ventilation/perfusion mismatch. A study of OSAHS patients found that the severity of nocturnal arterial oxygen desaturation was related to several factors, including the awake supine PaO_2, the percentage of sleeptime spent in apnea, and the expiratory reserve volume (ERV) (91). Patients with a baseline PaO_2 of 55 to 60 mm Hg are on the steep part of the oxyhemoglobin saturation curve. A small fall in PaO_2 results in significant desaturation. While apnea duration is an obvious factor in the severity of desaturation, the length of the ventilatory period between events also is important. Some patients do not completely resaturate between events, as they quickly return to sleep and the airway closes again. Long event duration and short periods between apneas mean the percentage of total sleep

time (TST) spent in apnea is high. The clinical significance of a low ERV may be less obvious. The ERV is the difference between the functional residual capacity (FRC) and the residual volume (RV). The FRC (end-expiratory volume) is reduced in obesity secondary to low compliance of the chest wall/abdomen. The RV (volume at maximal exhalation) is increased if patients have any degree of obstructive airway disease (airtrapping). Thus a low ERV means that the patient has low oxygen stores at the start of apnea (a low FRC) and significant ventilation/perfusion mismatch at low lung volumes (identified by a high RV). Clinically, the groups of OSAHS patients with severe desaturation include patients with a low PO_2 for any reason (severe obesity, daytime hypoventilation, and COPD). In fact, some patients can have significant desaturation after events as short as 10 to 15 seconds. The severity of desaturation also depends on sleep stage. In most OSAHS patients, the longest apneas and most severe desaturations occur in REM sleep. Some studies also have suggested that at equivalent apnea length, the severity of desaturation is worse in obstructive than central apnea (92).

In evaluating pulse oximetry, the clinician should also remember that patients with a high carboxyhemoglobin level (heavy smoking) will have a falsely high SaO_2, as the devices do not differentiate carboxyhemoglobin and oxyhemoglobin. In addition, if a long averaging time is utilized, this may impair the ability of an oximeter to detect brief arterial oxygen desaturations.

EPIDEMIOLOGY OF OBSTRUCTIVE SLEEP APNEA HYPOPNEA SYNDROME

Prevalence and Progression

The importance of OSAHS to public health has been underscored by population-based studies that have shown an unexpectedly high prevalence of the disorder coupled with other studies linking even mild degrees of sleep-disordered breathing to increased cardiovascular risk (93). Prevalence is defined as the proportion of a population with a condition. The Wisconsin-based cohort study of state employees less than 65 years of age found a prevalence of sleep-disordered breathing (SDB) defined as an AHI >5 per hour (with hypopneas based on a definition of discernable change in airflow and ≥4% desaturations) to be 9% in women and 24% in men (94). The sleep apnea hypopnea syndrome, defined as the presence of both SDB and self-reported sleepiness, was present in 2% of women and 4% of men. Bixler et al. found a 17% and 7% incidence of an AHI >5 and 15 per hour in men, respectively (95,96). Higher prevalence rates may be present in referral or clinical populations. It is estimated that in Western countries up to 5% have an undiagnosed OSAHS (elevated AHI and symptoms) (93). There is also evidence that OSAHS severity can progress with time. Analysis of 8-year follow-up of 282 participants of the Wisconsin cohort study showed a mean increase from 2.6 events per hour to 5.1 (94). In obese individuals with a body mass index (BMI) over 30, the mean AHI increased from 4.8 to 10.1 per hour. However, not all studies of untreated patients with OSAHS have also shown progression.

Age

The prevalence of OSAHS appears to be higher in the elderly than in middle-aged populations. A study of in-home polysomnography (PSG) in the elderly (age >65) found the prevalence of OSAHS defined as an AHI >10 per hour to be 70% in men and 56% in women (97). Here hypopneas were based on changes in flow, independent of changes in the SaO_2. This is a prevalence of about three times that in middle-aged populations. There is evidence from the Sleep Heart Health Study that the SDB prevalence increases from age 40 to around 60 (93,98). After that, the prevalence appears to plateau. In older adults, the AHI may be less correlated with excessive sleepiness and increased cardiovascular risk. Enright and co-workers (99) studied a large group of subjects over age 65 with questionnaires and echocardiography, ultrasound of the carotids, and EKG. Snoring was very common, but interestingly, reported snoring seemed to decrease after age 75. Loud snoring, observed apneas, and daytime sleepiness were not associated with hypertension or the prevalence of cardiovascular disease. Thus, SDB in the elderly may be different from younger age groups and not correlate with cardiovascular disease (100). On the other hand, decreased snoring reports could be secondary to a lower frequency of having a bed partner or hearing deficits in the elderly.

Ethnicity

Some studies have suggested that OSAHS is more common in African-American than Caucasian populations (101,102). However, this finding was not present in another study which controlled for differences in age and BMI (98). In any case, one can say that the prevalence of OSAHS is at least as high in African-American populations and may be higher. Ip and co-workers (103) found a similar prevalence of OSAHS in a Chinese population as that found in Caucasians. The fact that OSAHS is common in Asian areas where obesity is much less common has led to the hypothesis that craniofacial characteristics of the Asian population might predispose to OSAHS (104). While increasing BMI was still associated with an increased prevalence of OSAHS in the study of Chinese patients, the association was not as strong as typically seen in Caucasian populations (103). The lack of obesity in Asian patients should certainly not discourage evaluation for possible sleep apnea.

RISK FACTORS FOR THE DEVELOPMENT OF THE OBSTRUCTIVE SLEEP APNEA HYPOAPNEA SYNDROME

Obesity

There seems little doubt of the association between increased BMI and the OSAHS. What is interesting is that once patients reach a certain point, even modest weight gain or loss can create relatively large worsening or improvement in the AHI. Peppard et al. (105), in a longitudinal study, found that in persons with an AHI <15 per hour at baseline, a 10% increase in body weight resulted in a sixfold risk of developing moderate to severe OSAHS (AHI >15 per hour) relative to patients with stable body weight. Others have shown that a 10% to 15% weight loss can be clinically significant (106,107). Of note, weight loss may reduce the AHI, but often not to normal levels. Other forms of treatment may still be necessary. Recurrence of sleep apnea after initial improvement from weight loss has been reported in the absence of later weight gain (108). One might suspect that the distribution of obesity as well as the total BMI might be important for the risk of sleep apnea. Some studies have suggested that neck circumference is a better predictor than BMI alone (109).

Male Gender

Population studies of OSAHS have consistently found a two to three times greater prevalence in men than women (93). The reasons for this difference remain uncertain despite many investigations. Androgen replacement therapy in hypogonadal males has induced sleep apnea (110,111). This suggests that the presence of testosterone itself increases the risk in men. Possible explanations of the sex differences include difference in upper-airway size or shape, differences in upper-airway muscle activity, or differences in stability of respiratory drive during state and changes. On the average, women actually have a smaller upper-airway size. A recent study found more severe hypopnea in men after an applied resistive load and greater tendency for airway collapse (112). Malhotra and co-workers (113) suggested that increased pharyngeal length of the male upper-airway may predispose to collapse in men. However, another study found no significant difference between upper-airway resistance or collapsibility in normal men and women (114). The same group found that gender differences in upper-airway size or compliance during sleep could be explained by gender differences in neck circumference (115). Following apnea–hypopnea termination there is a period of increased ventilation. If a patient falls asleep quickly the PcO_2 may be below or near the apneic threshold (the level triggering ventilation). As previously addressed, falling ventilatory drive may predispose to upper-airway closure or narrowing. Women appear less likely to develop hypocapnic-induced apnea–hypopnea during NREM sleep (116). In summary, the explanation for the difference in the prevalence of OS-AHS between men and women remains controversial. The effects of hormonal status in women will be discussed below.

Menopause

SDB is more common in post- than premenopausal women, but a number of factors are possible explanations for this difference, including increased age, higher BMI, or hormonal status (94). The Sleep Heart Health Study analysis of women over 50 found that the incidence of an AHI >15 per hour in women on hormone replacement therapy (HRT) was approximately one-half that of the nonusers (117). There was a higher prevalence of SDB in non-HRT users even when other factors, such as age and BMI, were considered. The risk was especially high in the 50- to 59-year-old group. The Wisconsin cohort study also found an increased risk for having an AHI >5 and >15 per hour in postmenopausal women compared with premenopausal women when adjusted for age and BMI (118). The risk was higher for postmenopausal women who were not on HRT than those who were. This suggests that a reduction in estrogen and progesterone may predispose to SDB.

Alcohol Consumption

Some, but not all, studies have shown an increase in snoring, the AHI, and arterial oxygen desaturation following alcohol consumption (119–122). In many studies, alcohol was administered before bedtime. The results may not apply to alcohol consumption earlier in the evening. One study found no effect of alcohol on breathing during sleep in premenopausal women (121). In animal studies, ethanol preferentially decreases hypoglossal nerve activity (innervates the genioglossus) compared to phrenic nerve activity (123). In a study of mask occlusion in normal subjects, ethanol ingestion delayed the time to arousal during NREM sleep (124). Most occlusions were performed in the early part of the night when the alcohol level would have been higher. However, studies of the effects of alcohol on sleep apnea have not always shown an increase in the duration of apnea–hypopnea (122). This may be related to low ethanol levels during the later part of the night or analysis of events in all stages of sleep. Alcohol does suppress REM sleep and, in this sense, could reduce the longer events associated with REM sleep during the early part of the night. However, more severe desaturations and presumably longer events do occur in some patients in the early portion of the night if bedtime alcohol is consumed (119).

Hypothyroidism

Hypothyroidism has been thought to be associated with sleep apnea (125–128). There are no large cohort stud-

ies evaluating the prevalence of sleep apnea in hypothyroid subjects. Obesity may be a significant confounding factor. Pelttari et al. (127) examined 26 patients with hypothyroidism and 188 euthyroid control subjects, finding that 50% of hypothyroid patients and 29% of control subjects had significant respiratory events. Rajagopal and coworkers (125) studied eleven patients with newly diagnosed hypothyroidism. Nine patients had SDB. The obese patients had a much higher AHI. After 3 to 12 months of thyroid replacement, the AHI significantly decreased from 78 to 12 per hour without a change in body weight. However, restoration of the euthyroid condition in patients with OSAHS does not reliably reverse sleep apnea in all patients. Moreover, initiation of even low doses of thyroid replacement in untreated patients with OSAHS and coronary artery disease has been reported to cause nocturnal angina (126). Therefore, effective treatment of OSAHS should be begun when low-dose gradual thyroid replacement is initiated. After the euthyroid state is attained, a repeat sleep study can determine if continued treatment of OSAHS (other than thyroid replacement) is required. While some physicians order thyroid function tests on all OSAHS patients, this may not be cost effective (129). Postmenopausal women with OSAHS (who are at higher risk for hypothyroidism) or OSAHS patients without predisposing OSAHS risk factors, might warrant thyroid studies. The reason hypothyroidism exacerbates OSAHS is unclear and possibly multifactorial. Upper-airway muscle myopathy, narrowing of the upper airway by mucoprotein deposition in the tongue (macroglossia), and abnormalities in ventilatory control are possible mechanisms.

Acromegaly

Growth hormone excesses resulting in acromegaly are also associated with sleep apnea. Grunstein et al. (130) noted that 60% of unselected acromegaly patients have sleep apnea. Weiss and co-workers found that 75% of a group with acromegaly had OSAHS (131). Independent predictors of OSAHS included increased activity of acromegaly (higher growth hormone), increased age, and a greater neck circumference. Potential pathophysiologic mechanisms of this association, include macroglossia and increased muscle mass of the upper airway. Since central sleep apnea (CSA) is also noted in acromegalic patients (130), alterations in central ventilatory control may also play a role. Isono (132) studied pharyngeal characteristics of acromegalics and found collapse at the base of the tongue to be especially prominent. Patients with acromegaly may also have excessive daytime sleepiness (EDS) without SDB that may respond to treatment of the growth hormone excess (133).

Nasal Congestion

Patients commonly complain of worsening sleep or snoring during periods of nasal congestion. Young et al. (134)

analyzed a subset of the Wisconsin Sleep Cohort Study population to determine if there was a relationship between snoring and nasal congestion. The odds ratio for habitual snoring adjusted for age, BMI, and smoking was 3.0 greater in those with a history of nasal congestion. This was not explained by the presence of sleep apnea. That is, the odds ratio was similar for snorers with and without associated sleep apnea. Another analysis of a subset of the cohort that had sleep studies was performed (135). Participants who reported nasal congestion due to allergy were 1.8 times more likely to have an AHI >15 per hour ($P<0.05$).

CLINICAL SYMPTOMS AND SIGNS

Patients with OSAHS usually present to physicians either because of the symptoms they experience, such as daytime sleepiness or because of the observation of their sleep behavior (snoring, choking, or apnea) by a bedmate (136). Common complaints are listed in Table 18-3. The spectrum and severity of complaints may not correlate well with the severity noted on PSG. Patients may have very severe sleep apnea and minimal daytime sleepiness. It is said that many women with sleep apnea complain of fatigue more than sleepiness.

The Epworth sleepiness scale (ESS) is a convenient method to quantify the propensity to fall asleep during daily life. Subjects respond to eight questions as to how likely they are to fall asleep in a given situation. The score of each question ranges from 0 to 3 (137). A score of 0 to 10 is considered normal. The mean ESS in categories of mild, moderate, and severe OSAHS in one study were 11, 13, and 16.2, respectively. Patients with sleepiness that interferes with driving or work definitely have a significant problem. There also are a number of OSAHS patients who complain of insomnia rather than daytime sleepiness (138). These patients may have other conditions, such as depression, or may have difficulty attaining deep sleep because of frequent awakenings from airway obstruction. Some studies have also found complaints of erectile dysfunction common in men with SDB (139). In taking a history, the physician must also consider the many other causes of excessive daytime sleepiness (EDS). These include insufficient sleep, depression, narcolepsy, the restless legs syndrome (RLS), periodic limb movements in sleep (PLMS), idiopathic hypersomnia, and sleep disturbance from medical diseases or medications (140). It is also not unusual for patients to have more than one problem.

The physical examination may be helpful in giving a general impression of an increased risk for OSAHS. Systematic studies of the utility of physical examination or upper-airway endoscopy have varied in their results (141, 142). Patients often have a dependent soft palate (free palate edge hidden behind the tongue), long uvula, large tongue, and small or posteriorly placed mandible. The neck circumference is frequently increased to over 17 inches in circumference. However, the absence of upper-airway findings suggestive of occlusion should not discourage evaluation of a clinical suspicion of sleep apnea. A minority of patients with OSAHS (<15%) will have physical findings suggestive of right heart failure, including jugular venous distension and pedal edema.

DIAGNOSIS AND POLYSOMNOGRAPHIC FINDINGS

A number of studies have sought to develop systematic prediction rules to improve the sensitivity and specificity of physician impression in suspecting OSAHS (106,143,144). Flemons and co-workers found that a model using neck circumference, the presence of hypertension (high blood pressure or taking antihypertensive medication), habitual snoring, and bed partner reports of nocturnal gasping/choking respirations to be the best predictor of the presence of OSAHS as defined on nocturnal PSG (143). Netzer and co-workers (144) used the "Berlin questionnaire" to identify patients at risk for sleep apnea syndrome. Patients with persistent symptoms in two or three domains including snoring, sleepiness or fatigue, and obesity or hypertension were found to likely have OSAHS.

The gold standard for the diagnosis of the OSAHS is attended PSG with EEG, electro-occulography (EOG), and electromyography (EMG) recording to detect the presence and stage of sleep, as well as monitoring of airflow, respiratory effort, arterial oxygen saturation, and usually leg EMG (145,146). The technologist is available to replace defective monitoring leads and assure the quality of signals. A split- or partial-night study usually employs at least 2 hours of recorded sleep for diagnosis followed by a positive pressure titration. This practice, while cost effective, may result in an underestimation of the severity of illness, as limited supine or REM sleep may be recorded during the diagnostic portion. Typical polysomnographic findings

▶ **TABLE 18-3. Symptoms of OSAHS**

Excessive daytime sleepiness
Frequent awakenings
Nonrestorative (nonrefreshing sleep)
Intellectual changes
Difficulty falling asleep
Morning headaches
Erectile dysfunction
Personality change
Nocturnal behavior
Loud snoring
Breathing pauses
Choking/gasping/snorting
Body movements
Nocturia

▶ **TABLE 18-4. Polysomnographic Findings in the OSAHS**

Increased wake after sleep onset and stage 1
Reduced stage 3 and 4 sleep
Reduced REM sleep
Increased respiratory arousals
Snoring
Mixture of obstructive and mixed apneas, obstructive hypopneas, central apnea may occur
AHI: mild 5 to < 15/h, moderate 15–30/h, severe >30/h
AHI supine > AHI nonsupine a common pattern
AHI REM > AHI NREM common
Apnea duration REM > NREM
Variable amounts of arterial oxygen desaturation
Lowest Sao_2 during REM sleep
Cyclic variation in heart rate

in OSAHS patients are listed in Table 18-4. Some patients have a much higher AHI in the supine position or during REM sleep (147,148). Arterial oxygen desaturation is also typically worse in those circumstances. Many sleep centers report a total AHI and AHI values for NREM and REM sleep separately. The AHI for supine and nonsupine sleep is also often reported to help identify positional sleep apnea.

Patients with OSAHS often have substantial abnormalities in indexes of sleep quality. These include reduced stage 3, 4, and REM sleep and increased wake after sleep onset and stage 1 sleep. The arousal index is usually increased secondary to increases in respiratory and spontaneous arousals. Respiratory arousals are defined as the arousals at or closely following apnea and hypopnea. If RERAs are determined, these are also included in respiratory-arousal calculations. In general, there is a high correlation between the AHI and the respiratory arousal index especially for patients with moderate to severe OSAHS (149). The patients with the highest high arousal indexes have the most decreased stage 3, 4, and REM sleep. Some have argued

that computing arousal indexes adds little information to the AHI, except in milder cases. This may also depend on the criteria for arousal and whether the RDI includes the RERA index or is simply equal to the AHI. The correlation between respiratory variables (AHI) and the EEG indexes (arousal index) from PSG and subjective and objective sleepiness is discussed below.

Attended PSG has a number of potential disadvantages, including cost, limited availability in some locales, long waiting periods for a study, and the fact that some patients may sleep poorly in the lab environment. There can be night-to-night variability in some patients (150,151) possibly related to the amount of REM or supine sleep or other factors, such as nasal congestion. Patients who do not drink their usual consumption of alcohol or take their usual narcotics could have a milder than normal study.

Efforts have been made to study the ability of less sophisticated and/or unattended monitoring methods (Table 18-5) to diagnose OSAHS. These include full PSG performed in the home (portable PSG), attended or unattended cardiopulmonary studies (airflow, respiratory effort, oxygen saturation, and EKG or heart rate), and attended or unattended single or dual bioparamater studies (oximetry or oximetry and airflow). Recently, the American Thoracic Society, the American College of Chest Physicians, and the American Academy of Sleep Medicine joined forces to study the diagnostic utility of alternate methods to diagnose OSAHS other than attended PSG. A large systematic literature review was performed (152). Based on the evidence from this review, clinical parameters were written by a committee composed of a representative from each organization (153). There was sufficient evidence to recommend only the cardiopulmonary type of study in the attended setting as a routine diagnostic approach. Review of raw data by the interpreting physician was suggested to validate the findings. It was also recommended that symptomatic patients with a negative limited study have full PSG. The guidelines also noted that a cardiopulmonary study would not qualify a patient for Medicare

▶ **TABLE 18-5. Types of Diagnostic Studies**

Level of Study	Name	Monitoring
Level 1	Attended PSG	EEG, EOG, chin EMG, EKG, airflow, respiratory effort, Sao_2, leg EMG
Level 2	Unattended PSG (comprehensive portable monitoring)	Same as level 1
Level 3	Cardiopulmonary study (attended or unattended)	Airflow, respiratory effort, EKG or heart rate, Sao_2
	Modified portable sleep apnea testing	
Level 4	Continuous single or dual bioparameter (attended or unattended)	Oximetry (Sao_2); oximetery + airflow

reimbursement of CPAP (at least 2 hours of sleep documented by EEG monitoring is required). If most patients studied with a cardiopulmonary study require a subsequent in CPAP titration with PSG, this approach has little advantage over a single split-PSG study. However, for patients in locales where PSG is not available or where there is a long wait for a study, limited studies may be of important value.

CONSEQUENCES OF OBSTRUCTIVE SLEEP APNEA HYPOPNEA SYNDROME

Mortality

Decreased survival is the most important potential consequence of any disorder. In patients with OSAHS, the frequent coexisting conditions, such as hypertension and obesity, make analysis of the impact of OSAHS on survival difficult. An early retrospective study by He et al. (154) showed a decreased survival in untreated patients with an apnea index (AI) >20 per hour. Patients with an AI >20 per hour who were treated with tracheostomy or CPAP did not have a decreased survival. The causes of death in the patients were not documented. The study was retrospective and patients were not randomized to treatment or no treatment, so selection bias could explain differences. However, it is unlikely that a randomized long-term trial of treatment versus observation is now possible for ethical reasons. Lavie et al. (155) reviewed the results on 1,620 patients diagnosed with OSAHS between 1976–1988. Fifty-seven patients had died by 1990, with 53% of the deaths due to respiratory and cardiovascular causes. Excess mortality was noted in men of 30 to 50 years of age, but not in patients over 70 years of age. The Sleep Heart Health Study has documented an increased risk of developing cardiovascular disease, even with mild increases in the AHI (28). However, there have been no large long-term studies showing that treatment of OSAHS improves survival.

Excessive Daytime Sleepiness and Neurocognitive Dysfunction

EDS is a cardinal manifestation of the OSAHS. However, the severity of this symptom is extremely variable. Chronic sleep deprivation/fragmentation from respiratory events is believed to be the major cause of sleepiness, although hypoxemia may also play a role. Normal subjects subjected to sleep fragmentation without hypoxemia develop subjective and objective daytime sleepiness (14,15). However, attempts at finding abnormalities demonstrated on PSG that correlate with subjective or objective sleepiness have been disappointing. Johns and co-workers found the ESS (subjective) to correlate with the RDI in a group of 165 patients with OSA ($r = 0.439$) and slightly less with the minimum SaO_2 ($r = -0.404$) (137). Guilleminault and co-workers

(156) found no PSG variable that correlated with sleepiness, as assessed by the MSLT. Roehrs and co-workers analyzed data from 466 patients using multiple regression analysis and found daytime sleepiness, as assessed by the MSLT, had a slightly higher correlation with the respiratory arousal index (RAI) ($r = -0.36$) than indexes of hypoxemia ($r = -0.34$) (157). Cheshire et al. (158) found the AHI to correlate with impaired cognitive function testing but not objective daytime sleepiness. Bennett and co-workers (10) found that the AHI, cortical arousal index (central and frontal EEG), sleep disturbance based on a neural network model, and a BMI correlated with objective daytime sleepiness. Of note, correlations with the indexes of sleep disturbance were higher than the AHI, but not that much higher. The BMI (based on video recording rather than EEG) and the neural network had the highest correlation coefficients. Certainly, routine EEG analysis based on sleep staging or EEG arousals may not be sensitive enough to detect all the adverse effects of respiratory disturbance. For example, noncortical arousals from respiratory events or other causes may result in daytime sleepiness (159). It may also be possible that long periods of airflow limitation with high respiratory effort without discrete arousal could be associated with symptoms. This pattern certainly occurs in children (160) who develop behavioral changes without frequent discrete arousals. There is also evidence from several studies that hypoxemia may be a factor associated with impaired cognition in patients with OSAHS (10,158,161).

Automobile Accidents and Sleep Apnea

The true increase in risk of patients with OSAHS of having an automobile accident is difficult to determine. However, studies have found a two to three times greater risk in untreated patients with OSAHS (162,163). Clearly, not all patients with sleep apnea are at high risk of having an auto accident. It appears that the presence of sleep apnea plus a history of a previous accident (or frequent falling asleep at the wheel) identifies a group of patients with especially high risk. The decision of whether to report a patient with OSAHS to a motor vehicle licencsing agency is a difficult one. A balance between patient confidentiality and protection of the public is required. A committee of the American Thoracic Society has issued the following reasonable recommendations (164): "In those jurisdictions in which conditions such as excessive daytime sleepiness caused by sleep apnea may be construed as reportable events, we recommend reporting to licensing bureaus if: (a) the patient has excessive daytime sleepiness, sleep apnea, and a history of a motor vehicle accident or equivalent level of clinical concern; and (b) one of the following circumstances exists: (i) the patient's condition is untreatable or is not amenable to expeditious treatment (within 2 months of diagnosis); or (ii) the patient is not willing to accept treatment or is unwilling to restrict driving until effective treatment has been instituted." The committee also noted that it is the physician's responsibility to notify every patient with sleep apnea that driving when sleepy is unsafe. Some form of written documentation that the patient understands this warning is prudent.

It is of concern that large financial tort settlements have been brought successfully against some physicians for failure to report a person with a medical condition who was subsequently involved in a serious traffic accident. Each state has its own laws and local medical societies have guidelines. However, in the end, the decision rests with the judgment of the treating physician. In some states, reporting is done to a health agency rather than directly to the motor vehicle licensing agency. Note that reporting does not always result in the loss of the patient's license.

To date there is no objective test that can quantify a patient's degree of driving impairment. The MSLT quantifies sleepiness, but does not predict the patient's ability to stay awake. The maintenance of wakefulness test (MWT) is a better test of the ability to remain awake, but it does not assess alertness or the ability to drive. There have been promising attempts at developing driving simulators, but the results of these performance tests have not correlated with actual driving ability (165). Studies have shown that the risk of traffic accidents does appear to be reduced with nasal CPAP therapy (if patients are compliant) (166).

Arterial Hypertension

Normal persons and patients with hypertension, but without sleep apnea, have a nocturnal fall in blood pressure. However, 20% to 40% of patients with OSA fail to have the normal nocturnal fall in systemic blood pressure ("nondippers") (167). During apnea, blood pressure tends to rise slightly and then to rise abruptly at apnea termination (Fig. 18-10) secondary to arousal from sleep and sympathetic activation and parasympathetic withdrawal. There is continued controversy about whether OSAHS can cause daytime (diurnal) hypertension. Animal models of simulated OSA suggest that it can (168). The evidence in humans is less definitive. Several studies have found that OSAHS is very common in adult populations with hypertension (>30%) (169). This association does not prove causality

as patients with hypertension and OSAHS share common potentially causative factors, such as obesity. Carlson et al. (170) found that age, obesity, and sleep apnea were independent and additive risk factors for the presence of hypertension (170). The Wisconsin cohort study has shown that the presence of even mild OSA increases the risk for the presence of hypertension, after adjusting for confounding factors such as obesity, age, and smoking (171). The Sleep Heart Health Study also found a modest increased risk of having hypertension when even mild levels of OSA were present (28). Even if sleep apnea does not cause hypertension, it may well worsen the physiologic impact of the disorder or impair treatment efficacy. For example, Verdeechia et al. (172) found that hypertensive patients who failed to have a 10% nocturnal fall in blood pressure had greater left ventricular hypertrophy.

If sleep apnea is effectively treated, does hypertension improve? This question has been approached by a number of studies that have determined the effect of nasal continuous positive airway pressure (CPAP) on nocturnal and daytime blood pressure in patients with OSAHS. Becker and co-workers (173) found that effective treatment of sleep apnea with nasal CPAP for 9 weeks or more lowered both nocturnal and daytime blood pressure by about 10 mm Hg using a placebo-controlled study (Fig. 18-11). Other investigations have shown smaller (174,175) or no effects on daytime blood pressure (176,177). These conflicting results may reflect inadequate CPAP treatment (poor adherence), too short a treatment interval, or less severe sleep apnea populations. In general, most hypertensive patients with sleep apnea will still continue to require antihypertensive medications when treated with CPAP. However, 24-hour control of blood pressure may improve on CPAP treatment.

Pulmonary Hypertension

Both hypoxemia and acidosis cause constriction of the pulmonary arteries. Hence, it is not surprising that the episodes of pulmonary hypertension occur during sleep in patients with OSAHS. It has been said that OSAHS patients with normal daytime blood gases usually have normal or only mildly increased daytime pulmonary pressures (178). Sajkov and co-workers (179) described a group of

FIGURE 18-10. This tracing shows the swings in arterial blood pressure associated with obstructive apnea (respiratory effort tracings not shown). At apnea termination there is a steep increase in blood pressure. (From Berry RB, *Sleep medicine pearls*, 2nd ed. Philadelphia: Hanley and Belfus, 2003:191. With permission.)

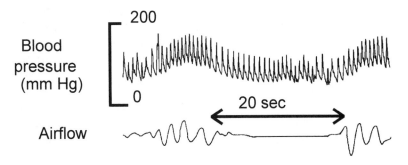

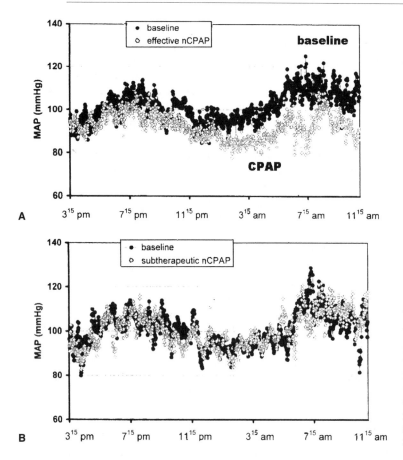

FIGURE 18-11. (A) The 24-hour blood pressure at baseline (black dots) is reduced after CPAP treatment (gray dots). The greatest reductions are during the night and in the morning. (B) There is no difference between baseline and subtherapeutic CPAP. (From Becker HF, Jerrentrup A, Ploch T, et al. Effect of nasal continuous positive airway pressure treatment on blood pressure in patients with obstructive sleep apnea. *Circulation.* 2003;107:68–73. With permission.)

OSAHS patients without hypoxemic lung disease with mean pulmonary pressures up to 30 mm Hg (normal <20 mm Hg). The affected group seemed to have a greater increase in pulmonary pressures in response to an increase in cardiac output or hypoxemia. The authors hypothesized that remodeling of the pulmonary vascular bed was responsible. In two studies, positive airway pressure treatment reduced both nocturnal and daytime pulmonary arterial pressure in patients with OSAHS (180,181). The improvement was not necessarily secondary to improvement in daytime oxygenation. One study found a decrease in pulmonary vascular reactivity to hypoxia with positive airway pressure use (181).

Arrhythmias

In normal individuals, the heart rate is lower during NREM sleep than wakefulness. This is thought to be due to parasympathetic predominance during sleep (182). In patients with OSAHS, the heart rate varies in cycles: slowing with apnea onset, increasing slightly during apnea, and increasing more dramatically in the postapneic period (Fig. 18-12). Although these cycles are referred to as brady/tachycardia, the heart rate often remains between 60 and 100 in many patients. Guilleminault reported on 400 patients with sleep apnea (183). Some type of arrhythmia was seen in 48%, 20% had more than two PVCs per

minute during sleep, 7% had severe bradycardia with less than 30 beats per minute, 3% had nonsustained ventricular tachycardia, and 5% and 3% had Mobitz type I and type II second-degree block, respectively. Sinus arrest from 2.5 to 13 seconds was noted in 11%. A recent prospective study of 45 recently diagnosed OSAHS patients used Holter monitoring for 18 hours after diagnosis and again after 2 to 3 days of CPAP (184). Only 8 of the 45 had significant rhythm disturbances, including ventricular tachycardia, atrial fibrillation, supraventricular tachycardia, and second- or third-degree heart block. In seven of these eight patients CPAP resulted in the abolition of changes.

Early studies attributed the slowing of heart rate during apnea to increased vagal tone and hypoxia (185). The slowing was diminished by atropine and supplemental oxygen. The increased vagal tone during apnea is the result of hypoxic stimulation of the carotid body during absent ventilation. With resumption of respiration, inflation of the lungs decreases vagal tone and the hypoxic influences on sympathetic tone are unmasked (tachycardia). More recent studies have not consistently found a reduction in heart rate in the last part of apnea (186). One investigation suggested that the individual differences in the effect of apnea on heart rate may be secondary to differences in the response of the carotid body to hypoxia (187).

The cycles of heart rate slowing may have little significance, except in cases of significant bradycardia or heart block. One study documented a reversal of atrioventricular

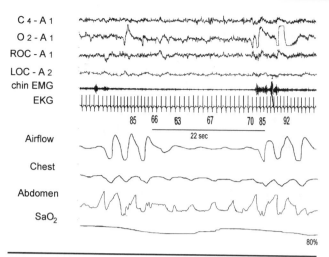

C 4 - A 1
O 2 - A 1
ROC - A 1
LOC - A 2
chin EMG
EKG

85 66 63 67 70 85 92

22 sec

Airflow

Chest

Abdomen

SaO₂

80%

FIGURE 18-12. This tracing shows changes in heart rate during an obstructive apnea. There is a slowing at the start of apnea, a minor increase during apnea, and a more rapid increase at apnea termination. The instantaneous heart rate is shown below the EKG channel. (From Berry RB, *Sleep medicine pearls.* 2nd ed. Philadelphia: Hanley and Belfus, 2003:195. With permission.).

conduction block on CPAP treatment (188). However, the periods of tachycardia and elevated blood pressure postapnea increase myocardial oxygen demand at the same time that hypoxemia exists, predisposing to ischemia and possibly tachyarrhythmias. In normal individuals, sleep usually is a time of reduced tachyarrhythmias and ischemia. Patients with OSAHS may not enjoy the same protection. Premature ventricular contractions (PVCs) are not uncommon in patients with OSAHS patients. However, in some patients, the PVC frequency is actually lower during sleep. Shepard (189) found no correlation between the SaO₂ at desaturation and PVC frequency during sleep unless the SaO₂ was less than 60% (189).

Heart rate variability has recently been used as a tool to study the balance of parasympathetic and sympathetic tone in patients with OSAHS. During wakefulness, OSAHS patients show less heart rate variability than normal individuals. This is thought secondary to an increase in sympathetic tone that is still present during the day. After successful treatment with CPAP, the heart rate variability may increase, suggesting a drop in sympathetic activity. Khoo and co-workers (190) found that CPAP treatment of OSAHS improved vagal heart rate control and that the degree of improvement varied directly with the amount of adherence with CPAP use.

Even if arrhythmias do not worsen during sleep, untreated OSAHS might worsen arrhythmia control. Kanagala and co-workers (191) found that patients with untreated OSAHS had a higher recurrence of atrial fibrillation after cardioversion than patients without a polysomnographic diagnosis of sleep apnea. Appropriate treatment with CPAP in OSAHS was associated with a lower recurrence of atrial fibrillation. As patients with

OSAHS may have nocturnal bradycardia and paroxysmal tacharrhythmias, one group investigated the effects of atrial pacing. An unexpected finding was that atrial overdrive pacing actually reduced the number of central and obstructive apneas (192). The mechanism for this action is unknown.

Coronary Artery Disease and Increased Atherosclerosis

The Sleep Heart Health Study of a large prospective cohort of patients found evidence of a modest increase in risk of having self-reported coronary artery disease at even low levels of sleep apnea (28). Peker and co-workers found an increase in mortality in patients with coronary artery disease who had untreated OSA (193).

There have also been a growing number of studies showing changes in blood components or indicators of inflammation in OSAHS that may be associated with an increased risk of atherosclerosis or thrombosis. In OSAHS an increase in the early morning hematocrit (194) and fibrinogen levels (195) decreased after CPAP treatment. The levels of vascular endothelial growth factor (VEGF) (196), amount of neutrophil (197,198), and platelet activation (199) are also reduced with CPAP treatment of patients with OSAHS. Inflammation is now believed to play a role in atherosclerosis or plaque rupture. The level of C-reactive protein (a marker of inflammation) is reduced with CPAP treatment (200,201). One study found a reduction in both leptin (a hormone secreted by adipose tissue) and visceral fat on CPAP treatment (202). Increased visceral fat is associated with an increased risk of cardiac disease.

Congestive Heart Failure

Studies have suggested that SDB is common in patients with congestive heart failure (CHF) (203,204). One should not assume that complaints of disturbed nocturnal sleep are simply secondary to heart failure. Sin et al. (204) retrospectively evaluated a group of patients with significant left ventricular (LV) failure referred to the sleep laboratory and found that risk factors for OSA included an increased BMI for men and increased age for women. In patients with CHF and OSA, the negative intrathoracic pressure, hypoxemia, and increased sympathetic tone associated with the apneas are believed to negatively impact ventricular function (182). Treatment of OSAHS with nasal CPAP in patients with cardiomyopathy was found to improve the ejection fraction and symptoms in two studies (205,206). This appears to occur because of a reduction in sympathetic tone and a decrease in ventricular afterload (182).

Stroke and Obstructive Sleep Apnea Hypopnea Syndrome

A number of studies have shown a high prevalence of SDB in patients soon after a cerebral infarction (stroke) (207,

208). This raises questions about the temporal relationship. Does brain damage from a cerebral infarction cause sleep apnea or did sleep apnea precede the stroke? If so, is the presence of sleep apnea an independent risk factor for the development of a stroke? The Sleep Heart Health Study did show an increased risk of developing a stroke if OSA is present (28). Again a major confounding problem is the fact that there are many overlapping risk factors and associations for stroke and OSAHS. If there is a causal role for OSAHS in stroke, what are the mechanisms? As noted previously, OSAHS may predispose to atherosclerosis, hypertension, and early morning hemoconcentraion. These factors would increase the risk of stroke. During sleep apnea there are increases in intracranial pressure (ICP) (209) and decreases in cerebral blood flow (210). There is an increase in ICP with each apneic event, and the rise tends to be correlated to the length of apnea. The increase in ICP is thought secondary to increases in CVP, systemic pressure, and cerebral vasodilation from rises in Pco_2 during events. As cerebral perfusion is proportional to the mean arterial pressure (MAP)—ICP, increases in ICP may reduce perfusion pressure, even if MAP also rises. Studies of cerebral blood flow velocity using Doppler monitoring have shown that flow velocity increases in early apnea and then has approximately a 25% fall below baseline at end apnea (210).

There is some evidence that the presence of OSAHS in patients who have suffered a stroke is a bad prognostic sign regardless of whether OSAHS precedes or follows the stroke. Good and co-workers (211) found that the Barthel index (a multifaceted scale measuring mobility and activities of daily living that is used to assess patients after stroke) was significantly lower in patients with OSAHS and stroke compared with those with no evidence

of OSAHS after stroke. The presence of OSAHS was determined at discharge, and the Barthel index was lower at 3 and 12 months in the OSA-stroke group. Future studies are needed to determine if treatment of OSAHS after stroke improves the outcome or prevents recurrence of stroke.

OBSTRUCTIVE SLEEP APNEA HYPOPNEA SYNDROME IN CHILDREN

The major differences in the presentation and characteristics of OSAHS between children and adults are listed in Table 18-6 (160,212–215). While very obese children can present with symptoms similar to adults, the typical history in childhood OSAHS is one of hyperactivity or developmental delay (213) combined with abnormal sleep behaviors observed by the parents. These include snoring, labored breathing, diaphoresis, or frequent movements during sleep. As adenotonsillar hypertrophy is the most common cause, the peak age of childhood OSAHS is 4 to 6 years. Children with congenital abnormalities can present much earlier or later.

In pediatric sleep monitoring, absent airflow of any length (usually at least two respiratory cycles) is considered abnormal. In addition, the occurrence of even one obstructive apnea perhoor (AI>1) is considered abnormal. However, the most common pattern in pediatric sleep monitoring is "obstructive hypoventilation." This pattern consists of long periods of airflow limitation, increased inspiratory effort, increased end-tidal Pco_2, and variable amounts of arterial oxygen desaturation. Traditional monitoring (thermistor flow) often demonstrates few changes except for an elevation in end-tidal Pco_2 and perhaps no or

▶ **TABLE 18-6. Differences between Children and Adults with OSAHS**

	Children	*Adults*
Clinical findings		
Peak age	Preschool (4–6 years)	60–70
Sex ratio	M = F	M > F
Etiology	Adenotonsillar hypertrophy	Obesity/upper airway structural shape
Weight	Failure to thrive to obese	Obese
Excessive daytime sleepiness	Uncommon	Common
Neurobehavioral	Hyperactivity, developmental delay	Impaired vigilance
PSG		
Definition of abnormal	AI >1/hr	AHI >5/h
Obstruction pattern	Obstructive hypoventilation apnea in REM	Obstructive apnea/ hypopnea; higher AHI in REM sleep
Sleep architecture	Normal	Reduced stage 3,4 and REM sleep
Sleep stage with OSA	REM	REM > NREM
Cortical arousal	Low rates <50% of apneas	High rates 60–80% of apnea/hypopnea

mild drops in the SaO$_2$. Paradoxic motion of the chest and abdomen may be noted (moving in opposite directions). Nasal pressure monitoring shows airflow limitation (flattening) and reduced, but stable, flow. This common pattern is the reason that end-tidal Pco$_2$ in an integral part of most pediatric sleep studies (115,212,214).

While the major cause of OSAHS in children is adenotonsillar hypertrophy, tonsil size does not correlate with findings on sleep studies. One child with large tonsils may be without symptoms while another with modest tonsil enlargement may have significant symptoms. Other upper airway characteristics are likely responsible. Of note, symptoms can recur in later life after initial improvement following tonsillectomy and adenoidectomy.

FUTURE DIRECTIONS

While major progress has been made at educating the general public and primary care physicians about the signs and symptoms of OSAHS much work remains. An even bigger challenge is to find methods to diagnose and treat patients in the large population with sleep apnea using the relatively limited number of sleep centers. New validated algorithms of diagnosis and treatment are needed. In addition, more information about the health risks of untreated sleep apnea is needed. This is especially essential for cases where the affected individual is not sleepy. Some studies suggest minimal benefit of CPAP treatment of nonsleepy OSA patients in the short term (216). However, most physicians recommend treatment of moderate to severe OSAHS even without symptoms based on the belief that effective treatment will reduce the risk of cardiovascular consequences for untreated sleep apnea. Evidence to support this belief is needed. Such information would allow patients and physicians to make good treatment decisions.

REFERENCES

1. Burwell C, Robin E, Whaley R, et al. Extreme obesity associated with alveolar hypoventilation—a pickwickian syndrome. *Amer J Med.* 1956;21:811–818.
2. Guilleminault C, Tilikan A, Dement WC. The sleep apnea syndromes. *Annu Rev Med.* 1976;27:465–484.
3. Gulleminault C. Obstructive sleep apnea: the clinical syndrome and historical perspective. *Med Clin N Amer.* 1985;69:1187–1203.
4. Remmers JE, Degroot WJ, Sauerland EK, et al. Pathogenesis of upper airway occlusion during sleep. *J Appl Physiol.* 1978;44:931–938.
5. Berry RB. Nasal and esophageal pressure monitoring. In: Lee-Chiiong TL, Sateia MJ, Caraskadon MA, eds. *Sleep Medicine.* Philadelphia: Hanley and Belfus, 2002:661–671.
6. Block AJ, Boysen PG, Wynne JW, et al. Sleep apnea, hypopnea, and oxygen desaturation in normal subjects. *N Engl J Med.* 1979;300:513–517.
7. Gould GA, Whyte KF, Rhind GB, et al. The sleep hypopnea syndrome. *Amer Rev Respir Dis.* 1988;137:895–888.

8. Redline S, Sander M. Hypopnea, a floating metric: implications for prevalence, morbidity estimates, and case finding. *Sleep.* 1997;20:1209–1217.
9. Redline S, Kapur VK, Sanders MH, et al. Effects of varying approaches for identifying respiratory disturbances on sleep apnea assessment. *Amer J Respir Crit Care Med.* 2000;161:369–374.
10. Bennett LS, Langford BA, Stradling JR. Sleep fragmentation indices as predictors of daytime sleepiness and nCPAP response in obstructive sleep apnea. *Amer J Respir Crit Care Med.* 1998;158:778–786.
11. Berg S, Haight JS, Yap V, et al. Comparison of direct and indirect measurements of respiratory airflow: implications for hypopneas. *Sleep.* 1997;20:60–64.
12. Guilleminault C, Stoohs R, Clerk A, et al. A cause of excessive daytime sleepiness: the upper-airway resistance syndrome. *Chest.* 1993;104:781–787.
13. Berry RB, Gleeson K. Respiratory arousal from sleep: mechanisms and significance. *Sleep.* 1997;20:654–675.
14. Bonnet MH. Performance and sleepiness as a function of frequency and placement of sleep disruption. *Psychophysiology.* 1986;23:263–271.
15. Roehrs T, Merlotti L, Petrucelli N, et al. Experimental sleep fragmentation. *Sleep.* 1994;17:438–443.
16. American Sleep Disorders Association—The Atlas Task Force. EEG arousals: scoring rules and examples. *Sleep.* 1992;15:174–184.
17. Norman RG, Ahmed MM, Walsleben JA, et al. Detection of respiratory events during NPSG: nasal cannula/pressure sensor versus thermistor. *Sleep.* 1997;20:1175–1184.
18. Monserrat JP, Farré R, Ballester E, et al. Evaluation of nasal prongs for estimating nasal flow. *Amer J Respir Crit Care Med.* 1997;155:211–215.
19. Chada TS, Watson H, Birch S, et al. Validation of respiratory inductance plethysmography using different calibration procedures. *Amer Rev Respir Dis.* 1982;125:644–649.
20. Cantineau JP, Escourrous P, Sartene R, et al. Accuracy of respiratory inductive plethysmography during wakefulness and sleep in patients with obstructive sleep apnea. *Chest.* 1992;102:1145–1151.
21. Kryger MH. Monitoring respiratory and cardiac function. In: Kryger MH, Roth T, Dement WC, eds. *Principles and practice of sleep medicine.* Philadelphia, WB Saunders, 2000:1217–1230.
22. American Academy of Sleep Medicine Task Force. Sleep-related breathing disorders in adults: recommendation for syndrome definition and measurement techniques in clinical research. *Sleep.* 1999;22:667–689.
23. Aappa I, Norman RG, Krieger AC, et al. Non-invasive detection of respiratory effort related arousals (RERAs) by a nasal cannula/pressure transducer system. *Sleep.* 2000;23:763–771.
24. Loube DI, Gay PC, Strohl KP, et al. Indications for positive airway pressure treatment of adult obstructive sleep apnea patients. A consensus statement. *Chest.* 1999;115:863–866.
25. Meoli AL, Casey KR, Clark RW. Clinical practice review committee—AASM. hypopnea in sleep disordered breathing in adults. *Sleep.* 2001;24:469–470.
26. Whitney C, Gottlieb DJ, Redline S, et al. Reliability of scoring respiratory disturbance indices and sleep staging. *Sleep.* 1998;21:749–757.
27. Drinnan MJ, Murray A, Griffiths CJ, et al. Interobserver variability in recognizing arousal in respiratory sleep disorders. *Amer J Respir Crit Care Med.* 1998;15:358–362.
28. Shahar E, Whitney CW, Redline S, et al. Sleep-disordered breathing and cardiovascular disease: cross-sectional results of the Sleep Heart Health Study. *Amer J Respir Crit Care Med.* 2001;163:19–25.
29. Douglas NJ. Upper airway resistance syndrome is not a distinct syndrome. *Amer J Resp Crit Care Med.* 161:1410–1415.
30. Guilleminault C, Chowdhuri S. Upper airway resistance syndrome is a distinct syndrome. *Amer J Respir Crit Care Med.* 2001;161:1413–1416.
31. Rees K, Kingshott RN, Wraith PK, et al. Frequency and significance of increased upper airway resistance during sleep. *Amer J Resp Crit Care Med.* 2000;162:1210–1214.
32. Mathur R, Douglas NJ. Frequency of EEG arousals from nocturnal sleep in normal subjects. *Sleep.* 1995;18:330–333.

33. Sullivan CE, Berthon-Jones M, Issa FG. Remission of severe obesity-hypoventilation syndrome after short-term treatment during sleep with nasal continuous positive airway pressure. *Amer Rev Respir Dis*. 1983;128:177–181.

34. Rapoport DM, Garay SM, Epstein H, et al. Hypercapnia in the obstructive sleep apnea syndrome. *Chest*. 1986;89:627–635.

35. Berger KI, Ayappa I, Chatr-amontri B, et al. Obesity hypoventilation syndrome as a spectrum of respiratory disturbances during sleep. *Chest*. 2001;120:1231–1238.

36. Shivaram U, Cash ME, Beal A. Nasal continuous positive airway pressure in decompensated hypercapnic respiratory failure as a complication of sleep apnea. *Chest*. 1993;104:770–774.

37. Piper AJ, Sullivan CE. Effects of short-term NIPPV in the treatment of patients with severe obstructive sleep apnea and hypercapnia. *Chest*. 1994;105:434–440.

38. Berthon-Jones M, Sullivan CE. Time course of change in ventilatory response to CO_2 with long-term CPAP therapy for obstructive sleep apnea. *Amer Rev Respir Dis*. 1987;135:144–147.

39. Rajagopal KR, Abbrecht PH, Jabbari B. Effects of medroxyprogesterone acetate in obstructive sleep apnea. *Chest*. 1986;90:815–821.

40. Bradley TD, Rutherford R, Lue F, et al. Role of diffuse airway obstruction in the hypercapnia of obstructive sleep apnea. *Amer Rev Respir Dis*. 1986;134:920–924.

41. Chan CS, Grunstein RR, Bye PTP, et al. Obstructive sleep apnea with chronic airflow limitation: comparison of hypercapnic and eucapnic patients. *Amer Rev Respir Dis*. 1989;140:1274–1278.

42. Goldstein RS, Ramcharan V, Bowes G, et al. Effect of supplemental nocturnal oxygen on gas exchange in patients with severe obstructive lung disease. *N Engl J Med*. 1984;310:425–429.

43. Fletcher EC, Schaaf JW, Miller J, et al. Long-term cardiopulmonary sequelae in patients with sleep apnea and chronic lung disease. *Amer Rev Respir Dis*. 1987;135:525–533.

44. Sampol G, Sagalés MT, Roca A, et al. Nasal continuous positive airway pressure with supplemental oxygen in coexistent sleep apnea-hypopnea syndrome and severe chronic obstructive pulmonary disease. *Eur Respir J*. 1996;9:111–116.

45. Horner RL. Motor control of pharyngeal musculature and implications for the pathogenesis of obstructive sleep apnea. *Sleep*. 1996;19:827–853.

46. Badr MS. Pathophysiology of upper airway obstruction during sleep. *Clinics in chest medicine*. 1998;19(1):21–32.

47. Schwab RJ, Gefter WB, Hoffman EA, et al. Dynamic upper-airway imaging during wake respiration in normal subjects and patients with sleep disordered breathing. *Amer Rev Respir Dis*. 1993;148:1385–1400.

48. Leiter JC. Upper-airway shape: is it important in the pathogenesis of obstructive sleep apnea? *Amer J Respir Crit Care Med*. 1996;153:894–898.

49. Isono S, Remmers JE, Tanakka A, et al. Anatomy of pharynx in patients with obstructive sleep apnea and normal subjects. *J Appl Physiol*. 1997;82:1319–1326.

50. Gleadhill IC, Schwartz AR, Schubert N, et al. Upper airway collapsibility in snorers and in patients with obstructive hypopnea and apnea. *Amer Rev Respir Dis*. 1991;143:1300–1303.

51. Tangel DJ, Messanotte WS, Sandberg EJ, et al. Influences of NREM sleep on activity of tonic vs. inspiratory phasic muscles in normal men. *J Appl Physiol*. 1992;73:1058–1066.

52. Tangel DJ, Mezzanotte WS, White DP. Influences of NREM sleep on activity of palatoglossus and levator palatini muscles in normal men. *J Appl Physiol*. 1995;78:689–695.

53. Tangel DJ, Messanotte WS, White DP. Influence of sleep on tensor palatini EMG and upper-airway resistance in normal men. *J Appl Physiol*. 1991;70:2574–2581.

54. Hudgel DW, Martin RJ, Johnson B, et al. Mechanics of the respiratory system and breathing pattern during sleep in normal humans. *J Appl Physiol*. 1984;56:133–137.

55. Pillar G, Malhotra A, Fogel RB, et al. Upper airway muscle responsiveness to rising PCO(2) during NREM sleep. *J Apply Physiol*. 2000;89:1275–1282.

56. Malhotra A, Pillar G, Fogel RB, et al. Genioglossal but not palatal muscle activity relates closely to pharyngeal pressure. *Amer J Respir Crit Care Med*. 2000;162:1058–1062.

57. Horner RL, Innes JA, Murphy K, et al. Evidence for reflex upper-airway dilatory muscle activation by sudden negative airway pressure in man. *J Physiol (London)*. 1991;436:15–29.

58. Wheatley JR, Tangel DJ, Mezzanotte WS, et al. Influence of sleep on response to negative airway pressure of tensor palatini muscle and retropalatal airway. *J Appl Physiol*. 1993;75:2117–2124.

59. Horner RL, Innes JA, Morrell MJ, et al. The effect of sleep on reflex genioglossus muscle activation by stimuli of negative airway pressure in humans. *J Physiol (London)*. 1994;476:141–151.

60. Wheatley JR, Mezzanotte WS, Tangel DJ, et al. The influence of sleep on genioglossal muscle activation by negative pressure in normal men. *Amer Rev Respir Dis*. 1993;148:597–605.

61. Mezzanotte WS, Tangel DJ, White DP. Waking genioglossal electromyogram in sleep apnea patient versus normal controls (a neuromuscular compensatory mechanism). *J Clin Invest*. 1992:1571–1579.

62. Fogel RB, Malhotra A, Pillar G, et al. Genioglossal activation in patients with obstructive sleep apnea versus control subjects. *Amer J Resp Crit Care Med*. 2001;164:2025–2030.

63. Berry RB, White DP, Roper J, et al. Awake negative pressure reflex response of the genioglossus in OSA patients and normal subjects. *J Appl Physiol*. 2003;94:1875–1882.

64. Mortimore IL, Douglas NJ. Palatal muscle EMG Response to negative pressure in awake sleep apneic and control subjects. *Amer J Respir Crit Care Med*. 1997;156:867–873.

65. Malhotra A, Pillar G, Edwards J, et al. Upper airway collapsibility: Measurement and sleep effects. *Chest*. 2001;120:156–161.

66. Mezzanotte WS, Tangel DJ, White DP. Influence of sleep onset on upper-airway muscle activity in apnea patients versus normal controls. *Amer J Respir Crit Care Med*. 1996;153:1880–1887.

67. Penzel T, Moller M, Becker HF, et al. Effect of sleep position and sleep stage on the collapsibility of the upper airways in patients with sleep apnea. *Sleep*. 2001;24:90–95.

68. Boudewyns A, Punjabi N, Van de Heyning PH, et al. Abbreviated method for assessing upper-airway function in obstructive sleep apnea. *Chest*. 2000;118:1031–1041.

69. Berry RB, McNellis M, Kouchi K, et al. Upper airway anesthesia reduces genioglossus activity during sleep apnea. *Amer J Resp Crit Care Med*. 1997;156:127–132.

70. Carlson DM, Onal E, Carley DW, et al. Palatal muscle electromyogram activity in obstructive sleep apnea. *Amer J Resp Crit Care Med*. 1995;152:1319–1322.

71. Badr MS, Toiber F, Skatrud JB, et al. Pharyngeal narrowing/occlusion during central apnea. *J Appl Physiol*. 1995;78:1806–1815.

72. Hoffstein V, Zamel N, Phillipson EA. Lung volume dependence of cross-sectional area in patients with obstructive sleep apnea. *Amer Rev Respir Dis*. 1984;130:175–178.

73. Stanchina ML, Malhotra A, Fogel RB, et al. The influence of lung volume on pharyngeal mechanics, collapsibility, and genioglossus muscle activation during sleep. *Sleep*. 2003;26:851–856.

74. Van de Graaff WB. Thoracic influences on upper-airway patency. *J Appl Physiol*. 1988;65:2124–2131.

75. Hudgel DW, Devadda P. Decrease in functional residual capacity during sleep in normal humans. *J Appl Physiol*. 1984;57:1319–1322.

76. Morrell MJ, Arabi Y, Zahn B, et al. Progressive retropalatal narrowing preceding obstructive apnea. *Amer J Respir Crit Care Med*. 1998;158:1974–1981.

77. Dempsey JA, Skatrud JB. A sleep-induced apneic threshold and its consequences. *Amer Rev Respir Dis*. 1986;133:1163–1170.

78. Iber C, Davies SF, Chapman RC, et al. A possible mechanism for mixed apnea in obstructive sleep apnea. *Chest*. 1986;89:800–805.

79. Badr MS, Kawak A. Post-hyperventilation hypopnea in humans during NREM sleep. *Respir Physiol*. 1996;103:137–145.

80. Gould GA, Gugger M, Molloy J, et al. Breathing pattern and eye movement density during REM sleep in humans. *Amer Rev Respir Dis*. 1988;138:874–877.

81. Wiegand L, Zwillich CW, Wiegand D, et al. Changes in upper-airway muscle activation and ventilation during phasic REM sleep in normal men. *J Appl Physiol*. 1991;71:488–497.

82. O'Malley EB, Norman RG, Farkas DF, et al. The addition of frontal EEG leads improves detection of cortical arousal following obstructive respiratory events. *Sleep*. 2003;26:435–439.

83. Kimoff RJ, Cheong TH, Olha AE, et al. Mechanisms of apnea termination in obstructive sleep apnea. Role of chemoreceptor

and mechanoreceptor stimuli. *Amer J Respir Crit Care Med.* 1994; 149:707–714.

84. Berry RB, Kouchi KG, Bower JL, et al. Effect of upper airway anesthesia on obstructive sleep apnea. *Amer J Respir Crit Care Med.* 1995; 151:1857–1861.

85. Cala SJ, Sliwinski P, Cosio MG, et al. Effect of topical upper airway anesthesia on apnea duration through the night in obstructive sleep apnea. *J Appl Physiol.* 1996;81:2618–2626.

86. Berry RB, Kouchi KG, Der DE, et al. Sleep apnea impairs the arousal response to airway occlusion. *Chest.* 1996;109:1490–1496.

87. Gora J, Trinder J, Pierce R, et al. Evidence of a sleep-specific blunted cortical response to inspiratory occlusion in mild obstructive sleep apnea syndrome. *Amer J Resir Crit Care Med.* 2002;166:1225–1234.

88. Montserrat JM, Kosmas EN, Cosio MG, et al. Mechanism of apnea lengthening across the night in obstructive sleep apnea. *Amer J Respir Crit Care Med.* 1996;154:988–93.

89. Berry RB, Asyali MA, McNellis MI, et al. Within-night variation in respiratory effort preceding apnea termination and EEG delta power in sleep apnea. *J Appl Physiol.* 1998;85:1434–1441.

90. Findley LJ, Ries AL, Tisi GM. Hypoxemia during apnea in normal subjects: mechanisms and impact of lung volume. *J Appl Physiol.* 1983;55:1777–1783.

91. Bradley TD, Martinez D, Rutherford R, et al. Physiological determinants of nocturnal arterial oxygenation in patients with obstructive sleep apnea. *J Appl Physiol.* 1985;59:1364–1368.

92. Series F, Cormier Y, La Forge J. Influence of apnea type and sleep stage on nocturnal postapneic desaturation. *Amer Rev Respir Dis.* 1990;141:1522–1526.

93. Young T, Peppard PE, Gottlieb DJ. Epidemiology of obstructive sleep apnea. *Amer J Respir Crit Care Med.* 2002;165:1271–1239.

94. Young T, Palta M, Leder R, et al. The occurrence of sleep-disordered breathing among middle-aged adults. *N Engl J Med.* 1993;328:1230–1235.

95. Bixler E, Vgontzas A, Ten Have T, et al. Effects of age on sleep apnea in men. *Amer J Respir Cir Care Med.* 1998;157:144–148.

96. Bixler E, Vgontzas A, Teh Have T, et al. Prevalence of sleep disordered breathing in women. *Amer J Respir Cir Care Med.* 2001;163:608–613.

97. Ancoli-Israel S, Klauber MR, Kripke DF. Sleep disordered breathing in community dwelling elderly. *Sleep.* 1991;14:486–495.

98. Young T, Shahar E, Nieto FJ, et al. Predictors of sleep disordered breathing in community dwelling adults: The Sleep Heart Health Study. *Arch Intern Med.* 2002;162:893–900.

99. Enright PL, Newman AB, Wahl PW, et al. Prevalence and correlates of snoring and observed apneas in 5,201 older adults. *Sleep.* 1996;19:531–538.

100. Young T. Sleep-disordered breathing in older adults. Is it a condition distinct from that in middle-aged adults? *Sleep.* 1996:529–530.

101. Ancoli-Israel S, Klauber M, Stepnowksy C, et al. Sleep-disordered breathing in African-American elderly. *Amer J Respir Crit Care Med.* 1995;152:1946–1949.

102. Redline S, Tishler PV, Hans MG, et al. Racial differences in sleep-disordered breathing in African-Americans and Caucasians. *Amer J Resp Crit Care Med.* 1997;153:186–192.

103. Ip M, Lam B, Lauder I, et al. A community study of sleep disordered breathing in middle-aged Chinese men in Hong Kong. *Chest.* 2001;119:62–69.

104. Li KK, Kushida C, Powell NB, et al. Obstructive sleep apnea syndrome: a comparison between far-east Asian and white men. *Laryngoscope.* 2000;110:1689–1693.

105. Peppard PE, Young T, Palta M, et al. Longitudinal study of moderate weight change and sleep-disordered breathing. *JAMA.* 2000;284:3015–3021.

106. Smith PL, Gold AR, Meyers DA, et al. Weight loss in mildly to moderately obese patients with obstructive sleep apnea. *Ann Intern Med.* 1985;103:850–855.

107. Schwartz AR, Gold AR, Schubert N, et al. Effect of weight loss on upper airway collapsibility in obstructive sleep apnea. *Amer Rev Respir Dis.* 1991;144:494–498.

108. Pillar G, Peled R, Lavie P. Recurrence of sleep apnea without concomitant weight increase years after weight reduction surgery. *Chest.* 1994;106:1702–1704.

109. Flemons WW. Obstructive sleep apnea. *N Engl J Med.* 2002;347:498–504.

110. Matsumoto AM, Sandblom RE, Schoene RB, et al. Testosterone replacement in hypogonadal men: effects on obstructive sleep apnea, respiratory drives, and sleep. *Clin Endocrinol* (Oxford). 1985:22:713–721.

111. Sandbloom RE, Matsumoto AM, Schoene RB, et al. Obstructive sleep apnea syndrome induced by testosterone administration. *N Engl J Med.* 1983;308:508–510.

112. Pillar G, Malhotra A, Foge R, et al. Airway mechanism and ventilation in response to resistive loading during sleep: influence of gender. *Amer J Respir Crit Care Med.* 2000;162:1627–1632.

113. Malhotra A, Huang Y, Fogel RB, et al. The male predisposition to pharyngeal collapse. *Amer J Resp Crit Care Med.* 2002;166:1388–1395.

114. Rowley JA, Zhou X, Vergine I, et al. Influence of gender of upper airway mechanics: upper airway resistance and Pcrit. *J Appl Physiol.* 2001;91:2248–2254.

115. Rowley JA, Sanders CS, Zahn BR, et al. Gender differences in upper-airway compliance during NREM sleep: role of neck circumference. *J Appl Physiol.* 2002;92:2535–2541.

116. Zhou XS, Shahabuddin S, Zahn BR, et al. Effect of gender on the development of hypocapnic apnea/hypopnea during NREM sleep. *J Appl Physiol.* 2000;89:192–199.

117. Shahar E, Redline S, Young T, et al. Hormone replacement therapy and sleep disordered breathing. *Amer J Respir Crit Care Med.* 2003;167;1186–1192.

118. Young T, Finn L, Austin D, et al. Menopausal status and sleep disordered breathing in the Wisconsin Sleep Cohort Study. *Amer J Respir Crit Care Med.* 2003;167:1181–1185.

119. Issa FG, Sullivan CE. Alcohol, snoring and sleep apnea. *J Neurol Neurosurg Psych.* 1982;45:353–359.

120. Mitler MM, Dawson A, Henriksen SJ, et al. Bedtime ethanol increases resistance of upper-airways and produces sleep apnea in asymptomatic snoreres. *Alcohol Clin Exp Res.* 1988;12:801–805.

121. Block AJ, Hellard DW, Slayton PC. Effect of alcohol ingestion on breathing and oxygenation during sleep. Analysis of the influence of age and sex. *Amer J Med.* 1986;80:595–600.

122. Scanlan MF, Roebuck T, Little PJ, et al. Effect of moderate alcohol upon obstructive sleep apnea. *Eur Respir J.* 2000;16:909–913.

123. St John WM, Bartlett D, Jr, Knuth KV, et al. Differential depression of hypoglossal nerve activity by alcohol. Protection by pretreatment with medroxyprogesterone acetate. *Amer Rev Respir Dis.* 1986;133:46–48.

124. Berry RB, Bonnet MH, Light RW. Effect of ethanol on the arousal response to airway occlusion during sleep in Normal subjects. *Amer Rev Respir Dis.* 1982;145:445–452.

125. Rajagopal KR, Abbrecht PH, Derderian SS, et al. Obstructive sleep apnea in hypothyroidism. *Ann Intern Med.* 1984;101:491–494.

126. Grunstein RR, Sullivan CE. Sleep apnea and hypothyroidism: Mechanisms and management. *Amer J Med.* 1988;85:775–779.

127. Pelttari L, Rauhala E, Polo O, et al. Upper airway obstruction in hypothyroidism. *J Intern Med.* 1994;236:177–181.

128. Lin CC, Tsan KW, Chen PJ. The relationship between sleep apnea syndrome and hypothyroidism. *Chest.* 1992;102:1663–1667.

129. Winkelman JW, Goldman H, Piscatelli N, et al. Are thyroid function studies necessary in patients with suspected sleep apnea? *Sleep.* 1996;19:790–793.

130. Grunstein RR, Ho KY, Sullivan CE. Sleep apnea in acromegaly. *Ann Intern Med.* 1991;115:527–532.

131. Weiss V, Sonka K, Pretl M, et al. Prevalence of the sleep apnea syndrome in acromegaly population. *J Endocrinol Invest.* 2000;23:515–519.

132. Isono S, Saeki N, Tanaka A, et al. Collapsibility of passive pharynx in patients with acromegaly *Amer J Respir Crit Care Med.* 1990:64–68.

133. Astrom C, Christensen L, Gjerris F, et al. Sleep in acromegaly before and after treatment with adenomectomy. *Neuroendocrinology.* 1991;53:328–331.

134. Young T, Finn L, Palta M. Chronic nasal congestion is a risk factor of snoring in a population-base cohort study. *Arch Intern Med.* 2001;161:1514–1519.

135. Young T, Finn L, Kim H. Nasal obstruction as a risk factor for sleep-disordered breathing. The University of Wisconsin Sleep and Respiratory Research Group. *J Allergy Clin Immunol.* 1997;99:S757–S762.

136. Strohl KP, Redline S. Recognition of obstructive sleep apnea. *Amer J Respir Crit Care Med.* 1996;154:279–289.

137. Johns MW. Daytime sleepiness, snoring, and obstructive sleep apnea. The Epworth sleepiness scale. *Chest.* 1993:103:30–36.

138. Krakow B, Melendez D, Ferreira E, et al. Prevalence of insomnia symptoms in patients with sleep-disordered breathing. *Chest.* 2001;120:1923–1929.

139. Seftel AD, Strohl KP, Loye TL, et al. Erectile dysfunction and symptoms of sleep disorders. *Sleep.* 2002;25:643–647.

140. Douglas NJ. "Why am I sleepy": Sorting the somnolent. *Amer J Respir Crit Care Med.* 2001;163:1310–1313.

141. Woodson BT, Nauanuma H. Comparison of methods of airway evaluation in obstructive sleep apnea syndrome *Otolaryngol Head Neck Surg.* 1999;210:460–463.

142. Zonato AI, Bittencourt LR, Martinho FL, et al. Association of systematic head and neck physical examination with severity of obstructive sleep apnea hypopnea syndrome. *Laryngoscope.* 2003;113:973–980.

143. Flemons WW, Whitelaw WA, Brant R, et al. Likelihood ratios for a sleep apnea clinical prediction rule. *Amer J Respir Crit Care Med.* 1994;150:1279–1285.

144. Netzer NC, Stoohs RA, Netzer CM, et al. Using the Berlin Questionnaire to identify patients at risk for the sleep apnea syndrome. *Ann Intern Med.* 1999;132:485–491.

145. American Sleep Disorders Association Report. Standards of Practice Committee. Practice parameters for the indications for polysomnography and related procedures. *Sleep.* 1997;20:406–422.

146. Chesson AL, Ferber R, Fry J, et al. The indications for polysomnography and related procedures. *Sleep.* 1997;20:423–487.

147. Oksenberg A, Silverberg DS, Arons E, et al. Positional versus non-positional obstructive sleep apnea patients. *Chest.* 1997;112:629–639.

148. Kass JE, Akers SM, Bartter TC, et al. Rapid-eye-movement-specific sleep-disordered breathing: a possible cause of excessive daytime sleepiness. *Amer J Respir Care Med.* 1996;154:167–169.

149. Collard P, Dury M, Delguste P, et al. Movement arousals and sleep related breathing in adults. *Amer J Respir Crit Care Med.* 1996;154:454–459.

150. Le Bon O, Hoffman G, Tecco J, et al. Mild to moderate sleep respiratory events: one negative night may not be enough. *Chest.* 2002;118:353–359.

151. Quan SF, Griswold ME, Iber C, et al. Sleep Heart Health Study (SHHS) Research group. Short term variability of respiration and sleep during unattended nonlaboratory polysomnography. *Sleep.* 2002;25:843–849.

152. Flemons W, Hudgel D, Littner M, et al. A systematic review of portable monitoring for investigating adult patients with suspected sleep apnea. *Chest.* 2003;124:1543–1579.

153. Chesson AL, Berry RB, Pack A. practice parameters for the use of portable monitoring devices in the investigation of suspected obstructive sleep apnea in adults. *Sleep.* 2003;26(7):907–913.

154. He J, Kryger MH, Zorick FJ, et al. Mortality and apnea index in obstructive sleep apnea. *Chest.* 1988;94:9–14.

155. Lavie P, Herer P, Peled R, et al. Mortality in sleep apnea patients: a multivariate analysis of risk factors. *Sleep.* 1995;18:149–157.

156. Guilleminault C, Partinen M, Quera-Salva A, et al. Determinants of daytime sleepiness in obstructive sleep apnea. *Chest.* 1988;94:32–37.

157. Roehrs T, Zorick F, Wittig R, et al. Predicators of objective level of daytime sleepiness in patients with sleep-related breathing disorders. *Chest.* 1989;95:1202–1206.

158. Cheshire K, Engleman H, Deary I, et al. Factors impairing daytime performance in patients with sleep apnea/hypopnea syndrome. *Arch Intern Med.* 1992;152:538–541.

159. Martin SE, Wraith PK, Deary IJ, et al. The effect of nonvisible sleep fragmentation on daytime function. *Amer J Respir Crit Care Med.* 1997;155:1596–1601.

160. Marcus CL. Sleep-disordered breathing in children. *Amer J Respir Crit Care Med.* 2001;164:16–30.

161. Findley LJ, Barth JT, Powers DC, et al. Cognitive impairment in patients with obstructive sleep apnea and associated hypoxemia. *Chest.* 1986;90:686–690.

162. Findley LJ, Unverzagt ME, Suratt PM. Automobile accidents involving patients with obstructive sleep apnea. *Amer Rev Respir Dis.* 1988;138:337–340.

163. Cassel W, Ploch C, Becker D, et al. Risk of traffic accidents in patients with sleep disordered breathing: reduction with nasal CPAP. *Eur Respir J.* 1996;9:2602–2611.

164. American Thoracic Society Official Statement. Sleep apnea, sleepiness, and driving risk. *Amer J Respir Crit Care Med.* 1994;150:1463–1473.

165. George CFP, Boudreau AC, Smiley A. Simulated driving performance in patients with obstructive sleep apnea. *Amer J Respir Crit Care Med.* 1996;154:175–181.

166. George CF. Reduction in motor-vehicle collisions following treatment of sleep apnea with nasal CPAP. *Thorax.* 2001;56:508–512.

167. Suzuki M, Guilleminault G, Otsuka K, et al. Blood pressure "dipping" and "non-dipping" in obstructive sleep apnea syndrome patients. *Sleep.* 1996;19:382–387.

168. Brooks D, Horner RL, Kozar LF, et al. Obstructive sleep apnea as a cause of systemic hypertension. Evidence from a canine model. *J Clin Invest.* 1997;99:106–109.

169. Kales A, Bixler EO, Cadieux RJ, et al. Sleep apnea in a hypertensive population. *Lancet.* 1984;3:1005–1008.

170. Carlson JT, Hedner JA, Ejnell H, et al. High prevalence of hypertension in sleep apnea patients independent of obesity. *Amer J Resp Crit Care Med.* 1994;150:72–77.

171. Peppard PE, Young T, Palta M, et al. Prospective study of the association between sleep-disordered breathing and hypertension. *N Engl J Med.* 2000;342:1378–1384.

172. Verdecchia P, Schillaci G, Guerrieri M, et al. Circadian blood pressure changes and left ventricular hypertropy in essential hypertension. *Circulation.* 1990;81:528–536.

173. Becker HF, Jerrentrup A, Ploch T, et al. Effect of nasal continuous positive airway pressure treatment on blood pressure in patients with obstructive sleep apnea. *Circulation.* 2003;107:68–73.

174. Pepperell JCT, Ramdassingh-Dow S, Crosthwaite N, et al. Ambulatory blood pressure after therapeutic and subtherapeutic nasal continuous positive airway pressure for obstructive sleep apnea: a randomized parallel trial. *Lancet.* 2002;359:204–210.

175. Faccendia J, Mackay TW, Bood NA, et al. Randomized placebo-controlled trial of continuous positive airway pressure on blood pressure in the sleep apnea-hypopnea syndrome. *Amer J Resp Crit Care Med.* 2001;163:344–348.

176. Engleman HM, Gough K, Martin SE, et al. Ambulatory blood pressure on and off continuous positive airway pressure therapy for the sleep apnea-hypopnea syndrome: Effects in "non-dippers." *Sleep.* 1996;19:378–371.

177. Dimsdale JE, Loredo JS, Profant J. Effect of continuous positive pressure on blood pressure placebo trial. *Hypertension.* 2000; 35:144–147.

178. Weitzenblum E, Krieger J, Apprill M, et al. Daytime pulmonary hypertension in patients with obstructive sleep apnea syndrome. *Amer Rev Respir Dis.* 1988;138:345–349.

179. Sajkov D, Cowie RJ, Thornton AT, et al. Pulmonary hypertension and hypoxemiain obstructive sleep apnea syndrome. *Amer J Respir Crit Care Med.* 1994;149:416–422.

180. Chaouat A, Weitzenblum E, Kessler R, et al. Five-year effects of nasal continuous positive airway pressure in obstructive sleep apnoea syndrome. *Eur Respir J.* 1997;10:2578–2582.

181. Sajkov D, Wang T, Saunders NA, et al. Continuous positive airway pressure treatment improves pulmonary hemodynamics in patients with obstructive sleep apnea. *Amer J Respir Crit Care Med.* 2002;165:152–158.

182. Leung RST, Bradley TD. Sleep apnea and cardiovascular disease. State of the art. *Amer J Resp Crit Care Med.* 2001;164:2147–2165.

183. Guilleminault C, Connoly SJ, Winkle RA. Cardiac arrhythmia and conduction disturbances during sleep in 400 patients with sleep apnea syndrome. *Amer J Cardiol.* 1983;52:490–494.

184. Harbison J, O'Reilly P, McNicholas WT. Cardiac rhythm disturbances in obstructive sleep apnea syndrome: effects of nasal continuous positive airway pressure therapy. *Chest.* 2000;118:591–595.

185. Zwillich C, Devlin T, White D, et al. Bradycardia during sleep apnea. Characteristics and mechanisms. *J Clin Invest.* 1982;69:1286–1292.

186. Weiss JW, Remsburg S, Garpestad E, et al. Hemodynamic consequences of obstructive sleep apnea. *Sleep.* 1996;19:388–397.

187. Sato F, Nishimura M, Sinano H, et al. Heart rate during obstructive sleep apnea depends on individual hypoxic chemosensitivity of the carotid body. *Circulation.* 1997;96:274–281.

188. Becker H, Brandenburg U, Peter JH, et al. Reversal of sinus arrest and atrioventricular conduction block in sleep apnea during nasal continuous positive airway pressure. *Amer J Resp Crit Care Med.* 1995;151:215–218.

189. Shepard JW, Jr, Garrison MW, Grither DA, et al. Relationship of ventricular ectopy to oxyhemoglobin desaturation in patients with obstructive sleep apnea. *Chest.* 1985;88:335–340.

190. Khoo MC, Belozeroff V, Berry RB, et al. Cardiac autonomic control in obstructive sleep anea: effects of long term CPAP therapy. *Amer J Respir Crit Care Med.* 2001;164:807–812.

191. Kanagala R, Murali NS, Friedman PA, et al. Obstructive sleep apnea and the recurrence of atrial fibrillation. *Circulation.* 2003;107:2589–2594.

192. Garrigue S, Bordier P, Jais P, et al. Benefit of atrial pacing in sleep apnea syndrome. *N Engl J Med.* 2002;346:404–412.

193. Peker Y, Hender J, Kraiczi H, et al. Respiratory disturbance index: an independent predictor of mortality in coronary artery disease. *Amer J Respir Crit Care Med.* 2000;162:81–86.

194. Kreiger J, Sforza E, Barthelmebs M, et al. Overnight decreases in hematocrit after nasal CPAP with patients with OSA. *Chest.* 1990;97:729–730.

195. Chin K, Ohi M, Kita H, et al. Effects of NCPAP therapy on fibrinogen levels in obstructive sleep apnea syndrome. *Amer J Respir Crit Care Med.* 1996;153:1972–1976.

196. Lavie L, Kraiczi H, Hefetz A, et al. Plasma vascular endothelial growth factor in sleep apnea syndrome: effects of nasal continuous positive air pressure treatment. *Amer J Respir Crit Care Med.* 2002;165(12):1624–1628.

197. Dyugovskaya L, Lavie P, Lavie L. Increased adhesion molecules expression and production of reactive oxygen species in leukocytes of sleep apnea patients. *Amer J Respir Crit Care Med.* 2002;165:934–939.

198. Schulz R, Mahmoudi S, Hattar K, et al. Enhanced release of superoxide from polymorphonuclear neutrophils in obstructive sleep apnea. Impact of continuous positive airway pressure therapy. *Amer J Respir Crit Care Med.* 2000;162:566–570.

199. Bokinsky G, Miller M, Ault K, et al. Spontaneous platelet activation and aggregation during obstructive sleep apnea and its response to therapy with nasal continuous positive airway pressure. A preliminary investigation. *Chest.* 1995;108(3):625–630.

200. Shamsuzzaman AS, Winnicki M, Lanfranchi P, et al. Elevated C-reactive protein in patients with obstructive sleep apnea. *Circulation.* 2002;105:2462–2464.

201. Yokoe T, Minoguchi K, Matsuo H, et al. Elevated levels of C-reactive protein and interleukin-6 in patients with obstructive sleep apnea syndrome are decreased by nasal continuous positive airway pressure. *Circulation.* 2003;107(8):1129–1134.

202. Shimizu K, Chin K, Nakamura T, et al. Plasma leptin levels and cardiac sympathetic function in patients with obstructive sleep apnoea-hypopnoea syndrome. *Thorax.* 2002;57:429–434.

203. Javaheri S, Parker TJ, Wexler L, et al. Occult sleep-disordered breathing in stable congestion heart failure. *Ann Intern Med.* 1995;122:487–492.

204. Sin D, Fitzgerald F, Parker J. Risk factors for central and obstructive sleep apnea in 450 men and women with congestive heart failure. *Amer J Respir Crit Care Med.* 1999;160:1101–1106.

205. Malone S, Liu PP, Holloway R, et al. Obstructive sleep apnea in patients with dilated cardiomyopathy: effects of continuous positive airway pressure. *Lancet.* 1991;33:1480–1484.

206. Kaneko Y, Floras JS, Usui K, et al. Cardiovascular effects of continuous positive airway pressure in patients with heart failure and obstructive sleep apnea. *N Engl J Med.* 2003;348:1233–1241.

207. Turkington P, Bamfor J, Wanklyn P, et al. Prevalence and predictors of upper-airway obstruction in the first 24 hours after acute stroke. *Stroke.* 2002;33:2037–2041.

208. Para O, Arboix A, Bechichi S, et al. Time course of sleep-related breathing disorders in first-even stroke or transient ischemic attack. *Amer J Respir Crit Care Med.* 2000;161:375–380.

209. Sugita Y, Susami I, Yoshio T, et al. Marked episodic elevation of cerebral spinal fluid pressure during nocturnal sleep in patients with sleep apnea hypersomnia syndrome. *Electroencephalogr Clin Neurophysiol.* 1985;60:214–219.

210. Balfors EM. Impairment of cerebral perfusion during obstructive sleep apneas. *Amer J Respir Crit Care Med.* 1994;150:1587–1591.

211. Good DC, Henkle JQ, Gelber D, et al. Sleep disordered breathing and poor functional outcome after stroke. *Stroke.* 1996;27:252–259.

212. American Academy of Pediatrics. Clinical practice guideline: diagnosis and managment of childhood obstructive sleep apnea syndrome. *Pediatrics.* 2002;109:704–712.

213. Chervin RD, Archbold KH, Dillon JE, et al. Inattention, hyperactivity, and symptoms of sleep-disordered breathing. *Pediatrics.* 2002;109:449–456.

214. Carroll JL, Loughlin GM: Obstructive sleep apnea in infants and children: diagnosis and management. In: Ferber R, Kryger M, eds. *Principles and practice of sleep medicine in the child.* Philadelphia, WB Saunders, 1995:193–230.

215. American Thoracic Society. Standards and indications for cardiopulmonary sleep studies in children. *Amer J Respir Crit Care Med.* 1996;153:866–878.

216. Barbe F, Mayoralas LR, Duran J, et al. Treatment with continuous positive airway pressure is not effective in patients with sleep apnea but no daytime sleepiness. A randomized, controlled trial. *Ann Intern Med.* 2001;134:1015–1023.

Obstructive Sleep Apnea: Treatment Overview and Controversies

Nancy A. Collop

WHO TO TREAT?

Defining what constitutes obstructive sleep apnea (OSA) can be challenging. Possible definitions might include: use of a polysomnographically defined threshold respiratory disturbance index (RDI) or apnea–hypopnea index (AHI); combining an RDI or AHI with an assessment of subjective sleepiness; or use of an RDI or AHI with some evidence of end-organ dysfunction such as hypertension. Different definitions will be useful depending upon the purpose. When deciding to treat individual patients, there are a number of considerations that may come into account, which will be outlined in this chapter. The comments in the beginning of the chapter pertain to adult OSA; later sections will deal with pediatric OSA.

Apnea–Hypopnea Index

The severity of OSA has been defined by use of AHI criteria alone (1). There are inherent problems with such an approach. First, there are substantial differences in how different sleep laboratories define respiratory events. One study showed that the definition of a hypopnea was not the same in 45 different accredited sleep laboratories (2). Another study showed that scoring studies with three different definitions of hypopnea would result in an extra case of OSA being diagnosed for every 14 to 31 patients tested, depending on which definition was used (3). Yet another study showed that there was tremendous variability among sleep laboratories in the scoring of individual sleep studies (4). It is therefore unlikely that two sleep laboratories would agree upon respiratory scoring, and an RDI in one sleep laboratory may be a very different parameter than in another sleep laboratory.

A second related issue is that not all sleep laboratories measure respiratory variables in the same way. The most obvious difference is that many sleep laboratories have changed the way that they measure airflow from using nasal and oral thermistors (NT)—qualitative heat-sensitive devices—to nasal cannula-pressure transducers (NCPT), more sensitive devices that monitor pressure swings. The latter have been shown to detect more subtle sleep-disordered breathing (SDB) events (5,6). Again, the main controversy revolves around the scoring of the more subtle sleep disturbances, hypopneas. NCPT will sense more subtle decreases in airflow and, if there is an

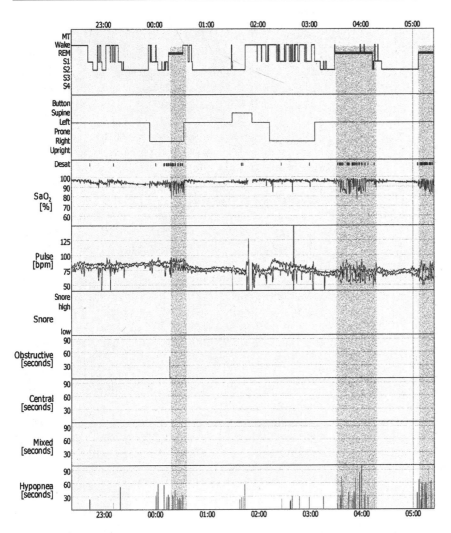

FIGURE 19-1. Hypnogram of REM-related OSA. The highlighted areas show the REM periods during the night and, as can be seen, most obstructive events occur during REM (S1, stage 1; S2, stage 2; S3, stage 3; S4, stage 4; SaO_2, oxygen saturation).

associated arousal from sleep or oxygen desaturation, it would be scored with a NCPT, whereas it may not be scored if using a NT. It has been suggested that an AHI of 18 using a NCPT to score events has the best discriminant ability, in comparison to the usual AHI of 5 or 10 with a NT (7).

To summarize, using a polysomnographically defined AHI alone is fraught with problems relating to lack of widespread standards for equipment and scoring of sleep studies.

Rapid Eye Movement/Positional Obstructive Sleep Apnea

Another issue relates to treating disease that may be confined or particularly severe in one stage of sleep (usually REM), but is not that significant, based on total sleep time (TST). REM-related OSA is an understudied phenomenon. It is a well known that obstructive SDB is worse (longer events and lower oxygen desaturations) in REM sleep because of a more collapsible upper airway (muscle atonia) and a blunted response to chemical stimuli (8). It is clear that some patients have most of their SDB during this stage

of sleep (Fig. 19-1). This phenomenon of REM-related OSA seems to be more common in women (9). This is likely due to inherent differences in the upper airway between men and women (10). There are conflicting data as to whether REM-related OSA alone can result in significant daytime sleepiness (11,12). It has been shown that pulmonary artery pressures are more elevated during REM- than NREM-related events, even after adjusting for oxygen saturation levels (13). However, there are no data as to whether REM-related OSA can cause long-term morbidity or mortality. Therefore, there is little to guide us as to how to treat this condition.

Similarly to REM-related OSA, it is commonly observed that patients have worsening of both frequency and number of SDB events when they are in the supine position. There are a subgroup of patients that only have OSA when supine (14). They tend to be both thinner and younger than "nonpositional" OSA patients, which leads one to wonder if, with time, some of these patients may progress to the "nonpositional" status. Although there are significantly more data on this phenomenon than on REM-related OSA, there is little data on long-term effects in those patients

▶ **TABLE 19-1. Common Symptoms Associated with Adult OSA**

Daytime sleepiness
Chronic fatigue
Morning headaches
Restless sleep
Insomnia
Nasal and/or sinus congestion
Impotence

whose SDB is predominantly in the supine position. There are treatment options aside from nasal continuous positive airway pressure (CPAP) in these patients, as will be discussed below.

Symptoms

Sleepiness

Another way to determine the "severity" of a patient's OSA, aside from measurement of events during polysomnography (PSG), is to evaluate their degree of symptomatology (Table 19-1). Since many patients with OSA are sleepy, one method of evaluating the severity of disease is by either subjectively or objectively measuring sleepiness. Subjective measures of sleepiness include validated patient questionnaires like the Stanford sleepiness scale (15) or the Epworth sleepiness scale (ESS) (16,17) (Fig. 19-2). These scales allow the physician to see how sleepy the patient feels and loosely correlate this with the degree of sleepiness as measured by objective measures (18). The multiple sleep latency test (MSLT) and the maintenance of wakefulness test (MWT) are two such objective measures of sleepiness. The MSLT measures how long it takes the patient to fall asleep during a series of four to five daytime naps following overnight PSG documenting adequate sleep the prior night. If the mean sleep latency is less than 5 minutes, that is consistent with severe daytime sleepiness present. If the mean sleep latency is from 5 to 10 minutes, this also considered abnormal and suggestive of excessive sleepiness. Mean sleep latencies greater than 10 minutes are considered normal. Interestingly, it has been shown that even with effective treatment, many patients with OSA will not "normalize" their MSLTs (19,20).

The MWT the ability of the patient to stay awake rather than fall asleep. This test is often used for patients with sleep disorders working in occupations that require vigilance, such as truck drivers and airplane pilots. The test is performed similarly to an MSLT, except that the patient is monitored for sleep onset over a 20- to 40-minute period. Normative values suggest that a patient should be able to stay awake for 20 minutes (21). Unfortunately, comparison studies of Epworth and MWT have not shown good concordance in OSA (22).

It has been shown that at-fault motor vehicle accidents occur more frequently in patients with OSA (23,24). One may assume that significant sleepiness might select out those who drive as part of their profession, but one study showed that 8.6% of professional truck drivers had OSA (25). Simulated driving tests in OSA patients have shown worse performance compared to controls, which can be improved with the use of CPAP (26,27). It may be possible to stratify OSA patients for driving risk utilizing these devices; however, the results to date are conflicting (28,29). At any rate, it is imperative that physicians screening patients for OSA query patients about falling asleep or nodding while driving (30).

In summary, subjective or objective measures of sleepiness may be helpful in assisting the clinician to determine who to treat, especially if the degree of SDB is low.

Other

Many patients referred to sleep clinics for sleep apnea are referred by their bed partner. The theory behind this is simple, but unproven. Most sleep apnea patients are male (3:1 by most epidemiologic studies). Women, in general are lighter sleepers, therefore, a snoring bed partner with apneas will be more likely to disrupt their sleep. Indeed the "spousal arousal syndrome" has been described (31). In addition, bed partner observation of breath pauses is one of the most sensitive historical items for OSA (32). It has been shown also, however, that if patients are referred by their spouse, they are less likely to be compliant with CPAP (33).

Although daytime sleepiness is the most common and clearly the most prominent complaint of OSA sufferers,

1. Sitting and reading
2. Watching television
3. Sitting, inactive in a public place (e.g., theatre or a meeting)
4. As a passenger in a car for an hour without a break
5. Lying down to rest in the afternoon when circumstances permit
6. Sitting and talking to someone
7. Sitting quietly after a lunch without alcohol
8. In a car, while stopped for a few minutes in traffic

FIGURE 19-2. Epworth sleepiness scale. The patient is asked how likely are they to doze off or fall asleep in the following situations. Answers are broken down via a Likert scale with 0, would never doze; 1, slight chance of dozing; 2, moderate chance of dozing; and 3, high chance of dozing.

other symptoms have been described. Chronic fatigue and tiredness, rather than true sleepiness, may be more common in females (34). Insomnia may be an underappreciated prevalent symptom of OSA (35). Morning headaches are found more frequently in patients with OSA, compared to other sleep disorders, presumably related to the hypoxemia and, concomitant hypercapnia (36). Hypercapnia causes vasodilation of cerebral vessels, which may predispose to headaches. Sinus disease has been linked to SDB. Allergy sufferers are 1.8 times more likely to have SDB (37). Impotence is well described in OSA. In one study of over 1,000 men with erectile dysfunction, almost 44% had an apnea–hypopnea index >5 (38). The reason for impotence in OSA is not well understood, although one study did suggest it could be related to nerve dysfunction (39). Signs and symptoms of OSA, aside from sleepiness, may be present and should be looked for in the assessment of individual patients.

Cardiovascular Disease

In the past decade, a number of cardiovascular diseases have been shown to occur frequently in association with OSA (Table 19-2). Although these are mostly associations, epidemiologic studies would suggest that many of these associations are more than coincidental. Perhaps the most studied cardiovascular disease associated with OSA is systemic hypertension. It has been shown that approximately 30% of patients in essential hypertension clinics have OSA (40–42), and it is estimated that 50% to 60% of OSA patients have hypertension (43). The difficulty with showing causality, i.e., that OSA can cause hypertension, lies in the fact that the population that has hypertension is similar to the population that has OSA: middle-aged, overweight males. Animal models have been instructive in showing that both recurrent apneas and/or hypoxemia during sleep will result in elevated blood pressure over time (44–46). Two large epidemiologic studies, one longitudinal and the other cross-sectional, showed an increasing dose response for the severity of OSA, defined by apnea–hypopnea index and the presence of hypertension (47,48). Another study showed that patients with refractory hypertension, defined by persistent elevation of blood pressure, despite the use of three or more antihypertensives, had a very high prevalence of OSA—96% of men and 65% of women (49). However, despite this suggestive evidence, there are conflict-

ing studies as to whether treatment of OSA improves hypertension (50). This is likely due to a number of factors including: the patient populations studied (normal blood pressure versus hypertensive), the use of antihypertensive medication, assessment of treatment compliance (both CPAP and medications), small study size, and lack of placebo control (51). Therefore, although the link between hypertension and OSA is well substantiated, reversal of the hypertension with treatment of the OSA is not yet proved.

Another cardiovascular disease associated with OSA is pulmonary hypertension. This has been shown to be present in approximately 15% to 20% of patients with OSA (52,53). In OSA patients, it tends to be mild (average mean pulmonary artery pressures of 20 to 25 mm Hg) or exercise induced. It is controversial whether pulmonary hypertension can occur in OSA independent of obesity or underlying lung disease (54,55). It has been shown, however, that treatment of OSA can improve pulmonary hemodynamics (56,57). The long-term effects of pulmonary hypertension on the course of OSA patients is unknown.

Aside from systemic and pulmonary hypertension, other cardiovascular diseases have been associated with OSA, including coronary artery disease (CAD) and stroke. It has been shown that patients with OSA have elevated risk markers such as C-reactive protein (58), leptin (59), and homocysteine (60), all of which have been associated with increased risk for cardiovascular disease. Case control studies of male and female patients who have had recent acute coronary syndrome show an association between the conditions with significantly elevated odds ratios (61,62). Nocturnal arrhythmias are also common in OSA patients. The risk of arrhythmia with OSA appears to be related to severity. Analysis of electrocardiographic recordings during sleep studies in >450 patients showed a 58% (versus 42% in non-OSA patients) prevalence of arrhythmias in patients with OSA, with most arrhythmias occurring in those with AHI >40 per hour (63). Bradycardia, sinus pauses, and nocturnal paroxysmal asystole are the most common arrhythmias seen, and these increase in frequency with increasing severity of the syndrome. Nonsustained supraventricular tachycardias may also occur in patients with severe OSA, however, ventricular arrhythmias are very uncommon (64). Treatment of OSA with CPAP improves most nocturnal arrhythmias (65).

The risk for stroke appears to be even more compelling than the risk for CAD in OSA patients. In the Sleep Heart Health study in which overnight PSG was done in >6,000 adults, the relative odds ratio of self-reported stroke was elevated when comparing the upper apnea–hypopnea index quartiles to the lower ones (1.58) (66). It has also been shown that the prevalence of SDB is very high in patients with recent stroke or transient ischemic attack (TIA), in some series as high as 95% (67,68). Patients with concomitant OSA and stroke have been shown to have early neurologic worsening and oxygen desaturation compared to controls (69).

▶ **TABLE 19-2. Cardiovascular Diseases Associated with Adult OSA**

Systemic hypertension
Pulmonary hypertension
Coronary artery disease
Nocturnal arrhythmias
Stroke

In conclusion, deciding on when to treat a patient with SDB requires several considerations: (1) the severity of the condition as defined by the disordered breathing indexes or oxygen desaturation, understanding that there is considerable variability from one sleep laboratory to the next; (2) the symptoms the patient has, and how those symptoms impact on day-to-day functioning; (3) the presence of concomitant diseases, particularly cardiovascular diseases, namely, systemic hypertension, pulmonary hypertension, heart disease, and stroke.

OVERVIEW OF TREATMENT OPTIONS

This section will provide a brief overview of the various treatments that have been attempted in OSA (Table 19-3). Later chapters will provide a more in-depth review of specific treatments.

Positive Pressure Devices

Nasal CPAP has become the current treatment of choice for the majority of adult patients with OSA. The mechanism by which nasal CPAP works is predominantly by creating a "pneumatic splint" in the upper airway, hence, preventing collapse (70). Other effects of CPAP include diminishing muscle tone in the upper airway and increasing functional residual capacity (71,72). The pressure required by an individual patient is usually determined during a sleep study, in which the pressure is gradually increased until obstructive events and snoring are eliminated and oxygen saturation is maintained above 90%. Nasal CPAP has been shown to be very successful in the treatment of OSA. Approximately 95% of patients can be definitively treated with this device, including patients with mild disease (73). Nasal CPAP has been shown to improve many aspects of the OSA syndrome including daytime sleepiness (74) and quality of life (75), and following initiation of CPAP OSA patients have fewer hospitalizations (76). An excellent review of all the randomized trials comparing CPAP with placebo or other treatments in adults is published in the Cochrane Library (77). This review concluded that although CPAP is more effective than placebo in improving sleepiness, multiple quality of life measures, and health status, further work is required to determine which specific groups of patients are most likely to benefit, how much benefit can be obtained, and at what cost.

The biggest drawback to nasal CPAP is adherence to nightly usage. Originally, physicians had to depend upon patient report regarding usage. However, with the advent of CPAP machines containing timers to measure hours of usage, it was found that the apparatus is used an average of 5 hours per night (78–80). Depending on the definition of compliance to therapy, 46% to 89% of patients continue to use their nasal CPAP after obtaining it (81–83). A number of techniques have been used to try to improve adherence to CPAP. However, no one measure has been shown to consistently do so. Such efforts include: giving patients proper instruction and follow-up on the use of the apparatus (84,85), assuring mask fit and comfort is maximal (86), and humidification to decrease dryness (87). Some studies suggest that autotitrating devices (see below) may also improve compliance (88,89).

Recently, new nasal CPAP devices have been developed that adjust to provide the minimal pressure needed to eliminate obstructive events. Autotitrating CPAP (auto-CPAPs) utilizes flow and pressure transducers to sense the patients' airflow patterns and adjust the pressure up or down accordingly. It has been shown that with such a device, the patient may spend as much as two-thirds of the night below the prescribed pressure and that sleep architecture is unchanged compared with standard nasal CPAP (90). These devices do not disrupt sleep and may improve compliance (88,89). Currently these devices are more expensive than standard CPAP and this additional cost is often not covered by insurance.

Some patients are intolerant of nasal CPAP, or (rarely) cannot be adequately treated with even high pressures (>16 cm of H_2O). Nasal bilevel ventilation may be used to treat OSA patients recalcitrant to standard nasal CPAP. These devices deliver a different pressure during inspiration and expiration. Only one trial has examined whether bilevel ventilation could improve adherence to therapy over standard nasal CPAP and no advantage was found (91). Several studies on patients with concomitant OSA and hypercapnia that could not be adequately treated with nasal CPAP alone showed dramatic improvement in symptoms and arterial blood gases following treatment with nasal bilevel ventilation (92–94). These studies, however, had no control groups. It has been suggested that nasal bilevel ventilation be reserved for OSA patients who have a concomitant hypoventilatory syndrome, such as a

▶ **TABLE 19-3. Treatments for Adult OSA**

Positive airway pressure
  CPAP
  Auto-CPAP
  Bilevel nasal ventilation

Surgery
  Tracheotomy
  Uvulopalatopharyngoplasty
  Nasal/sinus surgery
  Genioglossal advancement/hyoid myotomy
  Maxillomandibular advancement

Oral appliances

Weight loss

Medications

Conservative treatment
  Positional therapy
  Treatment of nasal/allergic condition

neuromuscular disease, and require more ventilation during the night or for patients who require very high CPAP pressure, but can not tolerate it.

Surgery

A tracheotomy is the surgical procedure performed to create a tracheostomy, a percutaneous opening into the trachea. In the OSA patient, the tracheostomy tube can be plugged during the waking hours and opened at night to allow ventilation to bypass the upper airway. This is the only surgical procedure that is consistently effective in the treatment of OSA. Unfortunately, it may be a difficult procedure for both the anesthesiologist and surgeon because the patients often have very large necks and pose difficult airway-management problems. A tracheotomy is now performed in OSA patients only when they have life-threatening disease secondary to cor pulmonale, arrhythmias, and/or severe hypoxemia that cannot be controlled with conventional modes of treatment (i.e., nasal CPAP).

Uvulopalatopharyngoplasty (UPPP) is the most common surgery for OSA in adults. This surgery enlarges the airway by removing redundant tonsillar tissue, trimming tonsillar pillars, and excising the uvula and posterior palate. This surgery was first introduced in 1952, for snoring and later described in 1981, for treatment of OSA (95,96). The "cure" rate of UPPP is usually quoted as <50% (97). However, the problem with the statistics on this and other surgical procedures is the lack of controlled studies. Variables differing between studies include body mass index (BMI), number of patients studied, severity of OSA, differences in surgical methods, and use of follow-up sleep studies (98). There are no good long-term predictors of success, although some studies have suggested lower BMI and lower AHI (99,100). It has been shown that patients who obstruct their airway at the tongue base do very poorly with UPPP—a <10% response rate (101). One small series showed that 31% of patients undergoing UPPP actually had higher AHIs following surgery (102).

Improving OSA by surgical correction of a nasopharyngeal anatomic obstruction has been investigated. Surgical approaches have included correction of the nasal valve area, septoplasty, and turbinate reduction. One small study ($n = 6$) examined the effect of correction of nasal valve obstruction. It showed both subjective and objective improvement in snoring and daytime somnolence (103). Two uncontrolled studies showed septoplasty or turbinate reduction had some positive effects on SDB. In one, 77% (47/113) of patients who snored had improvement or elimination of snoring postoperatively (104). The second study of patients with mild OSA used cephalometrics (measurements made from a standardized lateral head radiograph) preoperatively and showed those with abnormal cephalometric distances did not respond to improvement of their nasal airway (105). In a study of a diverse group of patients (94 adults and 55 children) with SDB, who underwent a variety of surgical procedures (including uvulopalatopharyngoplasty, midline laser glossectomy, and nasal surgery) significant improvement (defined as 75% reduction in AHI or a postoperative AHI below 10) occurred in only 48% of the adults (106). Nasal surgery has also been used in an attempt to decrease CPAP requirements. In one study, the AHI was not significantly improved and snoring improved in only 34% (107).

It appears from this group of surgical series that surgical improvement of the nasal airway may be most effective to improve OSA in those patients without skeletal anatomic abnormalities. Surgery may also improve snoring and decrease CPAP levels in some patients with an abnormal nasopharynx.

There are a variety of other procedures that have been used in OSA, either separately or in conjunction with UPPP. In 1989, maxillomandibular advancement (MMA) was described for use as a treatment for OSA. In this procedure, both the maxilla and mandible are advanced, with the mandible usually advanced slightly more to open the posterior airspace. The initial reported success rate was 96%. However, in most of the cases, the MMA was done after the patient had other procedures, such as UPPP (108). A later study of over 300 patients who underwent separate procedures involving various combinations based on the site of obstruction, had response rates, depending on what types of surgery were performed, from 66.7% to 97.8% (109). Hyoid advancement is also frequently done as part of these upper airway reconstruction surgeries (110). In general, surgery is considered second line to nasal CPAP in the treatment of OSA.

Oral Appliances

There are a variety of fixed or adjustable oral appliances invented to treat OSA. These devices alter the oral cavity to increase airway size and improve patency. The most common appliances are those which advance the mandible. For most of these devices, construction requires dental impressions, bite registration, and fabrication in a dental laboratory. In studies of these devices, the higher the AHI, the less likely the patient was to have a substantial benefit (111,112). Oral appliances are a reasonable first line approach to mild OSA, but are considered second line to nasal CPAP in moderate to severe cases.

Weight Loss

Obesity is commonly associated with OSA, and it is well documented that even minor amounts of weight loss can significantly decrease AHI (113). Weight loss improves many aspects of OSA, including increasing the size of the upper airway, decreasing the compliance of the upper airway, and improving oxygen saturation (114). The downsides of weight loss as a treatment modality include low success rates, the long-term nature of weight loss regimens, and successful maintenance of weight loss.

Pharmacologic Treatment

Protriptyline (Vivactil) has been shown to be partially effective in treating mild OSA (115,116). A double-blind trial in five men showed improvement in daytime somnolence, nocturnal oxygenation, and the REM apnea index. The mechanism of action in protriptyline is likely a combination of decreasing REM sleep and improving upper-airway stability. Another study compared fluoxetine (Prozac) to protriptyline and found equivalence between the two drugs in decreasing NREM AHI, yet found that fluoxetine resulted in fewer side effects (117). One study of paroxetine, a selective serotonin reuptake inhibitor (SSRI), found a modest decrease in the AHI during NREM, but not REM sleep (118). A study of OSA in the English bulldog found that a combination of trazodone and L-tryptophan reduced the AHI during both NREM and REM sleep and improved sleep quality (119). However, to date, no serotonergic medication has improved sleep quality in OSA patients. Medroxyprogesterone acetate (Provera) has been shown to induce hyperventilation (120) and has been studied as treatment for OSA. One study suggests that it may be useful for patients with obesity–hypoventilation syndrome, as it can lower Pco_2 and reduce AHI in that patient population (121). However, other studies, with small numbers of patients, have shown no significant improvement (122,123). Furthermore, potentially serious side effects including thromboembolism, gynecomastia and impotence in men, and menometrorrhagia in women preclude widespread usage.

Hypothyroidism and acromegaly have been associated with the development of OSA. Treatment of hypothyroidism with thyroxine replacement may improve and, in some cases, eliminate OSA, even if obesity is present (124). This may occur because of improvement in ventilatory drive as well as reduction in the upper-airway tissues following treatment of myxedema. Likewise, treatment of acromegaly with bromocriptine also improves OSA (125).

Therefore, there is currently little role for use of medications in the initial treatment of OSA. Alerting medications, like modafinil, have been used in some clinical trials to improve residual daytime sleepiness in OSA (126,127). This usage of modafinil has been in an environment of closely monitored research, however, and the outcome in less controlled circumstances is unknown. Such a use in general practice is controversial (128,129).

Conservative Treatment

Some patients with milder forms of OSA may benefit from more conservative forms of treatment. It has been shown that patients with positional OSA will benefit from keeping off their back (by sewing a soft ball in the back of the pajama top). This type of manuever decreases AHI and improves symptoms (130). Treatment of nasal allergies has also been shown to improve OSA in one study (131). However, caution is recommended in utilizing these less effective forms of therapy as the data on long-term outcomes is unknown.

CHOOSING A TREATMENT

A lack of long-term outcome data on patients with OSA limits our ability to know how aggressively to treat, although this syndrome has been apparent in the medical literature since 1966 (132), and a variety of treatment options are available. Whether treatment actually prolongs life or whether no treatment will result in earlier mortality is unknown. Therefore our choice of treatment for individual patients is often based on maximizing quality of life and minimizing adverse effects.

Weight loss should be uniformly recommended in all overweight patients with OSA. A discussion of weight loss regimens are outside the scope of this chapter, but suffice it to say that patients who are successful in losing weight, have fewer obstructive events (114). Unfortunately, most patients who do initially lose weight will not maintain this weight loss and even those who do may redevelop OSA (133). Despite these deficiencies, in the author's opinion, weight loss should be recommended in all overweight OSA patients due to its overwhelming general health benefits. However, if patients are successful in losing weight, they should be followed indefinitely, for aging and weight gain may precipitate a recurrence.

Nasal CPAP is the most efficacious treatment currently available for OSA. There are a large number of studies examining its effects with regards to elimination of SDB events; symptomatology; improvement in blood pressure, hospitalizations, and medical costs; motor vehicle accidents; and neuropsychologic testing. Unfortunately, these outcome studies have tremendous variability with regards to the number of patients studied, use of a control group, and the composition of the control (e.g., placebo pill and placebo CPAP) and length of study. Most clinicians have seen dramatic improvements in some OSA patients with use of nasal CPAP, however, improvement is not uniform.

Nasal CPAP is the current treatment of choice for the majority of OSA patients. On one end of the spectrum, highly symptomatic patients with high AHI (>30) likely benefit most from treatment. In fact, studies of moderate to severe OSA have shown improved mood, vigilance, executive functions, and quality of life (134–136). Importantly though, there are also studies that have shown milder forms of OSA (AHI <30) also reap benefit from use of nasal CPAP (137,138). It has been suggested, based on a consensus statement, that CPAP treatment is indicated for all OSA patients with an AHI >30, regardless of symptoms (139). Justification of this is based on the hypertension data, which suggests that untreated OSA may contribute to the development of hypertension (see above). Treatment with CPAP is also indicated for those with lower AHI (5 to 30) who have symptoms of hypersomnia, impaired cognition, mood disorders, insomnia, or known cardiovascular diseases, like hypertension, ischemic heart disease, or stroke.

However, CPAP therapy is not for everyone. Young patients, nonobese patients, and claustrophobic patients may be better candidates for some of the alternative treatments. Nonobese patients should be evaluated for a potentially reversible anatomic defect, such as retrognathia, tonsillar hypertrophy, or elongated palate/uvula. Surgery may be more appropriate in this select population. Most studies on surgery have shown that preselection of patients by choosing the most likely site of obstruction improves surgical outcome. The presence of obesity often complicates surgical success results, with decreased effectiveness and increased BMIs. Age also seems to have an impact, with younger patients tending to have improved outcomes. With the advent of "upper-airway reconstruction," younger patients, even if obese, may have a reasonable amount of success with surgical intervention versus the alternative of a lifetime of nasal CPAP.

Other special groups that may be better served by avoiding CPAP include those with mild positional OSA. Positional therapy is as effective as CPAP in improving symptoms in some small studies. Caution, however, is recommended in use of this therapy in any patient with compounding risk factors, such as cardiovascular disease, because there are no outcome data for this approach. Oral appliances have also been shown to be effective in treating positional OSA as well as other milder forms of OSA (140). Insurance companies are beginning to reimburse for the fabrication and visits associated with the cost of an oral appliance. These devices are favored in mild OSA or in patients with more moderate OSA, of intolerant CPAP and who are not surgical candidates.

There are no good answers for what to do with patients with REM-related OSA. The author's approach is to treat if the patient is symptomatic or has cardiovascular disease. This approach becomes problematic if the patient is intolerant of CPAP—is it reasonable to recommend surgery in this population? No outcome data is available. These cases have to be approached on a case-by-case basis. Theoretically, use of a SSRI or tricyclic antidepressant may help reduce REM-related events because of their REM suppressant effects. However, to date, there is no study examining this.

On the other end of the spectrum, are there patients, in this CPAP era who should undergo tracheostomy for OSA? I usually recommend tracheostomy only in cases of life threatening disease, namely, those with right-sided or biventricular heart failure, malignant arrhythmias or respiratory failure, who either cannot be adequately treated with CPAP or bilevel positive airway pressure (BPAP) or who are not able to adhere to positive airway pressure (PAP) therapy on a consistent basis.

When to use bilevel ventilation is also relatively unexplored in the literature. As noted earlier, most physicians would agree that its use be considered in those patients who cannot maintain their ventilation during sleep and who require an added inspiratory boost. It has not been shown that switching to BPAP will improve tolerance or adherence to treatment. However, this is also not well studied. The author's approach to BPAP in the uncomplicated OSA patient is to use it if the patient requires pressures >15 cm of H_2O, but cannot tolerate the high pressure. Some success in switching to BPAP in that population has been observed.

PEDIATRIC OBSTRUCTIVE SLEEP APNEA

The prevalence of pediatric OSA is estimated at 2% for children between the ages of 2 and 18 (141). Although obesity appears to be a risk factor, most children are otherwise healthy and have adenotonsillar hypertrophy. The symptoms in children also differ from adults. Although daytime sleepiness and fatigue are reported in children, behavioral problems, hyperactivity, and neurocognitive deficits are more common in children with OSA compared with controls (142–144). Cardiovascular complications have also been described, including right ventricular dysfunction and elevated blood pressure (145,146).

Pediatric OSA can be confirmed with PSG. The criteria are different from adults, with an apnea index of >1 per hour considered abnormal (147). However, many children do not have frank apneas and instead have partial obstructive hypoventilation. It has been recommended that PET_{CO_2} >53 mm Hg or PET_{CO_2} >45 mm Hg for 60% or more of TST also be considered abnormal (148,149).

There is a shortage of sleep laboratories that can accommodate children. Therefore a multitude of other screening techniques have been tried including questionnaires, home video, audiotaping, and screening oximetry. Unfortunately, none of these appear to have sufficient sensitivity and specificity to be recommended for widespread use (150). Therefore, in a child with behavioral problems, hyperactivity, or daytime sleepiness, PSG should be considered, especially if obesity, tonsillar and/or adenoidal hypertrophy, or other upper-airway anatomic abnormalities are present.

In contrast to adults, the treatment of choice for the majority of pediatric OSA cases is adenotonsillectomy. There are some specific groups who are at increased risk for postoperative morbidity: children <3 years of age, severe OSA, and those with underlying medical disorders (151–153). Weight loss and nasal CPAP are also used in pediatric OSA for those cases not improving after adenotonsillectomy or in patients that not surgical candidates. Craniofacial surgeries are also an option in selected children with anatomic abnormalities.

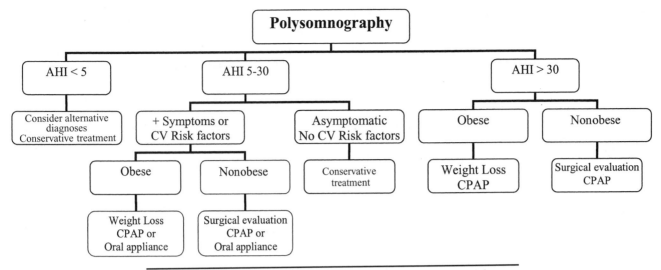

FIGURE 19-3. Flowchart outlining treatment for uncomplicated adult OSA.

CONCLUSIONS

In Fig. 19-3, a simple flowchart has been developed as a guide for treatment of uncomplicated adult OSA. This chart may not be applicable to patients with very severe disease that might require tracheostomy, patients with concomitant obesity hypoventilation or other hypoventilatory syndromes, or other similar complicating problems. As noted, guidance for treatment of adult OSA is limited in terms of availability of outcome information. Therefore, I believe the approach should be to improve a patient's quality of life and decrease cardiovascular morbidity. Nasal CPAP remains the treatment of choice for the vast majority of patients with adult OSA.

Pediatric OSA has a presentation, diagnostic criteria, and treatment different from adult OSA. Suspicion for pediatric OSA should ideally prompt PSG and, if abnormal, an adenotonsillectomy for the majority of cases.

REFERENCES

1. Sleep-related breathing disorders in adults: recommendations for syndrome definition and measurement techniques in clinical research. The Report of an American Academy of Sleep Medicine Task Force. *Sleep.* 1999;22(5):667–689.
2. Moser N, Phillips B, Berry D, et al. What is hypopnea, anyway? *Chest.* 1994;105(2):426–428.
3. Tsai W, Flemons W, Whitelaw W, et al. A comparison of apnea-hypopnea indices derived from different definitions of hypopnea. *Amer J Respir Crit Care Med.* 1999;159(1):43–48.
4. Collop N. Scoring variability between polysomnography technologists in different sleep laboratories. *Sleep Med.* 2002;3(1):43–47.
5. Norman R, Ahmad M, Walsleben J, et al. Detection of respiratory events during NPSG: nasal cannula/pressure sensor versus thermistor. *Sleep.* 1997;20:1175–1184.
6. Montserrat J, Farre R, Ballester R, et al. Evaluation of nasal prongs for estimating airflow. *Amer J Respir Crit Care Med.* 1997;155:475–480.
7. Hosselet J, Ayappa I, Norman R, et al. Classification of sleep-disordered breathing. *Amer J Respir Crit Care Med.* 2001;163(2):398–405.
8. Smith C, Henderson K, Xi L, et al. Neural-mechanical coupling of breathing in NREM sleep. *J Appl Physiol.* 1997;83:1923–1932.
9. O'Connor C, Thornley K, Hanly P. Gender differences in the polysomnographic features of obstructive sleep apnea. *Amer J Respir Crit Care Med.* 2000;161(5):1465–1472.
10. Collop N. Men are from Mars, women are from Venus, lessons to be learned from the differences between the sexes. *Chest.* 2001;120(5):1432–1433.
11. Kass J, Akers S, Bartter T, et al. Rapid-eye-movement-specific sleep disordered breathing: a possible cause of excessive daytime sleepiness. *Amer J Respir Crit Care Med.* 1996;154(1):167–169.
12. Punjabi N, Bandeen-Roche K, Marx J, et al. The association between daytime sleepiness and sleep-disordered breathing in NREM and REM sleep. *Sleep.* 2002;25(3):307–314.
13. Niijima M, Kimura H, Edo H, et al. Manifestation of pulmonary hypertension during REM sleep in obstructive sleep apnea syndrome. *Amer J Respir Crit Care Med.* 1999;159:1766–1772.
14. Oksenberg A, Silverberg D, Arons E, et al. Positional vs. nonpositional obstructive sleep apnea patients: anthropometric, nocturnal polysomographic and multiple sleep latency test data. *Chest.* 1997;112(3):629–639.
15. Hoddes E, Zarcone V, Smythe H, et al. Quantification of sleepiness: a new approach. *Psychophysiology.* 1973;10:431–436.
16. Johns MW. A new method for measuring daytime sleepiness: the Epworth sleepiness scale. *Sleep.* 1991;14:540–545.
17. Johns MW. Reliability and factor analysis of the Epworth sleepiness scale. *Sleep.* 1992;15:376–381.
18. Chung K. Use of the Epworth Sleepiness Scale in Chinese patients with obstructive sleep apnea and normal hospital employees. *J Psychosom Res.* 2000;49(5):367–372.
19. Bedard M-A, Montplaisir J, Malo J, et al. Persistent neuropsychological deficits and vigilance impairment in sleep apnea syndrome after treatment with continuous positive airways pressure (CPAP). *J Clin Exp Neuropsychol.* 1993;15:330–341.
20. Engleman HM, Martin SE, Deary IJ, et al. Effect of continuous positive airway pressure treatment on daytime function in sleep apnoea/hypopnoea syndrome. *Lancet.* 1994;343:572–575.
21. Doghramji K, Mitler MM, Sangal RB, et al. A normative study of the maintenance of wakefulness test (MWT). *Electroencephalogr Clin Neurophysiol.* 1997;103(5):554–562.
22. Sangal RB, Sangal JM, Belisle C. Subjective and objective indices of sleepiness (ESS and MWT) are not equally useful in patients with sleep apnea. *Clin Electroencephalogr.* 1999;30(2):73–75.
23. Findley L, Unverzagt M, Suratt P. Automobile accidents involving patients with obstructive sleep apnea. *Amer Rev Respir Dis.* 1988;138:337–340.
24. George C, Smiley A. Sleep apnea and automobile crashes. *Sleep.* 1999;22:790–795.
25. Diaz J, Guallar J, Arnedo A, et al. The prevalence of sleep

apnea-hypopnea syndrome among long-haul professional drivers. *Arch Bronchopneumol.* 2001;37:4771–4776.

26. Risser M, Ware J, Freeman F. Driving simulation with EEG monitoring in normal and obstructive sleep apnea patients. *Sleep.* 2000;23:393–398.

27. George C, Boudreau A, Smiley A. Effects of nasal CPAP on simulated driving performance in patients with obstructive sleep apnoea. *Thorax.* 1997;52:648–653.

28. Turkington P, Sircar M, Allgar V, et al. Relationship between obstructive sleep apnoea, driving simulator performance and risk of road traffic accidents. *Thorax.* 2001;56:800–805.

29. Telakibi T, Parinene M, Hublin C, et al. Obstructive sleep apnea syndrome among city bus drivers: diagnostic implications and driving capacity. *Sleep.* 2002;25:A225.

30. American Thoracic Society. Sleep apnea, sleepiness and driving risk. *Amer J Respir Crit Care Med.* 1994;150:1463–1473.

31. Beninati W, Harris CD, Herold DL, et al. The effect of snoring and obstructive sleep apnea on the sleep quality of bed partners. *Mayo Clin Proc.* 1999;74(10):955–958.

32. Rowley JA, Aboussouan LS, Badr MS. The use of clinical prediction formlas in the evaluation of obstructive sleep apnea. *Sleep.* 2000;23:929–937.

33. Hoy C, Vennelle M, Kingshott R, et al. Can intensive support improve continuous positive airway pressure use in patients with the sleep apnea/hypopnea syndrome? *Amer J Respir Crit Care Med.* 1999;159:1096–1100.

34. Chervin R. Sleepiness, fatigue, tiredness and lack of energy in obstructive sleep apnea. *Chest.* 2000;118(2):372–379.

35. Krakow B, Melendrez D, Ferreira E, et al. Prevalence of insomnia symptoms in patients with sleep-disordered breathing. *Chest.* 2001;120(6):1923–1929.

36. Loh N, Dinner D, Foldvary N, et al. Do Patients with obstructive sleep apnea wake up with headaches? *Arch Intern Med.* 1999;159:1765–1768.

37. Young T, Finn L, Kim H. Nasal obstruction as a risk factor for sleep-disordered breathing. The Univeristy of Wisconsin Sleep and Respiration Research Group. *J Allergy Clin Immunol.* 1997;99(2):S757–S762.

38. Hirshkowitz M, Karacan I, Arcasoy M, et al. Prevalence of sleep apnea in men with erectile dysfunction. *Urology.* 1990;36(3):232–234.

39. Fanfulla F, Malaguti S, Montagna T, et al. Erectile dysfunction in men with obstructive sleep apnea: an early sign of nerve involvement. *Sleep.* 2000;23(6):775–781.

40. Kales A, Bixler E, Cadieux R, et al. Sleep apnoea in a hypertensive population. *Lancet.* 1984;II:1005–1008.

41. Lavie P, Ben-Yosef R, Rubin A. Prevalence of sleep apnea syndrome among patients with essential hypertension. *Amer Heart J.* 1984;108:33–36.

42. Fletcher E, DeBehnke R, Lovoi M, et al. Undiagnosed sleep apnea in patients with essential hypertension. *Ann Intern Med.* 1985;103:190–195.

43. Silverberg D, Oksenberg A, Iana A. Sleep-related breathing disorders are common contributing factors to the production of essential hypertension but are neglected, underdiagnosed and undertreated. *Amer J Hypertens.* 1997;10:1319–1325.

44. Kimoff R, Makino H, Horner R, et al. A canine model of obstructive sleep apnea. *J Appl Physiol.* 1994;76:1810–1817.

45. Brooks D, Horner R, Kimoff R, et al. Effect of obstructive sleep apnea vs sleep fragmentation on responses to airway occlusion. *Amer J Respir Crit Care Med.* 1997;155:1609–1617.

46. Fletcher E. Effect of episodic hypoxia on sympathetic activity and blood pressure. *Respir Physiol.* 2000;119:189–197.

47. Peppard P, Terry Y, Pala M, et al. Prospective study of the association between sleep-disordered breathing and hypertension. *N Engl J Med.* 2000;342:1378–1384.

48. Nieto F, Yound T, Lind B, et al. Association of sleep-disordered breathing, sleep apnea and hypertension in a large community-based study. *JAMA.* 2000;283:1829–1836.

49. Logan A, Perlikowske S, Mente A, et al. High prevalence of unrecognized sleep apnea in drug-resistant hypertension. *J Hypertens.* 2001;19:2271–2277.

50. Fletcher E. Cardiovascular effects of CPAP in obstructive sleep apnea. *Sleep.* 2000;23(Suppl. 4);S154–S157.

51. Parait G, Ongaro G, Bonsignore M, et al. Sleep apnoea and hypertension. *Curr Opin Nephrol Hypertens.* 2002;11:201–214.

52. Chaouat A, Weitzenblum E, Krieger J, et al. Pulmonary hemodynamics in the obstructive sleep apnea syndrome. *Chest.* 1996;109:380–386.

53. Sanner B, Doberauer C, Konermann M, et al. Pulmonary hypertension in patients with obstructive sleep apnea syndrome. *Arch Intern Med.* 1997;157:2483–2487.

54. Badu E, Achkar A, Pascal S, et al. Pulmonary arterial hypertension in patients with sleep apnoea syndrome. *Thorax.* 2000;55:934–939.

55. Sajkov D, Cowie R, Thornton A, et al. Pulmonary hypertension and hypoxemia in obstructive sleep apnea syndrome. *Amer J Respir Crit Care Med.* 1994;149:416–422.

56. Alchanatis M, Tourkohoriti G, Kakouros S, et al. Daytime pulmonary hypertension in patients with obstructive sleep apnea: The effect of CPAP on pulmonary hemodynamics. *Respiration.* 2001;689:566–572.

57. Sajkov D, Wang T, Saunders N, et al. CPAP treatment improves pulmonary hemodynamics in patients with obstructive sleep apnea. *Amer J Respir Crit Care Med.* 2002;165:152–158.

58. Shamsuzzaman AS, Winnicki M, Lanfranchi P, et al. Elevated C-reactive protein in patients with obstructive sleep apnea. *Circulation.* 2002;105:2462–2464.

59. Phillips B, Kato M, Narkiewicz K, et al. Increases in leptin levels, sympathetic drive, and weight gain in obstructive sleep apnea. *Amer J Physiol Heart Circ Physiol.* 2000;279:H234–H237.

60. Lavie L, Perelman A, Lavie P. Plasma homocysteine levels in obstructive sleep apnea: Association with cardiovascular morbidity. *Chest.* 2001;120:900–908.

61. Mooe T, Tabben T, Wiklund U, et al. Sleep-disordered breathing in men with coronary artery disease. *Chest.* 1996;109:659–663.

62. Mooe T, Tabben T, Wiklund U, et al. Sleep-disordered breathing in women: occurrence and association with coronaty artery disease. *Amer J Med.* 1996;101:251–256.

63. Hoffstein V, Mateika S. Cardiac arrhythmias, snoring, and sleep apnea. *Chest.* 1994:106:466–471.

64. Roche F, Xuong AN, Court-Fortune I, et al. Relationship among the severity of sleep apnea syndrome, cardiac arrhythmias, and autonomic imbalance. *Pacing Clin Electrophysiol.* 2003;26(3):669–677.

65. Harbison J, O'Reilly P, McNicholas W. Cardiac rhythm disturbances in the obstructive sleep apnea syndrome: effects of nasal continuous positive airway pressure therapy. *Chest.* 2000;118(3):591–595.

66. Shahar E, Whitney C, Redline S, et al. Sleep-disordered breathing and cardiovascular disease: cross-sectional results of the Sleep Heart Health Study. *Amer J Respir Crit Care Med.* 2001;163:19–25.

67. Bassetti C, Aldrich M. Sleep apnea in acute cerebrovascular diseases: final report on 128 patients. *Sleep.* 1999;22:217–223.

68. Wessendorf T, Teschler H, Wang Y, et al. Sleep-disordered breathing among patients with first-ever strokes. *J Neurol.* 2000;247:41–47.

69. Iranzo A, Santamaria J, Berenguer J, et al. Prevalence and clinical importance of sleep apnea in the first night after cerebral infarction. *Neurology.* 2002;59:911–916.

70. Sullivan C, Berthon–Jones M, Issa F, et al. Reversal of obstructive sleep apnoea by continuous positive airway pressure applied through the nares. *Lancet.* 1981;1:862–865.

71. Strohl K, Redline S. Nasal CPAP therapy, upper airway muscle activation and obstructive sleep apnea. *Amer Rev Respir Dis.* 1986;134:555–558.

72. Abbey N, Cooper K, Kwentus J. Benefit of Nasal CPAP in obstructive sleep apnea is due to positive pharyngeal pressure. *Sleep.* 1989;12(5):420–422.

73. Redline S, Adams N. Strauss M, et al. Improvement of mild sleep-disordered breathing with CPAP compared with conservative therapy. *Amer J Respir Crit Care Med.* 1998;157:858–865.

74. Engleman H, Cheshire K, Deary I, et al. Daytime sleepiness, cognitive performance and mood after CPAP for the sleep apnoea/hypopnea syndrome. *Thorax.* 1993;48:911–914.

75. D'Ambrosio C, Bowman T, Mohsenin V. Quality of life in patient with obstructive sleep apnea. Effect of nasal CPAP—a prospective study. *Chest.* 1999;115:123–129.

76. Peker Y, Hedner J, Johansson A, Bende M. Reduced hospitalization with cardiovascular and pulmonary disease in obstructive sleep apnea patient on nasal CPAP treatment. *Sleep.* 1997;20(8):645–653.

77. White J, Cates C, Wright J. Continuous positive airways pressure for

obstructive sleep apnoea (Cochrane Review). The Cochrane Library, Issue 2, 2003. Oxford: Update Software.

78. Engleman H, Martin S, Douglas N. Compliance with CPAP therapy in patients with the sleep apnea/hypopnea syndrome. *Thorax.* 1994;49:263–266.

79. Reeves-Hoche M, Meck R, Zwillich C, et al. Nasal CPAP: an objective evaluation of patient compliance. *Amer J Respir Crit Care Med.* 1994;149:149–154.

80. Engleman H, Asgari-Jirhandeh N, McLeod A, et al. Self reported use of CPAP and benefits of CPAP therapy: a patient survey. *Chest.* 1996;109:1470–1476.

81. Hoffstein V, Viner S, Mateika S, et al. Treatment of obstructive sleep apnea with nasal CPAP: patient compliance, perception of benefits and side effects. *Amer Rev Respir Dis.* 1992;145:841–845.

82. Kreiger J. Long-term compliance with CPAP therapy in obstructive sleep apnea patients and in snorers. *Sleep.* 1996;19(9 Suppl.):136–143.

83. Meurice J, Dore P, Paquesteau J, et al. Predictive factors of long-term compliance with nasal continuous positive airway pressure treatment in sleep apnea syndrome. *Chest.* 1994;105:429–433.

84. Chervin R, Theut S, Bassetti C, et al. Compliance with nasal CPAP can be improved by simple interventions. *Sleep.* 1997;20:284–289.

85. Likar L, Panciera T, Erickson A, et al. Group education sessions and compliance with nasal CPAP therapy. *Chest.* 1997;111:1273–1277.

86. Jones D, Braid G, Wedzicha J. Nasal masks for domiciliary positive pressure ventilation: patient usage and complications. *Thorax.* 1994;49:811–812.

87. Richards G, Cistulli P, Ungar R, et al. Mouth leak with nasal continuous positive airway pressure increases nasal airway resistance. *Amer J Respir Crit Care Med.* 1996;154:182–186.

88. Stradling J, Barbour C, Pitson D, et al. Automatic nasal continuous positive airway pressure titration in the laboratory: patient outcomes. *Thorax.* 1997;52:72–75.

89. Meurice J, Marc I, Series F. Efficacy of auto-CPAP in the treatment of obstructive sleep apnea/hypopnea syndrome. *Amer J Respir Crit Care Med.* 1996;153:794–798.

90. Scharf M, Brannen D, McDannold M, et al. Computerized adjustable vs. fixed NCPAP treatment of obstructive sleep apnea. *Sleep.* 1996;19:491–496.

91. Reeves-Hoche M, Hudgel D, Meck R, et al. Continuous versus bilevel positive airway pressure for obstructive sleep apnea. *Amer J Respir Crit Care Med.* 1995;151:443–449.

92. Piper A, Sullivan C. Effect of short-term NIPPV in the treatment of patients with severe obstructive sleep apnea and hypercapnia. *Chest.* 1994;105:434–440.

93. Laursen S, Dreijer B, Hemmingsen C, et al. Bi-level positive airway pressure treatment of obstructive sleep apnoea syndrome. *Respiration.* 1998;65:114–119.

94. Schafer S, Hewig S, Hasper E, et al. Failure of CPAP therapy in obstructive sleep apnea apnoea syndrome: Predictive factors and treatment with bilevel-positive airway pressure. *Respir Med.* 1998;92:208–215.

95. Ikematsu T. Study of snoring. Therapy. *J Jpn Otol Rhinol Laryngol Soc.* 1964;64:434–435.

96. Fujita S, Conway W, Zorick F, et al. Surgical correction of anatomic abnormalities of obstructive sleep apnea syndrome: uvulopalatopharyngoplasty. *Otolaryngol Head Neck Surg.* 1981;89:923–934.

97. Shepard J, Olsen D, et al. Uvulopalatopharyngoplasty for treatment of OSA. *Mayo Clin Proc.* 1990;65:1260–1267.

98. Pirsig W, Verse T. Long-term results in the treatment of obstructive sleep apnea. *Eur Arch Otorhinolaryngol.* 2000;257:570–577.

99. Janson C, Gislason T, Bengtsson H, et al. Longterm followup of patients with obstructive sleep apnea treated with uvulopalatopharyngoplasty. *Arch Otolaryngol Head Neck Surg.* 1997;123:257–262.

100. Larrson L, Carlsson-Nordlander B, Scanborg E. Four year followup after uvulopalatopharyngoplasty in 50 unselected patients with obstructive sleep apnea syndrome. *Laryngoscope.* 1994;104:1362–1368.

101. Millman RP, Carlisle CC, Rosenberg C, et al. Simple predictors of uvulopalatopharyngoplasty outcome in the treatment of obstructive sleep apnea. *Chest.* 2000;118(4):1025–1030.

102. Sasse S, Mahutte C, Kickeo M, et al. The characteristics of five patient with obstructive sleep apnea whose apnea-hypopnea index deteriorated after uvulopalatopharyngoplasty. *Sleep Breath.* 2002;6(2):77–83.

103. Dayal V, Phillipson E. Nasal surgery in the management of sleep apnea. *Ann Otorhinolaryngol.* 1985;94:550–554.

104. Fairbanks D. Effect of nasal surgery on snoring. *South Med J.* 1985;78(3):268–270.

105. Series F, Pierre S, Carrier G. Surgical correction of nasal obstruction in the treatment of mild sleep apnea: importance of cephalometry in predicting outcome. *Thorax.* 1993;48:360–363.

106. Nishimura T, Morishima N, Hasegawa S, et al. Effect of surgery on obstructive sleep apnea. *Acta Otolaryngol.* 1996;(Suppl. 523):231–233.

107. Friedman M, Tanyeri H, Lim J, et al. Effect of improved nasal breathing on obstructive sleep apnea. *Otolaryngol Head Neck Surg.* 2000;122(1):71–74.

108. Waite P, Wooten V, Lachner J, et al. Maxillomandibular advancement surgery in 23 patients with obstructive sleep apnea syndrome. *J Oral Maxillofac Surg.* 1989;47:1256–1261.

109. Riley R, Powell N, Guilleminault C. Obstructive sleep apnea syndrome: A review of 306 consecutively treated surgical patients. *Otolaryngol Head Neck Surg.* 1993;108:117–125.

110. Vilaseca I, Morello A, Montserrat JM, et al. Usefulness of uvulopalatopharyngoplasty with genioglossus and hyoid advancement in the treatment of obstructive sleep apnea. *Arch Otolaryngol Head Neck Surg.* 2002;128(4):435–440.

111. Schmidt-Nowara W, Lowe A, Wiegand L, et al. Oral appliances for the treatment of snoring and obstructive sleep apnea: a review. *Sleep.* 1995;18:501–510.

112. Engleman H, McDonald J, Graham D, et al. Randomized crossover trial of two treatments for sleep apnea/hypopnea syndrome. CPAP and mandibular repositioning splint. *Amer J Respir Crit Care Med.* 2002;166:855–859.

113. Browman C, Sampson M, Yolles S, et al. Obstructive sleep apnea and body weight. *Chest.* 1984;85:435–436.

114. Schwartz A. Gold A, Schubert N, et al. Effect of weight loss on upper airway collapsibility in obstructive sleep apnea. *Amer Rev Respir Dis.* 1991;144:494–498.

115. Smith P, Haponick E, Allen R, et al. The effects of protriptyline in sleep-disordered breathing. *Amer Rev Resp Dis.* 1983;127:8–13.

116. Brownell L, West P, Sweatmen P, et al. Protriptyline in obstructive sleep apnea. *N Engl J Med.* 1982;307(17):1037–1042.

117. Hanzel D, Proia N, Hudgel D. Response of obstructive sleep apnea to fluoxetine and protriptyline. *Chest.* 1991;100:416–421.

118. Kraiczi H, Hedner J, Dahlof P, et al. Effect of serotonin uptake inhibition on breathing during sleep and daytime symptoms in obstructive sleep apnea. *Sleep.* 1999;22:61–67.

119. Veasey S, Fenik P, Panckeri K, et al. The effects of trazodone with L-tryptophan on sleep disordered breathing in the English bulldog. *Amer J Respir Crit Care Med.* 1999;160:1659–1667.

120. Skatrud J, Dempsey J, Kaiser D. Ventilatory response to medroxyprogesterone acetate in normal subjects: time course and mechanism. *J Appl Physiol.* 1978;61:618–623.

121. Strohl K, Hensley M, Saunders N, et al. Progesterone administration and progressive sleep apneas. *JAMA.* 1981;245:1230–1232.

122. Rajapagopal K, Abbrecht P, Jabbari B. Effects of medroxyprogesterone acetate in obstructive sleep apnea. *Chest.* 1986;90:815–821.

123. Cook W, Benich J, Wooten S. Indices of severity of obstructive sleep apnea syndrome do not change during medroxyprogesterone acetate therapy. *Chest.* 1989;96:262–266.

124. Hart T, Radwo S, Blackard W, et al. Sleep apnea in active acromegaly. *Arch Int Med.* 1985;151:194–198.

125. Zeimer D, Dickson B. Preliminary report: relief of sleep apnea in acromegaly by bromocriptine. *Amer J Med Sci.* 1988;295:49–51.

126. Pack A, Black J, Schwartz J, et al. Modafinil as adjunct therapy for daytime sleepiness in obstructive sleep apnea. *Amer J Respir Crit Care Med.* 2001;164(9):1675–1681.

127. Kingshott R, Vennelle M, Coleman E, et al. Randomized, double-blind, placebo-controlled crossover trial of modafinil in the treatment of residual excessive daytime sleepiness in the sleep apnea/hypopnea syndrome. *Amer J Respir Crit Care Med.* 2001;163(4):918–923.

128. Pollack C. Con: modafinil has no role in management of sleep apnea. *Amer J Respir Crit Care Med.* 2003;167(2):106–108.

129. Black J. Pro: modafinil has a role in management of sleep apnea. *Amer J Respir Crit Care Med.* 2003;167(2):105–106;108.
130. Jokic R, Klimaszewski A, Crossley M, et al. Positional treatment vs CPAP in patient with positional obstructive sleep apnea syndrome. *Chest.* 1999;115:771–781.
131. Craig T, Teets S, Lehman E, et al. Nasal congestion secondary to allergic rhinitis as a cause of sleep disturbance and daytime fatigue and the response to topical nasal corticosteroids. *J Allergy Clin Immunol.* 1998;101:633–637.
132. Gastaut H, Tassinari CA, Duron B. Polygraphic study of the episodic diurnal and nocturnal (hypnic and respiratory) manifestations of the Pickwick syndrome. *Brain Res.* 1966;1(2):167–186.
133. Pillar G, Peled R, Lavie P. Recurrence of sleep apnea without concomitant weight increase 7.5 years after weight reduction surgery. *Chest.* 1994;106(6):1702–1704.
134. Derderian S, Bridenbaugh H, Rajagopal K. Neuropsychological symptoms in obstructive sleep apnea improve after treatment with nasal CPAP. *Chest.* 1988;94:1023–1027.
135. Platon M, Sierra J. Changes in psychopathological symptoms in sleep apnea patients after treatment with nasal CPAP. *Intern J Neurosci.* 1992;62:173–195.
136. Engleman H, Martin S, Deary I, et al. Effect of CPAP treatment on daytime function in sleep apnea/hypopnea syndrome. *Lancet.* 1994;343:572–575.
137. Redline S, Adams N, Strauss M, et al. Improvement of mild sleep-disordered breathing with CPAP compared with conservative therapy. *Amer J Respir Crit Care Med.* 1998;157:858–865.
138. Guilleminault C, Kim YD, Palombini L, et al. Upper airway resistance syndrome and its treatment. *Sleep.* 2000;23(Suppl. 4):S197–S200.
139. Loube D, Gay P, Strohl K, et al. Indications for positive airway pressure treatment of adult obstructive sleep apnea patients. *Chest.* 1999;115:863–866.
140. Yoshida K. Influence of sleep posture on response to oral appliance therapy for sleep apnea syndrome. *Sleep.* 2001;24(5):538–544.
141. Redline S, Tishler P, Schluchter M, et al. Risk factors for sleep-disordered breathing in children: Associations with obesity, race and respiratory problems. *Amer J Respir Crit Care Med.* 1999;159:1527–1532.
142. Guilleminault C, Korobkin R, Winkle R. A review of 50 children with obstructive sleep apnea syndrome. *Lung.* 1981;159:275–287.
143. Ali N, Pitson D, Stradling J. Sleep disordered breathing: effect of adenotonsillectomy on behaviour and psychological functioning. *Eur J Pediatr.* 1996;155:56–62.
144. Rosen C. Clinical features of obstructive sleep apnea hypoventilation syndrome in otherwise healthy children. *Pediatr Pulmonol.* 1999;27:403–409.
145. Tal A, Leiberman A. Margios G, et al. Ventricular dysfunction in children with obstructive sleep apnea: Radionuclide assessment. *Pediatr Pulmon.* 1988;4:139–143.
146. Marcus C, Greene M, Carroll J. Blood pressure in children with obstructive sleep apnea. *Amer J Respir Crit Care Med.* 1998;157:1098–1103.
147. American Thoracic Society. Standard and indications for cardiopulmonary sleep studies in children. *Amer J Respir Crit Care Med.* 1996;153:866–878.
148. Rosen C, D'Andrea L, Haddad G. Adult criteria for obstructive sleep apnea do not identify children with serious obstruction. *Amer Rev Respir Dis.* 1992;146:1231–1234.
149. Marcus C, Omlin K, Basinki D, et al. Normal polysomnographic values for children and adolescents. *Amer Rev Respir Dis.* 1992;146:1235–1239.
150. American Academy of Pediatrics. Technical report: diagnosis and management of childhood obstructive sleep apnea syndrome. *Pediatrics.* 2002;109:1–20.
151. McColley S, April M, Carroll J, et al. Respiratory compromise after adenotonsillectomy in children with obstructive sleep apnea. *Arch Otolaryngol Head Neck Surg.* 1992;118:940–943.
152. Price S, Hawkins D, Kahlstrom E. Tonsil and adenoid surgery for airway obstruction: Perioperative respiratory morbidity. *Ear Nose Throat J.* 1993;72:526–531.
153. Rosen G, Muckle R, Mahowald M, et al. Postoperative respiratory compromise in children with obstructive sleep apnea syndrome: can it be anticipated? *Pediatrics.* 1994;93:784–788.

Positive Airway Pressure Treatment for Sleep Apnea

Richard B. Berry and Mark H. Sanders

HISTORY OF POSITIVE AIRWAY PRESSURE

Sullivan and co-workers published the original description of nasal continuous positive airway pressure (nasal CPAP) for the treatment of obstructive sleep apnea (OSA) in adults in 1981 (1). Prior to that report, the only effective treatment for moderate to severe OSA was a tracheostomy. Today positive airway pressure (PAP) is the mainstay of treatment for moderate to severe OSA in adults (2–6). Patients with mild OSA (7–12), the upper-airway resistance syndrome (13), or even heavy snoring (14,15) have also been treated successfully with positive pressure. Since the original description of CPAP, other methods for delivering PAP have been developed including bilevel PAP (16), autoadjusting positive pressure (APAP) (17–19), and expiratory pressure relief (Cflex). Many types of interfaces for the delivery of positive pressure including nasal masks (14,20,21), nasal prong interfaces (22), masks covering both nose and mouth (23–25), and oral interfaces (26) have been developed. However, even after many technological improvements, the overall therapeutic efficacy of PAP is still critically dependent on a knowledgeable physician directing care and an organized and responsive structure of support personnel (27).

MECHANISMS OF ACTION

It is currently believed that PAP maintains upper airway patency primarily by the "pneumatic splint mechanism." This refers to a simple dilation of the airway by intraluminal pressure that is positive compared to atmospheric pressure. Both computed axial tomography (CAT) and magnetic resonance imaging (MRI) have clearly shown that positive pressure increases upper-airway cross-sectional area and volume (28–30). The major configurational change appears to be an expansion of the airway in the lateral directions. Upper airway muscle activity tends to actually decrease once the upper airway is splinted open (28,31,32), suggesting that the effect of CPAP on upper-airway patency, in general, does not depend on upper-airway muscle activity. A second possible mechanism is an indirect action on the upper airway mediated by an increase in lung volume induced by PAP. Upper-airway size increases as lung volume increases (33). One explanation for this effect is that as lung volume increases there is a downward traction on the trachea (tracheal tug) and other upper-airway structures (34). By an undefined mechanism, possibly related to stretching or stiffening of upper airway walls, this pull tends to open the airway. A study of one patient with OSA found a decrease in the AHI with negative pressure around the chest and abdomen (35). However, another study found that an increase in functional residual capacity (FRC) by subatmospheric pressure via a negative pressure body suit did not decrease the frequency of obstructive events (36). A third study found little decrease in upper-airway resistance with the application of negative extra-thoracic pressure (37). It appears that most of the effect of CPAP on the upper airway is a direct consequence of the "pneumatic splint." Of note, one study did find a decrease in obstructive events when only expiratory positive airway pressure (EPAP) was applied (38). Thus, pneumatic splinting, even when confined to expiration, has some benefit.

Positive Pressure Modes—An Overview

Continuous positive airway pressure (CPAP) stabilizes the upper airway by maintaining a nearly constant positive pressure in both inspiration and exhalation (Fig. 20-1). In bilevel pressure, there are two independently adjusted pressures (16). A higher pressure is provided during inspiration (inspiratory positive airway pressure or IPAP) and a lower pressure during exhalation (EPAP). The IPAP–EPAP pressure difference is the amount of pressure support pro-

vided to assist inspiration. For example, a bilevel PAP of 15/5 cm H_2O provides an IPAP of 15, an EPAP of 5, and a pressure support of 10 cm H_2O. Bilevel pressure has two potential advantages over CPAP. First, airway patency can be maintained with a lower pressure during exhalation. A notable number of patients find CPAP uncomfortable, especially during exhalation, and may find the lower expiratory pressure more tolerable. Second, the IPAP–EPAP difference provides pressure support for inspiration and can augment ventilation. This feature is potentially very useful in patients who hypoventilate during sleep or benefit from pressure support because of lung disease, muscle weakness, or chest wall deformity, such as kyphoscoliosis. Whereas one study failed to find that bilevel PAP increased compliance compared to CPAP (39), individual patients may accept bilevel PAP treatment, but not CPAP. There may also be subsets of patients with OSA who tend to prefer bilevel PAP. A study by Resta and co-workers (40) suggested that bilevel PAP may be a better treatment than CPAP in the subsets of patients with OSA who have chronic obstructive pulmonary disease (COPD) or the obesity hypoventilation syndrome (OHS) (38). Of note, although uncommonly used in patients with OSA, bilevel devices can also be used with a back-up rate (spontaneous timed or ST mode). If the patient's respiratory rate exceeds the back-up rate, the bilevel devices functions as usual, in the spontaneous (S) mode. If the patient's respiratory rate drops below the back-up rate, the machine will cycle to IPAP. The duration of IPAP and EPAP are determined as in the spontaneous (S) mode. The machines will also cycle from IPAP to EPAP if no exhalation is sensed once the IPAP max time is reached. The bilevel PAP timed mode (T) is very rarely used in sleep apnea, but can be used to treat hypoventilation. In this mode, the device delivers IPAP–EPAP cycles only at the set rate. The relative proportion of IPAP–EPAP for the machine breath is that set by the clinician. One study suggested that OSA patients who continue to hypoventilate may benefit from bilevel in the timed mode (41). However, this study did not compare the efficacy of the ST and timed modes.

A common feature of both CPAP and bilevel PAP treatment is that a fixed level of pressure(s) is delivered during the entire night. This requires that an "optimal" level of

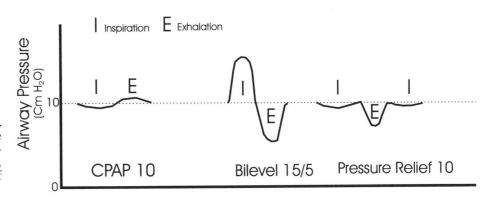

FIGURE 20-1. Positive pressure modes. Continuous positive airway pressure (CPAP), bilevel PAP, and CPAP with pressure relief (Cflex) are illustrated.

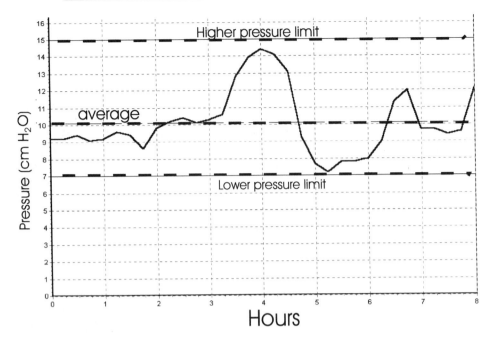

FIGURE 20-2. An example of pressure versus time for APAP treatment over a night. The device titrated between upper and lower pressure limits set by the clinician. The average pressure is lower than an optimal fixed pressure. In this case, treatment with a fixed pressure would require a CPAP of 14 to 15 cm H_2O. (From Berry RB: *Sleep medicine pearls.* 2nd edn, Philadelphia, Hanley and Belfus, 2003:153. With permission.)

fixed pressure(s) must be sufficient in all body positions and sleep stages. However, it has been recognized since the early days of positive pressure treatment that higher pressure is typically needed in the supine position (42–44). This has been well documented in systematic comparisons. In addition, higher pressure may be needed during REM sleep in many patients (42). Alternatively, some patients might require substantially less pressure in the lateral sleeping position or with the head elevated (44). Thus, a fixed pressure(s) may deliver higher than needed pressure to some patients during variable portions of the night. In theory, the average nightly pressure would be lower if only the minimum pressure required to maintain upper-airway patency was administered at any given time during sleep. It has been postulated that a lower average overnight pressure would increase adherence in some patients. Attended PAP titration to determine the optimal pressure is also a labor-intense procedure that may not be available in all circumstances. These difficulties associated with fixed PAP treatment and attended PAP titration resulted in the development of autotitrating and autoadjusting APAP devices (17–19,45–49). One or more of the following respiratory variables are typically monitored by a given APAP device: airflow magnitude (46), inspiratory airflow flattening (airflow limitation) (48), airway vibration/snoring, (47), and airway impedance (49). The algorithms for pressure change vary between different devices. Pressure changes are made gradually to avoid inducing arousal. For example, the presence of snoring could prompt a pressure increase of 0.5 cm H_2O over 1 minute. If none of the monitored variables is detected, the devices also begin to slowly lower pressure. Thus, APAP devices deliver the lowest effective pressure required in a given circumstance. The clinician sets the lower and upper pressure limits, and the de-

vice will deliver pressure as needed between these two limits (Fig. 20-2). High mask or mouth leak can simulate physiologic events and result in errors in APAP titration. One report of a large experience with the APAP devices estimated that leak exceeded 0.4 L per second (24 lpm) in about 10% of supervised nights and 15% of unsupervised nights (17). The devices also cannot differentiate between central and obstructive apnea. In many published studies of APAP, patients with central apnea or congestive heart failure (CHF) (increased incidence of Cheyne–Stokes breathing—central apnea) were excluded (18). The use of APAP devices as an alternative to traditional PAP titration will be discussed in the titration section. The evidence that APAP can increase adherence to PAP will be reviewed in the section on PAP adherence.

The newest method of PAP delivery is a variant of CPAP, expiratory pressure relief (Cflex), which allows the airway pressure to fall during expiration in proportion to expiratory airflow. The airway pressure returns to the prescribed CPAP level at end exhalation. Patients may select one of three levels of pressure relief, e.g., different relationships between expiratory flow and the amount of pressure decrease. This treatment may be useful in pressure-intolerant patients. To date, no information has been published regarding the impact on adherence to treatment. As will be discussed in later sections, pressure intolerance is not the most common PAP side effect.

INTERFACES FOR POSITIVE AIRWAY PRESSURE

Developing an optimal interface between the airflow–generator or blower and patient has been the source of

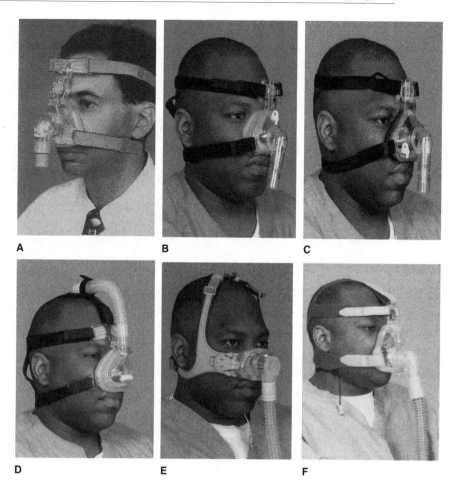

FIGURE 20-3. Six mask interfaces used for PAP treatment. (A) Ultramirage nasal mask (ResMed); (B) Comfort Classic (Respironics); (C) Profile Light (gel material) (Respironics); (D) Aclaim (Fisher-Paykel); (E) Vista (Res Med); (F) Full face Ultra Mirage Series 2 (Res Med). (A, From Berry RB. In: Johnson JT, Gluckman JL, Sanders MH, eds. Management of *obstructive sleep apnea*, United Kingdom, Martin Dunitz, 2001:95. With permission; F, From Berry RB. *Sleep medicine pearls.* 2nd edn. Philadelphia, Hanley and Belfus, 2003:155. With permission.)

tremendous challenge. The PAP industry has recognized this problem and currently a large variety of alternatives are available (Fig. 18-3 and 18-4). However, finding an adequate interface remains a significant problem. Mask discomfort (pain from pressure on the nose, cheeks, or upper lip), air leak (noise, eye irritation), and shift in mask position with body position changes all may impair sleep quality. In the original description of CPAP, small cannula-like tubes were placed in the nostrils and held in place with polymer (1). Later, the idea of a nasal mask was introduced (14,20,21). In many patients, mouth leaks are not problematic when using a nasal interface because the positive pressure in the nasopharynx moves the soft palate forward against the tongue, sealing off the oral cavity. Otherwise, the patient must maintain, or be assisted to maintain a closed mouth (chin strap), or utilize an oronasal mask, which simultaneously applies pressure to the nasal and oral airways.

Typically, a given type of mask is produced in a series of sizes (small, medium, large), but these rarely provided good fits for all facial structures. Material used for the mask are either compliant and bulge out from pressure against the face (Fig. 20-3A,B,D, and F) or are composed of a soft gel material (Fig. 20-3C). A particular challenge is obtaining a good seal over the bridge of the nose. Leaks of air

in this area typically irritate the eyes (50). Patients without upper teeth may have limited structural support for the upper lip area. In some of these patients, wearing dentures at night may help. To resolve these mask problems, several versions of interfaces have been developed to provide a seal in the nares, such as nasal pillows (Fig. 20-4A) or nasal prongs (Fig. 20-4B)(22). Two other advantages for this type device are that patients can read with the interface in place and typically feels less claustrophobic. Another method of handling similar problems is the design of "mini masks" that fit only over the tip/lower portion of the nose (Fig. 20-3E).

If patients have significant nasal congestion or obstruction, they may find breathing through a nasal mask with the mouth closed very uncomfortable. For this reason oronasal or full face masks covering both the nose and mouth (Fig. 20-3F) have been developed (23–25). These masks incorporate valves that allow inspiration of room air should the pressure source fail. They also have head straps that allow quick removal as a precaution against vomiting or other events requiring rapid mask removal. One problem with these full face masks is that they are required to form a good seal over a larger area of face. Thus, obtaining a good mask fit in all patients has been a problem. The full face mask can be especially useful in patients with mouth

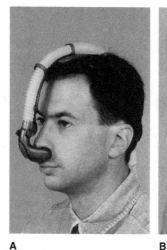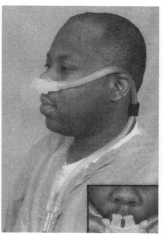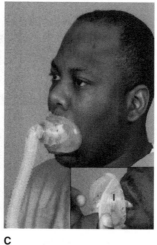

A   B   C

FIGURE 20-4. Three alternate interfaces for PAP treatment. (A) Breeze with nasal pillows (Mallincrokdt); (B) Nasal Aire (InnoMed); (C) Oracle (oral interface) by Fisher-Paykel. (A, From Berry RB. In: Johnson JT, Gluckman JL, Sanders MH, eds. *Management of obstructive sleep apnea*, United Kingdom: Martin Dunitz, 2001:95. With permission; (B) and (C) From Berry RB. *Sleep medicine pearls.* 2nd edn. Philadelphia, Hanley and Belfus, 2003:146,155. With permission.)

leak and also tend to prevent the drying of the upper airway. In some patients initially requiring a full face mask, intensive medical or surgical treatment of the nasal airway may allow eventual conversion to a nasal mask. Recently, oral interfaces (Fig. 20-4C) have also been developed for PAP (26). The nose is completely bypassed but aggressive humidification is required to prevent dryness. Nasal leak can be a problem with oral interfaces just as a mouth leak can complicate treatment with a nasal mask.

Because all modern CPAP equipment uses a single hose between blower and mask, some mechanism to wash out the exhaled CO_2 is needed. This is commonly performed by placing a small orifice or slit(s) in the nasal or full face mask. Of note, the amount of leak (intentional leak) can increase considerably with increases in pressure. While the possibility of rebreathing has been a concern if the mask is operating at lower pressures (less intentional leak), this does not appear to be a significant clinical problem. Most patients have some degree of unintentional leak and the orifices are large enough to provide adequate washout at low pressures. On the other hand, the amount of intentional leak at high pressures can be up to 40 L per minute with some masks.

ANCILLARY POSITIVE AIRWAY PRESSURE OPTIONS

The RAMP option is available on most CPAP and bilevel devices (4). This allows the patient to select a "ramp time" during which the pressure slowly increases from a low initial value (typically 4 cm H_2O) to the prescription pressure. This provides a window of time during which lower than the target pressure is applied and offers the patient an opportunity to fall asleep. The pressure from which a ramp may start to climb may be adjusted on some types of devices. This is a useful option because some patients prefer an initial pressure higher than 4 cm H_2O. While the RAMP option makes sense, it has never been shown to increase

adherence. Many PAP devices also offer mask-off alarms to alert the patient that the mask has been pulled off. The utility of this feature has never been systematically studied. Altitude compensation and adjustment for variable voltage sources also is available now on many PAP units. Altitude compensation may be automatic or user selectable. This is a valuable feature because the same blower speed at higher altitudes delivers less pressure because of the decreased air density (51).

Currently, all but the lowest priced PAP devices offer some method of objectively monitoring patient use (adherence) (52,53). As will be discussed later, the capacity to objectively monitor PAP use is essential for optimal clinical care. The most basic method is a simple run-time meter (recording time the device is turned on). The average hours per night the machine is turned on can be calculated by the change in the meter values divided by the number of elapsed days. More advanced machines can monitor actual use ("time at pressure" or time with varying blower speed) and computer chip technology has allowed recording of an electronic diary of the exact dates and times the machine was used (Fig. 20-5). This feature allows the physician to detect skipped days or early removal of the PAP device (the 4 AM trip to the bathroom). Some devices also will record estimates of persistent events or leak information. This stored machine information can be assessed through memory cards, modems, or direct transfer of information from the unit to a computer.

The use of humidification has been another frequently useful development. Initially, cold passover humidification (air simply blown across a water reservoir) was available. However, more moisture can be delivered with heated humidification and, currently, stand-alone heated humidifiers or models incorporated into the PAP device (integrated humidifier) are available. Studies have shown that nasal CPAP results in some drop in the relative humidity of air in the upper airway. Mouth leak causes a more dramatic drop in mask humidity via a unidirectional escape of water vapor out of the mouth (54,55) (Fig. 20-6). In fact,

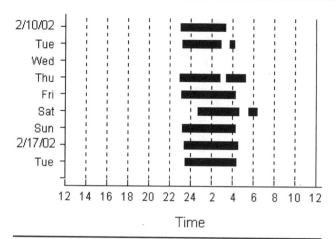

FIGURE 20-5. This is a typical graphical display of PAP device usage (time at pressure) over a period of time. The patient usually stopped using PAP after 4 AM. The electronic use diary also shows that the PAP device was not used at all on February 12, 2002. On questioning, the patient admitted he stopped using the device after returning from the bathroom in the early morning hours. (From Berry RB. *Sleep medicine pearls.* 2nd edn. Philadelphia, Hanley and Belfus, 2003:142. With permission.)

the symptom of mouth dryness usually implies some degree of mouth leak. Dryness of the nasal mucosa results in a large increase in nasal resistance (55). This tends to cause more mouth opening and greater leak. In order to prevent this cycle, adequate humidification of air is required. One study found that heated but not cold humidity prevented changes in nasal resistance secondary to large mouth leak (55). Humidification by preventing dryness may also reduce the nasal congestion some patients experience when using CPAP. In one study, humidification increased average nightly use and patient satisfaction with CPAP treatment (heated > cool > none) (56). Those patients who benefited the most were those with symptoms of nasal congestion or dryness at baseline. This study could be criticized for the fact that the subjects were not blinded to the fact that no humidity was used in the control arm. Medical devices can have an appreciable placebo effect. Another study found that prophylactic use of humidity to all comers did not improve satisfaction with the initial attended PAP titration

in the sleep laboratory (57). Thus, there is conflicting evidence on whether or not humidity should be used on every patient. It seems prudent to target humidification toward patients most likely to benefit (nasal congestion dryness and mouth leak). Certainly care of humidifiers (cleaning and filling with water) requires some extra patient effort. Adherence data on the use of humidifiers is not available.

PATIENT SELECTION FOR POSITIVE AIRWAY PRESSURE

There are three major reasons to treat OSA (58): (1) To decrease symptoms including excessive daytime sleepiness (EDS) (5) and associated morbidity such as an increased risk of autoaccidents (59,60), (2) to prevent long-term cardiovascular and cerebrovascular consequences of OSA (61–67), and (3) to improve bed partner sleep (alleviate socially unacceptable snoring) (68). Several controlled studies have demonstrated that PAP is effective in decreasing subjective and objective sleepiness and improving the quality of life in symptomatic patients with moderate to severe disease (5,6). In general, while PAP can be effective in some mild OSA patients (or those with isolated snoring), this group tends to be much less adherent to PAP treatment (7–12). Patient preference should also be considered. Some patients with milder disease may not want upper-airway surgery or an oral appliance. In these cases, choices are limited to conservative treatment (weight loss, etc.) or positive pressure.

The indication for PAP treatment of asymptomatic patients is more controversial. In one 6-week study, there was no benefit with regard to sleepiness, quality of life, or cognitive test performance in moderate to severe cases of OSA (AHI >30 per hour) when patients were not sleepy (69). In this study, there was also no improvement in blood pressure, a finding that conflicts with the results of some other studies (66,67). In addition, the severity of arterial oxygen desaturation was not specified. The results may not then be applicable to all patient groups. Social reasons for effective treatment can be very compelling for some patients.

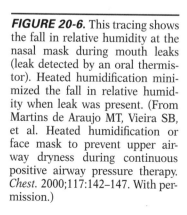

FIGURE 20-6. This tracing shows the fall in relative humidity at the nasal mask during mouth leaks (leak detected by an oral thermistor). Heated humidification minimized the fall in relative humidity when leak was present. (From Martins de Araujo MT, Vieira SB, et al. Heated humidification or face mask to prevent upper airway dryness during continuous positive airway pressure therapy. *Chest.* 2000;117:142–147. With permission.)

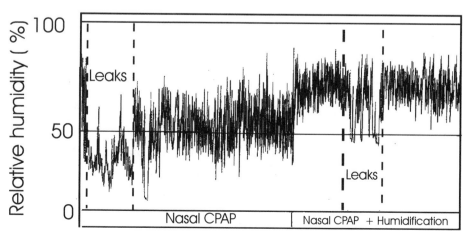

Some increased risk of developing cerebrovascular or cardiovascular disease exists even at low AHI levels (64,65). However, no prospective controlled study has yet demonstrated that CPAP treatment will decrease the risk of long-term consequences. The risk of long-term consequences of untreated OSA in a given patient cannot be estimated with certainty. However, the presence of more severe arterial oxygen desaturation or comorbid conditions [coronary artery disease, congestive heart failure, prior cerebrovascular accidents (CVA)] may well increase risk.

Medicare guidelines for reimbursement of PAP treatment have recently been revised (70). For patients with an AHI of 5 to 14 per hour, symptoms or signs of significant impairment are required. The qualifying impairments include daytime sleepiness, insomnia, hypertension, prior CVA, or a mood disorder. For patients with an AHI of 15 per hour or more, no associated findings are required. Of note, the Medicare definition of hypopnea is stringent. A hypopnea is defined as a 30% or greater reduction in flow followed by a 4% or greater desaturation. Arousals are not considered in this definition of hypopnea. No associated desaturation is required for an apnea.

In summary, one can argue that all patients with moderate to severe OSA, with or without symptoms, should be offered PAP treatment. Most would also offer PAP to symptomatic patients with mild OSA as an alternative to other treatments. For moderate to severe OSA patients without symptoms, the most compelling reasons for treatment would be social acceptance and prevention of long-term consequences. Scientific evidence (see later section) is accumulating that asymptomatic patients with significant cardiovascular comorbidity probably have the most to gain from PAP treatment.

POSITIVE PRESSURE TITRATION

The pressure used for PAP treatment is usually determined by a positive pressure titration (Table 20-1). Pressure is incrementally increased until an optimal pressure is reached. Standards for positive pressure titration have

▶ **TABLE 20-1. Essentials of Positive Pressure Titration**

Patient education about positive pressure
Mask fitting (before study)
CPAP training—acclimatization period (identify problems early)
Titration to eliminate apnea, hypopnea, snoring, desaturation, and RERAs in all body positions and sleep stages (including supine REM)
Reduction in the AHI <5/h if possible, at least <10/h

been published by a number of organizations (71,72). Attended polysomnography (PSG), including electroencephograph (EEG) monitoring has been the standard of care for titration. This allows a determination of sleep stage and body position (42–44). The sleep technologist is available for adjustment in mask seal and to minimize discomfort and patient complaints. Episodes of significant arterial oxygen desaturation that sometimes occur even when airflow is adequate (commonly during REM sleep) (73) or significant arrhythmias can be recognized and addressed. PAP titration is a labor-intensive process and usually a technologist can titrate only one or two patients at a time.

While airflow can be monitored with a thermistor or nasal pressure cannula under the mask, most sleep centers today monitor a flow signal generated by the positive pressure device (sometimes called machine flow, CPAP flow, Vest, or Cflow). This signal provides accurate information about the magnitude of flow and airflow limitation (flattened airflow profile). Some airflow signals may also provide snoring information, depending on the filtering and frequency response of the measuring device in the machine. An estimated leak signal as well as machine pressure are also available (74). Use of the leak signal will be discussed in the following section.

It has been recognized that both snoring and airflow limitation usually imply persistent high upper-airway resistance (75,76) and are clues that a higher pressure may be needed. In Fig. 20-7, a small increase in CPAP eliminates snoring and evidence of airflow limitation in the flow

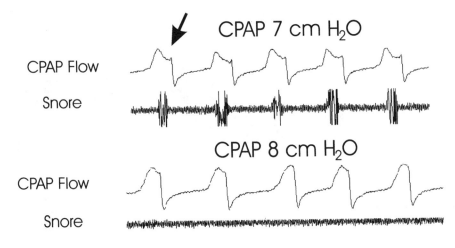

FIGURE 20-7. These tracings shows that an increase in CPAP of only 1 cm H_2O was needed to eliminate snoring. Notice that the increase in pressure also eliminated the subtle flattening in the inspiratory part of the flow signal from the CPAP device (arrow). (From Berry RB. *Sleep medicine pearls.* 2nd edn. Philadelphia, Hanley and Belfus, 2003:125. With permission.)

signal. The end point (goal) of titration varies somewhat, but ideally includes elimination (or near elimination) of obstructive apnea, hypopnea, snoring, arterial oxygen desaturation, and respiratory effort–related arousals (RERAs), which are those events associated with arousals secondary to increased respiratory effort that do not meet criteria for obstructive hypopneas (77). As esophageal pressure is not typically measured, RERAs are usually inferred from evidence of airflow limitation or snoring preceding an arousal. Some centers also try to eliminate all evidence of airflow limitation (77). Central apneas and mild airflow limitation may be acceptable as long as there is no associated sleep disturbance or significant oxygen desaturation. The goal of most centers is to have an AHI <5 per hour in all body positions and sleep stages. The highest pressures are usually needed during supine REM sleep. Unfortunately, supine REM sleep may not be recorded in every patient.

Bilevel pressure titration protocols vary, but two methods are popular (16). One can increase IPAP=EPAP until obstructive apneas are abolished. Further increases in IPAP are administered until hypopnea/snoring is eliminated. Alternatively, one could start with 6/4 to 8/4 and then sequentially increase IPAP and EPAP as needed. In general, apnea requires an increase in EPAP (Fig. 20-8). A common error is to attempt to stabilize the airway with EPAP that is too low or an IPAP–EPAP differential that is too high.

Initially, PAP titrations were performed during an entire night that followed a previous diagnostic study. This allowed an entire night for diagnosis and estimation of severity. Frequently, the patient could be educated by a physician about the nature of his problem, treatment alternatives, and the nature of PAP treatment before the PAP titration. However, because of limited resources and to expedite treatment, split- or partial-night studies were introduced (78–82). The first portion of the night is for diagnosis and the second part for the PAP titration. Obviously this approach allows less time for each goal, diagnosis, and PAP

> **TABLE 20-2. Suggested Criteria for Split Titration**

2 h of recorded sleep in diagnostic portion (so patient will qualify for Medicare payment of CPAP)
AHI > 40/h
AHI 20–40 /h with significant desaturation or other factors
At least 3 or more hours remaining for PAP titration

titration. Several studies have assessed the ability of a split-night approach to determine an effective level of PAP and guidelines for patient selection have been published by the AASM (71). In general, around 60% to 80% of patients can be handled adequately by the split-night approach. Criteria for patients to have a split study are listed in Table 20-2. The rationale for these criteria is that severe patients usually do not require either REM sleep or the supine position to manifest the severity of their problem. The severity of mild to moderate cases may be underestimated when adequate amounts of supine or REM sleep are not included in the diagnostic portion of the study. In addition, there appears to be more uncertainty in the optimal level of PAP in milder cases studied for only part of the night. Certainly, enough time must be left for an adequate PAP titration, once the diagnosis of OSA has been made. The split-study approach requires education, mask fitting, and, optimally, some brief period of PAP adaptation before lights out. If a patient does not meet criteria during the first part of the night, the entire study is performed as a diagnostic one. Autotitrating devices offer an alternative to traditional PAP titration (18,19, 83–88). Information stored in the device memory can be analyzed and a pressure can be chosen for fixed CPAP. A common method is to choose the 90th or 95th percentile pressure (pressure exceeded only 10% or 5% of the time, respectively) as the prescription pressure. This assumes periods of high leak have been eliminated from analysis. The devices could be used in an attended setting as a technologist extender. Interventions for mask leak, arterial oxygen desaturation, or arrhythmia would then be

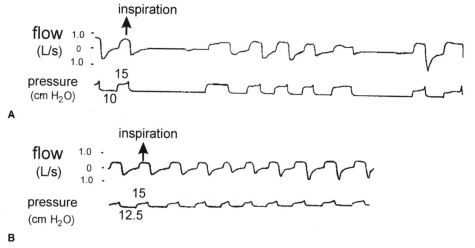

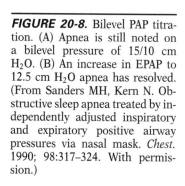

FIGURE 20-8. Bilevel PAP titration. (A) Apnea is still noted on a bilevel pressure of 15/10 cm H_2O. (B) An increase in EPAP to 12.5 cm H_2O apnea has resolved. (From Sanders MH, Kern N. Obstructive sleep apnea treated by independently adjusted inspiratory and expiratory positive airway pressures via nasal mask. *Chest.* 1990; 98:317–324. With permission.)

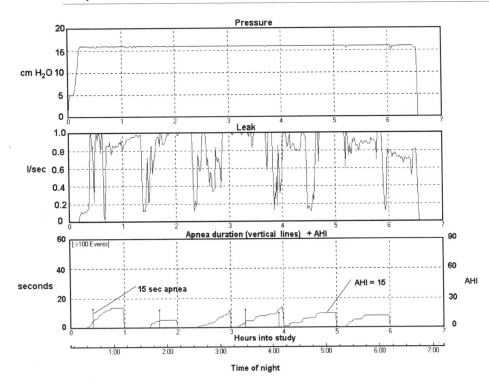

FIGURE 20-9. This is the tracing of a single night of inadequate APAP titration. There were very high leaks and the machine titrated up to 15 cm H_2O (the clinician set upper pressure limit). In addition, one can see that there were appreciable residual events.

possible. In this setting the ability of the devices to provide an adequate titration [low residual apnea-hypopnea index (AHI)] have been well documented (18,19,84,85). Of note, most studies excluded patients with congestive heart failure (CHF) or significant lung disease. The ability of APAP devices to perform in the unattended setting in CPAP naive patients (18,86–88) has been less well documented. Nevertheless, adequate titration can probably be obtained in many patients. Simply looking at a data summary can be misleading. Most devices allow the ability to look at single-night data in detail (pressure, leak, residual events versus time) (Fig. 20-9). Periods of high leak and the frequently associated increase in pressure can be appreciated. High leak can result in many devices promptly increasing pressure until the upper pressure limit is reached. In Fig. 20-9, a single night tracing on APAP shows high leak (>0.4 L per second). Patients with suboptimal or inconclusive APAP titrations should have an attended lab PAP titration.

Other methods of determining a CPAP level for chronic treatment have been investigated. Hoffstein and co-workers (89,90) developed a prediction equation for optimal CPAP based on the AHI and neck circumference. CPAP pressure = −5.121 + 0.13 * BMI + 0.16 * NC + 0.04 * AHI. This equation incorporates the body mass index [BMI = weight in kilograms/ (height in meters)^2], the neck circumference in centimeters (NC) at the cricothyroid membrane, and the apnea + hypopnea index (AHI). For example, a patient with a BMI of 27, neck circumference of 19 inches, and AHI of 60 per hour would be predicted to require a CPAP of 14.5 cm H_2O. This equation can

be used to guide empiric treatment, but the confidence limits are fairly wide. Some protocols have also used patient- or spouse-adjusted pressure as an alternative to attended pressure titration (91) with good results.

Common Problems and Decision Making in Positive Airway Pressure Titration

While most sleep centers have established PAP titration protocols, the skill of the technologist is still important. PAP titration remains an "art as well as a science." Establishing a good patient–technologist relationship will help the patient relax and hopefully adapt to the discomforts of the study. Some of the common problems encountered during PAP titration are listed in Table 20-3, along with possible solutions. Education about OSA and PAP should always be performed before lights out. Most centers also have mask fitting and a period of PAP acclimatization while the patient is awake. This is very useful for identifying an inadequate mask seal, significant patient apprehension, pressure intolerance, and significant nasal obstruction. The technologist might change the mask, use humidification, use bilevel pressure/or a very slow upward titration of CPAP, based on reaction to this brief trial of PAP. During titration it may be necessary to temporarily reduce pressure to allow a return to sleep.

Mask or mouth leaks can cause difficulties during both attended manual or unattended autotitration of PAP. As pressure is titrated upward during the night, mask or mouth leak may develop. If high leak is noted, the technologist can zoom in on the mouth area with the low light

▶ **TABLE 20-3. Problems During Continuous Positive Airway Pressure Titration and Typical Solutions**

Claustrophobia	Desensitization
	Nasal pillows, nasal prong interface
Mask leak	Careful mask fitting before study
	Adjust straps, change mask size or type
Nasal congestion	Full face mask
	Heated humidity
	Decongestant
Pressure Intolerance	Avoid rapid increase in pressure
	Temporary reduction in pressure to allow return to sleep
	Bilevel pressure
	Cflex
	Elevation of head of bed, side sleep position to decrease required pressure

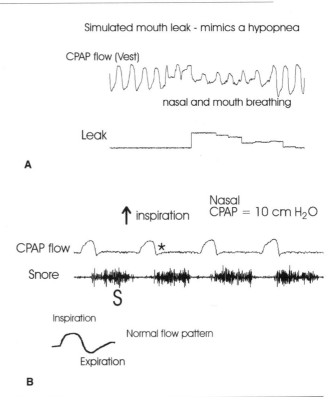

FIGURE 20-10. (A) This tracing was obtained when a patient breathing on nasal CPAP was asked to breathe partially through the mouth (nasal and mouth breathing). One can see what looks like a hypopnea. (B) This tracing shows airflow (inspiration up) with a truncated expiratory phase (*) compared with normal shape shown below. Expiratory leak was confirmed by evidence of expiratory snoring in the snore sensor tracing (S). The technician closely inspected the patient by zooming in on the face with a low-light camera. The patient's mouth was vibrating during exhalation. (From Berry RB. *Sleep medicine pearls.* 2nd edn. Philadelphia, Hanley and Belfus, 2003:126,132. With permission.)

camera to see if the mouth is open. Widely fluctuating leak without pressure change or body movement also suggests that an oral leak is present. Mouth leak can mimic hypopneic events (Fig. 20-10A), prevent airway stabilization, or result in arousal from sleep. If mainly expiratory leak is present, the expiratory portion of the airflow signal may be truncated (Fig. 20-11B). If leak is not recognized, the technologist may increase pressure in response to events rather than address the cause of the leak. A mask leak requires mask adjustment, and a mouth leak may be addressed by use of a chin strap or full face mask. If nasal congestion is causing the mouth leak, heated humidity may also be useful.

Central apneas may appear and are often a significant challenge. Some patients develop central apneas following arousals from high upper-airway resistance. An increase in pressure is indicated. Others develop central apneas following spontaneous arousals from pressure intolerance or leaks. In this case, a lowering of pressure may be attempted if central apneas persist.

Of note, some central apneas after treatment of OSA with tracheostomy were not uncommon and resolved with continued treatment. Treatment emergent central apneas may occur in some patients during CPAP titration if the Pco_2 is reduced to near the apneic threshold (the Pco_2 level required to stimulate respiratory effort during sleep). In this case, any brief increase in ventilation, such as occurs after an arousal, may trigger a central apnea. The treatment of Cheyne–Stokes type central apnea is discussed in later sections.

Factors Affecting Optimal Pressure

Because a single night or a partial night is utilized to establish an optimal pressure, the possibility of varying PAP requirements must be considered. Some studies have suggested a possible increase in upper-airway size (92) and decrease in the optimal pressure (93) with chronic CPAP treatment secondary to a reduction in upper-airway edema. However, others have found the pressure to be fairly constant (94). Table 20.3 lists factors that have been demonstrated to alter the pressure required to keep the airway open. Posture has already been mentioned. One study found that elevation of the head of the bed or the lateral sleep position could alter the optimal pressure by up to 5 cm H_2O (44). Weight loss/gain has also been demonstrated to alter pressure requirements (95). Snoring at home on CPAP is a useful clue that higher pressure may be needed. Many authors have stated that ethanol use can also increase the pressure required. However, two studies have not found this to be the case (96,97). Ethanol use is still to be discouraged, as patients might fail to apply the mask or remove it during the night, although it does increase the arousal threshold to respiratory stimuli (98).

Nasal congestion also could conceivably alter the required pressure. One must remember that the pressure at

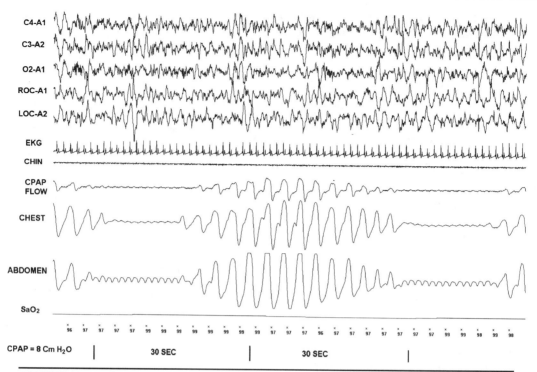

FIGURE 20-11. This tracing shows Cheyne–Stokes central apnea during treatment with CPAP of 8 cm H$_2$O. In this patient, no level of pressure reduced the apnea + hypopnea index to below 20 per hour. However, above 8 cm H$_2$O, all the persistent events were central apneas. Machine flow is the flow signal from the positive pressure device. While these central apneas persisted, they did not result in significant desaturation or arousal.

the collapsible areas of the upper airway rather than at the mask is the critical pressure. It is also possible that increased mask or mouth leaks can render a given pressure less effective at keeping the airway open (99). Mask pressure can be less than machine pressure (set pressure) when high leaks are present.

SIDE EFFECTS OF POSITIVE AIRWAY PRESSURE AND POSSIBLE SOLUTIONS

Studies have enumerated the many side effects associated with PAP treatment (100–108). If left untreated, side effects from PAP may cause a lower chance of acceptance and lower rates of adherence (104). Side effects and possible interventions are listed in Table 20-4. Many side effects are secondary to the mask interface. In one study, intolerance of the mask was the most common reason for discontinuing CPAP treatment (102). Obtaining an adequate mask fit may require trials of several different brands and types of masks. Adequate mask positioning is also essential, as is elimination of overtightening of head straps. Often moving the mask up or down slightly will produce a better seal than further tightening. Poor mask fit leads to leaks that are both uncomfortable (especially into the eyes) and may result in an inadequate pressure. Overtightening of head straps can result in severe skin abrasion especially on the

bridge of the nose ("CPAP divot"). Turning in bed can also change mask position, resulting in loss of mask seal. Improvements in mask material and flexibility in the mask–hose connection have attempted to reduce these problems. Masks today use either a deformable gel material or thin material that balloons out against the face under pressure. Nasal prongs (nasal pillows) can sometimes provide a useful alternative for patients unable to get a good seal around the nasal bridge. Adequate care of masks (cleaning) and replacement of masks when old (and less flexible) are also necessary.

Nasal symptoms including congestion, rhinorrhea, pain, dryness, and epistaxis are all potential problems with positive pressure treatment. Nasal congestion can often be improved with the use of heated humidification and/or treatment with nasal steroids, nonsedating antihistamines, or decongestants at bedtime. Some patients with intractable nasal congestion can be handled with use of a full face mask or oral interface (23–25). If all else fails, referral for surgical treatment of nasal obstruction is another approach (109,110). Recently, less morbid procedures to reduce turbinate size have been used with some success. While heated humidity generally is more effective in preventing dryness (55), an occasional patient will prefer cool humidification. A full face mask may also prevent a loss humidity from mouth leaks (54). Rhinorrhea may develop during CPAP treatment or immediately following

TABLE 20-4. Positive Airway Pressure Side Effects and Possible Interventions

Positive Pressure Side Effects	Interventions
Mask side effects	
Air leaks	Proper mask fitting
Conjunctivitis	Proper mask application (education)
Discomfort	Different brand/type of mask
Noise	
Skin breakdown	Avoid overtightening; intervene as above for leaks
	Alternate between different mask types
	Nasal prongs/ pillows
	Tape barrier for skin protection
Unintentional mask removal	Low pressure alarm
	Consider increase in pressure
Nasal symptoms	
Congestion/obstruction	Nasal steroid inhaler
	Antihistamines (if allergic component)
	Night time topical decongestants (oxymetazoline)
	Nasal saline
	Humidification (heated)
	Full face (oronasal) mask
Epistaxis	Nasal saline
Pain	Humidification (heated)
Rhinitis/rhinorrhea	Nasal ipratropium bromide
Other problems	
Mouth leaks	Humidification (prevent increased nasal resistance)
Mouth dryness	Treatment of nasal congestion
	Chin strap (?)
	Full face mask
	Lower pressure/bilevel pressure
Pressure intolerance	Ramp
	Bilevel pressure
	Autotitrating device
	Lower prescription pressure; accept higher AHI
	Lower pressure + adjunctive measures (elevated head of bed, side sleeping position, weight loss)

cessation of treatment. This is usually controlled with intranasal ipratropium bromide or humidification.

Although PAP devices have the ability to compensate for leak, large mouth leaks may compromise the ability to deliver pressure and maintain an open airway (99). Mouth leaks can also result in arousal and severe dryness, as noted above. Mouth leaks seem to be especially problematic in patients with prior surgery of the palate (111). To prevent mouth leaks one can use chin straps or full face masks. The efficacy of chin straps has never been documented but may work in an occasional patient. Some patients may have less mouth leak with bilevel pressure (especially those with ex-

piratory mouth leak). In others, using APAP by lowering the average nightly treatment pressure may decrease the tendency for mouth leak. For patients with nasal congestion, treatment with nasal steroids or vasoconstrictors and using humidification may reduce the tendency for mouth leak.

Machine noise was once a common problem, but newer blowers are generally much quieter. One could recommend a longer tubing and removal of the blower unit from the bedroom. Another worrisome side effect is the noise or discomfort from the stream of air exiting from the controlled leak orifice in the mask or mask/hose interface. This intentional leak can sometimes also bother the bedmate. New designs in the controlled leak have addressed this problem.

Intolerance to the level of positive pressure is also a common side effect, especially at higher treatment pressures. There are several approaches to handle the problem. The RAMP option has already been described. Other approaches are to use bilevel PAP, autoadjusting CPAP, expiratory pressure relief, or simply to use a lower than optimal pressure for a few weeks. Patients who complain of difficulty exhaling or those with obstructive lung disease may find bilevel pressure more comfortable (40). There has been conflicting evidence concerning the ability of autoadjusting APAP to improve adherence to treatment in unselected patients. Three studies found an increase in adherence with APAP compared to fixed CPAP (112–114) whereas three failed to do so (115–117). Perhaps this is not surprising when one considers that pressure intolerance is often not the biggest patient complaint. In addition, in some patients there is relatively little variability in the pressure applied over a night. A patient with optimal pressure of 10 cm H_2O and an average pressure of 8 cm H_2O might not notice much difference on APAP. Series and co-workers (118) found that the patients most likely to benefit from APAP were those with large variability in pressure over the night. In a recent study, Massie et al. (119) found that APAP used in patients requiring an optimal CPAP greater than 10 cm H_2O had significantly better compliance on APAP. However, of note, the mean improvement in adherence was only about 1/2 hour. In any case, individual patients may tolerate APAP much better than CPAP. Recently, the use of pressure relief during exhalation has been added to traditional fixed-pressure CPAP. The patient may select one of three levels of pressure relief. The amount the airway pressure drops during exhalation depends on the amount of flow. The greater the flow, the more the machine pressure is allowed to drop. The airway pressure returns to the set CPAP level at end expiration. Preliminary experience shows this approach may improve patient satisfaction. However, no data have yet been published to document an increase in adherence with this type of PAP.

Some patients find sensations of claustrophobia a severe problem when using PAP. Education and a period of CPAP adaptation prior to CPAP titration may help. Using nasal pillows or nasal prong interfaces may also reduce the feeling of claustrophobia in a few patients.

A systematic program of desensitization can also be effective (120), although it usually requires the assistance of counselors trained in the technique, as well as a motivated patient.

FACTORS DETERMINING ACCEPTANCE AND ADHERENCE

Acceptance is usually defined as patient willingness to take a PAP device home and use it for at least 1 week (121). The term adherence has become preferred over compliance and is used in much of the recent literature. The methods that have been employed to quantify adherence vary considerably, as does the definition of adequate adherence. However, one commonly used definition of an adherent patient is one using PAP for more than 4 hours per night for over 70% of days (52,108). This definition is unsatisfactory, as it is likely that a significant proportion of patients require more than 4 hours per night of use for maximal benefit from treatment (122). Estimates of acceptance vary from 5% to 50% and of those initially using PAP, up to 12% to 25% discontinue PAP by 3 years (121,123). Estimates of adherence have varied widely, with the highest figures of 70% to 80% reported by programs with a systematic program for PAP treatment (108).

Rational design of a system to improve acceptance and adherence to PAP requires understanding the factors that determine why patients either do not accept or adhere poorly to PAP treatment (121). Not all studies agree but, in general, more disease severity, more symptoms, self versus spouse referral, and more perceived benefit for PAP predict success (124,125). In one study, prior uvulopalatopharyngoplasty (UPPP) and problems with the nose or pharynx were more common in patients who stopped CPAP treatment than in those who were adherent (126). In other types of disease with demanding treatment regimens, cognitive constructs have been useful in determining adherence. Patients who place a high value on health, feel they are in control, do not believe that chance rules their life, and have high self-efficacy are better treatment risks. One study of psychologic correlates of adherence found that patients who by nature engaged in active coping strategies with new and difficult situations used CPAP more (127).

Studies of the pattern of adherence have also provided valuable information. Early intervention is important. Weaver and co-workers (128) found that a difference in the pattern of use by compliant and noncompliant patients is noted as early as day 4 of treatment. Patients complying over the first 1 to 3 months tend to continue to accept positive pressure treatment.

▶ **TABLE 20-5. Methods to Improve Positive Airway Pressure Adherence**

Education about OSA and PAP by
Staff
Video
Printed information
Involvement of significant other/spouse
Extended in-hospital (2–3 nights) stay
Subsequent mask and headgear adjustment or change
PAP help line
Unsolicited telephone follow-up
Early interventions for side effects and concerns
Objective monitoring of adherence
Early and regular clinic visits

METHODS TO INCREASE ADHERENCE

Some procedures that have been recommended to increase adherence are listed in Table 20-5. Of note, most systematic evaluations of interventions to improve adherence have not studied individual components but rather a "package" approach. The monitoring of objective adherence is now recommended, as several studies have demonstrated that patients overestimate their actual usage (52,53). Time at pressure or time of actual usage is preferred, although there appears to be good correlation between machine usage time and time at pressure for the majority of patients.

Education about OSA and CPAP is now a standard part of most programs (by staff, video, printed material, group sessions) (129). Involvement of the spouse in education and follow-up appointments has also been recommended (125). In many European centers, patients actually spend several extra nights in the hospital during the initial CPAP use (108). While this is not practical in fee-for-service health care systems, early follow-up and interventions to handle side effects are suggested. If the initial choice of mask and headgear are not satisfactory despite adjustments, a different size or type should be tried. Unfortunately, there continues to be some resistance to this intervention by home health care agencies because they may be only reimbursed for one mask every 6 months. Regular attendance at PAP clinics, where objective adherence is checked and education is repeated, has been shown to be effective. Even simple telephone follow-up has been shown to increase adherence (130). Today, many PAP devices have the ability to store information on memory cards that can be mailed in or transmit data via modem. A significant portion of PAP training and follow-up can be performed by nurses or respiratory therapists. However, physician involvement is especially important with respect to convincing the patient of the need for treatment and benefits of adequate adherence.

BENEFITS OF POSITIVE AIRWAY PRESSURE TREATMENT TO OBSTRUCTIVE SLEEP APNEA PATIENTS

There are many benefits and changes that occur after successful PAP treatment of OSA (Table 20-6). On the first night of PAP titration, some patients exhibit a large increase in both slow-wave and REM sleep (rebound from prior deprivation) and often will note improvement in sleepiness after only one night of CPAP (131). However, in 1997, Wright et al. (132) challenged the effectiveness and widespread use of PAP treatment of OSA because of the lack of placebo-controlled evidence that PAP improved symptoms and quality of life. Since that time, placebo-controlled studies have documented that PAP improves subjective and objective sleepiness and quality of life (5,6). Improvements in subjective sleepiness (Epworth sleepiness scale), maintenance of wakefulness test (MWT), and sleep latency are more robust than improvements in the multiple sleep latency test (MSLT) at detecting improvements after PAP (133–135). The Epworth sleepiness scale quantifies a patient's propensity to fall asleep in 8 commonly encountered situations (133). Many clinicians find it a useful tool to follow the symptomatic response to PAP treatment (134). Improvement in sleepiness (5,131) and neurocognitive function (136) can occur quickly, although many patients require up to 6 months for the peak benefit (137). Studies of quality of life have usually found improvements in vitality scales on PAP (138).

PAP treatment reverses many of the effects of OSA that are believed to increase the risk of coronary artery disease or CVAs or worsen coexisting heart failure. Reductions in nocturnal systemic and pulmonary arterial pressures on PAP have been well documented. It has been known for some time that many patients with OSA do not have the normal nocturnal fall in blood pressure, as blood pressure rises at each event termination ("nondippers"). PAP reduces this effect by preventing apnea and hypop-

nea (139,140). Of even greater importance is the finding that PAP can reduce daytime blood pressure as well (65,66, 141). For example, Becker and co-workers (66) found that CPAP treatment resulted in a mean drop in nocturnal and daytime blood pressure of about 10 mm Hg. The authors contended that similar long-term changes in blood pressure are believed to reduce coronary heart disease event risk by 37% and stroke risk by 56%. The failure of some studies to detect a drop in daytime blood pressure with PAP (142,143) may have been secondary to inadequate adherence, too short treatment time, inadequate ambulatory blood pressure-monitoring methods, or selection of patients with mild intermittent hypoxia.

Patients with OSA also have nocturnal increases in pulmonary arterial pressure secondary to hypoxic vasoconstriction. It has been said that OSA patients with normal daytime blood gases usually have normal or only mildly increased daytime pulmonary pressures (144,145). However, studies have shown that PAP reduces both nocturnal and daytime pulmonary arterial pressure (146,147). The improvement is not necessarily secondary to improvement in daytime oxygenation. One study found a decrease in pulmonary vascular reactivity to hypoxia with PAP use (147).

Patients with OSA have daytime as well as nocturnal increases in sympathetic tone. Several studies have shown that PAP can reduce daytime sympathetic activity (148–150). The increased sympathetic activity is believed to be one reason that OSA patients have reduced heart rate variability. PAP treatment has also been shown to increase heart rate variability OSA (151).

A growing number of studies show changes in blood components or indicators of inflammation in OSA that may be associated with an increased risk of atherosclerosis or thrombosis. PAP treatment reduces the early morning hematocrit (152) and fibrinogen levels (153). The levels of vascular endothelial growth factor (VEGF) (154), amount of neutrophil (155,156) and platelet activation (157) are also reduced with PAP. Inflammation is now believed to play a role in atherosclerosis or plaque rupture. The level of C-reactive protein (a marker of inflammation), is reduced with PAP treatment (158,159). Untreated OSA is associated with nocturnal naturesis probably due, at least in part, to an increased secretion of atrial naturetic peptide (160). PAP also decreases the naturesis and, clinically, patients may report a decrease in nocturia. PAP may also influence the distribution of fat. One study found a reduction in leptin (a hormone secreted by adipose tissue) and a reduction in visceral fat on PAP treatment (161). Increased visceral fat is associated with an increased risk of cardiac disease.

Recently, there has been tremendous interest in the effects of PAP on patients with heart failure. In patients with CHF and OSA, treatment with PAP increased the ejection fraction and reduced the level of dyspnea in patients with stable but severe failure (162,163). The use and benefits of

▶ **TABLE 20-6. Effects and Benefits of PAP Treatment: Benefits and Effects of Positive Airway Pressure**

Improved sleep quality
Decreased subjective and objective daytime sleepiness
Improved cognitive function (some studies)
Improved quality of life measures (vitality)
Decreased sympathetic tone
Increased heart rate variability
Decreased nocturnal and daytime blood pressure (most studies)
Decreased nocturnal and daytime pulmonary arterial pressure
Changes in possible mediators or markers of vascular disease
   Decreased fibrinogen level
   Decreased WBC and platelet activation
   Decreased C-reactive protein

PAP in patients with Cheyne–Stokes breathing and central sleep apnea will be discussed later.

POSITIVE AIRWAY PRESSURE IN OBSTRUCTIVE SLEEP APNEA–SPECIAL CIRCUMSTANCES

Hypoventilation with Obstructive Sleep Apnea

The two groups of patients with OSA who have daytime hypoventilation are those with the obesity hypoventilation syndrome (hypoventilation not secondary to lung disease) and those with coexistent OSA and obstructive airways disease (OSA + COPD), the so-called "overlap syndrome" (164). These patient groups are also likely to have more severe arterial oxygen desaturation (165). Chronic treatment with CPAP can reduce the daytime arterial carbon dioxide tension ($Paco_2$) in these groups (166–168). The ventilatory response to CO_2 typically shifts to the left without a change in slope (167). This suggests a change in set point. Whereas chronic CPAP treatment will improve the daytime $Paco_2$ in some of these patients, most physicians treat patients with OSA and hypoventilation with bilevel PAP. This treatment augments ventilation as well as maintains upper-airway patency during sleep. However, if the IPAP–EPAP gradient is narrow, as might occur when the EPAP required to prevent apnea is very high ($\geq$18 cm H_2O), the pressure support, which is available to augment ventilation (the amount IPAP exceeds EPAP), is reduced for devices delivering a maximum pressure of 20 cm H_2O. There are bilevel pressure devices capable of delivery pressures up to 30 cm H_2O, but mask and mouth leak may be problematic at these high pressures.

Patients with OSA and hypoventilation can present with acute hypercapnic respiratory failure (acute on chronic respiratory acidosis). Treatment with mask PAP and oxygen can often avoid the need for intubation (169). In very severe patients, one group reported on the use of volume-controlled ventilation with mask (170). One problem with this approach is that many volume ventilators are not leak tolerant. The addition of supplemental oxygen to PAP is usually required for adequate oxygenation in acutely ill patients. Patients with coexistent OSA and obstructive lung disease and those with the obesity hypoventilation syndrome (low daytime Po_2) may also require supplemental oxygen, as well as PAP, for chronic treatment (171). The challenges of using supplemental oxygen with PAP are discussed.

Supplemental Oxygen and Positive Airway Pressure

During CPAP titration some patients will exhibit significant arterial oxygen desaturation despite what appears to be adequate airflow (73). This is more common during REM sleep and in patients who are obese or have abnormal awake arterial blood gases. Presumably, desaturation is present because of hypoventilation and/or ventilation–perfusion mismatch. Hypoventilation may be related to a fundamental abnormality of ventilatory control or neuromuscular/chest wall abnormality (including obesity) sometimes complicated by a persistently high upper-airway resistance. Hypoxemia persisting despite maintenance of upper-airway patency during sleep may also be associated with ventilation–perfusion mismatch due to underlying lung disease or low functional residual capacity (severe obesity). If hypoxemia persists despite apparently normal airflow, one can try the following interventions. CPAP can be increased to eliminate unrecognized residual high upper-airway resistance, CPAP can be changed to bilevel pressure to increase tidal volume, or supplemental oxygen can be added. As noted, certain patient groups are more likely to require supplemental oxygen as well as PAP. When adding supplemental oxygen, one must remember that high flow from the device will dilute the added oxygen. Thus, a patient with an adequate saturation on 2 L per minute of oxygen by nasal cannula when awake may require a higher oxygen flow on PAP. High flows [and low effective oxygen concentration (FiO_2)] are especially likely when there is a high degree of unintentional leak (mask and mouth). One must also remember that the intentional leak devices built into masks have fixed orifices. Increases in pressure will increase the intentional leak and possibly mask leak, and thus the total flow delivered (reduced effective concentration of oxygen). Thus, increases in pressure may require an increase in the flow of supplemental oxygen to maintain a satisfactory arterial oxygen saturation, in some cases.

POSITIVE AIRWAY PRESSURE FOR CENTRAL SLEEP APNEA

Central sleep apnea (CSA) syndrome is usually diagnosed when the majority of events are central in nature. The group is heterogeneous but can be classified according to the presence or absence of daytime hypercapnia (172). In the hypercapnic CSA syndrome (central hypoventilation, chest wall disease, neuromuscular disease) there may be discrete central apneas or simply nocturnal hypoventilation. The daytime elevation in $Paco_2$ worsens with sleep. In the past, negative-pressure ventilators (cuirass, body wrap) were frequently used. Unfortunately, obstructive apnea may occur with these devices, as upper-airway muscle contraction and ventilation assistance may not be synchronized. Today, nasal or full face mask bilevel PAP are more frequently used (173,174). The EPAP is adjusted to maintain upper-airway patency. Some patients may require a timed back-up rate (ST mode). In more severe cases, volume-cycled ventilation with mask or tracheostomy may be necessary.

▶ **TABLE 20-7.** Summary of Acute Treatment Study for Cheyne–Stokes Breathing—Central Sleep Apnea

	Acute Study				
	Control	*Oxygen*	*CPAP*	*Bilevel*	*ASV[a]*
AHI (/h)	44.5 ± 3.4	28.2 ± 3.4	26.8 ± 4.6	14.8 ± 2.3	6.3 ± 0.9
Treatment mean values and ranges ( )	—	2 lpm	9.25 (7.5–10) cm H_2O	IPAP (11–15) EPAP (5–6) Mean: IPAP–EPAP 13.5/5.3 cm H_2O Back-up rate 13–18/min	EPAP 4–6 IPAP–EPAP difference was 4–10 cm H_2O

[a] ASV, adaptive servo ventilation.
Adapted from Teschler H, Dohring J, Wang YM, et al. Adaptive pressure support servo-ventilation: a novel treatment for Cheyne–Stokes respiration in heart failure. *Amer J Respir Crit Care Med.* 2001;164:614–619 with permission.

Nonhypercapnic CSA includes Cheyne–Stokes breathing (CSB) and the idiopathic CSA syndrome. Both groups develop central apnea because the sleeping $Paco_2$ is below the apneic threshold ($Paco_2$ level triggering ventilation). CSB is the most common form of central sleep apnea (CSB–CSA). It occurs in 30% to 40% of patients with moderate to severe congestive heart failure (175–176). These patients have periods of central apnea or hypopnea alternating with hyperventilation in a crescendo–decrescendo pattern. Patients with CSB–CSA have lower daytime and nocturnal $Paco_2$ levels than patients with similar cardiac function, but without CSB. The lower $Paco_2$ levels are thought secondary to higher pulmonary capillary pressure (stimulation of J receptors). The lower the cardiac output, the longer the ventilatory phase between apneas. Patients with CSB–CSA may not complain of daytime sleepiness, but often complain of disturbed sleep and nocturnal dyspnea. The goals of treatment include improved sleep (reduced events, arousals, and desaturations), improved cardiac function (177), and increased survival (178). Treatment of CHF-associated CSB always begins with optimization of CHF treatment (beta blockers, ACE inhibitors, and diuretics). If CSB persists, successful treatment of CSB with both PAP (177) and oxygen (179) has been reported. Of note, CPAP titration may reduce events acutely but rarely to the low levels usually seen in OSA. One randomized trial of 3 months of CPAP treatment (177) found a reduction in the AHI (43.2 ± 4.9 per hour to 14.7 ± 4.8 per hour) and improvement in the ejection fraction ($21.2 \pm 3.8\%$ to $28.9 \pm 4.2\%$). Neither the AHI nor the ejection fraction improved in the control group. In this study, CPAP was started at 5 cm H_2O and increased slowly over several nights to a mean of 10.1 ± 0.5 cm H_2O. Of note, studies of shorter duration have not always shown a clear benefit with CPAP treatment. Another study suggested a benefit for transplant-free survival in patients with CHF and CSB–CSA who were treated with CPAP (178). A large multicenter trial is in progress to confirm this finding (180). In some patients, a reduction in CSB may occur only after several weeks of treatment. CPAP appears to work acutely by inducing a mild increase in $Paco_2$ and

improving oxygenation. Chronically, CPAP may improve CSB by improving cardiac function. A recent acute study (181) compared one night of oxygen, CPAP, bilevel PAP, and a new form of ventilation (adaptive servo-ventilation or ASV). ASV uses a fixed level of EPAP and a varying level of IPAP. The IPAP–EPAP difference increases during periods of low ventilation and decreases during periods of high ventilation. The bilevel PAP in this study included a back-up rate (spontaneous rate –2 breaths per minute). The results are shown in Table 20-7. Only treatment with ASV reduced the AHI to levels commonly seen with PAP treatment of OSA, although all improved CSB.

CSB–CSA can coexist with OSA. These patients often have mixed apneas with a long central portion. The nadir in desaturation following the mixed apneas is typically delayed because of an increased circulation time. During PAP titration, pure CSB–CSA often appears once pressure is high enough to eliminate the obstructive component. In Fig. 20-11, a tracing shows CSB on a CPAP of 8 cm H_2O. During the diagnostic portion of the study, mixed apneas were seen.

In summary, there is no consensus on the best way to treat CSB–CSA or to titrate PAP for this disorder. A reasonable approach is to increase pressure until obstruction is abolished. If further increases in pressure do not eliminate CSB, then a reasonable goal would be treatment with 10 to12 cm H_2O (or higher if needed to maintain airway patency). If persistent significant arterial oxygen desaturation secondary to central apneas persists on PAP, some physicians add oxygen as well.

PAP has also been used as a treatment for idiopathic CSA (182,183). This syndrome is diagnosed when a majority of events are central, but no disorder such as neurologic disease or CHF is present. These patients usually have a low daytime $Paco_2$ and increased ventilatory responses. The mechanism by which PAP decreases central apnea in these patients is unknown. In some patients upper-airway stabilization may prevent RERAs that are followed by hyperventilation and a central apnea on returning to sleep. In others, PAP may induce a mild increase in the $Paco_2$, which may stabilize ventilation. In one case report, CPAP helped but bilevel worsened events in patients with idiopathic CSA (184).

POSITIVE AIRWAY PRESSURE IN CHILDREN

Adenotonsillectomy is the most common treatment for OSA in children. This surgery is effective in the majority of cases. In cases where this treatment is not effective, where only minimal adenotonsillar tissue is present, if there are specific surgical contraindications, or for those who prefer nonsurgical alternatives, PAP has been used with success (185,186). Children with craniofacial malformations, severe obesity, and those with hypoventilation are the most frequent candidates for PAP. Older children generally tolerate PAP. Young children or older children with learning or behavioral problems may require desensitization or behavior techniques to accept this treatment. Letting children play with the mask, try it on during the day, and wear it for short periods of time for several days to a week prior to the initial titration is an important technique for improving acceptance. The involvement of a dedicated caregiver and close attention to adherence is essential. The side effects of PAP treatment are similar to those in adults. One case of midface hypoplasia has been reported (187). Therefore, chronic overtightening of the mask should be avoided and attention to facial development is required. As pressure requirements may change with growth, periodic assessment of pressure requirements is also prudent. Some centers use bilevel PAP rather than CPAP routinely in an attempt to improve acceptance. Use of bilevel PAP would definitely be preferred in patients with hypoventilation.

FUTURE CHALLENGES FOR POSITIVE AIRWAY PRESSURE TREATMENT

Not long ago, the sleep medicine community was called upon to demonstrate the clinical value of CPAP (132). During the subsequent years, data have accumulated that demonstrate objective and meaningful benefits conferred on noteworthy subsets of OSA patients in terms of quality of life, daily function, specific measures of performance, and physiologic measures of cardiovascular function and health. In addition, data have been provided demonstrating public health benefits reflected by reduced motor vehicle accidents (59,60). Untreated OSA in the community is associated with an increase health care burden (188). Much remains to be learned, however, regarding long-term outcomes of this therapy and, in a similar vein, optimal identification of those patients who are most likely to accrue health benefits. In considering the utility and future of PAP therapy, health care providers and administrators must consider the five "C's" of PAP:

1. **Compliance (aka Adherence).** The common dialog in which clinicians engage regarding patients with poor

versus adequate compliance might lead one to the erroneous conclusion that we know what constitutes acceptable utilization of PAP modalities. However, further reflection on the poorly understood nature of the relationship between sleep and function will lead to the conclusion that we are currently not in a position to precisely define a duration or frequency of usage that alleviates symptoms, normalizes function, and prevents poor outcome. For example, recent data suggest that the modest degrees of sleep restriction that are prevalent in society are associated with meaningful functional impairment (122). Thus, assuming little or no value in "sleep" without PAP (and this is by no means currently known), it may be inappropriate to accept 4 hours of PAP use as adequate. Before we can confidently demand a requisite usage of PAP by our patients, we must first ourselves obtain compelling, evidence-based information to support our recommendations and expectations. It is also essential to define the complex elements and interactions that determine whether an individual patient will use PAP in the prescribed manner. Only with knowledge of these factors can we identify patient-specific issues that promote suboptimal adherence and, having identified the problem, only then can we begin to develop a solution.

2. **and** 3. **Comfort and Convenience.** Anyone who has slept with a PAP device will recognize that it engenders encumbrance and inconvenience. It will probably never be as easy to put an interface on one's nose, mouth or both as it is to simply go to bed. It is nonetheless imperative that the technologies continue to improve to reduce the size and noise of devices, to reduce the burden on bed partners as well as patients. Similarly, the interfaces must continue to evolve in order to provide a wide range of choices for patients. It is likely that a positive attitude is important. This includes the health care provider as well as the patient and family. If the health care provider appears unconvinced of the merits of PAP, the patient is unlikely to be a believer and is, therefore, a poor risk for successful home therapy.

4. **Consequences.** Considerable information regarding the cardiovascular and neurocognitive consequences of OSA has become available in the last decade. We have begun to learn how PAP interacts with cardiovascular physiology but, at present, can only infer how this might translate into long-term outcomes. Such data, as well as those related to the long-term impact on relevant neurocognitive functions, are essential if we are to make a justifiable argument for CPAP therapy to many of our patients (especially those with minimal symptoms).

5. **Cost.** The issue of health care costs spans a wide spectrum of considerations. Certainly it is important to maintain the cost of PAP devices within a range of affordability. However, we must learn more about the health care costs of untreated OSA and the impact of PAP therapy. We must assess the cost savings if any, with regard to fewer hospitalizations, provider visits,

and productivity. It is important to continue to explore innovative ways to minimize the costs associated with diagnosing and managing OSA in a manner that will maximize utilization of resources and patient satisfaction.

REFERENCES

1. Sullivan CE, Issa FG, Berthon-Jones M, et al. Reversal of obstructive sleep apnoea by continuous positive airway pressure applied through the nares. *Lancet.* 1981;1:862–865.
2. Loube DI, Gay PC, Strohl KP, et al. Indications for positive airway pressure treatment of adult obstructive sleep apnea patients. A consensus statement. *Chest.* 1999;115:863–866.
3. ATS Statement. Indications and standards of use of nasal continuous positive airway pressure (CPAP) in sleep apnea syndromes. *Amer J Respir Crit Care Med.* 1994;150:1738–1745.
4. Strollo PJ Jr, Sanders MH, Atwood CW. Positive pressure therapy. *Clin Chest Med.* 1998;19:55–68.
5. Jenkinson C, Davies RJO, Mullins R, et al. Comparison of therapeutic and subtherapeutic nasal continuous positive airway pressure for obstructive sleep apnea: a randomized prospective parallel trial. *Lancet.* 1999;353:2100–2105.
6. Ballester E, Badia JR, Hernandex L, et al. Evidence of the effectiveness of continuous positive airway pressure in the treatment of sleep apnea/hypopnea syndrome. *Amer J Respir Crit Care Med.* 1999;159:495–501.
7. Engleman HM, Kingshott RN, Wraith PK, et al. Randomized placebo controlled crossover trial of continuous positive airway pressure for mild sleep apnea. *Amer J Respir Crit Care Med.* 1999;159:461–467.
8. Redline, Adams N, Strauss ME, et al. Improvement of mild sleep-disordered breathing with CPAP compared with conservative therapy. *Amer J Respir Crit Care Med.* 1998;157:858–865.
9. Barnes M, Houston D, Worsnop CJ, et al. A randomized controlled trial of continuous positive airway pressure in mild obstructive sleep apnea. *Amer J Resp Crit Care Med.* 2002;165:773–780.
10. Rosenthal L, Gerhardstein R, Lumley A, et al. CPAP therapy with mild OSA: Implementation and treatment outcome. *Sleep Med.* 2000;1:215–220.
11. Engleman HM, Martin SE, Deary IJ, et al. Effect of CPAP therapy on daytime function in patients with mild sleep apnoea/hypopnoea syndrome. *Thorax.* 1997;52:114–119.
12. Monasterio C, Vidal S, Duran J, et al. Effectiveness of continuous positive airway pressure in mild obstructive sleep apnea-hypopnea syndrome. *Amer J Respir Crit Care Med.* 2001;164:939–949.
13. Guilleminault C, Stoohs R, Clerk A, et al. A cause of excessive daytime sleepiness: the upper airway resistance syndrome. *Chest.* 1993;104:781–787.
14. Berry RB, Block AJ. Positive nasal airway pressure eliminated snoring as well as obstructive sleep apnea. *Chest.* 1984;85:15–20.
15. Rauscher H, Formanerk D, Zick A. Nasal continuous positive airway pressure for nonapneic snoring? *Chest.* 1995;107:58–61.
16. Sanders MH, Kern N. Obstructive sleep apnea treated by independently adjusted inspiratory and expiratory positive airway pressures via nasal mask. *Chest.* 1990;98:317–324.
17. Teschler H, Berthon-Jones M. Intelligent CPAP systems: clinical experience. *Thorax.* 1998;53:S49–S54.
18. Berry RB, Parish JM, Hartse KM. The use of auto-titrating CPAP for treatment of adults with obstructive sleep apnea. *Sleep.* 2002;25:148–173.
19. Littner M, Hirshkowitz M, Davila D, et al. Standards of practice committee of the American Academy of Sleep Medicine Practice parameters for the use of auto-titrating continuous positive airway pressure devices for titrating pressures and treating adult patients with obstructive sleep apnea syndrome. An American Academy of Sleep Medicine Report. *Sleep.* 2002;15;25:143–147.
20. Sanders MH. Nasal CPAP effect on patterns of sleep apnea. *Chest.* 1984;86:839–844.
21. Rapoport DM, Sorkin B, Garay SM, et al. Reversal of the "Pickwickian Syndrome" by long-term use of nocturnal nasal airway pressure. *N Engl J Med.* 1982;931–933.
22. Massie CA, Hart RW. Clinical outcomes related to interface type in patients with obstructive sleep apnea/hypopnea syndrome who are using continuous positive airway pressure. *Chest.* 2003;123:1112–1118.
23. Prosise GL, Berry RB. Oral-nasal continuous positive airway pressure as a treatment for obstructive sleep apnea. *Chest.* 1994;106:180–186.
24. Sanders MH, Kern NB, Stiller RA, et al. CPAP therapy via oronasal mask for obstructive sleep apnea. *Chest.* 1994;106:774–779.
25. Mortimore IL, Whittle AT, Douglas NJ. Comparison of nose and face mask CPAP therapy for sleep apnea. *Thorax.* 1998;53:290–292.
26. Smith PL, O'Donnell CP, Schwartz AL. A physiologic comparison of nasal and oral positive airway pressure. *Chest.* 2003;123:689–694.
27. Berry RB. Improving CPAP compliance. Man more than machine. *Sleep Med.* 2000;1:175–178.
28. Kuna ST, Bedi DG, Ryckman C. Effect of nasal airway positive pressure on upper airway size and configuration. *Amer Rev Respir Dis.* 1988;138:969–975.
29. Abbey NC, Block AJ, Green D, et al. Measurement of pharyngeal volume by digitized magnetic resonance imaging. Effect of nasal continuous positive airway pressure. *Amer Rev Respir Dis.* 1989;140:717–723.
30. Schwab RJ, Pack AI, Gupta KB, et al. Upper airway and soft tissue structural changes influences by CPAP in normal subjects. *Amer J Respir Crit Care Med* 1996;154:1106–1016.
31. Alex CG, Aronson RM, Onal E, et al. Effects of continuous positive airway pressure on upper airway and respiratory muscle activity. *J Appl Physiol.* 1987;62:2026–2030.
32. Strohl KP, Redline S. Nasal CPAP therapy, upper airway muscle activation and obstructive sleep apnea. *Amer Rev Respir Dis.* 1986;134:555–558.
33. Hoffstein V, Zamel N, Phillipson EA. Lung volume dependence of cross-sectional area in patients with obstructive sleep apnea. *Amer Rev Respir Dis.* 1984;130:175–178.
34. Van de Graaff WB. Thoracic influences on upper airway patency. *J Appl Physiol.* 1988;65:2124–2131.
35. Series F, Cormier Y, Lampron N, et al. Increasing functional residual capacity may reverse obstructive sleep apnea. *Sleep.* 1988;11:349–353.
36. Abbey NC, Cooper KR, Kwentus JA. Benefit of nasal CPAP in obstructive sleep apnea is due to positive pharyngeal pressure. *Sleep.* 1989;12:420–422.
37. Series F, Cormier Y, Couture J, et al. Changes in upper airway resistance with lung inflation and positive airway pressure. *J Appl Physiol.* 1990;68:1075–1079.
38. Mahadevia AK, Onal E, Lopata M. Effects of expiratory positive airway pressure on sleep-induced respiratory abnormalities in patients with hypersomnia sleep apnea syndrome. *Amer Rev Respir Dis.* 1983;128:708–711.
39. Reeves-Hoché. MK, Hudgel DW, Meck R, et al. Continuous versus bilevel positive airway pressure for obstructive sleep apnea. *Amer J Resp Crit Care Med.* 1995;151:443–449.
40. Resta O, Guido P, Picca V, et al. Prescription of nCPAP and nBIPAP in obstructive sleep apnea syndrome: Italian experience in 105 subjects. A prospective two centre study. *Respir Med.* 1998;92:820–827.
41. Schafer H, Ewig S, Hasper E, et al. Failure of CPAP therapy in obstructive sleep apnea syndrome: predictive factors and treatment with bilevel positive airway pressure. *Respir Med.* 1998;92:208–215.
42. Pevernagie DA, Sheard JW, Jr. Relations between sleep stage, posture and effective nasal CPAP levels in OSA. *Sleep.* 1992;15:162–167.
43. Oksenberg A, Silverberg DS, Arons E, et al. The sleep supine position has a major effect on optimal nasal continuous positive airway pressure. *Chest.* 1999;116:1000–1006.
44. Neill AM, Angus SM, Sajkov D, et al. Effects of sleep posture on upper airway stability in patients with obstructive sleep apnea. *Amer J Respir Crit Care Med.* 1997;155:199–204.
45. Loube DI. Technologic Advances in the treatment of obstructive sleep apnea syndrome. *Chest.* 1999;116:1426–1433.
46. Ficker JH, Wiest GH, Lehnert G, et al. Evaluation of an auto-CPAP device for treatment of obstructive sleep apnea. *Thorax.* 1998;53:643–648.
47. Lofaso F, Lorino AM, Duizabo D, et al. Evaluation of an auto-CPAP device based on snoring detection. *Eur Respir J.* 1996;9:1795–1800.

48. Lloberes P, Ballester E, Montserrat JM, et al. Comparison of manual and automatic CPAP titration in patients with sleep apnea/hypopnea syndrome. *Amer J Respir Crit Care Med.* 1996;154:1755–1758.

49. Randerath W, Parys K, Feldmeyer, et al. Self-adjusting continuous positive airway pressure therapy based on the measurement of impedance—A comparison of two different maximum pressure levels. *Chest.* 1999;116:991–999.

50. Stauffer JL, Fayter NA, MacLurg BJ. Conjunctivitis from nasal CPAP apparatus. *Chest.* 1984;86:802.

51. Fromm RE, Jr, Varon J, Lechin AE, et al. CPAP machine performance and altitude. *Chest.* 1995;108:1577–1580.

52. Kribbs NB, Pack AI, Kline LR, et al. Objective measurement of patterns of nasal CPAP use by patients with obstructive sleep apnea. *Amer J Resp Crit Care Med.* 1993;147:887–895.

53. Reeves-Hoche MK, Meck R, Zwillich CW. Nasal CPAP: an objective evaluation of patient compliance. *Amer J Respir Crit Care Med.* 1994;149:149–154.

54. Martins de Araujo MT, Vieira SB, et al. Heated humidification or face mask to prevent upper airway dryness during continuous positive airway pressure therapy. *Chest.* 2000;117:142–147.

55. Richards GN, Cistulli PA, Ungar RG, et al. Mouth leak with nasal continuous positive airway pressure increases nasal airway resistance. *Amer J Respir Crit Care Med.* 1996;154:182–186.

56. Massie CA, Hart RW, Peralez K, et al. Effects of humidification on nasal symptoms and compliance in sleep apnea patients using continuous positive airway pressure. *Chest.* 1999;116:403–408.

57. Wiest GH, Harsch IA, Fuchs FS, et al. Initiation of CPAP therapy for OSA: Does prophylactic humidification during CPAP titration improve initial patient acceptance and comfort? *Respiration.* 2002;69:406–412.

58. Pack AI, Maislin G. Who should get treated for sleep apnea? *Ann Intern Med.* 2001:134:1065–1066.

59. Cassel W, Ploch C, Becker D, et al. Risk of traffic accidents in patients with sleep disordered breathing: reduction with nasal CPAP. *Eur Respir J.* 1996;9:2602–2611.

60. George CF. Reduction in motor-vehicle collisions following treatment of sleep apnea with nasal CPAP. *Thorax.* 2001;56:508–512.

61. He J, Kryger MH, Zorick FJ, et al. Mortality and apnea index in obstructive sleep apnea. *Chest.* 1988;94:9–14.

62. Peppard PE, Young T, Palta M, et al. Prospective study of the association between sleep-disordered breathing and hypertension. *N Engl J Med.* 2000;342:1378–1384.

63. Peker Y, Hedner J, Norum J, et al. Increased incidence of cardiovascular disease in middle-aged men with obstructive sleep apnea: a 7-year follow-up. *Amer J Respir Crit Care Med.* 2002;166:159–165.

64. Nieto FJ, Young TB, Lind BK, et al. Association of sleep-disordered breathing, sleep apnea, and hypertension in a large community based study. Sleep Heart Health Study. *JAMA.* 2000;283:1829–1985.

65. Shahar E, Whitney CW, Redline S, et al. Sleep disordered breathing and cardiovascular disease: cross-sectional results of the Sleep Heart Health Study. *Amer J Resp Crit Care Med.* 2001;163:19–25.

66. Becker HF, Jerrentrup A, Ploch T, et al. JH. Effect of nasal continuous positive ariway pressure treatment on blood pressure in obstructive sleep apnea. *Circulation.* 2003;107:68–73.

67. Pepperell JCT, Ramdassingh-Dow S, Crosthwaite N, et al. Ambulatory blood pressure after therapeutic and subtherapeutic nasal continuous positive airway pressure for obstructive sleep apnea: a randomized parallel trial. *Lancet.* 2002;359:204–210.

68. Beninati W, Harris CD, Herold DL, et al. The effect of snoring and obstructive sleep apnea on sleep quality of bed partners. *Mayo Clin Proc.* 1999;74:955–958.

69. Barbe F, Mayoralas LR, Duran J, et al. Treatment with continuous positive airway pressure is not effective in patients with sleep apnea but no daytime sleepiness. *Ann Intern Med.* 2001;134:1015–1023.

70. Medicare Coverage Issues Manual. Centers for Medicare and Medicaid Services. Transmittal 151.60-17 Continuous Positive Airway Pressure (CPAP), January 14, 2002.

71. American Sleep Disorders Standard of Practice Committee, Chesson A. Chairman. Practice parameters for the indications for polysomnography and related procedures. *Sleep.* 1997;20:406–422.

72. American Thoracic Society. Indications and standards for use of nasal continuous positive airway pressure (CPAP) in sleep apnea syndromes. *Amer J Respir Crit Care Med.* 1994;50:1738–1745.

73. Krieger J. Weitzenblum E, Monassier JP, et al. Dangerous hypoxemia during continuous positive airway pressure treatment of obstructive sleep apnea. *Lancet.* 1983;2:1429–1430.

74. Berry RB. *Sleep medicine pearls, 2003,* Philadelphia: Hanley and Beflus, 2003;130–133.

75. Condos R, Norman RG, Krishnasamy I, et al. Flow limitation as a noninvasive assessment of residual upper-airway resistance during continuous positive airway pressure therapy of obstructive sleep apnea. *Amer J Respir Crit Care Med.* 1994;150:475–480.

76. Montserrat JM, Ballester E, Olivi H. Time course of stepwise CPAP titration. *Amer J Respir Crit Care Med.* 1995;152:1854–1859.

77. American Academy of Sleep Medicine Task Force. Sleep-Related breathing disorders in adults: recommendation for syndrome definition and measurement techniques in clinical research. *Sleep.* 1999;22:667–689.

78. Meurice JC, Paquereau J, Denjean A, et al. Influence of correction of flow limitation on continuous positive airway pressure efficiency in sleep apnea/hypopnea syndrome. *Eur Respir J.* 1998;11:1121–1127.

79. Sanders MH, Kern NB, Costantino JP, et al. Adequacy of prescribing positive airway pressure therapy by mask for sleep apnea on the basis of a partial-night trial. *Amer Rev Respir Dis.* 1993;147:1169–1174.

80. Iber C, O'Brien C, Schluter J, et al. Single night studies in obstructive sleep apnea. *Sleep.* 1991;14:383–385.

81. Fleury B, Rakotonanahary D, Tehindrazanarivelo AD, et al. Long-term compliance to continuous positive airway pressure therapy (nCPAP) setup during a split-night polysomnography. *Sleep.* 1994;17:512–515.

82. Yamashiro Y, Kryger MH. CPAP titration for sleep apnea using a split night protocol. *Chest.* 1995;107:62–66.

83. Gagnadoux F, Rakotonanahary D, Martins de Araujo MT, et al. Evaluation of an auto-CPAP device for treatment of obstructive sleep apnea. *Sleep.* 1999;22:1095–1097.

84. Teschler H, Berthon-Jones M, Thompson AB, et al. Automated continuous positive airway pressure titration for obstructive sleep apnea syndrome. *Amer J Resp Crit Care Med.* 1996;154:734–740.

85. Teschler H. Automatic nasal continuous positive airway pressure titration in the laboratory: patient outcomes. *Thorax.* 1997;52:72–75.

86. Series F. Accuracy of unattended home CPAP titration in the treatment of obstructive sleep apnea. *Amer J Resp Crit Care Med.* 2000;162:94–97.

87. Stradling J, Barbour C, Pitson DJ, et al. Automatic nasal CPAP in the laboratory; patient outcomes. *Thorax.* 1997;52:72–75.

88. Fletcher EC, Stich J, Yang KL. Unattended home diagnosis and treatment of obstructive sleep apnea without polysomnography. *Arch Fam Med.* 2000;9:168–174.

89. Hoffstein V, Mateika S. Predicting nasal continuous positive airway pressure. *Amer J Respir Crit Car Med.* 1994;150:486–488.

90. Miljeteig H, Hoffstein V. Determinants of continuous positive airway pressure for treatment of obstructive sleep apnea. *Amer Rev Respir Dis* 1993;147:1526–1530.

91. Fitzpatrick MF, Alloway CED, Wakeford TM, et al. Can patients with obstructive sleep apnea titrate their own continuous positive airway pressure? *Amer J Respir Crit Care Med.* 2003:167:716–722.

92. Mortimore IL, Kochhar P, Douglas NJ. Effect of chronic continuous positive airway pressure (CPAP) therapy on upper airway size in patients with sleep apnoea/hypopnea syndrome. *Thorax.* 1996;51:190–192.

93. Jokic R, Klimaszewski A, Sridhar G, et al. Continuous positive airway pressure requirement during the first month of treatment in patients with severe obstructive sleep apnea. *Chest.* 1998;114:1061–1069.

94. Teschler H, Farhat AA, Exner V, et al. AutoSet nasal CPAP titration: constancy of pressure, compliance and effectiveness at 8 month follow-up. *Eur Respir J.* 1997;10:2073–2078.

95. Schwartz AR, Gold AR, Schubert N, et al. Effect of weight loss on upper airway collapsibility in obstructive sleep apnea. *Amer Rev Respir Dis.* 1991;144:494–498.

96. Berry RB, Desa MM, Light RW. Effect of ethanol on the efficacy of nasal continuous positive airway pressure as a treatment for obstructive sleep apnea. *Chest.* 1991;99:339–343.

97. Teschler H, Berthon-Jones M, Wessendorf T, et al. Influence of moderate alcohol consumption on obstructive sleep apnoea with and

without AutoSet nasal CPAP therapy. *Eur Respir J.* 1996;9:2371–2377.

98. Berry RB, Bonnet MH, Light RW. Effect of ethanol on the arousal response to airway occlusion during sleep in normal subjects. *Amer Rev Respir Dis* 1992;145:445–490.

99. Meurice JC, Marc I, Carrier G, et al. Effects of mouth opening on upper airway collapsibility in normal sleeping subjects. *Amer J Resp Crit Care Med.* 1996;153:255–259.

100. Nino-Murcia G, McCann CC, Bliwise DL, et al. Compliance and side effects in sleep apnea patients treated with nasal continuous positive airway pressure. *West J Med.* 1989;150:165–169.

101. Waldhorn RE, Herrick TW, Nguyen MC, et al. Long term compliance with nasal continuous positive airway pressure therapy of obstructive sleep apnea. *Chest.* 1990;97:33–38.

102. Rolfe I, Olson LG, Sanders NA. Long-term acceptance of continuous positive airway pressure in obsructive sleep apnea. *Amer Rev Respir Dis* 1991;144:1130–1133.

103. Hoffstein V, Viner S, Mateika S, et al. Treatment of obstructive sleep apnea with nasal continuous positive airway pressure. Patient compliance, perception of benefits, and side effects. *Amer Rev Respir Dis.* 1992;145:841–845.

104. Engleman HM, Martin SE, Douglas NJ. Compliance with CPAP therapy in patients with the sleep apnea/hypopnea syndrome. *Thorax.* 1994;49:263–266.

105. Meslier N, Lebrun T, Grillier-Lanoir V, et al. A French survey of 3,225 patients treated with CPAP for obstructive sleep apnea: benefits, tolerance, compliance, and quality of life. *Eur Respir J.* 1998;12:185–192.

106. McArdle N, Devereux G, Heidarnejad H, et al. Long term use of CPAP therapy for sleep apnea/hypopnea syndrome. *Amer J Respir Crit Care Med.* 1999;159:1108–1114.

107. Sin DD, Mayers I, Man GCW, et al. Long-term compliance rate to continuous positive airway pressure in obstructive sleep apnea. *Chest.* 2002;121:430–435.

108. Pépin JL, Krieger J, Rodenstein D, et al. Effective compliance during the first 3 months of continuous positive airway pressure. A European prospective study of 121 patients. *Am J Respir Crit Care Med.* 1999;160:1124–1129.

109. Powell NB, Zonato AI, Weaver AM, et al. Radiofrequency treatment of turbinate hypertrophy in subjects using continuous positive airway pressure: a randomized, double-blind, placebo-controlled clinical pilot trial. *Laryngoscope.* 2001;111:1783–1790.

110. Friedman M, Tanyeri H, Lim JW, et al. Effect of improved nasal breathing on obstructive sleep apnea. *Otolaryngol Head Neck Surg.* 2000;122:71–74.

111. Mortimore IL, Bradley PA, Murray JA, et al. Uvulopharyngopalatoplasty may compromise nasal CPAP therapy in sleep apnea syndrome. *Amer J Respir Crit Care Med.* 1996;154:1759–1762.

112. Meurice JC, Marc I, Series F. Efficacy of auto-CPAP in the treatment of obstructive sleep apnea/hypopnea syndrome. *Amer J Respir Crit Care Med.* 1996;153:794–798.

113. Konermann M, Sanner BM, Vyleta M, et al. Use of conventional and self-adjusting nasal continuous positive airway pressure for treatment of severe obstructive sleep apnea syndrome. *Chest.* 1998;113:714–718.

114. Hudgel DW, Fung C. A long-term randomized, cross-over comparison of auto-titrating and standard nasal continuous positive airway pressure. *Sleep.* 2000;23:645–648.

115. d'Ortho PM, Grillier-Lanoir V, Levy P, et al. Constant vs automatic continuous positive airway pressure therapy. *Chest.* 2000;118:1010–1017.

116. Teschler H, Wessendorf TE, Farhat AA, et al. Two months autoadjusting versus conventional nCPAP for obstructive sleep apnoea syndrome. *Eur Resp J.* 2000;15:990–995.

117. Randerath WJ, Galetke W, David M, et al. Prospective randomized comparison of impedance-controlled auto-continuous positive airway pressure (APAPFoT) with constant CPAP. *Sleep Med.* 2001;2:115–124.

118. Series F, Marc I. Importance of sleep stage and body position dependence of sleep apnea in determining benefits to auto-CPAP therapy. *Eur Resp J.* 2001;18:170–175.

119. Massie CA, McArdle N, Hart RW, et al. Comparison between automatic and fixed positive airway pressure therapy in the home. *Amer J Respir Crit Care Med.* 2003;167:20–23.

120. Edinger JD, Radtke RA. Use of in vivo desensitization to treat a patient's claustrophic response to nasal CPAP. *Sleep.* 1993;16:678–680.

121. Engleman HM, Wild MR. Improving CPAP use by patients with the sleep apnea/hypopnea syndrome. *Sleep Med Rev.* 2003;7:81–99.

122. Dinges DF, Pack F, Williams K, et al. Cumulative sleepiness, mood disturbance, and psychomotor vigilance performance decrements during a week of sleep restricted to 4-5 hours per night. *Sleep.* 1997;20:276–277.

123. Rauscher H, Popp W, Wanke T, et al. Acceptance of CPAP therapy for sleep apnea. *Chest.* 1991;100;1019–1023.

124. Meurice JC, Dore P, Paquereau J, et al. Predictive Factors of long-term compliance with nasal continuous positive airway pressure treatment in sleep apnea syndrome. *Chest.* 1994;105:429–433.

125. Hoy CJ, Vennelle M, Kingshott RN, et al. Can intensive support improve continuous positive airway pressure use in patients with the sleep apnea/hypopnea syndrome? *Amer J Respir Crit Care Med.* 1999;159:1096–1100.

126. Janson C, Noges E, Svedberg-Brandt S, et al. What characterizes patients who are unable to tolerate continuous positive airway pressure (CPAP) treatment? *Respir Med.* 2000;94:145–149.

127. Stepnowsky CJ, Bardwell WA, Moore PJ, et al. Physiologic coorelates of compliance with continuous positive airway pressure. *Sleep.* 2002 25:758–762.

128. Weaver TE, Kribbs NB, Pack AI, et al. Night to night variability in CPAP use over the first three months of treatment. *Sleep.* 1997;20:278–283.

129. Likar LL, Panciera TM, Erickson AD, et al. Group education sessions and compliance with nasal CPAP therapy. *Chest.* 1997;111:1273–1277.

130. Chervin RD, Theut S, Bassetti C, et al. Compliance of nasal CPAP can be improved by simple interventions. *Sleep.* 1997;20:284–289.

131. Rajagopal KR, Bennet LL, Dillard TA, et al. Overnight nasal CPAP improves hypersomnolence in sleep apnea. *Chest.* 1986;90:172–176.

132. Wright J, Johns R, Wart I, et al. Health effects of obstructive sleep apnoea and the effectiveness of continuous positive airways pressure: a systematic review of the research evidence. *BMJ.* 1997;314:851–860.

133. Johns MW. A new method for measuring daytime sleepiness: the Epworth Sleepiness Scale. *Sleep.* 1991;14:540–545.

134. Hardinge FM, Pitson DJ, Stradling JR. Use of the Epworth Sleepiness Scale to demonstrate response to treatment for nasal continuous positive airway pressure in patients with obstructive sleep apnea. *Respir Med.* 1995;89:617–620.

135. Poceta JS, Timms RM, Jeong D, et al. Maintenance of wakefulness test in obstructive sleep apnea syndrome. *Chest.* 1992;101:893–897.

136. Henke KG, Grady JJ, Kuna ST. Effect of nasal continuous positive airway pressure on neuropsychological function in sleep apnea-hypopnea syndrome. A randomized, placebo-controlled trial. *Amer J Respir Crit Care Med.* 2001;163:911–917.

137. Meurice JC, Paquereau J, Neau JP, et al. Long-term evolution of daytimes somnolence in patients with sleep apnea/hypopnea syndrome treated by continuous positive airway pressure. *Sleep.* 1997;20:1162–1166.

138. Sin DD, Mayers I, Man GC, et al. Can continuous positive airway pressure therapy improve the general health status of patients with obstructive sleep apnea? A clinical effectiveness study. *Chest.* 2002;122:1679–1685.

139. Akashiba T, Minemura H, Yamamoto H, et al. Nasal continuous positive airway pressure changes blood pressure "non-dippers" to "dippers" in patients with obstructive sleep apnea. *Sleep.* 1999;22:849–853.

140. Hla KM, Skatrud JB, Finn L, et al. The effect of sleep-disordered breathing on BP in untreated hypertension. *Chest.* 2002;122:1125–1132.

141. Faccenda JF, MacKay TW, Boon NA, et al. Randomized placebo-controlled trial of continuous positive airway pressure on blood pressure in the sleep apnea-hypopnea syndrome. *Amer J Resp Crit Care Med.* 2001;163:344–348.

142. Dimsdale JE, Loredo JS, Profant J. Effect of continuous positive airway pressure on blood pressure: a placebo trial. *Hypertension.* 2000;35:144–147.

143. Engleman HM, Gough K, Martin SE, et al. Ambulatory blood

pressure on and off continuous positive airway pressure therapy for the sleep apnea/hypopnea syndrome: Effects in "non-dippers." *Sleep.* 1996;19:378–381.

144. Weitzenblum E, Krieger J, Apprill M, et al. Daytime pulmonary hypertension in patients with obstructive sleep apnea syndrome. *Amer Rev Respir Dis.* 1988;138:345–349.

145. Sajkov D, Cowie RJ, Thornton AT, et al. Pulmonary hypertension and hypoxemia in obstructive sleep apnea syndrome. *Amer J Respir Crit Care Med.* 1994;149:416–422.

146. Chaouat A, Weitzenblum E, Kessler R, et al. Five-year effects of nasal continuous positive airway pressure in obstructive sleep apnoea syndrome. *Eur Respir J.* 1997;10:2578–2582.

147. Sajkov D, Wang T, Saunders NA, et al. Continuous positive airway pressure treatment improves pulmonary hemodynamics in patients with obstructive sleep apnea. *Amer J Respir Crit Care Med.* 2002;165:152–158.

148. Hedner J, Darpo B, Ejnell H, et al. Reduction in sympathetic activity after long-term CPAP treatment in sleep apnoea: cardiovascular implications. *Eur Respir J.* 1995;8:222–229.

149. Waradekar NV, Sinoway LI, Zwillich CW, et al. Influence of treatment on muscle sympathetic nerve activity in sleep apnea. *Amer J Respir Crit Care Med.* 1996;153:1333–1338.

150. Narkiewicz K, Kato M, Phillips BG, et al. Nocturnal continuous positive airway pressure decreases daytime sympathetic traffic in obstructive sleep apnea. *Circulation.* 1999;100:2332–2335.

151. Khoo MCK, Belozeroff V, Berry RB, et al. Cardiac autonomic control in obstructive sleep apnea: effects of long term CPAP therapy. *Amer J Resp Crit Care Med.* 2001;164:807–812.

152. Kreiger J, Sforza E, Barthelmebs M, et al. Overnight decreases in hematocrit after nasal CPAP with patients with OSA. *Chest.* 1990;97:729–730.

153. Chin K, Ohi M, Kita H, et al. Effects of NCPAP therapy on fibrinogen levels in obstructive sleep apnea syndrome. *Amer J Respir Crit Care Med.* 1996;153:1972–1976.

154. Lavie L, Kraiczi H, Hefetz A, et al. Plasma vascular endothelial growth factor in sleep apnea syndrome: effects of nasal continuous positive air pressure treatment. *Amer J Respir Crit Care Med.* 2002;165(12):1624–1628.

155. Dyugovskaya L, Lavie P, Lavie L. Increased adhesion molecules expression and production of reactive oxygen species in leukocytes of sleep apnea patients. *Amer J Respir Crit Care Med.* 2002;165:934–939.

156. Schulz R, Mahmoudi S, Hattar K, et al. Enhanced release of superoxide from polymorphonuclear neutrophils in obstructive sleep apnea. Impact of continuous positive airway pressure therapy. *Amer J Respir Crit Care Med.* 2000;162:566–570.

157. Bokinsky G, Miller M, Ault K, et al. Spontaneous platelet activation and aggregation during obstructive sleep apnea and its response to therapy with nasal continuous positive airway pressure. A preliminary investigation. *Chest.* 1995;108(3):625–630.

158. Shamsuzzaman AS, Winnicki M, Lanfranchi P, et al. Elevated C-reactive protein in patients with obstructive sleep apnea. *Circulation.* 2002;105:2462–2464.

159. Yokoe T, Minoguchi K, Matsuo H, et al. Elevated levels of C-reactive protein and interleukin-6 in patients with obstructive sleep apnea syndrome are decreased by nasal continuous positive airway pressure. *Circulation.* 2003;107(8):1129–1134.

160. Krieger J, Follenius M, Sforza E, et al. Effects of treatment with nasal continuous positive airway pressure on atrial naturetic peptide and arginine vasopressin release during sleep in patients with sleep apnea. *Clin Sci. (London).* 1991;80:443–449.

161. Shimizu K, Chin K, Nakamura T, et al. Plasma leptin levels and cardiac sympathetic function in patients with obstructive sleep apnoea-hypopnoea syndrome. *Thorax.* 2002;57:429–434.

162. Malone S, Liu PP, Holloway R, et al. Obstructive sleep apnea in patients with dilated cardiomyopathy: effects of continuous positive airway pressure. *Lancet.* 1991;338:1480–1484.

163. Kaneko Y, Floras JS, Kengo U, et al. Cardiovascular effects of continuous positive airway pressure in patients with heart failure and obstructive sleep apnea. *N Engl J Med.* 2003;348:1233–1241.

164. Bradley TD, Rutherford R, Lue F, et al. Role of diffuse airway obstruction in the hypercapnia of obstructive sleep apnea. *Amer Rev Respir Dis.* 1986;134:920–924.

165. Sanders MH, Newman AB, Haggerty CL, et al. Sleep Heart Health Study. Sleep and sleep-disordered breathing in adults with predominantly mild obstructive lung disease. *Amer J Resp Crit Care Med.* 2003;167:7–14.

166. Sullivan CE, Berthon-Jones M, Issa FG. Remission of severe obesity-hypoventilation syndrome after short-term treatment during sleep with nasal continuous positive airway pressure. *Amer Rev Respir Dis.* 1983;128:177–181.

167. Berthon-Jones M, Sullivan CE. Time course of change in ventilatory response to CO2 with long-term CPAP therapy for obstructive sleep apnea. *Amer Rev Respir Dis.* 1987;135:144–147.

168. Rapoport DM, Garay SM, Epstein H, et al. Hypercapnia in the obstructive sleep apnea syndrome. *Chest.* 1986;89:627–635.

169. Shivaram U, Cash ME, Beal A. Nasal continuous positive airway pressure in decompensated hypercapnic respiratory failure as a complication of sleep apnea. *Chest.* 1993;104:770–774.

170. Piper AJ, Sullivan CE. Effects of short-term NIPPV in the treatment of patients with severe obstructive sleep apnea and hypercapnia. *Chest.* 1994;105:434–440.

171. Sampol G, Sagalés MT, Roca A, et al. Nasal continuous positive airway pressure with supplemental oxygen in coexistent sleep apnea-hypopnea syndrome and severe chronic obstructive pulmonary disease. *Eur Respir J.* 1996;9:111–116.

172. Bradley TD, McNicholas WT, Rutherford R, et al. Clinical and physiologic heterogeneity of the central sleep apnea syndrome. *Amer Rev Respir Dis.* 1986;134:217–221.

173. Hill NW, Eveloff SE, Carlisle CC, et al. Efficacy of nocturnal nasal ventilation in patients with restrictive thoracic disease.

174. Claman DM, Piper A, Sanders M. Nocturnal noninvasive positive pressure ventilatory assistance. *Chest.* 1996;110:1581–1588.

175. Sin DD, Fitzgerald F, Parker JD, et al. Risk factors for central and obstructive sleep apnea in 450 men and women with congestive heart failure. *Amer J Respir Crit Care Med.* 1999;160:1101–1106.

176. Javaheri S, Parker TJ, Wexler L, et al. Occult sleep-disordered breathing in stable congestive heart failure. *Ann Intern Med.* 1995;122(7):487–492.

177. Naughton MT, Liu PP, Bernard DC, et al. Treatment of congestive heart failure and Cheyne–Stokes respiration during sleep by continuous positive airway pressure. *Amer J Respir Crit Care Med.* 1995;151:92–97.

178. Sin DD, Logan AG, Fitzgerald FS, et al. Effects of continuous positive airway pressure on cardiovascular outcomes in heart failure patients with and without Cheyne–Stokes respiration. *Circulation.* 2000;102:61–66.

179. Hanly PJ, Millar TW, Steljes DG, et al. The effect of oxygen on respiration and sleep in patients with congestive heart failure. *Ann Int Med.* 1989;111:777–782.

180. Bradley TD, Logan AG, Floras JS. CANPAP Investigators. Rationale and design of the Canadian continuous positive airway pressure trial for congestive heart failure patients with central sleep apnea–CANPAP. *Can J Cardiol.* 2001;17:677–684.

181. Teschler H, Dohring J, Wang YM, et al. Adaptive pressure support servoventilation: a novel treatment for Cheyne-Stokes respiration in heart failure. *Amer J Respir Crit Care Med.* 2001;164:614–619.

182. Issa FG, Sullivan CE. Reversal of central sleep apnea using nasal CPAP. *Chest.* 1986;90:165–171.

183. Hoffstein V, Slutsky AS. Central sleep apnea reversed by continuous positive airway pressure. *Amer Rev Respir Dis.* 1987;135:12101–12212.

184. Hommura F, Nishimura M, Oguri M, et al. Continuous versus bilevel positive airway pressure in a patient with idiopathic central sleep apnea. *Amer J Respir Crit Care Med.* 1997;155:1482–1485.

185. Marcus CL, Ward SL, Mallory GB, et al. Use of nasal continuous positive airway pressure as treatment of childhood obstructive sleep apnea. *J Pediatr.* 1995:127:88–94.

186. American Academy of Pediatrics. Clinical practice guideline: Diagnosis and management of childhood obstructive sleep apnea syndrome.

187. Li KK, Riley RW, Guilleminault C. An unreported risk in the use of home nasal continuous positive airway pressure and home nasal ventilation in children: mid-face hypoplasia. *Chest.* 2000;117:916–918.

188. Ronald J, Delaive K, Roos L, et al. Health care utilization in the 10 years prior to diagnosis in obstructive sleep apnea patients. *Sleep.* 1999;22:225–229.

Chapter 21

Obstructive Sleep Apnea: Surgical Treatment

Kasey K. Li

The exact etiologic factors of obstructive sleep apnea syndrome (OSA) have not been clearly elicited. However, it is well recognized that disproportionate anatomy of the upper airway exists in OSA, leading to obstruction during sleep (1,2). Although continuous positive airway pressure (CPAP) is the current mainstay of treatment, there are clear limitations with its use. Patient compliance remains a major problem and the long-term use of CPAP is an unrealistic expectation for many patients (3–5). Surgery has always played an integral part in the management of OSA. In fact, the first treatment of OSA was the use of tracheostomy to bypass upper-airway obstruction in "Pickwickian" patients (6). Although tracheotomy remains the most successful surgical treatment, patient acceptance is extremely low due to the associated morbidity and social implications.

In 1979, Fijita et al. (7) reported the use of uvulopalatopharyngoplasty (UPPP) for the treatment of OSA. Although the procedure has proved to be an excellent method for improving the oropharyngeal airway obstruction, only approximately 40% of patients respond successfully to this procedure (8). The lack of success is primarily due to other untreated sites of obstruction in the airway. There are potentially three major regions of obstruction: the nose, palate (oropharynx) and tongue base (hypopharynx). In addition, the lateral pharyngeal wall has been increasingly recognized as one of the major factors in upper airway collapse (9). Certain craniofacial features identified by cephalometric analysis have also been suggested as risk factors (10,11). In the early 1980s, several investigators reported that mandibular deficiency contributed to the development of OSA. With the increased recognition that hypopharyngeal airway obstruction is a major contributing factor of OSA, genioglossus and hyoid advancement were later developed to improve treatment outcomes (12,13). Subsequently, mandibular advancement by surgical means has been shown to improve airway obstruction (14,15). To maximize the extent of mandibular advancement, concurrent maxillary advancement was subsequently advocated (16). Today, many surgical procedures have been developed to expand the airway and/or to reduce the collapsibility of the airway (Table 21-1).

Despite the availability of numerous surgical procedures for the treatment of OSA, proper selection of the procedure(s) that would be the most beneficial for an individual patient remains difficult. Moreover, the complex interplay of the soft and hard tissues that contributes to upper-airway obstruction, the crucial role of this anatomic region to speech and swallowing, as well as the subsequent

▶ **TABLE 21-1.** **Common Obstructive Sleep Apnea Surgical Procedures**

Bypass all upper airway obstructions
Tracheotomy

Selectively improve upper-airway obstruction:
Nasal reconstruction
Uvulopalatopharyngoplasty
Laser-assisted uvulopalatoplasty
Uvulopalatal flap
Genioglossus advancement
Hyoid advancement
Maxillomandibular advancement
Temperature-controlled radiofrequency (RF) tongue base reduction

edematous response after surgical intervention present a formidable challenge to the sleep surgeon. Therefore, a logical and systematic approach to clinical evaluation, treatment planning, surgical execution, and perioperative management is necessary to maximize safety and improve outcomes.

CLINICAL EVALUATION

Clinical evaluation must include the overall body habitus (height, weight, and neck circumference), since it has been shown that the surgical outcomes can be influenced by these factors (17). Obviously, a detailed examination should be focused in the head and neck region to identify the potential sites of upper-airway obstruction, including the nose, soft palate, lateral pharyngeal walls, and tongue base. The presence of nasal septal deviation, turbinate hypertrophy, nasal valve collapse, elongation of the soft palate/uvula, tonsillar hypertrophy, enlargement of the tongue, and narrowing of the maxilla/mandible or mandibular/midface deficiency (small or hypoplastic) are many of the common findings in patients with OSA.

Fiberoptic Nasopharyngolaryngoscopy

Airway examination by a fiberoptic scope is highly recommended in patients with OSA. This evaluation enables the examiner to directly visualize the entire upper airway from the nose to the larynx. The dimension of the nasal, retropalatal, and retroglossal airway can be fully assessed. Furthermore, the prominence of the tongue base and the lateral pharyngeal wall and the pattern of obstruction, as well as their collapsibility, can be evaluated with the Muller's maneuver (Fig. 21-1) (18).

Lateral Cephalometric Radiograph

Many airway imaging methods are currently available. Computed tomography (CT) or magnetic resonance (MR)

can precisely assess the dimension of the upper airway (9,19). However, due to cost constraints, none can be widely used in clinical practice, except the lateral cephalometric radiograph. Although lateral cephalometric radiograph is only a static two-dimensional method of evaluating a dynamic three-dimensional area, it is a valuable study to identify abnormal facial skeletal anatomy that may contribute to airway obstruction, as well as the relation of the hard and soft tissues of the airway (Fig. 21-2). Furthermore, lateral cephalometric radiograph provides useful information on the posterior airway space behind the soft palate and the tongue base. The posterior airway space measurement on lateral cephalometric radiograph has been shown to correlate with the volume of hypopharyngeal airway on three-dimensional CT scans (20).

SURGICAL PLANNING

Since multiple sites of obstruction can be involved in OSA, surgical intervention must take place at different levels. Therefore, individual procedures for specific area(s) of obstruction have been developed. The ultimate goal of surgical management is to improve the entire upper airway, achieving total upper-airway reconstruction. Consequently, the identification of the sites of obstruction based on clinical examination, fiberoptic nasopharyngoscopy, and lateral cephalometric radiographs is essential for proper surgical planning.

OVERVIEW OF SURGICAL PROCEDURES

Tracheostomy

As stated earlier, tracheotomy is the first surgical treatment for OSA (6). Tracheotomy differs from all other surgical interventions for OSA because it bypasses the entire upper airway, thus achieving a success rate that is unsurpassed by any other procedures. However, due to poor patient acceptance, it is now performed only in patients with severe OSA when nasal continuous positive airway pressure (CPAP)/bilevel positive airway pressure (BPAP) or other surgical treatments have failed, or as a temporary measure for airway protection while the patient is undergoing other airway reconstructive procedures.

Nasal Reconstruction

The patency of the nasal airway is important for normal respiration; furthermore, nasal obstruction has been implicated in OSA (21). Nasal obstruction during sleep may result in increased oral breathing and mouth opening, thus leading to airway obstruction due to rotation of the

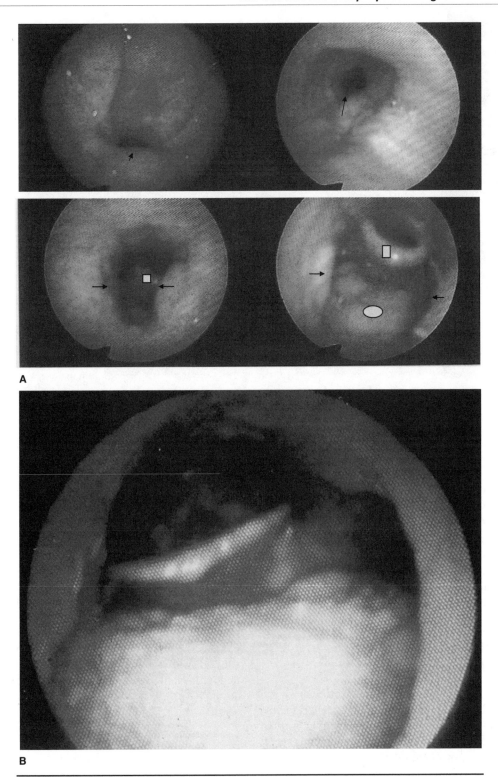

FIGURE 21-1. (A) Fiberoptic view of the upper airway. Upper left and right views showing significant narrowing of the retropaloatal airway (arrows demonstrate the soft palate). Lower left and right views showing hypertrophic tonsillar tissues obstructing the hypopharyngeal airway, the prominent tongue base, and retrodisplacement of the epiglottis (square demonstrates the epiglottis; oval demonstrates the tonguebase; arrows demonstrate the tonsils). (B) Fiberoptic view of the hypopharyngeal airway during passive respiration.

(continued)

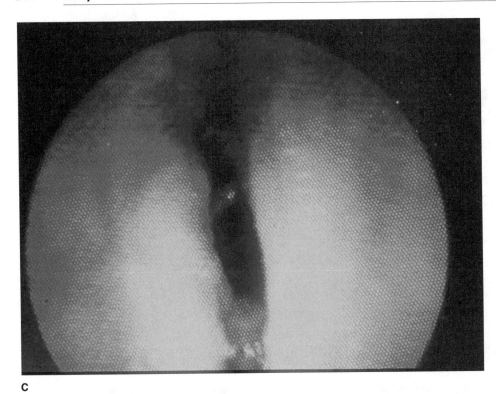

c

FIGURE 21-1. (*continued*) (C) Fiberoptic view of the hypopharyngeal airway during Muller's maneuver (note the significant lateral wall collapse).

mandible and retrodisplacement of the tongue base back to the pharynx. Nasal obstruction may also inhibit the optimal use of nasal CPAP. Therefore, the use of nasal surgery to improve nasal CPAP use should be considered. Three anatomic areas of the nose that require examination are the alar cartilage/nasal valve region, the septum, and the turbinates (Table 21-2). One of the least invasive procedures to improve nasal breathing has been the use of temperature-controlled radiofrequency energy to reduce hypertrophic turbinates (22). This technique alone may potentially improve nasal CPAP use.

Oropharyngeal Reconstruction

Uvulopalatopharyngoplasty (UPPP)

Popularized by Fijita (7), UPPP improves oropharyngeal obstruction (Table 21-3). This procedure was originally thought to be an alternative to tracheotomy in OSA. It is easily performed under general anesthesia and consists of the removal of a portion of the soft palate, uvula, and a limited amount of the lateral pharyngeal wall (Fig. 21-3). The

tonsillar tissues are also removed if present. The temptation to improve results by removing an excessive amount of the tissues should be resisted because the potential complications will dramatically increase. Since UPPP only addresses the oropharyngeal obstruction, its success rate is only approximately 40% (8).

Uvulopalatal Flap (UPF)

The uvulopalatal flap (UPF) is a modification of the UPPP (Fig. 21-4) (23). The goal of the modification is to reduce the potential complications of UPPP, including nasopharyngeal incompetence, nasopharyngeal stenosis, and dysphagia. The procedure involves the retraction of the uvula superiorly toward the hard-soft palate junction after a limited removal of the uvula, lateral pharyngeal wall, and mucosa. This results in widening of the oropharyngeal airway.

Laser-assisted Uvulopalatoplasty (LAUP)

LAUP was introduced by Kamimi as an office-based surgical procedure for the treatment of snoring (24). The

▶ **TABLE 21-2. Considerations for Nasal Reconstruction**

Nasal valve dysfunction
Nasal septal deviations
Turbinate hypertrophy – refractory to medical management

▶ **TABLE 21-3. Considerations for UPPP/UPF**

Long soft palate
Redundant lateral pharyngeal wall
Excess tonsillar tissues

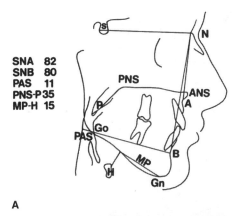

SNA 82
SNB 80
PAS 11
PNS-P 35
MP-H 15

A

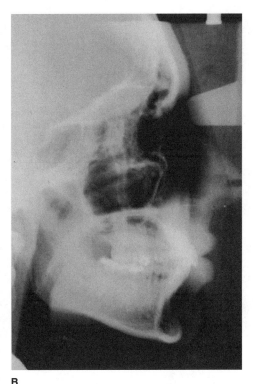

B

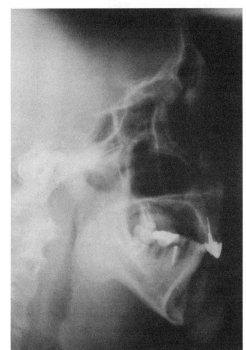

C

FIGURE 21-2. (A) Cephalometric analysis used for evaluation of patients with OSAS. SNA 82° (SD ± 2), maxilla to cranial base; SNB 80° (SD ± 2), mandible to cranial base; PAS 11 mm (SD ± 1), posterior airway space; PNS-P 37 mm (SD ± 3), length of soft palate; MP-H 15.4 mm (SD ± 3), distance of hyoid from inferior mandible. (B) Normal cephalometric radiograph. (C) Abnormal cephalometric radiograph. Note the mandibular deficiency, elongated soft palate, and the decreased posterior airway space.

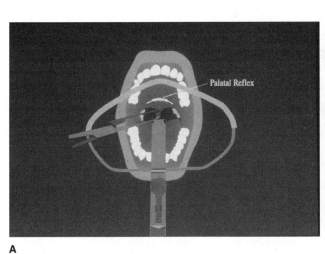

A

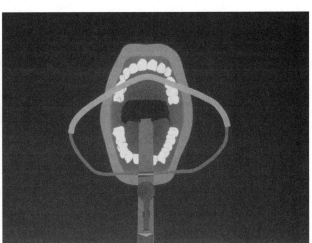

B

FIGURE 21-3. (A) The uvulopalatopharyngoplasty (UPPP) technique. Redundant soft palate and tonsillar tissues are being removed. (B) The completed UPPP.

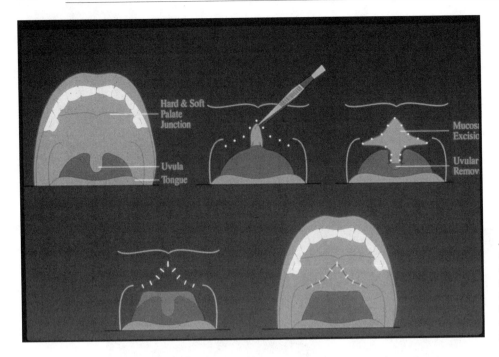

FIGURE 21-4. The reversible uvulopalatal flap (UPF) technique. The uvula is retracted superiorly to identify mucosal crease of muscular sling. The mucosa on proposed flap site is removed and the wound is sutured.

procedure involves removal of the uvula and a portion of the soft palate by carbon dioxide laser incisions and vaporization. Most of the uvula is amputated and the soft palate, 1 to 2 cm lateral to the uvula, is incised and vaporized. In addition, mucosal or tonsillar pillar tissue is vaporized as needed.

Although many studies have evaluated the efficacy of LAUP in the treatment of OSA, most of the studies are flawed by methodologic discrepancies or statistical inadequacies, such as ill-defined criteria for response and lack of adequate follow-up. A recent American Academy of Medicine paratice parameter paper stated that there was insufficient efficacy to recommend the LAUP in the treatment of OSA (25).

Hypopharyngeal Reconstruction

Genioglossus Advancement (GA)

The tongue and the lateral pharyngeal wall can significantly obstruct the airway during sleep. Genioglossus advancement was the first procedure to specifically address tongue obstruction in OSA (Table 21-4) (12). The initial rationale for this surgical approach was based on the findings that patients with OSAS have decreased posterior airway space and increased distance between the mandible and the hyoid. These measurements, along with the polysomnographic data, have been shown to improve after surgery. With increasing understanding that the genioglossus muscle plays an important role in nocturnal airway obstruction (26,27), an improved incorporation of the genioglossus muscle in the advanced portion of the

mandible was developed (28). GA does not alter the shape of the mandible, but only brings the attachment of the genioglossus forward. This advancement places tension on the tongue musculature, thus limiting the posterior displacement during sleep. The current GA procedure is performed completely intraorally. The mucosal incision is made just below the mucogingival junction and a subperiosteal flap is reflected to expose the anterior mandible and mental nerves. The genial tubercle and genioglossus muscle can be identified by finger palpation in the floor of the mouth and with the aid of the lateral cephalometric radiograph. A rectangular osteotomy is made to incorporate the geniotubercle. The geniotubercle is advanced and partially rotated to prevent retraction back into the floor of the mouth (Fig. 21-5).

Hyoid Advancement (HA)

The rationale for altering the hyoid position for the treatment of tongue base obstruction is that anatomically, the

▌ **TABLE 21-4. Considerations for Genioglossus/
Hyoid Advancement**

Evidence of hypopharyngeal obstruction
Macroglossia
Mandibular deficiency/microgenia
Tongue base prominence on fiberoptic nasopharyngoscopy
Retrodisplacement of epiglottis on fiberoptic nasopharyngoscopy
Reduced posterior airway space (<10 mm) by cephalometrics
Increased mandible–hyoid distance (>20 mm) by cephalometrics

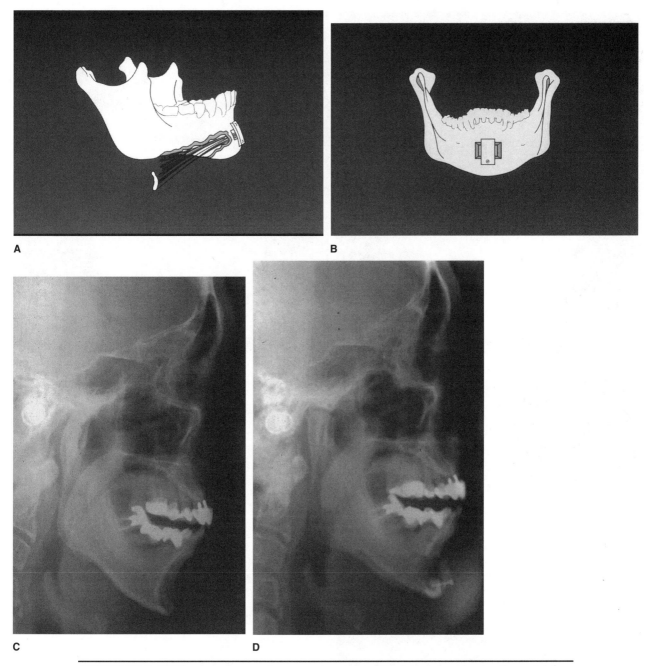

A

B

C

D

FIGURE 21-5. (A) The genioglossus advancement procedure. The lateral view showing the geniotubercle advanced anteriorly. (B) The anterior view showing the advanced geniotubercle rotated to allow bony overlap, and immobilized with a titanium screw. (C) Lateral cephalometric radiograph demonstrating obstruction of the upper airway. (D) Lateral cephalometric radiograph demonstrating improvement of the obstruction after genioglossus advancement.

hyoid complex is an integral part of the hypopharynx. Anterior movement of the hyoid complex improves the posterior airway space and numerous reports have supported the concept that surgical intervention at the hyoid level improves the hypopharyngeal airway (Table 21-4) (29,30). Initially, HA was routinely performed with GA for hypopharyngeal reconstruction (13). Currently, HA is not always performed simultaneously with GA. This is due to the fact that many patients with OSA have diffuse airway obstruc-

tion, and GA is generally combined with UPPP/UPF. The added insult to the infrahyoid region by combining the GA and HA may result in increased edema, which may increase the risk of postoperative airway compromise. We have also found that the hypopharyngeal airway obstruction is resolved with only GA in some patients, thus an HA may not always be necessary. Furthermore, in some elderly patients (>60 years old), airway edema following simultaneous GA and HA can result in prolonged

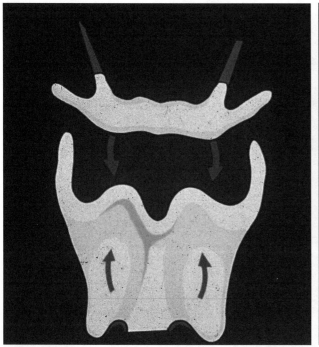

A

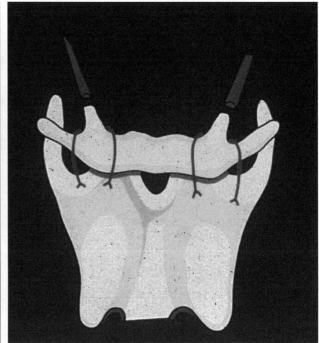

B

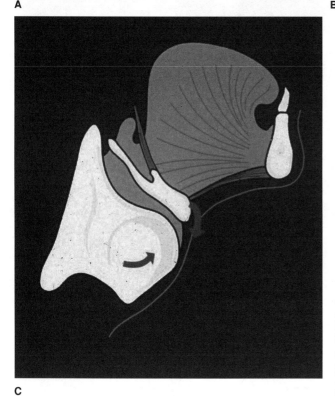

C

FIGURE 21-6. (A) The hyoid advancement procedure. The hyoid bone is isolated, and the inferior body dissected clean. The majority of the suprahyoid musculature remains intact. (B) The hyoid is advanced over the thyroid lamina and immobilized with sutures placed through the superior aspect of the thyroid cartilage. (C) Lateral view of the hyoid advancement showing the advancement of the hyoid bone.

dysphagia that may require days to recover. For these reasons we perform HA in some patients only as a separate surgical step. The original description of the HA involves suspending the hyoid to the anterior mandible. The technique has subsequently been modified and currently involves suspension of the hyoid to the superior thyroid cartilage (Fig. 21-6) (31). The current procedure still improves the hypopharyngeal airway but is less invasive (31).

The surgical approach is through a horizontal skin incision above the hyoid bone. The dissection is carried inferiorly along the suprahyoid musculature to the body of the hyoid. The body of the hyoid is isolated, which involves removing the infrahyoid muscles from the body of the hyoid. The suprahyoid muscles are left intact. If the hyoid lacks mobility, the stylohyoid ligament is amputated from the lesser cornu. The hyoid is suspended anteriorly to the superior thyroid cartilage with four permanent sutures.

Maxillomandibular Advancement (MMA)

As stated earlier, the contributing causes that lead to OSA are multifactorial. However, maxillofacial abnormality is a well-recognized predictor of OSA (10,11,32,33). MMA was initially advocated based on the finding that maxillofacial skeletal abnormality, i.e., maxillary and/or mandibular deficiency are frequently found in patients with OSA, and that maxillomandibular deficiency results in diminished airway dimension, which leads to nocturnal obstruction. MMA achieves enlargement of the pharyngeal and hypopharyngeal airway by physically expanding the skeletal framework. In addition, the forward movement of the maxillomandibular complex improves the tension and collapsibility of the suprahyoid and velopharyngeal musculature. Recent evidence further suggests that MMA improves lateral pharyngeal wall collapse (Fig. 21-7) (34), which has been shown to be a major contributor in OSAS (1,9,35).

MMA can be performed as the initial surgical treatment, or reserved as the "last resort" when other procedures have insufficiently improved the patient (Table 21-5) (36). The debate continues on whether patients should undergo less invasive procedures such as UPPP/UPF with GA/HA first, or a single-stage reconstruction consisting of MMA alone or in conjunction with other "adjunctive" procedures (37,38). In the author's experience, although the less invasive procedures are often attempted first, some patients have elected to proceed directly to MMA. These patients usually have either have severe sleep apnea or significant maxillomandibular deformity.

Although patients with maxillomandibular deficiency are considered "good" candidates for MMA, it should also be considered in patients without "disproportionate" maxillofacial features as well (39). This is because recent evidence suggests that previous concerns of MMA resulting in compromised facial aesthetics have been insignificant in most patients (39,40). It may be that most of the patients with OSA are middle-age adult, and most of them are showing signs of facial aging due to soft tissue sagging. MMA achieves facial skeletal expansion, thus enhancing the facial aesthetics by improving soft tissue support (39,40).

▶ **TABLE 21-5. Maxillomandibular Advancement Treatment**

Considerations
  Failure of other forms of treatment including medical and surgical
  Sufficient health to undergo and recover from surgery

As the primary treatment option
  Morbid obesity
  Significant facial-skeletal deficiency
  Severe OSA with minimally redundant soft palate

Surgical decision is usually based on the surgeon's preference, experience, the patient's body habitus, airway/skeletal anatomy, the severity of OSA, the patient's desire, and other comorbid factors (41).

MMA involves moving the maxilla and mandible forward. In order to maximize the airway expansion, a significant advancement of the maxillomandibular complex is required. However, it is important to achieve maximal advancement while maintaining a stable dental occlusion and a balanced aesthetic appearance. Although the MMA procedure has been used for many years to correct skeletal facial deformities and malocclusions, it must be emphasized that performing MMA for the treatment of OSA is quite different from procedures for the treatment of dentofacial deformity.

The maxillary procedure involves a Le Fort I osteotomy above the apices of the upper teeth. The maxilla is mobilized and advanced approximately 10 to 12 mm, which is usually the physiologic limitation of the soft tissue. The maxilla is stabilized with rigid fixation, utilizing small titanium plates. For proper alignment of the maxilla in relation to the mandible and the face, it is important to ensure an acceptable postoperative dental occlusion and aesthetics. The mandibular procedure involves a sagittal split technique. The medial and lateral cortex of the mandible is separated at the ramus region, while preserving the inferior alveolar nerve. The dentated mandibular segment is advanced the same distance as the maxilla; thus, occlusion is restored. Rigid fixation is achieved with four positional screws on each side (occasionally plates are also used to ensure rigidity) (Fig. 21-7).

Evolving Procedure—Maxillomandibular Expansion (MME)

Traditionally, correction of the maxillomandibular abnormality has been primarily in the saggital plane. The correction of transverse deficiency of the maxilla and/or mandible as a potential treatment of OSA has received little attention.

Constriction of the maxilla has been suggested as a possible risk factor of OSA (42–44). Indeed, the relationship of nasal resistance and maxillary morphology has long been recognized. The positive impact of maxillary expansion on nasal breathing is also well known in the orthodontic literature. Different investigators have demonstrated that patients with constricted maxilla have elevated nasal resistance, which can be improved by maxillary expansion. Other investigators have validated these findings, albeit that the beneficial effect of maxillary expansion on nasal resistance may not be uniformly achieved in all patients. It appears that patients with greater degrees of nasal resistance tend to have greater improvement after maxillary expansion (45–50). There is limited evidence suggesting that maxillary expansion improves OSA (51). The author has performed expansion of the maxilla and mandible (MME) for the treatment of OSA with early promising results (52).

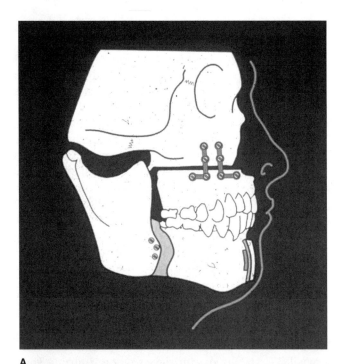

A

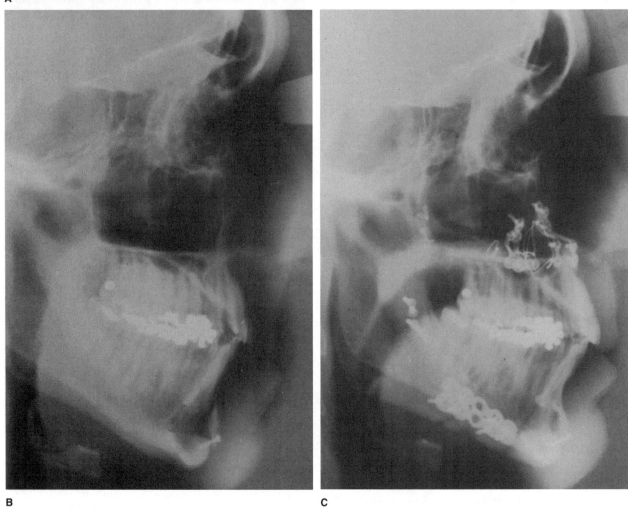

B   C

FIGURE 21-7. (A) The maxillomandibular advancement procedure (lateral view). Lefort I maxillary osteotomy with rigid plate fixation and a bilateral sagittal split mandibular osteotomy with bicortical screw fixation. (B) Lateral cephalometric radiograph prior to MMA. (C) Lateral cephalometric radiograph after MMA. Note the improvement of airway dimension throughout the upper airway.

Thus far, six patients have undergone MME with improvement of mean apnea–hypopnea index (AHI) from 13.2 ± 15.6 to 4.5 ± 5.8 events per hour and improvement of the mean lowest oxygen saturation (LSAT) from 88.2 ± 2.9% to 91.3 ± 3.3%. No complications were encountered and the follow-up period was 18.1 ± 9.8 months. MME may be a new treatment of OSA, which is less invasive than MMA. Clearly, further investigation is warranted.

Temperature-controlled Radiofrequency (TCRF) Tongue Base Reduction

Low-wave radiofrequency (RF) energy achieves therapeutic ablation of tissue in a minimally invasiveness fashion. RF tissue ablation has been previously evaluated in different medical and surgical specialties (53,54). RF energy is produced from a generator and is delivered through a needle electrode. The energy current causes ionic agitation of the tissue around the electrode, which results in frictional heating of the tissue. Therefore, the electrode itself does not get hot and the heat actually emanates from the tissue. Tissue injury occurs when the temperature reaches beyond 47° C, which is when the cell proteins undergo denaturation. The size of the lesion (area of tissue injury) created is dependent on the current intensity, the duration of energy delivery, and the size of the needle electrode (55). Typically, the lesion is in the shape of an ellipse, with the long axis of the lesion being two times the length of the needle electrode and the transverse axis being two-thirds of the long axis. Since the RF energy disbursement is proportional to 1/radius(4), heat dissipation is limited and excessive tissue injury is minimized. Furthermore, when the temperature reaches 90°–100°C, char formation on the electrode leads to an increase in the impedance and results in disruption of current flow, thus serving as a second layer of protection. These factors allow RF ablation to create a predictable tissue injury pattern, thus minimizing potential complications.

The initial investigation of the application of RF energy to the upper airway was on the porcine tongue (56). Microscopic examination of the treated tongue tissue demonstrated a typical pattern of injury with interstitial edema and focal hemorrhage 24 hours after treatment. Three weeks after treatment, there was fibrosis and chronic inflammation, characterizing early scar formation. The measurements of treated area over time demonstrated progressive volume reduction of 26.3% up to 10 days. Furthermore, the lesion correlated with the amount of RF energy delivered.

A prospective study of RF tongue base reduction was conducted in18 patients. After a mean total energy of 8,490 joules per patient delivered over a mean of 5.5 treatments, the mean RDI improved from 39.6 to 17.8 with an improved LSAT from 81.9% to 88.3%. The tongue volume was reduced by a mean of 17%, based on MRI. There were no changes in speech or swallowing and complications included a superficial tongue ulceration that resolved spontaneously, persistent pain on swallowing that resolved after several weeks, and a tongue abscess that required drainage (57). Other investigators have confirm the beneficial effect of RF for the treatment of OSA (58,59). However, it must be emphasized that the use of RF alone is usually ineffective in managing OSA. In addition, long-term follow-up has shown that there can be relapse of OSA in some patients (60). Clearly, larger studies will be necessary to validate the effectiveness of this treatment modality. Currently, RF is used as an adjunctive treatment along with other surgical procedures.

PERIOPERATIVE MANAGEMENT

Due to the risk of general anesthesia in patients with an already compromised airway, in conjunction with the potential for postoperative airway edema and the coexisting medical conditions, diligence and compunction must be practiced in the perioperative management of patients with OSA. If a patient can tolerate nasal CPAP on a short-term basis, it should be attempted shortly prior to surgery to reverse sleep debt and prevent REM rebound in the postoperative period. The team approach concept of anesthesia induction and intubation is always practiced with both the anesthesiologist and the surgeon present. In patients who have a difficult airway, such as those with significant obesity, increased neck circumference (>46 cm), or associated skeletal deformities (mandibular deficiency and low hyoid bone), awake fiberoptic intubation or tracheotomy should be considered. All patients should be extubated awake in the operating room immediately following surgery. All patients undergoing multiple procedures (UPPP/UPF combining with GA/Ha), or who have significant cardiovascular disease, are monitored in the ICU immediately after surgery. Postoperative airway protection with nasal CPAP or humidified oxygen (35%) via face tent are used on all patients, and oximetry monitoring is performed throughout the hospitalization. Blood pressure is monitored closely and hypertension is treated aggressively with intravenous antihypertensive medications to minimize postoperative bleeding and edema.

The use of narcotics after general anesthesia in OSA patients with postoperative airway edema must be done with caution. A strict protocol consisting of intravenous morphine sulfate (MS) or meperidine HCL administered by a nurse in graduated doses (e.g., MS 1 to 5 mg q 1 to 3 hours as necessary) in the ICU while monitoring respiratory rate has been utilized at our center. All nurses caring for OSA patients must be educated about sleep apnea and the use of narcotics. Patients are transferred to the ward on the second postoperative day and intramuscular meperidine HCL and oxycodone elixir are used. Oral hydrocodone is used following discharge. Discharge criteria include a stable airway, adequate oral intake of fluids, and satisfactory pain control. Patients are urged to use nasal CPAP following discharge from the hospital, and humidified oxygen is prescribed for 2 weeks for patients with severe OSA who cannot tolerate nasal CPAP.

STAGED SURGICAL APPROACH

Clearly, the most logical surgical approach would be to minimize surgical interventions and avoid unnecessary surgery while achieving a cure. Since UPPP/UPF, GA/HA are all rather limited procedures without significant surgical morbidity, these procedures are usually first attempted to improve OSA. After a healing period of 4 to 6 months, a postoperative polysomnogram (PSG) is obtained to evaluate outcome. In patients with persistent OSA, MMA can then be performed. UPPP/UPF combining with GA/HA is usually considered as a phase I operation, whereas MMA is considered as a phase II operation.

Clearly, not all patients undergo UPPP/UPF and GA/HA before MMA. Patients with severe OSA, morbid obesity, or significant maxillomandibular deficiency, or patients who wish to have the best chance for cure with a single operation can certainly be considered as candidates for MMA without undergoing other procedures. Therefore, it is important to review all possible treatment options and explain the rationale for upper-airway reconstruction. In the author's opinion, combining all of the procedures in a single operation should be cautioned due to the potential for unnecessary surgery, as well as the increased surgical morbidity and postoperative airway compromise.

SURGICAL TREATMENT OUTCOMES

Phase I Surgery (UPPP/UPF and GA/HA)

Early publication has demonstrated that a majority of the patients with OSA will require intervention at the oropharyngeal and hypopharyngeal levels. Data are available on 239 patients who had undergone phase I surgery (61). The overall cure rate was 61% (145/239 patients). The surgical results were comparable to nasal CPAP results. The mean preoperative AHI was 48.3, with a postoperative mean AHI of 9.5 (nasal CPAP RDI 7.2, p = NS). The LSAT improved from 75% to 86.6% (nasal CPAP LSAT 86.4%, p = NS). There was a higher cure rate with mild to moderately severe disease (approximately 70%) as compared to severe disease (42%). Most of the patients who failed phase I therapy had severe OSA (mean RDI 61.9) and morbid obesity (mean BMI 32.3 kg/m^2).

The postoperative morbidity was low. The mean hospital stay was 2.1 days. The complications associated with genioglossus advancement and hyoid suspension were infection (<2%), injury of tooth roots requiring root canal

therapy (<1%), permanent paresthesia and anesthesia of the mandibular incisors (<6%), and seroma (<2%). Major complications, such as mandibular fracture, alteration of speech, or alteration of swallow or aspiration were not encountered.

Phase II Surgery (MMA)

Approximately 400 MMA procedures have been performed for the treatment of OSA at Stanford. An analysis of 175 patients between 1988 and 1995 demonstrated 166 patients have had a successful outcome, with a cure rate of 95% (if using the criteria of achieving the AHI less than 20 events per hour *and* greater than 50% reduction). The mean preoperative AHI was 72.3 events per hour. The mean postoperative AHI was 7.2 events per hour. The mean LSAT improved from 64.0% to 86.7%. Eighty-six patients who failed phase I surgery, underwent MMA. The cure rate in this group was 97% (83/86 patients).

To date, 59 patients (49 men) have had long-term follow-up results (62). The mean age was 47.1 years. The mean BMI was 31.1 kg/m^2. Nineteen patients had only subjective (quality of life) results. These patients refused long-term PSG due to various reasons, including inconvenience, time consuming, and cost. Sixteen of the 19 patients continued to report subjective success with minimal to no snoring, no observed apnea, and no recurrence of excessive daytime sleepiness (EDS). All patients reported stable (unchanged) weight to mild weight gain (<5 kg). Three patients reported recurrence of snoring and EDS. Long-term PSG data were available in 40 patients (33 men). The mean age was 45.6 years. The mean BMI was 31.4 kg/m^2. The preoperative AHI and LSAT were 71.2 events per hour and 67.5%, respectively. The 6 months postoperative AHI was 9.3 events per hour and the LSAT was 85.6%. The mean follow-up period was 50.7 months, and long-term AHI and LSAT were 7.6 events per hour and 86.3%, respectively.

Due to different factors, such as the individual patient's lifestyle and treatment expectations, the subjective outcomes can be highly variable and may not correlate with the objective outcomes. To evaluate the patient's perspective on the outcomes after MMA, a study using a questionnaire was conducted. Six months after MMA, questionnaires were sent to 56 patients who had undergone MMA for persistent OSA after UPPP/UPF and GA/HA (63). Forty-two (75%) patients (36 men) completed and returned the questionnaires. The mean age was 46.3 years and the mean BMI was 32.1 kg/m^2. The mean AHI improved from 58.7 to 10.0 events per hour. The mean LSAT improved from 76.3% to 87.3%. Thirty-seven patients (88%) were cured, and all 42 patients reported improved sleep quality with a mean visual analog scale of 8.7 (VAS 0 to 10). Temporary postoperative paresthesia of the inferior alveolar nerve distribution occurred in all of these patients; however, only four patients (10%) did not report either total or near total recovery within 6 months. No major infection was encountered. Minor infection involving the mandibular osteotomy sites occurred in three patients (7%), which completely resolved with local care and oral antibiotics. Although the questionnaires identified ten patients with changes in speech, the changes were extremely subtle and insignificant; nine of the patients marked 0 on the VAS (mean VAS 0.08). Five patients reported changes in swallowing; the VAS scores were 0.5, 0.9, 1.0, 2.7, and 6.9 (mean VAS 2.4).

The perceived pain and suffering following UPPP/UPR and GA/HA (mean VAS 5.9) was found to be similar to MMA surgery (mean VAS 5.1). Eighteen patients felt that the pain and suffering following phase I surgery was worse. However, sixteen patients felt that the pain and suffering was worse following MMA. The remaining eight patients felt that the postoperative recovery was not significantly different between the two phases. Forty patients (95%) were satisfied with their results and would go through the reconstruction all over again.

Two patients (5%) responded that they would not go though the reconstruction again in retrospect. The first patient was a 54-year-old man with the complaint of severe daytime fatigue and sleepiness. Polysomnographic findings were consistent with severe OSA (AHI 56, LSAT 86%). Despite total upper-airway reconstruction, he continued to have significant symptoms of daytime sleepiness, and the postoperative PSG demonstrated persistent OSAS (AHI 35.7, LSAT 91%). The second patient was a 43-year-old man with severe OSAS (AHI 76.2, LSAT 82%). Although an improvement was achieved following the completion of airway reconstruction (AHI 20, LSAT 77.5%), he continued to have complaints of daytime sleepiness that affected his daily activity. This patient also reported significant changes in his swallowing (VAS 6.9), which contributed to the dissatisfaction.

Fourteen (25%) patients (all men) did not respond to the questionnaire. They were younger (mean age 41.4 years) and less obese (mean BMI 28.4 kg/m^2). The severity of OSA was similar; however, the cure rate was higher in this group, with 13 patients (93%) achieving an AHI ≤20. The mean AHI improved from 57.1 to 9.3 events per hour. The mean LSAT improved from 79.9% to 87.9%.

CONCLUSION

The evidence is overwhelming that OSA adversely affects the patient's quality of life and well being. Although nasal CPAP can be an effective treatment for the majority of patients, it is clearly limited by patient compliance. Even in "compliant" patients, the effectiveness may only be 50% of ideal. Although surgical therapy has been viewed as a treatment alternative in patients who are intolerant of conservative treatments, it is undeniable that outcome data have demonstrated that surgical therapy is highly successful in the management of OSA. A thorough preoperative evaluation to identify the type of airway abnormality is mandatory. The utilization of a logical and stepwise surgical protocol can result in improved clinical outcomes, while minimizing complications and avoiding unnecessary operations.

REFERENCES

1. Schwab RJ, Gefter WB, Hoffman EA. Dynamic upper airway imaging during awake respiration in normal subjects and patients with sleep disordered breathing. *Amer Rev Respir Dis.* 1993;148:1385–1400.
2. Rojewski TE, Schuller DE, Clark RW, et al. Videoendoscopic determination of the mechanism of obstruction in obstructive sleep apnea. *Otolaryngol Head Neck Surg.* 1984;92:127–131.
3. Kribbs NB, Redline S, Smith PL, et al. Objective monitoring of nasal CPAP usage in OSAS patients. *Sleep Res.* 1991;20:270–271.
4. Reeves-Hoche MK, Meck R, Zwillich CW. Nasal CPAP: an objective evaluation of patient compliance. *Amer J Respir Crit Care Med.* 1994;149:149–154.
5. Waldhorn RE, Herrick TW, Nguyen MC, et al. Long-term compliance with nasal continuous positive airway pressure therapy of obstructive sleep apnea. *Chest.* 1991;99:855–860.
6. Kuhlo W, Doll E, Franck MD. Erfolgreiche Behandlung eines Pickwick Syndroms durch eine Dauertrachekanuele. *Dtsch Med Wochenschr.* 1969;94:1286–1290.
7. Fijita S, Conway W, Zorick F, et al. Surgical correction of anatomic abnormalities of obstructive sleep apnea syndrome: Uvulopalatopharyngoplasty. *Otolaryngol Head Neck Surg.* 1981;89:923–934.
8. Sher AE, Schechtman KB, Piccirillo JF. The efficacy of surgical modifications of the upper airway in adults with obstructive sleep apnea syndrome. *Sleep.* 1996;19:156–177.
9. Schwab RJ, Gupta KB, Gefter WB, et al. Upper airway and soft tissue anatomy in normal subjects and patients with sleep-disordered breathing. *Amer J Respir Crit Care Med.* 1995;152:1673–1689.
10. Jamieson A, Guilleminault C, Partinen M, et al. Obstructive sleep apnea patients have craniomandibular abnormalities. *Sleep.* 1986;9:469–477.
11. Partinen M, Guilleminault C, Quera-Salva M, et al. Obstructive sleep apnea and cephalometric roentgenograms. *Chest.* 1988;93:1199–1205.
12. Riley RW, Guilleminault C, Powell NB, et al. Mandibular osteotomy and hyoid bone advancement for obstructive sleep apnea: A case report. *Sleep.* 1984;7:79–82.
13. Li KK. Lower pharyngeal airway surgery: Hyoid suspension/advancement. In: Fairbanks DNF, Mickelson SA, Woodson BT, eds. *Snoring and obstructive sleep apnea.* 3rd edn. Philadelphia: Lippincott Williams & Wilkins, 2003.
14. Bear SE, Priest JH. Sleep apnea syndrome: correction with surgical advancement of the mandible. *J Oral Surg.* 1980;38:543–549.
15. Powell N, Guilleminault C, Riley R, et al. Mandibular advancement and obstructive sleep apnea syndrome. *Bull Eur Physiopathol Respir.* 1983;19:607–610.
16. Li KK, Riley RW, Powell NB, et al. Overview of phase II surgery for obstructive sleep apnea syndrome. *ENT J.* 1999;78:851–857.
17. Li KK, Powell NB, Riley RW, et al. Morbidly obese patients with severe obstructive sleep apnea syndrome: Is airway reconstructive surgery a viable option? *Laryngoscope.* 2000;110:982–987.
18. Sher AE, Thorpy MJ, Shrintzen RJ, et al. Predictive value of Muller maneuver in selection of patient for uvulopalatopharyngoplasty. *Laryngoscope.* 1985;95:1483–1487.
19. Chen NH, Li KK, Chuang ML, et al. Airway assessment by volumetric CT in snorers and subjects with obstructive sleep apnea. *Laryngoscope.* 2002;112:721–726.
20. Riley RW, Powell NB. Maxillofacial surgery and obstructive sleep apnea syndrome. *Otolaryngol Clin N Amer.* 1990;23:809–826.
21. Olsen K. The role of nasal surgery in the treatment of obstructive sleep apnea. *Op Tech Otolaryngol Head Neck Surg.* 1991;2:63–68.
22. Li KK, Powell NB, Riley RW, et al. Radiofrequency volumetric tissue reduction for treatment of turbinate hypertrophy: a pilot study. *Otolaryngol Head Neck Surg.* 1998;119:569–573.

23. Powell NB, Riley RW, Guilleminault C, et al. A reversible uvulopalatal flap for snoring and obstructive sleep. *Sleep.* 1996;19:593–599.

24. Kamami YV. Laser CO2 for snoring-preliminary results. *Acta Otorhinolaryngol Belg.* 1990;44:451–456.

25. Littner M, Kushida CA, Hartse K, et al. Practice parameters for the use of laser-assisted uvulopalatoplasty: an update for 2000. *Sleep.* 2001;24:603–619.

26. Remmers JE, Degroot WJ, Sauerland EK, et al. Pathogensis of upper airway occlusion during sleep. *J Appl Physiol.* 1978;44:931–938.

27. Mezzanotte WS, Tangel DJ, White DP. Waking genioglossal electromyogram in sleep apnea patients versus normal controls (a neuromuscular compensatory mechanism). *J Clin Invest.* 1992;89:1571–1579.

28. Li KK, Riley RW, Powell NB, et al. Obstructive sleep apnea surgery: Genioglossus advancement revisited. *J Oral Maxfac Surg.* 2001;59:1181–1184.

29. Van de Graaf WB, Gottfried SB, Mitra J, et al. Respiratory function of hyoid muscles and hyoid arch. *J Appl Physiol.* 1984;57:197–204.

30. Patton TJ, Thawley SE, Water RC, et al. Expansion hyoid-plasty: A potential surgical procedure designed for selected patients with obstructive sleep apnea syndrome. Experimental canine results. *Laryngoscope.* 1983;93:1387–1396.

31. Riley RW, Powell NB, Guilleminault C. Obstructive sleep apnea and the hyoid: a revised surgical procedure. *Otolaryngol Head Neck Surg.* 1994;111:717–721.

32. Riley R, Guilleminault C, Powell N, et al. Palatopharyngoplasty failure, cephalometric roentgenograms, and obstructive sleep apnea. *Otolaryngol Head Neck Surg.* 1985;93:240–243.

33. DeBerry-Borowiecki B, Kukwa A, Blanks R. Cephalometric analysis for diagnosis and treatment of obstructive sleep apnea. *Laryngoscope.* 1988;98:226–234.

34. Li KK, Riley RW, Powell NB, et al. Obstructive sleep apnea and maxillomandibular advancement: An assessment of airway changes using radiographic and nasopharyngoscopic examinationa. *J Oral Maxillofac Surg.* 2002;60:526–530.

35. Suratt PM, Dee P, Atkinson RL, et al. Fluoroscopic and computed tomographic features of the pharyngeal airway in obstructive sleep apnea. *Amer Rev Respir Dis.* 1993;127:487–492.

36. Li KK, Powell N. Lower pharyngeal airway surgery: Maxillomandibular advancement. In: Fairbanks DNF, Mickelson SA, Woodson BT, eds. *Snoring and obstructive sleep apnea.* 3rd edn. Philadelphia: Lippincott Williams & Wilkins, 2003:182–189.

37. Prinsell JR. Maxillomandibular advancement surgery in a site-specific treatment approach for obstructive sleep apnea in 50 consecutive patients. *Chest.* 1999;116:1519–1529.

38. Hendler BH, Costello BJ, Silverstein K, et al. A protocol for uvulopalatopharyngoplasty, mortised genioplasty, and maxillomandibular advancement in patients with obstructive sleep apnea: An analysis of 40 cases. *J Oral Maxillofac Surg.* 2001;59:892–897.

39. Li KK, Riley RW, Powell NB, et al. Maxillomandibular advancement for persistent OSA after phase I surgery in patients without maxillomandibular deficiency. *Laryngoscope.* 2000;110:1684–1688.

40. Li KK, Riley RW, Powell NB, et al. Patient's perception of the facial appearance after maxillomandibular advancement for obstructive sleep apnea syndrome. *J Oral Maxillofac Surg.* 2001;59:377–380.

41. Li KK. Discussion on "A protocol for uvulopalatopharyngoplasty, mortised genioplasty, and maxillomandibular advancement in patients with obstructive sleep apnea: an analysis of 40 cases." *J Oral Maxillofac Surg.* 2001;59:898–899.

42. Seto BH, Gotsopoulos H, Sims MR, et al. Maxillary morphology in obstructive sleep apnea syndrome. *Eur J Orthod.* 2001;23:703–714.

43. Kushida C, Efron B, Guilleminault C. A predictive morphometric model for the obstructive sleep apnea syndrome. *Ann Int Med.* 1997;127:581–587.

44. Cistulli PA, Richards GN, Palmisano RG, et al. Influence of maxillary constriction on nasal resistance and sleep apnea severity in patients with Marfan's syndrome. *Chest.* 1996;110:1184–1188.

45. Timms DJ. The reduction of nasal airway resistance by rapid maxillary expansion and its effect on respiratory disease. *J Laryngol Otol.* 1984;98:357–362.

46. Timms DJ. Rapid maxillary expansion in the treatment of nocturnal enuresis. *Angle Orthod.* 1990;60:229–233.

47. White BC, Woodside DG, Cole P. The effect of rapid maxillary expansion on nasal airway resistance. *J Otolaryngol.* 1989;18:137–143.

48. Hartgerink DV, Vig PS, Abbott DW. The effect of rapid maxillary expansion on nasal airway resistance. *Amer J Orthod Dentofac Orthop.* 1987;92:381–389.

49. Warren DW, Hershey HG, Turvey TA, et al. *Amer J Orthod Dentofac Orthop.* 1987;91:111–116.

50. Kurol J, Modin H, Bjerkhoel A. Orthodontic maxillary expansion and its effect on nocturnal enuresis. *Angle Orthod.* 1998;68:225–232.

51. Cistulli PA, Palmisano RG, Poole MD. Treatment of obstructive sleep apnea syndrome by rapid maxillary expansion. *Sleep.* 1998;21:831–835.

52. Li KK, Guilleminault. Unpublished results. 2002.

53. Calkins H, Sousa J, El-Atassi R, et al. Diagnosis and cure of the Wolff–Parkinson–White syndrome or paroxysmal supraventricdular tachycardias during a single electrophysiologic test. *N Eng J Med.* 1991;324:1612–1618.

54. Sweet W, Wepsic J. Controlled thermocoagulation of trigeminal ganglion and rootlets for differential destruction of pain fibers: I. Trigeminal neuralgia. *J Neurosurg.* 1974;3:143–156.

55. Organ LW. Electrophysiologic principles of radiofrequency lesion making. *Appl Neurophysiol.* 1976/77;39:69–76.

56. Powell NB, Riley RW, Troell RJ, et al. Radiofrequency volumetric reduction of the tongue. *Chest.* 1997;111:1348–1355.

57. Powell NB, Riley RW, Guilleminault C. Radiofrequency tongue base reduction in sleep-disordered breathing: a pilot study. *Otolaryngol Head Neck Surg.* 1999;120:656–664.

58. Woodson BT, Nelson L, Mickelson S, et al. A multi-institutional study of radiofrequency volumetric tissue reduction for OSAS. *Otolaryngol Head Neck Surg.* 2001;125:303–311.

59. Stuck BA, Maurer JT, Verse T, et al. Tongue base reduction with temperature-controlled radiofrequency volumetric tissue reduction for treatment of obstructive sleep apnea syndrome. *Acta Otolaryngol.* 2002;122:531–536.

60. Li KK, Powell NB, Riley RW, et al. Temperature-controlled radiofrequency tongue base reduction for sleep-disordered breathing: long-term follow-up. *Oto Head Neck Surg.* 2002;127:230–234.

61. Riley RW, Powell NB, Guilleminault C. Obstructive sleep apnea syndrome: a review of 306 consecutively treated surgical patients. *Otolaryngol Head Neck Surg.* 1993;108:117–125.

62. Li KK, Riley RW, Powell NB, et al. Obstructive sleep apnea surgery: patients' perspective and polysomnographic results. *Otolaryngol. Head Neck Surg.* 2000;123:572–575.

63. Li KK, Powell NB, Riley RW, et al. Long-term results of maxillomandibular advancement surgery. *Sleep Breath.* 2000;4:137–139.

Chapter 22

Obstructive Sleep Apnea: Treatment with Oral Appliance

Wolfgang W. Schmidt-Nowara

INTRODUCTION

Oral appliances (OA) have been used for upper-airway management since the beginning of the last century (1). A dental device was proposed for snoring before the clinical problem of sleep apnea was known (Thomas Meade, 1990, personal communication). Thus, it is not surprising that oral appliances were investigated soon after the clinical problem of obstructive sleep apnea and the pathophysiology of upper-airway obstruction were described. Early clinical reports indicated that mandibular advancement (2,3) and retention of the tongue in an anterior position (4) could significantly reduce upper-airway obstruction in sleep. The next decade produced numerous case series that demonstrated not only the efficacy of the oral appliance concept, but also the safety and feasibility of long-term clinical use. An influential review and a practice parameter by the American Academy of Sleep Medicine firmly established oral appliance use in the therapy of snoring and obstructive sleep apnea (OSA) (5,6).

Ten years after the Academy's practice parameter, the scientific basis for OA therapy has significantly expanded.

In this chapter, the rationale for OA therapy and guidelines for their use will rely heavily on recent publications, including controlled treatment trials that indicate the efficacy, safety, and utility of OA relative to other OSA therapies.

CLINICAL EPIDEMIOLOGY

The prevalence of obstructive sleep apnea in middle-aged men and women is often stated to be 4% and 2%, respectively, but these numbers refer to the combination of 5+ and reported sleepiness (7). If symptoms are disregarded, the prevalences of apnea-hypopnea index (AHI) 5+ are 24% of men and 10% of women in the same population. The prevalence of frequent snoring is higher yet (8). Furthermore, the majority of OSA subjects identified in large surveys fit into the category of mild to moderate OSA (Table 22-1). If OA therapy is particularly suited to patients with mild to moderately severe OSA, as will be discussed below, it is clear that these represent the majority of potential cases from a population perspective.

▶ **TABLE 22-1. Distribution of OSA (AHI 5+) by Severity in Population Surveys**

AHI (%)		5–14	5–30	15+	30+
Wisconsin	Men	66	19		15
Cohort Study[a]	Women	72	18		10
Sleep Heart	Men	57		43	
Health Study[b]	Women	70		30	

[a]Terry Young, personal communication, June 2003.
[b]From Reference (22).

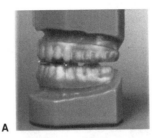
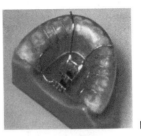
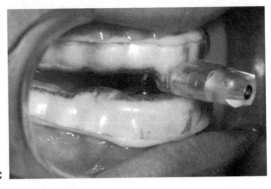

FIGURE 22-1. (A–C) A mandibular advancing oral appliance, custom type, with full occlusal coverage of both dental arches, minimal bite opening, and an adjustable advancement mechanism [(A and B), Klearway, Great Lakes Orthodontics Ltd., Tonawanda, NY. (C) Thornton Anterior Positioner (TAP), Airway Management Inc., Dallas, TX].

Based on these epidemiologic considerations, it appears that OA may be appropriate therapy for a substantial proportion of the OSA population. It is not known what percentage of OSA patients is currently receiving treatment with OA, but the ratio is estimated to be less than 20% and probably much less. It is interesting to speculate why such a small number of patients receive OA therapy. Possible explanations are a greater proportion of severe cases among patients presenting for clinical care, inadequate knowledge among OSA therapists, insufficient providers of OA therapy, and economic barriers to care. With change to be anticipated in each of these factors, OA therapy is likely to become an increasingly important component of OSA care in the future.

THE DATABASE

Types of Oral Appliances

The term oral appliance in this context is a device inserted into the oral cavity in order to modify the upper airway so as to relieve sleep-disturbed breathing (SDB). Similar "activator" appliances have long been used by dentists to modify dentition. The dominant OA design type consists of attachments to the mandibular and maxillary dental arches with varying degrees of bite opening and advance of the mandible relative to the maxilla (mandible advancing devices, MAD; Figs. 22-1 and 22-2). These OA may be in a fixed position with a predetermined advance, or adjustable, allowing advance according to the patient's response. Also in current use are devices that hold the tongue anterior in the oral cavity. Other approaches, such as palatal lifters and tongue depressors, have been tried and have failed. OA are typically fashioned in a laboratory from dental models, but so-called "boil and bite" types can be fitted to the patient in the clinic using manufactured templates.

Mechanism for Oral Appliances

Oral appliances are presumed to work by increasing the size of the airway. In fact there is abundant evidence to support this hypothesis. By direct inspection with videoendoscopy, or by radiographic imaging, i.e., cephalography or computed tomography (CT) or magnetic resonance imaging (MRI), mandible advancing OA have been shown to bring the tongue forward and increase pharyngeal volume. Interesting secondary effects are a stretching of the soft palate, an increase in the retropalatal space, and a change in the shape of the oral airway. These changes are readily understood by the anatomical relationships of the pharyngeal elements, including the ligamentous connections of the soft palate to the genioglossus and the genioglossus to the hyoid bone and mandible. Observations of the effect of OA on the airway have been made in waking patients, leaving some uncertainty regarding

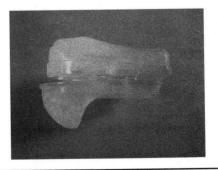

FIGURE 22-2. A mandibular advancing oral appliance, "boil and bite" type, with full occlusal coverage of the maxillary arch and limited contact of the lower arch, wider bite opening, and a multiposition advancement mechanism (Therasnore, Distar, Inc., Albuquerque, NM).

the status in sleep. However, Isono has shown similar airway effects of mandibular advancement in anesthetized subjects, suggesting that the airway in a relaxed state, including sleep, behaves as demonstrated during waking (9).

Additional explanations for the effect of OA have focused on the concepts of muscle tone, airway compliance, and mandibular posture. The displaced upper-airway muscles demonstrate increased tone by electromyography (EMG) (10). The critical closing pressure of the relaxed airway is decreased (opposing inspiratory collapse) with mandibular advance (11). By stabilizing mandibular posture, OA resist the naturally occurring downward rotation of the mandible with sleep and the accompanying retrusion of the genioglossus into the oropharynx (12).

Efficacy of Oral Appliance: Effect on Obstructive Sleep Apnea

Numerous studies have shown that OA therapy often, but not always, improves the manifestations of OSA. Typically most patients have reduced or abolished snoring, reduction in AHI, and improvement in oxygen saturation. These changes are accompanied by improved sleep parameters on polysomnography (PSG) and reduced sleepiness. In groups of patients, mean effects are typical of the selected studies in Table 22-2.

Comparison of treatment effects is complicated by the different definitions of "success." Recent studies define success as a relief of symptoms and a reduction of AHI to 10 to 15 per hour. The studies differ by the severity of patients studied, the type of OA, and the length of follow-up. Despite these differences, the findings are remarkably similar. One trend is the higher success rate with the modern adjustable and titratable appliances (Klearway, Table 22-2). Another trend is to attempt therapy in more severe patients. Initial studies were confined to cases of mild to moderate severity. More recent studies have demonstrated success in some severe cases, although

all studies show a lower success rate in such patients (13,14).

The studies cited in Table 22-2 are considered to be relatively higher quality because the study design includes control and randomization. Typically, the study design has been a crossover to CPAP with randomization of treatment order. For the purpose of efficacy, however, these studies do not differ from earlier case series in that the OA treatment effect is compared to a baseline measurement. One exception is a placebo-controlled study by Mehta, in which active treatment with a MAD was compared to placebo, consisting of the mandibular portion of the appliance (15). It is noteworthy that this study shows similar effects and leads to similar conclusions as the other studies (Table 22-2). Interestingly, the outcomes of the earlier case series, summarized in 1995 (Schmidt-Nowara (5) (Table 22-2), are similar to the more rigorous studies appearing later.

Comparisons of Oral Appliances to Continuous Positive Airway Pressure, Uvulopalatopharygoplasty, and between Different Oral Appliances

Many studies have compared OA to CPAP therapy (Table 22-3). The results are consistent: CPAP is uniformly efficacious in controlling snoring and OSA, whereas OA leave some fraction of patients inadequately treated. However, CPAP is not accepted by patients for long-term use as often as OA. The two effects approximately offset the differences and produce a relatively similar rate of effectiveness, i.e., the proportion of patients using a therapy with success. Furthermore, patients in these trials preferred OA therapy in all but one study (16). This discrepancy may be explained by a higher proportion of severe cases in the study favoring CPAP. Thus in the populations usually examined, i.e., mild to moderate OSA, CPAP acceptance is sufficiently low to produce a preference for OA therapy.

OA was compared to UPPP in one randomized controlled treatment trial with follow-up at 4 years. The findings were an increased number of cases with treatment

▶ **TABLE 22-2.** Efficacy of Oral Appliance on Obstructive Sleep Apnea: Selected Publications

| Author (Ref) | OA Type | N | AHI (Mean SD) | | Success (%) | OA Treatment Success Criteria |
			Untreated	Treated		
Clark (23)	Herbst	21	34 (14)	20 (13)	Not specified	
Engelman (16)	MAD[a]	48	31 (26)	15 (16)	47	AHI <10
Ferguson (24)	SnoreGuard	25	20 (14)	10 (7)	48	AHI <10, no symptom
Lowe (13)	Klearway	38	33 (13)	12 (10)	71	AHI <15, no symptom
Marklund (14)	MAD[a]	44	Not specified		64	AHI <10
Mehta (15)	MAD[a]	28	30 (11)	14 (11)	54	AHI <10
Ono (25)	TRD[a]	7	41 (18)	14 (11)	Not specified	
Pancer (26)	TAP[a]	75	44 (28)	12 (15)	51	AHI <10
Schmidt-Nowara (5)	Various	271	43	19	51	AHI <10

[a]MAD, mandibular advancement device; TRD, tongue retaining device; TAP, Thornton anterior positioner.

▶ **TABLE 22-3.** Comparison of Oral Appliance to Continuous Positive Airway Pressure, Selected Studies

Author (Ref)	OA Type	N	Study Design	Treatment Effectiveness[a]		Criteria
				CPAP (%)	OA (%)	
Ferguson (24)	MAD,[b] Snore Guard	25	Randomized Crossover	52	48	AHI<10 + no symptoms
Ferguson (27)	MAD, AMP[b]	20	Randomized Crossover	70	55	AHI<10 + no symptoms
Engleman (16)	MAD	48	Randomized Crossover	66	47	AHI<10

[a]Treatment effectiveness, demonstrated efficacy and long-term acceptance.
[b]MAD, mandibular advancement device; AMP, anterior mandibular positioner.

crossover in the surgery group due to inefficacy, and a better group result in the OA patients at 4 years (normal AHI at 1 and 4 years: OA, 78%, 63%; UPPP, 51%, 33%, $p<0.05$) (17). This study suggests that when CPAP is not tolerated or accepted, OA is the better alternative therapy.

Several studies have compared different oral appliances in controlled studies. The consistent finding is that mandibular advancing appliances are usually effective in reducing OSA and improving sleep, whereas soft palate lifters and a labial shield are ineffective.

Long-term Follow-up and Safety

Early case series suggested that MAD therapy was associated with increased salivation and minor discomfort, especially early in therapy, but dental complications and temporomandibular joint (TMJ) injury were uncommon. These somewhat haphazard observations were improved with more systematic follow-up studies (Table 22-4). Although the general impression of safety is not changed, the newer studies have demonstrated a significant occurrence of occlusal change with long-term use. In a careful follow-up study by Pantin of 132 patients after 1 to 3 years of treatment (18), the principal findings were TMJ, dental or myofacial pain in 25%, and a 14% rate of malocclusion developing with chronic use. Interestingly, most patients considered these changes minor and acceptable, manageable with exercises, and almost all patients chose not to discontinue OA therapy. Rose et al. (19) described a high rate of minor discomfort, which decreased with time of use. They also documented minor movement of teeth, but

only two patients described symptoms of malocclusion at a mean of 30 months. Robertson (20) performed systematic studies of lateral cephalograms at 6-month intervals in chronic OA users (20). These showed a significant tilting of incisors, forward at the mandible and backward at the maxilla, appearing after 12 to18 months of use. Again the effects were minor and usually tolerated.

DIAGNOSIS AND SELECTION FOR THERAPY

The diagnosis of OSA is described in other chapters. All patients presenting for OA therapy require an objective examination of breathing during sleep. Symptoms, whether elicited during interview or with a questionnaire, are not sufficiently sensitive to eliminate OSA. Even patients with no apparent sleep impairment, e.g., patients with a bed-partner's complaint of snoring, often have significant OSA that needs to be considered in the therapy.

The initial evaluation should include a history of dental and TMJ problems, including bruxing and orthodontic correction and previous experiences with appliances. TMJ symptoms are not an absolute contraindication to OA therapy, but may suggest a lower likelihood of tolerating mandibular advance. The examination should seek to identify adequate dentition for MAD attachment. One expert suggests a minimum of ten sound teeth in each arch (Lowe, personal communication, 1996). Mandibular protrusive mobility is required, although the amount is undefined.

The 1995 practice guidelines of the American Academy of Sleep Medicine continue to be appropriate for the

▶ **TABLE 22-4.** Side Effects of Oral Appliance Therapy

Author (Ref)	OA Type	N	Follow-Up Duration	Discomfort (%)	Occlusal Change (%)
Pantin (18)	MAD[a]	132	31 mo	25	14
Rose (19)	MAD	34	30 mo	47	6

[a]MAD, mandibular advancement device.

▶ **TABLE 22-5. Guidelines for Oral Appliance Therapy**[a]

Diagnosis of OSA must be evaluated with objective measures in all candidates for OA therapy
OA indicated as initial therapy for primary snoring or mild OSA if behavioral measures not effective
OA indicated in moderate to severe OSA if CPAP is not tolerated/ accepted and surgery not indicated
Follow-up sleep study after OA adjustment in more than mild OSA
Long-term dental follow-up

[a]Adapted from American Academy of Sleep Medicine Practice Parameter, Reference 6.

selection of OA therapy (Table 22-5). Patients with AHI <15 and/or predominantly low-grade obstruction, as in the upper-airway resistance syndrome, are included under mild OSA. Others suggest AHI <30 as the group with a high probability of success (13,14). When CPAP is not accepted, OA is considered preferable to surgery, because of Scandinavian studies demonstrating relatively lower success rates with UPPP (17).

The patient's symptoms and the goals of treatment should be considered when assigning initial therapy. Patients with substantial sleep disturbance may be better treated with CPAP and are more likely to accept this therapy than those who consider their sleep normal. Patients who primarily wish to satisfy the complaints of a bed partner are more likely to accept OA therapy.

Upper-airway imaging might be considered in the evaluation of patients before therapy, but it is not recommended in any form, since no reliable predictive information can be derived from such measurements. Some investigators have examined titration of mandibular position during sleep to aid patient selection, but such protocols require more work before they can be recommended for clinical use.

CLINICAL MANAGEMENT

Regardless of how patients initiate their search for snoring and OSA care, the dentist is the key provider. However, physicians should be involved in the diagnosis of OSA for reasons of licensing, liability, and access to medical insurance (21). When OA therapy is proposed, full disclosure of the procedures to implement therapy and follow-up care, as well as a prognosis of success, never 100%, must be provided to the patient. There is little science to guide the choice of appliance, particularly between different MADs, which are the most widely used and best evaluated OA type. For optimal comfort and maximum efficacy, an adjustable custom appliance should be used. A tongue device might be suitable for the patient without teeth and limited other options. The initial fitting is followed by a period of

adjustment or "titration" to a position that optimizes the trade-off between optimal effect and comfort. Knowledgeable professional input at this time is critical. An objective reassessment of OSA is appropriate after a symptom-based end point has been achieved. Reliance on symptoms alone will often result in suboptimal treatment. The type of reassessment depends on the clinical setting. If the symptoms are improved, oximetry may be a good choice, especially since it can be repeated at little cost when further adjustment is required.

All patients with OA therapy need long-term follow up by the treating dentist. Patients should be seen at 6- to 12-month intervals to evaluate potential alterations of the bite. These side effects can be managed with special exercises without discontinuing therapy. Wear and tear of the OA requires periodic service, especially of the soft lining layer that promotes adhesion and retention of the appliance.

PROGNOSIS

Since not all patients improve with OA, the outcome of treatment is uncertain until the adjustment period is completed. The expectation is that about 60% of patients will proceed to long-term care, the rate varying with initial severity. Limited data suggest that when OSA is adequately controlled, most patients will adhere to treatment for years (17). The principal reason for discontinuing therapy in various studies is lack of efficacy. If the treatment effect diminishes with time, a change in the underlying condition, possibly due to weight gain, should be suspected. In some patients the loss of effect occurs for no apparent reason, suggesting a change in airway properties, possibly tissue compliance. Further advance may restore the effect.

FUTURE DIRECTIONS

The principal challenge with OA therapy is to improve the rate of successful treatment. Since the limits are dictated by the range of mandibular mobility, it seems unlikely that a better appliance will change the current state-of-the-art. There may be an opportunity to improve titration protocols, although the limit of slow gradual titration was demonstrated in one trial when subjects stopped OA therapy because of impatience with the delay in achieving effective treatment (13). Improvements in the design of prefabricated appliances may make them more generally applicable and may lower the cost of OA therapy. Currently a good adjustable custom-made appliance and an experienced therapist provide the best chance of success. Beyond that, patient selection becomes the biggest challenge. No single criterion appears to be sufficiently predictive to preclude failed treatment, although OSA severity is the best. Predictors based on airway anatomy have not been useful, possibly because they do not adequately reflect airway function during sleep.

CLINICAL PEARLS

- Consider OA therapy for patients with mild to moderate OSA, particularly when the chief complaint is snoring.
- When moderate to severe patients fail CPAP, consider OA therapy, although the success rate will be less than 50%.
- After adjustment, evaluate OA treatment effect objectively; symptoms are not reliable.
- Use a dentist with experience in OA therapy. Untrained dentists have difficulty advancing the mandible to optimal effect for fear of complication.
- Advise the patient of potential tooth movement and insist on long-term dental follow-up.

REFERENCES

1. Robin P. Glossoptosis due to atresia and hypotrophy of the mandible. *Amer J Dis Child.* 1934;48:541–547.
2. Meier-Ewert K, Schafer H, et al. Treatment of sleep apnea by a mandibular protracting device. *Berichtsb* 7th *Eur Congr Sleep Res,* Munich, Germany, 1984:217.
3. Soll B, George P. Treatment of obstructive sleep apnea with a nocturnal airway patency appliance. *N Engl J Med.* 1985;313:386–387.
4. Cartwright R, Samelson C. The effects of a nonsurgical treatment for obstructive sleep apnea–the tongue-retaining device. *JAMA.* 1982;248:705–709.
5. Schmidt-Nowara W, Lowe A, Wiegand L, et al. Oral appliances for the treatment of snoring and obstructive sleep apnea: a review. *Sleep.* 1995;18:501–510.
6. American Sleep Disorders Association Standards of Practice Committee. Practice parameters for the treatment of snoring and obstructive sleep apnea with oral appliances. *Sleep.* 1995;18:511–513.
7. Young T, Palta M, Dempsey J, et al. The occurrence of sleep-disordered breathing among middle-aged adults. *N Engl J Med.* 1993;328:1230–1235.
8. Schmidt-Nowara W, Coultas D, Wiggins C, et al. Snoring in an Hispanic–American population: risk factors and association with hypertension and other morbidity. *Arch Intern Med.* 1990;150:597–601.
9. Isono S, Tanaka A, Sho Y, et al. Advancement of the mandible improves velopharyngeal patency. *J Appl Physiol.* 1995;79:2132–2138.
10. Lowe A, Fleetham J, Ryan F, et al. Effects of mandibular repositioning appliance used in the treatment of obstructive sleep apnea on tongue muscle activity. In: Suratt PM, Remmers JE, eds. *Sleep and respiration.* New York: Wiley–Liss, 1990:395–405.
11. Kato J, Isono S, Tanaka A, et al. Dose-dependent effects of mandibular advancement on pharyngeal mechanics and nocturnal oxygenation in patients with sleep-disordered breathing. *Chest.* 2000;117:1065–1072.
12. Miyamoto K, Ozbek M, Lowe A, et al. Mandibular posture during sleep in patients with obstructive sleep apnea. *Arch Oral Biol.* 1999;44:657–664.
13. Lowe A, Sjoholm T, Ryan C, et al. Treatment, airway and compliance effects of a titratable oral appliance. *Sleep.* 2000;23:S172–S178.
14. Marklund M, Franklin KA, Sahlin C, et al. The effect of a mandibular advancement device on apneas and sleep in patients with obstructive sleep apnea. *Chest.* 1998;113:707–713.
15. Mehta A, Qian J, Petocz P, et al. A randomized controlled study of mandibular advancement splint for obstructive sleep apnea. *Amer J Respir Crit Care Med.* 2001;163:1457–1461.
16. Engleman H, McDonald J, Graham D, et al. Randomized cross-over trial of two treatments for sleep apnea/hypopnea syndrome, continuous positive airway pressure and mandibular repositioning splint. *Am J Respir Crit Care Med.* 2002;166:855–859.
17. Walker-Engstrom M, Tegelberg A, Wilhelmsson B, et al. Four year follow-up of treatment with dental appliance or uvulopalatopharyngoplasty in patients with obstructive sleep apnea. *Chest.* 2002;121:739–746.
18. Pantin C, Hillman D, Tennant M. Dental side effects of an oral device to treat snoring and obstructive sleep apnea. *Sleep.* 1999;22:237–240.
19. Rose E, Staats R, Virchow C, et al. Occlusal and skeletal effects of an oral appliance in the treatment of obstructive sleep apnea. *Chest.* 2002;122:871–877.
20. Robertson CJ. Dental and skeletal changes associated with long-term mandibular advancement. *Sleep.* 2001;24:531–537.
21. Cooper N. Legal perspective: licensing and liability issues regarding the use of oral appliances in the treatment of obstructive sleep apnea. *Sleep Breath.* 2000;4:89–94.
22. Young T, Shahar E, Nieto J, et al. Predictors of sleep-disordered breathing in community-dwelling adults. *Arch Intern Med.* 2002;162:893–900.
23. Clark GT, Blumenfeld I, Yoffe N, et al. A cross-over study comparing the efficacy of continuous positive airway pressure with anterior mandibular positioning devices on patients with obstructive sleep apnea. *Chest.* 1996;109:1477–1483.
24. Ferguson KA, Ono T, Lowe AA, et al. A randomized crossover study of an oral appliance vs nasal-continuous positive airway pressure in the treatment of mild-moderate obstructive sleep apnea. *Chest.* 1996;109:1269–1275.
25. Ono T, Lowe A, Ferguson K, et al. A tongue-retaining device and sleep-state genioglossus muscle activity in patients with obstructive sleep apnea. *Angle Orthodont.* 1996;66:273–279.
26. Pancer J, Al-Faifi S, Al-Faifi M, et al. Evaluation of variable mandibular advancement appliance for treatment of snoring and sleep apnea. *Chest.* 1999;116:1511–1518.
27. Ferguson KA, Ono T, Lowe AA, et al. A short term controlled trial of an adjustable oral appliance for the treatment of mild-moderate obstructive sleep apnea. *Thorax.* 1997;52:362–368.

Chapter 23

Central Sleep Apnea

Atul Malhotra, Richard B. Berry, and David P. White

OVERVIEW

Cessation of breathing during sleep is defined as apnea (in adults greater than 10 seconds by convention), while reductions in breathing are called hypopneas (1,2). Cessation of breathing during sleep despite ongoing respiratory effort is associated with obstruction of the upper airway (obstructive apnea), whereas loss of ventilatory effort can also lead to loss of airflow (central apnea). The term *central sleep apnea* (CSA) is used to describe both the events and the clinical disorders characterized by repeated cessations of airflow during sleep resulting from temporary loss of ventilatory effort (Fig. 23-1). Although this chapter is focused on CSA, we acknowledge that central apneas are rarely seen in isolation. The majority of patients with central apneas will also have some obstructive apnea, and vice versa (3). By extension, it follows that the mechanisms responsible for the different types of apnea must overlap (4). A diagnosis of the CSA syndrome is usually made when the majority of events are central in nature (arbitrarily $> \approx 50\%$).

As will be discussed, the CSA syndromes are a heterogeneous group of disorders (5) that can be broadly classified on the basis of arterial carbon dioxide levels during wakefulness (hypercapnic versus eucapnic/hypocapnic; see Table 23-1).

VENTILATORY CONTROL AND PATHOPHYSIOLOGIC MECHANISMS

Ventilatory Control

Control of ventilation is dependent on both metabolic (automatic, i.e., chemoreceptors, stretch receptors), as well as behavioral (wake-dependent) control systems. During NREM sleep, ventilation is critically dependent on the metabolic control system. Under metabolic control, ventilation can be stimulated through medullary brain stem centers by CO_2 (likely via H^+ concentration) and the carotid body by P_{O_2} and P_{CO_2}. During wakefulness,

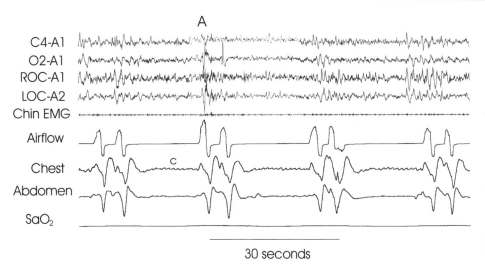

FIGURE 23-1. Idiopathic central apnea. The figure illustrates three apneas (cessation of airflow) without respiratory effort detectable in the chest and abdominal belts. Termination of the first apnea is associated with arousal (A). The small deflections in the chest tracing during apnea (C) do not reflect respiratory effort, but are secondary to cardiac pulsations.

an additional nonspecific "wakefulness drive" maintains ventilation even if the P_{CO_2} is reduced below the eucapnic level. However, during sleep the wakefulness drive is lost (6–8). With the onset of sleep, this loss of wakefulness drive plus other factors (e.g., upper-airway collapse) contribute to the normal rise in P_{CO_2} of 4 to 6 mm Hg above the eucapnic level during wakefulness. In addition, if the Pa_{CO_2} falls below a certain level (the apneic threshold) during NREM sleep, ventilatory effort ceases. The

apneic threshold is typically 2 to 6 mm Hg below the eucapnic sleeping Pa_{CO_2} level depending on the method used to determine this value. The apneic threshold usually corresponds roughly to the awake eucapnic P_{CO_2} level or slightly lower (8,9). This apnea threshold may, in part, explain the dysrhythmic breathing frequently seen at sleep onset (see below, *sleep transition central apneas*), even in normal individuals. Once a stable sleep stage is reached, ventilation should become regular under stable metabolic control.

▶ **TABLE 23-1. Classification of Central Sleep Apnea
Syndromes**

Hypercapnic Central Sleep Apnea
1. Central hypoventilation
a. Idiopathic central hypoventilation ("Ondine's curse")
b. Brain tumors
c. Cerebrovascular disease
d. Chronic narcotic use
e. Obesity hypoventilation syndrome
2. Neuromuscular disorders
a. Myasthenia gravis (neuromuscular junction)
b. Amyotrophic lateral sclerosis (motor neuron disease)
c. Post polio syndrome
d. Myopathies (eg acid maltase deficiency)
3. Chest wall syndromes (kyphoscoliosis)

Nonhypercapnic Central Sleep Apnea
1. Idiopathic
2. Treatment emergent
3. Sleep transition
4. Cheyne-Stokes breathing
a. Congestive heart failure
b. Neurologic disorders
5. Periodic breathing at high altitude

Ventilatory Control in Central Sleep Apnea

Since the CSA syndromes are heterogeneous, the pathophysiology is also quite varied (Table 23-2). In some patients with hypercapnic CSA, ventilatory control is abnormal. These individuals have low or absent hypoxic/hypercapnic responsiveness. Respiration during wakefulness is maintained by behavioral/wakeful stimuli plus weaker automatic mechanisms. However, during sleep, when these wakefulness-dependent mechanisms are no longer operative, there is little residual drive to ventilation because metabolic control is defective. As a result, hypoventilation and central apneas frequently ensue.

Based on the comments above, the slope of the ventilatory response to hypercapnia (frequently measured during wakefulness) may be an important variable in the development of central apneas during sleep (10,11). In patients with markedly diminished or absent chemosensitivity, some form of sleep-disordered breathing (SDB), frequently central apnea, would be expected. If carbon dioxide sensitivity is very low or absent, there would be little stimulus to ventilation during sleep and central apneas with sustained hypoventilation would be predictable. Patients with disorders such as central alveolar hypoventilation ("Ondine's curse") and the obesity-hypoventilation

▶ **TABLE 23-2. Pathophysiological Mechanisms of Central Sleep Apnea**

Hypercapnic central sleep apnea
  A. 'Won't breathe' — low or absent ventilatory response to Pco_2 and/or Po_2
     Abnormal ventilatory control centers
     Abnormal chemoreceptors
     Abnormal communication between chemoreceptors and control centers
     Brainstem defects
  B. 'Can't breathe'
     Motorneuron defects (brainstem/spinal cord)
     Motor nerve lesions
     Neuromuscular junction abnormalities
     Myopathy
     Increased respiratory impedance (chest wall disease, obesity)

Eucapnic/hypocapnic central sleep apnea (ultimate mechanism: Pco_2 is below the apneic threshold)
  A. Idiopathic Central Sleep Apnea
     High ventilatory drive (ventilatory response to Pco_2 or Pco_2)
     Small difference between the apneic threshold and sleeping eucapnic Pco_2
     High plant gain
     Long transition between wake and stable sleep
  B. Cheyne–Stokes respirations
     High ventilatory drive (ventilatory response to Pco_2 or Po_2)
     Small difference between the apneic threshold and sleeping eucapnic Pco_2
     Long circulation time (delay in ABG information to controllers)
     Increase in reflex stimulation of breathing (J receptors)— pulmonary congestion

(Pickwickian) syndrome would fall into this category (12). Similarly, recent reports have suggested a high prevalence of CSA among patients chronically taking narcotic medications (which can inhibit chemosensitivity) (13).

On the other hand, increased hypercapnic sensitivity can also lead to ventilatory instability during sleep (14). These "high drive" CSA patients often have low arterial Pco_2 levels during wakefulness and a high hypercapnic ventilatory response. The unusually steep hypercapnic responsiveness can lead to respiratory instability with a fluctuating pattern of ventilation in the wake–sleep transition. This is believed to be secondary to intermittent overventilation (yielding hypocapnia) alternating with underventilation (yielding hypercapnia). Such cycling ventilation probably results from the marked fluctuations in ventilation that occur with modest changes in $Paco_2$. Thus, elevated chemosensitivity contributes to cessations in airflow by producing ventilatory overshoots during which $Paco_2$ falls below the apnea threshold (6,15).

A unifying phenomenon in all forms of CSA is a complete loss of ventilatory drive. This can be recognized by an absence of electromyographic activity in the respiratory muscles or an absence of pleural pressure swings (estimated using esophageal pressure). In nonhypercapnic CSA, the basic mechanism underlying central apnea is that the Pco_2 falls below the apneic threshold. This can occur following an arousal (typically increasing ventilation) if sleep resumes before the Pco_2 rises above the apneic threshold (i.e., sleep transition apneas) or if there is ventilatory overshoot due to control instability. As an individual changes from wakefulness to stage 1 or 2 sleep, the Pco_2 level that was adequate to stimulate ventilation during wakefulness may be inadequate to do so during sleep and an apnea may occur. This apnea may arouse the individual, and the process repeats itself over and over. Thus there is ventilatory instability with oscillating levels of ventilatory drive. The causes of this instability include high ventilatory gain (hypercapnic responsiveness), high plant gain (efficient CO_2 excretion), delay in information reaching the controllers (long circulation time), and a $Paco_2$ level close to the apnea threshold.

The term loop gain is used to describe the net stability of the ventilatory control system. A high-loop gain refers to one that is intrinsically unstable, whereas a low-loop gain implies instrinsic stability. Loop gain is defined as the ratio of the response to the stimulus (ventilatory response/ventilatory disturbance) in a feedback control system, i.e., a large response to a minor perturbation is destabilizing. Thus, an intrinsically stable system would experience a minor response to a perturbation and continue relatively stably thereafter. On the other hand, an intrinsically unstable system may have a large response to a minor perturbation yielding subsequent instability. In the case of breathing, a robust ventilatory response to a trivial increase in $Paco_2$ would be destabilizing to the control system. This loop gain concept is useful in determining the various factors that can contribute to the development of CSA (16–19).

Pathophysiology of Cheyne–Stokes Respiration

The most common type of nonhypercapnic CSA is called Cheyne–Stokes respiration (Fig. 23-2). This disorder is characterized by a waxing and waning pattern of breathing most commonly seen in individuals with congestive heart failure (CHF) and left ventricular systolic dysfunction. This type of respiration is quite distinct, with a crescendo–decrescendo ventilatory pattern with a central apnea or hypopnea at the nadir. Thus, it is somewhat different from the aforementioned central apnea, which has a more abrupt onset and offset. Typically, the ventilatory phase between central apneas is longer in CSR than other types of repetitive central apneas due to a prolonged circulation time in CSR. Another difference is that arousal tends to occur at the peak of the ventilatory effort rather than at event

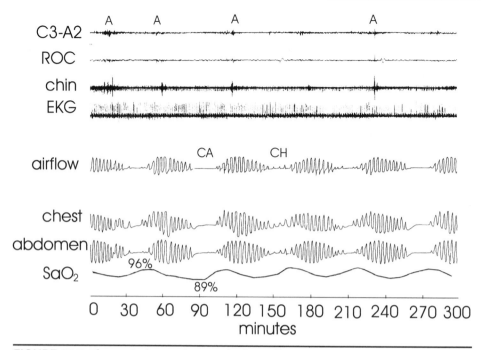

FIGURE 23-2. Cheyne–Stokes respiration. The figure illustrates a waxing and waning pattern of airflow and respiratory effort over the course of this 5-minute recording. Central apnea (CA) or central hypopnea (CH) occur at the nadirs in respiratory effort. Of note, the duration of each cycle is roughly 1 minute. The periods of ventilation between events are much longer than in idiopathic central apnea (Fig. 23-1). In addition, note the fall in oxygen saturation that occurs following each apnea. The time duration from end of apnea to the nadir in arterial oxygen saturation (Sao_2) desaturation is prolonged and reflects circulatory delay. Although difficult to see at this resolution, there is frequently arousal (A) from sleep at the peak of the hyperpnea with associated tachycardia. In idiopathic central apnea, arousal usually occurs at apnea termination (Fig. 23-1).

termination in CSR. The etiology of this breathing pattern in CSR has never been fully understood, but is probably a product of respiratory control system instability (high-loop gain with out-of-phase signal at the chemoreceptor) resulting from a prolonged circulation time and increased ventilatory responsiveness to rising Pco_2 (14). In an anesthetized animal, lengthening a normal circulation time can induce Cheyne–Stokes breathing. Such an increased circulation time may produce unstable ventilation due to the delay that occurs between mechanical changes in respiration (hyperpnea or hypopnea) and receptor stimulation resulting from changes in arterial blood gases. If a patient hypoventilates or has an apnea, a substantial period of time will pass before increasing Pco_2 or decreasing Po_2 is detected at the appropriate receptor. As a result, the apnea or hypopnea is prolonged. When the deoxygenated, hypercapnic blood does reach the receptor, ventilation is stimulated for a disproportionately long period of time because the corrected blood gases are again not presented to the receptor for an extended period of time. Thus, ventilation can wax and wane, with actual apneas occurring at the nadir of this cycle. Whether this is the mechanism of Cheyne–Stokes ventilation seen with CHF is speculative, because a severalfold increase in circulation time is necessary to produce such breathing dysrhythmias in an-

imals. This is probably a greater change than commonly occurs with heart failure. When groups of CHF patients with and without CSR have been compared, the groups do not systematically differ in circulation time (20). On the other hand, patients with CSR in CHF do have high ventilatory drive based on increased chemosensitivity and stimulation of ventilation through pulmonary stretch receptors (14). Thus, the group with CSR does generally have a lower awake arterial Pco_2 than CHF patients without CSR. One cause of the higher drive appears to be a higher wedge pressure (pulmonary arterial occlusion pressure). Presumably, pulmonary congestion results in stimulation of J receptors in the lung, which also increases ventilatory drive. Thus a prolonged circulation time probably must be combined with an increased ventilatory drive to yield Cheyne–Stokes breathing. Patients with congestive heart failure and CSR tend to maintain their waking eupnic Pco_2 levels during sleep, thus keeping the $Paco_2$ close to the apnea threshold (21). Thus, rather minor overshoots in ventilation could dramatically reduce ventilatory drive (21). These mechanisms (circulation time, CO_2 responsiveness, CO_2 set point) explain much of the variability in CSR occurrence in heart failure patients.

Cheyne–Stokes respiration has also been reported in patients with neurologic disease, primarily cerebrovascular disorders (22). However, the actual ventilatory pattern in these patients has been less well characterized than in CHF patients and the mechanisms remain poorly understood. In many cases, a cardioembolic etiology for the cerebrovascular event has not been carefully excluded, leading many to suspect underlying cardiac dysfunction in such patients. In addition, fluctuations in the level of consciousness in stroke patients have been associated with central apneas (state instability), similar in mechanism to the sleep-transition apneas described earlier. Other mechanisms leading to increased ventilatory drive have also been proposed to explain CSR in stroke patients. A reduction in or loss of tonic inhibition of ventilation could lead to this instability, but has not been fully characterized. Thus, the major mechanisms of Cheyne–Stokes respirations in cerebrovascular disease remain to be elucidated.

Pathophysiology of Hypercapnic Central Sleep Apnea—Effects of Sleep Stage

As noted above, some hypercapnic CSA patients have a defect in central drive. This may be caused by abnormal chemoreceptors [the sensors detecting Pco_2 (or H^+) and Po_2], poor communication of this information to the controllers, or a defect in generation of ventilatory rhythm. In some of these patients, the wakefulness drive is sufficient to maintain ventilation during wakefulness but hypoventilation and/or central apnea occurs during sleep. In other patients with hypercapnic CSA, the central drive is intact but other abnormalities compromise ventilation during sleep. These include defects in the neural motor circuits, respiratory muscles, or the chest wall. In this group, high ventilatory drive and accessory respiratory muscle activation may partially compensate for these problems during wakefulness. However, the loss of the wakefulness drive with sleep onset may result in the worsening of hypoventilation and/or frank central apnea (7). Of note, the majority of the patients with hypercapnic CSA have the most severe hypoventilation during REM sleep. During this sleep stage, ventilation is under both metabolic and nonmetabolic control and there is generalized skeletal muscle hypotonia. Those patients with compromised respiratory muscles or chest wall abnormalities are frequently dependent on the accessory muscles of respiration to maintain ventilation. When these muscles develop the atonia characteristic of REM sleep, the diaphragm alone may be unable to maintain adequate ventilation. On the other hand, there does exist the rare patient with central defects in ventilatory control who experiences improvements in respiration during REM sleep, as compared with NREM sleep. This phenomenon is thought to result from the nonmetabolic influences on ventilation that occur in REM sleep, but not NREM sleep (23). However, this is very uncommon.

DEFINITIONS AND CLASSIFICATION OF CENTRAL SLEEP APNEA SYNDROMES

Patients with predominantly central sleep apnea constitute fewer than 10% of apneic individuals in most sleep laboratory populations, with some recent data suggesting only about 4%. As a result, only a small number of studies with more than a few such patients have been reported, which makes knowledge of this disorder limited. Most of this chapter is dedicated to a discussion of patients with CSA who breathe normally during the day. However, any patient with hypoventilation during wakefulness will almost certainly have further hypoventilation (with central apneas) at night. As stated, the CSA syndromes are a heterogeneous group of disorders that can be classified into the hypercapnic and nonhypercapnic types (Table 23-1) (24).

HYPERCAPNIC CENTRAL SLEEP APNEAS AND SLEEP HYPOVENTILATION SYNDROMES

Patients with hypercapnic CSA usually have daytime hypercapnia that worsens with sleep. Some authors have used the term sleep hypoventilation syndrome to highlight the fact that most such patients hypoventilate during sleep but actually have few discrete central apneas (1). These hypercapnic patients can be further separated into a "won't breathe" group with defects in central drive but intact motor nerves, spinal cord, respiratory muscles, and lungs and a "can't breathe" group with normal drive but defects distal to the ventilatory control centers (Table 23-2). The former group comprises the central hypoventilation syndromes. Although uncommon, one form of this syndrome can present in infancy [congenital central hypoventilation syndrome (CCHS)] (25,26). In others, the neural pathways from these medullary respiratory neurons to the motorneurons of the ventilatory muscles are interrupted, which may occur after cervical cordotomy (27–29). Because the brainstem is the primary source of both ventilatory pattern generation and the processing of respiratory afferent input from chemoreceptors and intrapulmonary receptors, any disease process affecting this area could influence ventilation during sleep (30). Damage to the brainstem, particularly the medullary area, may lead to hypoventilation during wakefulness but more commonly affects ventilation during sleep early in the disease. Other processes, such as tumor, infarction, hemorrhage, or encephalitis, can damage the medullary area, leading to breathing dysrhythmias during sleep, with central apneas being a prominent feature (31).

The second group of hypoventilation syndromes (unimpaired drive—"can't breathe") are commonly classified anatomically, including lesions of the upper motor neurons [e.g., amyotrophic lateral sclerosis (ALS) which can involve both upper and lower motor neurons), spinal cord

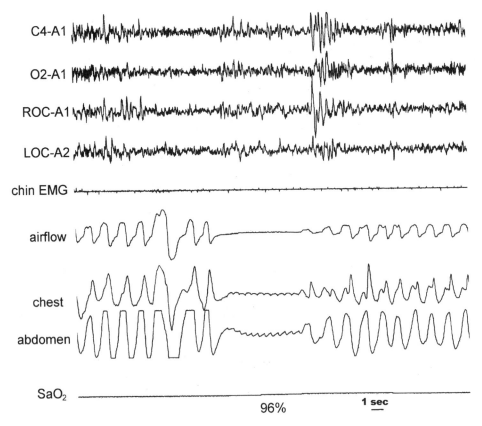

C4-A1

O2-A1

ROC-A1

LOC-A2

chin EMG

airflow

chest

abdomen

SaO₂   96%   **1 sec**

FIGURE 23-3. Sleep-transition apnea. This figure illustrates the importance of the apnea threshold during sleep. One large breath soon after sleep onset leads to the cessation of airflow without respiratory effort. Presumably the one large breath drove the Pco_2 below the apnea threshold, leading to cessation of output from the respiratory pattern generator.

(e.g., trauma), anterior horn cells (e.g., poliomyelitis), lower motor neurons (e.g., phrenic nerve C3–C5), neuromuscular junction (e.g., myasthenia gravis), and the respiratory muscles themselves (e.g., polymyositis, acid maltase deficiency). Mechanical impairment of the chest wall (e.g., kyphoscoliosis) and lung parenchyma can also lead to hypercapnic respiratory failure. Whereas these disorders may be characterized by central apneas during sleep, the principal problem is nocturnal hypoventilation, particularly during REM sleep, which leads to substantial hypoxia and hypercapnia with their associated sequelae. Thus, the hypercapnic CSA syndromes include a spectrum of disease from hypoventilation to frank cessation in breathing.

Finally, as stated previously, any neurologic disorder affecting the ventilatory control system could influence ventilatory patterns during sleep, possibly leading to central apneas. Thus, patients with autonomic dysfunction, such as the Shy–Drager syndrome, familial dysautonomia, or diabetes mellitus, may have central apneas, although the precise mechanisms leading to such apneas have not been determined.

NONHYPERCAPNIC CENTRAL SLEEP APNEA

Patients with nonhypercapnic CSA have normal or low daytime Pco_2. Syndromes falling under this category include idiopathic CSA and CSA with Cheyne–Stokes respiration (Table 23-1). We have also included sleep-transition CSA and treatment-emergent CSA for completeness, although these are really forms of isolated CSA rather than true CSA syndromes (Fig. 23-3 and 23-4). Sleep-transition central apneas may occur in normal individuals at sleep onset, when there is a waxing and waning of ventilation. These sleep-transition apneas occur when there is state instability (transitions from sleep to wake), with concomitant fluctuations in Pco_2. Therefore, any process that leads to frequent sleep–wake transitions over the course of the night [e.g., insomnia, periodic limb movements (PLMs), obstructive apneas, spontaneous arousals] may increase the number of central apneas. Treatment-emergent central apneas occur during titration of continuous positive airway pressure (CPAP) in obstructive sleep apnea (OSA) patients (Fig. 23-4). Although this has been studied minimally and the explanation remains obscure, CPAP does lower the resistance in the upper airway, which can lead to falls in Pco_2. If the Pco_2 falls below the apnea threshold, central apneas will ensue (32). Increased lung volume on CPAP may also activate stretch receptors that can inhibit ventilation (33). Clinical experience suggests that this form of central apnea generally resolves with ongoing therapy. A similar phenomenon has been observed in OSA patients following tracheostomy, wherein some individuals will experience central apneas that eventually resolve (34). Patients with idiopathic CSA have no other identifiable

CPAP = 10 cm H₂O

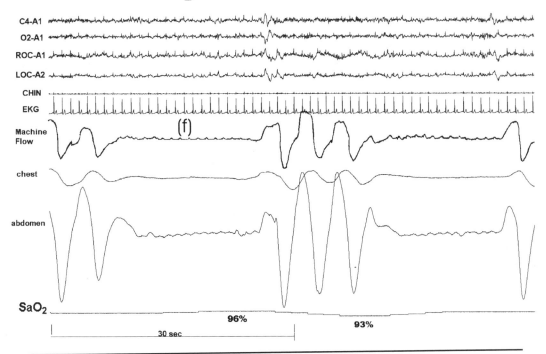

FIGURE 23-4. Treatment-emergent central sleep apnea. The figure shows the absence of respiratory effort during the cessation of airflow with associated desaturations. The resumption of breathing is associated with arousal from sleep. In this case, the central apneas occurred after initiation of positive pressure therapy. Also of note are small fluctuations (f), visible in flow channel during the central apnea, that likely represent cardioballistic flow, since they occur at the same frequency as the R wave in the electroencephalogram.

disorder (i.e., diagnosis of exclusion). However, this syndrome is relatively rare.

The most common type of nonhypercapnic central sleep apnea is Cheyne–Stokes respiration (CSR) (35,36). Increasing data suggest deleterious effects from this breathing pattern on cardiac function and survival as well as improvements in cardiovascular function with treatment of the CSR (37–40).

CENTRAL SLEEP APNEA SYNDROMES—CLINICAL ASPECTS, DIAGNOSIS, AND TREATMENT

Hypercapnic Central Sleep Apnea

Depending on the underlying cause, the clinical presentation of these individuals can be quite varied (Table 23-3; Fig. 23-5). They are occasionally detected based on an unexplained low-baseline saturation (either on a polysomnogram or in a hospitalized patient). In other instances, an elevated bicarbonate level is observed on routine chemistries. More extreme presentations include cor pulmonale (peripheral edema and right heart failure) or hypercapnic respiratory failure. Another common presenta-

tion is major hypoxemia and hypercapnia secondary to a minor respiratory infection. In the case of neuromuscular disease, these patients frequently present with systemic fatigue and/or weakness and are subsequently found to have respiratory muscle involvement. On further questioning, these patients frequently complain of positional dyspnea, specifically profound orthopnea in the case of diaphragm weakness.

The diagnostic approach for these patients is straightforward based on the history and physical examination as well as some basic laboratory testing. Patients with a clinical presentation compatible with a profound pulmonary parenchymal abnormality or neuromuscular weakness are usually readily apparent. Similarly, obesity hypoventilation syndrome can be suspected based on morbid obesity. An arterial blood gas during wakefulness can be very useful in these individuals to confirm a chronic respiratory acidosis. An elevated P_{CO_2}, with a low normal pH, and a preserved A-aD_{O_2} gradient are highly suggestive of a hypoventilation syndrome with normal lung parenchyma. In cases of suspected diaphragmatic weakness, physical examination can be quite revealing, with the development of respiratory paradox in the supine posture. In more subtle cases, the performance of a sniff test (under fluoroscopy to assess paradoxical motion), esophageal balloon

▶ **TABLE 23-3. Clinical Presentations of Sleep-Disordered Breathing Syndromes**

CSA
  Hypercapnic
    Respiratory failure (acute or chronic)
    Neuromuscular weakness
    Low saturation or elevated bicarbonate
    Polycythemia
    Cor pulmonale
  Idiopathic
    Daytime sleepiness
    Minimal snoring
    Insomnia
    Nocturnal awakenings
  CSR
    Orthopnea
    Paroxysmal nocturnal dyspnea
    Recurrent awakenings
    Nonrestorative sleep
    Witnessed apneas

OSA
  Obesity
  Snoring
  Excessive daytime sleepiness
  Non-restorative sleep
  Hypertension

maximal expiratory pressure (MEP)] can help assess the severity of underlying neuromuscular disease. Although measurement of hypercapnic and hypoxic ventilatory response curves can be quite helpful for research purposes, these tests are rarely done clinically due to a lack of specific therapies targeting these abnormalities. A final test that is sometimes used clinically is the $P_{0.1}$ (or P_{100}) (41). This test measures the pressure generated by an individual during a sudden unsuspected airway occlusion during the first 100 milliseconds of spontaneous tidal inspiration. Although not definitive, a low value is compatible with low central drive and generally suggests the category of "won't breathe" for a particular individual.

Polysomnography (PSG) may be helpful clinically in some of these hypercapnic CSA patients. However, it remains controversial whether this expensive test is necessary for patients with neuromuscular disease and known hypercapnia. This decision regarding diagnostic testing is in part determined by the treatment approach being used. In some instances, the institution of nocturnal ventilation may be performed using empiric settings with satisfactory results. Due to the potential impact of accessory respiratory muscle atonia during REM sleep, the respiratory system mechanics can change substantially from wakefulness to the various stages of sleep. Thus, we often do recommend polysomnograms to determine the extent of the abnormalities during sleep and to determine the optimal bilevel positive pressure settings during sleep. In many cases, nocturnal hypoventilation is observed, rather than frank central apneas; however, the extent to which this observation changes management is unclear.

The treatment of hypercapnic CSA depends to a large extent on the etiology. In those instances where reversible or treatable abnormalities are found, specific treatments

study, or diaphragm ultrasound is occasionally necessary. Spirometry measured in the supine and upright posture can be quite helpful if a marked decline in vital capacity is observed while in the supine posture. Respiratory muscle forces [maximal inspiratory pressure (MIP), and

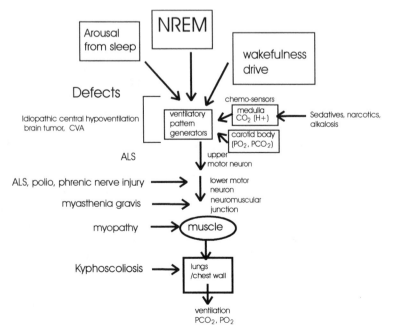

FIGURE 23-5. The various mechanisms important in the pathogenesis of hypercapnia CSA. Loss of output from the ventilatory pattern generator and disruption of this neuromuscular pathway can lead to hypoventilation and CSA.

should be instituted (e.g., steroid myopathy, polymyositis). Although alleviation of hypoxemia (supplementary nasal oxygen) may be beneficial in some alveolar hypoventilation patients with CSA, these patients are probably in the minority (42). Because respiratory stimulants have generally been ineffective, mechanical ventilation treatments are generally used in this population. For the hypercapnic patient with alveolar hypoventilation during wakefulness and worsening hypoventilation during sleep with central apneas, nocturnal ventilation is the most appropriate approach. Initially, such ventilation was accomplished only by tracheostomy with a mechanical respirator, diaphragmatic pacing, or negative-pressure (cuirass) ventilators. However, more recent experience indicates that nocturnal ventilation can be accomplished satisfactorily with a nasal or nasal–oral mask and a pressure-cycled ventilator or, less commonly, a volume-cycled ventilator. If a bilevel pressure device is used, the level of expiratory positive airway pressure (EPAP) is adjusted to keep the upper airway patent, and the inspiratory positive airway pressure (IPAP)–EPAP difference (pressure support) is adjusted to augment nocturnal ventilation. A frequent mistake in such patients is the administration of excessive EPAP in the absence of upper airway instability. EPAP levels above 5 cm H_2O are frequently unnecessary in neuromuscular disease patients and can substantially limit patient tolerance and adherence. Many of these patients require a backup rate for optimum treatment [spontaneously timed (ST mode)]. With advancing technology, the ease of administration of nocturnal ventilation has improved substantially, as has patient acceptance. Although rigorous randomized controlled data are as yet unavailable to prove the efficacy of these treatments, nasal bilevel positive airway pressure has become the treatment of choice for hypercapnic CSA (43–45). Finally, end-stage patients may require tracheostomy and volume-cycled ventilation, if they choose to proceed with this therapy.

NONHYPERCAPNIC CENTRAL SLEEP APNEA–CLINICAL ASPECTS, DIAGNOSIS, AND TREATMENT

Cheyne–Stokes Respiration

Patients with Cheyne–Stokes ventilation during wakefulness, whether from heart failure or other causes, will continue this respiratory pattern during sleep with frequent apneas. In addition, a number of reports suggest that many patients with CHF without obvious breathing abnormalities during wakefulness may have CSR during sleep. In fact, several studies suggest that up to 45% of patients with CHF (left ventricular ejection fraction <40%) have more than 10 apneas plus hypopneas per hour of sleep. Thus Cheyne–Stokes breathing during sleep in patients with CHF is likely quite common. However, because of recent changes in therapy for CHF (beta blockade, aldosterone antagonism, more aggressive diuresis, and blood pressure lowering), the prevalence of Cheyne–Stokes respirations in well-treated CHF is not known with certainty. This is further complicated by the fact that the prevalence studies that do exist are primarily from sleep referral centers, leading to a potential lack of generalizability of these data to the broader heart failure population. Thus, further research is clearly needed in this area.

The existing data also suggest a reduced survival in individuals with left ventricular failure and Cheyne–Stokes respiration when compared with patients in heart failure who breathed rhythmically. Lanfranchi et al. (46) performed a multivariate analysis of potential predictors of mortality in a CHF population. This study included numerous demographic, hemodynamic, exercise, and autonomic variables that are traditionally regarded as major predictors of mortality in CHF. The authors concluded that only two variables had independent predictive value: AHI and left atrial size. Because the equipment used in this study did not include a measurement of sleep *per se*, the AHI was based on hours of recording, leading some to question the applicability of these findings. However, despite this limitation, the results strongly suggest that CSR has independent predictive value.

The clinical presentation of CSR is quite variable and can be subtle (see Table 23-3). As a result, the majority of these patients remain undiagnosed. Complaints such as paroxysmal nocturnal dyspnea or disturbed sleep in CHF patients should prompt consideration of this diagnosis. Although classically considered a symptom of CHF itself, nocturnal awakenings with shortness of breath (i.e., paroxysmal nocturnal dyspnea) are commonly related to the breathing instability itself. The characteristic breathing pattern (crescendo–decrescendo respiration) is not commonly observed during wakefulness. This is largely related to the behavioral influences that determine ventilatory pattern during wakefulness. Occasionally, the breathing instability will emerge during exercise, presumably when behavioral influences on breathing pattern are minimized (47). Finally, Sin et al. determined the characteristics predicting the presence of CSR among patients with CHF in a sleep-disorders clinical population (Fig. 23-6). The authors found four variables to have independent predictive value: male gender, age, hypocapnia, and atrial fibrillation (36). Whether these same factors are applicable in other clinical settings (e.g., outside of a referral sleep clinic) remains to be determined.

Whether PSG is required to make the diagnosis of CSR also remains unclear. In instances where a waxing and waning breathing pattern is apparent during physical examination, no further testing is required. Pulse oximetry has been used in some instances to assess cyclical changes in saturations; however, published data on this technique are rather limited. In the United States, the need for objective documentation of breathing abnormalities in order

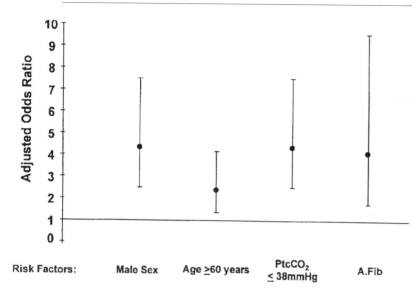

FIGURE 23-6. The various risk factors that predict the occurrence of CSR in patients with CHF. Male gender, age, hypocapnia, and atrial fibrillation are useful risk factors to keep in mind when assessing these patients. (Reproduced with permission from Sin D, et al. Risk factors for central and obstructive sleep apnea in 450 men and women with congestive heart failure. *Amer J Respir Crit Care Med.* 1999; 160:1101–1106).

to obtain reimbursement for positive airway pressure therapy is also a consideration. Thus, in some instances, PSG is required even when the diagnosis is fairly clear based on clinical factors. As in Fig. 23-2, PSG reveals the characteristic oscillations in breathing pattern in the respiratory belts and in the airflow channel. The oxygen saturation characteristically cycles as well, with the delay in desaturation being a function of cardiac output. The length of the ventilatory period between apneas is inversely proportional to the cardiac output. There are typically repeated arousals from sleep, which are classically at the peak of the hyperpneas, although not invariably. Bursts of tachycardia are also commonly seen with each arousal, emphasizing the ongoing sympathoexcitation that occurs in association with this disease. Of note, CSR is usually confined to stage 1 and 2 sleep. If these patients are able to reach stage 3 and 4 sleep or REM sleep, CSR usually abates or diminishes. This is probably secondary to the increase in PCO_2 during stage 3 and 4 sleep and or nonmetabolic influences on ventilation during REM sleep. Decreased chemoresponsiveness in REM sleep likely plays a role as well. At this time, overnight PSG remains the gold standard for the diagnosis of CSR until newer technologies emerge.

Both central and obstructive apneas have been reported in patients with CHF. This may be dependent on the characteristics of the individual's upper airway (size, collapsibility), with obstructive events resulting from decreased upper-airway muscle tone at the nadir of the respiratory cycle in an individual with a susceptible pharyngeal airway. In reality, the distinction between patients with central and obstructive events in this population is not absolute. Some patients who exhibit pure CSR in the lateral sleeping position have mixed (terminal obstructive portion) or obstructive apnea when sleeping in the supine position (increased upper-airway closure) (48). Central apneas and CSR may emerge during CPAP therapy for OSA when the obstructive component is eliminated with positive airway pressure (PAP). An example of a mixed apnea in a patient with snoring, daytime sleepiness, OSA, and underlying CSR is shown in Fig. 23-7. In this patient with mixed apnea during the diagnostic portion of the study, a pure Cheyne–Stokes morphology emerged during CPAP titration. The clues that CSR coexists with OSA are that there is a long delay in the nadir of the oxygen saturation (prolonged circulation time), a crescendo–decrescendo ventilatory pattern may be noted between apneas, and mixed apneas may contain a long central portion (48).

The treatment of CSR is somewhat controversial. A number of therapies have been recommended, including the treatment of the underlying CHF itself, oxygen, theophylline, nasal CPAP, and some newer positive pressure devices designed specifically to treat CSR (see below). Aggressive treatment of the underlying cardiac failure is frequently overlooked by sleep physicians. In many instances, patients who are apparently optimally treated medically would benefit from further diuresis or increased doses of beta-adrenoceptor blocker and/or afterload reduction (49). Rigorous studies have demonstrated the resolution of CSR in some patients with intensive hemodynamic management. Thus, medical therapy should be intensified, if possible, prior to other interventions.

The use of oxygen to treat CSR has also raised considerable controversy. Several studies have found improvement in breathing pattern (reduced AHI) and sleep quality (50,51) when patients with CSR were treated with oxygen. While some have argued that oxygen may have cardiodepressant effects mediated by oxidant radicals (52), others argue that such effects are largely theoretical. Some recent data suggest reduced sympathoexcitation with oxygen administration during volitional apneas (53). However, the hemodynamic benefits of oxygen therapy in CSR, if any, have not been clearly established (54). As a result, the judicious use of oxygen is considered by most to be a second-or third line treatment for CSR in CHF.

Theophylline has also received considerable attention in the treatment of CSR (55). There are a number of

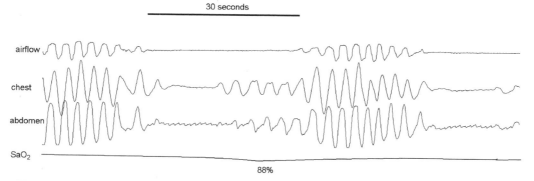

FIGURE 23-7. Mixed apnea in a patient with combined obstructive sleep apnea and Cheyne–Stokes respiration associated with heart failure. Note that the nadir in SaO_2 (88%) occurs "before apnea termination." In fact, this desaturation belongs to the previous event (prolonged circulation time). The airflow shows a crescendo–decrescendo pattern with relatively many breaths between apneas. When this patient was placed on low levels of CPAP, the obstructive portion was abolished and typical Cheyne-Stokes respiration was noted.

theoretical reasons why this agent may work; however, the exact mechanism of action remains unclear. Theophylline treatment reduces, but does not eliminate, CSR events. The majority of available data suggesting efficacy for this agent are from short-duration studies. However, in the short term, the methylxanthine class of medications has major inotropic effects on the heart. Because most long-term studies of inotropic agents in CHF have suggested deleterious effects on outcome, there is concern about this possibility with methylxanthines (e.g., via increased ventricular arrhythymias). Thus, theophylline is not commonly used to treat CSR with CHF since long-term efficacy and toxicity data are lacking.

Nasal CPAP is emerging as the treatment of choice for CSR with CHF. A number of studies have revealed stabilization of breathing pattern with chronic nasal CPAP therapy (1 to 3 months) (40). Although some studies have found an acute reduction in the AHI in CSR patients, this is rarely to the same extent as seen with OSA. In fact, a few studies have found no acute effect (54). It appears that nasal CPAP has an acute beneficial effect in most patients but some require chronic treatment of 1 to 3 months for a reduction in CSR. The mechanisms through which CPAP works are likely complex, but reflect some combination of reduced cardiac preload, reduced left ventricular afterload, suppressed catecholamines, blunted arousals, reduced extravascular lung water (reduced gain), and improved oxygenation (see Table 23-4) (56). Because CPAP does not generally completely stabilize the breathing pattern acutely, an empiric pressure of 10 to 12 cm H_2O via nasal mask is generally used for the treatment of CSR (54). This level of pressure has been found to be hemodynamically beneficial in many CHF patients. Of note, if CSR patients are not sleepy, they may find sleeping with CPAP difficult. Thus, in some centers, the pressure is slowly increased over several nights. In cases where ongoing obstructive events are detected despite this level of pressure, a higher pressure may be required. Preliminary data have also been published

showing CPAP-induced improvements in sleep quality, left ventricular ejection fraction, catecholamine levels, cardiac arrhythmias, and, most recently, transplant-free survival (37–40) (Fig. 23-8). However, all published studies are quite small, leading to no definitive conclusions thus far. Ongoing research including the CANPAP (Canadian Positive Airway Pressure) study are examining the role of CPAP in the treatment of CSR with CHF in a large randomized multicenter trial (57).

Newer devices (e.g., adaptive servo-ventilation) have been developed by industry to stabilize breathing pattern in CSR in a more acute fashion than standard devices (58,59). As stated previously, nasal CPAP usually reduces, but does not eliminate, CSR acutely. The substantial time delay makes some patients reluctant to use the device due to the lack of immediate benefit. The concept underlying the newer devices is to stabilize breathing patterns on the night of titration, thus improving sleep quality acutely, perhaps yielding improved patient adherence with therapy as

▶ **TABLE 23-4. Mechanisms of Hemodynamic Improvement with Continuous Positive Airway Pressure in Cheynes–Stokes Respiration**

1. Reduced cardiac preload via increased caval resistance (decreased venous return)
2. Increased lung compliance via reduced extravascular lung water
3. Reduced left ventricular afterload via less wall stress (decreased transmural pressure)
4. Reduced catecholamines
5. Reduced inspiratory fall in pleural pressure (affects Nos.1 and 3)
6. Improved hypoxemia
7. Sleep consolidation, blunted arousals
8. Reduced myocardial oxygen consumption through smaller chamber
9. Reduced mitral regurgitation, if present

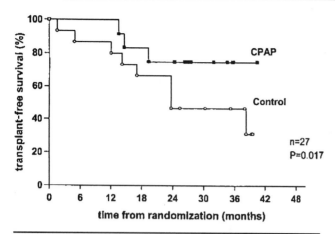

FIGURE 23-8. The figure illustrates the improvement in survival observed among patients with CHF and CSR who were adherent with CPAP therapy as compared with control patients not treated with CPAP. (From Sin D, Logan A, Fitzgerald F, et al. Effects of continuous positive airway pressure on cardiovascular outcomes in heart failure patients with and without Cheyne–Stokes respiration. *Circulation.* 2000; 102:61–66. With permission).

a result of the more immediate perceived benefits. This hypothesis remains untested, but is the subject of a number of ongoing studies. In addition, the hemodynamic benefits of these newer devices must be rigorously evaluated, since they may or may not provide the same benefits as CPAP. Thus, newer devices for the treatment of CSR are evolving, but are not yet ready for routine clinical use. The positive pressure treatment of CSR is discussed in detail in the chapter on positive pressure.

Two other treatments deserve mention, although neither are likely applicable clinically. They are added dead space and carbon dioxide inhalation (60,61). The use of added dead space has been shown to stabilize breathing in CSR due to damped oscillation in the P_{CO_2} value. Similarly, carbon dioxide inhalation can raise the arterial CO_2 tensions well above the apnea threshold and lead to a more stable breathing pattern. However, neither added dead space nor inhaled CO_2 are well tolerated clinically. Moreover, the hemodynamic benefits of these approaches have not been well studied. Thus, these approaches are valuable as a proof of concept, but cannot be recommended for clinical use.

In summary, CSR in CHF may be of major clinical importance due to its high prevalence, the deleterious effects on patient outcome, and the improvements in hemodynamics with positive pressure therapy.

IDIOPATHIC CENTRAL SLEEP APNEA

Patients with hypocapnia or normocapnia during wakefulness, who experience the cessation of respiratory effort during sleep in the absence of the characteristic pattern of CSR or sleep transition apnea, fall into the category of idiopathic CSA. By definition, this disorder is a diagnosis of exclusion. Patients with idiopathic central sleep apnea may present with complaints of either insomnia or hypersomnolence. In general, they are thinner and snore less than patients with OSA. Idiopathic CSA is uncommon with these patients, probably representing less than 5% of all cases of sleep apnea. The frequency and duration of central apneas in the nonhypercapnic group required to produce these clinical symptoms are difficult to determine from the currently available literature. In fact, investigators are actually still uncertain about which variables should be monitored to predict clinical outcomes in this disorder. Despite the limitation of the available data, five central events per hour of sleep are currently considered the upper limit of normal. Although this number is somewhat arbitrary, we must await new information before a more meaningful definition can be chosen.

As expected, arterial oxygen desaturation does occur with central apneas. The extent to which desaturation occurs during a given apnea is likely to be related to the P_{O_2} when ventilation ceased, the duration of the apnea, and the lung volume at which the apnea occurred. Whether ventilatory effort is occurring (obstructive apnea) or not (central apnea) may also have a minor effect on the rate of desaturation. Obstructive sleep apnea (OSA) patients do generally desaturate to a greater extent than central apnea patients. This is probably a function of longer apnea duration, reduced lung volume [supine functional residual capacity (FRC) lower in patients with OSA due to obesity], and the presence of ventilatory efforts in the obstructive apnea patient.

The impact of breathing instability on sleep disruption is well known. However, little information is available specifically addressing idiopathic CSA in this role. An improvement in sleep efficiency and a trend toward more time in deeper (stages 3 and 4) and rapid eye movement (REM) sleep has been reported after treatment of CSA, which does imply that sleep was disrupted by the apneas (62). In fact, the six reported patients had a mean of 209 apnea-associated awakenings and arousals in a single night before therapy. Another group also found a reduction in what is generally considered a normal percentage of stages 3 and 4 sleep and an increase in stages 1 and 2 sleep in patients with approximately 50% central apneas. In general, most central apneas occur during stage 1 and 2 sleep. If patients can reach stage 3 and 4 sleep, central apnea tends to abate, possibly secondary to higher P_{CO_2} and less frequent arousals in that sleep stage.

In some cases, it can be challenging to separate the phenomenon of central apneas leading to insomnia (recurrent arousals) from the converse: insomnia leading to central apneas (sleep transition type). This distinction can be a difficult one clinically since components of both coexist. In many cases, however, this "chicken or egg" argument becomes largely academic since therapy will often address both problems.

The diagnosis of idiopathic CSA generally requires a full-night recording of standard polysomnographic variables with a particular focus on respiratory effort. To prove that an apnea is indeed central, it must be documented that there is no respiratory effort throughout the event. This is most effectively and consistently accomplished with an esophageal balloon. Recognizing the difficulty of clinically using an esophageal balloon, other strategies have been employed. Most evidence suggests that respiratory inductive plethysmography (RIP), calibrated or uncalibrated, can adequately assess respiratory effort. If there is a complete absence of thoraco-abdominal motion (RIP or strain gauges) throughout an apnea, this strongly suggests that the event is central in origin. Although some evidence suggests that chest–abdominal wall motion as a measure of effort may overestimate the frequency of central apnea (1), rarely will the patient be misclassified using this methodology. A third option to assess effort would be diaphragmatic electromyography (EMG) although this is frequently difficulty to obtain and, therefore, cannot always be relied upon. Finally, classic teaching has suggested that cardioballistic artifacts in the oronasal flow signal indicate a patent airway and, therefore, a central apnea. However, this technique is somewhat controversial (63). Central hypopneas are usually indistinguishable from obstructive hypopneas using standard monitoring techniques. As a result, central apneas, not hypopneas, are usually documented to make a definitive diagnosis of CSA.

As mentioned, five central apneas per hour of sleep are currently considered the upper limit of normal and a greater frequency implies an abnormal state. In patients with components of both OSA and CSA, the primary abnormality is frequently difficult to determine. As a result, no definitive event percentage can be provided that will always indicate a central process. For research purposes, generally 75% to 85% of events must be central for patient inclusion, although occasionally a lower percentage has been used. As obstructive apneas are considerably more common, and current diagnostic methodologies tend to overestimate central apnea frequency, to use 80% central events as a threshold would seem reasonable. However, this value can be adjusted according to the clinical scenario.

Because this disorder is rare, few well-controlled studies of treatment exist (32). In addition, the patients with this disorder appear to be heterogeneous; therefore, treatment to some extent must be individualized. However, therapeutic options are available for CSA patients with insomnia, restless sleep, waking hypersomnolence, and mild-to-moderate nocturnal hypoxemia. First, if any of the conditions known to be associated with central apnea are present (eg, nasal obstruction or pharyngeal collapse), the abnormality should be treated aggressively and the central apnea reassessed. Second, some recent data suggest that these central apneas may resolve spontaneously in some

patients. As a result, in patients without severe symptoms, expectant follow-up may be appropriate. Third, if the problem persists or if no known predisposing abnormality can be found, several pharmacologic approaches can be attempted. Acetazolamide is a carbonic anhydrase inhibitor known to induce bicarbonaturia, yielding metabolic acidosis and likely a shift in the P_{CO_2} apnea threshold to a lower value. It has been used to treat CSA in some previous studies. For example, in a small series ($n = 6$), acetazolamide (250 mg four times per day) reduced central apnea substantially in all participants when used over a short period of time (1 to 2 weeks) (62). Long-term use of the medication was assessed in only two individuals and was successful in one and failed in the other. However, a more recent study of 14 patients with central apnea suggests that acetazolamide may lead to a more sustained improvement in apnea frequency and symptoms (primarily hypersomnolence) (64). Of note, subsequent discontinuation of acetazolamide did not lead to an immediate return of symptoms or events (65). On the other hand, several studies have reported the development of obstructive apneas after acetazolamide administration in patients previously demonstrated to have central events. The explanation for this remains obscure but may relate to the respiratory-stimulating activity (increased loop gain) of acetazolamide in an individual with a pharyngeal airway predisposed toward collapse during sleep. When little ventilatory effort is present, the apneas appear central. However, when respiration is stimulated, obstructive events develop. Clearly, follow-up sleep studies are necessary in patients being treated with acetazolamide.

Isolated reports of the use of other medications such as theophylline, naloxone, and medroxyprogesterone acetate, imply that these drugs have little efficacy in the treatment of central apnea (66). Clomipramine (a tricyclic antidepressant), on the other hand, was found to be successful in several patients in whom it was tried. Theophylline improved apnea in a patient with a damaged brainstem. However, none of these drugs has been studied systematically, so firm recommendations regarding their use cannot be made. Our experience suggests that most pharmacologic approaches have limited efficacy.

Nasal CPAP has been shown to be an effective therapy for some idiopathic CSA patients (67,68). There are several possible mechanisms explaining why CPAP might be effective. First, pharyngeal airway collapse or closure during sleep may initiate a reflex inhibition of ventilation in some patients and therefore a central apnea. With nasal CPAP, airway closure is prevented, and such reflex apneas abolished. Therefore, in obese, snoring patients in whom predominantly central apneas are observed, nasal CPAP may be an effective form of therapy. Others authors have attributed the reduction of central apnea by CPAP to a CPAP-induced increase in arterial P_{CO_2}. As a result, the sleeping P_{CO_2} was kept above the apnea threshold. One study suggested that in some patients CPAP may be more beneficial than bilevel pressure (69). Thus, a wide range of

▶ **TABLE 23-5.** Treatment of CSA

A. Hypercapnic CSA
   Ventilatory stimulants—usually not effective
   Noninvasive (mask) positive pressure ventilation
   Negative pressure ventilation, diaphragmatic pacing
   Oxygen—selected cases
   Tracheostomy with volume-cycled ventilation

B. Hypocapnic/Eucapnic
   1. Idiopathic
      Acetazolamide
      Nasal CPAP
      Oxygen
      Hypnotics??
   2. CSR
      Medical treatment of CHF
      Nasal CPAP
      Oxygen

CSA patients may respond to CPAP, although the final role of this therapeutic modality in central apnea must await further investigation.

A number of studies suggest that oxygen may be a useful method of treating idiopathic CSA. One group of investigators observed that central apneas were completely eliminated with oxygen administration in two patients during a short-nap study (70). Another study evaluating the effects of low-flow oxygen in nine obese patients with a large component of central apneas reported a considerable reduction in these central events (71). However, the frequency of obstructive apneas increased somewhat. Although the mechanism by which oxygen administration reduces central apneas has not yet been established, three explanations seem possible. First, there is a potential destabilizing influence of the hypoxic ventilatory response on respiratory control. As at altitude, with hypoxemia, an individual will hyperventilate, yielding hypocapnia and alkalosis. Hypocapnia, when below the apnea threshold, may inhibit respiration during sleep. Thus, cycling ventilation may develop with central apneas occurring at the nadir of this periodic breathing. With administration of oxygen, the hypoxemic influence on ventilation may be reduced and breathing regularized. Second, hypoxia, in some studies, has been shown to be a central ventilatory depressant. If respiration is depressed by hypoxia, then central apneas may occur. In theory, oxygen administration in this situation could reduce apneas. Third, oxygen administration can lead to slight elevations in arterial carbon dioxide concentrations via a variety of different mechanisms. In normal individuals, the Haldane effect, the release of carbon dioxide from hemoglobin in the context of oxygen administration, may be the predominant mechanism leading to elevations in $Paco_2$ (72). Regardless, if carbon dioxide tension elevates to a value above the apneic threshold, one would predict the cessation of central apneas. Whatever

the mechanism, low-flow oxygen may be an effective treatment for some cases of idiopathic central sleep apnea.

An alternative approach is probably worthy of consideration. In the patient with CSA in whom hypoxemia is not a major issue but sleep is seriously disrupted, a hypnotic agent might prove useful. If the patient can sleep through the apneas, often deeper stages of sleep (stages 3 and 4) can be attained and apneas diminished. Thus, sleep quality is improved, and the remaining apneas may be of little consequence. However, because hypnotics could inhibit ventilation and worsen the problem in some patients, this therapeutic modality must be approached cautiously. In patients with the overlap of insomnia and central apneas, this therapeutic approach may be most appealing. However, chronic hypnotic therapy remains controversial due to limited data regarding efficacy (73) and potential hypnotic side effects (74,75).

SUMMARY

Although CSA is less common than OSA, the frequent overlap of these two syndromes mandates thorough knowledge of both by the practicing clinician. The various syndromes of CSA fall into distinct categories depending on the presence of hypercapnia, cardiac dysfunction, and sleep–wake state instability. A systematic approach to these patients can frequently yield a satisfactory clinical outcome (Table 23-5). Through further research into the basic mechanisms of ventilatory control, new treatments such as effective ventilatory stimulants are likely to evolve.

REFERENCES

1. AASM. Sleep-related breathing disorders in adults: recommendations for syndrome definition and measurement techniques in adults. *Sleep.* 1999;22(5):667–689.
2. Lavie P, Pillar G, Malhotra A. *Sleep disorders diagnosis, management and treatment: a handbook for clinicians.* Martin Dunitz, 2002:1–185.
3. Badr MS, Roiber F, Skatrud JB, et al. Pharyngeal narrowing/occlusion during central sleep apnea. *J Appl Physiol.* 1995; 78:1806–1815.
4. Onal E, Lopata M, TOC. Pathogenesis of apneas in hypersomnia-sleep apnea syndrome. *Amer Rev Respir Dis.* 1982;125(2):167–74.
5. Bradley TD, McNicholas WT, Rutherford R, et al. Clinical and physiologic heterogeneity of the central sleep apnea syndrome. *Amer Rev Respir Dis.* 1986;134:217–221.
6. Nakayama H, Smith CA, Rodman JR, et al. Effect of ventilatory drive on carbon dioxide sensitivity below eupnea during sleep. *Amer J Respir Crit Care Med.* 2002;165(9):1251–1260.
7. Orem J. The nature of the wakefulness stimulus for breathing. *Progr Clin Biol Res.* 1990;345:23–30,31.
8. Skatrud JB, Dempsey JA. Interaction of sleep state and chemical stimuli in sustaining rhythmic ventilation. *J Appl Physiol.* 1983;55(3):813–822.
9. Meza S, Mendez M, Ostrowski M, et al. Susceptibility to periodic breathing with assisted ventilation during sleep in normal subjects. *Sleep.* 1993;85(5):1929–1940.
10. Wilcox I, Grunstein RR, Collins FL, et al. The role of central chemosensitivity in central apnea of heart failure. *Sleep.* 1993;16 (8 Suppl.):S37–38.

11. Solin P, Roebuck T, Johns DP, et al. Peripheral and central ventilatory responses in central sleep apnea with and without congestive heart failure. *Amer J Respir Crit Care Med.* 2000;162(6):2194–2200.

12. Rapoport DM, Garay SM, Epstein H, et al. Hypercapnia in the obstructive sleep apnea syndrome. A reevaluation of the "Pickwickian syndrome." *Chest.* 1986;89(5):627–635.

13. Farney RJ, Walker JM, Cloward TV, et al. Sleep-disordered breathing associated with long-term opioid therapy. *Chest.* 2003;123(2):632–639.

14. Javaheri S. A mechanism of central sleep apnea in patients with heart failure. *N Engl J Med.* 1999;23:985–987.

15. Naughton M, Benard D, Tam A, et al. Role of hyperventilation in the pathogenesis of central sleep apneas in patients with congestive heart failure [see comments]. *Amer Rev Respir Dis.* 1993;148(2):330–338.

16. Younes M, Ostrowski M, Thompson W, et al. Chemical control stability in patients with obstructive sleep apnea. *Amer J Respir Crit Care Med.* 2001;163(5):1181–1190.

17. Wellman D, Malhotra A, Fogel R, et al. Respiratory system loop gain measured in normal men and women using proportional assist ventilation. *J Appl Physiol.* 2002;in press.

18. Khoo MC. Using loop gain to assess ventilatory control in obstructive sleep apnea. *Amer J Respir Crit Care Med.* 2001;163(5):1044–1045.

19. Khoo MC, Kronauer RE, Strohl KP, et al. Factors inducing periodic breathing in humans: a general model. *J Appl Physiol.* 1982;53(3):644–659.

20. Leung RST, Bradley TD. Sleep apnea and cardiovascular disease. *Amer J Resp Crit Care Med.* 2001;164:2147–2165.

21. Xie A, Skatrud JB, Puleo DS, et al. Apnea-hypopnea threshold for CO_2 in patients with congestive heart failure. *Amer J Respir Crit Care Med.* 2002;165(9):1245–1250.

22. Bassetti C, Aldrich MS, Chervin RD, et al. Sleep apnea in patients with transient ischemic attack and stroke: a prospective study of 59 patients. *Neurology.* 1996;47(5):1167–1173.

23. Orem J. Excitatory drive to the respiratory system in REM sleep. *Sleep.* 1996;19(10 Suppl.):S154–S156.

24. Bradley TD. Crossing the threshold: implications for central sleep apnea. *Amer J Respir Crit Care Med.* 2002;165(9):1203–1204.

25. Hunt CE, Silvestri JM. Pediatric hypoventilation syndromes. *Curr Opin Pulmon Med.* 1997;3(6):445–448.

26. Shea SA, Andres LP, Shannon DC, Ventilatory responses to exercise in humans lacking ventilatory chemosensitivity. *J Physiol.* 1993;468:623–640.

27. Krieger AJ. Sleep apnea produced by cervical cordotomy and other neurosurgical lesions in man. In: Guilleminault C, Dement WC, eds. *Sleep apnea syndromes.* New York: Liss, 1978:273–294.

28. Lahuerta J, Buxton P, Lipton S, et al. The location and function of respiratory fibres in the second cervical spinal cord segment: respiratory dysfunction syndrome after cervical cordotomy. *J Neurol Neurosurg Psych.* 1992;55(12):1142–1145.

29. Tranmer BI, Tucker WS, Bilbao JM. Sleep apnea following percutaneous cervical cordotomy. *Can J Neurol Sci.* 1987;14(3):262–267.

30. Bradley TD, Day A, Hyland RH, et al. Chronic ventilatory failure caused by abnormal respiratory pattern generation during sleep. *Amer Rev Respir Dis.* 1984;130(4):678–681.

31. Schulz R, Fegbeutel C, Althoff A, et al. Central sleep apnoea and unilateral diaphragmatic paralysis associated with vertebral artery compression of the medulla oblongata. *J Neurol.* 2003;250(4):503–505.

32. Xie A, Rankin F, Rutherford R, et al. Effects of inhaled CO_2 and added dead space on idiopathic central sleep apnea. *J Appl Physiol.* 1997;82(3):918–926.

33. Rice AJ, Nakayama HC, Haverkamp HC, et al. Controlled versus assisted mechanical ventilation effects on respiratory motor output in sleeping humans. *Amer J Respir Crit Care Med.* 2003;168(1):92–101.

34. Guilleminault C, Cummiskey J. Progressive improvement of apnea index and ventilatory response to CO_2 after tracheostomy in obstructive sleep apnea syndrome. *Amer Rev Respir Dis.* 1982;126(1):14–20.

35. Javaheri S, Parker TJ, Liming JD, et al. Sleep apnea in 81 ambulatory male patients with stable heart failure. *Circulation.* 1998;97(21):2154–2159.

36. Sin D, Fitzgerald F, Parker J. Risk factors for central and obstructive sleep apnea in 450 men and women with congestive heart failure. *Amer J Respir Crit Care Med.* 1999;160:1101–1106.

37. Sin D, Logan A, Fitzgerald F, et al. Effects of continuous positive airway pressure on cardiovascular outcomes in heart failure patients with and without Cheyne-Stokes respiration. *Circulation.* 2000;102:61–66.

38. Naughton MT, Benard DC, Rutherford R, et al. Effect of continuous positive airway pressure on central sleep apnea and nocturnal Pco_2 in heart failure. *Amer J Respir Crit Care Med.* 1994;150(6 Pt 1):1598–1604.

39. Naughton MT, Benard DC, Liu PP, et al. Effects of nasal CPAP on sympathetic activity in patients with heart failure and central sleep apnea. *Amer J Respir Crit Care Med.* 1995;152(2):473–479.

40. Naughton MT, Liu PP, Bernard DC, et al. Treatment of congestive heart failure and Cheyne-Stokes respiration during sleep by continuous positive airway pressure. *Amer J Respir Crit Care Med.* 1995;151(1):92–97.

41. Whitelaw WA, Derenne JP. Airway occlusion pressure. *J Appl Physiol.* 1993;74(4):1475–1483.

42. McNicholas WT, Carter JL, Rutherford R, et al. Beneficial effect of oxygen in primary alveolar hypoventilation with central sleep apnea. *Amer Rev Respir Dis.* 1982;125(6):773–775.

43. Shneerson JM, Simonds AK. Noninvasive ventilation for chest wall and neuromuscular disorders. *Eur Respir J.* 2002;20(2):480–487.

44. Make BJ, Hill NS, Goldberg AI, et al. Mechanical ventilation beyond the intensive care unit. Report of a consensus conference of the American College of Chest Physicians. *Chest.* 1998;113(5 Suppl.):289S–344S.

45. Waldhorn RE. Nocturnal nasal intermittent positive pressure ventilation with bi-level positive airway pressure (BiPAP) in respiratory failure. *Chest.* 1992;101(2):516–521.

46. Lanfranchi PA, Braghiroli A, Bosimini E, et al. Prognostic value of nocturnal Cheyne–Stokes respiration in chronic heart failure. *Circulation.* 1999;99:1435–1440.

47. Leite JJ, Mansur AJ, de Freitas HF, et al. Periodic breathing during incremental exercise predicts mortality in patients with chronic heart failure evaluated for cardiac transplantation. *J. Amer Coll Cardiol.* 2003;41(12):2175–2181.

48. Dowdell WT, Javaheri S, McGinnis W. Cheyne-Stokes respiration presenting as sleep apnea syndrome. *Amer Rev Respir Dis.* 1990;141:871–879.

49. Solin P, Bergin P, Richardson M, et al. Influence of pulmonary capillary wedge pressure on central apnea in heart failure. *Circulation.* 1999;99(12):1574–1579.

50. Javaheri S. Pembrey's dream: the time has come for a long-term trial of nocturnal supplemental nasal oxygen to treat central sleep apnea in congestive heart failure. *Chest.* 2003;123(2):322–325.

51. Krachman SL, Ge DA, Berger TJ, et al. Comparison of oxygen therapy with nasal continuous positive airway pressure on Cheyne-Stokes respiration during sleep in congestive heart failure. *Chest.* 1999;116(6):1550–1557.

52. Mak S, Azevedo ER, Liu PP, et al. Effect of hyperoxia on left ventricular function and filling pressures in patients with and without congestive heart failure. *Chest.* 2001;120(2):467–473.

53. Andreas S, Bingeli C, Mohacsi P, et al. Nasal oxygen and muscle sympathetic nerve activity in heart failure. *Chest.* 2003;123(2):366–371.

54. Bradley TD, Floras JS. Sleep apnea and heart failure. *Circulation.* 2003;107:1822–1826.

55. Javaheri S, Parker TJ, Wexler L, et al. Effect of theophylline on sleep-disordered breathing in heart failure. *N Engl J Med.* 1996;335:562–567.

56. Malhotra A, Muse VV, Mark EJ. Case records of the Massachusetts General Hospital. Weekly clinicopathological exercises. Case 12-2003. An 82-year-old man with dyspnea and pulmonary abnormalities. *N Engl J Med.* 2003;348(16):1574–1585.

57. Bradley TD, Logan AG, Floras JS. Rationale and design of the Canadian continuous positive airway pressure trial for congestive heart failure patients with central sleep apnea—CANPAP. *Can J Cardiol.* 2001;17(6):677–684.

58. Teschler H, Dohring J, Wang YM, et al. Adaptive pressure support servo-ventilation: a novel treatment for Cheyne-Stokes respiration in heart failure. *Amer J Respir Crit Care Med.* 2001;164(4):614–619.

59. Pittman S, Hill P, Malhotra A, et al. Stabilizing Cheyne Stokes respiration associated with congestive heart failure using computer assisted positive airway pressure. *Comp Cardiol.* 2000;27:201–204.

60. Khayat RN, Xie A, Patel AK, et al. Cardiorespiratory effects of added dead space in patients with heart failure and central sleep apnea. *Chest.* 2003;123(5):1551–1560.
61. Steens RD, Millar TW, Su X, et al. Effect of inhaled 3% CO2 on Cheyne-Stokes respiration in congestive heart failure. *Sleep.* 1994;17(1):61–68.
62. White DP, Zwillich CW, Pickett CK, et al. Central sleep apnea. Improvement with acetazolamide therapy. *Arch Intern Med.* 1982;142(10):1816–1819.
63. Morrell MJ, Badr MS, Harms CA, et al. The assessment of upper airway patency during apnea using cardiogenic oscillations in the airflow signal. *Sleep.* 1995;18(8):651–658.
64. DeBacker WA, Verbraecken J, Willemen M, et al. Central apnea index decreases after prolonged treatment with acetazolamide. *Amer J Respir Crit Care Med.* 1995;151(1):87–91.
65. Verbraecken J, Willemen M, De Cock W, et al. Central sleep apnea after interrupting long-term acetazolamide therapy. *Respir Physiol.* 1998;112(1):59–70.
66. Hudgel DW, et al. Pharmacologic treatment of sleep-disordered breathing. *Amer J Respir Crit Care Med.* 1998;158(3):691–699.
67. Issa FG, Sullivan CE. Reversal of central apnea using nasal CPAP. *Chest.* 1986;90:165–171.
68. Hoffstein V, Slutsky AS. Central sleep apnea reversed by continuous positive airway pressure. *Amer Rev Respir Dis.* 1987;135:1210–1212.
69. Hommura F, Nishimura M, Oguri M, et al. Continuous versus bilevel positive airway pressure in a patient with idiopathic central sleep apnea. *Amer J Respir Crit Care Med.* 1997;155(4):1482–1485.
70. Martin RJ, Sanders MH, Gray BA, et al. Acute and long-term ventilatory effects of hyperoxia in the adult sleep apnea syndrome. *Amer Rev Respir Dis.* 1982;125(2):175–180.
71. Gold AR, Bleecker ER, Smith PL. A shift from central and mixed sleep apnea to obstructive sleep apnea resulting from low-flow oxygen. *Amer Rev Respir Dis.* 1985;132(2):220–223.
72. Malhotra A, Schwartz DR, Ayas N, et al. Treatment of oxygen-induced hypercapnia. *Lancet.* 2001;357(9259):884–885.
73. Bonnet MH, Dexter JR, Arand DL. The effect of triazolam on arousal and respiration in central sleep apnea patients. *Sleep.* 1990;13:31–41.
74. Nowell PD, Mazumdar S, Buysse DJ, et al. Benzodiazepines and zolpidem for chronic insomnia: a meta-analysis of treatment efficacy. *JAMA.* 1997;278(24):2170–2177.
75. Barbone F, McMahon AD, Davey PG, et al. Association of road-traffic accidents with benzodiazepine use. *Lancet.* 1998;352(9137):1331–1336.

Diencephalic and Brainstem Sleep Disorders

David Surhbier

ENCEPHALITIS LETHARGICA

Introduction

Between 1917 and 1925, an epidemic due to an encephalitic illness was first described as encephalitis lethargica (EL) by a Greek psychiatrist named Constantin Von Economo (1). Thirteen patients with a syndrome of somnolence, oculomotor dysfunction, and ptosis following symptoms of fever, headache, and nausea were first reported in Vienna during the winter of 1916 (2). An estimated 100,000 to 160,000 cases of EL are believed to have occurred throughout Western Europe and North America, with a mortality rate of approximately 40% (3,4).

After 1925, the number of new cases dramatically decreased and, to date, the disease is seen only in sporatic case reports. Von Economo identified three distinct clinical patterns of EL, correlated clinical symptoms with neuropathology of the midbrain, and described the neurologic sequelae, which was later named postencephalitic parkinsonism (PEP) (4). Although an infectious etiology is presumed to be the vector for EL, efforts to isolate a causative agent have failed. Furthermore, recent evidence has refuted the popular belief that the 1918 "Spanish" influenza A virus was the cause of the EL epidemic (5).

Howard and Lees (6) proposed a list of criteria that would support a clinical diagnosis of EL and reported the presence of oligoclonal immunoglobulin G (IgG) banding in the cerebrospinal fluid (CSF) of patients during the acute phase of the illness, thus offering evidence of a potential viral etiology. With the advent of magnetic resonance imaging (MRI), recently diagnosed cases of EL have demonstrated signal abnormality in the substantia nigra corresponding to autopsy findings initially reported by Von Economo in 1917 (7,8).

Clinical Characteristics

Von Economo categorized EL into three clinical patterns: somnolent–ophthalmoplegic, hyperkinetic, and amyostatic–akinetic (4). Somnolent-ophthalmoplegic ("sleepy sickness") form of EL was the most common of the three syndromes and presented with brief, nonspecific symptoms of malaise, headache, and mild fever. This was followed by the development of an increasing somnolent state resulting in the patient falling asleep during daily activities such as sitting, standing, eating, and even walking. The patient could easily be aroused, but would quickly lapse back into sleep if not continuously stimulated. The somnolence would persist for weeks to months frequently progressing to stupor, coma, and, in nearly 50% of cases, death. Associated symptoms included ptosis, ophthalmoplegia, nystagmus, oculogyric crisis, motor weakness, and rigidity.

The hyperkinetic form of EL was characterized by an agitated, emotionally labile mental state mimicking catatonic schizophrenia in association with myoclonic jerks of the extremities. Associated symptoms included severe neck and back discomfort, inversion of sleep patterns, and insomnia. As the condition progressed, involuntary movements similar to chorea developed, along with dystonic posturing of the limbs.

The amyostatic–akinetic form was the least common presentation of EL; however, it was associated with the highest percentage of neurologic sequelae. The clinical picture was similar to that of idiopathic Parkinson's disease (IPD), with symptoms of bradykinesia, rigidity, an expressionless face, mutism, inversion of sleep patterns, and ophthalmoplegia.

Postencephalitic parkinsonism represented a syndrome of delayed onset fatigue, weakness, rigidity, bent posture, and unsteady gait, which developed months to years after the acute phase of EL. Although similar to Parkinson's disease, Von Economo outlined clinical differences that distinguished PEP as a separate condition. The onset of symptoms in PEP could be at any age, including childhood, whereas IP occurred after age 50. The characteristic "pill rolling" tremor of IP was absent in cases of PEP. Finally, the progression of symptoms in PEP was rapid, often occurring in spurts versus the slow, progressive nature of IP.

Pathophysiology

Von Economo described EL as a "nonpurulent, nonhemorrhagic, acute inflammation of the grey matter" with pronounced involvement of the brainstem to include the substantia nigra and locus ceruleus. Microscopic features included a perivascular infiltration of lymphocytes in the Virchow–Robin spaces along with small, perivascular ring hemorrhages (4). Cases of PEP demonstrated extensive severe degeneration and gliosis of the substantia nigra and the presence of intracytoplasmic globose neurofibrillary tangles (NFT) in the remaining neurons. The presence of NFT and the absence of Lewy bodies distinguished PEP from IP (9–11). McCall et al., using reverse transcription-polymerase chain reaction for influenza RNA on archived CNS tissue from patients who died during the original EL epidemic, demonstrated negative findings in all cases (5).

Diagnosis

Howard and Lees reviewed four cases of EL and proposed a list of criteria to be used for clinical diagnosis (6). Two of the four cases represented the somnolent–ophthalmoplegic type and the other two were consistent with the hyperkinetic type. Symptoms considered as major criteria included: (a) signs of basal ganglia involvement, (b) oculogyric crisis, (c) ophthalmoplegia, (d) obsessive–compulsive behavior, (e) akinetic mutism, (f) central respiratory irregularities, and (g) somnolence and/or sleep inversion. A minimum of three features was suggested as requirement for diagnosis of EL.

CSF analysis demonstrates pleocytosis with cell count ranges of 2 to 1350 cells/mm^3. CSF protein and glucose are unremarkable. CSF culture for viral, bacterial, mycobacteria, and fungi are negative. CSF from three patients from the Howard and Lees study demonstrated the presence of oligoclonal IgG banding, which the authors postulated provided supportive evidence of a viral etiology for EL.

MRI has demonstrated bilateral hyperintense signal abnormality in the substantia nigra in two isolated case reports (Fig. 24-1) (7,8).

Electroencephalographic (EEG) findings during the acute phase of the illness demonstrate generalized, moderate-high voltage, slow-wave activity (6). Polysomnography (PSG) in an isolated case report was described as normal (7), but this has not been formally studied.

Treatment

No treatment was available during the initial EL outbreak, with patients experiencing a significant morbidity and mortality. Von Economo described 40% mortality, 26% incomplete recovery with neurologic deficit, 20% chronic disability, and only 14% spontaneous full recovery (4). In 1966, Oliver Sacks, a then consulting neurologist for Beth Abraham Hospital in New York, encountered survivors of

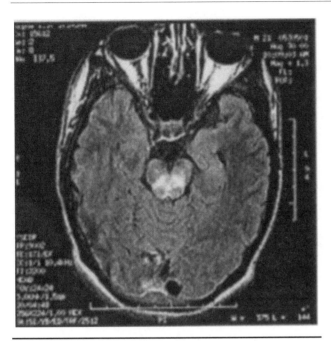

FIGURE 24-1. MRI of the brain demonstrating bilateral hyperintense signal abnormality in the substantia nigra reported in two cases of encephalitis lethargica (EL).

the 1917 epidemic and treated them with L-dopa. The dramatic clinical response of these patients became the subject of Sacks' book *Awakenings* (12). To date, dopamine and dopamine agonists (ropinirole) have been used to treat the extrapyramidal symptoms of PEP (8). Electroconvulsive therapy has been used with success in two cases of malignant catatonia secondary to encephalitis lethargica (13,14).

Future Directions

Encephalitis lethargica remains a mysterious disease without a recognized etiology. Perhaps further analysis of archived tissue of EL patients may provide insight into a possible cause.

FATAL FAMILIAL INSOMNIA

Introduction

In 1986, Lugaresi reported two family members who died of a progressive neurologic disorder manifested by insomnia, dysautonomia, ataxia, and myoclonus (15). At autopsy, these patients had atrophy of the mediodorsal and anterior ventral thalamic nuclei. In 1992, "fatal familial insomnia" (FFI) was identified as a prion disease with the discovery of a missense mutation at codon 178 of the prion protein (PrP) gene (PRNP) on chromosome 20 (16,17). This results in a protease-resistant PrP (PrP-Sc) that accumulates in the thalamus, inferior olive, and, to a lesser extent, the cortex, with particular involvement of the limbic structures (15,18). Currently, there are 27 known pedigrees of FFI

spanning several countries in Europe, Australia, Japan, China, and the United States (19–26). The disease is uniformly fatal without known treatment.

Clinical Characteristics

Affected individuals begin to develop symptoms between the ages of 36 and 62 years. Impairment of attention and vigilance are reported, along with an inability to initiate and maintain sleep. Autonomic dysfunction develops, manifested by hypertension, pyrexia in the evenings, increased tendency to perspire, tear, and salivate. As the insomnia and dysautonomia worsen, the patient experiences a hallucinatory state and exhibits behaviors related to the contents of a dream. Next to evolve are disturbances in gait, disequilibrium, dysmetria, signs of pyramidal tract involvement (hyperreflexic DTRs and presence of Babinski sign), and myoclonus. Later stages of the disease are marked by increasing bouts of stupor, persistent drowsiness, and myoclonus, inability to stand or walk, progressive dysarthria, dysphagia, and loss of sphincter control. Death occurs 8 to 72 months after the development of insomnia (mean duration of 18 months) (27).

Pathophysiology

Patients with FFI harbor a missense GAC–ACC mutation resulting in an asparagine-for-aspartic acid substitution at codon 178 of the PRNP gene (D178N) (17,18). This same mutation is also seen in pedigrees of familial Creutzfeldt–Jakob disease (CJD). The phenotype expression of the D178N mutation (FFI versus CJD) depends on a second intragenic polymorphism at codon 129. If the patient exhibits homozygosity for methionine (Met/Met) at codon 129, the patient develops FFI. If the patient is heterozygous with alleles for methionine and valine (Met/Val), the patient develops an FFI variant with longer symptom duration. If the patient is homozygous for valine (Val/Val), familial CJD develops. In FFI, the D178N mutation results in the coding for PrP-Sc (Fig. 24-2) (28,29).

The hallmark of this prion disease is the presence of PrP-Sc, an aberrant isoform of PrP, which is resistant to proteases. Deposition of this protein is noted in the mediodorsal and anterior ventral thalamus, caudate nucleus, limbic areas, and the neocortex. The amount of PrP-Sc deposition is much less than seen in other prion diseases, such as CJD. The amount of deposition increases with time in other cortical structures, but remains unchanged in the thalamus; however, the severity of neuronal loss in these structures suggests an increased vulnerability to injury from PrP-Sc in the thalamic neurons. The most consistent neuropathologic findings in FFI patients are observed in the thalamus. Of the magnocellular and parvicellular neurons located in the anterior ventral and mediodorsal nuclei, 50% to 80% are lost, with associated reactive astrogliosis. Severe neuronal loss with similar reactive astrogliosis is also observed in the

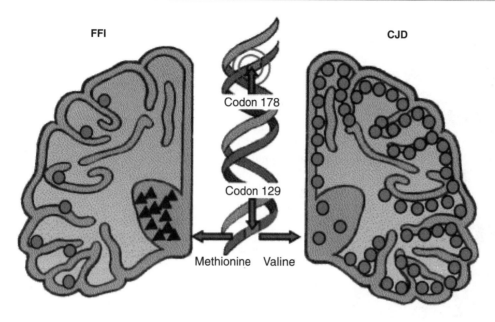

FIGURE 24-2. Illustratation of how the clinical phenotype of FFI and CJD depend not only on a mutation of condon 178, but also on the amino acid composition of condon 129. If the patient is homozygous for methionine, then FFI results. If the patient is homozygous for valine, then CJD results.

inferior olives. With longer disease duration, spongy degeneration of cortical layers II–IV and loss of the cerebellar Purinje and granule cells with reactive gliosis develop (15,18).

Diagnosis

Brain CT and MR imaging reveal nonspecific findings of cortical and cerebellar atrophy with associated ventricular dilation. These findings are more prominent in the later stages of the disease (30).

Proton emission tomography (PET) imaging with fluorine-18-labeled 2-fluorodeoxy-D-glucose [(18F)FDG] has demonstrated hypometabolism predominantly in the thalamus and cingulate cortex, as well as more widespread involvement of the frontal and temporal cortex, caudate

nucleus, and cerebellum in patients with prolonged disease. Currently, hypometabolism of the thalamus and cingulate cortex is considered the PET hallmark of FFI (Fig. 24-3) (31).

EEG and PSG monitoring demonstrates a progressive deterioration of normal sleep architecture and the development of aberrant behavior during rapid eye movement (REM) sleep. EEG background activity progressively changes from an initial organized alpha rhythm to a slowed, flat, monomorphic activity with bursts of 1- to 2-Hz periodic sharp waves correlated with myoclonus. PSG monitoring initially showed a reduction in total sleep time (TST) with a progressive loss of sleep spindles and K complexes. Abrupt episodes of REM sleep would interrupt the sleep cycle both with and without atonia. REM phases of longer duration were associated with complex

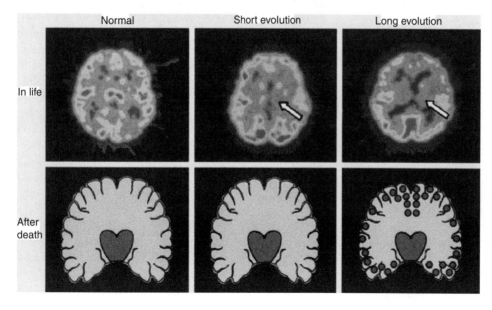

FIGURE 24-3. PET scan in a patient with fatal familial insomnia (FFI) demonstrating hypometabolism in the thalamus and cingulate cortex (a hallmark finding for this condition).

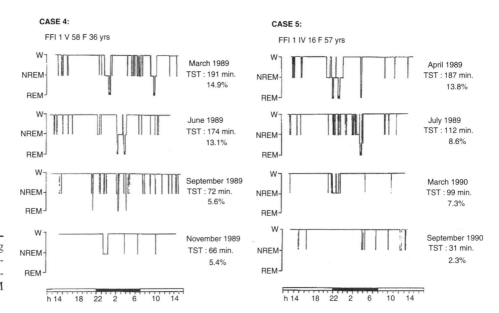

FIGURE 24-4. PSG illustrating the findings seen in fatal familial insomnia (FFI). Note the progressive loss of NREM and REM sleep.

behaviors of sitting up, looking around, speaking, and defensive posturing. Non-REM (NREM) sleep stages and eventually REM sleep are progressively lost (32). Figure 24-4 illustrates these findings.

Treatment

No treatment exists for FFI; the disease is uniformly fatal.

Future Directions

The selective lesions noted in patients with FFI serve to offer evidence of the role of the thalamus in sleep regulation, autonomic function, and instinctive behavior. Ablative lesions of the mediodorsal thalamus have already been demonstrated in animal models. This thalamic nucleus receives afferent fibers from the reticular nuclei (recognized as the source of spindle activity) as well as additional fibers from the cingulate cortex and hypothalamus—all of which are known to influence sleep. The mediodorsal and anterior nucleus together receive input from the limbic system (anterior cingulate and insular) as well as the amygdala and hypothalmus, structures involved in autonomic control. Thus, lesions of the thalamus serve to disconnect these various cortical areas, resulting in a shift toward persistent wake behavior and metabolic hyperactivity (33).

Future areas of research may be directed at understanding the role that thalamic injury plays in deterioration of normal sleep architecture and how this, in turn, results in morbidity and mortality. Finally, the search for treatment modalities will remain the foremost challenge in this disease.

SLEEPING SICKNESS (AFRICAN TRYPANOSOMIASIS)

Introduction

Human African trypanosomiasis (HAT) is an endemic parasitic disease exclusively located in intertropical Africa. The disease has reached epidemic proportions in four countries: Sudan, Uganda, the Democratic Republic of Congo, and Angola. It is estimated that 300,000 to 500,000 persons are infected with HAT (34–37). The trypanosome parasite is transmitted to man through the bite of the tsetse fly, where it propagates initially through the blood and lymphatics (stage I) before penetrating the blood–brain barrier and entering the CNS (stage II) (38). The disease was named for the observation that infected persons appear to be sleepy by day and restless at night. PSG monitoring has determined that HAT represents a disruption in the circadian rhythm of the sleep–wake cycle (39). Treatment for this condition exists, but therapy is complicated by the toxicity of the medications, developing resistance of the trypanosomes to the drugs, and logistic difficulties of diagnosing and providing care to individuals in developing countries.

Epidemiology

HAT is divided into two distinct epidemiologic diseases: West African and East African trypanosomiasis (40). The West African form results from infection with *Trypanosomi brucei gambiense,* which is transmitted through the bite of the tsetse fly (*G. palpalis*) located in the rain forests of Central and West Africa. The East African form results from infection with *T. brucei rhodesiense* transmitted through the bite of the tsetse fly (*G. morsitans*) located in the

evidence of elevated serum IgM for trypanosomes using the card-agglutination trypanosomiasis test (CATT) (38,42). Those testing positive are examined for lymphadenopathy and/or neurologic signs. Blood samples are taken to detect typanosomes. Patients with positive findings on physical or blood sampling are evacuated to the nearest hospital for lumbar puncture and appropriate treatment.

The most evident need for future research is in the area of newer, safer remedies. No drug for the treatment of HAT has been developed since melarsoprol in 1949. Clinical trials using combinations of existing drugs and experimental new drugs (diaminotriazine, DB-289, megazol) are ongoing (44).

KLEINE–LEVIN SYNDROME

Introduction

Kleine–Levin syndrome (KLS) is a rare complex of symptoms occurring predominantly in young males and is comprised of recurrent episodes of prolonged hypersomnia, excessive food intake, and abnormal behavior. In 1925, Willi Kleine, a German psychiatrist in reviewing five cases of episodic somnolence, described two patients with symptoms that now bear his name (48). In 1929, Max Levin, an American psychiatrist added a case report of a 19-year-old male with recurring sleep attacks of 1 to 6 weeks duration, waking only to eat large quantities of food and urinate/defecate (49). The term Kleine–Levin syndrome was first introduced in 1942, by Critchley and Hoffman who described two additional patients with periodic somnolence and morbid hunger (50). They suggested the syndrome reflected the sequelae of encephalitis, although conclusive evidence of this was not found.

Over the next two decades, isolated case reports entered the literature of male patients with the same series of symptoms of sleep disorder, compulsive eating, and behavior abnormalities followed by spontaneous recovery. In 1968, Duffy described the first female case of KLS (51). A comprehensive review of the clinical features of KLS were summarized by Orlosky in 1982 (52). Most recently, the PSG characteristics of 34 KLS patients were reviewed the sleep literature (53). A definitive etiology for KLS has not been established and, although various pharmacotherapies have been used to treat the symptoms, no definite therapy has been recognized.

Clinical Characteristics

Orlosky (52) reviewed the clinical features of 33 reported cases of KLS and categorized the symptoms into disturbances of behavior and disturbances of mood and thought (Table 24-1).

▶ **TABLE 24-1. Orlosky's Clinical Features of KLS**

	Cases (n = 33)	%
Behavior		
Lethargy	8	24
Hypersexuality	6	18
Apathy	5	15
Withdrawal	5	15
Truculence	5	15
Agitation	4	12
Social disinhibition	4	12
Inappropriate singing	4	12
Slurred speech	3	9
Poor hygiene	2	6
Muteness	2	6
Bizzare movements	2	6
Mood		
Irritability	19	58
Depression	7	21
Euphoria	7	21
Lability	1	3
Thought		
Confusion	24	73
Amnesia	13	39
Delusions	10	30
Vivid dreams	5	15
Auditory hallucinations	4	12
Visual hallucinations	3	9

In his review, Orlosky described a 19-year-old male who served as an archetype for the Kleine-Levin syndrome (52). This patient began to experience symptoms at the age of 12 years. He would develop excessive irritability and emotional lability. His ability to concentrate became impaired and his cognitive processing slowed. Within 24 hours, he developed the irresistible urge to sleep, sleeping continuously for periods of 4 to 6 days. During this time, he could be aroused, but appeared confused, drowsy, and withdrawn. He would awaken spontaneously only to urinate, defecate, or eat inordinate quantities of food. When awake, he exhibited whining and demanding behavior, frequently using profanity when urged to cooperate. He ate compulsively, preferring sweets. Occasionally, he engaged in bizarre behavior, such as rocking on his elbows and knees. These symptoms gradually resolved spontaneously with the patient returning to full function with only partial memory of his behavior during the acute phase of his attack. This phenomena recurred four separate times over a 7-year period and resulted in prolonged hospitalizations.

The American Sleep Disorders Association modified the definition of KLS and published diagnostic criteria as part of the International Classification of Sleep Disorders in 1990 (54). The criteria are as follows: (a) patient has complaint of excessive sleepiness, (b) episodes of somnolence last for at least 18 hours a day, (c) episodes recur at least once to twice yearly, lasting from 3 days to 3 weeks, (d) disorder occurs predominantly in adolescent males, (e) associated features includes one of the following symptoms: voracious eating, hypersexuality, disinhibited behavior, verbal response to strong stimuli, and absence of bladder incontinence, (f) somnolence not associated with other medical condition/sleep disorder, and (g) PSG demonstrates reduced stage 3 and 4 sleep, reduced sleep latency, and reduced REM latency.

Pathophysiology

There is no consensus opinion regarding the etiology or pathophysiology of Kleine–Levin syndrome. Most theories involve either structural or functional abnormality of the hypothalamus and diencephalon. Haugh (55) reported the case of a woman who exhibited symptoms of hyperphagia, aggressive behavior, and reversal of wake–sleep patterns who died of pancreatitis. At autopsy, she had the presence of a low-grade astrocytoma involving the hypothalamus. Snow et al. (56) reported a series of six patients who developed hypersomnolence following surgery for pituitary and hypothalamic tumors. However, KLS patients have not demonstrated any consistent abnormal findings in the diencephalon on either computed tomography (CT) or MRI of the brain.

Fenzi (57) reported a 9-year-old girl with clinical features of KLS who died as a result of pulmonary embolism, with evidence of perivascular inflammation infiltrates and microglial proliferation in the diencephalon and midbrain suggesting an encephalitis. Viral etiology was also suggested by Carpenter, based on postmortem results of microglial infiltration of the thalamus in a male patient with KLS who died during a symptomatic phase of the illness (58). KLS patients are often diagnosed with encephalitis due, in part, to the frequent association of fever and symptoms of upper respiratory infection prior to the onset of symptoms or exacerbations (59). However, despite this temporal relation, illness is not a obligate phenomena in all KLS cases, and multiple case series have failed to demonstrate pleocytosis on CSF analysis (53,60). A neuroendocrine-based theory of hypothalamic dysfunction has been suggested, based on aberrant secretion of various hormones in KLS patients (61,62). During symptomatic periods of hypersomnia, reduced cortisol levels and increased prolactin levels have been reported. Declining cortisol levels have been observed in normal individuals to be associated with slow-wave sleep (SWS). Prolactin secretion is inhibited by dopamine in the portal system, thus implying reduced dopamine release during acute attack of KLS. The impact of dopamine on promoting arousal and wakefulness is well documented (63). In addition, Koerber (64) reported elevated levels of 5-HT and 5-HIAA in the CSF of a KLS patients, suggesting an imbalance in the serotonergic pathways. However, a recent study

of five KLS patients by Mayer et al. (65) demonstrated no such endocrine abnormalities during symptomatic periods.

Human leukocyte antigen (HLA) analysis performed on KLS patients failed to demonstrate the HLA-DR2 haplotype seen in patients with narcolepsy, thus excluding immunogenetic similarity between the disorders. Furthermore, no association was demonstrated between KLS patients and the TpH (tryptophan hydroxlase) or the COMT (catechol-O-methytransferase) gene (60).

Diagnostic Testing

As referenced above, CT and MRI imaging series have not demonstrated characteristic abnormality in KLS patients (53,60,65). CSF analysis has been unremarkable (53,60). Hormone secretion patterns have yielded conflicting results (61–65).

PSG monitoring during symptomatic and asymptomatic periods, however, have demonstrated consistent trends. PSG during hypersomnolent attacks show reduced stage 3 and 4 sleep with increased stage 1 sleep. Sleep efficiency is also reduced due to frequent wakenings in stage 2 sleep. PSG monitoring during asymptomatic periods between attacks demonstrate normal sleep architecture (Fig. 24-7) (53,66).

Treatment

Various classes of medications have been used empirically to treat the symptoms of KLS. Stimulants (d-amphetamine, methylphenidate, and modafinil) have been used to promote wakefulness, but have shown only partial effectiveness (60,67).

Mood-stabilizing agents, such as lithium, have been reported as effective for both acute exacerbations of hypersomnolence and aberrant behavior, as well as reducing frequency of attacks (60,68,69). Anticonvulsants, such as carbamazepine and valproic acid, have also been reported effective in isolated case reports (70,71). References to light therapy and melatonin have also appeared in the literature (72).

Prognosis

KLS is a self-limited phenomena with spontaneous recovery of full cognitive and behavior function by early adulthood. Gadoth et al. (53), in their series of 34 KLS patients claimed to have not seen persistent KLS exacerbations beyond the age of 30 years.

Future Directions

Continued research into an association between the recognized altered sleep architecture in KLS patients and hypothalamic dysfunction may yield an understanding to this perplexing condition. While the mechanism of action of

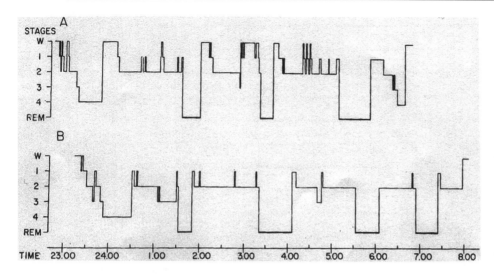

FIGURE 24-7. PSG illustrating the findings seen in Kleine–Levin syndrome (KLS). Note the reduction of stages 3 and 4 with an increase in stage 1, as well as reduced sleep efficiency, during an attack and normal PSG findings between attacks.

lithium is not fully known, its clinical effect is felt to be mediated in part to an enhancement of serotonin (5-HT) function (73). Serotonin is postulated to play a role in the induction of sleep and the prolongation of NREM sleep (74). This suggests that lithium may exert its effect by modifying sleep architecture by increasing stage 3 and 4 sleep found to be decreased in KLS patients. Carbamazepine reduces TST and significantly increases sleep latency, number of arousals, and periods of wakefulness (75). Valproic acid increased latency to REM sleep (75). The role of melatonin in entraining the sleep–wake cycle and its regulation by light also implies areas of future investigation in KLS patients.

PRADER–WILLI SYNDROME

Introduction

In 1956, five male and four females were reported by Prader, Labhardt, and Willi (76) with features of obesity, short stature, marked hypotonia, mental retardation, undescended testes in the males, and feeding difficulties in the newborn period. In 1963, Prader and Willi (77) subsequently reviewed a series of 14 cases. Holm (78) first proposed diagnostic criteria for the Prader–Willi syndrome (PWS) in 1981, which was subsequently modified into its final form in 1993 (79). PWS is a genetic disorder which results from one of three mechanisms: deletion of the 15q11-q13 region from the paternal chromosome, maternal uniparental disomy, or mutation/deletion in the imprinting center (80–85). PWS remains a relatively rare disorder, with an incidence of 1 in 10,000 to 15,000 (78). Uncontrolled eating habits and behavioral/psychiatric disturbance continue to be the most problematic issues facing families. PWS patients have evidence of sleep-disordered breathing (SDB), altered sleep architecture, and abnormal ventilatory responses to hypoxia and hypercarbia (86–89). Hypothalamic dysfunction is considered to be an essen-

tial component of these patients clinical phenotype and sleep disorder. Treatment with growth hormone replacement therapy has demonstrated benefits in growth, body composition, and physical strength (90).

Molecular Genetics

The Prader–Willi phenotype results from an inactivation of the 15q11-q13 region on the paternally donated chromosome. In approximately 70% of PWS patients, there is a deletion of this region from the chromosome (80). In addition, the homologous maternal allele is selectively inactivated (a phenomena known as *genetic imprinting*), thus leading to an absence of gene expression due to structural abnormality (81,82). A smaller percentage (25%) of the PWS population demonstrates the unique genetic phenomena of uniparental disomy (UPD) (82,83).

These patients have inherited two copies of the maternal chromosome without paternal contribution. Thus, without the presence of the chromosome donated from the father, normal imprinting occurs on the two maternal chromosomes, leading to a functional loss of gene expression. Finally, in approximately 5% of cases, a mutation in the imprinting control center may lead to a loss of gene expression from the paternal chromosome (84,85).

Clinical Characteristics

At birth, PWS infants are profoundly hypotonic with dysmorphic features to include dolicocephaly, small almond-shaped eyes, and tent-shaped mouth. The hands and feet are small. Significant feeding difficulty typically results in tube feeding (91). Early childhood is remarkable for global developmental delay and an excessive weight gain for age, beginning after 12 months. The hypotonia gradually improves with age, and PWS children achieve the ability to walk after the age of 2 years (91). Obesity develops due to hyperphagia. Weight control is difficult due to the child's obsession with food and hoarding behaviors. PWS children are of short stature due to growth hormone deficiency and exhibit hypogonadism, with delayed puberty (91,92). Characteristic behavior problems develop in the form of temper tantrums, violent outbursts, and obsessive–compulsive behaviors. They also tend to be argumentative and oppositional. The mean IQ of these patients is 70 (93). Sleep disturbances, such as excessive daytime somnolence and sleep apnea, are frequently reported.

Pathophysiology

Hypothalamic dysfunction has been hypothesized to be central to this condition. However, no consistent neuroanatomic lesions have been identified.

Supporting this hypothesis are the findings of reduced growth hormone (GH) secretion in PWS patients (94). Furthermore, a postmortem study of five PWS patients revealed relatively few oxytocin-secreting neurons in certain regions of the hypothalamus (95). Conversely, a subsequent study of five PWS patients demonstrated increased levels of oxytocin in the CSF (95). Despite the contraindication with postmortem data, the authors suggested that these findings implied hypothalamic dysfunction control of this peptide. In addition, MR imaging has demonstrated the absence, in some PWS individuals, of the presence of the "posterior pituitary bright spot," thought to be a marker of hypothalamic function (93).

Normal patterns of ventilation response to hypoxia and hypercarbia involve multiple brainstem structures, such as the locus ceruleus, red nucleus, and paramedian reticular nucleus (96–98). However, recent animal studies have suggested the hypothalamus may also modulate these responses (99). Arens et al. (100,101) demonstrated abnormal ventilatory control in PWS patients during wakefulness and sleep. It was shown that these patients failed to increase their minute ventilation (Ve) in rapidly developing O_2 desaturation. In addition, PWS patients failed to arouse from sleep in response to hypoxia and hypercapnia. These findings point to significantly impaired peripheral chemoreceptor activity.

Diagnosis

Excessive daytime somnolence and sleep apnea are frequently reported symptoms in PWS patients. However, results of multiple sleep latency test (MSLT) and PSG studies have been conflicting. Helbing-Zwanenburg et al. (102), Hertz et al. (103), Kaplan et al. (104), and Vela-Bueno et al. (105) found no evidence of obstructive sleep apnea (OSA) or abnormal apnea plus hyponea index. This is contrasted with the findings of Sforza et al. (106), Weinzheimer et al. (107), and Lammer and Desaga (108), who described PWS patient with severe sleep apnea requiring continuous positive airway pressure (CPAP) therapy. Richards et al. (109) also reported an increased apnea plus hypopnea index of

greater than 10 events per hour in 12 PWS patients. In addition to reports of SDB, changes in sleep architecture have also been documented. Vela-Bueno et al. (104) described five patients who had REM sleep occur at onset of sleep (SOREM). Manni et al. (89) reported three patients during nocturnal PSG and five patients during MSLT who demonstrated SOREM. Of interest, Vgontzas et al. (110) found a higher prevalence of hypersomnia and/or SOREM in PWS patients with UPD genotype.

Treatment

Growth hormone used in Prader–Willi patients has been shown to improve growth, body composition, physical strength, agility, and fat utilization (111). The standard dosing is 1 mg/m^2 per day. Recent work has shown continued benefits in growth, strength, and physical function after 48 months of therapy at this dosing (90).

Future Directions

Future research into the role of the hypothalamus' in ventilatory response in PWS patients may provide insight into the patterns of SDB noted in these patients. This could include assessing ventilatory response and apnea + hypopnea index (AHI) in patients treated with GH.

REFERENCES

1. Von Economo C. Encephalitis Lethargica. *Wien Klin Weshr.* 1917;30:581–583.
2. Von Economo C. Der schalf als lokalizations problem. In: D. Sarason ed. *Der Schalf* 1929. Munchen: JF Lehmanns Verlag, 1929:54–63.
3. Reid A, et al. *J Neuropathol Exp Neurol.* 2001;60(7):663–670.
4. Von Economo C. *Encephalitis lethargica: Its sequelae and treatment.* Newman KO, translator. London: Oxford University Press, 1931.
5. McCall S, et al. *J Neuropathol Exp Neurol.* 2001;60(7):696–704.
6. Howard RS, Lees AJ. Encephalitis Lethargica: a report of four recent cases. *Brain.* 1987;110:19–35.
7. Kun J, et al. Bilateral substantia nigra changes on MRI in a patient with encephalitis lethargica. *Neurology.* 1999;53:1860–1862.
8. Verschueren K, Crols A. Bilateral substantia nigra lesions on magnetic resonance imaging in a patient with encephalitis lethargica. *J Neurol Neurosurg Psych.* 2001;71:275.
9. Jellinger K. Pathology of Parkinson's disease. In: Fahn S, et al., eds. *Recent developments in Parkinson's disease.* New York: Raven Press, 1986.
10. Forno L. Pathology of parkinson's disease. In: Marsden CD, Fahn S, eds. *Neurology 2: Movement disorders.* London: Butterworth Scientific, 1982.
11. Hallervorden J. Anatomische Untersuchungen zur Pathogenese des postencephalitischen Parkinsonismus. *Dtsche Z Nervenheilk.* 1935;136:68–77.
12. Sacks O. *Awakenings.* London: Picador, 1991.
13. Dekleva KB, Husain MM. Sporadic encephalitis lethargica: a case treated successfully with ECT. *J Neuropsych Clin Neurosci.* 1995;7:237–239.
14. Shill HA, Stacy MA. Malignant catatonia secondary to sporadic encephalitis lethargica. *J Neurol Neurosurg Psych.* 200;69:402–403.
15. Lugaresi E, Medor R, Montagna P, et al. Fatal familial insomnia and dysautonomia with selective degeneration of the thalamic nuclei. *N Engl J Med.* 1986;315:997–1003.

16. Medori R, Montagna P, Tritschler HJ, et al. Fatal familial insomnia: a second kindred with mutation of prion protein gene at codon 178. *Neurology.* 1992;42:669–670.

17. Medori R, Tritschler HJ, LeBlanc A, et al. Fatal familial insomnia, a prion disease with a mutation at codon 178 of the prion protein gene. *N Engl J Med.* 1992;326:444–449.

18. Manetto V, Medori R, Cortelli-Montagna P, et al. Fatal familial insomnia: clinical and pathologic study of five new cases. *Neurology.* 1992;42:312–319.

19. Tabernero C, Polo JM, Sevillano MD, et al. Fatal familial insomnia: clinical, neuropathological, and genetic description of a Spanish family. *J Neurol Neurosurg Psych.* 2000;68:774–777.

20. Colombier C, Geraud G, Delisle MB, et al. Fatal familial insomnia: phenotypic changes determined by polymorphism of the codon 129. *Rev Neurol (Paris).* 1997;153:239–243.

21. Goldfarb LG, Haltia M, Brown P, et al. New mutation in scrapie amyloid precursor gene (at codon 178) in Finnish Creutzfeldt-Jakob kindred. *Lancet.* 1991;337:425.

22. Almer G, Hainfellner JA, Brucke T, et al. Fatal familial insomnia: a new Austrian family. *Brain.* 1999;122:5–16.

23. Harder A, Jendroska K, Kreuz F, et al. Novel twelve-generation kindred of fatal familial insomnia from Germany representing the entire spectrum of disease expression. *Amer J Med Genet.* 1999;87:311–316.

24. Silburn P, Cervenakova L, Varghese P, et al. Fatal familial insomnia: a seventh family. *Neurology.* 1996;47:1326–1328.

25. Reder At, Mednick AS, Brown P, et al. Clinical and genetic studies of fatal familial insomnia. *Neurology.* 1995;45:1068–1075.

26. Nagayama M, Shinohara Y, Furukawa H, et al. Fatal familial insomnia with a mutation at codon 178 of the prion protein gene: first report from Japan. *Neurology.* 1996;47:1313–1316.

27. Montagna P, Cortell P, Avoni P, et al. Clinical features of fatal familial insomnia: phenotypic variability in relation to a polymorphism at codon 129 of the prion protein gene. *Brain Pathol.* 1998;8:515–520.

28. Goldfarb LG, Petersen RB, Tabaton M, et al. Fatal familial insomnia and familial Creutzfeldt-Jakob disease: disease phenotype determined by a DNA polymorphism. *Science.* 1992;258:806–808.

29. Petersen RB, Goldfarb LG, Tabaton M, et al. A novel mechanism of phenotypic heterogeneity demonstrated by the effect of polymorphism on a pathogenic mutation in the PRNP (prion protein gene). *Mol Neurobiol.* 1994;8:99–103.

30. Montagna P, Gambetti P, Cortelli P, et al. Famial and sporatic fatal insomnia. *Lancet Neurol.* 2003;2(3):1105–1109.

31. Parani D, Cortelli P, Lacignani G, et al. (18F)FDG PET in fatal familial insomnia: The functional effects of thalamic lesions. *Neurology.* 1993;43:2565–2569.

32. Sforza E, Montagna P, et al. Sleep–wake cycle abnormalities in fatal familial insomnia. Evidence of the role of the thalamus in sleep regulation. *Electroencephalog Clin Neurophysiol.* 1995;94:398–405.

33. Hess WR. Das Schlafsyndrom als Folge diencephaler Reizung. *Helv Physiol Pharmacol Acta.* 1944;2:305–344.

34. Smith DH, Pepin J, Stich AHR. Human African trypanosomiasis: An emerging public health crisis. *Brit Med Bull.* 1998;54:341–355.

35. Moore A, Richer M. Re-emergence of epidemic sleeping sickness in southern Sudan. *Trop. Med. Intern Health.* 2001;6:342–347.

36. Stranghellini A, Josenando T. The situation of sleeping sickness in Angola: A calamity. *Trop. Med. Intern Health.* 2001;6:330–334.

37. Van Nieuwenhove S, Betu-Ku-Mesu VK, Diabakana PM, et al. Sleeping sickness resurgence in the DRC: the past decade. *Trop Med Intern Health.* 2001;6:335–341.

38. Buguet A, et al. The duality of sleeping sickness: focusing on sleep. *Sleep Med Rev.* 2001;5(2):139–153.

39. Buguet A, et al. Sleep–wake cycle in human African typanosomiasis. *J Clin Neurophysiol.* 1993;10:190–196.

40. Bouteille B, Dumas M. Human African trypanosomiasis: sleeping sickness. In: Chopra JS, Sawhhney IMS, eds. *Neurology in tropics.* New Delhi: Churchill Livingston, 1999:324–336.

41. Dumas M, Bisser S, Clinical aspects of human African trypanosomiasis. In: Dumas M, Bouteille B, Buguet A, eds. *Progress in human African trypanosomiasis, sleeping sickness.* Paris: Springer Verlag, 1999:215–233.

42. Kirchhoff L. Agents of African typanosomiasis. In: Mandell G, Bennett J, Dolin R, eds. *Principles and practice of infectious diseases.* Philadelphia: Churchill Livingstone, 2000:2853–2858.

43. Buguet A, et al. Reversal of the sleep/wake cycle disorder of sleeping sickness after trypanosomicide treatment. *J Sleep Res.* 1999;8:225–235.

44. Bouteille B et al. Treatment perspectives for human African typanosomiasis. *Fund Clin Pharmacol.* 2003;17(2):171–181.

45. Lapeyssonnie MJ. In: Musin L, ed. *Le vainqueur de la maladie du sommeil.* Les Presses de l'INAM, 1987.

46. Stanghellini A. Prophylactic strategies in human African typanosomiasis In: Dumas M, Bouteille B, Buguet A, eds. *Progress in human African trypanosomiasis, sleeping sickness.* Paris: Springer Verlag, 1999:235–252.

47. Ahmad K. Tsetse eradication programme under fire. *Lancet Infect. Dis.* 2003;3(1):4.

48. Kleine W. Periodische schlafsucht. *Monatsschr Psychiatr Neurol.* 1925;57:285–320.

49. Levin M. Nacolepsy (Gelineau's syndrome) and other varieties of morbid somnolence. *Arch Neurol Psych.* 1929;22:1172–1200.

50. Critchley M, Hoffman HL. The syndrome of the periodic somnolence and morbid hunger (Kleine–Levin Syndrome). *BMJ.* 1942;1:137–139.

51. Duffy JB, Davidson K. A female case of Kleine–Levin syndrome. *Br J Psych.* 1968;114:77–84.

52. Orlosky M. The Kleine–Levin syndrome: a review. *Psychosomatics.* 1982;23(6):609–621.

53. Gadoth N, et al. Clinical and polysomnographic characteristics of 34 patients with Kleine–Levin syndrome. *J Sleep Res.* 2001;10:337–341.

54. Diagnostic Classification Steering committee. International classification of sleep disorders: diagnostic and coding manual. Rochester, MN: American Sleep Disorders Association, 2000.

55. Haugh RM, Markesbery WR. Hypothalamic astrocytoma. Syndrome of hyperphagia, obesity, and disturbance of behavior and endocrine and autonomic function. *Arch Neurol.* 1983;40:560–563.

56. Snow, et al. Severe hypersomnolence after pituitary/hypothalmic surgery in adolescents: clinical characteristics and potential mechanisms. *Pediatrics.* 2002;110;6:e74.

57. Fenzi F. et al. Clinical features of Kleine–Levin syndrome with localized encephalitis. *Neuropediatrics.* 1993;24(5):292–295.

58. Carpenter S, Yassa R, Ochs R. A pathologic basis for Kleine–Levin syndrome. *Arch Neurol.* 1982;39(1):25–28.

59. Merriam AE. Kleine–Levin syndrome following acute viral encephalitis. *Biol Psych.* 1986;21:1301–1304.

60. Dauvilliers Y, et al. Kleine-Levin syndrome: an autoimmune hypothesis based on clinical and genetic analyses. *Neurology.* 2002;59(11):1739–1745.

61. Gadoth N, Dickerman Z, et al. Episodic hormone secretion during sleep in Kleine–Levin syndrome: Evidence for hypothalamic dysfunction. *Brain Develop.* 1987;9(3):309–315.

62. Chesson AL, Jr., Levine SN, et al. Neuroendocrine evaluation in Kleine-Levin syndrome: evidence of reduced dopaminergic tone during periods of hypersomnolence. *Sleep.* 1991;14(3):226–232.

63. Gaillard JM, Nicholson A, Pascoe P. Neurotransmitter systems. In: Kryger M, Roth T, Dement W, eds. *Principles and practice of sleep medicine.* Philadelphia: W.B. Saunders, 1989:208–209.

64. Koerber RK, et al. Increased cerebrospinal fluid 5-hydroxytryptamine and 5-hydroxyindoleacetic acid in Kleine–Levin syndrome. *Neurology.* 1984;34(12):1597–1600.

65. Mayer G. et al. Endocrinological and polysomnographic findings in Kleine-Levin syndrome: no evidence for hypothalamic and circadian dysfunction. *Sleep.* 1998;21(3):278–284.

66. Wilkus R, Chiles J. Electrophysiological changes during episodes of the Kleine–Levin syndrome. *J Neurol Neurosurg Psych.* 1975;38:1225–1231.

67. Critchley M. Periodic hypersomnia and megaphagia in adolescent males. *Brain.* 1962;85:627–656.

68. Goldberg M. The treatment of Kleine-Levin syndrome with lithium. *Can J Psych.* 1983;28:491–493.

69. Muratori F, Bertini N, Masi G. Efficacy of lithium treatment in Kleine–Levin syndrome. *Eur Psych.* 2002;17:232–233.

70. Mukaddes N, Kora M, Bilge S. Carbamazepine for Kleine–Levin Syndrome. *J Amer Acad Child Adolesc Psych.* 1999;38(7):791–792.

71. Crumley FE. Valproic acid for Kleine–Levin Syndrome. *J Amer Acad Child Adolesc Psych.* 1997;36(7):868–869.
72. Crumley FE. Light therapy for Kleine–Levin Syndrome. *J Amer Acad Child Adolesc Psych.* 1988;37:1245.
73. Price LH, Heninger GR. Lithium in the treatment of mood disorders. *N Engl J Med.* 1994;331:591–598.
74. Gaillard JM, Nicholson A, Pascoe P. Neurotransmitter systems. In: Kryger M, Roth T, Dement W, eds. *Principles and practice of sleep medicine.* Philadelphia: W. B. Saunders, 1989:206–207.
75. Bazil C, Pedley T. Neurophysiologic effects of antiepileptic drugs. In: Levy RH, Mattson RH, Meldrum BS, eds. *Antiepileptic drugs.* 4th edn. New York: Raven Press, 1995:79–89.
76. Prader A, Labhardt A, Willi H. Ein syndrom von adipositas, kleinwuchs, kryptorchismus und oligophrenie nach myotoniear-tigem. Zustandim Neugeborenenalter. *Schweizer Med Wochensch.* 1956;86:1260.
77. Prader A, Willi H. Das Syndrom von imbezillitat, adipositas, muskelhypotonie, hypogonadismus and diabetes mellitus mit 'myotonie'-anamnese. *Verhandl. 2nd Intern Kong Psych. Entwick-Storungen Kindersalter,* Vienna, Part 1. Basel and New York: Karger, 1961:353.
78. Holm VA. The diagnosis of Prader-Willi syndrome. In: Holm VA, Sulzbacher S, Pipes PL, eds. *The Prader–Willi syndrome.* Baltimore, MD: University Park Press; 1981:27–36.
79. Holm VA, Cassidy SB, Butler MG, et al. Prader-Willi Sydrome: Consensus diagnostic criteria. *Pediatrics.* 1993;91:398–402.
80. Ledbetter DH, Riccardi VM, Airhart SD, et al. Deletion of chromosome 15 as a cause of Prader–Willi syndrome. *N Engl J Med.* 1981;304:325–329.
81. Nicholls RD, Knoll JHM, Butler MG, et al. Genetic imprinting suggested by maternal heterodisomy in non-deletion Prader-Willi syndrome. *Nature (London).* 1989;342:281–285.
82. Robinson WP, Bottani A, Yagang X, et al. Molecular, cytogenetic and clinical investigations of Prader-Willi syndrome patients. *Amer J Hum Genet.* 1991;49:1219–1234.
83. Mascari MJ, Gottlieb W, Rogan PK, et al. The frequency of uniparental disomy in Prader-Willi syndrome. *N Engl J Med.* 1992;326:1599–1607.
84. Reis A, Dittrich B, Greger V, et al. Imprinting mutations suggested by abnormal methylation patterns in familial Angelman and Prader–Willi sydromes. *Amer J Hum Genet.* 1994;54:741–747.
85. Buiting K, Saitoh S, Gross S, et al. Inherited microdeletions in the Angelman and Prader-Willi sydromes define an imprinting center on human chromosome 15. *Nature Genet.* 1995;9:395–400.
86. Menendez A. Abnormal ventilatory responses in patients with Prader–Willi syndrome. *Eur J Pediatr.* 1999;158:941–942.
87. Schluter B, Buschatz D, et al. Respiratory control in children with Prader–Willi syndrome. *Eur J Pediatr.* 1997;156:65–68.
88. Vela-Bueno A, Kales A, et al. Sleep in the Prader-Willi syndrome. Clinical and polygraphic findings. *Arch Neurol.* 1984; 41;3:294.
89. Manni R, et al. Hypersomnia in the Prader–Willi syndrome: clinical-electrophysiological features and underlying factors. *Clin Neurophysiol.* 2001;112:800–805.
90. Carrel A, et al. Benefits of long-term GH therapy in Prader-Willi syndrome: a 4-year study. *J Clin Endo Metab.* 2002;(4): 1581–1585.
91. Dubowitz V. Prader-Willi syndrome. In: Dubowtiz V, ed. *Muscle disorders in childhood.* Philadelphia: W. B. Saunders, 1995:467–471.
92. Jones K. Prader-Willi syndrome. In: Jones K, ed. *Smith's recognizable patterns of human malformation.* 5th edn. Philadelphia: W. B. Saunders, 1997:202–203.
93. State M, Dykens E. Genetics of childhood disorders: XV. Prader-Willi syndrome: genes, brain and behavior. *J Amer Acad Child Adolesc Psych.* 2000;39(6):797–800.
94. Costeff H, Holm VA, Ruvalcaba R, et al. Growth hormone secretion in Prader–Willi syndrome. *Acta Paediatr Scan.* 1990;79:1059–1062.
95. Swaab DF, Purba JS, Hofman MA. Alterations in the hypothalamic paraventricular nucleus and its oxytocin neurons (putative satiety cells) in Prader-Willi syndrome: a study of five cases. *J. Clin Endocrinol Metab.* 1995;80:573–579.
96. Ackland GL, Noble R, Hanson R. Red nucleus inhibits breathing during hypoxia in neonates. *Respir Physiol.* 1997;110:251–260.
97. Moore PJ, Ackland GL, Hanson MA. Unilateral cooling in the region of locus ceruleus blocks the fall in respiratory output during hypoxia in anaesthetised neonatal sheep. *Exp Physiol.* 1996;81:983–994.
98. Carroll JL, et al. Ventral medullary neuronal responses to peripheral chemoreceptor stimulation. *Neuroscience.* 1996;73:989–998.
99. Dillon GH, Waldrop TG. Electrophysiological and morphological properties of the caudal hypothalamic hypoxic and hypercapneic sensitive neurons in vitro. *Soc Neurosci Abstr.* 1992;492:10A.
100. Arens R, Keens TG, et al. Hypoxic and hypercapneic ventilatory responses in Prader–Willi syndrome. *Appl Physiol.* 1994;77:2224–2230.
101. Arens R, Keens TG, et al. Arousal and cardiorespiratory responses to hypoxia in Prader-Willi syndrome. *Amer J Respir Crit Care Med.* 1996;153:283–287.
102. Helbing-Zwanenburg B, et al. The origin of excessive daytime sleepiness in the Prader-Willi syndrome. *J Intellect Disability Res.* 1993;37:533–541.
103. Hertz G, et al. Sleep and breathing patterns in patients with Prader-Willi syndrome: effects of age and gender. *Sleep.* 1993;16:366–371.
104. Kaplan J, et al. Sleep and breathing in patients with Prader-Willi syndrome. *Mayo Clin Proc.* 1991;66:1124–1126.
105. Vela-Bueno A, et al. Sleep in the Prader–Willi syndrome. Clinical and polygraphic findings. *Arch Neurol.* 1984;41:294–296.
106. Sforza E, et al. Sleep and breathing abnormalities in a case of Prader–Willi syndrome. The effects of acute continuous positive airway pressure treatment. *Acta Paediatr Scan.* 1991;80:80–85.
107. Weinzheimer HR, et al. Prader–Willi syndrom: extreme obstruktive Apnoen und PEEP-Maskenbeatmung (Abstract). *Monatsschr Kinderheilkd.* 1994;142:S58.
108. Lammer C, et al. Schlafapnoe und Prader–Willi syndrom (PWS). In: Mayer G, ed. *Jahruch schlafmedizin in Deutschland.* Munchen: MMV Medizin Verlag, 1994:83–87.
109. Richards, et al. The upper airway and sleep apnoea in the Prader Willi syndrome. *Clin Otolaryngol.* 1994;19:193–197.
110. Vgontzas AN, et al. Relationship of sleep abnormalities to patient genotypes in Prader–Willi syndrome. *Amer J Med Genet.* 1996a;67:478–482.
111. Carrel AL, et al. Growth hormone improves body composition, fat utilization, physical strength and agility, and growth in Prader-Willi syndrome: a controlled study. *J Pediatr.* 1999;134:215–221.

Sleep Patients with Other Medical Disorders

Psychiatric Disorders and Sleep

Andrew D. Krystal, Mugdha Thakur, and W. Vaughn McCall

INTRODUCTION

Psychiatric disorders and sleep are strongly interconnected. The effects they have on each other are complex and bidirectional. Individuals with psychiatric illness frequently experience sleep difficulties. In fact, disruptions of sleep are often among the key symptoms that define these illnesses. At the same time, many disorders of sleep are associated with psychiatric symptoms and some sleep disorders are correlated with an increased lifetime risk of experiencing an episode of psychiatric illness.

This link is also evident in the treatments used to address these two types of problems. A number of sleep disorders and psychiatric symptoms are treated with the same pharmacologic agents. For example, antidepressant medications are among the most frequently instituted insomnia treatments and are also used to treat the cataplexy,

hypnogogic/hypnopompic hallucinations, and sleep paralysis experienced by those with narcolepsy [1,2]. It is also the case that stimulant agents, which are a mainstay of the treatment of narcolepsy and other hypersomnias, are used in the treatment of depression and are the treatment of choice for attention deficit disorder [3,4]. To further complicate matters, sleep disorders may impede the response to psychiatric treatments or may be caused by psychiatric treatments, while treatments instituted to address sleep disorders may predispose individuals to psychiatric difficulties [5,6]. As if the link was not already complicated enough, there is evidence that sleep deprivation can lead to improvement in some psychiatric disorders while exacerbating others [7].

While a relationship with psychiatric disease exists for many sleep disorders, one of the best examples of this complex relationship is the link between insomnia and psychiatric problems. Insomnia is among the defining symptoms of depression, generalized anxiety, mania, panic disorder, and other psychiatric illness (8,9). In fact, those with comorbid psychiatric disorders represent the largest group of patients with insomnia (10). A growing body of literature indicates that those experiencing insomnia have a greater likelihood of having had a psychiatric disorder in the past, having a current comorbid psychiatric disorder, and developing a psychiatric disorder in the future (11–13). In addition, a number of the key treatments for depression and anxiety can lead to insomnia (14), while, at the same time, persistent insomnia following successful treatment of depression is associated with a greater risk of any psychiatric disorder, depression, and anxiety disorders (11).

These relationships present challenges for both scientists and clinicians. They mandate that those working with either psychiatric disorders or sleep be knowledgeable about both areas and understand the relationships between them. From a scientific perspective there are a number of key considerations. One issue is the difficulty in identifying what is "core" disease and what are secondary symptoms. As we will see, this becomes complicated by the fact that a secondary symptom could change the course of a disease.

From a clinical perspective, the interrelatedness of sleep and psychiatric disease has the implication of blurring the lines of distinction between these two areas. It may be detrimental to think of treating psychiatric disease or sleep disorders as separate entities. Patients with either type of disorder are likely to present with, develop, or have response to treatment affected by the other domain of problem.

This review is intended to be of benefit for both clinical practice and research by presenting the current literature on the relationships between psychiatric disorders and sleep. The chapter is organized by psychiatric disease, sequentially providing a basic review of the epidemiology, course, diagnostic criteria, differential diagnosis, relevant sleep issues, and treatment of a number of the major psychiatric disorders of greatest interest from a sleep perspective: anxiety disorders, mood disorders, schizophrenia, and alcohol dependence and abuse. For each type of disorder the discussion will focus on elucidating what is known about links to sleep and sleep disorders and how such issues may impact our understanding of the disease and clinical management.

ANXIETY DISORDERS

The subject of this section is a group of psychiatric disorders characterized by inappropriate or excessive activation of the "fight–flight" system. Individuals with these problems experience fear and worry, which are central nervous system aspects of this activation and peripheral effects reflecting activation of the sympathetic nervous system. This activation appears to potently disrupt sleep, as evidenced by the fact that anxiety disorders are the most common comorbid condition seen in insomnia patients. Epidemiologic studies have reported comorbid anxiety disorders in 24% and 36% of individuals diagnosed with insomnia (11,12). Anxiety disorders are also of particular interest because they have the type of reciprocal relationship with sleep disruption mentioned above. As a group, individuals diagnosed with insomnia have an increased likelihood of experiencing a subsequent anxiety disorder compared with individuals without insomnia (14% versus 7%) (12). In this section, we will discuss the subset of the anxiety disorders that is most typified by sleep disruption including generalized anxiety disorder, posttraumatic stress disorder (PTSD), and panic disorder. While sleep disruption may occur with all anxiety disorders, for some of the disorders disturbed sleep is not typical or predominant because potentially disruptive activation may be limited to specific circumstances, which may be isolated to daytime experience. This is most likely to occur in phobias and obsessive compulsive disorder (OCD), which will not be covered in this section. It is worth noting that, in such disorders, sleep difficulties can occur when the specific circumstance happens to relate to the bedroom, bedtime, or night-specific phenomena. For example, sleep may be disturbed in OCD patients who have a compulsion of repeatedly checking to make sure the doors are locked or the stove is off before being able to go to bed (15). Similarly, sleep disruption may occur in those with phobias of the dark, of being alone, or those with social phobia the night before a feared social circumstance is scheduled to occur. There is one study, which awaits replication, suggesting that the sleep of individuals with social phobias may, in general, be disturbed compared with normal controls (16).

Generalized Anxiety Disorder (GAD)

Overview, Epidemiology, and Course

A key distinguishing feature of generalized anxiety disorder (GAD) is persistence and chronicity of both central and peripheral symptoms of anxiety. Affected individuals experience excessive worry associated with a number of physical symptoms (see below) most days for extended periods of time. They are frequently identified as "worriers," who appear to have excessive concerns and while they are typically aware of this exaggerated response, they are unable to change.

The lifetime prevalence of GAD has been estimated to be 5% and patients often present with somatic complaints, which leads to their diagnosis and treatment (17,18). The chronicity of this condition is evident in that many patients diagnosed with GAD report anxiety all of their lives and there is a high rate of relapse following termination of treatment (60% to 80% in the first year) (17–19). There is currently no clear evidence for a genetic role in this disease (18).

Diagnostic Criteria for GAD

The following is the DSM-IV TR diagnostic criteria for 300.02 Generalized Anxiety Disorder (18).

A. Excessive anxiety and worry (apprehensive expectation), occurring more days than not for at least 6 months, about a number of events or activities (such as work or school performance).
B. The person finds it difficult to control the worry.
C. The anxiety and worry are associated with three (or more) of the following six symptoms (with at least some symptoms present for more days than not for the past 6 months). (*Note*: Only one item is required in children.)
  1. Restlessness or feeling keyed up or on edge
  2. Being easily fatigued
  3. Difficulty concentrating or mind going blank
  4. Irritability
  5. Muscle tension
  6. Sleep disturbance (difficulty falling or staying asleep, or restless unsatisfying sleep)
D. The focus of the anxiety and worry is not confined to features of an Axis I disorder; e.g., the anxiety or worry is not about having a panic attack (as in panic disorder), being embarrassed in public (as in social phobia), being contaminated (as in obsessive–compulsive disorder), being away from home or close relatives (as in separation anxiety disorder), gaining weight (as in anorexia nervosa), having multiple physical complaints (as in somatization disorder), or having a serious illness (as in hypochondriasis), and the anxiety and worry do not occur exclusively during posttraumatic stress disorder (PTSD).
E. The anxiety, worry, or physical symptoms cause clinically significant distress or impairment in social, occupational, or other important areas of functioning.
F. The disturbance is not due to the direct physiologic effects of a substance (e.g., a drug of abuse, a medication) or a general medical condition (e.g., hyperthyroidism) and does not occur exclusively during a mood disorder, a psychotic disorder, or a pervasive developmental disorder.

Differential Diagnosis

Anxiety is a useful and normal reaction in many circumstances, and it is important not to mistake normal anxiety in an individual in difficult circumstances for GAD (20). The most important distinguishing features are the chronic, excessive, and pervasive (related to many events or aspects of life) character of GAD. Similarly, at times, it may be difficult to distinguish GAD from anxiety that

is caused by psychic trauma (see PTSD below), a medication, or a medical condition. Another common area of diagnostic overlap occurs in many patients with GAD who present with a somatic complaint. Such patients illustrate the utility of asking about associated anxiety symptoms in those who present with the typical somatic symptoms of anxiety, including nausea, dry mouth, muscle soreness, twitching, or tension, urinary frequency, sweating, swallowing difficulties, and, most relevant to this chapter, insomnia (18).

Sleep Disturbance in GAD

The most common sleep difficulty in patients with GAD is insomnia. It is estimated that over 50% of those with GAD have difficulty sleeping (21). While it had long been held that anxiety led to difficulties falling asleep and not staying asleep, the available evidence, which includes both self-report and polysomnographic (PSG) data, suggests that both types of sleep difficulties are quite common (21,22). The viewpoint that sleep onset problems were characteristic of GAD derives from the correct observation that these patients frequently describe difficulties relaxing, shutting off their minds, or stopping worrying when they go to bed at night (15).

Treatment

The options for treatment of GAD that have been demonstrated to have efficacy versus placebo include a number of pharmacologic agents: benzodiazepines, the serotonin 1A receptor agonist buspirone, tricyclic antidepressants, selective serotonin reuptake inhibitors (SSRIs), venlafaxine (serotonin and norepinephrine reuptake inhibitor), and trazodone (some serotonin reuptake inhibition and serotonin 2 and 3 receptor antagonism) (21–23). There are very few studies comparing these treatments. One study suggested that trazodone, diazepam, and imipramine were equally efficacious (24). Another study suggests that venlafaxine might be more effective than buspirone (25). Another consideration is that depression is frequently comorbid with GAD, and this has led some to recommend that the antidepressants with demonstrated efficacy, namely, venlafaxine, paroxetine, and tricyclic antidepressants may be preferable in the long-term treatment of this condition (26).

There are no data available to provide specific guidance in the management of insomnia in patients with GAD. It might be assumed that sedating GAD treatments could be more expeditious at addressing insomnia in GAD, such as benzodiazepines, trazodone, and tricyclic antidepressants, although there is no evidence to suggest this at present. It also remains unknown when the addition of a second treatment targeted to the insomnia is indicated. Possibilities include a hypnotic agent, adjunctive sedating antidepressant, or cognitive–behavioral therapy for sleep.

Future Directions

Studies comparing the effectiveness of treatment options for GAD are needed. Another important unaddressed issue is whether insomnia in GAD is secondary to an underlying anxiety disorder, is a fundamental part of the syndrome, or is an autonomous process. No studies have yet been carried out to assess this issue. Such studies would require determining the frequency with which patients with GAD are left with residual insomnia when all of the other symptoms resolve. It will also be important to study traditional treatment plus placebo versus traditional treatment plus therapy targeted specifically to the associated insomnia.

Posttraumatic Stress Disorder (PTSD)

Overview, Epidemiology, and Course

It has been estimated that approximately 1% of individuals in the general population will experience PTSD in their lifetime (26a,27). However, this does not correspond to the number of people who have undergone what would be generally experienced as a severe, unexpected, and uncontrollable stressor. Only a subset (estimated to be 15% to 25%) of the individuals who experience the same event develop persistent difficulties that meet the criteria for this disease (see below) (27). The factors, which may lead some individuals to experience greater difficulties, are poorly understood.

It should also be noted that not all extreme events are believed to be likely to lead to the set of difficulties that characterize PTSD. The current definition according to the DSM-IV TR (see below) identifies several key aspects of events that tend to cause PTSD (18). These are: the threat of death or serious injury that is associated with a response of intense fear, helplessness, or horror. While these features may be useful, they are incompletely specified, since what defines "serious," "intense," "helplessness," and "horror" remain unclear and are not quantifiable phenomena.

The difficulties that individuals experience have been categorized into three types: avoidance and re-experiencing of the trauma and a persistent hyperarousal. Avoidance includes the development of general isolation and detachment, however, specific attempts to prevent encountering things that are reminiscent of the traumatic event are an important aspect of PTSD for many individuals. The re-experiencing symptoms include recurrent intrusive recollections, nightmares, flashbacks (where individuals have the experience of reliving the traumatic situation), and both central and peripheral hyperactivation in response to anything that is reminiscent of the trauma. The third type of difficulty, hyperarousal, includes disrupted sleep, along with irritability, exaggerated startle, and hypervigilance.

The available data on the natural history suggest that PTSD is typically a chronic condition. It has been estimated that 74% of affected individuals continue to have significant symptoms for more than 6 months (27). It has been further observed that even those who receive treatment continue to experience long-term PTSD-associated difficulties (28). The latter observation may reflect the striking limitation of empirically validated treatment options (see below).

Diagnostic Criteria for Posttraumatic Stress Disorder

DSM-IV TR diagnostic criteria for 309.81 posttraumatic stress disorder (18) are as follows

A. The person has been exposed to a traumatic event in which both of the following were present:
1. The person experienced, witnessed, or was confronted with an event or events that involved actual or threatened death or serious injury, or a threat to the physical integrity of self or others.
2. The person's response involved intense fear, helplessness, or horror. (*Note:* In children, this may be expressed, instead, by disorganized or agitated behavior.)

B. The traumatic event is persistently re-experienced in one (or more) of the following ways:
1. Recurrent and intrusive distressing recollections of the event, including images, thoughts, or perceptions. (*Note:* In young children, repetitive play may occur, in which themes or aspects of the trauma are expressed.)
2. Recurrent distressing dreams of the event. (*Note:* In children, there may be frightening dreams without recognizable content.)
3. Acting or feeling as if the traumatic event were recurring (includes a sense of reliving the experience, illusions, hallucinations, and dissociative flashback episodes, including those that occur on awakening or when intoxicated). (*Note:* In young children, trauma-specific re-enactment may occur.)
4. Intense psychologic distress at exposure to internal or external cues that symbolize or resemble an aspect of the traumatic event.
5. Physiologic reactivity on exposure to internal or external cues that symbolize or resemble an aspect of the traumatic event.

C. Persistent avoidance of stimuli associated with the trauma and numbing of general responsiveness (not present before the trauma), as indicated by three (or more) of the following:
1. Efforts to avoid thoughts, feelings, or conversations associated with the trauma
2. Efforts to avoid activities, places, or people that arouse recollections of the trauma
3. Inability to recall an important aspect of the trauma
4. Markedly diminished interest or participation in significant activities

5. Feeling of detachment or estrangement from others
6. Restricted range of affect (e.g., unable to have loving feelings)
7. Sense of a foreshortened future (e.g., does not expect to have a career, marriage, children, or a normal life span)
D. Persistent symptoms of increased arousal (not present before the trauma), as indicated by two (or more) of the following:
   1. Difficulty falling or staying asleep
   2. Irritability or outbursts of anger
   3. Difficulty concentrating
   4. Hypervigilance
   5. Exaggerated startle response
E. Duration of the disturbance [symptoms in criteria (B), (C), and (D)] is more than 1 month.
F. The disturbance causes clinically significant distress or impairment in social, occupational, or other important areas of functioning.

Differential Diagnosis

In considering a diagnosis of PTSD it is important to make sure that the symptoms that the patient is experiencing were not present prior to the trauma. In that case, other diagnoses are indicated. Another consideration in patients with predominantly re-experiencing symptoms is to rule out obsessive–compulsive disorder (OCD) (see below) (18). In OCD, obsessions are present, which are recurrent intrusive thoughts that can be similar to symptoms of PTSD, but are not related to an event. Similarly, flashbacks may at times be difficult to differentiate from hallucinations that can be seen in schizophrenia, delirium, psychotic mood disorders, substance intoxication, or withdrawal (18). The distinction rests on determining whether the onset began with a traumatic event, which is reflected in the flashback and evaluating the patient for the associated symptoms that typify these syndromes (e.g., in delirium and waxing and waning of consciousness). For schizophrenia there can be further overlap with PTSD, because the negative symptoms of schizophrenia (see below), may share features with the avoidance symptoms of PTSD, placing greater importance on the capacity to identify a traumatic event. However, in practice it is rarely difficult to differentiate these conditions.

Sleep Disturbance in Posttraumatic Sleep Disorder

Sleep difficulties are so prevalent in patients with PTSD that it has been suggested that disrupted sleep is a hallmark of this condition (29). It is widely believed that the reaction to trauma leads to a constellation of symptoms that frequently includes insomnia. To date, there is no evidence suggesting that preexisting insomnia is a predisposing factor for the development of the PTSD syndrome following an extreme event, although we are aware of no studies that

have specifically investigated this question. There is, however, one study suggesting that sleep complaints occurring at 1 month or longer after trauma were significant predictors of the presence of a diagnosis of PTSD at 1 year post-trauma. While this report is intriguing, it is of uncertain significance.

As is generally true of PTSD studies, the results of research on the sleep of patients with PTSD are confounded by the inclusion of vastly differing patient populations in terms of type of trauma and period of time since the trauma, comorbid conditions, and number of subjects. It is not surprising that the results are inconsistent. The predominant types of sleep problems reported by patients with PTSD are insomnia (trouble falling asleep or staying asleep) and nightmares.

A number of sleep laboratory studies have examined the sleep of patients with PTSD in an effort to explore the associated neurophysiologic changes. The most consistent findings suggest disruption of sleep in measures of the ability to stay asleep. A diminished sleep efficiency (time asleep divided by time in bed) has been reported in four studies, whereas an elevation in the time spent awake after initially falling asleep (WASO) has been noted in two reports (30–33). In one additional study, there was an association between an increase in WASO and nightmares (34). However, it should be noted that there are several studies that have not found evidence for sleep difficulties in the PSG in PTSD patients (35). This inconsistency may not be specific to PTSD, however. There is evidence among patients with insomnia complaints occurring in other settings that there is often a weak relationship between PSG and self-report measures of sleep.

Another frequent PSG finding in PTSD patients is an alteration in rapid eye movement (REM) sleep. The most frequently reported REM sleep aberration has been an increase in REM density (30,32,33). REM density has been regarded as a measure of the "intensity" of REM sleep and is derived by dividing the total number of eye movements that occur in REM by the total time spent in REM across the night. This finding may not reflect a physiologic alteration specific to PTSD, however, because REM density has also been reported to be elevated in those with major depression, which has a high-rate of comorbidity with PTSD (28). The elevation in REM density is currently of interest in terms of understanding the pathophysiology of PTSD and the fact that it is observed in both PTSD and depression is intriguing in this regard.

Treatment

Surprisingly few placebo-controlled studies of the treatment of PTSD have been carried out. The treatments that have been studied tend to be inconsistently found to have efficacy. This may reflect the high frequency of comorbid conditions, the heterogeneity of symptoms in those with PTSD, or differences in the effects of the many different types of traumatic events, all of which may increase the noise in the data and complicate the interpretation of results (36). Placebo controlled studies have best demonstrated the efficacy of the SSRIs sertraline and fluoxetine (37,38). There is also a study suggesting the efficacy of the anticonvulsant lamotrigine; however, further studies are needed (39).

As in the case of GAD, there are no placebo-controlled studies of treatment targeted to the sleep difficulties associated with PTSD. Agents that have been demonstrated to improve the capacity to stay asleep and fall asleep in primary insomnia (such as the FDA-approved hypnotic agents, primarily benzodiazepines and related compounds) would be expected to also improve sleep in patients with PTSD, although this remains to be demonstrated. Those agents with demonstrated efficacy in helping individuals stay asleep would be of particular interest given the prevalence of this problem in PTSD patients. Sedating antidepressants may also be of utility, although their efficacy for the treatment of insomnia in any setting is much less well established.

We have much less experience in other settings that can be brought to bear on the treatment of the nightmares that plague many patients with PTSD [roughly 60% of patients with PTSD report nightmares (40,41)]. One group has published two uncontrolled preliminary reports (one clinical retrospective chart review and an open-label study in five patients) suggesting that the alpha-1 adrenergic antagonist prazosin might improve the nightmares of PTSD patients (42,43). Future placebo-controlled studies will be needed to determine the efficacy of prazosin in this setting. There has also been a clinical retrospective study of the anticonvulsant topiramate, which provides very preliminary evidence of a positive effect on nightmares in PTSD patients (44).

Future Directions

Work is needed to develop treatments for both the sleep disruption and nightmares associated with PTSD. Placebo controlled trials of hypnotics and sedating antidepressants should be considered. While there is little to suggest that sleep disruption plays an important role in affecting the natural history of the disease, studies on the relationship of the development of sleep difficulties and the appearance of other PTSD symptoms may be of interest.

Panic Disorder

Overview, Epidemiology, and Course

Panic disorder is characterized by recurrent and unexpected acute episodes, or attacks, of extreme levels of fear and peripheral somatic symptoms of sympathetic system activation that are not provoked by environmental events.

Because these attacks so often lead to dread that another attack will occur, the presence of fear of future attacks and their possible consequences is considered a central feature of this syndrome (see below). There is often spreading fear that is caused by the tendency in some patients to become frightened of places or circumstances where panic attacks happen to have occurred.

The lifetime prevalence of panic disorder is estimated to be roughly 2% (18) with onset typically occurring between the ages of 18 and 35. As with PTSD and GAD, panic disorder is often a chronic condition (18). At times, agoraphobia (fear of being in places perceived as particularly unsafe if a panic attack should occur), may persist long after an individual has experienced their last panic attack. Like GAD, it is often the somatic symptoms that cause affected individuals to seek medical attention, frequently leading to extensive medical evaluations of the affected organ system that do not identify any underlying organic pathology.

Diagnostic Criteria for Panic Disorder

DSM-IV TR diagnostic criteria for 300.01 Panic Disorder (18) follow:

A. Both (1) and (2):
   1. Recurrent unexpected panic attacks defined as a discrete period of intense fear or discomfort, in which four (or more) of the following symptoms developed abruptly and reached a peak within 10 minutes:
      a. Palpitations, pounding heart, or accelerated heart rate
      b. Sweating
      c. Trembling
      d. Sensations of shortness of breath or smothering
      e. Feeling of choking
      f. Chest pain or discomfort
      g. Nausea or abdominal distress
      h. Feeling dizzy, unsteady, lightheaded or faint
      i. Derealization (feelings of unreality) or depersonalization (being detached from oneself)
      j. Fear of losing control or going crazy
      k. Fear of dying
      l. Paresthesias (numbness or tingling sensations)
      m. Chills or hot flashes
   2. At least one of the attacks has been followed by 1 month (or more) of one (or more) of the following:
      a. Persistent concern about having additional attacks
      b. Worry about the implications of the attack or its consequences (e.g., losing control, having a heart attack, "going crazy")
      c. A significant change in behavior related to the attacks

B. The panic attacks are not due to the direct physiologic effects of a substance (e.g., a drug of abuse, a medication) or a general medical condition (e.g., hyperthyroidism).

C. The panic attacks are not better accounted for by another mental disorder, such as social phobia (e.g., occurring on exposure to feared social situations), specific phobia (e.g., on exposure to a specific phobic situation), obsessive–compulsive disorder (e.g., on exposure to dirt in someone with an obsession about contamination), posttraumatic stress disorder (e.g., in response to stimuli associated with a severe stressor), or separation anxiety disorder (e.g., in response to being away from home or close relatives).

Differential Diagnosis

Isolated panic attacks may be spontaneous or elicited by medications, abused substances, or medical illnesses. Such circumstances differ from panic disorder, which is characterized by recurrent panic attacks. The most important differential diagnosis in clinical practice is the differentiation of organic medical disease from the somatic symptoms that may be experienced during panic attacks. It may also be difficult to distinguish those with phobias, in particular social phobia, from those experiencing panic disorder with agoraphobia. When these disorders are being considered, it is most useful to bear in mind that phobias, unlike panic disorder, are associated with anxiety triggered by specific circumstances, such as public speaking or particular interpersonal circumstances, in the case of social phobia (18). In panic disorder, the fears are focused around circumstances where a panic attack happened to occur or where it is felt to be a particularly unsafe place to be if an attack occurs.

Sleep Disturbance in Panic Disorder

A comparison of sleep complaints in panic disorder patients and normal controls (defined as having no psychiatric illness) found that those with panic disorder were significantly more likely to report sleep panic attacks (those reporting ever having an attack: panic disorder, 31% and controls 8%; recurrent attacks: panic disorder, 15% and controls, 0%) and recurrent difficulty staying asleep (panic disorder, 67% and controls, 23%) (45). Individuals with panic disorder report that the nocturnal panic attacks are much more of a problem for them than the difficulty staying asleep (15). The nocturnal panic events are typically sudden awakenings occurring in NREM sleep, much like night terrors, reinforcing their independence from awakenings secondary to nightmares, which generally occur out of REM (45). Once awake, the presentation of nocturnal panic is much like that of waking panic, with the associated fear and somatic symptoms (15). Of note, there is some reason to believe that the nocturnal panic may subsequently lead to the observed difficulty staying asleep and may also lead to a fear of going to bed and associated sleep deprivation (15,46). The resulting fear of going to bed may explain the curious association between nocturnal panic attacks and a response of anxiety to relaxation (45). Of further interest is the possibility that the sleep deprivation resulting from the fear of going to bed may exacerbate both daytime and sleep anxiety (15).

In terms of PSG findings in those with panic disorder, there appears to be some decrease in sleep efficiency and increase in sleep onset latency but, as in PTSD, these effects appear to be less than what would be expected on the basis of the patients' complaints (15). As mentioned above, the lack of concordance may be a general characteristic of insomnia and not specific to panic disorder. Unlike PTSD, there does not appear to be any alterations in REM physiology evident in the PSG in patients with panic disorder (15).

Treatment

The treatment of panic was initially dominated by heterocyclic antidepressants (primarily imipramine), and monoamine oxidase inhibitors (most commonly phenelzine), which were shown to have significant efficacy in a number of placebo-controlled trials. However, based on side-effect profile and nearly 30 placebo-controlled studies, SSRIs are now recommended for first-line use (47,48). Because those with panic disorder may be particularly prone to having problems tolerating the initial side effects of these agents, such as restlessness and sweating, it has been recommended to start with a lower dosage than usual or consider an initial short-course of benzodiazepines (49). In terms of other antidepressants, trazodone and bupropion appear to be relatively less effective in the treatment of panic disorder, and there is some evidence suggesting that venlafaxine may be efficacious. While benzodiazepines appear to have the most rapid onset of therapeutic effect and have been demonstrated to have efficacy in a number of placebo-controlled trials (particularly, alprazolam and clonazepam), other agents tend to be preferentially recommended because of dependence and withdrawal concerns, associated sedation, and lack of efficacy in the treatment of the frequently comorbid depression (49,50). The sedation associated with the benzodiazepine class of medications could be desirable in those with insomnia complaints and nocturnal panic, however, there is very little research on the treatment of those aspects of panic disorder with any agent. In this regard, there is one report of an open-label trial of imipramine in individuals with relatively frequent sleep panic attacks where a reduction in sleep attacks was found (51). An additional consideration of importance in the treatment of patients with panic disorder is the use of education and cognitive–behavioral therapy, which may be particularly relevant in longer-term therapy and when attempting to address associated agoraphobia (49).

Future Directions

Studies of the treatment of nocturnal panic are needed. In addition, it will be important to explore means to diminish the fear of going to bed that may develop. The suggestion that sleep disruption in patients with panic disorder occurs secondary to nocturnal panic attacks is of interest and will require better longitudinal studies of symptom development. A further area of interest is the relationship of sleep disruption and sleep deprivation with the course of the disease and both daytime and nighttime panic. Thus far, the interrelationships of panic and sleep have remained hypothetical and been the subject of minimal experimentation. As discussed in the introduction, panic disorder may be a disease for which there is a complex bidirectional relationship with sleep. The implicit scenario is that once a nocturnal panic attack occurs, there is a resultant sleep disruption and fear of sleep, causing sleep deprivation that increases anxiety and predisposes individuals to panic attacks both during the day and during sleep. This, in turn, worsens the sleep disruption, setting up a vicious cycle. Testing this hypothesis has important treatment implications. If true, it would suggest that the development of sleep difficulties may be intrinsic to the evolution of panic disorder and suggests that getting control of the disease may require that specific treatment be targeted to the sleep disruption and deprivation, in addition to addressing the panic attacks. Particular importance is conferred upon these considerations by the fact that the current first-line treatments for panic disorder, SSRIs, may disrupt sleep and, therefore, in some individuals, may perpetuate the process or hinder resolution. As in GAD, studies in which patients are randomized to traditional panic disorder treatment, such as an SSRI along with either placebo or a therapy directed at sleep difficulties, would be of interest.

MOOD DISORDERS

Mood disorders include both depressive disorders and bipolar spectrum disorders (18). These two broad categories are further divided into major depressive disorder, dysthymic disorder, and, bipolar I disorder, bipolar II disorder, and cyclothymic disorder. The prototypes of each of these groups, namely major depressive disorder and bipolar I disorder respectively, have sleep disturbance as a core symptom. These two groups will be the focus of the following section, as most of the research examining the relationship between mood and sleep disturbance has been done with these patient populations. As we outline below, the mood disorders are the group of psychiatric disturbances where there is the strongest evidence of a complex bidirectional relationship with sleep difficulties. This includes the types of relationships with insomnia observed with some of the anxiety disorders. However, the empirical support for these relationships is much more compelling for the mood disorders, and these disorders are unique in that manipulations of sleep have significant therapeutic efficacy in their treatment.

Epidemiology

Major Depression

Major depression is a highly prevalent condition that appears to be more frequent in women (lifetime prevalence of 10% to 25%) than in men (5% to 12%). There appears to be a complex relationship between age and risk of depression (18). Taking a broad view of this issue, the prevalence of depression is higher in persons younger than 45 years than in those older than 45 (18).

Bipolar I Disorder

Bipolar I disorder is much less prevalent, with a lifetime prevalence of only 0.4% to 1.6%, and equally affects both genders (18). In males with bipolar disorder, the first episode is more often manic, whereas females are more likely to have a major depressive episode first (18). Women are more likely to have their first or subsequent mood episode during the immediate postpartum period. The prevalence of mood disorders does not vary significantly by race or ethnicity (18).

Course

Major Depression

The course of major depression differs a great deal among affected individuals. The average age of onset of major depression is in the mid-20s, but the first episode of depression may occur at any age. The course is highly variable and generally the number of previous episodes predicts the likelihood of having another episode (18). For example, 50% to 60% of patients with a first episode of depression will have a second episode, and those with two episodes have a 70% chance of having a third episode of depression. After the third episode, the chance of having a fourth is 90%. In naturalistic studies of depression, 20% of patients continue to show no evidence of achieving remission, 40% show partial remission, and 40% have no evidence of mood disorder at the end of 1 year.

Bipolar I Disorder

In comparison with major depressive disorder, bipolar disorder tends to be a more recurrent disease. Patients with bipolar disorder tend to have more lifetime episodes than patients with depressive disorder (18). Studies of bipolar disorder done before the availability of good treatments suggest an average of four episodes occur in a 10-year period (18).

Diagnostic Criteria

Major Depression

The diagnosis of a major depressive episode requires the presence of five of the following nine symptoms over a period of at least 2 weeks. One of the five symptoms has to be either depressed mood (a) or loss of interest or pleasure (b):

1. Depressed mood, present most of the day, every day, as noted by subjective report or objectively.
2. Loss of interest or pleasure in all or almost all activities, most of the day, nearly every day.
3. Significant change in appetite nearly every day or significant change in weight (5% of body weight over a 1 month period).
4. Insomnia or hypersomnia nearly every day.
5. Observable psychomotor agitation or retardation present nearly every day.
6. Fatigue or lack of energy nearly every day.
7. Feelings of worthlessness or excessive guilt nearly every day.
8. Indecisiveness, diminished ability to concentrate, nearly every day.
9. Recurrent thoughts of death (not just fear of dying), recurrent suicidal ideation with or without intent or plan.

Bipolar Disorder

A bipolar I disorder is diagnosed when a patient has experienced at least one manic episode, with or without prior history of depressive episodes. A manic episode is a period of abnormally and persistently elevated, expansive, or irritable mood, lasting at least 1 week or any duration if hospitalization is necessary.

During the period of mood disturbance, three (or more) of the following symptoms are present to a significant degree (four symptoms, if the mood is irritable):

1. Grandiosity or inflated self-esteem.
2. Decreased need for sleep.
3. Pressure to keep talking or more talkative than usual.
4. Flight of ideas or a subjective feeling that thoughts are racing.
5. Distractibility (i.e., attention too easily drawn to irrelevant or unimportant external) stimuli.
6. Psychomotor agitation or an increase in goal-directed activity (at work, social or sexual).
7. Impulsivity with increased involvement in high-risk, high-reward activities with potential for painful consequences (e.g., expensive shopping sprees or sexual indiscretions).

Other Mood Disorders

Patients are diagnosed with dysthymia when they have depressive symptoms for a 2-year period without meeting criteria for major depression. Patients with bipolar II disorder never quite have a manic episode, but may have a period of "hypomania," which is similar in quality to mania but less intense. Patients who have alternating episodes of dysthymia and hypomania are classified as "cyclothymic."

Sleep Disturbances in Mood Disorders

Major Depression

Epidemiologic studies suggest that depression is present in up to 20% of patients with insomnia, compared to only 1% of those without insomnia (11,52). In a sample of primary care patients, the symptoms of sleep complaints and fatigue were strongly predictive of depression (53). Breslau et al. (12) also found the rates of major depression to be increased in young adults with sleep complaints, 31% for patients with insomnia, 25% for patients with hypersomnia, and 54% for those with both insomnia and hypersomnia versus 2.7% for those with no sleep complaints. During a 3-year follow-up period, the relative risk for a new onset of major depression in persons with insomnia or hypersomnia at baseline was significantly higher than those without sleep disturbances. Another study of older adults also showed insomnia to be predictive of a future episode of depression (54). It is also the case that subjects who reported sleep disturbance at baseline and again at a 1 year follow-up interview were more likely to become clinically depressed than those whose sleep disturbance had resolved (11). In a long-term prospective study of medical students, those who reported insomnia in medical school showed a higher subsequent relative risk of clinical depression than those who did not (55).

Thus, robust data suggests that insomnia is predictive of future depression. It has been argued, however, that insomnia is not a "risk factor" for depression by definition, since it is not phenomenologically distinct from the diagnostic cluster itself. Hence, it may be better termed a "precursor symptom" and, as such, out of all mood symptoms, it is the strongest predictor of the onset of a depressive episode (56).

During a depressive episode, sleep disturbance typically manifests as insomnia. There may be a decrease in total sleep time (TST) (middle or terminal insomnia and sometimes, initial insomnia), disturbing dreams, and nonrestorative sleep, often with daytime fatigue and sedation. The sleep disturbance may precede a mood episode by several weeks (6). During an "atypical" depressive episode, patients may have hypersomnia, rather than insomnia and an increase in appetite rather than a decrease in appetite (these unusual features have led to the term "atypical depression"). The excessive sleeping may be during the night or daytime, with at least 10 hours of sleep per day. Atypical features are two to three times more common in women. They are also more common in young patients with depression, in seasonal affective disorder (in which patients experience depression during the winter months), and in bipolar disorder.

Bipolar Disorder

Manic episodes are almost always characterized by a decreased need for sleep and decreased amount of total sleep. In fact, sleep reduction has been proposed as a final common pathway in the genesis of mania (57). These authors have proposed a bidirectional relationship between insomnia and mania, such that insomnia causes mania, which further causes insomnia, thus reinforcing a manic episode. In addition, experimental sleep deprivation in bipolar patients has been shown to precipitate mania (58,59). Although most treatments of mania include early and aggressive treatment of the sleep disturbance, it is not clear if this is necessary and/or sufficient for treatment of an acute manic episode. Interestingly, in bipolar patients, depressive episodes are more likely to be associated with hypersomnia than insomnia.

Polysomnographic Findings

Major Depression

REM Sleep Abnormalities

The earliest finding in the relationship between REM sleep and depression was the reduction of REM latency (60–63). This finding also has the strongest empirical support among the sleep disturbances of depression (64–69). In addition, increase in REM density (70–72), an increased percentage of REM sleep (69,70,73), and a longer duration of the first REM period (73–75) have all been reported.

Disturbances of Sleep Continuity and Slow-Wave Sleep (SWS)

Depressed patients show increased sleep latency, frequent wakefulness, and early morning awakening, with the net result of decreased sleep efficiency (64,70,73,76). Patients also show decreased amount of SWS (70,73,74,76), particularly in the first NREM period (74,77). The finding of decreased amounts of SWS among depressed patients as compared with normals has not always been consistent (67,68,78).

Bipolar Disorder

PSG studies of manic patients have yielded comparable findings to those of depressed patients (79,80). Bipolar depressed patients with hypersomnia do not always show decreased REM latency and have normal sleep latency on multiple sleep latency tests (MSLT) (81).

Pathophysiologic and Clinical Implications of Polysomnographic Findings

Relationship to Disease

Some uncertainty exists about whether these findings are pathophysiologically related to the changes that occur in the brain during an episode of depression (state marker) or whether they are markers of a predisposition toward mood disorders (trait marker). There is evidence to suggest that some sleep abnormalities, like increased REM density and decreased sleep efficiency, are more prominent in the acute stages of a depressive episode (82–84). On the other hand, certain elements of disrupted sleep may be present in patients with mood disorders, even when they are not experiencing an episode. In particular, reduced REM latency and decreased SWS can persist when the clinical signs and symptoms have remitted (82,85–88). Thus, these PSG findings may be trait markers for some patients with depressive disorders. In fact, there is data suggesting that family members of probands with depression and reduced REM latency may themselves have reduced REM and SWS deficits, even without a past history of a mood episode (85,89). Thus, it is possible that some of the sleep disturbances seen in those with major depression are traits that have familial transmission.

Potential Clinical Utility

The fact that there are PSG markers that appear to identify patients with mood disorders suggests the possibility that such markers have the potential to serve as a diagnostic tool that might be of utility in the clinical management of patients with mood disorders. Many studies have looked at the potential utility of sleep parameters as a tool for diagnosing mood disorders. Reduced REM latency has been shown to distinguish depressed patients from normal controls (90,91). REM density also has been shown to separate depressed patients from normals (92,93). A limitation of both these parameters is a lack of a consistent definition for both normal REM latency and density. A large meta-analysis was carried out to compare patients with depression, those with other psychiatric diagnoses, and normal controls (66). This study combined data from 177 PSG studies of psychiatric patients with a variety of diagnoses, including affective disorders, alcoholism, dementia, schizophrenia, anxiety disorders, and others. Patients with insomnia and narcolepsy were included for comparison. All patient groups showed significantly more sleep abnormalities than controls, with mood disorders patients having the most. Although patients with mood disorders showed less SWS and more sleep continuity disturbances compared with controls, these did not differ significantly from other psychiatric illnesses. In addition, reduced REM latency was seen in patients with eating disorders, schizophrenia, and borderline personality disorder. Interestingly, in controlled studies only, of the four groups in which REM density was measured, only the affective disorders group had increased REM density. It was also the only group with more total night REM sleep time. Other studies have reported shortened REM latency in alcoholism (94), PTSD (95,96), schizophrenia (97,98), panic disorder (93,99), and eating disorders (100,101). Although all of these diagnoses can have comorbid depression, this has not always accounted for the REM findings (99). Thus, it appears that PSG markers of depression could help in the differentiation of individuals with depression from normal controls. However, because the challenge in clinical practice is more often differentiating those with depression from other psychiatric diseases, where the same PSG findings appear to be present, the clinical utility of these physiologic markers appears to be limited (66).

Diagnosis and Treatment of Sleep Complaints in Mood Disorders

Major Depression

Diagnosis

Making the diagnosis begins with a review of the patient's mood; neurovegetative symptoms of depression including changes in sleep, appetite, concentration and psychomotor changes; and assessing cognitive symptoms, such as feelings of guilt, worthlessness, hopelessness, and most importantly, suicidal ideation. It is important also to carry out a careful history and physical examination to identify medications, medical disorders, or other psychiatric diseases that may precipitate an episode of depression or complicate management. A number of such considerations include medications like beta blockers, medical conditions, like stroke or myocardial infarction, and psychiatric diseases, like substance abuse or personality disorders.

Treatment

The treatment of depression involves three different modalities—psychotropic medications, psychotherapy, electroconvulsive therapy (ECT), or some combination of these. Generally speaking, greater severity and the presence of psychosis increase the likelihood of response to a biological treatment. Patients with milder forms of depression may respond to psychotherapy alone. Successful psychotherapy of depression is associated with reduction in insomnia severity (102).

ECT is the most effective antidepressant treatment. It is generally reserved for patients who have failed to respond to medications, or in whom the depression severity or lethality necessitates a rapid response. This is often the case in patients who are actively suicidal, psychotic, malnourished, dehydrated, or unable to care for themselves. In terms of sleep effects, ECT has been shown to lead to improvements in insomnia both in terms of self-report and PSG measures when used as a treatment for patients with depression (103).

For most patients with depression, medications are the first-line treatments. The older medications, namely tricyclic antidepressants (TCAs) and the monoaminooxidase inhibitors (MAOIs), are at least as effective as the newer agents, but are limited by their often-intolerable adverse event profile. However, one of the main side effects of the TCA group is sedation, and they have often been used in low doses to treat insomnia, although they have fallen out of favor for treatment of depression. Insomnia severity, as measured on standard depression rating scales, lessens in patients who are deemed responders to tricyclic antidepressants (TCA) (104). Furthermore, improvement in insomnia is typically among the earliest symptoms to change during TCA therapy (105), and this improvement in the insomnia complaint is mirrored PSG improvement, such as increased TST and SWS (106). Patients with atypical features, namely hypersomnia and increased appetite, respond better to MAOIs. The biggest drawback to using these agents is the risk of hypertensive crisis if used concomitantly with tyramine-containing foods or sympathomimetic drugs.

With respect to the PSG considerations discussed above, MAOIs are of particular interest because they are very potent suppressors of REM sleep (107–109). Notably, so is ECT and the tricyclic antidepressants (to varying degrees). This initially led to the thinking that REM suppression may be a necessary ingredient for antidepressant response. However, this has not always held true, especially for some of the newer antidepressants like nefazodone or bupropion, that appear to have no consistent effects on REM sleep.

The advent of SSRIs and the other classes of newer antidepressants (bupropion, venlafaxine, nefazodone, mirtazapine, and others) has changed the landscape of depression treatment. SSRIs and the other newer antidepressant medications have superceded the TCAs as first-line treatment in depression, largely because of more benign side effects, particularly a lower risk in death from overdose. One result of this transition from TCAs to newer, less sedating antidepressants is that there may be a greater likelihood that insomnia may not be treated during the acute episode of depression and that patients completing successful treatment for an episode of depression will experience residual insomnia. Indeed, insomnia is the most common residual symptom among patients who have otherwise been successfully treated with fluoxetine for depression (110). As described by Nierenberg et al. (110), 25% to 45% of patients who were otherwise deemed responders to antidepressant therapy (17-item HRSD <7) reported persistent insomnia.

Importance of Treating Insomnia Symptoms in Patients with Depression

There is some evidence that it may be very important to target treatment to addressing insomnia in patients with major depression. In a sample of 53 highly treatment-resistant depressed inpatients, Nolen et al. (111) found that coadministration of a short-acting hypnotic (lormetazepam) at the outset of antidepressant treatment (nortriptyline or maprotiline) for 30 days resulted in greater reductions in nonsleep depressive symptoms on the Hamilton Rating Scale for Depression (HRSD), as compared with coadministration of placebo. This study implies that the insomnia associated with depression induces or aggravates some of the symptoms of depression during wakefulness and that treatment of the insomnia may result in improvement in the symptoms during wakefulness. However, this study cannot rule out the possibility that residual daytime effects from the nighttime dose of lormetazepam might have directly impacted on symptoms of daytime anxiety.

McCall et al. (112) found that insomnia makes a unique contribution to poor quality of life (QOL) in depressed patients after controlling for all other symptoms of depression. They tested whether a complaint of insomnia was related to QOL as part of a larger study examining the relationship between depression severity and QOL in 88 depressed inpatients. They found that the single insomnia item in the 21-item Beck Depression Inventory (BDI) predicted poor patient-rated performance of their ability to function in their primary role, even after controlling for the effects of all 20 other nonsleep BDI items, with higher insomnia scores predicting poorer role functioning. Asnis et al. (113) compared 4 weeks of treatment with either placebo or the hypnotic zolpidem 10 mg at bedtime in 190 depressed outpatients with continuing insomnia despite otherwise successful treatment with at least 2 weeks of an SSRI (fluoxetine, sertraline, or paroxetine). Those patients randomized to zolpidem reported shorter sleep latency and longer TST across the 4 weeks. Although the nonsleep depression symptom items on the HRSD were not different between groups during randomized treatment, the patients receiving zolpidem reported better concentration, greater vitality on the SF-36, less daytime sleepiness, feeling more refreshed, and less difficulty doing daily activities.

Another consideration is that insomnia appears to be an independent risk factor for suicide, which is the most important safety consideration in managing patients with major depression. Observational studies of elderly persons in the community show that complaints of poor sleep quality are associated with an elevated incidence of suicide (114). Severe insomnia is an independent risk factor for suicide during the first 2 years of an episode of major depression (115,116). Insomnia is also a risk factor for suicidal ideation. Agargun et al. (117) described the severity of sleep disturbance and suicidal ideation in 113 patients with depression, as assessed by the Schedule for Affective Disorders and Schizophrenia (SADS). They found that a complaint of hypersomnia was associated with a higher SADS suicide score, compared with a no sleep complaint group. However, the insomnia group had suicide scores that were higher than either the no-complaint or the hypersomnia groups. Higher SADS suicide scores among depressed patients with insomnia may translate into higher rates of completed suicide. Fawcett et al. prospectively followed 954 patients with depression for 10 years and 32 of these completed suicide during follow up. "Global insomnia" was a significant predictor of suicide within the first year of follow-up, second only to "anhedonia." Taken together, these studies suggest an association between sleep difficulties and risk of suicide in patients with depression. While this is an important consideration, it remains unknown whether treatment of persistent insomnia would reduce that risk.

Several studies provide a preliminary indication that there may be other implications of residual insomnia following successful antidepressant therapy. These complications include a higher risk of relapse into a depressive episode (102) and possibly premature drop out from treatment (118,119).

In addressing the insomnia associated with depression, there are a number of possible options. A sedating antidepressant such as nefazodone or mirtazapine may be used as the antidepressant agent with the intention that the associated sedation will address the insomnia that is present. When a nonsedating antidepressant is used an adjunctive medication to treat insomnia, this is most commonly low-dose trazodone (120) or a sedative–hypnotic, such as zolpidem or zalpelon.

A further sleep-related consideration related to depression treatment is that many antidepressants may cause or exacerbate the sleep disorders restless legs syndrome (RLS) and periodic leg movements of sleep (PLMS). Antidepressants that are particularly likely to be associated with these conditions are the MAOIs and tricyclic antidepressants. These conditions and their treatments are further discussed elsewhere in this textbook.

Patients developing an element of psychophysiologic insomnia may benefit from behavior therapy. Cognitive–behavior therapy (CBT) of sleep is based on the understanding that although predisposing factors, such as individual vulnerability, and precipitating factors such as stress, lead to initial development of insomnia, poor sleep hygiene is critical in perpetuating sleep problems. This approach is designed, in part, to correct poor sleep habits that sustain the sleep problems and involves patient education, prescribed "time in bed," and elimination of sleep incompatible behaviors that occur in bed. The treatment takes place over several sessions to make adjustments to prescribed time in bed, to trouble-shoot, and to encourage compliance. CBT has been shown to produce significant sleep improvements within 6 weeks in treatment of primary insomnia, with maintenance of gains at 6-month follow-up (121).

Bipolar Disorder

The management of bipolar disorder tends to be more complicated, and should be carried out by a psychiatrist. Because of the complexity of this issue, we will discuss only the highlights and encourage readers to liaison with the psychiatric consultant caring for a specific patient. The first-line agents for treatment of bipolar manic episode are lithium and mood stabilizers, such as valproic acid and carbamezapine. Lithium increases SWS in manic patients and may also suppress REM sleep and increase REM latency (122). It has also been reported to precipitate RLS (123). During the treatment of an acute manic episode, benzodiazepines are frequently used early for their sedating and tranquillizing properties. Antipsychotic agents may be required for psychotic symptoms and may also benefit by their sedating action. Treatment of depressive episodes of bipolar disorder usually requires use of antidepressants, in addition to mood stabilizers.

Finally, for those patients with mood disorders and insomnia who do not respond to adequate treatment of the mood disorder, it is important to address the possibility of a concomitant primary sleep disorder, such as sleep apnea or narcolepsy, which often are complicated by comorbid depression and have overlapping symptoms.

Sleep Deprivation as a Treatment for Mood Disorders

One of the most interesting facts about the relationship between sleep and mood disorders is the robust antidepressant effect of sleep deprivation. Studies have shown response rates of 50% and higher for the antidepressant effect of a single night of sleep deprivation (124–126). The peak of antidepressant effect was seen the afternoon following a night of sleep deprivation (127). In fact, sleep deprivation can trigger a manic episode in patients with bipolar depression, further affirming its mood-elevating properties (58,128). Studies have suggested that sleep deprivation may be more effective for patients with more severe depression and may actually cause worsening of mood in remitted patients and controls (129,130). The major drawback to sleep deprivation becoming a clinically utilized treatment modality is the fact that its antidepressant effect is immediately reversed by recovery sleep, even a short nap (126,131). Chronic REM sleep deprivation has similar effect on mood, albeit less immediate, but these effects are not immediately reversed following recovery sleep (132). Partial sleep deprivation in the second half of the night also has immediate antidepressant effect, which is comparable to those of total sleep deprivation (133,134). Sleep phase advance has been suggested to aug-

ment the effects of total sleep deprivation and those of antidepressant medications (135,136). Neuroimaging studies (137,138) have led to the suggestion that effects of sleep deprivation are mediated by metabolic changes in the limbic structures.

Future Directions

We have developed increasing clarity on the relationship between mood disorders and sleep disturbances over the years, yet a lot of questions remain unanswered. Although they appear to be biologically linked, it is not clear if this is a causal link or just an association. Further, if there is causality, it is not yet clear whether insomnia promotes the development of depression or if depression promotes insomnia, or both. A key unanswered issue that awaits future studies is to determine if it is possible to prevent the onset of episodes of depression and relapse following successful treatment by targeting treatment to insomnia. These studies would require placebo-controlled trials of the treatment of insomnia in those who have successfully completed antidepressant therapy, but have residual insomnia and remain on antidepressant therapy. Longitudinal data are also needed to determine how often those who experience insomnia and do not receive or do not respond to treatment develop subsequent depression versus those who respond to therapy and remain insomnia free.

In terms of issues of causality, it will be very helpful to develop a greater understanding of the neurobiology and genetics of sleep and mood disorders. One interesting area in this regard are research studies of the hypothalamic–pituitary–adrenal (HPA) axis in insomnia and mood disorders. Of particular note is that elevated HPA activity in the form increased cortisol and ACTH levels has been reported in both primary insomnia and major depression (139). While not specific to these disorders and probably somewhat different in manifestation (the dexamethasone nonsuppression characteristic of severe major depression has not been reported in insomnia), this coincidence of findings suggests the possibility of common underlying neurohumoral mechanisms. It has also been hypothesized that elevated HPA activity might be the mediator of the increased risk of depression in insomnia patients via changes in brain structures, such as hippocampal atrophy, which is thought to be caused by elevated HPA activity and is associated with an increased depression risk (139).

Another promising area for future research includes investigating how to extend the duration of antidepressant benefit achieved by sleep deprivation and the mechanisms of this therapeutic effect. A related question is the mechanism by which sleep disruption may predispose individuals with bipolar disorder to develop mania. Further, we have very limited data on how to optimally treat the insomnia that occurs in individuals with mania or bipolar depression.

SCHIZOPHRENIA

Schizophrenia is a devastating illness that was first described in the mid-1800s. The term schizophrenia was coined by Eugen Bleuler (140), to express the presence of schisms between thought, behavior, and emotions in patients with this disorder. Over the years, much has been learned about the phenomenology, epidemiology, and pathophysiology of this disease. It has become clear, over time, that sleep disturbance is not a core symptom of this illness. However, investigations of the sleep of patients with schizophrenia have raised some interesting questions about the pathophysiology, diagnosis, prognosis, and treatment of this disease, which will be discussed in the following section.

Epidemiology

The lifetime prevalence of schizophrenia is estimated to be between 0.5% and 1%. Because it is a chronic illness, incidence rates are much lower, estimated at approximately 1 per 10,000 per year (18). The male to female ratio is roughly equal, although women are more likely to have a later onset, prominent mood symptoms, and better prognosis (18).

Course

Most patients with schizophrenia experience a prodromal phase, wherein there is gradual development of a variety of symptoms, including social withdrawal, deterioration in hygiene, loss of interest in work or school, or irritability. The subsequent emergence of symptoms such as delusions, hallucinations, and grossly disorganized behavior (see below) typically mark the point at which individuals receive the diagnosis of schziophrenia. The onset of schizophrenia occurs typically between the late teens and the mid-30s, although it can at times begin much later in life (18). The age of onset has pathophysiologic and prognostic implications. Patients with early onset tend to have poor premorbid functioning, are more often male, have lower educational achievement, have more structural brain abnormalities, more cognitive impairment, and a worse outcome. The late onset cases, on the other hand, tend to have a higher percentage of women, and better premorbid functioning in terms of occupational and marital history (18).

Studies of the course of schizophrenia highlight the variability of this illness. Complete remission is a rare outcome in schizophrenia. A proportion of patients tend to have a relatively stable course, whereas others have numerous acute psychotic exacerbations, necessitating hospitalization. A small percentage of patients require long-term institutionalization, because of severity of symptoms and lack of responsiveness to standard antipsychotic treatment (18).

Diagnostic Criteria

The diagnosis of schizophrenia requires the presence of two or more of the following characteristic symptoms, each present for a significant portion of time during a 1-month period (18):

1. Delusions
2. Hallucinations
3. Disorganized speech (e.g., frequent derailment or incoherence)
4. Grossly disorganized or catatonic behavior
5. Negative symptoms (i.e., affective flattening, alogia, or avolition)

Only one of these symptoms is required if delusions are bizarre or hallucinations consist of a voice keeping up a running commentary on the patient's thought or behavior, or two or more voices conversing with each other.

Further, the diagnosis requires that significant social/occupational dysfunction is present, and that other psychiatric diagnoses, medical diagnoses, and substance abuse have been ruled out. In addition, the duration of symptoms should be at least 6 months, with at least 1 month of characteristic symptoms above, with other periods of prodromal or residual symptoms.

Sleep Disturbances in Schizophrenia

The most common sleep complaint in acute psychotic episodes of schizophrenia is either early or middle insomnia (141). In fact, Van Kammel et al. have reported that severe insomnia is a prodromal symptom of acute psychotic decompensation. Schizophrenics may also experience nightmares and terrifying hypnagogic hallucinations. Because these patients avoid social interaction, many end up with reversal of sleep and wake, wherein they prefer to sleep in the day and stay up at night. In addition, many schizophrenic patients have comorbid substance abuse disorders and their sleep is further impacted by substance use.

Polysomnographic Findings

The perceptual distortions and bizarre thinking inherent in dreaming led to the early hypothesis that schizophrenia is an intrusion of a dream state and, thereby, REM sleep state, into wakefulness. Early PSG studies tested this hypothesis. The first study was by Dement in 1955 (142), which showed that the temporal distribution of REM during nocturnal sleep was normal in schizophrenics. Koresko et al. (143) compared seven hallucinating patients to four nonhallucinating patients and found little difference in REM time. These studies did not support the REM intrusion into wakefulness hypothesis of schizophrenia. What was found to be abnormal in schizophrenics, however, was REM rebound following REM sleep deprivation. Three studies (144–146) showed a REM rebound failure in acutely ill schizophrenics. This finding led to the hypothesis that REM rebound failure in schizophrenia is a result of REM phasic events (which appear to drive REM sleep) leaking into non-REM sleep and into wakefulness. It was speculated that these REM phasic events caused the thought disorder of schizophrenia. One study (147) attempted to test this hypothesis in schizophrenics. This study utilized surface recordings of phasic integrated potentials (PIPs) of the ocular muscles and middle ear muscle activity (MEMA) as indicators of ponto–geniculo–occipital (PGO) spikes activity. No abnormalities were found in the REM–NREM distribution of PIPs and MEMA in schizophrenic patients, in comparison with depressive patients, schizoaffective patients, and nonpsychiatric controls.

Eye movement density and REM latency have also been areas of interest in sleep research in schizophrenia. Although studies have found no difference in EM density between schizophrenic and nonschizophrenic patients, within the schizophrenia group, EM density is higher in hallucinating patients compared to nonhallucinating patients (148,149). Most polysomnographic studies have found a reduction in REM latency in schizophrenic patients (97,98,150,151).

In addition to REM sleep abnormalities, studies have also looked at NREM sleep abnormalities in schizophrenia. The most consistent finding has been a decrease in stage 4 sleep in schizophrenic patients relative to nonpsychiatric controls (152,153).

Overall, these findings do not provide any useful insights into the pathophysiology of schizophrenia. Most attention has been drawn to the issue of whether these findings help to explain the pathophysiologic differences between what has been referred to as the "positive" and "negative" symptoms of this disease. The positive symptoms loosely connote features of the disease that represent the presence of abnormal phenomena, like delusions, hallucinations, and disorganized thinking, whereas the negative symptoms are comprised of the loss of usual functions, such as affective flattening, alogia, avolition, and attentional deficits. Positive symptoms have been associated with short REM latency (154), increased EM density (148,149), reduced sleep efficiency (155), and increased sleep latency (156). Negative symptoms, on the other hand, have been associated with SWS deficits (157–159), and short REM latency (160).

It is notable that increased suicidality has been associated with greater REM sleep EM activity and more REM sleep time (161,162). While these findings are interesting, unfortunately, the reported associations between the PSG and symptom type have been inconsistently found and have not provided a useful physiologic framework.

In terms of potential diagnostic utility, the PSG abnormalities seen in schizophrenia are also seen in many other psychiatric conditions. For example, decreased REM latency as well as longer sleep onset latency is seen in schizoaffective disorder, depression, and mania (98,163).

Stage 4 sleep deficits are also seen in depression (76) and posttraumatic stress disorder (164). It is of research interest that these diseases share some PSG characteristics; however, this lack of specificity suggests that the PSG findings in schizophrenia are of minimal clinical utility.

Comorbid Sleep Disorders in Schizophrenia

As noted earlier, schizophrenics tend to have poor sleep hygiene and substance use that will tend to disturb their sleep. They also tend to have a high incidence of intrinsic sleep disorders. For example, in one study (165), 15% of schizophrenic patients were found to have sleep-disordered breathing (SDB), 11% had periodic limb movement (PLM) disorder, and 2% had both. As with any other patient with SDB, treatment with continuous positive airway pressure is indicated and effective. Likewise, treatment of PLM disorder should be carried out as described elsewhere in this textbook. One caveat is that caution should be used in prescribing dopaminergic agents as they can potentially worsen psychotic symptoms.

Management of Schizophrenia

Because of the complexities of managing schizophrenia, the involvement of a psychiatrist is critical. A comprehensive treatment plan includes antipsychotic medication, family therapy, including psychoeducation, rehabilitation of the patient in the community, and adequate routine medical care. The initial psychotic break almost invariably warrants hospitalization in order to complete a work up to rule out medical causes of psychosis and to initiate antipsychotic treatment. Because the older antipsychotic agents were fraught with tolerability issues, most important, the risk of tardive dyskinesia, they are not used as first-line agents in newly diagnosed schizophrenia. The newer or "atypical" agents including clozapine, risperidone, and olanzapine, are more efficacious in addressing positive as well as negative symptoms of schizophrenia and are much less likely to cause tardive dyskinesia. These agents are sedating, although less so compared to older antipsychotics, and are typically administered at bedtime to take advantage of their sedating properties. PSG studies of schizophrenic patients treated with clozapine (166,167) reveal its sedative–hypnotic effect in that it increases TST, decreases sleep latency, decreases WASO, and increases sleep efficiency.

The antipsychotic agents may take several weeks to achieve maximum benefit, and patients often end up being discharged from hospitals with some level of residual symptoms, including anxiety, which may also cause insomnia. In such instances, short-term judicious use of benzodiazepine agents may be considered, after ruling out SDB disorders and taking into account substance abuse comorbidity. Antipsychotic agents can also cause a syndrome identical to restless legs syndrome (RLS), which, in this context is called "akathisia," and is also characterized by intense subjective restlessness and a desire to move. It is caused by the dopamine receptor antagonism of the antipsychotic agents (which supports the therapeutic mechanism of dopamine agonists as RLS treatments, which would be effective but would be counterproductive in this setting). As well described with RLS, the symptoms can be very distressing to the patient, and can cause sleep disruption. The first step in addressing this problem is lowering the dose of the antipsychotic agent. Akathisia can also be treated with propranolol, or with amantadine when propranolol is contraindicated, e.g., in reactive airway disease.

Older or "typical" antipsychotics are reserved for patients who do not respond to the newer agents. These agents, including haloperidol, fluphenazine, and chlorpromazine, all cause sedation, decreased sleep latency, and decrease in WASO (168–170). Some patients, especially those with schizoaffective disorder or behavioral dyscontrol may need augmentation with mood stabilizers, which are usually also sedating.

Little attention has been paid to the management of sleep difficulties in patients with schizophrenia. Since many of the pharmacologic treatments of this condition are sedating, it is important to be cognizant of the possibility of sleep apnea, which is likely to be exacerbated by such medications. In terms of insomnia management, clinicians have the option of choosing more sedating antipsychotic agents in patients where insomnia is a prominent symptom. Since these medications tend to have a greater degree of unwanted side effects, such as weight gain and anticholinergic symptoms, it may be of utility to explore the use of sedative–hypnotic agents, although there are no studies of single- vs. dual-agent therapy that might help guide clinical practice in this regard.

Future Directions

Studies of the treatment of insomnia in patients with schizophrenia are needed to help determine optimal therapeutic strategies. It will also be of interest to carry out further research related to the intriguing finding that severe insomnia appears to herald the onset of acute episodes of illness. Studies are needed to determine if addressing the insomnia can prevent the onset of the episode, the mechanisms leading to the insomnia, and whether the insomnia plays a significant role in the course of this disease.

SUBSTANCE DEPENDENCE AND SUBSTANCE ABUSE

Overview

There are a wide range of substances that can affect brain function. The resulting effects are extremely varied and fre-

quently involve profound alterations of sleep. These effects may be due to the acute effects of the substances or may be the result of adaptations that can occur in the brain with repeated regular use of a substance over time (171). From the point of view of disease, the acute effects are termed the intoxication syndrome, while the problems stemming from the adaptive effects are referred to as dependence problems (see DSM-IV-TR definition below) (18). While the effects of intoxication vary among substances, dependence defines a set of effects that may be common to many substances including tolerance, where there is a perceived need to increase dosage over time due to loss of substance effect, and withdrawal, where adverse symptoms arise upon substance discontinuation. It is these latter effects of adaptation that lead individuals to have difficulty stopping the use of substances. Tolerance promotes use of higher dosages over time that increase the withdrawal symptoms, which are avoided by continued substance use. When these effects lead to significant distress or impairment, a diagnosis of substance dependence is indicated.

DSM-IV TR Criteria for Substance Dependence

A maladaptive pattern of substance use, leading to clinically significant impairment or distress, as manifested by three (or more) of the following, occuring at any time in the same 12-month period:

1. Tolerance, as defined by either of the following:
   a. A need for markedly increased amounts of the substance to achieve intoxication or desired effect
   b. Markedly diminished effect with continued use of the same amount of the substance
2. Withdrawal, as manifested by either of the following:
   a. Characteristic withdrawal syndrome for the substance (refer to criteria A and B of the criteria sets for withdrawal from the specific substances)
   b. The same (or a closely related) substance is taken to relieve or avoid withdrawal symptoms
3. The substance is often taken in larger amounts or over a longer period than was intended
4. There is persistent desire or unsuccessful efforts to cut down or control substance use
5. A great deal of time is spent in activities necessary to obtain the substance (e.g., visiting multiple doctors or driving long distances), use the substance (e.g., chain-smoking), or recover from its effects
6. Important social, occupational, or recreational activities are given up or reduced because of substance use
7. Substance use is continued despite knowledge of having a persistent or recurrent physical or psychologic problem that is likely to have been caused or exacerbated by the substance (e.g., current cocaine use despite recognition of cocaine-induced depression, or continued drinking despite recognition that an ulcer was made worse by alcohol consumption).

DSM-IV TR Criteria for Substance Withdrawal

A. The development of a substance-specific syndrome due to the cessation of (or reduction in) substance use that has been heavy and prolonged.

B. The substance-specific syndrome causes clinically significant distress or impairment in social, occupational, or other important areas of functioning.

C. The symptoms are not due to a general medical condition and are not better accounted for by another mental disorder.

It is quite common to confuse dependence with abuse [see DSM-IV TR definition below; (18)], where there is significant distress or impairment arising from repeated substance use, however, there is no evidence of dependence phenomena. In the case of abuse, there have not been adaptive brain changes that are manifested in tolerance and withdrawal problems. Instead, it is the repeated direct effects of the substance, the intoxication syndrome, that cause maladaptive problems in an individual's life.

DSM-IV TR Criteria for Substance Abuse

A. A maladaptive pattern of substance use leading to clinically significant impairment or distress, as manifested by one (or more) of the following, occurring within a 12-month period:

1. Recurrent substance use resulting in a failure to fulfill major role obligations at work, school, or home (e.g., repeated absences or poor work performance related to substance use; substance-related absences, suspensions, or expulsions from school; neglect of children or household)

2. Recurrent substance use in situations in which it is physically hazardous (e.g., driving an automobile or operating a machine when impaired by substance use)

3. Recurrent substance-related legal problems (e.g., arrests for substance-related disorderly conduct)

4. Continued substance use despite having persistent or recurrent social or interpersonal problems caused or exacerbated by the effects of the substance (e.g., arguments with spouse about consequences of intoxication, physical fights)

B. The symptoms have never met the criteria for substance dependence for this class of substance.

Difficulties with sleep may occur either with dependence (associated with tolerance and withdrawal phenomena) or abuse (part of an intoxication syndrome) of a number of substances. This section is concerned with this subset of substances in which the intoxication or withdrawal syndromes include a disturbance of sleep. Intoxication with caffeine, alcohol, amphetamines, cocaine, opioids, benzodiazepines, and barbiturates have been identified as having significant effects on sleep (18). The withdrawal syndromes of nicotine, caffeine, marijuana, alcohol, amphetamines, cocaine, opioids, benzodiazepines, and barbiturates also include alterations of sleep.

Awareness of these problems in clinical practice is important because patients suffering from abuse or dependence with one of the above substances will present with what looks like a sleep disorder. Considering that roughly 20% of general medical patients and 35% of psychiatric patients are believed to present with substance-related disorders, knowledge of the presentation, course, and differential diagnosis of these conditions will be of great value to sleep physicians, psychiatrists, and general practitioners (172). Unfortunately, all of the relevant substances cannot be adequately covered in a review of this scope. As a result, we will discuss only alcohol and its relationship to sleep, since problems with alcohol have the most greatest prevalence and there has been the research on the relationship of sleep difficulties and the course of alcohol dependence and abuse. We will review the literature suggesting that the difficulties with sleep caused by alcohol may also predispose individuals to drink or to relapse following successful abstinence. As we have seen, particularly with the mood and anxiety disorders, these data blur the boundary between sleep disorders and substance-related disorders. For substances other than alcohol, we limit ourselves to including the DSM-IV diagnostic criteria for their intoxication and withdrawal syndromes.

Alcohol

Background and Prevalence

Alcohol is the substance most frequently associated with dependence and abuse problems, with a lifetime prevalence estimated to be 14% in the United States in a 1984 publication (173). That alcohol is associated with the greatest prevalence of difficulties is largely due to the relative ease of access to alcohol compared with illegal substances or those legally available only via prescription, such as marijuana, cocaine, amphetamines, sedative–hypnotic medications, and opiates. A series of studies carried out in animals suggest that alcohol may have less physiologic abuse and dependence liability than some of these agents. These studies have examined the lengths to which animals will go to self-administer these substances and the extent to which they are reinforcing. The emerging picture is that cocaine and opiates are strongly and consistently reinforcing and self-administered, whereas for alcohol these attributes are dependent upon genetics. A propensity to consume alcohol until dependent and for pharmacologic effects can be selectively bred into rats. This is consistent with the evidence that only a subset of humans exposed to alcohol develop problems. In the United States 10% of men and 3% to 5% of women who drink alcohol experience problems (172). A genetic influence on the propensity to develop dependence and abuse problems is also evident in the varying prevalence of these problems in subpopulations. The observation that alcohol-related problems are relatively low in Asian countries and in women has been explained by an inherited form of an enzyme involved in the metabolism of alcohol that is less efficient at eliminating breakdown products (18). A genetic factor is also suggested by evidence that monozygotic twins are more likely to be concordant for alcohol problems than dizygotic twins (18).

Course

The peak prevalence of onset of alcohol dependence is between ages 20 and 35 (18). The course is typically characterized by multiple episodes of difficulties following by temporary remission. Relapse is often precipitated by a crisis and begins with a period of drinking that is not associated with problems (18). While the recidivism of the severely affected individuals may create the impression that alcohol abuse and dependence problems are intractable, many individuals respond well to treatment. In fact, 65% maintain abstinence for at least 1 year following treatment (18). Further, it has been estimated that at least 20% of alcohol-dependent individuals are able to refrain from drinking long-term without treatment.

Diagnosis

While patients with alcohol dependence and abuse are extremely frequently encountered in clinical practice, few present their difficulties to their doctors as resulting from alcohol use or disclose their degree of drinking (172). As a result, it is important for practitioners to be aware of the typical presentations and diagnostic features of alcohol dependence and intoxication.

Diagnostic Criteria for 303.00 Alcohol Intoxication

A. Recent ingestion of alcohol.
B. Clinically significant maladaptive behavioral or psychologic changes (e.g., inappropriate sexual or aggressive behavior, mood lability, impaired judgment, impaired social or occupational functioning) that developed during, or shortly after, alcohol ingestion.
C. One (or more) of the following signs, developing during, or shortly after, alcohol use:
   1. Slurred speech
   2. Incoordination
   3. Unsteady gait
   4. Nystagmus
   5. Impairment in attention or memory
   6. Stupor or coma
D. The symptoms are not due to a general medical condition and are not better accounted for by another mental disorder.

Diagnostic Criteria for 291.81 Alcohol Withdrawal

A. Cessation of (or reduction in) alcohol use that has been heavy and prolonged.
B. Two (or more) of the following, developing within several hours to a few days after criterion (A):
   1. Autonomic hyperactivity (e.g., sweating or pulse rate greater than 100)
   2. Increased hand tremor
   3. Insomnia
   4. Nausea or vomiting
   5. Transient visual, tactile, or auditory hallucinations or illusions
   6. Psychomotor agitation
   7. Anxiety
   8. Grand mal seizures
C. The symptoms in criterion (B) cause clinically significant distress or impairment in social, occupational, or other important areas of functioning.
D. The symptoms are not due to a general medical condition and are not better accounted for by another mental disorder. Specify if with perceptual disturbances.

Laboratory tests that may also be useful in diagnosis include blood alcohol levels, liver enzyme tests, and automated blood count (172). The most important consideration is to ask specifically about alcohol consumption. One tool that has been frequently recommended to identify those with problems are the four "CAGE" questions: (1) Cut down: Have you ever felt the need to cut down? (2) Annoyed: Have you felt annoyed by people criticizing your drinking? (3) Guilty: Have you ever felt guilty about your drinking? (4) Eye-opener: Have you felt the need for an eye-opener in the morning to get rid of a hangover? (174). Family history is important to obtain because of the evidence that there is a greater risk of abuse and dependence problems when individuals have genetically linked relatives with these problems.

Differential Diagnosis

Because of the incoordination, ataxia, and slurred speech, alcohol intoxication is most likely to be confused with neurologic diseases. The differential diagnosis of altered mental status may also be a consideration with extreme levels of intoxication. Withdrawal represents a much more difficult diagnostic challenge. The hallucinosis that may occur can lead to consideration of schizophrenia, or delirium of any its many causes. A complaint of difficulty sleeping may be the focus of the presentation due to the insomnia that is common in this setting. It may also be difficult at times to distinguish those in alcohol withdrawal from those with anxiety disorders and gastrointestinal disorders. Generalized anxiety is the most common consideration among the anxiety disorders, and is easily distinguished by its chronicity. When seizures occur in withdrawal, the differential diagnosis can be challenging when there have been recurrent episodes of postwithdrawal seizures. In all of the above situations, the most helpful considerations are whether other signs and symptoms of alcohol withdrawal are present and whether there is a recent history of alcohol use and discontinuation.

Sleep Effects

The consumption of alcohol at bedtime shortens sleep latency and increases the amount of NREM at the expense of REM sleep in the early portion of the night (175). Because of the short-duration of action of alcohol, it has been hypothesized to cause a withdrawal-like syndrome in the last half of the night, characterized by sleep disruption, increased REM, increased dreaming, and sympathetic arousal (172). The sleep-promoting effect that shortens sleep onset latency is responsible for its use as a sleeping aid by many individuals. While there have been no studies of the regular use of relatively low-dose alcohol at bedtime as a sleep aid, the general belief has been that it is not an effective treatment because of the likelihood of tolerance and the very short duration of benefit and subsequent sleep disruption.

An inability to fall asleep without alcohol is often observed as dependence develops and during withdrawal insomnia is typically experienced (18). These reflect adaptations that occur in the brain in response to the sleep-inducing effects of alcohol. PSG recorded in dependent individuals reflects the difficulties with sleep in the form of long sleep onset latency, decreased time asleep per hour in bed, and decreased TST (69,176).

Regular alcohol use may also lead to disruption of the usual circadian rhythm. This is because alcohol consumption may occur at any time of the day, leading to brief periods of sleep induction following by brief periods of wakefulness (172). Over time, the cumulative effects of this type of irregular sleep–wake schedule will tend to erode the day–night cycle. Also, following withdrawal, a period of prolonged sleep has been observed, which has been reported to be comprised of relatively minimal SWS and REM sleep (177).

The persistence of disrupted sleep during abstinence following a period of alcohol dependence is striking (178). Signs and symptoms of sleep disruption have been observed as much as 2 years following abstinence. The most consistent findings are shortened TST and a tendency for an elevated amount of REM sleep.

Effects of Sleep Difficulties on the Treatment of Alcohol Difficulties

The results of a series of studies suggest that the same types of disturbances of sleep that appear to be caused by alcohol appear to predict relapse. In a study in which individuals in recovery were given the opportunity to drink alcohol, those

with a self-report of sleep difficulties were more likely to choose the alcohol (172). PSG predictors of relapse that have been reported include diminished SWS, short REM latency, elevated percentage of REM sleep, increased number of eye movements per minute of REM sleep (REM density), increased sleep latency, and diminished sleep efficiency (sleep time divided by time in bed) (179,180). It should be noted that the REM sleep–related predictors of relapse, which are also observed at a greater frequency in depressed patients than the general population, were predictors of relapse in nondepressed alcoholics (180).

Studies demonstrate potential utility of such measures as predictors of relapse, however, which measures are more useful may vary with the period of the recovery process (172). Increased REM density during the initial period of abstinence was the best predictor of relapse at 3 to 4 months postabstinence. When sleep was studied at 5 months of abstinence, REM density was not predictive of relapse at 1 year: however, prolonged sleep latency and low amount of time asleep per hour in bed was a significant predictor of 1 year relapse (178). In another study, PSG-derived sleep onset latency measured at approximately 1 month after achieving abstinence was the best predictor of whether subjects would subsequently relapse (181).

Future Directions

These data suggest that the types of difficulties with sleep caused by alcohol dependence appear to predispose those in remission to relapse. However, the data paint an incomplete picture. There are relatively few studies and data are available only for a few points in time during the period of abstinence. It is better established that acute consumption of alcohol has a brief sleep induction effect, and withdrawal is associated with insomnia. Thus, alcohol dependence disrupts, sleep, and that sleep disruption seems to increase the likelihood of alcohol consumption leading to perpetuation of alcohol use–dependence and relapse. In this sense, the relationship of alcohol dependence and sleep disruption is much like the reciprocal relationships of sleep disruption and a number of the psychiatric disorders discussed above.

One unique feature of the relationship of sleep disruption to alcohol dependence is that there is evidence that some individuals begin drinking alcohol in order to treat difficulties sleeping. This adds a further layer of complexity to the relationship. While this may be a key issue in the relapse part of the relationship, referred to in the previous paragraph, it could suggest that a subset of individuals has a course of difficulty that begins with insomnia, which then leads to the initial regular consumption of alcohol, thereby setting off the cycle of dependence, remission, and relapse. From this perspective, alcohol dependence could be viewed as an attempt at self-medication that fails due to adaptive brain mechanisms that lead to the dependence phenomena. On this basis, effective treatment of insomnia is the obviously needed intervention. There are no studies that we are aware of that have credibly tested this hypothesis. In fact, for alcoholism in general, one of the most important unaddressed needs is to determine whether the treatment of insomnia in alcohol-dependent or recovering alcoholics will enhance the likelihood of abstinence and decrease their likelihood of relapse.

Another key unexplored issue is to determine the extent of interaction between predisposition to insomnia and alcoholism. While we know little about factors generally predisposing individuals toward insomnia, a particularly high-risk group for alcohol-dependence problems would be expected to be those with both predisposition to insomnia and genetic loading for alcoholism.

Considering the prevalence of alcohol-related problems and the frequency with which the course is marked by repeated relapses, these questions clearly deserve attention.

Amphetamines

Diagnostic Criteria for 292.89 Amphetamine Intoxication

A. Recent use of amphetamine or a related substance (e.g., methylphenidate).
B. Clinically significant maladaptive behavioral or psychological changes (e.g., euphoria or affective blunting, changes in sociability, hypervigilance, interpersonal sensitivity, anxiety, tension, or anger, stereotyped behaviors, impaired judgment, or impaired social or occupational functioning) that developed during, or shortly after, use of amphetamine or a related substance.
C. Two (or more) of the following, developing during, or shortly after, use of amphetamine or a related substance:
  1. Tachycardia or bradycardia
  2. Pupillary dilation
  3. Elevated or lowered blood pressure
  4. Perspiration or chills
  5. Nausea or vomiting
  6. Evidence of weight loss
  7. Psychomotor agitation or retardation
  8. Muscular weakness, respiratory depression, chest pain, or cardiac arrhythmias
  9. Confusion, seizures, dyskinesias, dystonias, or coma
D. The symptoms are not due to a general medical condition and are not better accounted for by another mental disorder.

Diagnostic Criteria for 292.0 Amphetamine Withdrawal

A. Cessation of (or reduction in) amphetamine (or a related substance) use that has been heavy and prolonged.

B. Dysphoric mood and two (or more) of the following physiologic changes, developing within a few hours to several days after criterion (A):
  1. Fatigue
  2. Vivid, unpleasant dreams
  3. Insomnia or hypersomnia
  4. Increased appetite
  5. Psychomotor retardation or agitation
C. The symptoms in criterion (B) cause clinically significant distress or impairment in social, occupational, or other important areas of functioning.
D. The symptoms are not due to a general medical condition and are not better accounted for by another mental disorder.

Benzodiazepines and Barbiturates

Diagnostic Criteria for 292.89 Sedative, Hypnotic, or Anxiolytic Intoxication

A. Recent use of a sedative, hypnotic, or anxiolytic.
B. Clinically significant maladaptive behavioral or psychologic changes (e.g., inappropriate sexual or aggressive behavior, mood lability, impaired judgment, impaired social or occupational functioning) that developed during, or shortly after, sedative, hypnotic, or anxiolytic use.
C. One (or more) of the following signs, developing during, or shortly after, sedative, hypnotic, or anxiolytic use:
  1. Slurred speech
  2. Incoordination
  3. Unsteady gait
  4. Nystagmus
  5. Impairment in attention or memory
  6. Stupor or coma
D. The symptoms are not due to a general medical condition and are not better accounted for by another mental disorder.

Diagnostic Criteria for 292.0 Sedative, Hypnotic, or Anxiolytic Withdrawal

A. Cessation of (or reduction in) sedative, hypnotic, or anxiolytic use that has been heavy and prolonged.
B. Two (or more) of the following, developing within several hours to a few days after criterion (A):
  1. Autonomic hyperactivity (e.g., sweating or pulse rate greater than 100)
  2. Increased hand tremor
  3. Insomnia
  4. Nausea or vomiting
  5. Transient visual, tactile, or auditory hallucinations or illusions
  6. Psychomotor agitation
  7. Anxiety
  8. Grand mal seizures

C. The symptoms in criterion (B) cause clinically significant distress or impairment in social, occupational, or other important areas of functioning.

D. The symptoms are not due to a general medical condition and are not better accounted for by another mental disorder.

Caffeine

Diagnostic Criteria for 305.90 Caffeine Intoxication

A. Recent consumption of caffeine, usually in excess of 250 mg (e.g., more than 2 to 3 cups of brewed coffee).

B. Five (or more) of the following signs, developing during, or shortly after, caffeine use:

1. Restlessness
2. Nervousness
3. Excitement
4. Insomnia
5. Flushed face
6. Diuresis
7. Gastrointestinal disturbance
8. Muscle twitching
9. Rambling flow of thought and speech
10. Tachycardia or cardiac arrhythmia
11. Periods of inexhaustibility
12. Psychomotor agitation

C. The symptoms in criterion (B) cause clinically significant distress or impairment in social, occupational, or other important areas of functioning.

D. The symptoms are not due to a general medical condition and are not better accounted for by another mental disorder (eg, an anxiety disorder).

Cocaine

Diagnostic Criteria for 292.89 Cocaine Intoxication

A. Recent use of cocaine.

B. Clinically significant maladaptive behavioral or psychologic changes (e.g., euphoria or affective blunting, changes in sociability, hypervigilance, interpersonal sensitivity, anxiety, tension, or anger, stereotyped behaviors, impaired judgment, or impaired social or occupational functioning) that developed during, or shortly after, use of cocaine.

C. Two (or more) of the following, developing during, or shortly after, cocaine use:

1. Tachycardia or bradycardia
2. Pupillary dilation
3. Elevated or lowered blood pressure
4. Perspiration or chills
5. Nausea or vomiting
6. Evidence of weight loss
7. Psychomotor agitation or retardation
8. Muscular weakness, respiratory depression, chest pain, or cardiac arrhythmias

9. Confusion, seizures, dyskinesias, dystonias, or coma

D. The symptoms are not due to a general medical condition and are not better accounted for by another mental disorder.

Diagnostic Criteria for 292.0 Cocaine Withdrawal

A. Cessation of (or reduction in) cocaine use that has been heavy and prolonged.

B. Dysphoric mood and two (or more) of the following physiologic changes, developing within a few hours to several days after criterion (A):

1. Fatigue
2. Vivid, unpleasant dreams
3. Insomnia or hypersomnia
4. Increased appetite
5. Psychomotor agitation or retardation

C. The symptoms in criterion (B) cause clinically significant distress or impairment in social, occupational, or other important areas of functioning.

D. The symptoms are not due to a general medical condition and are not better accounted for by another mental disorder.

Opiates

Diagnostic Criteria for 292.89 Opioid Intoxication

A. Recent use of an opioid.

B. Clinically significant maladaptive behavioral or psychologic changes (e.g., initial euphoria followed by apathy, dysphoria, psychomotor agitation or retardation, impaired judgment, or impaired social or occupational functioning) that developed during, or shortly after, opioid use.

C. Pupillary constriction (or pupillary dilation due to anoxia from severe overdose) and one (or more) of the following signs, developing during, or shortly after, opioid use:

1. Drowsiness or coma
2. Slurred speech
3. Impairment in attention or memory

D. The symptoms are not due to a general medical condition and are not better accounted for by another mental disorder.

Diagnostic Criteria for 292.0 Opioid Withdrawal

A. Either of the following: (1) cessation of (or reduction in) opioid use that has been heavy and prolonged (several weeks or longer); (2) administration of an opioid antagonist after a period of opioid use.

B. Three (or more) of the following, developing within minutes to several days after criterion (A):

1. Dysphoric mood
2. Nausea or vomiting
3. Muscle aches

4. Lacrimation or rhinorrhea
5. Pupillary dilation, piloerection, or sweating
6. Diarrhea
7. Yawning
8. Fever
9. Insomnia

C. The symptoms in criterion (B) cause clinically significant distress or impairment in social, occupational, or other important areas of functioning.
D. The symptoms are not due to a general medical condition and are not better accounted for by another mental disorder.

Marijuana (Cannabis)

Diagnostic Criteria for 292.89 Cannabis Intoxication

A. Recent use of cannabis.
B. Clinically significant maladaptive behavioral or psychologic changes (e.g., impaired motor coordination, euphoria, anxiety, sensation of slowed time, impaired judgment, social withdrawal) that developed during, or shortly after, cannabis use.
C. Two (or more) of the following signs, developing within 2 hours of cannabis use:
  1. Conjunctival injection
  2. Increased appetite
  3. Dry mouth
  4. Tachycardia
D. The symptoms are not due to a general medical condition and are not better accounted for by another mental disorder.

Nicotine

Diagnostic Criteria for 292.0 Nicotine Withdrawal

A. Daily use of nicotine for at least several weeks.
B. Abrupt cessation of nicotine use, or reduction in the amount of nicotine used, followed within 24 hours by four (or more) of the following signs:
  1. Dysphoric or depressed mood
  2. Insomnia
  3. Irritability, frustration, or anger
  4. Anxiety
  5. Difficulty concentrating
  6. Restlessness
  7. Decreased heart rate
  8. Increased appetite or weight gain
C. The symptoms in criterion (B) cause clinically significant distress or impairment in social, occupational, or other important areas of functioning.
D. The symptoms are not due to a general medical condition and are not better accounted for by another mental disorder.

SUMMARY AND CONCLUSIONS

There is clearly a linkage between psychiatric disorders and sleep. Psychiatric disorders are associated with sleep disturbances. Sleep disturbances predispose individuals to psychiatric disorders and may increase the likelihood of relapse. This circular relationship is based on relatively few studies, which are only correlational; clearly more research is needed. In particular, for each of the disorders discussed, what would be the most compelling piece of information is missing. We do not yet have any data establishing that treatment of the sleep difficulties typically caused by a psychiatric condition can change the course of that psychiatric condition. This is a needed area of future research.

At the same time, when we look at the strong relationships between these two areas, it becomes clear why many patients with sleep disorders seek psychiatric treatment and many patients with psychiatric disorders are found in sleep medicine clinics. While there is clearly a need for specialists in both areas to be knowledgeable about both types of disorders, these considerations suggest that it may be necessary to rethink how we define these groups of diseases.

This review points to a blurring between sleep disorders and psychiatric disorders. Both psychiatric and sleep disorders have typically been viewed as primary or secondary to another illness such as a psychiatric or medical disease. But the data suggest a breakdown of this idea. Is it reasonable to define insomnia occurring in the context of depression as secondary when the insomnia often precedes the depression, often continues to exist following what is identified as remission of depression, and predicts relapse of depression? Yet, it would not be reasonable to say that depression is secondary to insomnia. The currently available data do not support that conclusion. We need better longitudinal, pathophysiologic, and treatment data to understand the relationships between these diseases. It will be important to understand these types of interrelationships well enough to develop optimal treatment strategies, which will need to include a consideration of when to treat sleep, when to treat psychiatric disease, and when specific treatments targeted to both are needed. Another important scientific challenge will be to understand the mechanisms that mediate the interconnections between sleep and psychiatric disease, which may also be useful in developing improved treatment.

We currently have a chicken-and-egg problem. We are suggesting that the distinction of primary versus secondary may no longer be the best way to think about these disorders. If that is the case, what other options are there? There are a number of alternative explanations for the findings reviewed above. The mechanism of relationship may vary among the sleep and psychiatric disorders.

1. There are two independent problems with circular causality (e.g., insomnia may cause psychiatric disease

and at the same time psychiatric illness may lead to insomnia and that, in both cases, the resulting difficulty may exacerbate the causative condition).

2. Both types of difficulties are independent but tend to be comorbid and predictive due to a common genetic, environmental, or other type of factor that leads both of them to commonly occur in the same individual.

3. Insomnia is causative of psychiatric disorders and some individuals may be genetically or environmentally predisposed to developing sleep disruption. Such individuals might be particularly likely to experience insomnia when under stress, which then predisposes them to depression, which then exacerbates the insomnia. In this scenario, the mechanisms of relapse of psychiatric disease would both be residual insomnia and a propensity for insomnia to recur due to stressors.

4. Psychiatric disorders and sleep disruption are both "symptoms" and are manifestations of the same underlying disease and, therefore, tend to be comorbid and copredictive.

While there are no doubt many other interesting possibilities, future research is needed to better understand the complex relationships between sleep and psychiatric disorders. This promises to allow us to better treat these highly prevalent diseases, which represent major public health challenges.

REFERENCES

1. Walsh JK, Schweitzer PK. Ten-year trends in pharmacologic treatment of insomnia. *Sleep*. 1999;22:371–375.
2. Thorpy M. Current concepts in the etiology, diagnosis and treatment of narcolepsy. *Sleep Med*. 2001;2:5–17.
3. Santosh PJ, Taylor E. Stimulant drugs. *Eur Child Adolesc Psych*. 2000;9(Suppl. 1):I27–143.
4. Nierenberg AA, Dougherty D, Rosenbaum JF. Dopaminergic agents and stimulants as antidepressant augmentation strategies. *J Clin Psych*. 1998;59(Suppl. 5):60–63.
5. Baran AS, Richert AC. Obstructive sleep apnea and depression. *CNS Spectrosc*. 2003;8:128–134.
6. Bakshi R. Fluoxetine and restless legs syndrome. *J Neurol Sci*. 1996;142(1–2):151–152.
7. Giedke H, Schwarzler F. *Sleep Med Rev*. 2002;6:361–377.
8. American Psychiatric Association. *Diagnostic and statistical manual of mental disorders*. 4th edn. Washington, D.C: APA, 1994.
9. Obermeyer Wit, Benca RM. *Neurol Clin*. 1996;14:827–840.
10. Katz DA, McHorney CA. *Arch Intern Med*. 1998;158:1099–1107.
11. Ford DE, Kamerow DB. Epidemiologic study of sleep disturbance and psychiatric disorders: An opportunity for prevention? *JAMA*. 1989;262:1479–1484.
12. Breslau N, Roth T, Rosenthal L, et al. Sleep disturbance and psychiatric disorders: a longitudinal epidemiologic study of young adults. *Biol Psych*. 1996;39:411–418.
13. Ohayon MM, Roth T. *J. Psych Res*. 2003;37:9–15.
14. Ashton H. *Sleep*. 1994:175–211.
15. Uhde TW. Anxiety disorders. In: Kryger MH, Roth T, Dement WC, eds. *Principles and practice of sleep medicine*. 3rd edn. Philadelphia: W.B. Saunders, 2000:1123–139.
16. Stein MB, et al. *Psych Res*. 1993;49:251–256.
17. Wittchen HJ, et al. *Arch Gen Psych*. 1994;51:355–364.
18. American Psychiatric Association. *Diagnostic and statistical manual of mental disorders*. 4th ed. Text revision. Washington, D.C: APA, 2000.
19. Hales et al. *J Clin Psych*. 1997;58(Suppl. 3):76.
20. LeDoux J. *Biol Psych*. 1998;44:1129–1238.
21. Monti JM, Monti D. Sleep disturbance in generalized anxiety disorder and its treatment. *Sleep Med Rev*. 2000;4:263–276.
22. Reynolds CF, III, et al. EEG sleep in outpatients with generalized anxiety: a preliminary comparison with depressed outpatients. *Psych Res*. 1983;8:81–89.
23. Gelenberg AJ, Lydiard RB, Rudolph RL, et al. Efficacy of venlafaxine extended-release capsules in nondepressed outpatients with generalized anxiety disorder: a 6-month randomized controlled trial. *JAMA*. 2000;283:3082–3088.
24. Rickels K, Downing R, Schweizer E, et al. Antidepressants for the treatment of generalized anxiety disorder. A placebo-controlled comparison of imipramine, trazodone, and diazepam. *Arch Gen Psych*. 1993;50:884–895.
25. Davidson JR, DuPont RL, Hedges D, et al. Efficacy, safety, and tolerability of venlafaxine extended release and buspirone in outpatients with generalized anxiety disorder. *J Clin Psych*. 1999;60:528–535.
26. Gorman J. Treating generalized anxiety disorder. *J Clin Psych*. 2003;64(Suppl. 2):24–29.
26a. Helzer JE, et al. Post-traumatic stress disorder in the general population: findings of the Epidemiologic Catchment Area survey. *N Eng J Med*. 1987;317:1630–1634.
27. Breslau N. The epidemiology of posttraumatic stress disorder: What is the extent of the Problem? *J Clin Psych*. 2001;62(Suppl. 17):16–22.
28. Breslau N. Outcomes of posttramatic stress disorder. *J Clin Psych*. 2001;62(Suppl. 17):55–59.
29. Ross et al. Sleep disturbance as the hallmark of posttraumatic stress disorder. *Amer J Psych*. 1989;146:697–707.
30. Dow et al. Sleep and dreams in Vietnam PTSD and depression. *Biol Psych*. 1996;39:42–50.
31. Mellman TA, et al. Sleep events among veterans with combat-related posttraumatic stress disorder. *Amer J Psych*. 1995a;152:110–115.
32. Mellman TA, et al. Nocturnal/daytime urine noradrenergic measures and sleep in combat-related PTSD. *Biol Psych*. 1995b:174–179.
33. Mellman TA, et al. A polysomnogreaphic comparison of veterans with combat-related PTSD, depressed men, and non-ill controls. *Sleep*. 1997;20:46–51.
34. Woodward, et al. Laboratory sleep correlates of nightmare complaint in PSTD inpatients. *Biol Psych*. 2000b;48:1081–1087.
35. Hurwitz TD, Mahowald MW, Kuskowski M, et al. Polysomnographic sleep is not clinically impaired in Vietnam combat veterans with chronic posttraumatic stress disorder. *Biol Psych*. 1998;44:1066–1073.
36. Van Der Kolk BA, et al. Fluoxetine in posttraumatic stress disorder. *J Clin Psych*. 1994;55:517–522.
37. Brady et al. Efficacy and safety of sertraline treatment of posttraumatic stress disorder: a randomized controlled trial. *JAMA*. 2000;283:1837–1844.
38. Connor KM, et al. Fluoxetine in post-traumatic stress disorder. Randomized, double-blind study. *Br J Psych*. 1999;175:17–22.
39. Hertzberg MA, et al. A preliminary study of lamotrigine for the treatment of posttraumatic stress disorder. *Biol Psych*. 1999;45:1226–1229.
40. Horowitz et al. Signs and symptoms of posttraumatic stress disorder. *Arch Gen Psych*. 1980;37:85–92.
41. Van der Kolk BA, et al. A survey of nightmare frequencies in a veterans outpatient clinic. *Sleep Res*. 1980;9:229.
42. Taylor F, Raskind M. The [alpha]1-adrenergic antagonist prazosin improves sleep and nightmares in civilian trauma posttraumatic stress disorder. *J Clin Psychopharmacol*. 2002;22:82–85.
43. Rasking MA, Thompson C, Petrie EC, et al. Prazosin reduces nightmares in combat veterans with posttraumatic stress disorder. *J Clin Psych*. 2002;63:565–568.
44. Berlant J, van Kammen DP. Open-label topiramate as primary or adjunctive therapy in chronic civilian posttraumatic stress disorder: a preliminary report. *J Clin Psych*. 2002;63:15–20.

45. Mellman TA, Uhde TW. Sleep panic attacks: new clinical findings and theoretical implications. *Amer J Psych.* 1989;146:1204–1207.

46. Craske MG, Barlow DH. Nocturnal panic. *J Nerv Ment Dis.* 1989;177:160–167.

47. Coplan JD, et al. An algorithm-oriented treatment approach for panic disorder. *Psych Ann.* 1996;26:192–201.

48. Boyer W. Serotonin uptake inhibitors are superior to imipramine and alprazolam in alleviating panic attacks: A meta-analysis. *Intern Clin Psychopharmacol.* 1995;10:45–49.

49. Taylor CB. Treatment of anxiety disorders. In: Schatzberg AF, Nemeroff CB, eds. *Textbook of psychopharmacology.* 2nd edn. American Psychiatric Press, Washington D.C., 1998:775–789.

50. Gorman JM, Kent JM, Coplan JD. The current and emerging therapeutics of anxiety and stress disorders. In: Davis KL, Charney D, Coyle JT, Nemeroff C, eds. *Neuropsychopharmacology. The 5th generation of progress.* Philadelphia: Lippincott Williams & Wilkins, 2002:967–980.

51. Mellman TA, Uhde TW. Patients with frequent sleep panic: Clinical findings and response to medication treatment. *J Clin Psych.* 1990;51:513–516.

52. Mellinger GD, Balter MB, Uhlenhuth EH. Insomnia and its treatment. Prevalence and correlates. *Arch Gen Psych.* 1985;42:225–232.

53. Gerber PD, Barrett JE, Barrett JA, et al. The relationship of presenting physical complaints to depressive symptoms in primary care. *J Gen Internal Med.* 1992;7:170–173.

54. Livingston G, Blizard B, Mann A. Does sleep disturbance predict depression in elderly people? A study in inner London. *Br J Gen Practice.* 1993;43:445–448.

55. Chang PP, Ford DE, Mead LA, et al. Insomnia in young men and subsequent depression. *Amer J Epidemiol.* 1997;146:105–114.

56. Eaton WW, Badawi M, Melton B. Prodromes and precursors: epidemiological data for primary prevention of disorders with slow onset. *Amer J Psych.* 1995;152:967–972.

57. Wehr TA, Sack DA, Rosenthal NE. Sleep reduction as a final common pathway in the genesis of mania. *Amer J Psych.* 1987;144:201–204.

58. Wehr TA, Goodwin FK, Wirz-Justice A, et al. 48-hour sleep–wake cycles in manic-depressive illness: naturalistic observations and sleep deprivation experiments. *Arch Gen Psych.* 1982;39:559–565.

59. Zimanova J, Vojtechovsky M. Sleep deprivation as a potentiation of antidepressant pharmacotherapy. *Acta Nerv Super (Praha).* 1974;16:188–189.

60. Kupfer DJ, Foster FG. Interval between onset of sleep and rapid-eye-movement sleep as an indicator of depression. *Lancet.* 1972;2:684–686.

61. Hartmann E, Verdone P, Snyder F. Longitudinal studies of sleep and dreaming patterns in psychiatric patients. *J Nervous Mental Disorders* 1966;142:117–126.

62. Mendels J, Hawkins DR. Sleep and depression: a controlled EEG study. *Arch Gen Psych.* 1967;16:344–354.

63. Snyder F. Dynamic aspects of sleep disturbance in relation to mental illness. *Biol Psych.* 1969;1:119–130.

64. Gillin JC, Duncan WC, Pettigrew KD, et al. Successful separation of depressed, normal and insomniac subjects by EEG sleep data. *Arch Gen Psych.* 1979;36:85–90.

65. Kupfer DJ, Ulrich RF, Coble PA, et al. Electroencephalographic sleep of younger depressives. *Arch Gen Psych.* 1985;42:806–810.

66. Benca RM, Obermeyer WH, Thisted RA, et al. Sleep and psychiatric disorders: a meta-analysis. *Arch Gen Psych.* 1992;49:651–668.

67. Kupfer DJ, Reynolds CF, III, Ehlers CL. Comparison of EEG sleep measures among depressive subtypes and controls in older individuals. *Psych Res.* 1989;27:13–21.

68. Quitkin FM, Rabkin JG, Stewart JW, et al. Sleep of atypical depressives. *J Affect Disorders* 1985;8:61–67.

69. Emslie GJ, Rush AJ, Weinberg WA, et al. Children with major depression show reduced rapid eye movement latencies. *Arch Gen Psych.* 1990;47:119–124.

70. Waller DA, Hardy BW, Pole R, et al. Sleep EEG in bulimic, depressed and normal subjects. *Biol Psych.* 1989;25:661–664.

71. Jones DA, Kelwala S, Bell J, et al. Cholinergic REM sleep induction response correlation with endogenous depressive subtype. *Psych Res.* 1985;14:99–110.

72. Foster FG, Kupfer DJ, Coble PA, et al. Rapid eye movement sleep density. An objective indicator in severe medial-depressive syndromes. *Arch Gen Psych.* 1976;33:1119–1123.

73. Berger M, Doerr P, Lund RD, et al. Neuroendocrinological and neurophysiological studies in major depressive disorders: are there biological markers for the endogenous subtype? *Biol Psych.* 1982;17:1217–1242.

74. Borbely AA, Tobler I, Loepfe M, et al. All night spectral analysis of the sleep EEG in untreated depressives and normal controls. *Psych Res.* 1984;12:27–33.

75. Feinberg M, Gillin JC, Carroll BJ, et al. EEG studies of sleep in the diagnosis of depression. *Biol Psych.* 1982;17:305–316.

76. Kupfer DJ, Ulrich RF, Coble PA, et al. Application of automated REM and slow-wave sleep analysis. II: Testing the assumptions of the two-process model of sleep regulation in normal and depressed subjects. *Psych Res.* 1985;13:335–343.

77. Kupfer DJ, Reynolds CF III, Ulrich RF, et al. Comparison of automated REM and slow wave sleep analysis in young and middle-aged depressed subjects. *Biol Psych.* 1986;21:189–200.

78. Kupfer DJ, Frank E, Ehlers CL. EEG sleep in young depressives: First and second night effects. *Biol Psych.* 1989;25:87–97.

79. Linkowski P, Kerkhofs M, Rielaert C, et al. Sleep during mania in manic-depressive males. *Eur Arch Psychiatry Neurol Sci.* 1986; 235:339–341.

80. Hudson JI, Lipinski JF, Frankenburg FR, et al. Electroencephalographic sleep in mania. *Arch Gen Psych.* 1988;45:267–273.

81. Nofzinger EA, Thase ME, Reynolds CF, III, et al. Hypersomnia in bipolar depression: a comparison with narcolepsy using the multiple sleep latency test. *Amer J Psych.* 1991;148:1177–1181.

82. Thase ME, Fasiczka AL, Berman SR, et al. Electroencephalographic sleep profiles before and after cognitive behavioral therapy of depression. *Arch Gen Psych.* 1998;55:138–144.

83. Kerkhofs M, Hoffman G, De Martelaere V, et al. Sleep EEG recordings in depressive disorders. *J Affect Disorders.* 1985;9:47–53.

84. Schulz H, Lund RD, Cording C, et al. Bimodal distribution of REM sleep latencies in depression. *Biol Psych.* 1979;14:595–600.

85. Giles DE, Etzel BA, Reynolds CF, III, et al. Stability of polysomnographic parameters in unipolar depression: a cross-sectional report. *Biol Psych.* 1989;25:807–810.

86. Hauri PJ, Chernic D, Hawkins DR, et al. Sleep of depressed patients in remission. *Arch Gen Psych.* 1974;31:386–391.

87. Rush AJ, Erman MK, Giles DE, et al. Polysomnographic findings in recently drug-free and clinically remitted depressed patients. *Arch Gen Psych.* 1986;43:878–884.

88. Lee JH, Reynolds CF, III, Hoch CC, et al. Electroencephalographic sleep in recently remitted, elderly depressed patients in double-blind placebo maintenance therapy. *Neuropsychopharmacology.* 1993;8:143–150.

89. Giles DE, Kupfer DJ, Rush AJ, et al. Controlled comparison of electroencephalographic sleep in families of probands with unipolar depression. *Amer J Psych.* 1998;155:192–199.

90. Somoza E, Mossman D. Optimizing REM latency as a diagnostic test for depression using receiver operating characteristic analysis and information theory. *Biol Psych.* 1989;27:990–1006.

91. Giles DE, Roffwarg HP, Rush AJ. A cross-sectional study of the effects of depression on REM latency. *Biol Psych.* 1990;28:697–704.

92. King D, Akiskal HS, Lemmi H, et al. REM density in the differential diagnosis of psychiatric from medical-neurological disorders: a replication. *Psych Res.* 1981;5:267–276.

93. Lauer CJ, Garcia D, Pollmacher T, et al. All-night EEG sleep in anxiety disorders and major depression. In: Horne J, ed. *Sleep '90,* Bochum, Germany: Pontenagel Press, 1991.

94. Gillin JC, Smith TL, Irwin M, et al. Short REM latency in primary alcoholic patients with secondary depression. *Amer J Psych.* 1990;147:106–109.

95. Greenberg R, Pearlman CA, Gampel D. War neuroses and the adaptive function of REM sleep. *Br J Med Psychol.* 1972;45:27–33.

96. Kauffman CD, Reist C, Djenderedjian A, et al. Biological markers of affective disorders and post-traumatic stress disorder: a pilot study with desipramine. *J Clin Psych.* 1987;48:366–367.

97. Hiatt JF, Floyd TC, Katz PH, et al. Further evidence of abnormal non-rapid-eye-movement sleep in schizophrenia. *Arch Gen Psych.* 1985;42:797–802.

98. Zarcone VP, Benson KL, Berger PA. Abnormal rapid eye movement latencies in schizophrenia. *Arch Gen Psych.* 1987;44:45–48.

99. Uhde TW, Roy- Bryne P, Gillin JC, et al. The sleep of patients with panic disorder: a preliminary report. *Psych Res.* 1985;12: 251–259.

100. Katz JL, Kuperberg A, Pollack CP, et al. Is there a relationship between eating disorder and affective disorder? New evidence from sleep recordings. *Amer J Psych.* 1984;141:753–759.

101. Neil JF, Merikangas JR, Foster FG, et al. Waking and all-night sleep EEGs in anorexia nervosa. *Clin Electroencephalogr.* 1980;11:9–15.

102. Reynolds CF, III, Frank E, Houck PR, et al. Which elderly patients with remitted depression remain well with continued interpersonal psychotherapy after discontinuation of antidepressant medication? *Amer J Psych.* 1997;154:958–962.

103. Coffey CE, McCall V, Hoelscher TJ. Effects of ECT on polysomnographic sleep: a pilot prospective study. *Convulsive Ther.* 1988;4: 269–279.

104. Fontaine R, Ontiveros A, Elie R, et al. A double-blind comparison of nefazodone, imipramine, and placebo in major depression. *J Clin Psych.* 1994;55:234–241.

105. DiMascio A, Weissman MM, Prusoff BA, et al. Differential symptom reduction by drugs and psychotherapy in acute depression. *Arch Gen Psych.* 1979;36:1450–1456.

106. David J. Kupfer. The sleep EEG in diagnosis and treatment of depression. *Depression: basic mechanisms, diagnosis, and treatment.* New York: Guilford Press, 1986:102–125.

107. Bowers M, Kupfer DJ. Central monoamine oxidase inhibition and REM sleep. *Brain Res.* 1971;35:561–564.

108. Wyatt RJ, Fram DH, Buchbinder R, et al. Treatment of intractable narcolepsy with a monoamine oxidase inhibitor. *N Eng J Med.* 1971;285:987–991.

109. Wyatt RJ, Fram DH, Kupfer DJ, et al. Total prolonged drug-induced REM sleep suppression in anxious-depressed patients. *Arch Gen Psych.* 1971;24:145–155.

110. Nierenberg AA, Keefe BR, Leslie VC, et al. Residual symptoms in depressed patients who respond acutely to fluoxetine. *J Clin Psych.* 1999;60:221–225.

111. Nolen WA, Haffmans PM, Bouvy PF, et al. Hypnotics as concurrent medication in depression. A placebo-controlled, double-blind comparison of flunitrazepam and lormetazepam in patients with major depression, treated with a (tri)cyclic antidepressant. *J Affect Disorders.* 1993;28:179–188.

112. McCall WV, Reboussin BA, Cohen W. Subjective measurement of insomnia and quality of life in depressed inpatients. *J Sleep Res.* 2000;9:43–48.

113. Asnis GM, ChakrabURTTY A, DuBoff EA, et al. Zolpidem for persistent insomnia in SSRI-treated depressed patients. *J Clin Psych.* 1999;60:668–676.

114. Turvey CL, Conwell Y, Jones MP, et al. Risk factors for late-life suicide: A prospective, community-based study. *Amer J Geriatr Psych.* 2002;10:398–406.

115. Fawcett J, Scheftner WA, Fogg L, et al. Predictors of early suicide: Identification and appropriate intervention. *J Clin Psych.* 1988;49: 7–8.

116. Fawcett J, Scheftner WA, Fogg L, et al. Time-related predictors of suicide in major affective disorder. *Amer J Psych.* 1990;147:1189–1194.

117. Agargun MY, Kara H, Solmaz M. Sleep disturbances and suicidal behavior in patients with major depression. *J Clin Psych.* 1997;58:249–251.

118. Fawcett J, Edwards JH, Kravitz HM, et al. Alprazolam: an antidepressant? Alprazolam, desipramine, and an alprazoloam-desipramine combination in the treatment of adult depressed outpatients. *J Clin Psychopharmacol.* 1987;7:295–310.

119. Dominguez R, Jacobson AF, Goldstein BJ, et al. Comparison of triazolam and placebo in the treatment of depressed patients. *Curr Ther Res.* 1984;36:856–865.

120. Scharf MB, Sachais BA. Sleep laboratory evaluation of the effects and efficacy of trazodone in depressed insomniac patients. *J Clin Psych.* 1990;51:13–17.

121. Edinger JD, Wohlgemuth WK, Radtke RA, et al. Cognitive behavioral therapy for treatment of chronic primary insomnia: a randomized controlled trial. *JAMA.* 2001;285 (14):1856–1864.

122. Kupfer DJ, Reynolds CF, III, Weiss BL, et al. Lithium carbonate and sleep in affective disorders: Further considerations. *Arch Gen Psych.* 1974;30:79–84.

123. Terao T, Terao M, Yoshimura R, et al. Restless legs syndrome induced by lithium. *Biol Psych.* 1991;30:1167–1170.

124. Post RM, Kotin J, Goodwin FK. Effects of sleep deprivation on mood and central amine metabolism in depressed patients. *Arch Gen Psych.* 1976;33:627–632.

125. Pflug B, Tolle R. Disturbance of the 24-hour rhythm in endogenous depression by sleep deprivation. *Interm Pharmacopsych.* 1971;6:187–196.

126. Van den Burg W, Van den Hoofdakker RH. Total sleep deprivation on endogenous depression. *Arch Gen Psych.* 1975;32:1121–1125.

127. Wu JC, Bunney WE. The biological basis of antidepressant response to sleep deprivation and relapse: review and hypothesis. *Amer J Psych.* 1990;147:14–21.

128. Wehr TA. Sleep loss as a possible mediator of diverse causes of mania. *Br J Psych.* 1991;159:576–578.

129. Naylor MW, King CA, Lindsay KA, et al. Sleep deprivation in depressed adolescents and psychiatric controls. *J Amer Acad Child Adolesc Psych.* 1993;32:753–759.

130. Pilcher JJ, Huffcutt AI. Effects of sleep deprivation on performance: A meta-analysis. *Sleep.* 1996;194:318–326.

131. Weigand M, Berger M, Zulley J, et al. The influence of daytime naps on the therapeutic effect of sleep deprivation. *Biol Psych.* 1987;22:386–389.

132. Vogel GW, Thurmond A, Gibbons P, et al. REM sleep reduction effects on depressive syndromes. *Arch Gen Psych.* 1975;32:765–777.

133. Sack DA, Dancan W, Rosenthal NE, et al. The timing and duration of sleep in partial sleep deprivation therapy of depression. *Acta Psych Scand.* 1988;77:219–224.

134. Schilgen B, Tolle R. Partial sleep deprivation as therapy for depression. *Arch Gen Psych.* 1980;37:267–271.

135. Berger M, Vollmann J, Hohagen F, et al. Sleep deprivation combined with consecutive sleep phase advance as a fast-acting therapy in depression: an open pilot trial in medicated and unmedicated patients. *Amer J Psych.* 1997;154:870–872.

136. Sack DA, Nurnberger J, Rosenthal NE, et al. Potentiation of antidepressant medications by phase advance of the sleep–wake cycle. *Amer J Psych.* 1985;142:606–608.

137. Wu JC, Gillin JC, Buschbaum MS, et al. Effect of sleep deprivation on brain metabolism of depressed patients. *Amer J Psych.* 1992;149:538–543.

138. Ebert D, Feistel H, Barocka A. Effects of sleep deprivation on the limbic system and the frontal lobes in affective disorders: a study with Tc-99m-HMPAO SPECT. *Psych Res.* 1991;40:247–251.

139. Vgontzas AN, Bixler EO, Hung-Mo L, et al. Chronic insomnia is associated with nyctohemeral activation of the hypothalamic-pituitary-adrenal axis: clinical implications. *J Clin Endocrin Metabolism.* 2001;86:3787–3794.

140. Bleuler E. *Dementia praecox.* New York: International University Press, 1950:168–169.

141. Van Kammen DP, Van Kammen WB, Peters JL, et al. CSF MHPG, sleep and psychosis in schizophrenia. *Clin Neuropharmacol.* 1986;9(Suppl. 4):575–577.

142. Dement W. Dream recall and eye movements during sleep in schizophrenics and normals. *J Nerv Ment Dis.* 1955;122:263–269.

143. Koresko R, Snyder F, Feinberg I. "Dream time" in hallucinating and non-hallucinating schizophrenic patients. *Nature (London).* 1963;199:1118–1119.

144. Zarcone VP, Azumi K, Dement W, et al. REM phase deprivation and schizophrenia: II. *Arch Gen Psych.* 1975;32:1431–1436.

145. Gillin JC, Buchsbaum MS, Jacob LS, et al. Partial sleep deprivation, schizophrenia and field articulation. *Arch Gen Psych.* 1974;30:653–662.

146. Jus K, Gagnon-Binette M, Desjardins D, et al. Effets de la deprivation du sommeil rapid pendant la premiere et la seconde partie de la nuit chez les schizophrenes chroniques. *La Vie Med Can Fr.* 1977;6:1234–1242.

147. Benson KL, Zarcone VP. Testing the REM sleep phasic event intrusion hypothesis of schizophrenia. *Psych Res.* 1985;15:163–173.

148. Feinberg I, Koresko RL, Gottlieb F. Further observations on electrophysiological sleep patterns in schizophrenia. *Comp Psych.* 1965;6:21–24.

149. Benson Kl, Zarcone VP. REM sleep eye movement activity in schizophrenia and depression. *Arch Gen Psych.* 1993;50:474–482.

150. Jus K, Bouchard M, Jus AK, et al. Sleep EEG studies in untreated long-term schizophrenic patients. *Arch Gen Psych.* 1973;29:386–390.

151. Stern M, Fram D, Wyatt R, et al. All night sleep studies of acute schizophrenics. *Arch Gen Psych.* 1969;20:470–477.

152. Feinberg I, Braum N, Koresko RL, et al. Stage 4 sleep in schizophrenia. *Arch Gen Psych.* 1969;21:262–266.

153. Caldwell DF, Domino EF. Electroencephalographic and eye movement patterns during sleep in chronic schizophrenia patients. *Electroencephalogr Clin Neurophysiol.* 1967;22:414–420.

154. Lauer CJ, Schreiber W, Pollmacher T, et al. Sleep in schizophrenia: a polysomnographic study on drug-naïve patients. *Neuropsychopharmacology.* 1997;16:51–60.

155. Neylan TC, Van Kammen DP, Kelley ME, et al. Sleep in schizophrenic patients on and off haloperidol therapy. *Arch Gen Psych.* 1992;49:643–649.

156. Zarcone VP, Benson KL. BPRS symptom factors and sleep variables in schizophrenia. *Psych Res.* 1997;66:111–120.

157. Van Kammen DP, Van Kammen WM, Peters J, et al. Decreased slow-wave sleep and enlarged lateral ventricles in schizophrenia. *Neuropsychopharmacology.* 1988;1:265–271.

158. Keshavan MS, Pettegrew JW, Reynolds CF, et al. Biological correlates of slow wave sleep deficits in functional psychoses: ^{31}P-magnetic resonance spectroscopy. *Psych Res.* 1995;57:91–100.

159. Keshavan MS, Miewald J, Haas G, et al. Slow-wave sleep and symptomatology in schizophrenia and related psychotic disorders. *J Psych Res.* 1995;29:303–314.

160. Taylor SF, Tandon R, Shipley JE, et al. Sleep-onset REM periods in schizophrenic patients. *Biol Psych.* 1991;30:205–209.

161. Keshavan MS, Reynolds CF, Montrose D, et al. Sleep and suicidality in psychotic patients. *Acta Psych Scand.* 1994;89:122–125.

162. Lewis CF, Tandon R, Shipley JE, et al. Biological predictors of suicidality in schizophrenia. *Acta Psych Scand.* 1996;94:416–420.

163. Hudson JL, Lipinski JF, Keck PE, et al. Polysomnographic characteristics of schizophrenia in comparison with mania and depression. *Biol Psych.* 1993;34:191–193.

164. Benson KL, King A, Gordon D, et al. Sleep patterns in borderline personality disorder. *J Affect Disorders* 1990;18:267–273.

165. Benson KL, Zarcone VP. Sleep abnormalities in schizophrenia and other psychotic disorders. In: Oldham JM, Riba MS, eds. *Review of psychiatry.* Vol 13. Washington, DC: American Psychiatric Press, 1994:677–705.

166. Hinze-Selch D, Mullington J, Orth A, et al. Effects of clozapine on sleep: A longitudinal study. *Biol Psych.* 1997;42:260–266.

167. Wetter TC, Lauer CJ, Gillich G, et al. The electroencephalographic sleep pattern in schizophrenic patients treated with clozapine or classical anti-psychotic drugs. *J Psych Res.* 1996;30:411–419.

168. Nofzinger EA, Van Kammen DP, Gilbertson MW, et al. Electroencephalographic sleep in clinically stable schizophrenic patients: two-weeks versus six-weeks neuroleptic free. *Biol Psych.* 1993;33:829–835.

169. Hartmann E, Cravens J. The effects of long term administration of psychotropic drugs on human sleep, IV: The effects of chlorpromazine. *Psychopharmacology (Berlin).* 1973;33:203–218.

170. Brannen JO, Jewett RE. Effects of selected phenothiazines on REM sleep in schizophrenics. *Arch Gen Psych.* 1969;21:284–290.

171. Hyman SE, Nestler EJ. Initiation and adaptation: A paradigm for understanding psychotropic drug action. *Amer J Psych.* 1996;153:151–162.

172. Gillin JC, Drummond SPA. Medication and substance abuse. In: Kryger MH, Roth T, Dement WC, eds. *Principles and practice of sleep medicine.* 3rd edn. Philadelphia: W.B. Saunders, 2000:1176–1195.

173. Robins LN, Helzer JE, Weissman MM, et al. Lifetime prevalence of specific psychiatric disorders in three sites. *Arch Gen Psych.* 1984;41:949–958.

174. Koob G, LeMoal M. Drug abuse: hedonic homeostatic dysregulation. *Science.* 1997;278:52–58.

175. Lobo LL, Tufik S. Effects of alcohol on sleep parameters of sleep-deprived healthy volunteers. *Sleep.* 1997;20:52–59.

176. Adamson J, Burdick JA. Sleep of dry alcoholics. *Arch Gen Psych.* 1973;28:146–149.

177. Kotorii T, Nakazawa Y, Yokoyama T. Terminal sleep following delirium tremens in chronic alcoholics—polysomnographic and behavioral study. *Drug Alcohol Depend.* 1982;10:125–134.

178. Drummond SPA, Gillin JC, Smith TL, et al. The sleep of abstinent pure primary alcoholic patients: natural course and relationsip to relapse. *Alcohol Clin Exp Res.* 1988;22:1796–1802.

179. Allen RP, Wagman AM, Funderburk FR, et al. Slow wave sleep: a predictor of individual differences in response to drinking? *Biol Psych.* 1980;15:345–348.

180. Gillin JC, Smith TL, Irwin M, et al. Increased pressure for rapid eye movement sleep at time of hospital admission predicts relapse in nondepressed patients with primary alcoholism at 3-month follow-up. *Arch Gen Psych.* 1994;51:189–197.

181. Brower KJ, Aldrich MS, Hall JM. Polysomnographic and subjective sleep predictors of alcoholic relapse. *Alcohol Clin Exp Res.* 1998;22:1864–1871.

Sleep Disorders, Dementia, and Related Degenerative Disorders

Bradley F. Boeve and Michael H. Silber

INTRODUCTION

The interrelationships between cognition, dementia, movement disorders, and sleep disorders are increasingly being recognized. Yet, the clinical characterization of patients with cognitive impairment or dementia has largely reflected data gathered during wakefulness, with little attention given to the nocturnal hours and the effects of untreated sleep disorders on cognition. Movement disorders can profoundly affect sleep and wakefulness by inducing insomnia, excessive sleepiness, or disturbances of nocturnal respiration. Conversely, sleep can alter the manifestations of a movement disorder by suppressing some dyskinesias, activating others, and sometimes providing post-sleep benefit by reducing symptoms in the early morning. Some abnormal movements are at least partially suppressed by sleep, including tremor, chorea, dystonia and tics, whereas others are activated by sleep, including periodic limb movements (PLMs), sleep starts, rhythmic movement disorder, bruxism, and REM sleep behavior disorder (RSBD). Certain sleep disorders may be providing etiologic clues to the pathophysiology of brain disease that until only recently were largely ignored.

In this chapter, we will discuss the pertinent data that exists in the literature regarding sleep-related symptoms and disorders and their relationships to the major degenerative, vascular, and prion disorders of the brain that affect cognition and movement [this review is updated from reference (1)]. We will also present comments from personal or institutional experience, as some may find this information useful.

SLEEP DISORDERS AND DEMENTIA

Overview

Over the past 15 years, neuropathologic studies using immunocytochemical techniques have led to significant changes in our understanding of the etiologic underpinnings of dementing illnesses. Alzheimer's disease (AD) is the most common cause of irreversible dementia, and includes about 60% to 80% of patients with dementia. Dementia with Lewy bodies (DLB) is now considered the second most common irreversible cause of dementia, accounting for approximately 15% to 25% of cases. Recent data suggest Parkinson's disease (PD) with dementia and DLB have the same neuropathologic substrate of limbic and cortical Lewy bodies, but the relationship between the two disorders has not been clearly defined. The frontotemporal dementia category of disorders accounts for approximately 10% to 15% of untreatable dementia cases. Pick's disease, corticobasal degeneration (CBD), and dementia lacking distinctive histology (DLDH) are often manifested by features reflecting frontal and/or temporal cortical dysfunction, and can be considered under the term frontotemporal dementia (FTD). Multi-infarct dementia, classically thought to be the second most common etiology of dementia, is now considered within the spectrum of vascular dementia. The prevalence of vascular dementia is debated, with recent studies suggesting pure vascular dementia probably accounts for less than 20% of cases with dementia. Creutzfeldt–Jakob disease (CJD), fatal familial insomnia (FFI), and Gerstmann–Straussler–Scheinker syndrome comprise the primary human prion disorders.

Importantly, most of the literature on sleep disturbances in dementia involve patients clinically diagnosed with AD. However, a significant minority of patients with typical AD clinical features do not have AD when examined postmortem, and instead have the non-AD disorders noted above. Others have a combination of two or more conditions. The literature on sleep disturbances in dementia has, therefore, very likely included cases with non-AD disorders and thus the findings may not be specific for AD. Furthermore, sleep-related issues may be quite different from one disorder to another. We will, therefore, review sleep-disordered breathing (SDB), movement disorders and parasomnias, insomnia, and circadian rhythm disorders as they pertain to patients with dementia. We will then review specific sleep disorders associated with specific dementing conditions.

Sleep-Disordered Breathing and Dementia

Obstructive Sleep Apnea

The relationships between obstructive sleep apnea (OSA), cognitive status, and dementia are still being defined. Although there appears to be an association between OSA and dementia, there is conflicting data on whether OSA *causes* dementia (2–9). Since there is a marked increase in intracranial pressure and change in cerebral perfusion during apneic events (10,11), one would expect that if OSA is causally related to dementia at all, that vascular dementia would be most likely related. Evidence accumulated over the past 10 years indicates that untreated OSA in the nondemented population causes cognitive impairment, excessive daytime sleepiness (EDS), and diminished mood and quality of life. Treatment of OSA [particularly with nasal continuous positive airway pressure (CPAP)] improves cognitive performance, EDS, mood, and quality of life (QoL) (12–22). Neuropsychologic analyses have

revealed that in patients with OSA, cognitive flexibility, attention, processing speed, and memory all improve with CPAP therapy (13,23,24). There are instances in which patients have been diagnosed with delirium (25,26), dementia (not otherwise specified) (7), and a degenerative-dementing illness (27) who were found to have untreated OSA, and delirium or dementia disappeared with CPAP therapy. *Hence, OSA should be considered one of the treatable contributors to and causes of delirium and dementia.* The frequency of such cases is not known, but the fact that some individuals have significant functional and neuropsychometric improvement with CPAP therapy, and the high prevalance of OSA in the elderly (2,3), underscore the need to consider OSA in any patient with cognitive impairment. Furthermore, as CPAP therapy has now been shown to improve the sleep quality in bed partners of patients with OSA (28), caregivers of patients with dementia and OSA could enjoy improved quality of sleep/quality of life with their bed partners' use of CPAP therapy.

There are no published data on whether cognition improves with CPAP therapy in patients with OSA and a coexisting dementing illness, nor whether CPAP therapy is tolerated in demented individuals. No published data exists on the effects of CPAP therapy on the bed partners/caregivers of patients with OSA and dementia.

However, experience at our center has revealed the following regarding patients with dementia and OSA:

- A minority of patients experience significant functional and mild to moderate neuropsychometric improvement with CPAP therapy.
- A significant proportion of patients tolerate CPAP therapy and use it nightly.
- Some patients with positional OSA tolerate positional therapy and experience mild clinical improvement.
- Some caregivers of patients experience less fragmented sleep and less daytime somnolence while their bed partners with dementia use CPAP therapy.

Clearly, well-designed, prospective studies in patients with dementia and OSA are needed to better understand the clinical and financial implications of the evaluation and management of OSA in the cognitively impaired elderly.

Central Sleep Apnea

Central sleep apnea (CSA) is known to occur in patients with primary cardiac and primary central nervous system dysfunction. The dysregulation of the brainstem respiratory neuronal networks is presumed to be responsible for CSA in degenerative dementing illnesses and likely contributes similarly in vascular dementia. The frequency of CSA in the degenerative and vascular dementing conditions is not known, but in our experience this is far less common than OSA in those with mild to moderate dementia. Like in CSA related to cardiac dysfunction, management can be quite challenging. Nasal CPAP therapy, bilevel positive airway pressure (BPAP) therapy, supplemental oxygen, benzodiazepines, or a combination of two or three of these can provide symptomatic improvement in some cases. Therapeutic trials may require two nights of polysomnography (PSG) to determine which single treatment or combination of therapies provide the maximal benefit.

Movement Disorders/Parasomnias and Dementia

Restless Legs Syndrome

Restless legs syndrome (RLS) is a common condition characterized by unpleasant limb sensations that are precipitated by rest and relieved by activity. It is worse in the evening and often results in insomnia. The incidence and prevalence of RLS in patients with AD and other dementing conditions are not known, nor are there any studies that address the safety and efficacy of various agents in this population. A recent study suggests almost 10% of individuals 65 to 83 years of age have RLS, thus a significant proportion of demented individuals likely have the disorder (29). As is always the case in dementia, histories from patients may be inaccurate by virtue of their illness. Since the diagnosis of RLS is based on the clinical history, one must often rely on the bed partner's determination of the degree of restlessness at night rather than solely basing one's impression on the patient's recall of typical RLS symptoms. Our clinical experience suggests that RLS occurs with relative frequency in patients with AD, DLB, PD with dementia, FTD, and vascular dementia.

Several agents (e.g., carbidopa/levodopa, pramipexole, ropinirole, and gabapentin) appear to be generally well-tolerated and efficacious. In some patients, dopaminergic agents have a stimulating effect and may lead to insomnia. The dopaminergic agents should be used with caution in patients with psychotic features, as these agents can escalate psychosis, although in our experience, these agents rarely do so when used at the low doses that are effective for RLS.

Patients with cognitive impairment and RLS +/− periodic limb movements in sleep (PLMS) can be challenging to treat. Since iron deficiency—as reflected by ferritin levels below 50 μg/L—can precipitate or aggravate RLS (30), one must consider iron deficiency in patients with a recent history of surgery, peptic ulcer, or colon lesion, and in those with RLS symptoms that are refractory to medical therapy. Iron deficiency can reflect inadequate iron intake since cognitively impaired individuals may forget to eat certain meals or may have difficulty preparing meals with adequate nutrition. The cause of the iron deficiency should be sought when indicated and treated if possible; iron replacement therapy should be considered, realizing that such therapy is often poorly tolerated in the elderly.

The goal of iron therapy should ideally be to raise the concentration of serum ferritin to greater than 50 μg/L.

Periodic Limb Movements of Sleep

About 80% of patients with RLS also have accompanying PLMS, although PLMS can occur in patients with no RLS symptoms. PLMS are stereotyped repetitive flexion movements of the legs that occur semirhythmically at intervals of usually 20 to 40 seconds and may cause sufficient arousals to fragment sleep and result in daytime hypersomnolence. PLMS occur with high frequency in normal elderly individuals (31). As in the other primary sleep disorders, the incidence and prevalence of PLMS in patients with dementia are not known. In our experience, PLMS are relatively common in this population, but it can be difficult to determine by history alone if PLMS are clinically significant or not. PSG may be diagnostically helpful in hypersomnolent patients with dementia even when their bed partners are unaware of the presence of PLMS. However, the PLMS must result in arousals on PSG before they should be considered potentially significant. As in RLS, treatment with carbidopa/levodopa, pramipexole, ropinirole, or gabapentin is generally efficacious and well-tolerated. Again, the dopaminergic agents should be titrated gingerly in patients with psychotic features, as these agents can aggravate psychosis.

REM Sleep Behavior Disorder

REM sleep behavior disorder (RBD) is characterized by simple or complex limb movements and/or vocalizations during rapid eye movement (REM) sleep, and such behaviors typically mirror the content of the dream when a patient is awakened and questioned (32,33). Behaviors can be violent, and patient and bed partner injuries can occur. The frequency and severity of RBD is variable between patients and during the course of symptoms in individual patients, but when RBD is associated with a neurodegenerative disorder, the symptoms often tend to wane as the degenerative illness progresses (33). Differentiating RBD from nocturnal wandering can usually be done by taking a careful history. RBD is more short-lived, involves more vigorous limb movements and vocalizations, dream content often involve chasing or attacking themes and mirrors behaviors, and tends to occur more in the second half of the night when more REM sleep typically occurs. In contrast, nocturnal wandering is typically more prolonged, less violent, not associated with any apparent dream, and has a pacing or rummaging quality. When the diagnosis is in question, or when the potential for injury is present, PSG is warranted and should be performed with additional EMG leads on the arms and with synchronous video monitoring.

The association of RBD with neurodegenerative disease is well established. Until recently, RBD had generally been considered a nonspecific manifestation of the neurodegenerative process. However, there is growing evidence that RBD occurs in a disproportionally greater frequency in certain neurodegenerative disorders, namely DLB, PD, and multiple system atrophy (MSA) (see below) (34,35). These disorders are known collectively as "synucleinopathies" due to the prominent immunoreactivity to α-synuclein on autopsied brain tissue. We have hypothesized that RBD associated with a degenerative dementing or parkinsonian disorder often reflects an underlying synucleinopathy (34,35). All autopsied cases of RBD plus dementia and/or parkinsonism reported thus far have had Lewy body disease or MSA, which supports this contention. Importantly, RBD typically precedes the development of dementia or parkinsonism by years and sometimes decades. Therefore, the presence of RBD may reflect the earliest clinical manifestation of an evolving neurodegenerative disorder.

Ensuring safety in the sleep environment is the simplest recommendation for managing RBD (i.e., remove all potentially injurious objects away from the bed, place mattress on floor next to bed, etc.). Clonazepam is the drug of choice and is usually effective in the 0.25 to 1.0 mg per night dose range (33,36). As benzodiazepines can precipitate or aggravate OSA, it is important to ensure that no OSA exists before using this agent, or ensure nasal CPAP therapy is successfully treating OSA if this is present. There is often concern expressed by clinicians about using this long-acting benzodiazepine in patients with dementia, but in our experience with over 40 patients with dementia and clinically significant RBD, clonazepam has been tolerated quite well with few or no cognitive side effects in the vast majority of cases. Recent reports have indicated that melatonin can alleviate RBD (37–39), but the mechanism by which this agent improves RBD has not be elucidated. Other agents with reported efficacy include donepezil (40), carbamazepine (41), triazolam (33), clozapine (33), and quetiapine (1).

Insomnia/Circadian Rhythm Disorders and Dementia

Insomnia

The incidence and prevalence of insomnia in patients with dementing illnesses are not known (42–44). There is some discrepancy in the literature regarding whether time spent in slow wave sleep (SWS) is impaired in the earlier stage of dementia (45). Nonetheless, there does seem to be increased magnitude of changes in sleep architecture with increasing severity of dementia (46). Reduced time in SWS represents greater time spent in stages of sleep considered to be nonrestorative.

Sleep disturbances may lead to nocturnal awakenings and nocturnal wandering, which can cause considerable caregiver burden (42,47,48). In addition to severity of dementia, nursing home placement has been found to be strongly related to the inability for patients to stay in bed at night (49,50). Nocturnal wandering in dementia may reflect insomnia secondary to night/day reversal, medication effects, emotional distress, the need to find the bathroom, under- or overstimulation during the day, the experience of pain, (51), or restless legs syndrome (see above). Patients with dementia may be unable to explain why they are awake at night and, therefore, it is the responsibility of caregivers, physicians, and health care providers to carefully examine the entire context in which the behavior occurs in order to determine its cause. First and foremost, evaluating for pain, medical conditions, or medication side effects is essential.

Caution should be exercised when prescribing medications used to treat insomnia since these can worsen OSA and daytime symptoms of sleepiness (52) and may worsen cognitive impairment, thus causing increased disability. If insomnia is considered to be an isolated disturbance that is not attributable to other causes, such as those identified above, then agents such as trazodone, melatonin, zolpidem, or zaleplon may be considered.

Circadian Dysrhythmia

Although precise data on the incidence and prevalence of circadian dysrhythmia in the demented population do not exist, several groups have observed a high frequency of sleep fragmentation and circadian dysrhythmia in the institutionalized elderly (43,44,53,54). The symptoms of insomnia and hypersomnia can reflect a primary circadian dysrhythmia. Degenerative changes in the suprachiasmatic nucleus of the hypothalamus and decreased melatonin production are thought to be contributing factors in the circadian dysrhythmic abnormalities in patients with AD and other dementing conditions (55–58).

These anatomic and physiologic changes form the basis for the two primary management strategies that have been employed—exogenous melatonin and phototherapy. Data from relatively small numbers of patients with dementia suggest that melatonin can improve sleep continuity and lengthen total sleep time (TST) (59,60), which formed the basis for the melatonin for sleep disturbance in Alzheimer's disease treatment trial (see below). Phototherapy has shown some promise in the management of circadian dysrhythmia in demented individuals, although the optimal timing and duration of phototherapy and illumination intensity have not yet been determined (61–64).

Hypersomnia and Dementia

The incidence and prevalence of hypersomnia in the various dementing conditions are not known, but hypersomnia is clearly quite evident in patients with dementia residing at chronic care facilities. Hypersomnia often reflects untreated OSA, CSA, PLMS, circadian dysrhythmia, or some combination of these. Although there are only sparse published reports of hypersomnia directly related to an underlying degenerative dementing disorder, experience at our center indicates some individuals with DLB, PD with dementia, or FTD have objective evidence of hypersomnolence as measured by the multiple sleep latency test (MSLT), which is not associated with another primary sleep disorder. Low dose methylphenidate (5 mg or less) has been shown to improve alertness in very old patients residing in nursing homes (65). In our experience, methylphenidate, as well as modafinil, has been moderately helpful in managing hypersomnolence in demented patients without inducing untoward neurobehavioral or cardiovascular side effects. However, caregivers must be counseled on the potential emergence or exacerbation of agitation, wandering, and other problematic behaviors if alertness is improved with psychostimulant therapy.

The anatomic and physiologic underpinnings of hypersomnia in dementing conditions have not been defined, although one could hypothesize that degeneration of hypocretin-secreting neurons could contribute to hypersomnolence in some patients. Preliminary data on autopsied patients with Alzheimer's disease +/− Lewy body disease but no recorded hypersomnolence, has shown hypocretin-1 levels in the cerebrospinal fluid (CSF) are not reduced (66). Additional analyses involving CSF hypocretin-1 quantification in hypersomnolent as well as alert patients with dementia will address whether hypocretin-1 deficiency plays any role in dementia-related hypersomnolence.

Specific Dementia Disorder—Sleep Disorder Associations

Alzheimer's Disease (AD) and Circadian Dysrhythmia

The literature suggests circadian dysrhythmias are particularly common in patients with AD. A multicenter placebo-controlled trial, sponsored by the Alzheimer's Disease Cooperative Study group (funded by the National Institute on Aging), sought to determine the safety and efficacy of low-dose and high-dose melatonin for sleep disturbances (particularly circadian dysrhythmias) in AD (67). There were no significant differences in nocturnal sleep time, sleep efficiency, wake-time after sleep onset (WASO), or day–night sleep ratio between the low-dose and high-dose melatonin and placebo groups. However, one subject had a dramatic response to melatonin. The authors concluded that melatonin was not an effective soporific agent in AD patients, although it was well-tolerated and occasional patients may respond well (67).

Dementia with Lewy Bodies (DLB) and REM Sleep Behavior Disorder

We first reported the association of RBD and DLB in 1997, and subsequent studies have clearly shown RBD occurs with relative frequency in DLB, although the prevalence is not yet known (68–78). RBD is now regarded as a supportive feature for the diagnosis of DLB (79). Most of the patients described in these reports began experiencing RBD some years or decades before their cognitive symptoms evolved.

There is growing evidence that the neuropsychologic profile of impairment in patients with dementia and RBD is distinct and likely reflecting underlying Lewy body disease. We performed neuropsychologic testing in 37 patients with degenerative dementia +/− parkinsonism and RBD and demonstrated impaired visual perceptual–organizational skills, constructional praxis, and verbal fluency (71). There were no significant differences in neuropsychologic performance, or in the frequency of clinical features, between patients with or without parkinsonism. Thirty-four (92%) cases met criteria for clinically possible or probable DLB (80). Three patients were autopsied: all had limbic with or without neocortical Lewy bodies. We concluded that the clinical and neuropsychometric features of patients with and without parkinsonism were similar, and hypothesized that the underlying pathology in these patients was DLB (71).

A subsequent analysis in which the neuropsychometric profile of 31 patients with RBD/dementia was compared to 31 cases of autopsy-proved AD revealed a striking double dissociation. The RBD/dementia groups had worse impairment on measures of attention, visual perceptual organization, and letter fluency, whereas the AD group had significantly worse performance on confrontation naming and verbal memory (75). We concluded that patients with RBD and degenerative dementia have a significantly different pattern of cognitive performance from AD and the pattern of cognitive differences from AD is similar to that reported between DLB and AD. These data therefore suggested that the dementia associated with RBD may represent DLB (75).

We recently reported on the neuropsychometric features in patients with dementia and RBD who did not have parkinsonism or visual hallucinations (81). Neurocognitive data from groups of patients with a similar dementia severity were compared in those with clinically probable DLB, dementia, and RBD without visual hallucinations or parkinsonism, and definite AD. The neurocognitive profiles between the probable DLB and dementia with RBD groups did not differ and, when compared to the AD group, both groups had worse visual perceptual organization and sequencing and better confrontation naming and verbal memory. We concluded that patients with dementia and RBD, who do not have parkinsonism or visual hallucinations, have a dementia syndrome that is neuropsychologically indistinguishable from that of probable DLB, and the features of both of these groups differ from AD (81). Therefore, in the absence of visual hallucinations or parkinsonism, the presentation of dementia and RBD may indicate underlying Lewy body disease. This study suggests that early detection of evolving DLB may be possible, and emphasizes the utility of probing for RBD in the clinical interview and of neuropsychological testing.

The sensitivity and specificity of RBD for DLB in the setting of dementia has not yet been determined, but detailed antemortem analyses and the lack of any pathologically confirmed cases of RBD in pure AD, Pick's disease, FTD, or vascular dementia suggests that RBD may be predictive of underlying DLB in most patients with dementia (34,35,71,82). Therefore, a careful sleep history and neuropsychologic testing may provide diagnostically relevant information in the evaluation of patients with dementia.

Clinicopathologic studies in patients with RBD plus a neurodegenerative disease support the hypothesis that RBD plus dementia and/or parkinsonism often reflects an underlying synucleinopathy (34,35,82). A patient with a 20-year history of RBD but no cognitive or motor findings throughout his clinical course was found to have brainstem Lewy bodies at autopsy (83). Schenck et al. (84,85) reported a man with a 15-year history of RBD before dementia evolved, and autopsy revealed limbic Lewy bodies as well as Alzheimer changes. Turner et al. (86,87) have provided detailed clinical and pathologic descriptions of their case with RBD and dementia, in which Lewy body disease was identified. In an updated analysis in which 12 autopsied patients with RBD plus dementia were characterized, all had limbic +/− neocortical Lewy body disease (82). Therefore, to date, all of the patients with RBD plus dementia have had Lewy body pathology identified at autopsy (78,82,85–88). If future analyses support the RBD/synucleinopathy association, the presence of RBD in patients with dementia could have significant clinical diagnostic as well as pathophysiologic implications (35).

Frontotemporal Dementia (FTD)

No specific sleep disorders have been identified in patients with FTD. Thus, the comments in the previous sections may apply to FTD as well.

Vascular Dementia (VaD)

Although one might expect that OSA is particularly associated with VaD (see earlier) and perhaps even be a cause of VaD in some patients, there is no evidence supporting these contentions. Comments in earlier sections are, therefore, also likely applicable to VaD.

Fatal Familial Insomnia (FFI)

Fatal familial insomnia (FFI) is a familial autosomal dominant prion disorder associated with the D178N mutation and methionine–methionine genotype at codon 129 in the prion protein gene on chromosome 20 (89–91). Since the D178N mutation and valine–valine genotype at codon 129 are associated with familial Creutzfeldt–Jakob disease

(CJD), it appears that the polymorphism at codon 129 confers the topographic distribution of brain pathology and, hence, the clinical features. Specifically, the methionine–methionine genotype at codon 129 of FFI is associated with dorsomedial and anteroventral thalamic dysfunction, whereas the valine–valine genotype of CJD is associated with more generalized cortical involvement. Florid sleep–wake dysregulation and prominent nocturnal insomnia are the clinical hallmarks of FFI.

Although the initial characterization of FFI centered on the insomnia (89,92), the phenotypic variability has expanded greatly to include other features, such as dementia, parkinsonism, ataxia, dysarthria, dysautonomia, hallucinations, and even hypersomnolence (93,94). No gender predilection has been observed. The age of onset has varied from 30 to 70 years and the duration from onset to death has ranged from a few months to almost 4 years (91,94).

PSG reveals severe disruption of the sleep–wake cycle, markedly reduced SWS and REM sleep, markedly reduced sleep efficiency, and limb jerks without periodicity. Some degree of REM sleep without atonia has also been reported (89,95).

Since FFI appears to have incomplete penetrance (91), the disorder should be considered in any patient with a prominent sleep–wake disturbance associated with other cognitive, motor, or autonomic findings regardless of family history. Sporadic cases with fatal insomnia and no identifiable mutation in the prion protein have also been reported (95,96).

Management is symptomatic as no curative treatment exists.

SLEEP DISORDERS AND PARKINSONISM

Overview

The principal degenerative parkinsonian disorders with notable sleep-related issues are Parkinson's disease (PD), MSA, progressive supranuclear palsy (PSP), CBD, and spinocerebellar ataxia type 3 (SCA-3). The Lewy bodies and Lewy neurities of PD, and oligodendroglial inclusions of MSA, are immunoreactive to α-synuclein immunocytochemistry and the disorders are therefore considered "synucleinopathies." The globose neurofibrillary tangles and tufted astrocytes of PSP and astrocytic plaques and oligodendroglial coiled bodies of CBD are immunoreactive to tau immunocytochemistry, and these disorders are therefore considered "tauopathies." SCA-3, also known as Machado–Joseph disease (MJD), is one of the polyglutamine disorders.

In this section, we will briefly review SDB, movement disorders and parasomnias, and insomnia and circadian rhythm disorders as they pertain to patients with parkinsonism, in general. There are far more data on specific sleep disorder–parkinsonian disorder associations, which will be reviewed in more detail.

Sleep-Disordered Breathing and Parkinsonism

There is remarkably little data on the frequency, diagnosis, and management of OSA in PD. Experience at our center has led to observations similar to those noted for patients with OSA and dementia (see earlier), in which many patients tolerate and experience significant functional improvement with CPAP therapy, and many spouses experience less fragmented sleep and less daytime somnolence while their bed partners with parkinsonism use CPAP therapy. For those with positional OSA, it is important for patients to have sufficient mobility (ie, adequate dopaminergic therapy during the night in patients with PD) to roll off their back.

Even less data exists on CSA, central neurogenic hypoventilation, and respiratory dysrhythmias in patients with PD. Management strategies are similar to those described previously.

Most, if not all, patients with nocturnal stridor and parkinsonism have underlying MSA; this association will be discussed below.

Movement Disorders/Parasomnias and Parkinsonism

Restless legs syndrome, periodic limb movements in sleep, REM sleep behavior disorder, as they pertain to the relevant parkinsonian disorders, will be discussed later.

Insomnia/Circadian Dysrhythmias and Parkinsonism

Insomnia can be caused by a primary sleep disorder (e.g., RLS), psychophysiologic and sleep hygiene factors, medications, and from the parkinsonism, with the resulting inability to turn in bed. The frequencies of insomnia and circadian dysrhythmias have not been assessed in detail in the parkinsonian disorders.

Hypersomnia and Parkinsonism

Most data on hypersomnia in parkinsonism relates to PD or as an apparent side effect of dopamine agonists in PD, which will be discussed in the section on PD.

Specific Sleep Disorder—Parkinsonian Disorder Associations

Parkinson's Disease (PD) and Restless Legs Syndrome

One of the most common primary sleep disorders that is experienced by PD patients is restless legs syndrome (RLS). RLS may be more common in PD than age-matched controls (97), although this has not been assessed adequately with current criteria. However, RLS is sufficiently common in an older population for this to be considered carefully in the PD patient with insomnia. PLMs may also be present, sometimes causing sleep fragmentation (98). The management of uncontrolled RLS in PD can be challenging, as most patients are already taking levodopa, often in doses considerably higher than those used to treat RLS. Not uncommonly, this results in the daytime augmentation phenomenon, in which RLS paradoxically worsens during the day. Often a change from levodopa to a dopamine agonist, such as pramipexole or ropinirole, is needed, but this may result in less optimal control of motor symptoms. Alternatively, addition of an opioid, a benzodiazepine or gabapentin before bed may help.

Parkinson's Disease and REM Sleep Behavior Disorder

Numerous PD patients with clinically suspected and PSG-confirmed RBD have been reported (33,37,99–107). In a series of 148 RBD patients, 12.8% had PD (16). In a study of 93 patients with RBD, 57% had underlying neurologic disease and 27% had PD (33). In a questionnaire study of 75 patients with PD, 15% met clinical criteria for PD (105). A study of 33 patients with PD revealed RBD in 11 (33%) (107). Less than one-half would have been diagnosed clinically by relying on the history of a home observer. In addition, eight other patients showed REM sleep without atonia, but no observed dream enactment behavior in the laboratory. Thus, 58% of the patients had motor dyscontrol in REM sleep. Retrospective case series have demonstrated that RBD symptoms often commence before any other symptoms of PD (102). In a series of 25 PD patients with RBD, symptoms of RBD were the initial manifestation of PD in 52% of patients, occurring a median of 3 years earlier (33). A prospective study of 29 male patients older than 50 years with apparently idiopathic RBD, showed that 38% had developed signs of parkinsonism a mean of 3.7 years later (108). Schenck et al. (109) have recently reported on their updated experience in patients with idiopathic RBD, in which 65% have developed parkinsonism and/or dementia. A single patient with RBD and no signs of parkinsonism or dementia was shown at autopsy to have Lewy body disease (83). Two studies using positive emission tomography (PET) and SPECT scans have shown reduced presynaptic dopaminergic activity in the striatum of patients with idiopathic RBD, suggesting that at least some of these patients may have been in an asymptomatic stage of PD (110,111). Management of RBD is similar to that described in the section on DLB.

In an interesting paper, Arnulf et al. (106) investigated the relationship between hallucinations and sleep disorders by performing PSG and MSLT studies in ten patients with PD and visual hallucinations (PD + VH) and ten PD patients without hallucinations (PD − VH) (106). PSG revealed RBD in all PD + VH cases and 6 PD − VH cases. MSLT studies showed approximately one-half in each group had EDS and one or more sleep onset REM periods (SOREMPs) occurred in 80% of the PD + VH patients compared to 20% of the PD − VH patients. Two patients reported hallucinations, which were immediately preceded by REM sleep; delusions were also present in some. The authors conclude that visual hallucinations and delusions in patients with PD may reflect dream imagery and suggest that the psychosis in PD reflects a narcolepsy-like REM sleep disorder (106). Clearly these relationships warrant further study as they have implications for pathophysiology as well as treatment.

Parkinson's Disease and Hypersomnia

Daytime sleepiness is common in PD, but somewhat surprisingly, this does not appear to correlate closely with the severity of parkinsonian symptoms at night. Depression needs always to be considered, as the vegetative symptoms may mimic EDS. However, the major causes are obstructive sleep apnea syndrome (OSAS), the effects of antiparkinsonian medications, and a possible intrinsic disorder of sleepiness linked to PD itself.

Despite respiratory function tests demonstrating upper airway obstruction during wakefulness in PD (112), remarkably little data is available on the prevalence of OSA in PD. In a single study, OSA did not appear to be more common in PD than in controls (113). Nevertheless, OSA is sufficiently common in older patients that a careful history of snoring, snort arousals, and observed apneas should be taken in any sleepy PD patient. If present, management of OSA is similar to that in a patient without PD.

Recent evidence suggests the possibility of an intrinsic disorder of excessive somnolence related to the pathology of PD itself. A community-based study of PD patients showed that 27% complained of daytime sleepiness. Compared to those without sleepiness, somnolence did not appear to be related to nocturnal sleeping complaints or to the use of dopamine agonists. The sleepy patients had more severe parkinsonism, lower cognitive functioning, and more hallucinations (114). An 18-year-old untreated patient with juvenile PD and daytime sleepiness had a mean initial sleep latency on a MSLT of 6.3 minutes with 3/5 sleep onset REM periods (SOREMS), despite adequate nocturnal sleep time and efficiency on PSG (104). The patient did not have cataplexy or hallucinations and was HLA DQB1*0602 negative. PSGs and MSLTs were performed in 27 PD patients on medication (but not pramipexole or ropinerole) (115). The mean sleep latency on MSLT (11.0 minutes) did not differ from age-matched controls, but mean latencies were <5 minutes in 19% of patients. Shorter latencies correlated with higher sleep efficiency and nocturnal TST. One or more SOREM was seen in 22% of patients. The mean MSLT latencies were shorter in this subgroup, the disease duration was longer, and more experienced daytime or nocturnal hallucinations. The use of selegiline, but no other dopaminergic agents, was associated with shorter mean latencies and more SOREMS. As noted above, ten treated PD patients with vivid hallucinations were compared to ten PD patients without hallucinations (106). Six hallucinating patients had mean initial sleep latencies on MSLT <10 minutes compared to five patients without hallucinations. Five hallucinating and one nonhallucinating patient had two or more SOREMS on MSLT. The hallucinating patients with SOREMS had shorter mean sleep latencies. These reports have led to the suggestion that PD may be associated with an intrinsic, narcolepsy-like disorder of sleepiness, more common in patients with more advanced disease.

In 1999, a report appeared describing episodes of sudden, overwhelming sleepiness while driving in seven PD patients treated with pramipexole (1 to 4.5 mg daily) and in one treated with ropinerole (16 mg daily) (116). The episodes ceased after discontinuation or lowering the dose of the agents. No sleep studies were performed. This report led to considerable concern that non-ergot dopamine agonists could cause "sleep attacks." However, other case reports of sleepiness induced by bromocriptine, pergolide, and levodopa indicate that any dopaminergic agent may induce hypersomnolence (117). In a study of 236 PD patients, episodes of sudden, irresistible sleepiness correlated on multivariate analysis with the use of ropinerole and bromocriptine (118). A retrospective chart review of patients receiving pramipexole during a clinical trial showed no significant difference in the frequency of hypersomnia in patients taking the drug compared to placebo. However, in the open-label phase of the study, 38% of 37 patients complained of moderate or severe sleepiness. Two patients underwent MSLT testing; both showed short mean initial sleep latencies that improved after discontinuation of the drug (119). In contrast, no "sleep attacks" were identified in a study of 55 patients and sleepiness measured by the Epworth Sleepiness Scale (ESS) was not associated with any medication, and specifically not with pramipexole (120). A multicenter study of 638 PD patients revealed no correlation between sleepiness and any specific dopaminergic medication. Falling asleep at the wheel, without warning, occurred in only 0.7% of drivers (121). A PSG recorded on a single PD patient with sudden episodes of sleep, but not taking nonergot dopaminergic agents, revealed a rapid transition from wakefulness to stage 2 NREM sleep (122).

The entire notion of "sleep attacks" is controversial; most patients with any cause of sleepiness will experience a prodrome of drowsiness before falling asleep, although this may not always happen. There is little evidence to suggest that the sleepiness induced by dopaminergic agents is different from that caused by other problems, such as OSAS (117). Dopamine is generally associated with arousal, and the mechanism of paradoxical drowsiness is unknown. Down-regulation of dopaminergic input has been suggested (116). The frequency of drug-induced sleepiness in PD is unknown; careful, large studies excluding other causes of hypersomnolence will be needed.

A recent study showed that sleepiness in a large cohort of PD patients correlated with L-dopa dose, the use of agonists, and disease severity (123). However, together, these three factors accounted for only 9% of the sleepiness, suggesting the presence of other, as yet undetermined factors.

Other causes of sleepiness should be considered before deciding that it is due to medication or the disease itself. While larger studies are awaited, dopaminergic agents should be used at the lowest effective dose, patients should be warned about this potential side effect before commencing treatment, and questions about sleepiness should be routinely asked at return visits. Should sleepiness develop, the dose should be reduced, other causes sought, and driving restricted until the problem is elucidated (117). Stimulant therapy with modafinil or classic stimulants, such as methylphenidate, should be considered if hypersomnolence persists (124). A recent placebo-controlled trial of sleepy PD patients showed significant decreases in the ESS with modafinil, but no change in the maintenance of wakefulness test (125).

Multiple System Atrophy (MSA) and Nocturnal Stridor

The most characteristic respiratory sleep disorder in MSA is nocturnal stridor. Nocturnal stridor was noted to be present in 13% of 203 pathologically proved cases of MSA (126), but the actual frequency may be higher. It may present at any stage of the disease and occasionally be the presenting feature (127). The patient's sleeping partner will describe a strained, high-pitched, harsh inspiratory sound, and will often be able to distinguish it from previously noted snoring. Sometimes stridor may also be present during wakefulness. Awake laryngoscopy may be normal, but sometimes shows restriction of abduction of the cords, paradoxical movement, and eventually complete paramedian fixation with markedly reduced size of the aperture. Occasionally only one cord is involved initially, with later progression to both (128).

The pathogenesis of the symptom is controversial and both peripheral and central factors may play a role. Abduction of the cords is caused by contraction of the posterior cricoarytenoid (PCA) muscles innervated by branches of the recurrent laryngeal nerves, whose nuclei are found in nucleus ambiguus in the medulla. Pathologic studies of the PCA muscles in MSA with stridor have yielded contradictory results. Definite neurogenic atrophy was found in two out of three cases in one series (129), neither of two in a second (130), and in all six in a third (131). The recurrent laryngeal nerve has been reported as normal in one case (130), has revealed axonal loss in one of two cases (129), and reduced fiber count in six cases compared to controls (131). Loss of neurons in the caudal two-thirds of nucleus ambiguus has been reported in three cases (132,133), while the nucleus was reported as normal in two other cases (129). However, surface (134) and wire electrode (135)

recordings during sleep of the PCA, as well as the adductor thyroarytenoid (TA) and cricothyroid (CT) muscles, have shown paradoxical activity in the TA and CT muscles during stridorous inspiration. Merlo et al. (136) used concentric needle electrodes to study seven patients with MSA and stridor and found no denervation changes but tonic electromyographic (EMG) activity suggestive of dystonia in the TA and PCA muscles (136). These studies suggest a possible central cause, with abnormally enhanced adduction as a contributory factor.

Because some patients with vocal cord dysfunction die in their sleep (137–140), tracheostomy has been the standard recommended treatment (128,140). In one study (132), five of eight patients with vocal cord paralysis, who did not undergo tracheostomy, died suddenly, with a mean of 1.1 years after diagnosis, while 9 of 11 patients who underwent tracheostomy were alive a maximum of 5 years later. In a study of 30 patients, those with stridor had a significantly shorter survival from the time of the sleep evaluation (137). Nine of eleven with stridor died a median of 1.8 years after the sleep evaluation. Tracheostomy had been performed in both survivors. However, tracheostomy did not entirely prevent death, as two of four patients with tracheostomy died; both 1 year after presentation. One was noted to be hypoxemic and the other hypercapnic on presentation. Six of 19 patients without stridor died, 2 from pneumonia and 3 from respiratory failure—a mean of 2.4 years after presentation.

A recommendation to perform tracheostomy is tempered by the experiences that many patients, unaware themselves of stridor, are unconvinced of its necessity and fear it will result in decreasing QoL. Nasal continuous positive airway pressure (nCPAP) has been used with variable results; in three patients, stridor was eliminated without recurrence after 6 months (141), but in another study all five patients treated with nCPAP died (137). A single study of unilateral injection of botulinum toxin into the thyroarytenoid muscle reported improvement of the stridor and reduction in tonic EMG activity in the muscle 1 month later in three of four patients (136). In the absence of prospective studies, we recommend that a PSG be performed if stridor or OSA are suspected. If stridor is present, tracheostomy should be strongly considered, especially if the vocal cords move abnormally on laryngoscopy or daytime stridor is heard. If the patent declines tracheostomy, nCPAP should be used at a pressure that eliminates stridor. However, care should be taken to ensure as near perfect compliance as possible and that stridor does not recur. The possibility of centrally mediated nocturnal hypoventilation developing should also be kept in mind.

Obstructive and central sleep apnea syndrome (137,142,143), central neurogenic hypoventilation, and respiratory dysrhythmias are also important components of MSA. Periodic breathing in the erect position, Cheyne–Stokes breathing, apneustic breathing (138), cluster breathing (144), and irregular breathing (145) have been reported. Alveolar hypoventilation, resulting in hypercapnic respiratory failure during sleep, and sometimes wakefulness, occurs in some patients and may be the cause of death (131,146). A blunted CO_2 response curve has been reported (140). Pathologic involvement of the neuronal circuitry in the pons and medulla controlling respiration is presumed to underlie these abnormalities.

Multiple System Atrophy and REM Sleep Behavior Disorder

Numerous cases of RBD plus MSA have been described (33,101,103,137,142,143,147–152), and three cases of autopsy-confirmed MSA have been reported (78,82). Although the incidence and prevalence of RBD in MSA is not known, RBD does appear to be present in most MSA patients. In a series of 21 consecutive cases not referred specifically for sleep symptoms, REM sleep without atonia was found in 20 of 21 (95%) with abnormal motor behavior recorded in the laboratory in 19 patients (90%) (143). Of 39 consecutive patients with MSA, 33 referred for neurologic and 6 for sleep symptoms, relatives reported agitated sleep talking or motor behavior in 27 (69%), whereas 35 (90%) had increased muscle tone in REM sleep (142). RBD can occur in both male and female RBD patients, in contrast to PD patients with RBD who are predominantly male (33,142). As in PD, RBD symptoms may be the initial manifestation of MSA (33,142). The presence of RBD has been used to predict the presence of MSA in patients presenting with autonomic failure (153).

Management of RBD in MSA patients is similar to that in other neurodegenerative disorders, with an important caveat. While clonazepam is certainly effective for most patients with RBD, it should probably not be used in patients with autonomic respiratory instability or untreated stridor, and only with caution in patients with gait disturbances due to ataxia or parkinsonism.

Progressive Supranuclear Palsy

Progressive supranuclear palsy (PSP) is a neurodegenerative disorder characterized by a rigid akinetic parkinsonian syndrome with prominent axial rigidity and lack of responsiveness to levodopa, early gait instability with falls, supranuclear (especially downward) vertical gaze palsies, pseudobulbar palsy, and frontal cognitive features.

Sleep disturbances appear to be an integral part of PSP, but the frequency of sleep complaints is uncertain. A questionnaire study of 437 patients with a clinical diagnosis of PSP revealed that 50% of patients more than 3 years after diagnosis reported changed sleeping patterns or difficulty sleeping (154).

A number of studies have shown consistent abnormalities in sleep architecture. A PSG study of six PSP patients compared with age- and sex-matched controls revealed decreased TST, decreased sleep efficiency (mean 50.9%),

increased WASO, and increased percentage of stage 1 sleep. The percentage of REM sleep was decreased with decreased REM period duration (155). The PSGs of ten PSP patients were compared to published norms, also showing decreased TST, decreased percentage sleep efficiency (mean 58%), increased WASO, decreased percentage REM sleep, and decreased REM period duration. Percentage of stage 2 sleep was increased (156). A characteristic feature is the reduction in abundance and amplitude of sleep spindles (155,156).

The question whether RBD occurs in PSP is of interest, both in view of its high frequency in PD and MSA, and the abnormalities in REM sleep architecture and in brainstem nuclei noted in PSP. PSG-confirmed RBD has been reported in only two cases of clinically diagnosed PSP (33,157), suggesting that it is a rare phenomenon. The EMG tone in REM sleep appeared to be normal in an EEG study of four patients (158). Montplaisir et al. (155) found that phasic EMG tone comprised 3% and atonia 99.2% of REM time in six patients, findings not significantly different from those of age- and sex-matched controls. The apparent rarity of motor disturbances of REM sleep in PSP is puzzling. It has been postulated that REM sleep without atonia may be a common feature of the alpha-synucleinopathies, but rare in the tauopathies (34).

Nocturnal respiratory disturbances do not appear to be common in PSP. In an oximetry study of 11 patients, infrequent decreases of 4% or more in oxyhemoglobin saturation were noted in three patients, but all were at a frequency of less than 4 per hour (159). Aldrich et al. (156) noted 2 of 10 patients had sleep apneas, 1 predominantly central and 1 predominantly obstructive. PLMs have been reported in 2 of 10 patients (156).

The pathophysiology of the sleep disturbances is presumably linked to the extensive brainstem pathology. The profound sleep maintenance insomnia noted in PSP could be due to immobility, but appears to be more severe than that seen in patients with similar neurodegenerative illnesses, such as PD (156). Involvement of the locus ceruleus or other pontomesencephalic nuclei may play a role. The reduction in spindle density and amplitude may be related to interruption of pontine tegmental connections to the thalamic nucleus reticularis. The decrease in REM time could also be due to involvement of REM-generating systems in the pontine tegmentum, including the pedunculopontine nuclei.

Corticobasal Degeneration

Corticobasal degeneration (CBD) is a neurodegenerative disorder characterized by progressive asymmetric rigidity and apraxia associated with other findings reflecting cortical (e.g., alien limb phenomenon, cortical sensory loss, myoclonus) and basal ganglia (e.g., dystonia, tremor) dysfunction (160).

Few sleep-related issues have been reported in CBD. Although REM sleep without atonia (considered by some as "subclinical RBD") has been reported in CBD (161), clinical RBD appears uncommon if present at all (34,35,82). Unilateral PLMs during sleep have been reported (162). In our experience, OSA, RLS, and PLMs occur with some frequency in CBD, and many patients benefit from therapy. Nasal CPAP therapy can be challenging to use, however, due to the significant apraxia characteristic of the disease and associated difficulties with manipulating the headgear.

Spinocerebellar Ataxia 3/Machado–Joseph Disease

The spinocerebellar ataxias (SCA) are a group of neurologic disorders that can be subclassified into the polyglutamine disorders, the channelopathies, and the gene expression disorders (163). SCA-3, otherwise known as Machado–Joseph disease (MJD), is caused by a polyglutamine expansion on chromosome 14q21, and a wide spectrum of clinical manifestations has been observed (163).

SCA-3 is the only SCA that has been associated with any sleep disorder. REM sleep behavior disorder has been noted in SCA-3 patients (164–166), suggesting that RBD is not entirely specific to the synucleinopathies. The SCA-3 gene has been implicated in the pathogenesis of RLS (167). Management of RBD and RLS is similar to that in other disorders.

REFERENCES

1. Boeve B, Silber M, Ferman T. Current management of sleep disturbances in dementia. *Cur Neurol Neurosci Rep.* 2001;2:169–177.
2. Ancoli-Israel S, Kripke D, Klauber M, et al. Sleep-disordered breathing in community-dwelling elderly. *Sleep.* 1991;14:486–495.
3. Ancoli-Israel S, Klauber M, Butters N, et al. Dementia in the institutionalized elderly: relation to sleep apnea. *J Amer Geriat Soc.* 1991;39:258–263.
4. Bliwise D, Yesavage J, Tinklenberg J, et al. Sleep apnea in Alzheimer's disease. *Neurobiol Aging.* 1989;10:343–346.
5. Bliwise D. Sleep apnea, dementia, and Alzheimer's disease: a minireview. *Bull Clin Neurosci.* 1989;54:123–126.
6. Bliwise D. Cognitive function and sleep disordered breathing in aging adults. In: Sleep and respiration in aging adults: Proceedings of the Second International Symposium on Sleep and Respiration; League City, Texas: Elsevier, 1991.
7. Bliwise D. Is sleep apnea a cause of reversible dementia in old age? *J Amer Geriatr Soc.* 1996;44:1407–1408.
8. Hoch C, Reynolds C, Kupfer D, et al. Sleep-disordered breathing in normal and pathologic aging. *J Clin Psych.* 1986;47:499–503.
9. Pond C, Mant A, Eyand E, et al. Dementia and abnormal breathing during sleep. *Age Ageing.* 1990;19:247–252.
10. Siebler M, Daffertshofer M, Hennerici M, et al. Cerebral blood flow velocity alterations during obstructive sleep apnea syndrome. *Neurology.* 1990;40:1461–1462.
11. Hayakawa T, Terashima M, Kayukawa Y, et al. Changes in cerebral oxygenation and hemodynamics during obstructive sleep apneas. *Chest.* 1996;109:916–921.
12. Engelman H, Martin S, Deary J, et al. Effect of continuous positive airway pressure treatment on daytime function in sleep apnea/hypopnea syndrome. *Lancet.* 1994;343:572–575.
13. Engelman H, Kingshott R, Wraith P, et al. Randomized placebo-controlled crossover trial of continuous positive airway pressure for mild sleep apnea/hypopnea syndrome. *Amer J Respir Crit Care Med.* 1999;159:461–467.
14. Ferguson K, Ono T, Lowe A, et al. A randomized crossover study of an oral appliance vs nasal continuous positive airway pressure in the treatment of mild-moderate obstructive sleep apnea. *Chest.* 1996;109:1269–1275.
15. Borak J, Cieslicki J, Koziej M, et al. Effect of CPAP treatment on psychological status in patients with severe obstructive sleep apnea. *J Sleep Res.* 1996;5:123–127.
16. Grenberg G, Watson R, Deptula D. Neuropsychological dysfunction in sleep apnea. *Sleep.* 1987;10:254–362.
17. Jenkinson C, Stradling J, Petersen S. Comparison of three measures of quality of life outcome in the evaluation of continuous positive airway pressure for sleep apnea. *J Sleep Res.* 1997:199–204.
18. Jenkinson C, Davies R, Mullins R, et al. Comparison of therapeutic and subtherapeutic nasal continuous positive airway pressure for obstructive sleep apnea: a randomized prospective parallel trial. *Lancet.* 1999;353:2100–2105.
19. Kullen A, Stepnowsky C, Parker L, et al. Cognitive impairment and sleep disordered breathing. *Sleep Res.* 1993;22:224.
20. Montplaisir J, Bedard M, Richer F, et al. Neurobehavioral manifestations in obstructive sleep apnea syndrome before and after treatment with continuous positive airway pressure. *Sleep.* 1992;15:517–519.
21. Redline S, Adams N, Strauss M, et al. Improvement of mild sleep disordered breathing with CPAP compared with conservative therapy. *Amer J Respir Crit Care Med.* 1998;157:858–865.
22. Weaver T, Chugh D, Maislin G, et al. Changes in functional status after 3 months of CPAP treatment. *Amer J Respir Crit Care Med.* 1998;157:A53.
23. Kribbs N, Pack A, Kline L, et al. Effects of one night without nasal CPAP treatment on sleep and sleepiness in patients with obstructive sleep apnea. *Amer Rev Respir Dis.* 1993;147:1162–1168.
24. Bedard M, Montplaisir J, Malo J, et al. Persistent neuropsychological deficits and vigilance impairment in sleep apnea syndrome after treatment with continuous positive airway pressure (CPAP). *J Clin Exp Neuropsychol.* 1993;15:330–341.
25. Munoz X, Marti S, Sumalla J, et al. Acute delirium as a manifestation of obstructive sleep apnea syndrome. *Amer J Resp Crit Care Med.* 1998;158:1306–1307.
26. Lee J. Recurrent delirium associated with obstructive sleep apnea. *Gen Hosp Psych.* 1998;20:120–122.
27. Scheltens P, Visscher F, Van Keimpema A, et al. Sleep apnea syndrome presenting with cognitive impairment. *Neurology.* 1991;41:155–156.
28. Beninati W, Harris C, Herold D, et al. The effect of snoring and obstructive sleep apnea on the sleep quality of bed partners. *Mayo Clin Proc.* 1999;74:955–958.
29. Rothdach A, Trenkwalder C, Haberstock J, et al. Prevalence and risk factors of RLS in an elderly population: The MEMO Study. *Neurology.* 2000;54:1064–1068.
30. Sun E, Chen C, Ho G, et al. Iron and the restless legs syndrome. *Sleep.* 1998;21:371–377.
31. Ancoli-Israel S, Kripke D, Klauber M, et al. Periodic limb movements in sleep in community-dwelling elderly. *Sleep.* 1991;14:496–500.
32. Schenck C, Mahowald M. REM sleep behavior disorder: clinical, developmental, and neuroscience perspectives 16 years after its formal identification in SLEEP. *Sleep.* 2002;25:120–138.
33. Olson E, Boeve B, Silber M. Rapid eye movement sleep behavior disorder: demographic, clinical, and laboratory findings in 93 cases. *Brain.* 2000;123:331–339.
34. Boeve BF, Silber MH, Ferman TJ, et al. Association of REM sleep behavior disorder and neurodegenerative disease may reflect an underlying synucleinopathy. *Mov Disord.* 2001;16(4):622–630.
35. Boeve B, Silber M, Ferman T, et al. REM sleep behavior disorder in Parkinson's disease, dementia with Lewy bodies, and multiple system atrophy. In: Bedard M, Agid Y, Chouinard S, Fahn S, Korczyn A, Lesperance P, eds. *Mental and behavioral dysfunction in movement disorders.* Totowa, NJ: Human Press, 2003:383–397.
36. Schenck C, Mahowald M. A polysomnographic, neurologic, psychiatric and clinical outcome report on 70 consecutive cases

with REM sleep behavior disorder (RBD): sustained clonazepam efficacy in 89.5% of 57 treated patients. *Cleveland Clin J Med.* 1990;57(Suppl.):10–24.

37. Kunz D, Bes F. Melatonin as a therapy in REM sleep behavior disorder patients: An open-labeled pilot study on the possible influence of melatonin on REM-sleep regulation. *Mov Disord.* 1999;14:507–511.

38. Takeuchi N, Uchimura N, Hashizume Y, et al. Melatonin therapy for REM sleep behavior disorder. *Psych Clin Neurosci.* 2001;55:267–269.

39. Boeve B, Silber M, Ferman T. Melatonin for treatment of REM sleep behavior disorder in neurologic disorders: results in 14 patients. *Sleep Med.* 2003;4:281–284.

40. Ringman J, Simmons J. Treatment of REM sleep behavior disorder with donepezil: a report of three cases. *Neurology.* 2000;55:870–871.

41. Bamford C. Carbamazepine in REM sleep behavior disorder. *Sleep.* 1993;16:33–34.

42. Swearer J, Drachman D, O'Donnell B, et al. Troublesome and disruptive behaviors in dementia. *J Amer Geriat Soc.* 1988;36:784–790.

43. Vitiello M, Prinz P. Alzheimer's disease: sleep and sleep/wake patterns. *Clin geriat med.* Philadelphia: W.B. Saunders, 1989.

44. Vitiello M, Bliwise D, Prinz P. Sleep in Alzheimer's disease and the sundown syndrome. *Neurology.* 1992;42 (Suppl. 6):83–94.

45. Vitiello M, Prinz P, Williams D, et al. Sleep disturbances in patients with mild stage Alzheimer's disease. *J Gerontol.* 1990;45:M131–M138.

46. Prinz P, Vitaliano P, Vitiello M, et al. Sleep, EEG and mental function changes in senile dementia of the Alzheimer type. *Neurobiol Aging.* 1982;3:361–370.

47. Pollack C, Perlick D, Linser J, et al. Sleep problems in community elderly as predictors of death and nursing home placement. *J Community Health.* 1990;15:123–125.

48. Little J, Satlin A, Sunderland T, et al. Sundown syndrome in severely demented patients with probable Alzheimer's disease. *J Geriatr Psych Neurol.* 1995;8:103–106.

49. Severson MA, Smith GE, Tangalos EG, et al. Patterns and predictors of institutionalization in community-based dementia patients. *J Amer Geriatr Soc.* 1994;42(2):181–185.

50. Smith G, Tangalos E, Ivnik R, et al. Tolerance weighted frequency indices for non-cognitive symptoms of dementia. *Amer J Alzheimer Dis.* 1995:2–10.

51. Carlson D, Fleming K, Smith G, et al. Management of dementia-related behavioral disturbances: a nonpharmacologic approach. *Mayo Clin Proc.* 1995;70:1108–1115.

52. Reynolds C, Kupfer D, Hoch C, et al. Sleeping pills in the elderly: Are they ever justified? *J Clin Psych.* 1985;46:9–12.

53. Bliwise D, Carroll J, Lee K, et al. Sleep and "sundowning" in nursing home patients with dementia. *Psych Res.* 1993;48:277–292.

54. Ancoli-Israel S, Klauber M, Jones D, et al. Variations in circadian rhythms of activity, sleep, and light exposure related to dementia in nursing-home patients. *Sleep.* 1997;20:18–23.

55. Czeisler C, Dumont M, Duffy J, et al. Association of sleep–wake habits in older people with changes in output of circadian pacemaker. *Lancet.* 1992;340:933–936.

56. Swaab D, Fliers E, Partman T. The suprachiasmatic nucleus of the human brain in relation to sex, age and senile dementia. *Brain Res.* 1985;342:37–44.

57. Sack R, Lewy A, Erb D, et al. Human melatonin production declines with age. *J Pineal Res.* 1986;3:379–388.

58. Stopa E, Volicer L, Kuo-Leblanc V, et al. Pathologic evaluation of the human suprachiasmatic nucleus in severe dementia. *J Neuropathol Exp Neurol.* 1999;58:29–39.

59. Singer C, MacArthur A, Hughes R, et al. High dose melatonin and sleep in the elderly. *Sleep Res.* 1995;24A:151.

60. Brusco LI, Fainstein I, Marquez M, et al. Effect of melatonin in selected populations of sleep-disturbed patients. *Biol Signals Receptors.* 1999;8(1–2):126–131.

61. Hozumi S, Okawa M, Mishima K, et al. Phototherapy for elderly patients with dementia and sleep–wake rhythm disorders—A comparison between morning and evening light exposure. *Japan J Psych Neurol.* 1990;44:813–814.

62. Lyketsos C, Lindell Veiel L, Baker A, et al. A randomized, controlled trial of bright light therapy for agitated behaviors in dementia patients residing in long-term care. *Intern J Geriatr Psych.* 1999;14:520–525.

63. Satlin A, Volicer L, Ross V, et al. Bright light treatment of behavioral and sleep disturbances in patients with Alheimer's disease. *Amer J Psych.* 1992;149:1028–1032.

64. Van Someren E, Kessler A, Mirmiran M, et al. Indirect bright light improves circadian rest-activity rhythm disturbances in demented patients. *Biol Psych.* 1997;41:955–963.

65. Gurian B, Rosowsky E. Low-dose methylphenidate in the very old. *J Geriatr Psych. Neurol.* 1990;3:152–154.

66. Boeve B, Krahn L, Silber M, et al. Normal CSF hypocretin-1 levels in autopsy-proven Alzheimer's disease +/− Lewy body disease. *Neurology.* 2003;60:A34.

67. Singer C, Tractenberg R, Kaye J, et al. A multicenter, placebo-controlled trial of melatonin for sleep disturbance in Alzheimer's disease. *Sleep.* 2003;26:893–901.

68. Ferman T, Boeve B, Silber M, et al. Hallucinations and delusions associated with the REM sleep behavior disorder/dementia syndrome. *J Neuropsych Clin Neurosci.* 1997;9:692.

69. Boeve B, Silber M, Petersen R, et al. REM sleep behavior disorderand degenerative dementia with or without parkinsonism: A syndrome predictive of Lewy body disease? *Neurology.* 1997;48 (Suppl. 2):358–359.

70. Silber M, Boeve B, Petersen R, et al. REM sleep behavior disorder and dementia: a syndrome possibly predictive of Lewy body disease. *Sleep.* 1998;21:196.

71. Boeve BF, Silber MH, Ferman TJ, et al. REM sleep behavior disorder and degenerative dementia: an association likely reflecting Lewy body disease. *Neurology.* 1998;51(2):363–370.

72. Ferman TJ, Boeve BF, Smith GE, et al. The REM sleep behavior disorder/dementia syndrome: neuropsychological differences when compared to Alzheimer's disease. *Neurology.* 1998;50(Suppl. 4):A282.

73. Boeve BF, Silber MH, Ferman TJ, et al. Further data supporting underlying Lewy body disease in the RBD/dementia syndrome. *Neurobiol Aging.* 1998;19:S205.

74. Ferman TJ, Boeve BF, Smith GE, et al. RBD/dementia syndrome: a non-Alzheimer dementia. *Clin Neuropsychol.* 1998;12:257.

75. Ferman TJ, Boeve BF, Smith GE, et al. REM sleep behavior disorder and dementia: cognitive differences when compared with AD. *Neurology.* 1999;52(5):951–957.

76. Boeve B, Silber M, Ferman T, et al. Association of REM sleep behavior disorder and neurodegenerative disease. *Sleep.* 1999;22(Suppl. 1):S72.

77. Boeve B, Silber M, Ferman T, et al. Association of REM sleep behavior disorder and neurodegenerative disease may reflect an underlying synucleinopathy. *Mov Disord.* 2000;15:227–228.

78. Boeve B, Silber M, Ferman T, et al. Association of REM sleep behavior disorder and neurodegenerative disease may reflect an underlying synucleinopathy. *Mov Disord.* 2001;16:622–630.

79. McKeith IG, Perry EK, Perry RH. Report of the second dementia with Lewy body international workshop: diagnosis and treatment. Consortium on Dementia with Lewy Bodies. *Neurology.* 1999;53(5):902–905.

80. McKeith IG, Galasko D, Kosaka K, et al. Consensus guidelines for the clinical and pathologic diagnosis of dementia with Lewy bodies (DLB): report of the consortium on DLB international workshop. *Neurology.* 1996;47(5):1113–1124.

81. Ferman T, Boeve B, Smith G, et al. Dementia with Lewy bodies may present as dementia with REM sleep behavior disorder without parkinsonism or hallucinations. *J Internat Neuropsychol Soc.* 2002;8:907–914.

82. Boeve B, Silber M, Parisi J, et al. Synucleinopathy pathology and REM sleep behavior disorder plus dementia or parkinsonism. *Neurology.* 2003: in press.

83. Uchiyama M, Isse K, Tanaka K, et al. Incidental Lewy body disease in a patient with REM sleep behavior disorder. *Neurology.* 1995;45:709–712.

84. Schenck CH, Garcia-Rill E, Skinner RD, et al. A case of REM sleep behavior disorder with autopsy-confirmed Alzheimer's disease: Postmortem brain stem histochemical analyses. *Biol Psych.* 1996;40(5):422–425.

85. Schenck CH, Mahowald MW, Anderson ML, et al. Lewy body variant of Alzheimer's disease (AD) identified by postmortem ubiquitin

staining in a previously reported case of AD associated with REM sleep behavior disorder [letter]. *Biol Psych.* 1997;42(6):527–528.

86. Turner RS, Chervin RD, Frey KA, et al. Probable diffuse Lewy body disease presenting as REM sleep behavior disorder. *Neurology.* 1997;49(2):523–527.

87. Turner R, D'Amato C, Chervin R, et al. The pathology of REM sleep behavior disorder with comorbid Lewy body dementia. *Neurology.* 2000;55:1730–1732.

88. Boeve B, Silber M, Parisi J, et al. Neuropathologic findings in patients with REM sleep behavior disorder and a neurodegenerative disorder. *Neurology.* 2001;56:A299.

89. Lugaresi E, Medori R, Montagna P, et al. Fatal familial insomnia and dysautonomia with selective degeneration of thalamic nuclei. *N Engl J Med.* 1986;315(16):997–1003.

90. Lugaresi E, Tobler I, Gambetti P, et al. The pathophysiology of fatal familial insomnia. *Brain Pathol.* 1998;8(3):521–526.

91. Collins S, McLean CA, Masters CL. Gerstmann–Straussler–Scheinker syndrome, fatal familial insomnia, and kuru: a review of these less common human transmissible spongiform encephalopathies. *J Clin Neurosci.* 2001;8(5):387–397.

92. Manetto V, Medori R, Cortelli P, et al. Fatal familial insomnia: Clinical and pathologic study of five new cases. *Neurology.* 1992;42(2):312–319.

93. Harder A, Jendroska K, Kreuz F, et al. Novel twelve-generation kindred of fatal familial insomnia from Germany representing the entire spectrum of disease expression. *Amer J Med Genet.* 1999;87(4):311–316.

94. Kovacs GG, Trabattoni G, Hainfellner JA, et al. Mutations of the prion protein gene phenotypic spectrum. *J Neurol.* 2002; 249(11):1567–1582.

95. Scaravilli F, Cordery RJ, Kretzschmar H, et al. Sporadic fatal insomnia: a case study. *Ann Neurol.* 2000;48(4):665–668.

96. Parchi P, Capellari S, Chin S, et al. A subtype of sporadic prion disease mimicking fatal familial insomnia. *Neurology.* 1999; 52(9):1757–1763.

97. Menza MA, Rosen RC. Sleep in Parkinson's disease: the role of depression and anxiety. *Psychosomatics.* 1995;36:262–266.

98. Wetter TC, Collado-Seidel V, Pollmacher T, et al. Sleep and periodic leg movement patterns in drug-free patients with Parkinson's disease and multiple system atrophy. *Sleep.* 2000;23(3):361–367.

99. Silber M, Ahlskog J. REM sleep behavior disorder in parkinsonian syndromes. *Sleep Res.* 1992;21:313.

100. Silber M, Dexter D, Ahlskog J, et al. Abnormal REM sleep motor activity in untreated Parkinson's disease. *Sleep Res.* 1993;22:274.

101. Schenck CH, Bundlie SR, Ettinger MG, et al. Chronic behavioral disorders of human REM sleep: a new category of parasomnia. *Sleep.* 1986;9(2):293–308.

102. Tan A, Salgado M, Fahn S. Rapid eye movement sleep behavior disorder preceding Parkinson's disease with therapeutic response to levodopa. *Mov Disord.* 1996;11:214–216.

103. Sforza E, Krieger J, Petiau C. REM sleep behavior disorder: clinical and physiopathological findings. *Sleep Med Rev.* 1997;1:57–69.

104. Rye D, Johnston L, Watts R, et al. Juvenile Parkinson's disease with REM sleep behavior disorder, sleepiness, and daytime REM onset. *Neurology.* 1999;53:1868–1872.

105. Comella C, Nardine T, Diederich N, et al. Sleep-related violence, injury, and REM sleep behavior disorder in Parkinson's disease. *Neurology.* 1998;51:526–529.

106. Arnulf I, Bonnet AM, Damier P, et al. Hallucinations, REM sleep, and Parkinson's disease: a medical hypothesis. *Neurology.* 2000;55(2):281–288.

107. Gagnon J-F, Medard M-A, Fantini M, et al. REM sleep behavior disorder and REM sleep without atonia in Parkinson's disease. *Neurology.* 2002;59:585–589.

108. Schenck CH, Bundlie SR, Mahowald MW. Delayed emergence of a parkinsonian disorder in 38% of 29 older men initially diagnosed with idiopathic rapid eye movement sleep behaviour disorder. *Neurology.* 1996;46(2):388–393.

109. Schenck C, Bundlie S, Mahowald M. REM behavior disorder (RBD): delayed emergence of parkinsonism and/or dementia in 65% of older men initially diagnosed with idiopathic RBD, and an analysis of the minimum and maximum tonic and/or phasic electromyographic abnormalities found during REM sleep. *Sleep.* 2003;26:A316.

110. Eisensehr I, Linke R, Noachtar S, et al. Reduced striatal dopamine transporters in idiopathic rapid eye movement sleep behaviour disorder: comparison with Parkinson's disease and controls. *Brain.* 2000;123:1155–1160.

111. Albin R, Koeppe R, Chervin R, et al. Decreased striatal dopaminergic innervation in REM sleep behavior disorder. *Neurology.* 2000;55:1410–1412.

112. Hovestadt A, Bogaard JM, Meerwaldt JD, et al. Pulmonary function in Parkinson's disease. *J Neurol Neurosurg Psych.* 1989;52:329–333.

113. Apps MCP, Sheaff PC, Ingram DA, et al. Respiration and sleep in Parkinson's disease. *J Neurol Neurosurg Psych.* 1989;48:1240–1245.

114. Tandberg E, Larsen JP, Karlsen K. Excessive daytime sleepiness and sleep benefit in Parkinson's disease: a community-based study. *Mov Disord.* 1999;14(6):922–927.

115. Rye DB, Bliwise DL, Dihenia B, et al. Daytime sleepiness in Parkinson's disease. *J Sleep Res.* 2000;9(1):63–69.

116. Frucht S, Rogers JD, Greene PE, et al. Falling asleep at the wheel: Motor vehicle mishaps in persons taking pramipexole and ropinirole. *Neurology.* 1999;52(9):1908–1910.

117. Olanow CW, Schapira AH, Roth T. Waking up to sleep episodes in Parkinson's disease. *Mov Disord.* 2000;15(2):212–215.

118. Montastruc JL, Brefel-Courbon C, Senard JM, et al. Sleep attacks and antiparkinsonian drugs: a pilot prospective pharmacoepidemiologic study. *Clin Neuropharmacol.* 2001;24(3):181–183.

119. Hauser RA, Gauger L, Anderson WM, et al. Pramipexole-induced somnolence and episodes of daytime sleep. *Mov Disord.* 2000; 15(4):658–663.

120. Tracik F, Ebersbach G. Sudden daytime sleep onset in parkinson's disease: polysomnographic recordings. *Mov Disord.* 2001; 16(3):500–506.

121. Hobson DE, Lang AE, Martin WRW, et al. Excessive daytime sleepiness and sudden-onset sleep in Parkinson disease. A survey by the Canadian Movement Disorders Group. *JAMA.* 2002;287:455–463.

122. Pal S, Bhattacharya KF, Agapito C, et al. A study of excessive daytime sleepiness and its clincial significance in three groups of Parkinson's disease patients taking pramipexole, cabergoline and levodopa mono and combination therapy. *J Neural Transmission.* 2001;198:71–77.

123. O'Suilleabhain PE, Dewey RBJ. Contributions of dopaminergic drugs and disease severity to daytime sleepiness in Parkinson disease. *Arch Neurol.* 2002;59:986–989.

124. Adler CH, Caviness JN, Hentz JG, et al. Modafinil for the treatment of excessive daytime sleepiness in patients with Parkinson's disease. *Neurology.* 2001;56:A308.

125. Hogl B, Saletu M, Brandauer E, et al. Modafinil for the treatment of daytime sleepiness in Parkinson's disease: a double-blind, randomized, crossover, placebo-controlled polygraphic trial. *Sleep.* 2002;25:905–909.

126. Wenning G, Shlomo T, Magelhaes M, et al. Clinical features and natural history of multiple system atrophy: an analysis of 100 cases. *Brain.* 1994;117:835–845.

127. Martinovits G, Leventon G, Goldhammer Y, et al. Vocal cord paralysis as a presenting sign in the Shy-Drager syndrome. *J Laryngol Otol.* 1988;102(3):280–281.

128. Williams A, Hanson D, Calne DB. Vocal cord paralysis in the Shy-Drager syndrome. *J Neurol Neurosurg Psych.* 1979;42(2):151–153.

129. Bannister R, Gibson W, Michaels L, et al. Laryngeal abductor paralysis in multiple system atrophy. A report on three necropsied cases, with observations on the laryngeal muscles and the nuclei ambigui. *Brain.* 1981;104(2):351–368.

130. DeReuck J, Van Landegem W. The posterior crico-arytenoid muscle in two cases of Shy-Drager syndrome with laryngeal stridor. Comparison of the histological, histochemical and biometric findings. *J Neurol.* 1987;234(3):187–190.

131. Hayashi M, Isozaki E, Oda M, et al. Loss of large myelinated nerve fibres of the recurrent laryngeal nerve in patients with multiple system atrophy and vocal cord palsy. *J Neurol Neurosurg Psych.* 1997;62:234–238.

132. Isozaki E, Miyamoto K, Osanai R, et al. Clinical studies of 23 patients with multiple system atrophy presenting with vocal cord paralysis. *Clin Neurol.* 1991;31:249–254.

133. Lapresle J, Annabi A. Olivopontocerebellar atrophy with velopharyngeal paralysis: a contribution to the somatopy of the nucleus ambiguus. *J Neuropathol Exp Neurol.* 1979;38:401–406.

134. Isozaki R, Osanai R, Horiguchi S, et al. Laryngeal electromyography with separated surface electrodes in patients with multiple system atrophy presenting with vocal cord paralysis. *J Neurol.* 1994;241:551–556.

135. Plazzi G, Provini F, Montagna P. Video-polygraphic recording of sleep-related stridor. *Sleep Res.* 1996;25:439.

136. Merlo IM, Occhini A, Pacchetti C, et al. Not paralysis, but dystonia causes stridor in multiple system atrophy. *Neurology.* 2002;58:649–652.

137. Silber M, Levine S. Stridor and death in multiple system atrophy. *Mov Disord.* 2000;15:699–704.

138. Guilleminault C, Tilkian A, Lehrman K, et al. Sleep apnoea syndrome: States of sleep and autonomic dysfunction. *J Neurol Neurosurg Psych.* 1977;40:718–725.

139. Hughes RG, Gibbin KP, Lowe J. Vocal fold abductor paralysis as a solitary and fatal manifestation of multiple system atrophy. *J Laryngol Otol.* 1998;112(2):177–178.

140. Kavey N, Whyte J, Blitzer A, et al. Sleep-related laryngeal obstruction presenting as snoring or sleep apnea. *Laryngoscope.* 1989;99:851–854.

141. Iranzo A, Santamaria J, Tolosa E. Continuous positive air pressure eliminates nocturnal stridor in multiple system atrophy. Barcelona Multiple System Atrophy Study Group. *Lancet.* 2000;356:1329–1330.

142. Plazzi G, Corsini R, Provini F, et al. REM sleep behavior disorder in multiple system atrophy. *Neurology.* 1997;48:1094–1097.

143. Tachibana N, Kimura K, Kitajima K, et al. REM sleep motor dysfunction in multiple system atrophy: With special emphasis on sleep talk as its early clinical manifestation. *J Neurol Neurosurg Psych.* 1997;63:678–681.

144. Hanson DG, Ludlow CL, Bassich CJ. Vocal fold paresis in Shy-Drager syndrome. *Ann Otol Rhinol Laryngol.* 1983;92:85–90.

145. Isozaki E, Hayashi M, Hayashida T, et al. Vocal cord abductor paralysis in multiple system atrophy–Paradoxical movement of vocal cords during sleep. *Clin Neurol.* 1996;36(4):529–533.

146. Wenning G, Tison F, Ben Shlomo Y, et al. Multiple system atrophy: A review of 203 pathologically proven cases. *Mov Disord.* 1997;12:133–147.

147. Schenck CH, Bundlie SR, Patterson AL, et al. Rapid eye movement sleep behavior disorder. A treatable parasomnia affecting older adults. *JAMA.* 1987;257(13):1786–1789.

148. Quera Salva M, Guilleminault C. Olivopontocerebellar degeneration, abnormal sleep, and REM sleep without atonia. *Neurology.* 1986;36:576–577.

149. Tison F, Wenning G, Quinn N, et al. REM sleep behavior disorder as the presenting symptom of multiple system atrophy. *J Neurol Neurosurg Psych.* 1995;58:379–380.

150. Wright B, Rosen J, Buysse D, et al. Shy-Drager syndrome presenting as a REM behavioral disorder. *J Geriatr Psychiatry Neurol.* 1990;3:110–113.

151. Manni R, Morini R, Martignoni E, et al. Nocturnal sleep in multisystem atrophy with autonomic failure: Polygraphic findings in ten patients. *J Neurol.* 1993;240:247–250.

152. Coccagna G, Martinelli P, Zucconi M, et al. Sleep-related respiratory and haemodynamic changes in Shy-Drager syndrome: a case report. *J Neurol.* 1985;232:310–313.

153. Plazzi G, Cortelli P, Montagna P. REM sleep behavior disorder differentiates pure autonomic failure from multiple system atrophy with autonomic failure. *J Neurol Neurosurg Psych.* 1998;64:683–685.

154. Santacruz P, Uttl B, Litvan I, et al. Progressive supranuclear palsy. A survey of the disease course. *Neurology.* 1998;50:1637–1647.

155. Montplaisir J, Petit D, Decary A, et al. Sleep and quantitative EEG in patients with progressive supranuclear palsy. *Neurology.* 1997;49:999–1003.

156. Aldrich MS, Foster NL, White RF, et al. Sleep abnormalities in progressive supranuclear palsy. *Ann Neurol.* 1989;25:577–581.

157. Pareja J, Caminero A, Masa J, et al. A first case of progressive supranuclear pasy and pre-clinical REM sleep behavior disorder presenting as inhibition of speech during wakefulness and somniloquy with phasic muscle twitching during REM sleep. *Neurologia.* 1996;11:304–306.

158. Leygonie F, Thomas J, Degos JD, et al. Troubles de somneil dans la maladie de Steele-Richardson. *Rev Neurol.* 1976;132:125–136.

159. De Bruin VS, Machado C, Howard RS, et al. Nocturnal and respiratory disturbances in Steele-Richardson-Olszewski syndrome (progressive supranuclear palsy). *Postgrad Med J.* 1996;72:293–296.

160. Boeve B. Corticobasal Degeneration. In: Adler C, Ahlskog J, eds. *Parkinson's disease and movement disorders: diagnosis and treatment guidelines for the practicing physician.* Totowa, NJ: Human Press, 2000:253–261.

161. Kimura K, Tachibana N, Toshihiko A, et al. Subclinical REM sleep behavior disorder in a patient with corticobasal degeneration. *Sleep.* 1997;20:891–894.

162. Iriarte J, Alegre M, Arbizu J, et al. Unilateral periodic limb movements during sleep in corticobasal degeneration. *Mov Disord.* 2001;16:1180–1183.

163. Margolis R. The spinocerebellar ataxias: Order emerges from chaos. *Curr Neurol Neurosci Rept.* 2002;2:447–456.

164. Fukutake T, Shinotoh H, Nishino H, et al. Homozygous Machado-Joseph disease presenting as REM sleep behavior disorder and prominent psychiatric symptoms. *Eur J Neurol.* 2002;9:97–100.

165. Friedman J. Presumed rapid eye movement behavior disorder in Machado–Joseph disease (spinocerebellar ataxia type 3). *Mov Disord.* 2002;17:1350–1353.

166. Syed B, Rye D, Singh G. REM sleep behavior disorder and SCA-3 (Machado–Joseph disease). *Neurology.* 2003;60:148.

167. Schols L, Haan J, Riess O, et al. Sleep disturbance in spinocerebellar ataxias: Is the SCA3 mutation a cause of restless legs syndrome? *Neurology.* 1998;51:1603–1607.

Sleep and Epilepsy

Bradley V. Vaughn and O'Neill F. D'Cruz

INTRODUCTION

The dynamic interaction of sleep and epilepsy has been recognized since ancient times. In the 2nd century AD, Galen accounted the importance of sleep for patients with epilepsy by cautioning these patients against sleepiness (1). In the 4th century AD, Aristole drew the conclusion that "sleep is similar to epilepsy and in some way, sleep is epilepsy" (2). Although these early observations reveal the important aspects of the intricate relationship, we still have many unsolved mysteries in the interplay between sleep and epilepsy.

Individuals with epilepsy frequently complain of symptoms referrable to disturbed sleep. These complaints may come in the form of easily recognizable symptoms, such as daytime sleepiness or insomnia, or in more subtle complaints, such as an increase in seizure frequency. The clinician must be able to differentiate between dysomnia and disorders related to epilepsy and its treatment. Patients with epilepsy may also display unusual nighttime events due to nonepileptic parasomnias. These patients can provide a challenge to even the most astute clinicians.

In this chapter, we will explore the relationship of sleep and epilepsy through the reciprocal effects of these disorders, the differential diagnosis of nocturnal events, and the management of sleep complaints in the patient with epilepsy.

Epilepsy

The terms epilepsy and epileptic are derived from the Greek work *"epilambanien,"* which means to seize or to attack. Although, in the Greek era of medicine, patients were thought to be seized by demons, we have come to the understanding that epileptic seizures are the clinical manifestations of excessive hypersynchronus central neuronal activity and that epilepsy is a chronic condition of recurrent unprovoked epileptic seizures.

We typically divide epileptic seizures into partial seizures that are initiated in one location and potentially spread to other regions of the brain. Primary generalized seizures involve both hemispheres at the onset. Partial seizures may be classified as simple partial (retention of memory and consciousness), complex partial (impairment of memory or consciousness) or secondarily

▶ **TABLE 27-1.** Seizure Classification[a]

Partial seizures
Simple partial (without loss of consciousness)
   With motor symptoms
   With sensory symptoms
   With autonomic symptoms
   With psychic symptoms
   Compound forms
Complex partial (impaired consciousness)
   Simple partial onset followed by impairment of consciousness
   With impairment of consciousness at onset
   With or without automatisms
Secondary generalized

Generalized seizures of nonfocal origin
   Tonic–clonic
   Tonic
   Clonic
   Absence
   Atonic/akinetic
   Myoclonic
Unclassified seizures

[a]Adapted from the ILAE Commission on Classification (1981).

▶ **TABLE 27-2.** Epilepsy Classification[a]

Localization-related (focal)
Idiopathic, age related onset—genetic, often associated with normal
   intelligence
Symptomatic—seizures arise from a known lesion or site
Cryptogenic—No identified symptomatic cause

Generalized
   Idiopathic, with age-related onset
   Cryptogenic or symptomatic
   Symptomatic

Undetermined whether focal or generalized

Special syndromes

[a]Adapted from Commission on Classification (1989).

generalized. Primary generalized seizures begin diffusely across the brain, and may comprise various types of behavior. Absence seizures are characterized by brief staring episodes. Atonic seizures result in sudden loss of postural tone resulting in unprotected falls or head drops. Tonic seizures produce generalized increase in muscle tone during the clinical event. Clonic seizures are associated with repetitive jerking. Tonic–clonic seizures start with tonic activity that progresses to clonic activity; myoclonic seizures are single rapid jerks. A summary is given in Table 27-1.

The clinical diagnosis of epilepsy is made on the basis of recurrent unprovoked epileptic seizures. Individuals with epilepsy can have multiple types of seizures that subsequently are represented as a single form of epilepsy. Epilepsies can be divided into the focal onset epilepsies and the primary generalized epilepsies (Table 27-2). Both types of epilepsies can have specific relationships to the sleep–wake cycle.

In 1881, Gower studied the relationship of sleep–awake state to epilepsy, noting that 21% of patients had seizures solely during sleep (3). He noted other patients had seizures only during the awake state (42%), whereas a third group had seizures during both the awake and asleep states (37%). A later investigation, by Janz, revealed that some individuals have seizures primarily in the first 2 hours after awakening. Janz coined the term "awakening" epilepsies for these individuals and referred to seizures occurring without dependence on the sleep–awake state as diffuse epilepsies (4,5). Many patients with a primary generalized form of epilepsy, juvenile myoclonic epilepsy, have seizures soon after awakening. On the other hand, benign epilepsy of childhood with centrotemporal spikes and autosomal dominant nocturnal frontal lobe epilepsy are forms of focal onset epilepsies that primarily occur during sleep.

Nocturnal seizures may be associated with some of the most bizarre and obscure nighttime behaviors. The differentiation of a sleep-related phenomenon, nocturnal seizures, or psychogenic events could be difficult because of the frequent overlap of clinical descriptions (Table 27-3). Many times patients may not follow the "classical" patterns of parasomnia or epilepsy, and some patients may have a parasomnia provoked by another sleep disturbance or seizures. Thus, the diagnosis of these behaviors may require intensive investigation and monitoring of these difficult patients. The dilemma, for the physician, is to determine which procedures will yield clues of the underlying

▶ **TABLE 27-3.** Distinguishing Features of Nocturnal Events

Feature	NREM Parasomnia	REM Behavior Disorder	Nocturnal Seizures	Psychogenic Events	Rhythmic Movement Disorder
Time of occurrence	First third of night	During REM	Anytime	Anytime	Start of sleep
Memory of event	Usually none	Dream recall	Usually none	None	Variable
Stereotypical movements	No	No	Yes	No	Yes
PSG findings	Arousals from delta sleep	Excessive EMG tone during REM	Potentially epileptiform activity	Occur from awake state	Rhythmic movement artifact

etiology, without diverting attention to inaccurate or premature conclusions.

PREVALENCE

Epilepsy

Epilepsy is one of the most common neurologic conditions. The prevalence of epilepsy in the general population is approximately 1% to 2%. Epilepsy most frequently begins in childhood and the later adult years (6). Middle-age adults have the lowest incidence of epilepsy. Focal onset epilepsy is the predominant form of epilepsy beginning in the adult years, but has the greatest incidence in childhood and late adulthood. Primary generalized epilepsies most commonly begin during childhood or adolescence.

Sleep Complaints

Patients with neurologic disorders, in general, appear to have a greater prevalence for sleep disturbance than normal subjects. This increase in prevalence appears to extend to patients with epilepsy. Miller reported that over two-thirds of patients with epilepsy seen at a university center have complaints regarding sleep (7). Miller found 68% complained of feeling sleepy during the day, and 39% complained of difficulty falling asleep or staying asleep. Nearly 42% felt that their sleep issues interfered with their daytime performance. In a survey of 30 independently living adults with partial or generalized seizures and 23 normal controls, night awakenings were reported more frequently in those with epilepsy (8). Those who had at least one seizure a month were the most affected, and the majority of epileptic subjects described feeling mildly tired or very tired upon awakening. Using the Epworth Sleepiness Scale (ESS), Malow and colleagues (9) reported that 28% of 158 adult epilepsy patients surveyed had an elevated score (>10 points), with 44% of subjects reporting a moderate or high tendency to fall asleep while watching television (9). However, Manni (10) found only 11% of patients with epilepsy and 10% of controls had an ESS greater than ten (10). This partial increase in sleep complaints in patients with epilepsy may be related to the disruption of the central nervous system (CNS) involved in the regulation of sleep and the abilities of these individuals to perceive sleep–wake related symptoms. The combination of these factors raises the question of potential dysfunction in sleep physiology or the perception of the sleep and awake states.

Information regarding sleep physiology can be gleaned from review of polysomnography (PSG). Sleep architecture is frequently disrupted in patients with epilepsy. Touchon (11) showed that patients with epilepsy have greater sleep fragmentation and "instability." PSG investigation of individuals with epilepsy by Malow showed that nearly one-third of patients with medically refractory epilepsy had a respiratory disturbance index (RDI) of greater than 5 and approximately 10% of the patients had periodic limb movement index (PLMI) greater than 20 events per hour (12). In our own cohort of 25 patients with intractable epilepsy, we have found that 36% had an RDI greater than 10 and approximately 12% had PLMI over 15 events per hour. These studies involve relatively small numbers of patients and include a high percentage of patients continuing to have seizures despite medications.

Obstructive sleep apnea (OSA) may also influence the prevalence of epilepsy. Seizures as a direct result of apnea are rare. In one patient, an apnea in sleep reportedly caused a seizure after severe oxygen desaturation and cardiac arrest (13). Yet, Sonka found in their cohort that 4% of patients with OSA apnea had epilepsy (14). This prevalence exceeds that of the general population. Over three-fourths of these patients had seizures only during sleep and most of the events were generalized seizures. Although this study may be skewed by variances in referral patterns, the elevated prevalence raises the interesting question of sleep apnea provoking seizures or unmasking an underlying potential for seizures.

Nocturnal Events

Nocturnal events may be relatively common. Over 3% of adults and 10% to 30% of children have nocturnal events on a routine basis. These events can be divided into nocturnal seizures and nonepileptic events. Gowers found 21% of the institutionalized epilepsy patients to have seizures strictly while asleep and 42% to have seizures strictly while awake (3). These results are similar to Janz's and Billiard's studies of epileptic patients one century later (4,5,15). Nonepileptic nocturnal events are more common. Approximately 30% of children have disorders of arousal, such as sleepwalking or sleep terror events, and the reported prevalence in adults ranges from 2% to 5% (16,17). The prevalence of rapid eye movement (REM) sleep-related parasomnias, such as REM sleep behavior disorder (RBD) is unknown, but appears to increase with age (18).

DIFFERENTIAL DIAGNOSIS

The differential diagnosis of the patient with hypersomnia or insomnia and epilepsy should utilize the same framework as any other patient with a chronic condition and sleep complaints. The clinician should consider diagnoses that include sleep disorders, effects of medication, and circadian rhythm disorders, as well as sleep disturbance from epilepsy (Tables 27-4 and 27-5).

Preliminary studies of patients with epilepsy suggests that there is an increased prevalence of sleep disorders. This is especially true for sleep-related respiratory disturbances (12). These patients may also have other sleep disorders, such as periodic limb movements (PLMs) or restless

▶ **TABLE 27-4. Differential Diagnosis for Hypersomnia**

Intrinsic sleep disorders
  Obstructive sleep apnea
  Central sleep apnea
  Periodic limb movements of sleep
  Restless leg syndrome
  Narcolepsy
  Idiopathic hypersomnia
Extrinsic sleep disorders
  Inadequate sleep hygiene
  Insufficient sleep
Medication
  Somulent medications used during the day
  Activating medications disrupting sleep at night
  Drug interactions
Affective disorders
Circadian rhythm disturbance
Endocrine or metabolic dysfunction
Disruption of nocturnal sleep from epileptic focus
Nocturnal seizures

▶ **TABLE 27-5. Differential Diagnosis for Insomnia**

Intrinsic sleep disorders
  Psychophysiological insomnia
  Idiopathic insomnia
  Restless legs syndrome
  Obstructive sleep apnea
  Periodic limb movements
  Narcolepsy
Extrinsic sleep disorders
  Inadequate sleep environment
  Inadequate sleep hygiene
Medications
  Use of activating medications prior to bedtime (ethosuximide, felbamate, lamotrigine, zonisamide)
  Withdraw of somnogenic medications (barbiturates, benzodiazepines, etc.)
  Herbs or food supplements
  Caffeine
Epileptic related arousals
Affective disorders
Metabolic or endocrine dysfunction

legs syndrome (RLS), which disturb their sleep and produce daytime sequelea. Intrinsic dysfunction in the regulation of sleep, such as narcolepsy, can also produce similar symptoms.

Individuals with epilepsy are frequently treated with medications the side effects of which include somnolence or insomnia (Table 27-6). Most of the traditional anticonvulsants have sleepiness as a side effect (19). Although this is most notable for the barbiturates and benzodiazepines, others, such as carbamazepine, phenytoin, valproate, gabapentin, topitiramate, vigabatrin, levitiracetam, and oxcarbazepine can produce complaints of somnolence or fatigue. Medications such as felbamate, ethosuximide, lamotrigine, and zonisamide may induce insomnia. Drugs may actively change metabolic and en-

docrine features that promote appropriate sleep and wakefulness. Enzyme-inducing medications may increase the metabolism of medications used to treat hypersomnolence or insomnia.

Circadian rhythm disorders should be considered in patients with epilepsy. Many of these patients have relatively sedentary lifestyles and may have limited exposure to zeitgebers. In addition, these patients may experience brief shifts or attenuations in the circadian rhythms from seizures or medications (20).

The epileptic process may directly contribute to the sleep disturbance. Touchon (11) showed that patients had more frequent spontaneous arousals and awakenings prior to treatment with anticonvulsants. In animal studies, discharges from the amygdala or mesiotemporal

▶ **TABLE 27-6. Antiepileptic Medication Effects on Sleep**

Drug	Sleep complaint	Sleep efficiency	Total sleep time	Sleep latency	Arousals	Stage 1	Stage 2	Stage 3/4	REM sleep
Phenobarbital	Sleepiness	↓	No change	↓	↓	↑	↑	No change	↓
Phenytoin	Sleepiness	↓	No Change	↓	↓	↑	↑	↓	No change
Carbamazepine	Sleepiness	↑	No change	↓	↓	No change	No change	↑	?
Valproate	Sleepiness	No change	No change	No change	↑	↓	No change	↑	No change
Ethosuximide	Insomnia	↓	?	?	↑	↑	No change	↓	↑
Felbamate	Insomnia	↓			↑				
Gabapentin	Sleepiness	↑	↑		↓	↓		↑	↑
Lamotrigine	Insomnia	No change	No change	No change	No change	No change	No change	↓	↑
Topriamate	Sleepiness	?	?	?	?	?	?	?	?
Vigabatrin	Sleepiness	?	No change	No change	?	?	?	?	?
Tiagabine	Insomnia	?	?	?	?	?		?	?
Levitiracetam	Sleepiness	No change	No change	No change	No change	No change			No change
Zonisamide	Insomnia	?	?	?	?	?	↑	↓	?
Oxcarbazepine	Sleepiness	?	?	?	?	?	?	?	?

structures produce arousals. Frequent nocturnal seizures can also produce significant sleep disturbance. Patients with frontal lobe seizures may experience between five to twenty brief seizures in a single night (21). Thus, the ictal and interictal discharges may play a role in the patient's feeling unable to rest.

Events

Sleep-Related Events during Wakefulness

Sometimes diurnal events that occur as a result of a sleep disorder can be confused with epilepsy. This is most common for two sleep-related complaints, sleep attacks and cataplexy, but other sleep-related events, such as sleep paralysis and hypnagogic hallucinations, can also be confused with epileptic events. A careful history is most helpful in differentiating these events. Yet, for some patients, further investigation, including combined video–electroencephalographic and PSG recording can be useful.

Sleep Attacks

Sleep attacks, as irresistible bouts of sleep, may arise from a variety of underlying etiologies. These events usually occur with the patient sitting or lying, but are rare with the patient standing. Usually associated with narcolepsy or extreme sleep deprivation, these sudden onset events can be confused with seizures or psychogenic events. They may result from sedative medication or be due to underlying narcolepsy, idiopathic hypersomnolence, and other dysomnias.

REM Fragments: Cataplexy, Hypnagogic Hallucinations, Sleep Paralysis

Cataplexy can be easily confused with atonic seizures. The sudden loss of tone is similar for both events. However, cataplexy is usually paired with an emotional trigger and the electroencephalogram (EEG) retains normal background activity. Atonic seizures are usually not triggered by emotion and are frequently associated with EEG changes, such as a electrodecremental response.

Occasionally, patients will present with the description of other REM sleep fragmentary events as nocturnal behaviors. Patients with terrifying hypnagogic hallucinations may note recurrent scary imagery just as they are falling asleep. These events may be associated with screaming, yelling, or other frightened behavior. Patients have a clear memory for the events, and can recall the visual imagery, which distinguishes them from most epileptic events.

Patients with recurrent sleep paralysis may also present with complaints of unusual spells. These individuals will describe complete paralysis upon awakening with a sense of impending doom or of being chased. These episodes may last seconds to minutes and can be aborted by another individual touching the patient.

Nocturnal Events

Nocturnal Seizures

Sleep-related seizures could be easily confused with other parasomnias or psychiatric conditions, especially if the patients have no diurnal findings (Tables 27-3 and 27-7). Nocturnal seizures can present as a variety of events. The historical review from witnesses of the events may give cardinal clues to the etiology. Features of stereotypic behavior and a repetitive nature of the events point to a possible underlying epileptic disorder. Patients usually do not have memory for the seizures, and the seizures can occur at any time in the sleep period (day or night). Most nocturnal seizures occur in nonrapid eye movement sleep (NREM) sleep, whether they are of temporal or frontal onset (22). Rare REM-related seizures have been described involving recurrent dreams and dreams similarly to RBD (23). Other authors have described seizures involving recurrent dreams (24). Clear description of the behaviors is paramount. Patients can have a variety of nocturnal

▶ **TABLE 27-7. Differential For Nocturnal Events**

Nocturnal seizures
 Focal onset seizures
  Symptomatic
  Frontal lobe epilepsy
  Temporal lobe epilepsy
  Parietal lobe epilepsy
  Occipital lobe epilepsy
  Idiopathic (genetic preponderance)
  Benign focal epilepsy with centrotemporal spikes
  Benign occipital epilepsy of childhood
  Autosomal dominant nocturnal frontal lobe epilepsy
  Nocturnal temporal lobe epilepsy
  Unknown
 Generalized seizures
  Generalized tonic clonic seizures
  Myoclonic seizures
Disorders of arousals
 Sleepwalking
 Sleep terrors
REM-related events
 REM sleep behavior disorder
 Sleep paralysis
 Cataplexy
 Hypnagogic hallucinations
Overlap syndromes
Sleep transition abnormalities
 Sleep talking
 Sleep starts
 Rhythmic movement disorder
 Bruxism
Psychogenic events
 Panic attacks
 Dissociative disorders
 Conversion disorder
Other

behaviors, such as ambulation, confused wandering, or screaming, which appear similar to events of sleepwalking or sleep terrors. Some seizures have a repetitive nature that can be easily confused with rhythmic movement disorder. The overlap of these symptoms can make classification of these extraordinary events difficult.

Seizure-related Behavior

Nocturnal seizures can produce a wide range of behaviors. The behavioral expression of the seizure depends upon the location of the seizure discharge. Nearly any behavior that can be produced by the brain can be exhibited as a seizure (Table 27-8). Yet, the hallmark of seizures is the stereotypic nature. Each seizure should have similar behavior to the others. The frontal and temporal lobes are the most common sites for seizure foci, and these are areas more commonly involved in sleep-related epilepsies (25,26). Seizures involving the frontal lobes may evoke tonic posturing, complex bizarre motor activity, and even violent behavior. Temporal lobe seizures usually produce episodes of staring, psychic phenomena, and some complex behaviors. Temporal and frontal lobe seizures can also evoke a wide range of autonomic symptoms, such as bradycardia, asystole, tachycardia, emesis, and respiratory disturbances. Parietal onset seizures are more likely to evoke disturbances or distortion of sensory perception. Occipital lobe onset seizures are usually associated with visual phenomena, visual distortion, or eye movement. Benign occipital epilepsy of childhood is frequently associated with nocturnal seizures and headache and is frequently misdiagnosed as migraine. With the complexity of these behaviors, one can easily see an overlap in presentation among patients with seizures and parasomnias.

▶ **TABLE 27-8. Seizure Semiology**

Origin of Seizure	Possible Behaviors (Not Limited To)
Frontal	Posturing of extremities, vocalization, rocking, turning, ambulation, sitting up, pelvic thrusting, gestural automatisms, jerking of face or extremities
Temporal	Staring, an absence of other activity, autonomic events, olfactory and auditory hallucinations, out-of-body and psychic experiences, oralimentary automatisms, expressions of fear, rising epigastric sensation, belching
Parietal	Somatosensory events (tingling, electrical, wavelike, temperature change or numbness), feeling of movement in a portion of the body or vertigo, metamorphopsia
Occipital	Visual hallucinations (sparks, flashes or more formed images), hemianopsia, scotoma, visual distortion

Following the seizure, patients are frequently confused and disoriented. We have recorded wandering behavior, pronounced violence, rhythmic movement, snoring, and even psychosis as postictal events. The confusion may resolve over minutes or may only improve after the patient sleeps. Postictal somnolence is common and can make differentiating seizures from a parasomnia very difficult.

Memory loss or impairment of consciousness are required features for complex partial or generalized seizure. Amnesia indicates that both hippocampal structures were impaired from incorporating recent memories during the seizure. If one hippocampus is not impaired during the seizure, patients can have retained memory despite complex motor behavior. Patients without temporal lobe extension of their seizures can have retained memory for the events and, therefore, may have complex behaviors with retained memory. These patients are frequently mislabeled as having psychogenic disorders.

Nocturnal Paroxysmal Dystonia

Previously known as hypnogenic paroxysmal dystonia, this is characterized by repeated dystonic or dyskinetic episodes occurring at night (27–29). The movements can involve a single extremity or up to all four extremities and the neck. Occasionally patients may vocalize and frequently recall the event. They typically occur out of NREM sleep and demonstrate in two major forms: short duration (15 to 60 seconds) and long duration (up to 60 minutes). Patients may have multiple spells per night or may have clusters of spells with relatively quiescent periods. NPD is considered to be a form of frontal lobe epilepsy. Lugaresi has described an Italian form of inherited nocturnal frontal lobe epilepsy. This complex disorder may show episodes of nocturnal dystonia, paroxysmal arousals, and nocturnal wandering. Patients may demonstrate any combination of these behaviors with few EEG changes. Most patients respond to anticonvulsant medication.

Autosomal Dominant Nocturnal Frontal Lobe Epilepsy

This is a rare disorder originally described in Australia and, subsequently, in Italy (30–33) It has clinical characteristics of NPD and is passed in an autosomal dominant pattern. Patients have recurrent nocturnal events characterized by brief tonic movements, hypertonic activity, or brief arousals. The EEG frequently demonstrates no epileptic changes during the spells, and daytime EEGs are normal. The family history can be difficult to obtain, since the spells may not be recognized by or acknowledged to other family members. About one in four of these individuals will have daytime seizures. These patients frequently respond to anticonvulsant therapy. The Australian form of ADNFLE has been linked to chromosome 20q 13.2 to the CHRNA4 gene (31,32). An abnormality of the neuronal nicotinic acetylcholine receptor 4 subunit has been found in association with this disorder, yet augmentation of acetylcholine does not appear to alter the frequency or intensity of the seizures.

Benign Focal Epilepsy with Centrotemporal Spikes or Benign Rolandic Epilepsy

Also known as BECTS, this condition is another form of inherited nocturnal seizures. BECTS occurs in children between 5 to12 years of age. Patients typically present with episodes of hemifacial and body tonic activity, drooling, and speech impairment. These events occur approximately 20 minutes to 2 hours after going to bed. EEG usually demonstrates a high-amplitude centrotemporal spike and wave discharge associated with bifrontal positivity. Patients are easily treated with anticonvulsant medication as the seizures diminish with age.

Myoclonic Epilepsy

Epileptic-based myoclonus can occur soon after awakening. The rapid jerk of myoclonus can involve any portion of the body (4). Myoclonus associated with the awakening epilepsies frequently occurs soon after arousal. The jerks can occur in a rapid succession or as single events. Sleep deprivation will exacerbate the events. They should be differentiated from hypnic jerks, which occur at sleep onset and periodic limb movement of sleep (PLMS).

Continuous Spike and Wave during Sleep or Electrical Status during Sleep

Seizurelike electrical activity has been noted to replace normal EEG features of sleep. Patry (34) described six children in whom the background electrical activity was replaced with slow 1- to 2.5-Hz generalized spike and wave discharges (34). These children may not have significant nocturnal behavioral manifestations of the aberrant activity, but they are noted to have significant cognitive and psychological decline. Many of these children will have nocturnal and diurnal absence, focal motor, and generalized tonic-clonic seizures.

Sleep-related Events

Sleep-related events are frequently confused with epilepsy. The states of wakefulness, NREM sleep, and REM sleep are distinguished by features resulting from activation of several neuronal processes of the CNS (35). These state changes are neither concise nor instantaneous. Although the state change occurs in a systematic fashion, fragments or incomplete state change can be observed during the sleep transitions. Disorders of arousal that predominately occur from NREM sleep, such as sleepwalking or sleep terrors, and RBD can present as dramatic dream enactment. These parasomnia events are related to the state of sleep. These disorders can produce a mixture of sleep–wake states and thus the expression of abnormal behaviors during sleep (36). These phenomena are recognized as an overlapping of sleep–wake behaviors and explain some of these fascinating clinical syndromes (Table 27-7).

NREM Sleep Events

Disorders of arousal from NREM sleep are defined by the incomplete arousal from NREM stage 2 or NREM stages 3 and 4 (slow-wave) sleep (SWS). Events such as sleepwalking, sleep terrors, and confusional arousals are common in children and, to a lesser extent, in adults. The decrease in NREM events with increasing age raises the question that these disorders represent a maturational process of sleep–wake regulation. Frequently, patients with a NREM parasomnia disorder will have a family history (37). First-degree relatives of a patient with sleepwalking have a tenfold greater incidence of sleepwalking. Typically, NREM events are more common in the first half of the night and patients have no memory for the event (Table 27-3). Yet, these are not absolute rules since patients can have spells at anytime during the night and report memory of visual imagery and auditory perceptions.

These NREM parasomnia events can sometimes be difficult to distinguish from epilepsy. Stereotypic behavior is a characteristic historical feature for epilepsy. However, the stereotypic behavior may be relatively short, and the witnesses to the event may only see the nonstereotypic postictal behavior. Postevent somnolence, confusion, and lack of memory are features common to both epilepsy and NREM sleep events. For difficult patients, video–EEG combined with PSG may be necessary to delineate the underlying cause.

Sleepwalking

Sleep walking events are arousals, typically from SWS, occurring during the first one-third of the sleep period. Patients usually have little or no memory for the event and can include elaborate behaviors, such as dressing, unlocking locks, cleaning, cooking, and driving. A potential variant of this behavior is nocturnal eating disorder in which patients arise during the night and eat high-calorie food. The patients generally have eating habits different from their usual daytime habits and have no memory for the events. Occasionally, these events coincide with time periods of restricted caloric intake (37).

Sleep Terrors

Sleep terrors are a more intense form of sleepwalking since most patients with sleep terror also have sleepwalking events. The predominance of autonomic expression during sleep terrors helps distinguish these from other partial arousals from NREM sleep. The sudden arousal from SWS with a piercing scream or cry, accompanied by autonomic and behavioral manifestation of intense fear, is rarely forgotten by any witness. The onset of the event is abrupt, and patients have tachycardia, tachypnea, flushing, diaphoresis, and mydriasis. The patients are confused, disoriented, and attempts to intercede may result in harm to the person trying to wake the patient. Patients can become violent, resulting in injury to the patient and bed partners.

Confusional Arousals

Confusional arousals can occur at any arousal from NREM sleep and are characterized by disorientation, slow speech, and mentation or inappropriate behavior (38). Patients have memory impairment for the event, and the events can be induced with forced arousal. The course of these events usually improves with age, but usually remains stable in adults. These events can be very difficult to distinguish from postictal confusion.

REM Sleep-related Events

REM sleep, characterized by a low-amplitude fast EEG activity, rapid movements of the eye, and paralysis of the somatic muscles can occur in concert or as separate fragments (39). This fragmentation of REM sleep can present as symptoms of visual imagery (hypnogogic hallucinations), loss of muscle tone (cataplexy or sleep paralysis), or dream enactment (REM sleep behavior disorder). The later can be dangerous and frequently misdiagnosed as epilepsy or psychiatric events.

REM Sleep Behavior Disorder

Originally predicted by Jouvet in 1965, REM sleep behavior disorder (RBD) in humans was described in 1986, by Schenck and Mahowald (17,40). The disorder is characterized by intermittent loss of REM sleep EMG atonia and by the appearance of elaborate motor activity associated with dream mentation (Table 27-3). These nonstereotypic behaviors can include punching, kicking, leaping, running, talking, yelling, and any behavior that could occur during a dream, and bed partners are frequently injured. Patients usually have a vivid recall of the actual dreams that correlate to the witnessed behavior, but dream recall is not uniform. These events occur more commonly in the latter half of the night, but can occur any time that the patient enters REM sleep (17). RBD can be induced by medication, such as tricyclic antidepressants, monoamine oxidase inhibitors, and selective serotonin reuptake inhibitors, and acutely from alcohol withdrawal. In 40% of the chroinc form, an identifiable neurologic disorder such as strokes, posterior fossa tumors, demyelination, or degenerative disorders may prevent the induction of REM sleep-related atonia (17,41). Memory for the event and lack of stereotypic features distinguishes these events from epilepsy.

Other REM Sleep-related Events

A rare disorder, REM sleep sinus arrest can present as events of sudden arousal with the sense of impending doom. In these patients, the sense of panic and fear can be a symptom. These patients may have histories compatible with isolated nocturnal panic attacks. PGS will show sinus pauses of 2.5 seconds or greater during REM sleep. These patients need to be identified and referred for cardiac evaluation and pacemaker placement.

NREM–REM Overlap Syndromes

Some patients may demonstrate events that occur during both NREM and REM sleep. These patients have features that make differentiation of their events into solely related to NREM or REM sleep difficult. Patients may have some memory or no memory. The behaviors can be subtle or violent and may occur multiple times per night. Some of these patients have had significant central nervous system injury or degeneration or are experiencing toxic or metabolic derangement. The lack of memory and periods of confusion make these event difficult to distinguish from epileptic events.

Other Sleep-Related Behaviors

Sleep Talking

Sleep talking is the phenomena of utterances or even longer soliloquy during stage 2, SWS, or REM sleep. Sleep talking is more likely to occur in the first half of the night; however, it may occur at any time during the sleep period. Patients are more likely to have episodes during acute medical illness, stress, or new medications. Some patients may have sleep talking provoked by an underlying sleep disorder.

Rhythmic Movement Disorder

Patients with rhythmic movement disorder can present with complaints of rocking movements, which occur prior to sleep onset. The movements are stereotyped, involving large muscles, usually of the head and neck, and are sustained into light sleep. Movements may include head banging, body rocking, leg rolling, humming, and chanting. Some patients are relatively unaware of the movement, and others will describe the movement as a calming effect or as a compulsion prior to sleep. This behavior is frequently seen in infants and young children and those with mental handicaps or autism, and the prevalence diminishes with age. Typical episodes are seen on PSG as episodes of rhythmical movement preceding sleep onset and during NREM stage 1 sleep. The relatively normal appearance of the EEG immediately before and after the movement artifact is key to distinguishing this disorder.

Bruxism

Sleep bruxism can also occur as a rhythmical or repetitive movement during sleep (42). Grinding or clenching of the teeth during sleep may produce bizarre sounds and patients can even rarely vocalize with the episodes. Patients may have abnormal wear of the teeth, jaw pain, headache, or facial or tooth pain. They may have hundreds of events per night and the events increase with emotional stress. These events usually begin in the teen years and, occasionally, a familial pattern can be ascertained. The PSG demonstrates repetitive bouts of increased temporalis muscle activity, particularly occurring prior to sleep onset and continuing through NREM stage 2 sleep. Patients should have a dental evaluation and be considered for bite plates. Familial nocturnal facio-mandibular myoclonus can also mimic sleep bruxism, but, as opposed to bruxism, the muscle activation spreads from the masseter to the orbicularis oris and oculi muscles (43).

Psychogenic States

Psychogenic events can also occur at night. This broad class of behavioral phenomena denotes a lack of findings suggestive of epilepsy and can be subdivided into groups of psychologic classifications. These events can be considered under panic disorders, dissociative disorders, or conversion disorders. These patients typically wake up prior to the onset of the events. Unfortunately, some patients labeled as having psycogenic events can still have unrecognized epilepsy and, therefore, the diagnosis of nonepileptic seizures should always be considered with some skepticism.

In the general population, panic disorders range in prevalence between 1.0% to 3.0% of the general population, and as many as 2.5% of these panic attacks, may occur exclusively at night (44). PSG data demonstrate that panic attacks can occur at sleep onset or NREM stage 2, but the hallmark PSG feature is for the event to begin after awakening. Patients have an abrupt arousal from sleep, with subsequent associated tachycardia, tachypnea, diaphoresis, tremulousness, feelings of impending doom, and clear memory of the events (45,46). These events may be difficult to distinguish from epileptic autonomic events, even when captured on video–EEG.

Dissociative disorders can also present as nocturnal events. These fugue states may last for hours with loss of identity and memory (47). Patients usually have some diurnal symptoms and may have a history of physical or sexual abuse. They can occur in association with posttraumatic stress disorder (PTSD) (47,48). Simultaneous time-synchronized video monitoring frequently demonstrate wakefulness prior to the onset of the spells.

Conversion disorders also present as nocturnal events (49). Patients have significant underlying stressors or conflicts, which initiate or exacerbate the episodes. These events usually start in young adults, but may begin in the later adult years (50). Patients may have models to mimic epileptic spells. Although unintentional, events have a clear impact on the patient's ability to function. Most patients with nocturnal conversion disorders have arousals prior to their events, with variable memory for the events (Table 27-3). The lack of clear stereotypic nature and normal EEG features in the immediate postictal distinguish these events from epilepsy.

ETIOLOGY

Effects of Seizures and the Epileptic State on Sleep

Seizures in Sleep

Seizures acutely alter the mechanism involved in determining the sleep–wake state. The disruption caused by seizures frequently results in many patients having postictal somnolence and sleep disruption. Patients with nocturnal seizures are subjectively and objectively sleepy on the day following a seizure (51). The hypersynchronus electrochemical activity of seizures can acutely alter the regulation of nocturnal sleep. The changes produced by seizures most frequently result in sleep fragmentation and suppression of REM sleep. Early investigation by Baldy-Moulinier (52), showed that individuals with partial or generalized seizures had decreased amounts of REM sleep on nights with seizures. Touchon and colleagues showed (11), in a study of 77 subjects with primary or secondarily generalized tonic–clonic seizures, that subjects had reduced total sleep time (TST), a decreased percentage of REM sleep, increased wake time after sleep onset (WASO), and an increased stage 2 sleep on nights following generalized seizures as compared with seizure-free nights. They also reported that, in 80 subjects, recurrent partial seizures during sleep decreased the relative proportion of REM sleep. Besset (53) also found that patients with seizures had a reduction in TST and REM sleep, when compared with patients without seizures. Other investigators reported this REM-suppressing effect of seizures, as well as other effects on sleep organization. On nights when seizures occurred versus seizure-free nights, Bazil found nighttime seizures reduced sleep efficiency and REM and stages 2 and 4 sleep and prolonged REM latency and increased drowsiness as measured by the maintenance of wakefulness test. Bazil (51) also found by studying patients in an epilepsy monitoring unit that when seizures occurred during the day, REM sleep was significantly decreased the ensuing night, with deceased amount of stage 4 sleep. This finding demonstrates that seizures alter central nervous system sleep regulation effects for hours and that even diurnal seizures disrupt sleep regulation. Given the wealth of connections between the frontal and temporal lobes and diencephalic components of sleep regulation, disruption of sleep is expected.

Sleep also has an effect on seizures. Most seizures occur out of NREM sleep, with the highest rate per hour occurring from stage 2 sleep (54,55). Seizures are also noted to frequently occur in relationship to an awakening. This finding has raised significant debate if the seizure caused the arousal or the arousal promoted the seizure. REM sleep has the lowest rate of seizures. This antiseizure property appears to hold true for both the overall sleep time and the seizure rate per hour of REM sleep when compared with other states (55).

Effects of Interictal Epileptiform Discharges on Sleep

Although seizures acutely disrupt sleep, the epileptic process may promote sleep disruption. Sleep is disrupted in patients with epilepsy on seizure-free nights as compared with nonepileptic controls. Touchon (11) noted a decrease in sleep efficiency, increase in sleep stage shifts, and periods of wakefulness in patients with primary generalized epilepsy or complex partial seizures as compared with normal controls. Touchon (11) also noted that the disruption was greater in individuals with focal onset seizures. These individuals had more stage shifts, less deep sleep, and sleep fragmentation. Sleep fragmentation by awakenings was greater in untreated, newly diagnosed patients. Touchon reported that after treatment with carbamazepine for 1 month, the newly diagnosed epilepsy patients showed improvement in these parameters.

This sleep disruption may, in part, be related to the interictal discharge. The interictal discharge is the electrical signature typically associated with epilepsy between seizures. For primary generalized epilepsies, the interictal discharge is a brief seizure that is not long enough to produce a behavioral manifestation. These bursts of activity are decreased in occurrence with appropriate medication. However, interictal discharges, for focal onset epilepsies, are not brief representations of focal seizures, but distinct electrical events that are not altered by medication. The underlying etiology of interictal discharges in relation to focal onset seizures has yet to be understood. Needless to say, these discharges have an effect on neuronal function.

Interictal epileptiform discharges may disrupt sleep. Peled (56) showed that bursts of generalized spike–wave complexes can appear in stages 2 and 3 of NREM sleep and occur with K complexes and arousals. Some of these bursts produced nonconvulsive body movements resulting in significant sleep fragmentation and decreased amounts of REM sleep. Three patients treated with antiepileptic medications showed reduced paroxysmal events during sleep, increased REM sleep, increased sleep efficiency, and improvement in daytime sleepiness. Not all interictal discharges result in arousals. In temporal lobe epilepsy, Malow and colleagues (57) found that interictal discharges were rarely associated with arousals from sleep and were most prevalent with the onset of SWS. This study utilized surface electrodes and did not look at other features, such as autonomic arousals or other physiologic parameter shifts. In humans, interictal activity can be associated with limited physiologic changes. Interictal discharges have been reported to change the cardiac cycle times and, in animals, may produce significant changes in hypothalamic function (58,59). The relationship of these brief discharges to sleep has yet to be defined. The chaotic nature of these discharges, however, may disrupt various neuronal drivers and the microarchitecture involved in the regulation of sleep or its many physiologic features.

Sleep and Sleep Deprivation Effects on Epilepsy

The deprivation of sleep has long been a method used to trigger epileptic-related activity. The activation of interictal activity may be related to the promotion of the onset of sleep, but this point has yet to be resolved (60). Sleep may activate interictal activity in approximately one-third of epileptic patients and up to 90% of subjects with sleep–wake related, or state-dependent, epilepsies (61–63). Overnight studies of interictal activity demonstrate that the interictal activity increases with entrance into the deeper stages of NREM sleep (57). These interictal discharges are not only more frequent with the onset of the deeper stages of sleep, the discharges show greater spatial spread and variability in localization. These stages of sleep are physiologically linked to fewer neurons engaged in active membrane depolarization and thus more neurons in the resting membrane. In addition, there is greater synchronization of thalamocortical relay neurons. The greater number of neurons in the resting membrane state that occur in NREM sleep allows the synchronization ability of the thalamocortical neurons to facilitate these interictal discharges. Sleep deprivation was noted to increase the interictal discharges more in patients with generalized epilepsies (64). Discharges in patients with primary generalized epilepsies may represent a small seizure discharge. For most focal onset seizure disorders, however, interictal discharges do not represent small seizures and have little correlation to seizure control. Thus, those pathophysiologic mechanisms involved with sleep that increase generalized seizures may be different from those in focal onset seizures.

Sleep deprivation is frequently used in long-term epilepsy monitoring settings to promote seizures. Sleep deprivation exacerbates seizures in some patients with epilepsy whereas other patients have little exacerbation with sleep deprivation (4,5,65). Janz noted that sleep deprivation frequently provokes seizures in the awakening epilepsies. This also appears to be true for focal onset epilepsies. Rajna and Veres (65) found that in 9 of 14 patients with temporal lobe epilepsy, seizures are more likely to occur on the days following sleep deprivation. Sleep deprivation for these patients may occur from a variety of causes such as schedule limitations, medication effect, epilepsy, or other dysomnias. No matter the cause, these studies demonstrate the importance of correcting potential causes of sleep deprivation to improve seizure control.

Sleep Disorders in Epilepsy

Sleep disorders in epilepsy may have a significant impact on the epilepsy. This is well demonstrated in the relationship of obstructive sleep apnea (OSA) and epilepsy. Several investigators have shown in a significant proportion of patients that treatment of the OSA improved the seizure control. The first report of treatment of sleep apnea in a patient with epilepsy was in 1981, by Wyler and Weymuller (66). Their patient underwent tracheostomy and attained control of the generalized seizures and improvement in partial seizures. Subsequent reports suggest a range of benefits for patients with epilepsy once the sleep apnea is treated (67–70). In our original report, we showed that 40% of our cohort attained seizure freedom and another 10% had greater than 95% reduction in seizures with treatment of the OSA alone (71). The observations of improvement in seizure control promote the view that OSA increases the seizure frequency in patients with epilepsy. The underlying hypotheses have been focused on two primary etiologies: sleep loss and oxygen desaturation. OSA is known to cause sleep deprivation and sleep fragmentation. This direct sleep disruption deprives the patient from attaining restorative sleep as well as increases the time spent in stages of sleep vulnerable to seizure induction. OSA also produces oxygen desaturation. Although there was little correlation between the lowest oxygen desaturation and the improvement of seizure frequency in the reported case series, oxygen desaturation is noted to decrease potential seizure inhibitory mechanisms (72).

The apparent increased prevalence of sleep apnea in patients with epilepsy may be from several etiologies. These factors may be inherent in the epileptic disorder or from the treatment of the epilepsy. Disorders of the central nervous system (CNS) may affect the regulation of respiration during sleep and increase the risk of sleep apnea. This is seen in patients with other neurologic disorders such as Alzheimer's disease, strokes, cerebral palsy, and myotonic dystrophy (73–76). Therapeutic intervention for epilepsy also may increase the risk of sleep apnea. Valproate, vigabatrin, and gabapentin are well known to promote weight gain, thus increasing the likelihood for sleep apnea (77). In addition, benzodiazepines and barbiturates may cause suppression in responsiveness of carbon dioxide and oxygen desaturation and increase upper-airway musculature relaxation (78). Another form of therapy for epilepsy, vagus nerve stimulation, has been reported to potentially increase airway disturbance during sleep in some patients (79). This therapy may increase airway resistance from stimulation of the recurrent laryngeal nerve or by interfering with the respiratory sensory feedback. Although all of these studies are compelling, larger cohorts are needed to elucidate the true prevalence and age and gender distribution of sleep apnea in patients with epilepsy.

Seizures are reportedly more common in individuals with OSA and seizures are reported to increase the likelihood of disturbed breathing at night (12,80). No matter what the underlying etiology, treatment of this sleep disorder improved the neurologic condition. Thus, this reciprocal relationship of epilepsy and OSA show that treatment of either may improve the other disorder.

Effects of Anticonvulsants on Sleep

Antiepiletic medications diminish the brain's ability to initiate a seizure by altering central nervous system chemistry. These medications may act through changing receptor binding, altering ion-channel function, or affecting second messenger systems. Ideally, the medications would only act in the neuronal networks involved with the epileptic focus. However, these drugs are nonselective and bathe the entire brain. This nonselectivity and pervasiveness of agents that suppress neuronal functioning, led to a high incidence of patients complaining of sedation with therapy. Antiepileptic medications also affect the regulation of sleep architecture (Table 27-6) (26). One of the oldest anticonvulsant agents is phenobarbital. Phenobarbital increases the time the chloride channel is open during gamma aminobutyric acid (GABA) binding to its receptor, resulting in hyperpolarization of the neuronal membrane. This medication shortens sleep latency and decreases the number of arousals in patients with epilepsy, but this drug has little effect on SWS (81). Benzodiazepines increase the frequency of the chloride channel opening when GABA binds to the receptor. This produces a decrease in sleep latency and the number of awakenings, with an increase in the amount of stage 2 sleep and a decrease in the percentage of stages 3 and 4 sleep (26,82). Phenytoin, which alters sodium and calcium channel conductivity, increases the amount of light NREM sleep, but decreases sleep efficiency and sleep latency (81,83). Touchon (11) showed with carbamazepine, another medication that alters sodium channel conductivity, that newly diagnosed patients with epilepsy had an improvement in sleep fragmentation and reduced awakenings. Yet, Gigli reported (84) that in the acute phase use of controlled-release carbamazepine, patients with epilepsy had a reduction in REM sleep and an increase in the number of sleep stage shifts. These effects did not bear out in long-term follow-up. Ethosuximide appears to alter low-threshold calcium channel function, especially in the thalamic neurons. It decreases SWS and increases stage 1 NREM sleep in patients with epilepsy (85). Valproate, which increases GABA by inhibiting GABA transaminase, increases stage 3 and 4 sleep and decreases REM sleep in normal subjects (86). This increase in SWS was also observed by Ehrenberg in patients with PLMs given valproate (87). This high prevalence of untoward effects of the "traditional" antiepileptic medications directed the development of newer medications with fewer side effects and greater potency.

The first of these new antiepileptic medications released in the United States was felbamate. This medication was found to have stimulantlike effects in patients with epilepsy (88). Clinically, patients noted less sedation, but also complained of insomnia (89). Lamotrigine is also been reported to cause a dose-dependent insomnia, but PSG investigation of this medication showed it had little effect on sleep architecture with a mild increase in percent of REM sleep (90,91). Gabapentin has been reported to increase sleep efficiency SWS and REM sleep while decreasing arousals, but this medication can occasionally be associated with daytime sleepiness (92). Levetiracetam has also been reported to induce sleepiness and appears to increase stage 2 sleep, but decrease stage 4 sleep (93). Topiramate has been found to induce complaints of daytime fatigue, and its effects on sleep have not been extensively studied. In fact, most of the newer agents have not had extensive PSG investigation on mainstay groups of patients with epilepsy, not to mention subgroups such as the elderly or children. These studies obviously would be helpful for the clinician to direct therapy toward not only a specific epilepsy type, but a specific effect on sleep. Further development of medications to inhibit epileptic seizures and the underlying epileptic process may provide indirect improvement in sleep in the patient with epilepsy. The reduction of seizures and the "interictal" electrochemical disturbance may promote the return of more normal physiologic regulation. On the other hand, antiepileptic medications that may adversely affect sleep or indirectly contribute to sleep disorders may increase the likelihood of recurrent seizures. The next generation of antiepileptic medications must not only address the epileptic focus but re-establish normal neuronal processes, such as sleep.

CLINICAL MANAGEMENT

Patients with sleep complaints usually present as one of three major categories: excessive daytime sleepiness, insomnia, or unusual events at night. The clinician faced with the epileptic patient who has a sleep complaint should utilize a standard clinical approach with several key points. The clinician needs to obtain the typical detailed history, including information regarding the clinical course, the degree of impact on the patient, the sleep–wake pattern, report from bed partner on sleep activities, dietary and activity schedule, but also must focus on medications (including timing and dosage schedule, over-the-counter agents, and herbs), seizure frequency intensity, and impact upon the patient. The physician should look for potential causes of sleep disturbance from three groups: effect of epilepsy on sleep, effect of medication on sleep, and the presence of another sleep disorder.

Approach to the Epilepsy Patient with Daytime Sleepiness

Excessive daytime sleepiness (EDS) should be approached by the clinician considering a variety of causes. Daytime sleepiness is common in the epilepsy patient, but this symptom is frequently dismissed as an acceptable side effect of therapy (7,9). For many of these patients, our clinical experience has shown that multiple factors contribute to this symptom (Table 27-4). These patients may have a variety of opportunities to improve sleep.

Patients with chronic conditions frequently have maladaptive behaviors negatively impacting upon their sleep. These factors should be addressed with education regarding sleep hygiene. We have found that written materials and explaining the treatment plan to both the patient and a family member is a valuable method to circumvent lapses in memory. Although the Epworth Sleepiness Scale (ESS) has never been validated in patients with epilepsy, useful information can aid the clinician. Malow showed that elevated scores on the ESS in epilepsy patients were more commonly associated with symptoms of OSA and RLS than the number or type of antiepileptic medication or seizure frequency (9). Patients with symptoms, such as sleep-related respiratory problems, unrefreshing sleep, or other findings suggestive of nocturnal disturbance, should have an overnight PSG and be treated accordingly. Treatment of disorders, such as OSA, may improve the patient's sleep symptoms and seizure frequency. However, frequent nocturnal interictal discharges and nocturnal seizures may also cause significant sleep disruption and result in daytime sleepiness of patients with epilepsy (9). Extended EEG montage or video–EEG with PSG may be valuable to elucidate the extent of the sleep disruption. For these patients, sleep disruption may be treated with higher doses of antiepileptic medication prior to the sleep period. Affective disorders are also common in patients with epilepsy and may account for some of the symptoms of feeling fatigued and sleepy.

For some complex or treatment-resistant patients, multiple sleep latency testing (MSLT) may also quantitate the degree of daytime sleepiness and the occurrence of inappropriate REM sleep (94). We have found this testing to be helpful in assessing the degree of sleepiness and in with understanding the patient's perception of sleepiness. Patients with significant sleepiness but without an identifiable cause may be potential candidates for stimulant therapy. This requires careful monitoring and supervision by the clinician to note the impact both on the epileptic seizures and potential for drug interactions.

Antiepileptic drugs are frequently considered by patients and their physicians to be the cause of their sleepiness (95). Traditional anticonvulsants are more commonly associated with somnolence, although some of the newer agents also produce similar effects (Table 27-6). The course of antiepileptic medication use in patients with epilepsy should be for the clinician to start one medication at a low dose and titrate the dosage until either the patient is seizure free or develops intolerable side effects. The goal of the epileptologist is to have the patient attain complete seizure control with no side effects on the least number of medications. When antiepileptic medications are suspected of causing the daytime sleepiness, the medication dosage may be reduced during the day or completely withdrawn or substituted with a less sedating medication. Considering the potential for enhancement of sleep, sedating medications may be dosed so that the peak effect is during the usual sleep period. This technique is also helpful in the treatment of nocturnal seizures when the patient can tolerate much higher drug levels during sleep. This type of dosing schedule is usually achieved with regular release preparations. We have found that extended-release preparations have longer drug release time and do not allow the relatively rapid decline of the drug level prior to end of the sleep period. Reciprocal to sedating anticonvulsants, medications that are noted to be stimulating should be dosed higher at the beginning of the period of wakefulness and reduced prior to the expected sleep period.

Approach to the Patient with Epilepsy and Insomnia

Insomnia appears to disrupt approximately 40% of individuals with epilepsy (7). These patients also can in approached with standard sleep medicine paradigms is an effort to find potential factors contributing to the complaint (Table 27-5). At first glance, the issues of sleep schedule, sleep hygiene, and stimulus control need to be addressed. Reclusive or sedentary lifestyles may be clues to the sleep disruption. Some patients utilize caffeine to counteract the sedating symptoms of the antiepileptic medications. Patients should be warned not consume caffeine in the late afternoon and evening hours. Patients may have schedule limitations due to driving restrictions; thus, timing of exercise and meals needs to be reviewed. Sleep environment may also play a role. Patient with seizures may have anxiety regarding issues of their epilepsy or fear of recurrence of seizures during their sleep. They may sleep with the light on or sleep in uncomfortable settings. These individuals may benefit from education, reassurance, and counseling. For some patients, relaxation techniques, biofeedback, and stimulus control may also be helpful. Insomnia may occur on the basis of frequent arousals caused by epileptic activity. For these patients, higher doses of antiepileptic medication at night and optimization of seizure control may improve symptoms. Patients should be queried about symptoms suggesting RLS, PLMS, or OSA and referred for PSG study when these diagnoses are suspected. Depression or anxiety occur in over 40% of patients with epilepsy and contribute to the complaint of insomnia (96). Patients can be treated with antidepressant and antianxiety medications to benefit both the affective disorder and sleep disorder (97).

Some antiepileptic medications, such as felbamate, ethosuximide, zonisamide, and lamotrigine, can provoke insomnia. These medications may be necessary for control of the seizures, but may be given earlier in the evening or doses spread out through the day. Alternatively, a more sedating medication may be substituted or, if the insomnia-producing antiepileptic medication is required for seizure control. Patients undergoing medication tapers may also experience insomnia due to removal of sedating medication.

Sleep Disorders in Patients with Epilepsy

Patients with epilepsy can present with a wide variety of sleep disorders, including OSA, RLS, PLMS, narcolepsy, and idiopathic hypersomnolence. The diagnosis and treatment of these disorders may not only improve the sleep-related complaints and quality of life (QOL), but also seizure frequency. Patients with epilepsy can be effectively treated with CPAP positional therapy and surgery. Dental devices may be used if the patient does not have a history of ictal or postictal vomiting and the device is tightly fitted to avoid aspiration (79). Antiepileptic medications may be chosen to aid with both the epilepsy and sleep disorder. Gabapentin and carbamazepine have been reported to be beneficial in RLS and neuropathic pain disorders (98). In addition, clonazepam has been the mainstay of therapy for patients with RBD (25). As mentioned above, the side effects of certain antiepileptic medications may be used to counter the complaints of insomnia or EDS. Whatever the cause, improving the sleep and daytime alertness of individuals with epilepsy may have benefits reaching beyond traditional symptoms of sleep disorders.

Diagnosis of Nocturnal Epilepsy

The cornerstone of any evaluation of nocturnal events is the history and physical exam. Although there are no absolutes, the foundation of the evaluation is based on the accurate description of the behaviors. The observer needs to note stereotypic or repetitive nature, memory for the event, potential provoking factors and associated symptoms. Features in the history, such as frequency of events, time of events in the sleep period, family history of nocturnal events, seizures or parasomnias, and a history of recent stressors or spells during wakefulness are also important. The physical exam may provide clues to focal neurologic lesions that may increase the likelihood of certain disorders. Focal lesions in the cerebrum increase the risk epileptic seizures, whereas findings indicative of Parkinson's disease suggest the possibility of RBD. For epilepsy, historic features, such as stereotyped events, the occurrence of a seizure while awake, or family history of seizures add to the evidence supporting a diagnosis of nocturnal seizures. Zacconi (27) proposed that multiple events per night and a continuum of minor to major behaviors was more frequently seen in NFLE than NREM parasomnias. The physical exam is frequently normal, but findings may indicate cerebral insults or other evidence of potential increased risk for seizures. Many clinicians consider a response to anticonvulsant therapy as supporting evidence of the diagnosis of epilepsy. In our opinion, the response to anticonvulsant therapy should not be considered as supportive evidence, since anticonvulsants have diverse neuropharmacologic effects.

Traditional analog PSG has several technical disadvantages. The limited encephalographic electrode placement decreases the likelihood of capturing an epileptiform discharge. The common paper speed of 10 mm per second is also inadequate for observing many ictal epileptic events and does not allow identifying interictal abnormalities. For PSG evaluation of these patients, the paper speed needs to be increased and the array of cephalic electrodes increased. Although the American Academy of Sleep Medicine guidelines support paper speeds of 15 or 20 mm per second, most electroencephalographers prefer paper speeds of 30 mm per second (99).

Incorporation of a full 10- to 20-electrode array and paper speed of 30 mm per second are helpful in evaluating for seizures. Foldvary (100) found that a seven-channel EEG montage and increasing paper speed to 30 mm per second improved the accuracy of distinguishing epileptic events over the traditional four-channel, 10 mm per second recording (100). These settings and expanded electrode array allow for better differentiation of the epileptiform discharges from potential normal variants or artifacts.

EEG is frequently normal in individuals with sleep-related epilepsies. The absence of an epileptiform discharge does not rule out the possibility of epilepsy nor does the presence of an epileptiform discharge confirm the diagnosis of epilepsy. Sleep also plays a significant role in the prevalence, morphology, and location of interictal discharges. Interictal discharges are more common in NREM sleep, whereas REM sleep demonstrates some antiepileptic qualities (101,102). Capture of multiple events on video-EEG recording, comparison of the

behaviors, EEG, and other measures, such as prolactin levels, can lead to a greater chance of obtaining an accurate diagnosis. Epileptic seizures may occur without clear EEG changes. The ictal discharge is typically characterized by hypersynchronous activity (Fig. 27-1), but may be obscured at the surface EEG for multiple reasons. The electrical potential may be of limited amplitude or directed away from recording electrodes, or represent desynchronization of activity and thus be unable to be clearly seen. The surface EEG is also prone to be obscured by muscle activity, movement, and 60-Hz artifacts and distorted by the dura and skull configuration. Depth electrode studies have shown that surface EEG may show no evidence of an ictal discharge in the face of a well-documented discharge near the depth electrodes (103). Even depth electrodes may not demonstrate the electrographic discharge if not located near the seizure focus. Despite all of these limitations, video and EEG recording of multiple events still provides the best method for identification of seizures. The clinician needs to retain a valid skepticism, especially for patients who have stereotypic and reproducible events but lack electrographic changes.

Video–EEG monitoring provides an excellent opportunity for recording the actual event with concurrent EEG recording. Video–EEG monitoring is usually undertaken if further history suggests nonepileptic events, the patient fails three separate anticonvulsants, or the episodes change in character. The criteria for determining when someone should be monitored vary between laboratories

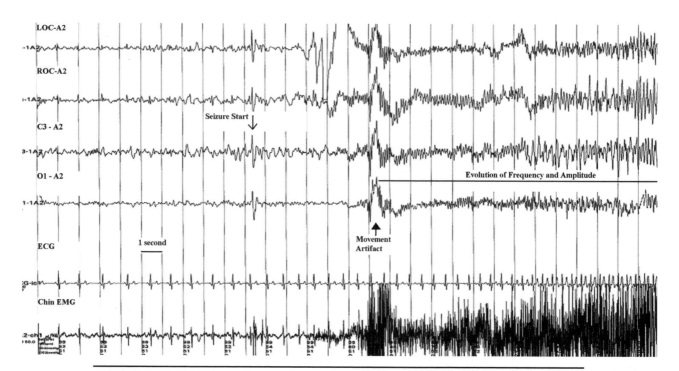

FIGURE 27-1. This PSG recording reveals an electrographic and behavioral seizure starting as a higher-amplitude spike followed by activity in the central lead, evident as a low-amplitude 2- to 3-Hz rhythm, building in frequency and amplitude to an 8-Hz rhythm, then slowing to about 3- to 4-Hz activity (right side of figure). Vertical lines are separated by 1 second.

▶ **TABLE 27-9. Indications for Video–EEG Monitoring**

1. Stereotypical or repetitive events
2. Multiple spells per night with a minimum of one event per week
3. Lack of response to medication trials
4. Other history suggestive of epileptic or nonepileptic events

(Table 27-9) (104,105). Mohan and Chen independently showed that 45% to 80% patients with seizure frequencies of one event or more per week had spells on monitoring (106,107). Nousianen (108) studied patients who had one spell per week and found 85% of patients had spells within 2 days of recording. Even with this intensive recording, some patients are difficult to diagnose.

Other Parasomnias with Epilepsy

Epilepsy has also been implicated as a cause for provoking other parasomnias. Montagna, Lugaresi, and Plazzi (109) noted nocturnal wandering is more likely to occur in patients who had a history of sleepwalking prior to the development of nocturnal epilepsy. They suggest that the epileptic-related arousals could provoke an arousal disorder.

Treatment of Nocturnal Epilepsy

Treatment of nocturnal seizures may be challenging. Even in the best of circumstances, seizures are frequently missed, but seizures during the night are typically not witnessed unless they involve significant motor components. Therefore, our most commonly used marker for medication effect is in question. If patients are having seizures only at night, clinicians should strive to utilize medications in which they can achieve drug levels in the brain relatively quickly and avoid daytime side effects. These typically come in the form of standard release forms, since extended-release medications may outlast the sleep period. The clinician may need to utilize multiple medications if the patient fails monotherapy trials. Sometimes the addition of a medium- or long-acting benzodiazepine as an adjunct to the anticonvulsant therapy may reduce the seizures. If the patient fails three anticonvulsants, confirmation of the diagnosis through video–EEG monitoring should be performed, and the patient should be referred to an epilepsy center.

PROGNOSIS

Patients with epilepsy and sleep disorders have an excellent chance of responding to therapy. Therapies that improve sleep disorders may improve seizure control and improve the patient's quality of life. As mentioned in the clinical management section, the clinician needs to ap-proach these patients in a logical manner to unfold the underlying etiologies that are contributing to sleep complaints. Although no large studies exist that demonstrate the responsiveness of these patients, some patients may be refractory to therapy. For many patients with nocturnal seizures, antiepileptic medications can improve, if not control, the seizures. Intractable epilepsy occurs in approximately one-fourth of individuals with epilepsy. The prevalence of intractable epilepsy in patients who have sleep-related epilepsy is unknown.

FUTURE DIRECTIONS

Sleep and epilepsy research is striving toward unfolding the mysteries of this relationship. Although seizures are the defining component of the epilepsies, further research is needed to completely characterize the effect the epileptic process has upon the regulation of sleep. As we learn the intricacies of the regulation of sleep, new variables in the potential effects of epilepsy are learned. The development of new antiepileptic therapies provides exciting avenues to improve sleep and seizure control. Whatever the method of treatment, we know we must strive to selectively treat the neurons participating in the seizure focus while not altering normal brain function. This will ultimately provide a path for us to unlock the mysteries of these exciting neuronal networks.

REFERENCES

1. Temkin O. *The falling sickness: a history of epilepsy from the Greeks to the beginning of modern neurology.* Revised 2nd edn. Baltimore, MD: Johns Hopkins Press, 1994.
2. Hett WS. (Translator). *Aristotle, on sleep and waking. On the soul, Parva naturalia, on breath.* Lobe Classical Library. Boston: Harvard Univ Press, 1957:457 A, 8–9.
3. Passouant P. Historical aspects of sleep and epilepsy. *Epilepsy Res.* 1991;2:19–30.
4. Janz D. The grand mal epilepsies and the sleep waking cycle. *Epilepsia.* 1962;3:69–109.
5. Janz D. Epilepsy and the sleep-waking cycle. In: Vinken PJ, Bruyn GW, ed. *The epilepsias, handbook of clinical neurology,* Vol 15. Amsterdam: North Holland, 1974:457–490.
6. Hauser WA, Annegers JF, Kurland LT. Incidence of epilepsy and unprovoked seizures in Rochester, Minnesota 1935–1984. *Epilepsia.* 1994;34:453–468.
7. Miller MT, Vaughn BV, Messenheimer JA, et al. Subjective sleep quality in patients with epilepsy. *Epilepsia.* 1996;36(Suppl 4):43.
8. Hoeppner JB, Garron, DC, Cartwright RD. Self reported sleep disorder symptoms in epilepsy. *Epilepsia.* 1984;5(4):434–437.
9. Malow BA, Bowes RJ, Lin X. Predictors of sleepiness in epilepsy patients. *Sleep.* 1997;20(12):1105–1110.
10. Manni R, Politini L, Sartori I, et al. Daytime sleepiness in epilepsy patients: evaluation by means of the Epworth Sleepiness Scale. *J Neurol.* 2000;247:716–717.
11. Touchon J, Baldy-Moulinier M, Billiard M, et al. Sleep organization and epilepsy. *Epilepsia.* 1991;2:73–81.
12. Malow BA, Fromes GA, Aldrich MS. Usefulness of polysomnography in epilepsy patients. *Neurology.* 1997;48(5):1389–1394.
13. Kryer M, Quesney LF, Holder D, et al. The sleep deprivation syndrome of the obese patient, a problem with periodic nocturnal upper airway obstruction. *Amer J Med.* 1974;56:531–538.

14. Sonka K, Juklichova M, Pretl M, et al. Seizures in sleep apnea patients: Occurrence and time distribution. *Sb Lekarsky.* 2000;1(3):229–232.

15. Billiard M. Epilepsies and the sleep–wake. In: Sterman MB, Shouse MN, Passouant P, eds. *Sleep and epilepsy,* New York: Academic Press, 1982:269–286.

16. Bixler EO, Kales A, Soldatos CR, et al. Prevalence of sleep disorders in the Los Angeles Metropolitan Area. *Amer J Psych.* 1979;136:1257–1262.

17. Klackenberg G. Incidence of parasomnias in children in a general population. In: Guilleminault C, ed. *Sleep and its disorders in children.* New York: Raven Press, 1987:99–113.

18. Schenck CH, Mahowald MW. Polysomnographic, neurologic, psychiatric, and clinical outcome report on 70 consecutive cases with the REM Sleep Behavior Disorder (RBD): sustained clonazepam efficacy in 89.5% of 57 treated patients. *Cleveland Clin J Med.* 1990;57:S10–24.

19. Sammarintino M, Sherwin A. Effect of anticonvulsants on sleep. *Neurology.* 2000;54(1):S16–S24.

20. Quigg M. Seizures and circadian rhythms. *Sleep and epilepsy: the clinical spectrum.* 1st edn. Amsterdam: Elsevier Science, 2002:127–142.

21. Zacconi M, Ferini-Strambi L. NREM parasomnias: arousals and differentiation from nocturnal frontal lobe epilepsy. *Clin Neurophysiol.* 2000;111(Suppl. 2):S129–135.

22. Malow BA, Bowes RJ, Ross D. Relationship of temporal lobe seizures to sleep and arousal: A combined scalp-intracranial electrode study. *Sleep.* 2000;23:231–234.

23. D'Cruz OF, Vaughn BV. Nocturnal seizures mimic REM behavior disorder. *Amer J Electro-Neurodiagnosis Technol.* 1997;37:258–264.

24. Epstein AR, Hill W. Ictal phenomena during REM sleep of a temporal lobe epileptic. *Arch Neurol.* 1966;15:367–375.

25. Mikati M, Holmes G. Temporal lobe epilepsy. *The treatment of epilepsy principles and practice,* 1993:513–524.

26. Van Ness, PC. Frontal and parietal lobe epilepsy. *The treatment of epilepsy principles and practice.* 1993:525–532.

27. Lugaresi E, Cirigonotta F. Nocturnal paroxysmal dystonia. In: Sternman MB, Shouse MN, Passouant P., eds. *Sleep and epilepsy.* New York: Academic Press, 1982:507–511.

28. Montplaisir J, Godbout R, Rouleau I. Hypnogenic paroxysmal dystonia: Nocturnal epilepsy or sleep disorder? *Sleep Res.* 1985;14:193.

29. Silvestri R, De Domenico P, Raffaele M, et al. Hypnogenic paroxysmal dystonia: a new type of parasomnia? *Functional Neurol.* 1988;3:95–103.

30. Phillips HA, Scheffer IE, Berkovic SF, et al. Localization of a gene for autosomal dominant nocturnal frontal lobe epilepsy to chromosome 20q 13.2 *Nature Genet.* 1995;10(1):117–118.

31. Steinlein OK, Mulley JC, Propping P, et al. A missense mutation in the neuronal nicotinic acetylcholine receptor alpha 4 subunit is associated with autosomal dominant nocturnal frontal lobe epilepsy. *Nature Genet.* 1995;11(2):201–203.

32. Steinlein OK, Magnusson A, Stoodt J, et al. An insertion mutation of the CHRNA4 gene in a family with autosomal dominant nocturnal frontal lobe epilepsy. *Human Mol Genet.* 1997;6(6):943–947.

33. Oldani A, Zucconi M, Asselta R, et al. Autosomal dominant nocturnal frontal lobe epilepsy. A video-polysomnographic and genetic appraisal of 40 patients and delineation of the epileptic syndrome. *Brain.* 1998;121:205–223.

34. Patry G, Lyagoubi S, Tassinari A. A subclinical "electrical status epilepticus" induced by sleep in children. *Arch Neurol.* 1971;24:242–252.

35. Scher MS, Dokianakis SG, Steppe DA, et al. Computer classification of state in healthy preterm neonates. *Sleep.* 1997;20(2):132–141.

36. Mahowald Mark W, Schenck Carlos H. *Parasomnia purgatory: The epileptic/non-epileptic parasomnia interface. Non-epileptic seizures.* New York: Butterworth-Heinemann, 1993;123–139.

37. Kales A, Soldatos CR, Bixler EO, et al. Hereditary factors in sleepwalking and night terrors. *Br J Psych.* 1980;137:111–118.

38. Guilleminautlt C. Sleep terrors and sleepwalking: In: Kryger MH, Roth T, Dement WC, eds. *Principles and practice of sleep medicine.* 2nd edn. section XII, chapter 56; 567–573. Philadelphia: W.B. Saunders, 1994:567–573.

39. Siegel JM. Brainstem mechanisms generating REM sleep. In: Kryger MH, Roth T, Dement WC, eds. *Principles and practice of sleep medicine,* 3rd edn. Philadelphia: W.B. Saunders, 2000:125–144.

40. Jouvet M, Delorme F. Locus coeruleus et sommeil paradoxal. *C R Soc Biol.* 1965;159:895–899.

41. Culebras A, Moore JT. Magnetic resonance findings in REM sleep behavior disorder. *Neurology.* 1989;39:1519–1523.

42. Hartmann Ernest. *Bruxism: Principles and practice of sleep medicine.* 2nd edn. Chap. 59. Philadelphia: W.B. Saunders, 1994:598–601.

43. Vetrugno R, Provini F, Plazzi G, et al. Familial nocturnal facio-mandibular myoclonus mimicking sleep bruxism. *Neurology.* 2002;58:644–647.

44. Shapiro CM. Nocturnal panic—an under recognized entity. *J Psychosom Res.* 1998;44:181–182.

45. Craske MG, Krueger MT. Prevalence of nocturnal panic in a college population. *J Anxiety Disorder.* 1990;4:125–139.

46. Lesser IM, Poland RE, Holcomb C, et al. Electroencephalographic study of nighttime panic attacks. *J Nerv Ment Disorders.* 1985;173:744–746.

47. Rice E, Fisher C. Fugue states in sleep and wakefulness: A psychophysiological study. *J Nervous Mental Dis.* 1976;163:79–87.

48. Mellman TA, Kulick-Bell R, Ashlock LE, et al. Sleep events among veterans with combat-related posttraumatic stress disorder. *Amer J Psych.* 1995;152(1):110–115.

49. Green SA. A case of functional sleep seizures. *J Nervous Mental Dis.* 1977;164:223–227.

50. Fakhoury T, Abou-Kahalil B, Newman K. Psychogenic seizures in old age: A case report. *Epilepsia.* 1993;34:1049–1051.

51. Bazil CW, Walczak TS. Effect of sleep and sleep stage on epileptic and nonepileptic seizures. *Epilepsia.* 1997;38:56–62.

52. Baldy-Moulinier M. Sleep organization in benign childhood partial epilepsies. *Benign localized and generalized epilepsies of early childhood.* Vol. 6. Amsterdam: Elsevier Science, 1992:121–124.

53. Besset A. Influence of generalized seizures on sleep organization. In: Stermna MB, Shouse MN, Passouant P, eds. *Sleep and Epilepsy,* New York: Academic Press, 1982:339–346.

54. Herman ST, Walczak TS, Bazil CW. Distribution of partial seizures during the sleep–wake cycle: differences by seizure onset site. *Neurology.* 2001;56(11):1453–1459.

55. Minecan D, Natarajan A, Marzec M, et al. Relationship of epileptic seizures to sleep stage and sleep depth. *Sleep.* 2002;25(8):899–904.

56. Peled R, Lavie P. Paroxysmal awakenings from sleep associated with excessive daytime somnolence a form of nocturnal epilepsy. *Neurology.* 1986;36(1):95–98.

57. Malow BA, Lin X, Kushwaha R, et al. Interictal spiking increases with sleep depth in temporal lobe epilepsy. *Epilepsia.* 1998;39(12):1309–1316.

58. Zaatreh MM, Quint SR, Tennison MB, et al. Heart rate variability during interictal epileptiform discharges. *Epilepsy Res.* 2003: in press.

59. Adamec R, Young B. Neuroplasticity in specific limbic system circuits may mediate specific kindling induced changes in animal affect—implications for understanding anxiety associated with epilepsy. *Neurosci Behav Rev.* 2000;24(7):705–723.

60. Dinner DS. Effect of sleep on epilepsy. *J Clin Neurophysiol.* 2002;19(6):504–513.

61. Ellinson RJ, Wilkin K, Bennett DR. Efficacy of sleep deprivation as an activation procedure in epilepsy patients. *J Clin Neurophysiol.* 1984;1:83–101.

62. Thomaides TN, Kerezoudi EP, Chaudhuri LR, et al. Study of EEG's following 24 hour sleep deprivation in patients with post traumatic epilepsy. *Eur Neurol.* 1992;32:79–82.

63. Degen R, Degen HE. Sleep and sleep deprivation in epileptology. *Epilepsy Res.* 1991;(Suppl. 2):235–260.

64. Arne-Bes MC, Calvet V, Thiberge M, et al. Effects of sleep deprivation in an EEG study of epileptics. In: Sternman BM, Shouse MN, Passouant P, ed. *Sleep and epilepsy.* New York: Academic Press, 1982:441–452.

65. Rajna P, Veres J. Correlations between night sleep duration and seizure frequency in temporal lobe epilepsy. *Epilepsia.* 1993;343(3):574–579.

66. Wyler AR, Weymuller EA. Epilepsy complicated by sleep apnea. *Ann Neurol.* 1981;9:403–404.

67. Devinsky O, Ehrenberg B, Bathlen GM, et al. Epilepsy and sleep apnea syndrome. *Neurology.* 1994;44:2060–2064.

68. Vaughn BV, D'Cruz OF, Beach R, et al. Improvement of epileptic seizure control with treatment of obstructive sleep apnea. *Seizure.* 1996;5:73–78.
69. Ezpeleta D, Garcia-Penna A, Peraita-Adrados R. Epilepsia y sindrome de apnea del sueno. *Rev Neurol.* 1998;26(151):389–392.
70. Koh S, Ward SL, Lin M, et al. Sleep apnea treatment improves seizure control in children with neurodevelopmental disorders. *Pediatr Neurol.* 2000;22:36–39.
71. Vaughn BV, Messenheimer JA, D'Cruz O, et al. Sleep apnea in patients with epilepsy. *Epilepsia.* 1993;34(Suppl 6):136.
72. Vaughn BV, D'Cruz OF. Obstructive sleep apnea in epilepsy. In: Lee-Chiong T, Mohsenin V, eds. *Clinics in chest medicine.* Philadelphia: Elsevier Science, 2003:239–248.
73. Turkington PM, Bamford J, Wanklyn P, et al. Prevalence and predictors of upper airway obstruction in the first 24 hours after acute stroke. *Stroke.* 2002;33(8):2037–2042.
74. Guilleminault C, Stoohs R, Quera-Salva MA. Sleep related obstructive and nonobstructive apneas and neurologic disorders. *Neurology.* 1992;42(Suppl. 6):53–60.
75. Bliwise DL, Yesavage JA, Tinklenberg JR, et al. Sleep apnea in Alzheimer's disease. *Neurobiol Aging.* 1989;10(4):343–346.
76. Kotagal S, Gibbons VP, Stith JA. Sleep abnormalities in patients with severe cerebral palsy. *Develop Med Child Neurol.* 1994;36(4):304–311.
77. Lambert MV, Bird JM. Obstructive sleep apnea following rapid weight gain secondary to treatment with vigabatrin (Sabril). *Seizure.* 1997;6(3):233–235.
78. Takhar J, Bishop J. Influence of chronic barbiturate administration on sleep apnea after hypersomnia presentation: case study. *J Psych Neurosci.* 2000;25(4):321–324.
79. Malow BA, Edwards J, Marzee M, et al. Effects of vagus nerve stimulation on respiration during sleep: a pilot study. *Neurology.* 2000;55(10):1450–1454.
80. Sharp S, D'Cruz OF. Seizures as a cause of sleep related respiratory disturbance. *Sleep.* 1998;21(Suppl. 3):77.
81. Wolf P, Roder-Wanner UU, Brede M. Influence of therapeutic phenobarbital and phenytoin medication on the polygraphic sleep of patients with epilepsy. *Epilepsia.* 1984;25(4):467–475.
82. Copinschi G, Van Onderbergen A, L'Hermite-Baleriaux M, et al. Effects of the short-acting benzodiazepine triazolam, taken at bedtime, on circadian and sleep related hormonal profiles in normal men. *Sleep.* 1990;13(3):232–244.
83. Roder-Wanner UU, Noachtar S, Wolf P. Response of polygraphic sleep to phenytoin treatment for epilepsy. A longitudinal study of immediate short-and long-term effects. *Acta Neurol Scand.* 1987; 76(3):157–167.
84. Gigli GL, Placidi F, Diomedi M, et al. Nocturnal sleep and daytime somnolence in untreated patients with temporal lobe epilepsy: changes after treatment with controlled release carbamazepine. *Epilepsia.* 1997;38(6):696–701.
85. Roder UU, Wolf P. Effects of treatment with dipropylacetate and ethosuximide on sleep organization in epileptic patients. In: Dam M, Gram L, Perry JH, eds. *Advances in epileptology: XII epilepsy international symposium.* New York: Raven Press, 1981:145–153.
86. Harding GF, Alford CA, Powell TE. The effect of sodium valproate on sleep, reaction times, and visual evoked potential in normal subjects. *Epilepsia.* 1985;25(6):597–601.
87. Ehrenberg BL, Eisensehr J, Corbett KE, et al. Valproate for sleep consolidation in periodic limb movement disorder. *J Clin Psychopharmacol.* 2000;20(5):574–578.
88. Ketter TA, Malow BA, Flamini R, et al. Felbamate monotherapy has stimulant-like effects in patients with epilepsy. *Epilepsy Res.* 1996;23(2):129–137.
89. Leppik IE. Felbamate. *Epilepsia.* 1995;36(Suppl. 2):S66–S72.
90. Sadler M. Lamotrigine associated with insomnia. *Epilepsia.* 1999;40(3):322–325.
91. Foldvary N, Perry M, Lee J, et al. The effects of lamotrigine on sleep in patients with epilepsy. *Epilepsia.* 2001;42(12):1569–1573.
92. Placidi F, Diomedi M, Scalise A, et al. Effect of anticonvulsants on nocturnal sleep in epilepsy. *Neurology.* 2000;54(5 Suppl. 1):S25–S32.
93. Bell C, Vanderlinden H, Hiersemenzel R, et al. The effects of levetiracetam on objective and subjective sleep parameters in healthy volunteers and patients with partial epilepsy. *J Sleep Res.* 2002;11(3):255–263.
94. Manni R, Tartara A. Evaluation of sleepiness in epilepsy. *Clin Neurophysiol.* 2000;111(Suppl. 2):S111–S114.
95. Salinski MC, Oken BS, Binder LM. Assessment of drowsiness in epilepsy patients receiving chronic antiepileptic drug therapy. *Epilepsia.* 1996;37(2):181–187.
96. Kanner AM, Palac S. Neuropsychiatric complications of epilepsy. *Curr Neurol Neurosci Rep.* 2002;2(4):365–372.
97. Dailey JW, Naritoku DK. Antidepressants and seizures: Clinical anecdotes overshadow neuroscience. *Biochem Pharmacol.* 1996;52(9):1323–1329.
98. Ehrenberg B. Importance of sleep restoration in co-morbid disease: Effect of anticonvulsants. *Neurology.* 2000;54(Suppl. 1):S33–S37.
99. Aldrich MS, Jahnke B. Diagnostic value of video-EEG polysomnography. *Neurology.* 1991;41:1060–1066.
100. Foldvary N, Caruso AC, Mascha E, et al. Identifying montages that best detect electrographic seizure activity during polysomnography. *Sleep.* 2000;23:221–229.
101. Shouse MN, Siegel JM, Wu MF, et al. Mechanisms of seizure suppression during rapid eye movement (REM) sleep in cats. *Brain Res.* 1989;505:271–282.
102. Sterman MB, Shouse MN, Passouant P, eds. *Sleep and epilepsy.* New York: Academic Press, 1982.
103. So NK, Gloor P, Quesney F, et al. Depth electrode investigations in patients with bitemporal epileptiform abnormalities. *Ann Neurol.* 1989;25:423–431.
104. Binnie CD, Rowan AJ, Overweg J, et al. Telemetric EEG and video monitoring in epilepsy. *Neurology.* 1981;31:298–303.
105. Delgado-Escueta AV, Enrile Bacsal, Treiman DM. Complex partial seizures on closed circuit television and EEG: A study of 691 attacks in 79 patients. *Ann Neurol.* 1982;11:292–300.
106. Chen LS, Mitchell WG, Horton EJ, et al. Clinical utility of video-EEG monitoring. *Pediat Neurol.* 1995;12(3):220–224.
107. Mohan KK, Markand ON, Salanova V. Diagnostic utility of video EEG monitoring in paroxysmal events. *Acta Neurol Scand.* 1996;94(5):320–325.
108. Nousianen U, Suomalainen T, Mervaala E. Clinical benefits of scalp-EEG studies in intractable seizure disorders. *Acta Neurol Scand.* 1992;85:181–186.
109. Montagna P, Lugaresi E, Plazzi G. Motor disorders in sleep. *Euro Neurol.* 1997;38(3):190–197.

Sleep and Cardiovascular Diseases

Lyle J. Olson, Anna Svatikova, and Virend K. Somers

INTRODUCTION

Cardiovascular disorders constitute the most common cause of morbidity and mortality in the industrialized world (1,2). Sleep disorders are also highly prevalent, estimated to affect more than 40 million individuals in the United States (3). Hence, disorders of sleep and cardiovascular disease frequently coexist. In recent years, an increased appreciation of cardiovascular pathophysiology has prompted more careful evaluation of the role of sleep in cardiovascular disease pathogenesis. Recognition and management of sleep disorders may offer an opportunity to enhance the quality of life and prognosis of patients with cardiovascular disease.

Sleep interacts with cardiovascular function and pathology in many different ways (4). Autonomic and hemodynamic changes occurring during normal sleep, such as sympathetic activation during rapid eye movement (REM) and blood pressure lowering during non-REM (NREM) sleep, may influence cardiovascular disease presentations either during sleep or in the hours imme-

diately following sleep. Physiologic responses to arousal from sleep, such as autonomic activation and increases in blood pressure and heart rate, may stress a compromised cardiovascular substrate. Sleep deprivation, both acutely and in the long-term, may also be accompanied by increased blood pressure and increased cardiovascular risk (5,6). Most acute cardiovascular presentations including acute myocardial infarction and sudden death manifest a peak occurrence in the early morning hours around the time of waking from sleep, again suggesting an interaction between sleep, waking, and cardiovascular events. However, the most important sleep disorder relating to cardiovascular disease is sleep apnea, which affects an estimated 15 to 20 million individuals in the United States and which will be the primary focus of this chapter (3,7). Sleep apnea may be considered as either obstructive sleep apnea (OSA) or central sleep apnea (CSA). These sleep-related breathing disorders may be conceptualized as either contributing to the initiation and progression of cardiovascular disease or as occurring secondary to existing cardiovascular disease conditions. The objective of this chapter is to critically review the epidemiology, differential diagnosis, etiology, diagnostic evaluation, management, and prognosis of sleep-related breathing disorders as they relate to cardiovascular disease.

CLINICAL EPIDEMIOLOGY

Obstructive Sleep Apnea

Many case-controlled and cross-sectional epidemiologic investigations have demonstrated an association between OSA and cardiovascular disease (8–12). However, confounding clinical factors have made it difficult to definitively establish a causal relationship, with the exception of systemic hypertension, in which the relationship appears more clear. In general, epidemiologic studies of sleep have not used uniform methods and criteria for either diagnosis or classification of the severity of SDB (7–11). Furthermore, as OSA may contribute to the manifestations of cardiovascular disease only after years of disordered nocturnal breathing, the optimal design for any epidemiologic investigation of OSA and cardiovascular risk would require long-term, prospective studies. Nevertheless, data from recent large cross-sectional epidemiologic studies support the concept of some association between the presence of OSA and the risk for hypertension, stroke, coronary artery disease, and congestive heart failure (CHF). For hypertension, stroke, and ischemic heart disease the risk appears modest, whereas the relative risk for CHF is highest (9). Smaller case-controlled studies also support a relationship between OSA and the risk for atrial fibrillation (13,14).

Systemic Arterial Hypertension

The Sleep Heart Health Study utilized home polysomnography (PSG) to investigate the relationship between sleep apnea and hypertension. In a cross-sectional analysis of 6,132 subjects, a modest independent association between OSA and hypertension was observed; the odds ratio for patients with the most severe OSA with apnea–hypopnea index (AHI) >30 was 1.37 and the prevalence of hypertension increased with greater severity of OSA (9). In a separate cross-sectional study, 1,069 subjects underwent laboratory-based PSG, which demonstrated a significant linear relationship between daytime blood pressure and the severity of the AHI (10,11). Most important, this study also prospectively demonstrated a dose–response relationship between AHI at baseline and the presence of hypertension at 4-year follow-up (Fig. 28-1) (11). This association was independent of baseline blood pressure, body mass index (BMI), age, gender, alcohol, and cigarette use. Thus, a substantial proportion of what is generally considered to be essential hypertension may be hypertension that is, to some degree, secondary to untreated OSA.

Ischemic Heart Disease

Cross-sectional epidemiologic studies indicate that OSA may be a risk factor for coronary artery disease, although the level of risk appears low. In the Sleep Heart Health Study cohort the odds ratio for coronary artery disease in the highest AHI quartile (AHI >11) was 1.27 that of the lowest quartile (AHI <1.4) (9). The slightly increased risk for ischemic heart disease in these patients may be related to the increased risk for hypertension.

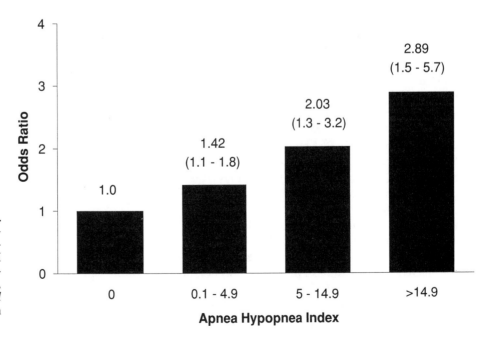

FIGURE 28-1. Odds ratio for development of hypertension at 4-year follow-up in relation to AHI in subjects from the Wisconsin Cohort Study. (From Peppard PE, Young T, Palta M, et al. *N Engl J Med.* 2000;342:1378–1384. With permission.)

Congestive Heart Failure

In the largest case series of patients with CHF studied by PSG, the frequency of OSA has ranged from 11 to 37% (12,15). In the Sleep Heart Health Study, the presence of OSA was associated with a 2.38 greater risk for coexistent CHF, which was independent of other recognized risk factors (9).

Arrhythmia

Cross-sectional epidemiologic and case-control studies indicate that the frequency of atrial fibrillation is increased in individuals with SDB, suggesting a role in arrhythmogenesis (12–16). A recent prospective, case-controlled study demonstrated that patients with untreated OSA had a significantly greater risk of recurrence of atrial fibrillation compared with individuals without OSA or with treated OSA, following cardioversion (13).

Stroke

OSA is very common in patients who have had a prior stroke, with a frequency ranging from 32% to 80% (17). The relationship between sleep apnea and cerebrovascular disease was also investigated in 6,424 patients in the Sleep Heart Health Study that demonstrated a significant increased risk for stroke in patients with OSA (9). The increased level of risk was proportional to the severity of OSA, with individuals in the highest AHI quintile having an odds ratio for stroke 1.58-fold greater than individuals in the lowest quintile.

Central Sleep Apnea

In contrast to OSA, central sleep apnea (CSA) is likely a consequence rather than a cause of CHF. As such, there is no clear causal relationship between CSA and increased risk for development of cardiovascular disease. However, in the setting of CHF, CSA appears to promote disease progression and increase risk for death (18–20). In patients with CHF, the frequency of CSA ranges from 30% to 50%, exceeding the frequency of OSA by a factor of three- to fourfold (15,20). In patients with asymptomatic left ventricular (LV) dysfunction and no history of CHF, one study reported a frequency of CSA of 55% (21). As there are approximately 5 million individuals with CHF in the United States, and as many as 3 to 5 million more with asymptomatic LV dysfunction, there may be 5 million individuals with LV dysfunction and CSA (1,22,23). An important caveat, however, is that much of the data on CSA prevalence was obtained prior to the widespread use of intensive pharmacotherapeutic strategies for CHF, including beta blockade. It is possible that beta blockers and other agents recently introduced into heart failure management, as well as more effective treatment of heart failure per se, may be associated with reduction in the prevalence of CSA in this population.

DIFFERENTIAL DIAGNOSIS

Sleep-disordered Breathing and Cardiovascular Disease

As SDB is highly prevalent in patients with known cardiovascular disease, the clinician should have a high index of suspicion for these disorders in any such individual. Although clinical symptoms and signs are often nonspecific, certain patient complaints and physical findings should prompt further investigation.

Fatigue is a frequent complaint and is often inappropriately attributed to structural heart disease or medications without consideration of possible sleep apnea. If snoring or apnea is witnessed by family members or a sleeping partner, this greatly increases the likelihood of the presence of sleep apnea (24). Nocturnal dyspnea, chest pain, and palpitations as well as snoring and apneic episodes should also raise suspicion of a sleep breathing disorder in patients with clinical cardiovascular disease. Sleep apnea should also be considered in the differential diagnosis of possible causes of resistance to conventional treatment strategies, particularly patients with refractory hypertension, intractable heart failure, and, perhaps also, recurrent atrial fibrillation.

Several cardiovascular syndromes have been associated with SDB (Table 28-1). Each of these syndromes is recognized to have multiple, different, specific underlying primary etiologies. For each of these syndromes, SDB should be considered in the differential diagnosis as either a primary or precipitating cause.

Systemic Arterial Hypertension

Hypertension affects 60 to 70 million North Americans and is a major risk factor for stroke, coronary artery disease, renal failure, and CHF (25,26). In only 5% to 10% of individuals is a primary underlying cause identified; however, OSA is increasingly recognized as a common identifiable cause of hypertension (26). The first formal acknowledgment

▶ **TABLE 28-1. Cardiovascular Disorders that May Be Associated with Obstructive Sleep Apnea**

Hypertension
Ischemic heart disease
Congestive heart failure
Stroke
Arrhythmias

of an important role of OSA in the management of hypertension was included in the sixth report of the Joint National Commission (JNC) guidelines for the diagnosis and management of hypertension, where OSA was identified as a potential cause of resistant hypertension (25). The most recent version of these guidelines, JNC VII, has listed OSA as the leading identifiable cause of hypertension (26).

The frequency of hypertension is increased in patients with OSA, and hypertensive patients have increased likelihood of concurrent OSA, suggesting a mechanistic link to daytime hypertension (8–11,26). Hypertension in patients with known OSA may be more difficult to control by standard therapy than in patients without OSA (26). Indeed, in patients in whom hypertension is refractory to therapy, the frequency of OSA has been reported to be very high (26). OSA should also be considered in the differential diagnosis of the "nondipper" hypertensive patient, i.e., one in whom blood pressure does not fall appropriately during sleep, particularly if the patient is obese (27). Hence, OSA should be considered in the differential diagnosis of all patients with hypertension as either the primary cause or an exacerbating factor.

Ischemic Heart Disease

Increased myocardial oxygen demand is promoted by increased heart rate, blood pressure, and contractility. In patients with coronary artery disease and OSA, nocturnal angina or silent ischemia may be precipitated by the physiologic events associated with repetitive apneas. In patients with frequent episodes of nocturnal angina, especially if daytime angina is controlled or minimal, the diagnosis of OSA should be considered.

Nocturnal myocardial ischemia is frequent in patients with OSA and coexistent in coronary artery disease, in whom nocturnal ST–T segment changes attributed to coronary ischemia have been reported (28, 29). Such episodes may often be provoked by oxygen desaturation and postapneic surges in heart rate and blood pressure and may be associated with angina or may be silent (28, 29). Hence, OSA appears to be both a risk factor for coronary artery disease and a hemodynamic stressor, that can precipitate acute ischemia in patients with known coronary artery disease.

Congestive Heart Failure

Orthopnea and paroxysmal nocturnal dyspnea are often attributed to CHF without consideration that these symptoms may be due to obstructive or central apneas or to apneas superimposed upon underlying structural heart disease. CSA is also strongly associated with LV dysfunction and CHF, and symptoms associated with the two disorders are indistinguishable as patient complaints for both disorders include hypersomnolence and nocturnal dyspnea. Indeed, some patients with CHF have combined OSA and

CSA (12,30). Discrimination of OSA from CSA is not possible without PSG. Although patients with OSA are more likely to be obese and to have a history of snoring, these features are not adequate to differentiate the two disorders. Heart failure patients with low end-tidal carbon dioxide levels and increased carbon dioxide sensitivity are probably more likely to have CSA (31).

Cardiac Arrhythmia

Specific arrhythmias, which can be attributed to sleep apnea, are difficult to identify because of the high rate of comorbid conditions in such patients, which may promote arrhythmia. However, it is likely that patients with OSA are at increased risk for both brady- and tachyarrhythmias.

Bradyarrhythmias associated with OSA include sinus bradycardia, sinus arrest, and high-grade atrioventricular block likely due to enhanced vagal tone prompted by the combination of apnea and hypoxemia, which activates the diving reflex (32,33). Hence, in patients with documented nocturnal bradyarrhythmia, OSA should be excluded prior to consideration of discontinuation of medications that slow heart rate or implantation of a pacemaker. While sleep apnea should always be considered in the differential diagnosis of patients who develop nocturnal bradyarrhythmias, it is also important to recognize that sleep apnea patients often have severe somnolence and may have sleep apnea–associated bradyarrhythmias that may manifest even during daytime hours.

Atrial fibrillation is the most common sustained tachyarrhythmia affecting Americans with prevalence estimated at 2 million individuals; it is associated with significant morbidity and mortality (34). Factors frequently implicated in the pathogenesis of atrial fibrillation include hypertension, thyroid disorders, and structural heart disease (34). OSA appears to confer increased risk for recurrence of atrial fibrillation. Moreover, the magnitude of hypoxemia on polysomnography (PSG) is significantly correlated with risk of recurrence; continuous positive airway pressure (CPAP) therapy significantly lowers the risk (13). These observations suggest that OSA is both a risk factor for the initial onset of atrial fibrillation and a precipitating cause of recurrence. Hence, in any patient who presents for evaluation and management of atrial fibrillation OSA should be considered in the differential diagnosis.

The relationship of CSA to both brady- and tachyarrhythmias has been less intensively studied than for OSA (35). Furthermore, CSA usually occurs in the setting of significant LV dysfunction either with or without CHF. Patients with LV dysfunction are at increased risk for many arrhythmias, especially atrial fibrillation and ventricular tachycardia. CSA has been associated with increased frequency of nonsustained ventricular tachycardia in patients with CHF (21,36). As CSA is an independent risk factor for adverse prognosis in CHF, the demonstrated association of CSA with nonsustained ventricular arrhythmia suggests that risk for sudden death may be increased.

Stroke

Cerebrovascular disease is the third leading cause of death and the most frequent cause of long-term disability in the United States (1). Stroke patients often report nonlocalizable cerebral symptoms, such as memory impairment, difficulty concentrating, hypersomnolence, and emotional lability, which are often attributed to cerebral infarction by patient and physician. However, these same symptoms are also typical of patients with SDB. This difficulty of differential diagnosis is further compounded by the fact that stroke and sleep apnea frequently coexist in the same patient.

Pulmonary Hypertension

Pulmonary hypertension may be either primary or secondary. There are numerous recognized causes of pulmonary hypertension; OSA may be a principal or an exacerbating cause. Acute hemodynamic changes in the pulmonary circulation associated with apnea have been well described. Several studies have reported an increased frequency of daytime pulmonary hypertension in patients with OSA (37,38). However, it is unknown whether nocturnal and apnea-associated pulmonary hypertension is associated with persistent daytime pulmonary hypertension. Moreover, few studies have excluded coexistent chronic obstructive pulmonary disease (COPD) with daytime hypoxemia, which confounds demonstration of a causal association.

In patients with pulmonary hypertension with or without cor pulmonale, the main differential diagnoses include left heart disease with increased left atrial pressure and parenchymal lung disease with chronic hypoxemia. In the absence of these disorders, OSA is an especially important consideration. It should also be seen as a potentially exacerbating factor as it may frequently coexist with other disorders and may be more amenable to therapeutic intervention.

Nonapneic Sleep Disorders and Cardiovascular Disease

Although the most compelling etiologic and prognostic interactions with cardiovascular disease are in the context of sleep-related breathing disorders, other aspects of physiologic sleep and disordered sleep may be relevant to cardiovascular disease. Freedom from acute cardiovascular events is not conferred by sleep, so that acute myocardial infarctions, cerebrovascular accidents, and sudden death may manifest while patients are asleep. The reasons for the occurrence of these events during sleep are unclear, although several factors may be involved.

During physiologic NREM sleep, blood pressure significantly falls and may be potentiated by the use of pharmacologic hypotensive agents. Maintenance of blood pressure homeostasis may be further blunted by autonomic dysfunction or excessive antihypertensive medication predisposing to impaired perfusion and, hence, ischemia during sleep. Indeed, in the elderly, hypertensives asymptomatic lacunar infarctions may be especially prevalent in those in whom blood pressure falls excessively during sleep (39). Autonomic and hemodynamic responses to REM sleep may also be implicated in cardiovascular presentations. REM may be associated with coronary vasospasm eliciting nocturnal angina and may often be a precursor to nocturnal anginal episodes in patients with existing coronary artery disease (40,41). Furthermore, REM may be associated with significant bradyarrhythmias (35).

The circadian distribution of cardiac and vascular events speaks directly to the potential influence of sleep on cardiovascular disease. Acute myocardial infarction and sudden death exhibit a peak occurrence between 6 and 11 AM (42); this circadian peak may be linked to the autonomic and hemodynamic effects of arousal from sleep, a circadian increase in sympathetic activation (43) and platelet adhesiveness (44) in the early morning, and the preponderance of REM sleep that occurs in the early morning just before waking (45).

Sleep deprivation may also make an important contribution to both acute cardiovascular events and chronic cardiovascular disease. Short-term sleep restriction is associated with increased blood pressure; longer-term sleep restriction may also be accompanied by evidence of systemic inflammation and impaired glucose tolerance (46–50). Decreased sleep duration may be implicated in hypertension and myocardial infarction (5,6,51). Thus, while sleep-related breathing disorders are an important potential component in the initiation, progression, and presentation of cardiovascular disorders, it is important to recognize the potential contribution of other sleep-related phenomena to cardiovascular pathophysiology and pathogenesis.

ETIOLOGY

The primary causes of OSA and CSA have been described elsewhere in this text; the focus of the discussion will be on the role of these disorders in promoting cardiovascular disease. As OSA appears to cause hypertension, it should contribute directly to cardiovascular and cerebrovascular morbidity and mortality, given the recognized relationship between hypertension and these disorders. It is also likely that there are mechanisms other than hypertension that link OSA to the pathogenesis of cardiovascular disease.

In normal sleep, pharyngeal muscle tone decreases and in susceptible individuals with a narrow pharynx, further narrows or occludes the upper airway. The consequences of obstructive apneas that underlie abnormal cardiovascular responses include repetitive exaggerated negative intrathoracic pressure, hypoxia, and arousal from sleep. These events promote mechanical, hemodynamic, neural, humoral, and inflammatory events, which may drive acute and chronic maladaptive responses that contribute to promote cardiovascular disease pathogenesis.

Cardiovascular Effects of Sleep and Arousal

NREM sleep typically accounts for 85% of total sleep time (TST) in healthy adults (50). During NREM sleep in healthy individuals, the cardiovascular system is in a state of hemodynamic and autonomic quiescence. Concurrent declines in central respiratory and sympathetic nervous outflow during NREM sleep may be attributed to central connections between respiratory-related and central cardiovascular neurons in the brainstem (52). In contrast, arousals from sleep are associated with abrupt increases in chemosensitivity, with augmented ventilation and abrupt increases in sympathetic neural activation (SNA), heart rate, and blood pressure, as well as withdrawal of vagal activity. Accordingly, arousal is a state of heightened respiratory and cardiovascular activity (53). Patients with SDB have frequent and recurrent episodes of apnea and hypoxia, which, in conjunction with the SNA of arousal, may contribute to the pathogenesis of cardiovascular disease.

Physiology of Obstructive Sleep Apnea

Acute Effects

Exaggerated and ineffective inspiratory effort against the occluded pharynx causes more negative intrathoracic pressure that increases LV afterload and myocardial transmural pressure due to the exaggerated differences between extra- and intracardiac pressure. Venous return to the right ventricle is increased with a shift of the ventricular septum, which impedes LV filling; LV relaxation may also be decreased, which further impairs LV filling (54–56). In sum, the increased LV afterload and decreased LV preload lead to diminished stroke volume.

Sympathetic outflow from the central nervous system (CNS) in patients with OSA is also modulated by altered lung mechanics and hypoxia. Vagally mediated afferent neural feedback during lung inflation inhibits sympathetic neural outflow; during apnea this effect is disinhibited (57). Hypoxia and hypercapnia associated with apnea promote further increased sympathetic neural outflow via activation of central and peripheral chemoreceptors (58). As the patient with OSA has recurrent episodes of apnea, there are acute surges in blood pressure in response to chemoreflex-mediated hypoxic stimulation of sympathetic activity (58). These responses are potentiated in hypertensive subjects (59). In addition to these neuronal effects, neurohumoral activation is also observed. Subjects

with OSA and normal LV function have been described to have elevated concentrations of plasma catecholamine (60), endothelin (61), and natriuretic peptides (62) prior to treatment with CPAP, with subsequent normalization after CPAP intervention.

The peak surges of heart rate and blood pressure coincide with the nadir of oxygen saturation, resumption of ventilation, and arousal from sleep. Increased vascular sympathetic nerve activity and concentration of circulating vasoconstrictors, such as catecholamines and endothelin, act concurrently to increase peripheral vascular resistance. On termination of apnea, stroke volume abruptly increases and, in the presence of the vasoconstricted peripheral circulation, is associated with dramatic surges in blood pressure (Fig. 28-2).

Chronic Effects

The adverse physiologic effects of OSA are also mediated by chronic alterations of autonomic, vascular, and endothelial function, which persist during wakefulness. Sympathetic neural activity is increased during wakefulness as well as sleep in OSA patients compared to controls (63,64) (Fig. 28-3). Increased SNA in normoxic, awake patients with OSA is likely due in part to tonic chemoreflex activation, because these patients have increased peripheral chemosensitivity and pressor responses to hypoxia (65,66). Chemoreflex deactivation with 100% oxygen lowers blood pressure, heart rate, and SNA in awake, healthy patients with OSA (65). CPAP reduces both nocturnal and daytime SNA, although this may require several months of therapy (63).

Normotensive awake normoxic OSA patients, free of known cardiovascular disease, also have faster heart rates, diminished heart rate variability, and excessive blood pressure variability in comparison with closely matched controls proved to be free of OSA (67). Both faster heart rates and blunted heart rate variability (68) predispose to the development of future hypertension, and increased blood pressure variability predisposes to end-organ damage. In most patients with essential hypertension, there is a nocturnal decrease of blood pressure (i.e., "dippers"). However, many OSA patients do not have a nocturnal decline in blood pressure ("nondippers"); this lack of decline of nocturnal blood pressure may be associated with increased cardiovascular risk (69).

In OSA, repetitive surges in blood pressure, sympathetic activity, and oxidative stress may promote vascular and endothelial injury. Subsequent to endothelial injury, atherosclerosis may be initiated by an inflammatory response with leukocyte accumulation and adhesion. Elevated plasma levels of adhesion molecules have been reported in patients with OSA (70) and are reduced by CPAP therapy (71). Inflammatory mediators have been associated with increased risk for cardiovascular events (72). C-reactive protein (CRP) is an inflammatory marker, not

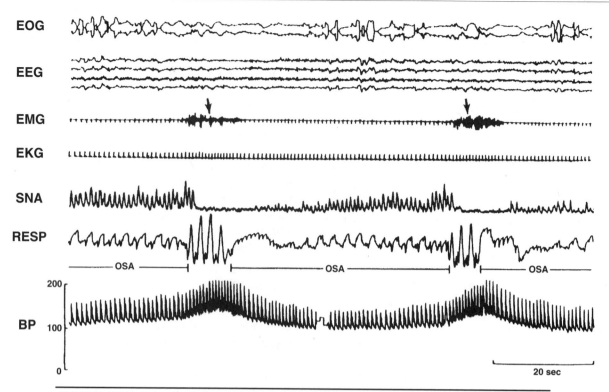

FIGURE 28-2. Recordings from PSG including electro-oculogram (EOG), electroencephalogram (EEG), electromyogram (EMG), electrocardiogram (EKG), sympathetic nerve activity (SNA), respiration (RESP), and blood pressure (BP) in patient with OSA during REM sleep. Arrows at EMG signify limb motion associated with sleep arousal. (From Somers VK, Dyken ME, Clary MP, Abboud FM. *J Clin Invest.* 1995;96:1897–1904. With permission.)

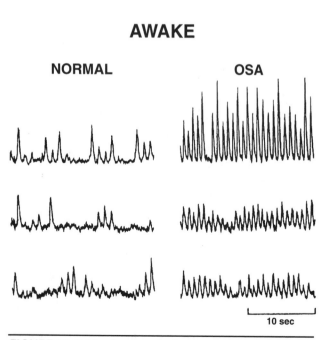

FIGURE 28-3. Muscle sympathetic nerve activity during wakefulness is increased in patients with OSA compared with normal subjects. (From Somers VK, Dyken ME, Clary MP, Abboud FM. *J Clin Invest.* 1995;96:1897–1904. With permission.)

only associated with increased risk of cardiac ischemic events, but one that may play a direct role in atherogenesis and thrombus formation. In patients with OSA, CRP is elevated compared to normal controls and is increased in proportion to the severity of the AHI (73) (Fig 28-4A and B). Mechanisms linking OSA to increased CRP may include repetitive hypoxemic episodes and sleep deprivation. Increased plasma interleukin (IL)-6 (74), IL-1 receptor antagonist (74), and CRP (74), and increased synthesis of fibrinogen (75) have been observed during hypoxic conditions at high altitude. Both sleep deprivation and excessive daytime sleepiness have also been associated with increased plasma levels of IL-6 (76).

Thus, OSA may act through multiple mechanisms to predispose to cardiac and vascular injury. These mechanisms are activated even in seemingly healthy OSA patients without overt cardiovascular disease. There are only limited data addressing the degree to which these abnormalities of neural, vasoactive, and inflammatory mechanisms can be corrected by effective treatment with CPAP. Nevertheless, there is preliminary evidence for a causal interaction between OSA and cardiovascular disease, in that successful treatment of OSA with CPAP reduces blood pressure in patients with hypertension (Fig. 28-5) (77) and improves LV ejection fraction in patients with heart failure (Fig. 28-6) (78).

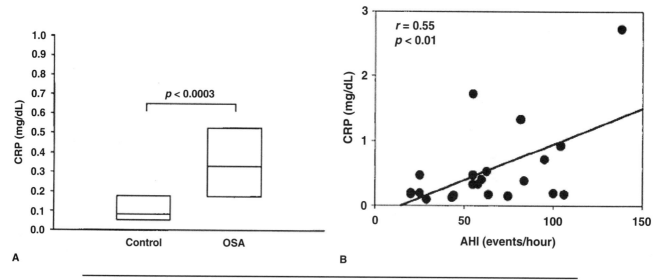

FIGURE 28-4. (A) Box plot demonstrating plasma CRP in patients ($n = 22$) with OSA and controls ($n = 20$). Horizontal line inside box indicates median. Bottom and top of box are 25th and 75th percentile, respectively. (B) Linear regression for CRP levels versus AHI. (From Shamsuzzaman AS, Winnicki M, et al. *Circulation.* 2002;105:2462–2464. With permission.)

Physiology of Central Sleep Apnea

CSA is a form of periodic breathing in which apneas and hypopneas alternate with ventilatory periods, forming a crescendo–decrescendo pattern of tidal volume. There is instability of ventilatory control associated with oscillation of the partial pressure of arterial carbon dioxide ($Paco_2$), which fluctuates above and below the apnea threshold, driven by alternating episodes of hyperventilation and apnea (Fig. 28-7). In general, the cardiovascular, autonomic, and neurohumoral consequences of CSA are less well characterized than for OSA. However, adverse consequences are likely similar to those previously characterized for OSA and include repetitive apnea-related hypoxemia and increased SNA associated with apnea and arousals (79,80).

Patients with CHF and CSA have lower $Paco_2$ during both sleep and wakefulness compared to subjects with CHF and no CSA (31,81–82). The mechanism for chronic hypocapnia in such individuals has not been completely elucidated. As systemic arterial oxygen saturation is not lower in affected patients compared with controls without CSA, the etiology cannot be ascribed to hypoxia (31,81–82). Patients with CHF are likely predisposed to CSA due to increased central chemoreceptor sensitivity, hyperventilation, prolonged circulation time, and altered baroreceptor function (31,81–83).

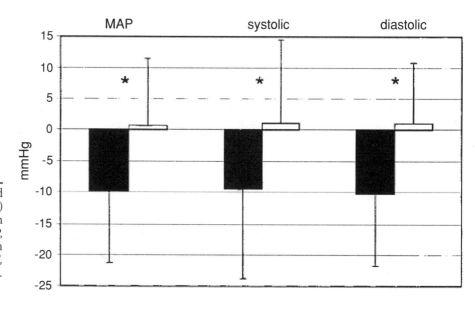

FIGURE 28-5. Change in blood pressure with effective (closed bars) and ineffective (open bars) CPAP in patients with OSA, (*p < 0.05). MAP, mean arterial blood pressure. (From Becker HF, Jerrentrup A, Ploch T, et al. *Circulation.* 2003;107:68–73. With permission.)

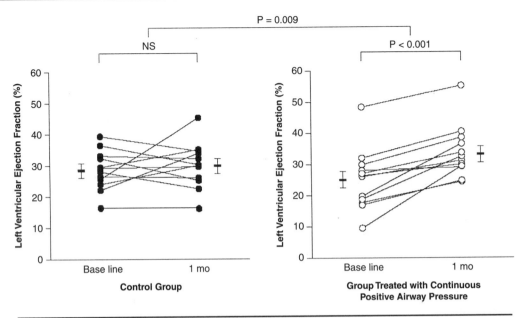

FIGURE 28-6. Effect of CPAP or control on LVEF in patients with CHF. LVEF was measured at baseline and at 30 days; all patients received standard pharmacotherapy. For controls, there was no significant change in LVEF from baseline to 1 month. LVEF increased in all subjects treated with CPAP (mean 25.0 ± 2.8 to 33.8 ± 2.4; $p < 0.001$). (From Kaneko Y, Floras JS, et al. *N Engl J Med.* 2003;348:1233–1241. With permission.)

Increased central and peripheral chemoreceptor sensitivity has been demonstrated in patients with CHF and CSA (84). Hyperventilation may also arise from afferent neural input from vagal stretch receptors stimulated by pulmonary congestion (85). Subjects with CHF and CSA have higher LV filling pressures as well as lower $Paco_2$ than patients without CSA (85). Prolongation of circulation time between the lungs and chemoreceptors in CHF associated with reduced cardiac output may also promote instability of ventilation because of delayed feedback control (83). Baroreflex regulation also likely contributes to instability of ventilatory control, as baroreflex deactivation augments the ventilatory response to stimulation of peripheral chemoreceptors (86). Baroreflex control is abnormal in patients with ventricular dysfunction, possibly enhancing chemoreflex gain. Hence, chemoreflex–baroreflex interactions may contribute to abnormal ventilatory control in patients with CSA and LV dysfunction.

Other factors that may contribute to the genesis of CSA in CHF patients include neurohumoral activation, recurrent hypoxia, changes in the state of consciousness, and upper-airway obstruction. Urinary catecholamine concentrations are increased in individuals with CHF and CSA compared with patients with CHF only (80); however, activation of other neurohumoral systems has not been described (80). Hypoxia associated with apnea may provoke arousals and thereby increase the ventilatory response to carbon dioxide (87). With onset of NREM sleep, the waking drive to breathe is diminished and the threshold for a ventilatory response to carbon dioxide is increased, resulting in central apnea; arousal during this phase of increased

$Paco_2$ may then be associated with hyperpnea, thereby initiating an oscillating breathing pattern. In some patients with CHF and OSA, the adverse hemodynamic effects of OSA appear to cause further deterioration in cardiac function overnight, leading to the development of CSA (88,89).

Central Sleep Apnea and the Progression of Congestive Heart Failure

Although the underlying mechanisms for the development of CSA have not been definitively established, CSA is especially evident in more severe cases of CHF. It is possible that CSA also contributes to the progression of CHF and may itself contribute to worse outcomes. Central apneas elicit increases in sympathetic nerve traffic (79) and patients with CSA and CHF have higher levels of urine and plasma norepinephrine as compared to CHF patients without CSA (80). Adrenergic activation induced by CSA would be expected to be deleterious in the setting of CHF, as would the significant pressor responses accompanying the repetitive apneas (90,91).

The presence of CSA even in patients with asymptomatic LV dysfunction and its association in these patients with increased arrhythmias, independent of measurements such as LV ejection fraction, exercise tolerance, or other variables, also suggests that CSA contributes to cardiovascular pathophysiology in patients with subclinical myocardial dysfunction (21). Whether asymptomatic LV dysfunction patients with CSA are more likely to progress to heart failure and whether CSA contributes to progression remains to be determined. Data suggestive of

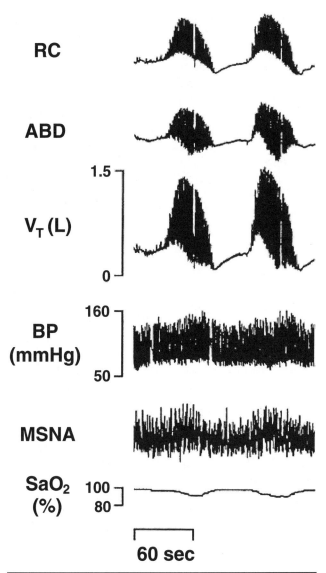

FIGURE 28-7. PSG recordings of CSA in a patient with CHF. There is an oscillating pattern of tidal volume (V_T) with hyperpnea alternating with apnea. Oxyhemoglobin desaturation ($Saco_2$) is associated with apneas. Central apneas are recognized by absence of rib cage (RC) and abdominal (ABD) motion. Each cardiac cycle is accompanied by increased muscle sympathetic nerve activity (MSNA). (From Bradley TD, Floras JS. *Circulation.* 2003;107:1822–1826. With permission.)

improved transplant-free survival in heart failure patients with CSA randomized to effective CPAP treatment support the concept of CSA as a contributing factor to worse CHF outcomes (92).

DIAGNOSTIC EVALUATION

The vast majority of patients with SDB and cardiovascular disease are undiagnosed due to limited physician awareness of the prevalence of sleep apnea. All patients with

TABLE 28-2. Associated Clinical Findings in OSA

Increased body mass index
Increased neck circumference
Small erythematous oropharynx
Systemic hypertension
Congestive heart failure
Pulmonary hypertension
Cor pulmonale
Atrial fibrillation

cardiovascular disease should be screened for signs and symptoms of these disorders.

Screening begins with a careful history; important features include hypersomnolence, witnessed snoring, and apnea. Interview of a sleeping partner greatly facilitates obtaining an accurate history of disordered nocturnal breathing. On physical examination, obesity, a large neck, and narrow upper airway, especially when associated with historic factors suggestive of sleep apnea, should prompt further evaluation (Table 28-2). Screening tools are established as useful aids for identification of patients with suspected SDB. As the frequency is quite high in patients with overt cardiovascular disease, it seems reasonable to have a low threshold for use of these tools. The Epworth Sleepiness Scale (ESS) provides a rapid, validated screening method with demonstrated utility in both clinical and research settings (24).

In-laboratory PSG remains the gold standard for diagnosis and resolves the differential diagnosis of obstructive versus central sleep apnea or mixed disorders and defines therapeutic intervention. However, specific clinical indications for PSG and threshold for treatment in patients with cardiovascular disease have not been clearly established. For this reason, the primary indications for PSG are identical to those for patients with suspected sleep apnea in whom there is no cardiovascular disease. Accordingly, patients with a history of hypersomnolence, snoring, apnea, and paroxysmal nocturnal dyspnea should be considered for PSG.

Because sleep-related breathing disorders are very common in patients with clinical cardiovascular disease, it also seems reasonable to have a low threshold for referral for PSG. However, in the absence of either symptoms (e.g., the nonsleepy sleep apneic) or proof of improved outcomes for cardiovascular disorders, the role for diagnosis and intervention is not clearly established. Moreover, there are insufficient numbers of PSG laboratories to investigate very large cardiovascular disease patient populations, and home-monitoring systems have not yet been demonstrated to be of sufficient diagnostic sensitivity and specificity. Studies from small patient samples showing benefits of diagnosis and treatment of OSA in patients with resistant hypertension (94) and improvements in LV ejection fraction in heart failure patients with OSA, who do not have daytime sleepiness (78), suggest that the presence of significant cardiovascular disease together with a reasonable suspicion for sleep apnea may justify evaluation even in the absence of significant daytime sleepiness. Until definitive evidence and consensus recommendations are available, it seems prudent to screen and investigate selected patients with cardiovascular disease, including refractory hypertension, recurrent or refractory CHF, nocturnal angina, and recurrent atrial fibrillation.

CLINICAL MANAGEMENT

Obstructive Sleep Apnea

For patients who are obese, weight loss is recommended as it reduces the AHI as well as improving other risk factors associated with cardiovascular disease. For nonobese individuals or those who are unable to lose weight, CPAP is the cornerstone of therapy. In patients who cannot tolerate CPAP, mandibular advancement devices or surgical interventions may be necessary.

Hypertension

Patients with OSA may be hypertensive during the night or daytime. Uncontrolled studies with CPAP or tracheostomy have demonstrated reductions of blood pressure at night in individuals who are normotensive during the day (94). The effects of CPAP on daytime blood pressure have also been assessed in patients with OSA who were normotensive during the day and not surprisingly demonstrated minimal effect (95,96). A single, nonrandomized study of CPAP therapy for patients with refractory hypertension has been reported; in this study, 2 months of therapy with CPAP was associated with significant reductions in nocturnal and daytime blood pressure (93). In patients with hypertension, a randomized study comparing therapeutic and subtherapeutic levels of CPAP has shown significant reductions not only in nighttime blood pressure but also in blood pressure recorded during the daytime (77) (Fig. 28-5).

Ischemic Heart Disease and Stroke

There have been a few uncontrolled reports describing the efficacy of CPAP for the relief of nocturnal angina in patients with coronary artery disease (97). However, no randomized studies have been reported. Similarly, there have been no controlled studies describing potential benefits of CPAP in stroke patients.

Congestive Heart Failure

Two small studies have demonstrated the efficacy of CPAP for the treatment of LV dysfunction associated with OSA

(78,98). The first of these studies was uncontrolled and limited to patients with nonischemic disease (98); the second study was randomized, controlled, and included subjects with either an ischemic or nonischemic etiology (78). Each study treated subjects with CPAP for 30 days, in addition to standard pharmacotherapy, and demonstrated significant improvement in left ventricular ejection fraction (LVEF) and functional status (Fig. 28-6). In addition to demonstrating of the beneficial effect of CPAP on LV function and symptoms, these studies provided evidence suggestive of a potential contribution of OSA to LV dysfunction. Whether CPAP improves morbidity and mortality outcomes in patients with CHF and OSA awaits completion of prospective, randomized, clinical trials.

Arrhythmia

A single study suggests that CPAP reduces the risk of recurrent atrial fibrillation in patients with OSA (13). In patients with recurrent atrial fibrillation who also have clinical features suggestive of OSA, PSG should be considered. In patients in whom OSA is identified, even if not sleepy, it seems reasonable to consider intervention with CPAP to lower risk for recurrence.

Central Sleep Apnea

There is no consensus regarding management of CSA associated with CHF in the absence of definitive therapies and long-term treatment trials demonstrating efficacy. Potential treatment goals would be to improve quality of life, improve cardiovascular function, and prolong life.

CSA is likely a consequence of CHF and, hence, optimum treatment of the underlying disease is the first step in management. CSA is related to left atrial pressure elevation, and reduction of intracardiac filling pressures have been associated with decreased frequency of apnea (85). Accordingly, standard pharmacotherapy of CHF, including diuretics, ACE inhibitors, digitalis, and beta blockade may attenuate CSA. Overdiuresis should be avoided as it may promote metabolic alkalosis, which may lower the threshold for CSA. Other therapies that may benefit patients with CHF and CSA include supplemental oxygen and noninvasive ventilation. Supplemental nocturnal oxygen has been demonstrated to alleviate hypoxia, decrease the frequency of apnea, and improve sleep architecture (99). It also reduces urinary norepinephrine levels and improves exercise tolerance (80). However, these benefits have not been associated with improved quality of life or objective improvement in cardiovascular function, morbidity, or mortality in short-term studies (80).

Controlled, short-term studies of noninvasive positive airway pressure support, including CPAP, bilevel, and adaptive-pressure support servoventilation, have been shown to reduce the frequency of apnea in subjects with CSA (100,101). In controlled studies evaluating cardiovascular outcomes, CPAP has also been demonstrated to increase LVEF, reduce mitral regurgitation, reduce excessive sympathetic neural activation, and improve quality of life (80,101).

Short-term studies with theophylline have demonstrated reduction of the frequency of apnea, although no benefit has been demonstrated for other clinical endpoints (102). Moreover, in the setting of chronic LV dysfunction, there are concerns about the potential proarrhythmic effects of chronic administration of a sympathomimetic agent. A single study reported reduction of the frequency of apnea with atrial overdrive pacing in subjects with a clinically indicated pacemaker for sinus node dysfunction who also had coexistent CSA or OSA (103). The mechanism of this apparent benefit was unclear, but may have been due to increased cardiac output with decreased pulmonary congestion.

PROGNOSIS

For hypertension, no studies characterizing the effect of SDB on prognosis have been reported. However, sleep apnea does appear to confer a more adverse prognosis for patients with ischemic heart disease, stroke, and CHF.

Obstructive Sleep Apnea

It is likely that OSA has adverse effects on prognosis in patients with LV dysfunction although prospective studies examining such a relationship have not been reported. In a well-matched case control study of coronary care unit patients with OSA, those who remained untreated had significantly increased mortality (104). Patients with stroke, who have OSA, may also have poorer prognostic outcomes (105).

Central Sleep Apnea

CSA is associated with increased arrhythmia risk (24) and more adverse prognosis in CHF (19). It is uncertain whether CSA is a manifestation of more severe cardiac dysfunction or whether it is an independent abnormality of ventilatory control with an adverse effect on the progression of underlying structural heart disease. However, several studies have reported that CSA is an independent risk factor for ventricular arrhythmia, death, or cardiac transplantation (19,20,36). Moreover, the frequency of disordered breathing events is directly related to prognosis (Fig. 28-8), and treatment with CPAP may enhance survival (20).

FUTURE DIRECTIONS

Sleep-related breathing disorders are underdiagnosed. It is important to educate practitioners, including primary care physicians and subspecialists, regarding the high prevalence of these disorders and their interaction with cardiovascular disease. Because of the number of patients with cardiovascular disease and the relative paucity of in-laboratory PSG facilities, reliable home-screening or outpatient techniques will need to be developed to facilitate identification and triage of high-risk patients for definitive PSG.

For both OSA and CSA, development of pharmacologic interventions that may attenuate apnea severity would be an important contribution to management of these disease conditions, particularly if any such medications are easily tolerated in patients with coexisting cardiovascular disease. The recent intriguing observation of overdrive pacing being accompanied by reduced numbers of both central and obstructive apneas suggests a potential future therapeutic strategy. However, additional studies are important

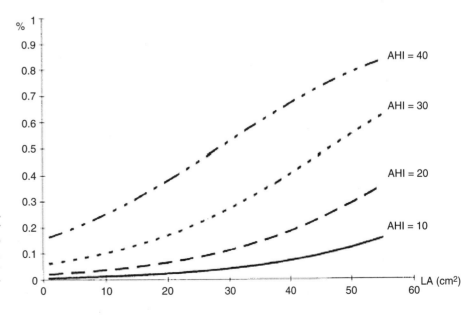

FIGURE 28-8. Mortality rates for patients with CSA according to AHI and left atrial (LA) area. (From Lanfranchi P, et al. *Circulation* 1999;99:1435–1440. With permission.)

to confirm these observations and perhaps to provide insights into potential mechanisms of benefit.

Obstructive Sleep Apnea

Cross-sectional and epidemiologic studies of OSA have demonstrated that asymptomatic disease is common (9). It may be important to reconsider the goals of CPAP therapy in patients with OSA and cardiovascular disease as the cardiovascular consequences of OSA become more apparent and may prove to be the most important. In principle, therapeutic intervention in asymptomatic individuals may lower the risk of atherogenesis and other cardiovascular disorders.

If OSA is an important risk factor for cardiovascular disease, carefully designed clinical studies will be needed to demonstrate the pathophysiologic basis of this relationship as well as the efficacy of therapy in patients who are not sleepy. Furthermore, if therapeutic intervention is associated with reduced cardiovascular morbidity, treatment indications may then be expanded to include asymptomatic patients. This, in turn, would require increased diagnostic efforts in patients at increased risk including obese patients and those with known cardiovascular disease or multiple risk factors.

Central Sleep Apnea

Clinical trials are underway to more definitively establish the efficacy of CPAP in the therapy of CHF (106). Adaptive servoventilation, investigational noninvasive ventilation that provides low-level CPAP and autotitrates, depending on tidal volume, appears to have promise, and may prove more efficacious than CPAP.

CLINICAL PEARLS

Risk factors for OSA in patients with heart failure

- Male gender
- Increased body mass index (men)
- Age (women)
- Refractory to standard therapy

Clues suggesting the presence of OSA in patients with cardiovascular disease

- Refractory hypertension
- Obesity
- Male gender
- Fatigue
- Snoring
- Witnessed apnea
- Nocturnal ischemia
- Nocturnal bradyarrhythmia
- Absence of nocturnal dip in blood pressure

Treatment options for CSA (Cheyne–Stokes respiration and CHF)

- Optimize pharmacotherapy of CHF (the foundation of treatment)
- Consider nocturnal supplemental oxygen
- CPAP/BiPAP

Investigational

- Adaptive sero-ventilation
- Pacing

ACKNOWLEDGMENTS

The authors are supported by: NIH HL-77478-02, HL-65176, HL-61560, HL-70602, HL-73211, M01-RR00585, the Dana Foundation, and the Mayo Foundation.

REFERENCES

1. American Heart Association. *Heart disease and stroke statistics—2003 update*. AHA website.
2. American Heart Association. *International cardiovascular disease statistics— 2003 update*. AHA website.
3. Report of the National Commission on Sleep Disorders Research. *Wake up America: A national sleep alert*. Washington, D.C.: U.S. Government Printing Office, 1995.
4. Verrier RL, Muller JE, Hobson JA. Sleep, dreams, and sudden death: the case for sleep as an autonomic stress test for the heart. *Cardiovasc Res*. 1996;31:181–211.
5. Kato M, Phillips BG, Sigurdsson G, et al. Effects of sleep deprivation on neural circulatory control. *Hypertension*. 2000;35:1173–175.
6. Ayas NT, White DP, Manson JT, et al. A prospective study of sleep duration and coronary heart disease in women. *Arch Internal Med*. 2003;163:205–209.
7. Young T, Palta M, Dempsey J, et al. The occurrence of sleep-disordered breathing among middle-aged adults. *N Engl J Med*. 1993;328:1230–1235.
8. Nieto FJ, Young TB, Lind BK, et al. Association of sleep-disordered breathing, sleep apnea, and hypertension in a large community-based study. Sleep Heart Health Study. *JAMA*. 2000;283:1829–1836.
9. Shahar E, Whitney CW, Redline S, et al. Sleep-disordered breathing and cardiovascular disease: cross-sectional results of the Sleep Heart Health Study. *Amer J Respir Crit Care Med*. 2001;163:19–25.
10. Young T, Peppard P, Palta M, et al. Population-based study of sleep-disordered breathing as a risk factor for hypertension. *Arch Internal Med*. 1997;157:1746–1752.
11. Peppard PE, Young T, Palta M, et al. Prospective study of the association between sleep-disordered breathing and hypertension. *N Engl J Med*. 2000;342:1378–1384.
12. Sin DD, Fitzgerald F, Parker JD, et al. Risk factors for central and obstructive sleep apnea in 450 men and women with congestive heart failure. *Amer J Respir Crit Care Med*. 1999;160:1101–1106.
13. Kanagala R, Murali NS, Friedman, PA, et al. Obstructive sleep apnea and the recurrence of atrial fibrillation. *Circulation*. 2003;107:2589–2594.
14. Mooe T, Gullsby S, Rabben T, et al. Sleep-disordered breathing: a novel predictor of atrial fibrillation after coronary artery bypass surgery. *Coronary Artery Dis*. 1996;7:475–478.
15. Javaheri S, Parker TJ, Liming JD, et al. Sleep apnea in 81 ambulatory male patients with stable heart failure: types and their prevalences, consequences, and presentations. *Circulation*. 1998;97:2154–2159.
16. Blackshear JL, Kaplan J, Thompson RC, et al. Nocturnal dyspnea and atrial fibrillation predict Cheyne-Stokes respirations in patients

with congestive heart failure. *Arch Internal Med.* 1995;155:1297–1302.

17. Yaggi H, Mohsenin V. Sleep-disordered breathing and stroke. *Clin Chest Med.* 2003;24:223–238.
18. Hanly PJ, Zuberi-Khokhar NS. Increased mortality associated with Cheyne-Stokes respiration in patients with congestive heart failure. *Amer J Respir Crit Care Med.* 1996;153:272–276.
19. Lanfranchi PA, Braghiroli A, Bosimini E, et al. Prognostic value of nocturnal Cheyne–Stokes respiration in chronic heart failure. *Circulation.* 1999;99:1435–1440.
20. Sin DD, Logan AG, Fitzgerald FS, et al. Effects of continuous positive airway pressure on cardiovascular outcomes in heart failure patients with and without Cheyne–Stokes respiration. *Circulation.* 2000;102:61–66.
21. Lanfranchi PA, Somers VK, Braghiroli A, et al. Central sleep apnea in left ventricular dysfunction: prevalence and implications for arrhythmic risk. *Circulation.* 2003;107:727–732.
22. Ho KK, Pinsky JL, Kannel WB, et al. The epidemiology of heart failure: The Framingham Study. *J Amer Coll Cardiol.* 1993;22:6A–13A.
23. Hunt HA, Baker DW, Chin MH, et al. ACC/AHA guidelines for the evaluation and management of chronic heart failure in the adult: executive summary. A report of the American College of Cardiology/American Heart Association Task Force on Practice Guidelines (Committee to Revise the 1995 Guidelines for the Evaluation and Management of Heart Failure). *Circulation.* 2001;104:2996–3007.
24. The report of an American Academy of Sleep Medicine Task Force. Sleep-related breathing disorders in adults. Recommendations for syndrome definition and measurement techniques in clinical research. *Sleep.* 1999;22:667–689.
25. Joint National Committee on Prevention Detection, Evaluation, and Treatment of High Blood Pressure. The sixth report of the Joint National Committee on Prevention, Detection, Evaluation and Treatment of High Blood Pressure. *Arch Internal Med.* 1997;157:2413–2446.
26. Joint National Committee on Prevention Detection, Evaluation, and Treatment of High Blood Pressure. The seventh report of the Joint National Committee on Prevention, Detection, Evaluation and Treatment of High Blood Pressure. *JAMA.* 2003;289:2560–2572.
27. Portaluppi F, Provini F, Cortelli P, et. al. Undiagnosed sleep-disordered breathing among male non-dippers with essential hypertension. *J Hypertens.* 1997;15:1227–1233.
28. Franklin KA, Nilsson JB, Sahlin C, et al. Sleep apnoea and nocturnal angina. *Lancet.* 1995;345:1085–1087.
29. Peled N, Abinader EG, Pillar G, et al. Nocturnal ischemic events in patients with obstructive sleep apnea syndrome and ischemic heart disease: effects of continuous positive air pressure treatment. *J Amer Coll Cardiol.* 199;34:1744–1749.
30. Tkacova R, Niroumand M, Lorenzi-Filho G, et al. Overnight shift from obstructive to central apneas in patients with heart failure: role of PCO(2) and circulatory delay. *Circulation.* 2001;103:238–243.
31. Javaheri S. A mechanism of central sleep apnea in patients with heart failure. *N Engl J Med.* 1999;341:949–954.
32. Zwillich C, Devlin T, White D, et al. Bradycardia during sleep apnea: characteristics and mechanism. *J Clin Invest.* 1982;69:1286–1292.
33. Somers VK, Dyken ME, Mark Al, et al. Parasympathetic hyperresponsiveness and bradyarrhythmias during apnea in hypertension. *Clin Autonomic Res.* 1992;2:172–176.
34. Fuster V, Ryden LE, Asinger RW, et al. ACC/AHA/ESC guidelines for the management of patients with atrial fibrillation: executive summary. *Circulation.* 2001;1204:2118–2150.
35. Guilleminault C, Connolly SJ, Winkle RA. Cardiac arrhythmia and conduction disturbances during sleep in 400 patients with sleep apnea syndrome. *Amer J Cardiol.* 1983;52:490–494.
36. Javaheri S. Effects of continuous positive airway pressure on sleep apnea and ventricular irritability in patients with heart failure. *Circulation.* 2000;101:392–397.
37. Sanner BM, Doberauer C, Konermann M, et al. Pulmonary hypertension in patients with obstructive sleep apnea syndrome. *Arch Internal Med.* 1997;157:2483–2487.
38. Bady E, Achkar A, Pascal S, et al. Pulmonary arterial hypertension in patients with sleep apnea syndrome. *Thorax.* 2000;55:934–939.
39. Kario K, Pickering TG, Matsuo T, et al. Stroke prognosis and abnormal nocturnal blood pressure falls in older hypertensives. *Hypertension.* 2001;38:852–855.
40. King MJ, Zir LM, Kaltman AJ, et al. Variant angina associated with angiographically demonstrated coronary artery spasm and REM sleep. *Amer J Med Sci.* 1973;265:419–422.
41. Nowlin JB, Troyer WG, Jr, Collins WS, et al. The association of nocturnal angina pectoris with dreaming. *Ann Internal Med.* 1965;63:1040–1046.
42. Guilleminault C, Connolly SJ, Winkle RA, et al. Cardiac arrhythmia and conduction disturbances during sleep in 400 patients with sleep apnea syndrome. *Amer J Cardiol.* 1883;52:490–494.
43. Muller JE, Kaufman PG, Luepker RV, et al. Mechanisms precipitating acute cardiac events. *Circulation.* 1997;96:3233–3239.
44. Ridker PM, Manson JE, Buring JE, et al. Circadian variation of acute myocardial infarction and the effect of low-dose aspirin in a randomized trial of physicians. *Circulation.* 1990;82:897–902.
45. Somers VK, Dyken ME, Mark AL, et al. Sympathetic-nerve activity during sleep in normal subjects. *N Engl J Med.* 1993;328:303–307.
46. Kato M, Phillips BG, Sigurdson G, et al. Effects of sleep deprivation on neural circulatory control. *Hypertension.* 2000;35:1173–1175.
47. Meunter NK, Watenpaugh DE, Wasmund WL, et al. Effects of sleep restriction on orthostatic cardiovascular control in humans. *J Appl Physiol.* 2000;88:966–972.
48. Vgontzas AN, Papanicalaou DA, Bixler EO, et al. Sleep apnea and daytime sleepiness and fatigue: relation to visceral obesity, insulin resistance, and hypercytokinemia. *J Clin Endocrinol Metab.* 2000;85:1151–1158.
49. Meier-Ewert HK, Ridker PM, Rifai N, et al. Effect of sleep loss on C-reactive protein, an inflammatory marker of cardiovascular risk. *J Amer Coll Cardiol.* 2004;43:678–688.
50. Spiegel K, Leproult R, Van Cauter E. Impact of sleep debt on metabolic and endocrine function. *Lancet.* 1999;354:1435–1439.
51. Tochibuko O, Ikeda A, Miyajima E, et al. Effects of insufficient sleep on blood pressure monitored by a new multibiomedical recorder. *Hypertension.* 1996;27:1318–1324.
52. Guyenet PG, Koshiya N, Huangfu D, et al. Central respiratory control of A5 and A6 pontine noradrenergic neurons. *Amer J Physiol.* 1993;264:R1035–R1044.
53. Mancia G. Autonomic modulation of the cardiovascular system during sleep. *N Engl J Med.* 1993;328:347–349.
54. Brinker JA, Weiss JL, Lappe DL, et al. Leftward septal displacement during right ventricular loading in man. *Circulation.* 1980;61:626–633.
55. Virolainen J, Ventila M, Turto H, et al. Effect of negative intrathoracic pressure on left ventricular pressure dynamics and relaxation. *J Appl Physiol.* 1995;79:455–460.
56. Tkacova R, Rankin F, Fitzgerald FS, et al. Effects of continuous positive airway pressure on obstructive sleep apnea and left ventricular afterload in patients with heart failure. *Circulation.* 1998;98:2269–2275.
57. Seals DS, Suwarno NO, Joyner MJ, et al. Respiratory modulation of muscle sympathetic nerve activity in intact and lung denervated humans. *Circ Res.* 1993;72:440–454.
58. Somers VK, Dyken ME, Clary MP, et al. Sympathetic neural mechanisms in obstructive sleep apnea. *J Clin Invest.* 1995;96:1897–1904.
59. Somers VK, Mark AL, Abboud FM. Potentiation of sympathetic neural response to hypoxia in borderline hypertensive subjects. *Hypertension.* 1988;11:608–612.
60. Dimsdale JE, Coy T, Ziegler MG, et al. The effect of sleep apnea on plasma and urinary catecholamines. *Sleep.* 1995;18:377–381.
61. Phillips BG, Narkiewicz K, Pesek CA, et al. Effects of obstructive sleep apnea on endothelin-1 and blood pressure. *J Hypertension.* 1999;17:61–66.
62. Baruzzi A Riva R, Cirignotta F, Zucconi M, et al. Atrial natriuretic peptide and catecholamines in obstructive sleep apnea syndrome. *Sleep.* 1991;14:83–86.
63. Narkiewicz K, Kato M, Phillips BG, et al. Nocturnal continuous positive airway pressure decreases daytime sympathetic traffic in obstructive sleep apnea. *Circulation.* 1999;100:2332–2335.
64. Narkiewicz K, van de Borne PJ, Cooley RL, et al. Sympathetic activity in obese subjects with and without obstructive sleep apnea. *Circulation.* 1998;98:772–776.

65. Narkiewicz K, van de Borne PJ, Montano N, et al. Contribution of tonic chemoreflex activation to sympathetic activity and blood pressure in patients with obstructive sleep apnea. *Circulation.* 1998;97:943–945.

66. Narkiewicz K, van de Borne PJ, Pesek CA, et al. Selective potentiation of peripheral chemoreflex sensitivity in obstructive sleep apnea. *Circulation.* 1999;99:1183–1189.

67. Narkiewicz K, Montano N, Cogliati C, et al. Altered cardiovascular variability in obstructive sleep apnea. *Circulation.* 1998;98:1071–1077.

68. Singh JP, Larson MG, Tsuji H, et al. Reduced heart rate variability and new-onset hypertension. Insights into pathogenesis of hypertension: The Framingham Heart Study. *Hypertension.* 1998;32:293–297.

69. Verdecchia P, Schillaci C, Borgioni C, et al. Gender, day-night blood pressure changes, and left ventricular mass in essential hypertension. Dippers and peakers. *Amer J Hypertension.* 1995;8:193–196.

70. El-Solh AA, Mador MJ, Sikka O, et al. Adhesion molecules in patients with coronary artery disease and moderate-to-severe obstructive sleep apnea. *Chest.* 2002;121:1541–1547.

71. Chin K, Nakamura T, Shimizu K, et al. Effects of nasal continous positive airway pressure on soluble cell adhesion molecules in patients with obstructive sleep apnea syndrome. *Amer J Med.* 200;109:562–567.

72. Ridker PM. High-sensitivity C-reactive protein: potential adjunct for global risk assessment in the primary prevention of cardiovascular disease. *Circulation.* 2001;103:1813–1818.

73. Shamsuzzaman AS, Winnicki M, Lanfranchi P, et al. Elevated C-reactive protein in patients with obstructive sleep apnea. *Circulation.* 2002;105:2462–2464.

74. Hartmann G, Tschop M, Fischer R, et al. High altitude increases circulating interleukin-6, interleukin-1 receptor antagonist and C-reactive protein. *Cytokine.* 2000;12:246–262.

75. Imoberdorf R, Garlick PJ, McNurlan MA, et al. Enhanced synthesis of albumin and fibrinogen at high altitude. *J Appl Phyiol.* 2001;90:528–537.

76. Shearer WT, Reuben JM, Mullington, JM, et al. Soluble TNF-alpha receptor 1 and IL-6 plasma levels in humans subjected to the sleep deprivation model of spaceflight. *J Allergy Clin Immunol.* 2001;107:165–170.

77. Becker HF, Jerrentrup A, Ploch T, et al. Effect of nasal continous positive airway pressure on blood pressure in patients with obstructive sleep apnea. *Circulation.* 2003;107:68–73.

78. Kaneko Y, Floras JS, Usui K, et al. Cardiovascular effects of continuous positive airway pressure in patients with heart failure and obstructive sleep apnea. *N Engl J Med.* 2003;348:1233–1241.

79. van de Borne P, Oren R, Abouassaly C, et al. Effect of Cheyne-Stokes respiration on muscle sympathetic nerve activity in severe congestive heart failure secondary to ischemic or idiopathic dilated cardiomyopathy. *Amer J Cardiol.* 1998;81:432–436.

80. Naughton MT, Benard DC, Liu PP, et al. Effects of nasal CPAP on sympathetic activity in patients with heart failure and central sleep apnea. *Amer J Respir Crit Care Med.* 1995;152:473–479.

81. Lorenzi-Filho G, Azevedo ER, Parker JD, et al. Relationship of PaCO2 to pulmonary wedge pressure in heart failure. *Eur Respir J.* 2002;19:37–40.

82. Naughton M, Benard D, Tam A, et al. Role of hyperventilation in the pathogenesis of central sleep apneas in patients with congestive heart failure. *Amer Rev Respir Dis.* 1993;148:330–338.

83. Leung RS, Bradley TD. Sleep apnea and cardiovascular disease. *Amer J Respir Crit Care Med.* 2001;164:2147–2165.

84. Solin P, Rebuck T, Johns DP, et al. Peripheral and central ventilatory responses in central sleep apnea with and without congestive heart failure. *Amer J Respir Crit Care Med.* 2000;162:2194–2200.

85. Solin P, Bergin P, Richardson M, et al. Influence of pulmonary capillary wedge pressure on central apnea in heart failure. *Circulation.* 999;99:1574–1579.

86. Somers VK, Mark AL, Abboud FM. Interactions of baroreceptor and chemoreceptor reflex control of sympathetic nerve activity in normal humans. *J Clin Invest.* 1991;86:1953–1957.

87. Khoo MC, Kronauer RE, Strohl, KP, et al. Factors inducing periodic breathing in humans: a general model. *J Appl Physiol.* 1982;53:644–659.

88. Alex CG, Onal E, Lopata M. Upper airway occlusion during sleep in patients with Cheyne-Stokes respiration. *Amer Rev Respir Dis.* 1986;133:42–45.

89. Tkacova R, Niroumand M, Lorenzi-Filho G, et al. Overnight shift from obstructive to central apneas in patients with heart failure: role of PCO(2) and circulatory delay. *Circulation.* 2001;103:238–243.

90. Lorenzi-Filho G, Dajani HR, Leung RS, et al. Entrainment of blood pressure and heart rate oscillations by periodic breathing. *Amer J Respir Crit Care Med.* 1999;159:1147–1154.

91. Trinder J, Merson R, Rosenberg JI, et al. Pathophysiological interactions of ventilation, arousals and blood pressure oscillations during Cheyne-Stokes respiration in patients with heart failure. *Amer J Respir Crit Care Med.* 2000;162:808–813.

92. Sin DD, Logan AG, Fitzgerald FS, et al. Effects of continuous positive airway pressure on cardiovascular outcomes in heart failure patients with and without Cheyne-Stokes respiration. *Circulation.* 2000;102:61–66.

93. Logan AG, Tkacova R, Perlikowski SM, et al. Refractory hypertension and sleep apnea: effects of continous positive airway pressure on blood pressure and baroreflex. *Eur Resp J.* 2003;21:241–247.

94. Fletcher EC, Miller J, Schaaf JW, et al. Urinary catecholamines before and after tracheosotomy in patients with obstructive sleep apnea and hypertension. *Sleep.* 1987;10:35–44.

95. Faccenda JF, Mackay TW, Boon NA, et al. Randomized, placebo-controlled trial of continous positive airway pressure on blood pressure in the sleep apnea-hypopnea syndrome. *Amer Rev Respir Crit Care Med.* 2001;163:344–348.

96. Engleman HM, Gough K, Martin SE, eta l. Ambulatory blood pressure on and off continuous positive airway pressure therapy for the sleep apnea/hypopnea syndrome: effects in "non-dippers." *Sleep.* 1996;19:378–381.

97. Philip P, Guillemenault C. ST segment abnormality, angina during sleep and obstructive sleep apnea. *Sleep.* 1993;16:558–559.

98. Malone S, Liu PP, Holloway R, et al. Obstructive sleep apnea in patients with dilated cardiomyopathy: Effects of continuous positive airway pressure. *Lancet.* 1991;338:1480–1484.

99. Hanly PJ, Millar TW, Steljes DG, et al. The effect of oxygen on respiration and sleep in patients with congestive heart failure. *Ann Internal Med.* 1989;111:777–782.

100. Naughton MT, Bernard DC, Rutherford R, et al. Effect of continuous positive airway pressure on central sleep apnea and nocturnal PCO2 in heart failure. *Amer Rev Resp Crit Care Med.* 1994;150:1598–1604.

101. Teschler H, Dohring J, Wang YM, et al. Adaptive pressure support servo-ventilation. A novel treatment for Cheynes-Stokes respiration in heart failure. *Amer J Resp Crit Care Med.* 2001;164:614–619.

102. Javaheri S, Parker TJ, Wexler L, et al. Effect of theophylline on sleep-disordered breathing in heart failure. *N Engl J Med.* 1996;335:562–567.

103. Garrigue S, Bordier P, Jais P, et al. Benefit of atrial pacing in sleep apnea syndrome. *N Engl J Med.* 2002;346:404–412.

104. Peker Y, Hedner J, Kraiczi H, et al. Respiratory disturbance index: An independent predictor of mortality in coronary artery disease. *Amer J Respir Crit Care Med.* 2000;162:81–86.

105. Dyken ME, Somers VK, Yamada T, et al. Investigating the relationship between stroke and obstructive sleep apnea. *Stroke.* 1996;27:401–407.

106. Bradley TD, Logan AG, Floras JS. Rationale and design of the Canadian Positive Airway Pressure Trial for patients with congestive heart failure and central sleep apnea: The CANPAP Trial. *Can J Cardiol.* 2001;17:677–684.

Chapter 29

Sleep and Pulmonary Diseases

W. McDowell Anderson, Arthur Andrews, and David G. Davila

INTRODUCTION

Disorders of the lung and chest wall have traditionally been classified according to their physiologic effects as measured by pulmonary function tests (PFT) (Table 29-1). Obstructive lung diseases have a disproportionate decrease in the forced expiratory volume that can be exhaled in 1 second (FEV_1) when divided by the total amount exhaled over more than 6 seconds, or forced vital capacity (FVC). This results in hyperinflation of the lung and elevation of the residual volume (RV), functional residual capacity (FRC), and total lung capacity (TLC) (Fig. 29-1). RV is the volume at maximal exhalation, FRC is the relaxed end-expiratory volume during tidal breathing, and TLC is the amount of air in the lung at the end of maximal inhalation. The RV is the first lung volume to increase (air trapping) with increases in the FRC and TLC in more severe obstructive airway disease. That is, in obstructive lung diseases, the TLC is either normal or increased. The hallmark of obstruction is a reduction in the FEV_1/FVC ratio on spirometry. In contrast, restrictive lung diseases, whether they be intrinsic to the lung parenchyma, such as interstitial fibrosis, or extrinsic, such as chest wall abnormalities, such as kyphoscoliosis, result in a reduced TLC and a normal FEV_1/FVC ratio. In severe parenchymal restrictive lung disease, the FRC and RV can be decreased as well as the TLC. In diseases associated with expiratory muscle weakness, the RV may be increased. Expiratory

muscles are required to exhale from FRC to RV. Of note, the vital capacity $=$ TLC $-$ RV can be decreased in both obstructive and restrictive lung disease. In obstruction, the RV increases more than the TLC. In restriction, the TLC decreases more that the RV. The differences in impact of disease on pulmonary function helps the clinician understand patient complaints during daytime activities as well as sleep.

Considerable research has been done to better understand the effects of sleep on obstructive lung diseases, such as chronic obstructive pulmonary disease (COPD). Improved monitoring has shown that sleep may have deleterious effects on oxygenation in sleep. This has enabled the development of noninvasive ventilation to improve morbidity and mortality during acute exacerbations of COPD, as well as chronic respiratory failure. Other than COPD, the clinician should understand the effects of sleep on other obstructive diseases, such as asthma and cystic fibrosis.

In contrast to COPD, intrinsic restrictive diseases of the lung, such as idiopathic pulmonary fibrosis (IPF), have not reached the same success in therapy, whereas the problems in sleep are well documented. The polio epidemics early in the last century led to expanded knowledge of how extrinsic lung diseases of the chest wall could lead to respiratory insufficiency. This prompted the development of noninvasive ventilation, even before invasive techniques, such as endotracheal intubation were instituted.

▶ **TABLE 29-1. A Clinical Classification of Interstitial Lung Diseases (Partial List)**

Collagen vascular diseases
Rheumatoid arthritis
Polymyositis
Scleroderma
Sjogren's syndrome
Systemic lupus erythematosus
Ankylosing spondylitis

Drug-induced
Nitrofurantoin
Sulfasalazine
Amiodarone
Gold
Cyclophosphamide (Cytoxan)
Carmustine (BCNU)
Methotrexate
Bleomycin
Busulfan
Procarbazine
Radiation

Primary diseases
Sarcoidosis
Eosinophilic granuloma
Vasculitis
Eosinophilic pneumonias
Diffuse alveolar hemorrhage
Lymphangioleiomyomatosis
Alveolar proteinosis
Acute respiratory distress syndrome

Occupational-environmental

Inorganic
Silicosis
Asbestosis
Beryllosis
Coal worker's pneumoconiosis

Organic
Hypersensitivity pneumonitis (farmer's lung, bird breeder's lung, etc.)

Unknown etiology
Idiopathic pulmonary fibrosis
Bronchiolitis-associated interstitial lung disease
Acute interstitial pneumonia (Hamman-Rich syndrome)
Bronchiolitis obliterans organizing pneumonia
Lymphocytic interstitial pneumonitis

These techniques have been applied not only to postpolio syndrome and respiratory failure, but also to the treatment of patients with most neuromuscular disorders.

OBSTRUCTIVE LUNG DISEASES

Sleep-related Ventilation and Oxygenation

Sleep is associated with a diminished responsiveness of the respiratory center to chemical, mechanical, and cortical inputs. These changes are more pronounced in REM sleep, during which there is more variability in respiratory rate and tidal volume (1). Therefore, one can expect the mandatory increase in $Paco_2$ and reduction in Pao_2 of 2 to 8 mm Hg and 3 to 10 mm Hg respectively. Regardless of the change in Pao_2, the Sao_2 only declines by less than 2% in this scenario, given the characteristics of the oxyhemoglobin dissociation relationship (2). In individuals with normal pulmonary function and at sea level, there is relatively little consequence to Sao_2. The impact of sleep in patients with COPD has been long-studied and, indeed, poses several challenging management considerations. Chronic bronchitis patients—the "blue bloaters"—are more likely to be hypoxemic and hypercapneic as compared to patients with advanced emphysema, the so-called "pink puffers" (3). Patients with COPD have been noted to demonstrate significant increases in mean pulmonary artery pressures and $Paco_2$ levels when going from wakefulness to sleep (4). The tendency for worsening nocturnal hypoxemia in these patients, coupled with the pulmonary vasculature's response of hypoxic vasoconstriction, predisposes to the development of pulmonary hypertension and cor pulmonale (5).

Clinical Epidemiology

COPD is now recognized as our nation's most rapidly growing health problem, ranking as the fourth most common killer (6). Patients with COPD must also endure the expected sleep-related increase in airways resistance, decreased intercostal muscle activity, and fall in FRC (1). Obstructive sleep apnea (OSA) and COPD often exist in the same patient in what is termed overlap syndrome. Chaouat and colleagues (7) prospectively studied 256 patients with confirmed OSA. Of these patients, 11% had evidence of obstruction on spirometry. The overlap patients were male, more hypoxemic, had higher $Paco_2$ levels, and were found to have more elevated rest and exercise mean pulmonary artery pressures. Suspicion for significant sleep-disordered breathing (SBD) in patients with COPD should be heightened in the following circumstances (8):

- Patients who desaturate during exercise
- Nonobese patients with moderate to severe COPD with progressive decline in arterial blood gases
- Hypercapneic patients with severe chronic bronchitis
- Pulmonary and systemic hypertension
- Congestive heart failure

Asthma and Other Obstructive Lung Diseases

Asthma affects 14 to 15 million persons in the United States and is the most common chronic disease in childhood (9). In a large study of nocturnal symptoms in 7,729 asthmatics in the United Kingdom, 74% reported awakening at least once per week and 64% awakened at least three times per week (10). Patients often underestimated the severity of

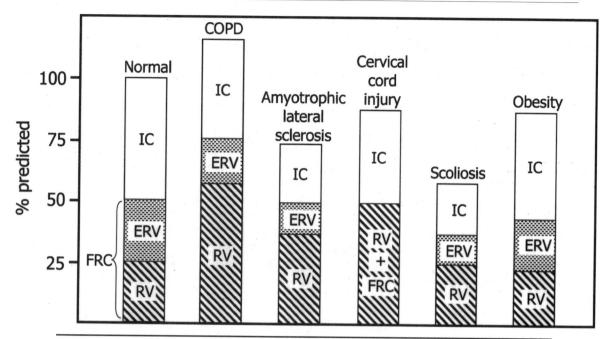

FIGURE 29-1. Lung volumes for a normal individual (far left) are compared with inflated lung volumes in a patient with COPD and reduced volumes in patients with various disorders of the thorax. IC, inspiratory capacity; FRC, functional residual capacity; ERV, expiratory reserve volume; RV, residual volume. (From Bergofsky EH. Respiratory insufficiency in mechanical and neuromuscular disorders of the thorax. In: Fishman AP, ed. *Pulmonary diseases and disorders.* New York, McGraw-Hill, 1980:1563. With permission.)

their asthma, were more prone to having allergies, and no particular asthma drug was associated with a lessening of symptoms (10). Serial measurements of peak expiratory airflow have shown that airflow obstruction in asthmatic patients peaks between 3:00 and 4:00 AM (11). As described in the next section, this is part of the reason why asthmatics are more likely to present to the emergency department between midnight and 8:00 AM, why 40% of their calls to physicians occur between 11 PM and 7:00 AM, and 42% to 53% of fatal asthma exacerbations occur at night (11–14).

A more extreme but much less common form of airway disease is cystic fibrosis (CF). It is the most common life-shortening autosomal recessive disorder in the white population (15). It affects approximately 30,000 persons in the United States. The resulting bronchiectasis, COPD, and chronic recurrent infection account for over 90% of fatalities.

Etiology

Chronic Obstructive Pulmonary Disease

The effects of hyperinflation on patients with COPD have been well documented. Factors, such as mechanical disadvantage from shortened diaphragmatic muscle fiber length, with resultant decrease in force of contraction, lead to an increased work of breathing. The excessive workload leads to respiratory muscle fatigue and potential failure

during periods of increased demands on the system. Patients with COPD have lower than normal PaO_2 and will have a greater fluctuation in SaO_2. These patients have been shown to be hypoxemic during sleep through the mechanisms of hypoventilation, OSA, reduction in FRC, and ventilation and perfusion (V/Q) mismatch (16). An increased incidence of SDB in these patients may further lead to significant nocturnal hypoxemia.

Asthma and Other Obstructive Lung Diseases

Whether nocturnal asthma is a distinct entity or just a manifestation of poorly controlled asthma, in general, is not clear. However, there are several mechanisms that have a role in worsening symptoms at night:

- Airway inflammation
- Circadian rhythm changes in parasympathetic tone and hormone levels
- Allergens and airway cooling
- Gastroesophageal reflux
- Mucociliary clearance
- Bronchial hyperactivity

Studies have shown that airway inflammation occurs specifically at night in asthmatics with increased airway eosinophils and neutrophils, superoxide, and cytokine concentrations, as well as activated lymphocyte and macrophage levels from bronchoalveolar lavage (BAL) samples and biopsies (17). Genetic factors may also play a role, such as in downregulation of the beta-2 adrenoreceptor number in the Gly16 polymorphism of this receptor (18).

Normal people have circadian changes in airway caliber, with mild nocturnal bronchoconstriction. This appears to be exaggerated in asthmatics. When subjects are given cholinergic blocking agents, such as inhaled ipratropium or intravenous atropine, this effect can be diminished (19,20). Sympathetic tone does not appear to be involved in these circadian changes (21). Control of allergen exposure has been a mainstay of asthma management. Controlling these factors at night, such as cleaning the bedroom or bedding, may enhance overall improvement in asthma and not just nocturnal symptoms. Avoiding these agents at night does not abolish the circadian changes in bronchoconstriction (21). Cold, dry air may further add nocturnal bronchoconstriction. When a small group of asthmatic patients breathed warm, humidified air (36° to 37°C, 100% saturation) compared with room air, bronchoconstriction could be abolished (22). Gastroesophageal reflux is highly prevalent in patients with asthma, but its role in producing daytime symptoms is not clear. While gastric acid can enhance previously mentioned bronchoconstriction, acid suppression with histamine type-2 blockers (23) or proton pump inhibitors (24) improves nighttime symptoms with minimal daytime effects (21). In addition, drugs such as theophylline, which are known to decrease distal esophageal sphincter (promoting reflux), actually improve nocturnal symptoms (25). Increased mucociliary clearance and bronchial hyperresponsiveness occur during sleep, but are not likely to be a major factor in producing symptoms over and above the previously described mechanisms.

CF results in mutations in the cystic fibrosis transmembrane conductance regulator (CFTR) gene, which results in defective chloride transport in the epithelial cells of the respiratory, hepatobiliary, gastrointestinal, and reproductive tracts, as well as the pancreas. This results in the clinical manifestations discussed below (15).

Diagnostic Evaluation

Ancillary Tests

Chest radiography is often of critical importance in the evaluation of pulmonary diseases. A stepwise approach to interpretation of a chest radiograph is often helpful. The large airways such as the glottis, trachea, and mainstem bronchi can be assessed for any suggestion of extrinsic compression by parenchymal or extraparenchymal masses or vascular structures. The remainder of the bronchial tree is evaluated for any evidence of intraluminal obstruction secondary to tumors or tenacious secretions, and diffuse enlargement and dilation as can be seen in bronchiectasis. The skeletal structures are reviewed for rib fractures

and spinal scoliosis and kyphosis, both of which may alter the mechanics of breathing. The cardiovascular structures, including the heart, pulmonary vasculature, and aorta, should be examined for signs of enlargement, engorgement, and dilation, respectively. Diaphragmatic contour and relative height may suggest the presence or lack of significant hyperinflation and paralysis. An increase in the retrosternal airspace (>3 cm) on the lateral view may also suggest hyperinflation. Pulmonary hypertension and right ventricular hypertrophy are indicated by prominent hilar vascular shadows and encroachment of the heart shadow on the retrosternal space as the right ventricle anteriorly enlarges (26). The pulmonary parenchyma may demonstrate lucencies representative of emphysematous changes or, indeed, deficient blood supply. Diffuse interstitial infiltrates in a peripheral distribution may point to interstitial lung disease. Asthma exacerbations with mucus plugging can lead to nodular densities and atelectasis, as well as the hyperinflation described above. The chest radiograph in CF reveals patchy infiltrates, bronchiectasis, and cystic areas resembling small abscesses.

The electrocardiogram (ECG) may supplement the clinician's suspicion for significant COPD, asthma, or other obstructive lung diseases. As many as 75% of patients with COPD have ECG abnormalities. Hyperinflation of the lungs leads to depression of the diaphragm and, therefore, clockwise rotation of the heart along its longitudinal axis (27). The end result would be deep S waves in the right precordial leads with poor R wave progression and QS waves in a pattern similar to that seen in anterior myocardial infarction. P pulmonale, defined as a P wave greater than or equal to 2.5 mm in the inferior leads resulting from right atrial enlargement due to hypertrophy or dilation, is often found in COPD. In the presence of cor pulmonale and right ventricular hypertrophy, the ECG may reflect right atrial enlargement with right axis deviation and a prominent R wave in lead V_1.

As previously described, PFTs are an essential part of the diagnosis of COPD as well as other obstructive lung diseases. They have a well-founded utility in establishing the severity of the impairment from disease and monitoring the response to treatment. The FEV_1 is the gold standard for the diagnosis of airflow obstruction (26). These patients also typically display a reduction in the FEV_1/FVC ratio, an increase in TLC and residual volume (RV), which suggests hyperinflation and air trapping, respectively (Fig. 29-1). Arterial blood gases (ABGs) reveal the expected hypoxemia. Hypercapnia develops as the disease progresses and is more common when the FEV_1 falls below 1 L.

Laboratory evaluation is important in the evaluation of patients with obstructive lung diseases and includes not only the ABG, as noted above, but also the carbon monoxide (CO) as measured by cooximetry. An evaluation of CO may be helpful in assessing further abuse of tobacco products and promote effective counseling. Erythrocytosis is more commonly seen when the arterial Pao_2 falls below

55 mm Hg. A normal hemoglobin in the face of severe obstruction on PFTs should prompt the physician to search for a source of blood loss. The appropriate patient with family history, early age onset, or the nonsmoker will need an alpha-1 antitrypsin level. If abnormal, then more specific genetic testing may be indicated. For patients with early obstructive airway disease but not limited to an early age at onset, sweat chloride analysis for cystic fibrosis may be warranted. More specific genetic testing for mutations of the CFTR gene can be obtained if results and clinical information are equivocal (15).

Nighttime Evaluation

The American Sleep Disorders Association (ASDA) recognizes four different levels of recording devices for the assessment of sleep apnea (28). Level I includes standard polysomnography (PSG) performed in the laboratory. Level II studies are performed outside of the lab and are capable of recording complete PSG without a technologist present (unattended). Level III devices can record respiratory effort, airflow, oxygen saturation, and pulse or ECG. Level IV devices record only one or two variables such as pulse, oximetry, and ECG.

PSG is the recommended test for the diagnosis of OSA and various disorders of sleep, such as periodic limb movements of sleep (PLMS), upper-airway resistance syndrome (UARS), REM behavior disorder (RBD), somnambulism, and parasomnias (28).

Interestingly, the sensitivity of PSG in the diagnosis of OSA has not been clearly shown, as PSG is usually assumed to be the gold standard of comparison. However, there can be substantial night-to-night variability in the apnea + hypopnea index on PSG studies. It is also well recognized that a negative overnight PSG does not completely exclude the diagnosis of obstructive sleep apnea. This is particularly the case for patients who have risk factors for SDB on clinical grounds. Meyer and colleagues (29) studied 11 such patients who met diagnostic criteria for OSA during a second study, with an increase in the apnea–hypopnea index (AHI) from 3.1 +/− 1.0 baseline, to 19.8 +/− 4.7 events per hour (mean +/− SEM, $p < 0.01$) on the repeat study. Studies have shown that 11.5% of patients with an AHI <5 on study night one have an increase to >5 on night two (30).

Level II and III devices refer to portable devices that are useful in situations where symptomatic patients who suggest OSA require prompt evaluation and treatment when PSG is not available. These devices have not been adequately studied in patients with COPD and are not yet recommended for routine clinical use (28).

Oximetry, the mainstay of level IV devices, measures the oxygen saturation of hemoglobin by distinguishing deoxyhemoglobin from oxyhemoglobin based on the differential absorption of light (31). The normal value for oxyhemoglobin saturation during sleep in healthy subjects is approximately 96.5% (+/−1.5%). There are no decreases reported in oxyhemoglobin saturation for different ethnic populations or sex, but it will decrease with altitude.

Historically, pulse oximetry was the key means to identify patients with Pickwickian syndrome with prolonged oxygen desaturation (Figs. 29-2 and 29-3) or severe sleep apnea syndrome with alveolar hypoventilation. The latter may be associated with a saw-toothed pattern (Fig. 29-4) (32). Over the last decade, multiple studies have evaluated the utility of pulse oximetry in screening for SDB. The term SDB encompasses OSA, central sleep apnea syndrome (CSAS), UARS, and sleep hypoventilation syndrome (SHVS). Sensitivities ranging from 31% to 98% and specificities from 41% to 100% have been reported. Williams and co-workers (33) used home oximetry and laboratory PSG to evaluate 40 patients suspected of having OSA. Sensitivity of oximetry was only 56%, whereas specificity was 100%. Epstein and Dorlac (34), retrospectively, reviewed overnight sleep studies on 100 consecutive patients. They used either a "deep" pattern of a 4% or greater decrease in SaO$_2$ to less than 90% or a "fluctuating pattern" without a definite criteria for change or nadir in the SaO$_2$ to identify events. Oximetry was considered abnormal when there were 10 or more oximetry events per hour. The fluctuating pattern had a greater sensitivity, whereas the deep pattern had a greater specificity in identifying OSA. If only mild patients were considered, the fluctuating pattern was still not as sensitive as PSG.

Overnight oximetry can be a useful screening test for SDB when there is a low clinical suspicion of sleep apnea. In a patient able to sleep efficiently for a sufficient time compared with what he or she would consider a routine night of sleep, a normal or negative oximetry can help exclude sleep apnea. Similarly, when there is a high degree of clinical suspicion for OSA and oximetry results are normal, further testing is required. The key characteristics of an abnormal overnight oximetry that suggests SDB are oscillatory variation in saturation and oscillatory desaturation (Fig. 29-4). Epstein and co-workers (34) suggest that this abnormality can be defined as a greater than 4% change in oxyhemoglobin saturation to less than or equal to 90% and a pattern of repetitive short-duration fluctuations in saturation and desaturations. Other investigators (35) have found that resaturations of greater than or equal to 3% SpO$_2$ within 10 seconds at the end of a respiratory event were a better detector of respiratory disturbance events. Low-baseline saturations that may slowly increase or decrease about baseline values without oscillations may be more indicative of gas-exchange abnormalities, such as those encountered in advanced COPD (Figs. 29-2 and 29-3). The desaturations, secondary to COPD, tend to last much longer and have a much lesser degree of slope in the waveform (32).

The accuracy of oximetry can be affected by factors such as vasoconstriction, hypotension, skin pigmentation, nail abnormalities, patient movement, and probe

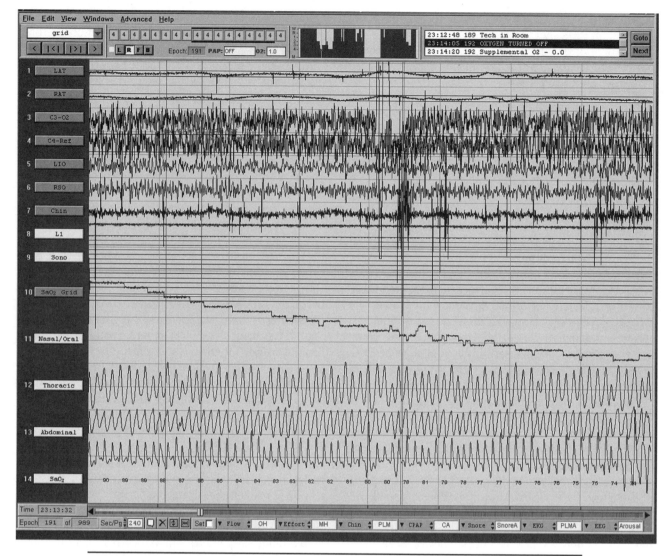

FIGURE 29-2. Periods of alveolar hypoventilation (gradual decline in Sao$_2$ channel 10) during sleep (30-second epoch) may go undetected as the nasal/oral flow (thermistor) and chest and abdominal effort (piezoelectric belts) signals remain essentially unchanged. Channels 1 and 2, left and right anterior tibialis electromyogram; channels 3 and 4, left and right central electroencephalogram; channels 5 and 6, left and right occipital electroencephalogram; channel 7, chin electromyogram; channels 8 and 9, not used; channel 10, oxygen saturation; channel 11, nasal and oral flow sensors; channels 12 and 13, thoracic and abdominal effort sensors; channel 14, numeric oxygen saturation.

positioning. Significantly different saturation data are obtained at various acquisition options. Davila and co-workers (36) studied 75 patients with suspected OSA with simultaneous pulse oxyhemoglobin saturation traces at three recording settings, or averaging times. These investigators found that faster recording settings (shorter averaging times or response times) resulted in lower levels of oxyhemoglobin saturation than slower settings (longer averaging times or response times) (Figs. 29-4 and 29-5). Several authors have also found significant differences in the saturation data obtained on-line real time (high sampling rates) and those values obtained from memory (low sampling rates) in unattended studies. Desaturation indexes obtained from memory have been found to be signifi-

cantly lower than those obtained on-line (36). Studies have confirmed lower sensitivities and higher specificities using longer averaging times settings (for example, 12 seconds) and memory display mode (36). Faster recording settings (shorter averaging times) and on-line display mode give rise to higher sensitivity and lower specificity. Therefore, the default settings must be known by the user and interpreter. Faster recording settings and on-line display is the methodology of choice.

Indeed, oximetry alone is not recommended for the evaluation of sleep apnea in place of PSG, given the lack of standardization in performance and interpretation. Oximetry is, however, comparatively inexpensive, less disruptive to sleep, and more readily available than PSG. It

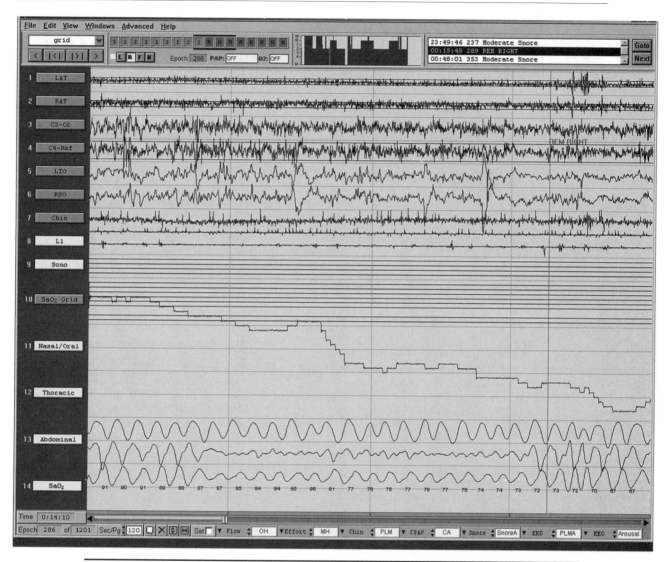

FIGURE 29-3. Periods of alveolar hypoventilation during sleep undetected by flow (thermistor) but demonstrated on the chest and abdominal effort channels (piezoelectric belts). Channels 1 and 2, left and right anterior tibialis electromyogram; channels 3 and 4, left and right central electroencephalogram; channels 5 and 6, left and right occipital electroencephalogram; channel 7, chin electromyogram; channels 8 and 9, not used; channel 10, oxygen saturation; channel 11, nasal and oral flow sensors; channels 12 and 13, thoracic and abdominal effort sensors; channel 14, numeric oxygen saturation.

has proved to be very useful in following the response to therapies for OSA, such as oral appliances.

Overnight pulse oximetry is also useful for determining the degree to which COPD patients desaturate during sleep. Patients with COPD and daytime hypoxemia (Po_2 <55 mm Hg) or Po_2 55–59 mm Hg with signs of end-organ damage have improved survival with continuous diurnal and nocturnal oxygen therapy. In the Nocturnal Oxygen Therapy Trial (NOTT) (37), 203 patients with hypoxemic COPD were randomized to continuous or 12-hour nocturnal supplemental oxygen. One-year follow-up demonstrated improved survival and decreased morbidity with continuous supplemental oxygen. However, there was no improvement in morbidity or mortality with

nocturnal oxygen therapy alone. COPD patients with FEV_1 less than 1 L may spend greater than 90% of the night with saturations well below 90% when breathing room air (3,4). Risk factors for nocturnal desaturation are $Paco_2$ greater than or equal to 45 mm Hg and Pao_2 less than 65 mm Hg on oxygen (3,4). However, the severity of nocturnal desaturation in COPD patients cannot be predicted with certainty. Hence, we can see the potential utility of overnight oximetry. The causes of the nocturnal desaturation include hypoventilation, coexisting sleep apnea, reduction in FRC, and altered ventilation-perfusion matching, as previously mentioned. The benefit of nocturnal oxygen therapy in patients with a daytime Po_2 >60 mm Hg, but nocturnal desaturation, is unproved. However, many clinicians will

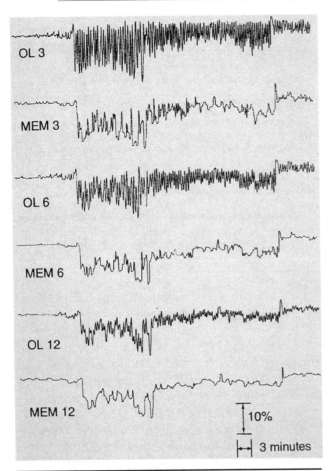

FIGURE 29-4. Cyclic desaturations in a patient with OSA depicted by oximetry. The oximetry data were recorded either online (OL) or from the oximeter's memory function (MEM) at three different recording settings (3,6, and 12 seconds) which equate to averaging time and response time. (From Davila DG, Richards KC, Marshal BL, et al: Oximeter performance: the influence of acquisition parameters. *Chest.* 2002;122:1654. With permission.)

prescribe oxygen treatment if there is prolonged desaturation or evidence of end-organ dysfunction (cor pulmonale).

Approximately 10% to 15% of patients with COPD have sleep apnea (1). In COPD patients with signs and symptoms of OSA and/or polycythemia or pulmonary hypertension with right heart dysfunction or right heart failure, a sleep study is indicated. The American Academy of Sleep Medicine (AASM) outlines other associated features and laboratory findings in many patients with SDB (38).

Asthma and Other Obstructive Lung Diseases

PSG has demonstrated decreased sleep efficiency, increased arousals and awakenings, decreased sleep time with associated daytime sleepiness, and impaired cognition in patients with asthma (21,25). The resulting sleep deprivation may be associated with impaired ventilatory

drive and contribute, along with other factors, to the worsening of hypoxemia and hypercapnia in severe acute attacks. In spite of these findings and in the absence of other symptoms of a specific sleep disorder, PSG is not indicated. Overnight oximetry may be used as described for COPD, to evaluate for nocturnal hypoxemia and plan home oxygen therapy.

Patients with cystic fibrosis may have more severe sleep disruption than in other obstructive lung diseases, with impaired daytime functioning. Dancey and associates (39) reported that 19 patients with severe CF had reduced sleep efficiency (71%) and frequent awakenings, as well as lower mean SaO_2 when compared with 10 healthy controls. Furthermore, the CF patients were sleepier, with reduced sleep latency on multiple sleep latency testing (MSLT) (6.7 minutes). These findings correlated with more reported fatigue and lower levels of happiness and activation as well as impaired cognitive function. Predicting nocturnal desaturation appears problematic, as spirometric parameters, awake SpO_2 were not found to be predictive in 70 patients with CF studied by Frangolias and colleagues (40). However, Milross reported that evening arterial PaO_2 did contribute to the ability to predict both sleep-related desaturation and elevated transcutaneous CO_2 in 32 stable CF patients in transitioning from NREM to REM sleep (41). Further studies are needed to determine if evening ABGs and/or nocturnal oximetry may be useful in the management of these patients with moderate to severe disease (15, 35–41).

Clinical Management

Chronic Obstructive Pulmonary Disease

As previously mentioned, long-term oxygen is the only therapy proved to extend survival in COPD patients (37). Many practitioners will prescribe nocturnal oxygen to COPD patients who demonstrate sustained oxygen desaturation at night to 88% or less (42). However, documentation of hypoxemia during sleep is not a proved justification for continuous oxygen therapy if hypoxemia is not present when the patient is awake and at rest. Nocturnal oxygen is indicated in those patients who qualify for long-term oxygen therapy while awake and in those patients with COPD who develop erythrocytosis, cor pulmonale, and right heart failure without awake hypoxemia (42,43). Treatment has been shown to reduce pulmonary artery pressure and reduce mortality.

Anticholinergics (ipratropium bromide), short- and long-acting beta agonists, and steroids are the foundation of therapy for COPD (6,17,19,21). They are helpful in improving nocturnal gas exchange given their impact on obstruction and gas trapping. The recently available long-acting anticholinergic tiotropium may also be a useful nocturnal bronchodilator.

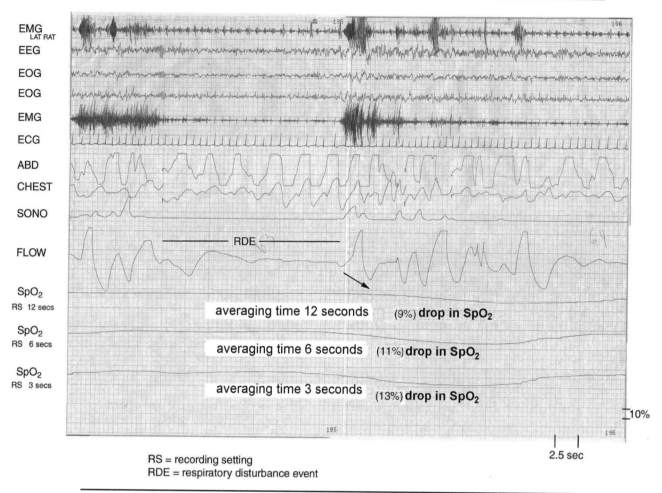

FIGURE 29-5. A respiratory disturbance event (RDE) with pulse oximetry monitoring at three different recording settings (RS) at averaging times of 3, 6, and 12 seconds Channels: EMG, electromyogram; EEG, electroencephalogram; EOG, electrooculogram; ECG, electrocardiogram; ABD (abdominal) and chest effort (piezoelectric belts); flow, thermistor sensors; SpO_2, oxygen saturation.

Theophylline has been of interest due to its known beneficial effects on diaphragmatic contraction, central respiratory stimulation, and reduction of airway obstruction and gas trapping (44). Berry and co-workers (44) compared a shorter-acting beta agonist with the combination of the beta agonist and sustained-action theophylline on sleep and breathing in patients with COPD. The addition of theophylline was found to improve morning FEV_1, non-REM SpO_2, and transcutaneous PCO_2, without impairing sleep quality. Unfortunately, sleep quality can be diminished in individual patients sensitive to the central stimulatory effects of theophylline (44).

Respiratory stimulants have been shown to have a short-lived impact on SDB. Progesterone has been studied in patients with COPD and hypoxemia and shown to be beneficial in reducing awake $PaCO_2$ after 4 weeks of therapy. Dolly and co-workers (45) performed a randomized, placebo-controlled study on the effects of medroxyprogesterone acetate (MPA) at 20 mg tid in patients with

COPD and SDB. Four weeks of therapy was associated with increased awake mean PaO_2 and reduced $PaCO_2$, but no change in numbers of apneas, hypopneas, desaturation events, or lowest SpO_2.

As stated earlier, COPD patients typically experience worsening hypoventilation and more profound desaturation in REM sleep. Protriptyline is a tricyclic antidepressant that reduces total REM sleep and may be helpful in patients with significant REM-associated SDB (16). However, the medication causes severe urinary hesitancy or retention in many older male patients.

Noninvasive ventilation (NIV) is often prescribed for patients with advanced COPD and respiratory failure, those with concomitant hypoventilation, and in patients with OSA intolerant of continuous positive airway pressure (CPAP) (46,47). Stable patients with overlap syndrome have been shown to benefit from NIV, as determined by de Miguel and colleagues (48). These investigators studied patients with eucapneic and hypercapneic overlap syndrome during 6 months of CPAP treatment. Significant increases in PaO_2, FEV_1, and FVC, with decreases in $PaCO_2$ resulted. Nasal bilevel positive airway pressure (BPAP) has been shown to decrease daytime $PaCO_2$ in patients with COPD (49). Other investigators have found no benefits from extended bilevel therapy in hypercapneic COPD patients. Automatic self-titrating CPAP (auto-CPAP) systems are designed to respond to changes in upper-airway resistance by variably increasing or decreasing the positive pressure in response to changes in pressure, flow, and/or the presence of snoring sounds (50). Therefore, the effectiveness would theoretically be equivalent to that of constant-pressure-treatment with a lower mean treatment pressure. Ficker et al. (51) evaluated auto-CPAP in comparison to conventional CPAP in the treatment of symptomatic OSA. There was no significant difference in mean AHI, sleep architecture, arousal index, Epworth Sleepiness Score (ESS), or vigilance tests. The mean pressure during auto-CPAP treatment was significantly higher than that used in conventional therapy. This mode of NIV has not been adequately tested in patients with COPD. Inappropriate ventilation could occur in these patients with a decreased capacity to trigger the device.

Acute exacerbations of COPD are often managed with NIV with a significant reduction in the requirements for intubation and mechanical ventilation. Brochard and colleagues (52) undertook a prospective, randomized study of 85 patients with COPD admitted to the intensive care unit for acute exacerbation. The standard treatment group was treated with up to 5 L per minute supplemental oxygen to maintain the SpO_2 greater than 90%, in addition to bronchodilators, antibiotics, and steroids. The group treated with NIV received similar therapy. The individuals treated with NIV experienced reduced morbidity, mortality, and length of hospital stay.

Asthma and Other Obstructive Pulmonary Diseases

The NIH defined asthma as a chronic inflammatory disease in the 1997 guidelines for diagnosis and therapy (9). With this designation, they have laid out a stepped approach to management centered around the decrease of acute and chronic airway inflammation and control of symptoms. Improvement in nocturnal asthma may be a marker of control in these two areas. The long-term goal of therapy is to prevent airway remodeling and fixed airway obstruction as measured by PFTs (17).

In the asthmatic patient with persistent nocturnal symptoms despite adequate inhaled corticosteroid therapy, specialized intervention in the form of long-acting medications, such as theophylline and long-acting beta agonists may be needed (9, 21, 25). Inhaled agents such as formoterol, bitolterol, and salmeterol have been shown to improve nocturnal symptoms, increase overnight peak flow rates, and improve sleep in asthma patients. While theo-phylline itself may have a deleterious effect on sleep quality, this side effect is somewhat balanced by the improvement in lung function in nocturnal asthma. One study comparing salmeterol with theophylline found only minor differences in sleep quality (slightly higher arousal rate on theophylline) (21).

No randomized controlled NIV trials have been published using NIV to treat acute or chronic asthma (53). However, multiple case series have demonstrated the effective use of NIV in acute situations, obviating the need for intubation. These studies lack appropriate controls to see if medical therapy alone would be equally efficacious. In contrast, patients with severe CF may have a benefit from chronic use of NIV (41, 53). Milross and associates (41) evaluated 13 patients with moderate to severe CF during sleep in random order, breathing room air, supplemental oxygen, or NIV with a bilevel device. Both oxygen and the bilevel device improved nocturnal SpO_2, but only the bilevel device attenuated the rise in $PaCO_2$. These results are promising but need confirmation in larger controlled studies over prolonged periods of time. This could be an effective bridge to lung transplantation (53).

Prognosis

Patients with COPD in combination with SDB would be expected to have increased morbidity and higher mortality, as each condition alone and ineffectively treated is associated with such outcomes. The cardiopulmonary consequences of those patients with overlap syndrome are well recognized. Fletcher and co-workers (46) prospectively followed 24 patients with OSA. Nineteen of these patients had concurrent lung disease. Over a mean follow-up of 27 months, the patients without lung disease were found to have less severe right-sided hemodynamic dysfunction, as determined by radionuclide-gated measures of right ventricular ejection fraction (RVEF) and pulmonary artery pressures.

The efficacy of anti-inflammatory treatment on the natural course of asthma is still debated, as the longest prospective studies available do not exceed 5 years (17). Inhaled corticosteroids can reduce the accelerated decline in both the pulmonary function and bronchial hyperresponsiveness in children and adults. While this improvement is incomplete, nocturnal symptoms also improve. It is not known whether long-term treatment with inhaled steroids (for 20 to 30 years) will succeed in the prevention of airway remodeling or result in significant side effects.

Management of CF is centered around pancreatic enzyme replacement (with reversal of secondary nutritional and vitamin deficiencies), clearance of lower-airway secretions, and treatment of pulmonary infections. A national group of CF treatment centers specializing in these principles has helped increase median survival from 14 years in 1969 to 30 years in 1995 (15).

RESTRICTIVE LUNG DISEASES

Interstitial Lung Diseases

As described earlier, restrictive lung diseases have traditionally been divided into intrinsic (Table 29-1) disorders involving the pulmonary parenchyma and those that involve the chest wall and neuromuscular systems (Table 29-2). Dyspnea is the predominate symptom and may begin abruptly or more insidiously with exertion. As in IPF, dyspnea is progressive and may be present for greater than 6 months before presentation. Patients may present with paroxysms of dry cough that are refractory to antitussive medications.

Sleep is disrupted in patients with interstitial lung disease. A decreased sleep efficiency and increased awakenings are not uncommon and may lead to complaints of fatigue or sleepiness, even in the absence of other sleep disorders such as OSA (54). This occurs along with a decrease in respiratory rate on falling asleep, as noted by McNicholas (55) in seven patients with interstitial lung disease. Furthermore, they have more time spent in stage 1 sleep, decreased REM, and increased arousals at a mean of 23.4 per hour when compared to age- and sex-matched control subjects who had a mean of 13.7 per hour (56,57). Clark et al. (54) showed further that in 48 patients, nocturnal hypoxemia was associated with decreased energy levels and impaired daytime social and physical functioning, and

▶ **TABLE 29-2.** **Classification of Extrinsic Lung Diseases and Conditions (Partial List)**

A. Myopathies
Muscular dystrophies—Duchenne, limb-girdle, myotonic
Acid maltase deficiency
Polymyositis
Myasthenia gravis

B. Neurological Disorders
Motor neuron diseases, ie, amyotrophic lateral sclerosis
Spinal muscular atrophies
Poliomyelitis
Hereditary sensory motor neuropathies
Phrenic neuropathies
Guillian-Barré syndrome
Multiple sclerosis
Traumatic brain injury and myelopathies
Stroke
Hypoventilation and congenital hypoventilation disorders

C. Skeletal Deformities
Kyphoscoliosis
Osteogenesis imperfecta
Ankylosing spondylitis

D. Other Conditions
Pregnancy
Altitude
Obesity

these effects were independent of pulmonary function, as measured by the FVC.

While not noted to have increased presence in patients with IPF (57), OSA was shown to have an increased incidence of 17% in 83 patients with sarcoidosis, an idiopathic granulomatous disease, when compared with the 3% incidence in controls. The frequency was elevated in males and in patients who had the skin findings of lupus pernio (58). Whether this could be related to mucosal airway involvement was not addressed in the study.

In patients with interstitial disease, physical examination reveals a rapid respiratory rate at rest in advanced disease. In IPF specifically, 80% of patients have inspiratory crackles or rales on auscultation. These may be present in the lower lung fields and extend to mid and upper lobes as the disease progresses. A loud P_2 may be auscultated over the heart as right ventricular enlargement and pulmonary hypertension ensue. Clubbing of the digits is noted in 25% to 50% of patients (56) and may be present in other interstitial diseases as well. As pulmonary hypertension develops, the clinician should note the development of leg edema (59).

Chest Wall and Neuromuscular Disorders

The development of chronic alveolar hypoventilation in this group of disorders separates them from the interstitial restrictive diseases, in which hypoventilation does not occur until very late in the course of the latter. The term hypoventilation defines the condition in which alveolar ventilation (V_A) is insufficient to meet the patient's metabolic demands, resulting in an inappropriately high arterial carbon dioxide tension ($Paco_2$) (60). The $Paco_2$ reflects the balance between CO_2 production by the body (V_{CO_2}) and its elimination through alveolar ventilation, as expressed in the equation:

$$Paco_2 = k(Vco_2/V_A)$$

where $Paco_2$ is the arterial carbon dioxide tension (mmHg), Vco_2 is the rate of metabolic production of carbon dioxide (milliliter per minute), V_A is a reflection of the total volume of gas breathed over time (minute ventilation, V_E), and k is a constant. Since an increased Vco_2 does not usually lead to chronic hypercapnea, we can say that a decreased V_A is the primary mechanism for the increased Pco_2 in this group of disorders. Martin and Sanders (60) divide them into "Won't breathe" with an inadequate drive from the central nervous system (CNS) respiratory centers (primary hypoventilation, certain strokes, CNS tumors, bulbar polio, and drug effects) versus "Can't breathe," because of muscular weakness or excessive work of breathing, as seen in most of the chest wall and restrictive disorders in Table 29-2.

During sleep, the minimal expected changes in ventilation, as described above, may be associated with marked aberrations in $Paco_2$ and Pao_2 in patients with alveolar hypoventilation. In normal individuals, V_E falls during NREM sleep and is quite variable during REM, which is associated with tonically decreased muscle tone and phasic decreases in phrenic nerve output. The increase in $Paco_2$ during sleep may be related to altered chemosensitivity, as both hypoxic and hypercapneic drives to breathe are diminished (61,62). There is also a decrease in upper-airway tone, which may further reduce V_E and result in increased $Paco_2$ (63). The REM-associated tonic decreases in muscle tone also involve the accessory and intercostal muscles. Patients with any severe lung disease may become dependent on these for aiding ventilation, even during wakefulness. Thus, they are at particular risk for developing hypoventilation, which initially may only develop as cyclic or sustained dips in Spo_2 during REM sleep, as recorded on overnight oximetry or full PSG (Figs. 29-2 and 29-3).

As with the interstitial lung diseases, dyspnea occurs on exertion and later at rest. Cough is not a significant symptom compared with IPF, when it can be disabling. As the $Paco_2$ levels increase, the patient may complain of CNS effects, such as altered mentation, hypersomnolence, and headache. Physical examination reveals relatively clear lung fields to auscultation as compared with the rales in patients with IPF or wheezing as noted in patients with asthma and COPD. However, the late findings of cor pulmonale are similar between each of the categories and is a final common pathway to respiratory failure.

Clinical Epidemiology

Interstitial Lung Diseases

IPF is defined by the American Thoracic Society (ATS) as a specific form of chronic fibrosing interstitial pneumonia, limited to the lung, with a characteristic histologic appearance (56). The etiology remains unknown, when other known causes of interstitial lung disease have been ruled out (Table 29-1). Males are affected more than females. This illness predominates in the elderly, age range 40 to 70, with two-thirds of patients over 60 years of age at time of presentation (56). Prevalence for middle-aged adults exceeds 2.7 per 100,000, while increasing to 175 per 100,00 in the older age group. The disease is progressive, leading to death from respiratory failure. From the time of diagnosis, survival has been found to be 3.2 to 5 years, with a median survival of 28.2 months from the onset of respiratory symptoms.

Other primary interstitial lung diseases such as pulmonary sarcoidosis have a variable incidence, based on ethnicity of patients; for example, African-Americans have a 10 to 17 times greater incidence than Caucasians (64). However, the disease occurs worldwide and this ethnic characteristic is not universal outside the United States. Prevalence rates per 100,000 vary from 64 in Sweden to 12 in Japan and 80 in African-Americans in New York City. Patients often present earlier in life than with IPF,

usually in the third to fourth decade. Table 29-1 lists additional primary diseases that are much less common. Eosinophilic granuloma (pulmonary Langerhans granulomatosis) occurs typically in young cigarette smokers. Respiratory bronchiolitis-associated interstitial lung disease (RBILD) occurs in smokers of any age; lymphangioleiomyomatosis (LAM) occurs predominately in women who are premenopausal and is rare (64).

Although asbestos insulation is no longer manufactured, it still remains a major health risk, as it may take 20–30 years for interstitial fibrosis, termed asbestosis, to develop. This represents the hallmark of the pneumoconioses or inhalational lung diseases. In contrast to the long time from exposure to asbestosis and the development of symptoms, patients with drug-induced injuries may have an acute onset of symptoms with rapid progression to respiratory failure.

Ventilatory Control, Neuromuscular, and Chest Wall Disorders

Disorders of ventilatory control can result in severe hypoventilation during sleep, even if the lung, respiratory muscles, and chest wall are normal. During wakefulness, ventilation is stimulated by the "waking stimulus" as well as chemoreflexes.

During NREM sleep, the wakefulness stimulus is lost and breathing is totally under metabolic control (hypoxia and hypercapnia stimulate breathing). Primary alveolar hypoventilation is a disorder of unknown etiology associated with chronic hypoxemia and hypercapnea with no other identifiable neurologic disorder (Table 29-2), respiratory muscle weakness, or chest wall disorder (65). It is thought to exist from a failure of the metabolic (or automatic) respiratory control system, which is manifested as a decrease in respiratory drive with elevated $Paco_2$. It is relatively rare in the isolated form, as seen in infants (Ondine's curse) (see Chapter 23). However, dysfunction of ventilatory control can be a significant component of other neuromuscular and chest wall disorders, where the degree of $Paco_2$ elevation appears to be out of proportion to the magnitude of impairment from the underlying neurologic or respiratory disease (66). When the abnormal control of ventilation is coupled with another disorder, such as weight in the obesity–hypoventilation syndrome, the incidence may rise to as high as 5% in morbidly obese men (67). This control abnormality may occur in as many as 4% to 10% of sleep laboratory populations of sleep apneic patients (68). The incidence in other specific disorders, as described individually below, is not known.

Specific Neuromuscular and Chest Wall Disorders

The number of intrinsic lung diseases are extensive (Table 29-1) and generally follow the evaluation discussed for IPF above. The extrinsic neuromuscular diseases and disorders represent distinct challenges for the sleep physician and a few are described in more detail.

Muscular Dystrophy

Duchenne's muscular dystrophy (DMD) is an X-linked recessive disorder of male subjects occurring in 30 per 100,000 patients (69–71). DMD is present at birth and manifests initially between the ages of 3 to 5 years with progression to immobility and death by 12 and 16 to 18 years, respectively. Muscle weakness, contractures, and progressive significant scoliosis decrease pulmonary function and lead to respiratory failure. Comorbidities include cardiomyopathies, aspiration of food, and acute gastric dilatation.

Sleep is altered in patients with DMD. Excessive daytime sleepiness (EDS) develops late in the course of the disease and may relate to SDB, increased number of nocturnal arousals, and a decrease in REM sleep. SDB may not occur until late in the illness. This includes central and obstructive sleep apnea, alveolar hypoventilation initially during REM sleep, and, as disease progresses, throughout sleep and then wakefulness (69). During PSG, the AHI correlates with the severity of EDS. Furthermore, the nocturnal oxygen desaturation corresponds to the awake spirometric measure of FEV_1 and awake ABG with $Paco_2$.

NIV may be initiated at the time of symptom onset, as presumptive therapy has not been shown effective (72). As described below, various nasal, oral, and orofacial interfaces are available with improved patient comfort. Mean survival of hypercapneic patients with DMD is 9.7 months. However, with NIV, nonrandomized studies show improved 1- and 5-year survival to be 85% and 73%, respectively (73). Vianello and colleagues (74) showed that over a 24-month follow-up, all five study patients were alive compared to only one of five in a comparable group of patients who refused NIV. After 6 months of follow-up, mean loss of FVC and maximal voluntary ventilation was considerably higher in nonventilated subjects (respectively, −0.23 L versus + 0.03 L and − 5 L per minute versus − 1.5 L per minute).

Myotonic Dystrophy

Mytonic dystrophy (MD) is distinct from the nondystrophic myotonias in that it is a multisystem disease (75). In addition to myotonia and muscle weakness, patients have cataracts, cardiac dysrrhythmias, hypersomnia, frontal balding, testicular atrophy, and other endocrine abnormalities. It is an autosomal dominant disorder and is the most common form of hereditary muscular dystrophy in adults. Respiratory muscles, especially the diaphragm, are involved as well as the pharyngeal and laryngeal muscles. There is an increased incidence of alveolar hypoventilation, especially in REM sleep, as well as central and obstructive sleep apnea. The degree of breathing dysfunction, however, is out of proportion to the amount of muscle weakness when compared with nonmyotonic patients with a similar degree of weakness, as measured by mouth pressures (76). Evidence suggests that other central mechanisms are abnormal, as EDS cannot be explained by the degree of OSA, hypercapnea, or sleep disruption (77). In this regard, Martinez-Rodriguez and colleagues (77) recently demonstrated abnormal hypothalamic function in six patients with MD type 1. All patients had abnormal MSLT results (mean sleep latency <5 minutes in 2, ≤8 in 4), were HLA-DQB1*0602 negative, and had decreased cerebrospinal fluid (CSF) levels of hypocretin, as has been reported in patients with narcolepsy. These findings support the need for stimulant medications in these patients. In an open-label study of 200 and 400 mg modafinil per day, Damian and associates (78) reported an increase in the mean sleep latency on MSLT from 7.3 to 22.7 minutes in nine patients with MD. In spite of these encouraging findings, a recent Cochrane Database Review (79) failed to find significant evidence to support the use of psychostimulants to treat hypersomnolence in MD.

Amyotrophic Lateral Sclerosis

Amyotrophic lateral sclerosis (ALS) is a chronic, progressive degenerative disease of the motor neurons of the spinal cord and motor cortex. Involvement of various respiratory neuron groups leads to a restrictive ventilatory impairment and ultimately to hypercapneic respiratory failure. Death is often related to respiratory events, and diaphragmatic dysfunction plays a significant role. Patients actually exhibit features of diaphragmatic paralysis, which results in daytime symptoms of dyspnea and orthopnea (73). These patients often have abnormal breathing during sleep, especially REM sleep, when there is variable decrease in phrenic nerve activity, and the intercostal and accessory inspiratory muscles are inhibited (73,80). In a subgroup of 21 patients with ALS, 13 were found to have decreased REM sleep and diaphragm dysfunction as compared with those who did not. Apneas and hypopneas were rare in both groups, but survival was decreased from 619 days to 217 in the diaphragm dysfunction group. NIV can help patients with ALS tolerate respiratory complications, but moderate or severe bulbar symptoms were more prevalent among intolerant patients than among tolerant patients (67% compared to 33%) (81). Median survival of ALS patients using NIV is approximately 10 to 15 months (73,80,81).

Poliomyelitis

Poliomyelitis is caused by an enterovirus that can result in respiratory failure by destruction of anterior horn cells in the spinal cord innervating respiratory muscles, neuronal destruction of the respiratory center in the medulla, or

was also noted to correlate with the degree of oxygen desaturation during sleep (106). Therefore, the presence of an increased chemical drive to breathe, associated with a greater awake SpO_2, appears to protect these patients from severe nocturnal desaturation.

Neuromuscular and Chest Wall Disorders

As described above, primary alveolar hypoventilation is thought to result from a failure of the chemoreceptors or of the brainstem neuronal networks that comprise the metabolic respiratory control system. These patients have a decreased responsiveness to hypoxemia and hypercapnea while awake. During sleep, the effects are increased due to the normal decreased responsiveness that occurs in NREM sleep and the more marked decreases that occur in REM sleep (61,65). In spite of these abnormalities in control of breathing, there are little, if any, pathologic findings at autopsy, in the absence of other neurologic disorders. As in primary alveolar hypoventilation, there is further evidence of a distinct and separate disorder of controlling ventilation in patients with OSA and obesity-related hypoventilation. This is demonstrated by their ability to voluntarily reduce their $PaCO_2$ during a 60- to 90-second spontaneous hyperventilation trial period (66). When any neurologic or respiratory disorder is present in patients with these disorders, or just normal sleep, the effects on hypercapnea are magnified.

Diagnostic Evaluation

Interstitial Lung Disease

The PFT remains the cornerstone of assessment of an individual patient's degree of impairment from any restrictive pulmonary disease. As described earlier, they also help differentiate these restrictive lung diseases from COPD and obstructive lung disease (Fig. 29-1). While the TLC is elevated in patients with COPD, it is reduced in interstitial lung disease. This difference is important to note, because the patient with moderate to severe COPD with a normal TLC may also have a concomitant restrictive disease, such as asbestosis. In addition to spirometry and lung volumes, the third component of full PFTs is the measurement of carbon monoxide diffusion (DL_{CO}). The DL_{CO} is reduced in interstitial diseases and some obstructive lung diseases. This decline may precede the decline in TLC or FVC.

IPF, as with most interstitial lung diseases, is most often associated with an abnormal chest radiograph (56,107,108). Basilar reticular opacities are usually present and may exist for years, in retrospect, before a diagnosis is made. This pattern is not specific to IPF and can be seen in all the interstitial lung diseases described above, as well as in collagen vascular diseases, such as scleroderma, rheumatoid arthritis, and mixed connective tissue disease. High-resolution computed tomography (HRCT)

has surpassed the chest radiograph in evaluation of these patients. This specialized form of CT scan uses 1- to 2-mm thick slices as compared to the standard 7- to 10-mm slices used in conventional scanning. When used with reconstruction algorithms that maximize spatial relationships, details such as the interface between a thickened interstitium and alveolar air can be appreciated. Predominately peripheral, subpleural, and bibasilar reticular abnormalities are seen in IPF, whereas a more homogenous pattern (ground glass) is seen in any disease causing alveolar filling, such as infectious pneumonia, lupus erythematosus, hypersensitivity pneumonitis or even congestive heart failure (CHF). The mediastinum is usually unremarkable in these diseases except for sarcoidosis, in which paratracheal and mediastinal adenopathy are common.

Laboratory evaluation includes arterial blood gases, which are frequently normal early in patients with IPF or reveal only mild hypoxemia when adjusted for age, or respiratory alkalosis, from the chronic hyperventilation. Early abnormalities may be seen in oxygenation when patients are exercised during cardiopulmonary exercise testing. This highlights the decreased diffusion, widened alveolar–arterial O_2 gradient, and associated ventilation to perfusion abnormality. Other lab tests are not specific, such as the rheumatoid factor and antinuclear antibody (ANA), which can be nonspecifically elevated in 10% to 20% of patients with IPF. However, titers are usually low (<1:160), for ANA (109).

PSG is not indicated in the routine evaluation of patients with interstitial lung disease. As shown in patients with sarcoidosis, an increased incidence of OSA may be present (58). PSG would thus be indicated in the appropriate patient with snoring, EDS, and/or witnessed apneas by a bed partner (see Chapter 18). Patients with IPF and snoring are more likely to have sleep disturbances, as described earlier, when the SpO_2 is less than 90% (56). Severe hypoxemia may occur even in the absence of OSA or changes in breathing pattern (104–106). Overnight oximetry may be the preferred mode of evaluation, reserving full PSG for the problem patient or one with symptoms of a specific sleep disorder (for example, sleep apnea).

Neuromuscular and Chest Wall Disorders

No routine specific test is available to document alveolar hypoventilation in the patient with normal arterial blood gases. Hypoxic and hypercapneic challenge tests can be performed, but may not add anything to clinical management. PFTs, as described, can help evaluate for impairment and help guide specific therapy, such as the use of bronchodilators. PSG is specifically helpful in the evaluation for OSA and guiding therapy with nocturnal nasal CPAP. When prolonged hypoventilation is noted on PSG (Fig. 29-2), severe OSA, neurologic disorder, respiratory disease, or obesity-related hypoventilation may be present. Measurement of respiratory muscle strength can be documented and followed as the inspiratory force created by taking a maximal inspiratory and expiratory breath against an occluded airway (110). In this technique, mouth pressures are measured with a pressure transducer in line with a mouthpiece, with nostrils occluded by a nose clip. Maximum inspiratory pressure is measured near RV after maximal expiration, while maximum expiratory pressure is measured at or near TLC. The patient maintains the effort over at least 1 second over three to six trials (110). For patients with neurologic disorders or when orthopnea is not felt to be cardiac in etiology, a sitting and supine spirometry can be measured. A decrease in the supine over the sitting FVC of 25% suggests severe impairment (110).

PSG is indicated in the evaluation of patients with symptoms of SDB, but not as a routine test for patients with neuromuscular or chest wall abnormalities. Overnight oximetry may show abnormal cyclic desaturations in REM sleep during early stages of disease, whereas sustained decreases in the SpO_2 (Figs. 27-2 and 27-3) would suggest sleep-associated alveolar hypoventilation, as may be seen in severe OSA, obesity-hypoventilation syndrome, or any of the specific diseases described previously (111,112). As described for IPF, patients with neuromuscular disorders may have poor sleep efficiency, abnormal sleep staging, and increased arousals, which can be assessed with PSG. Restless legs syndrome (RLS) and periodic limb movements of sleep (PLMS) (documented on PSG), thought to be significant factors contributing to sleepiness in these patients, may likely represent coincidental occurrence (113,114).

Clinical Management

General Principles

Changes in the classification of various interstitial lung diseases (Table 29-1) have prompted the need for open-lung biopsy to clarify the diagnosis (56,107,108). The importance of this has been questioned in the face of a clinical diagnosis in a patient with:

- Exclusion of secondary causes of IPF
- Pulmonary function studies showing evidence of restriction or impaired gas exchange
- Bibasilar reticular abnormalities with minimal ground-glass opacities on HRCT
- Absence of an alternative diagnosis on transbronchial biopsy or BAL (108).

Whereas steroids and immunosuppressive agents have been the traditional therapy, these have never been rigorously studied. Interferon gamma-1b has now been tested and shown to benefit a small group of patients (56,115). There is a multicenter study of over 300 patients that has been completed, but results are not yet available. Side effects, which could have an impact on sleep quality, include fever and chills, which are present in almost all pa-

tients, with a lesser incidence of muscle and bone pain, and migraine-like headaches.

Steroids and discontinuation of smoking still remain the preferred therapy in sarcoidosis, pulmonary Langerhans granulomatosis, and nonspecific interstitial pneumonitis (NSIP) (56). As therapy improves, dyspnea and cough, as well as sleep efficiency, should improve, however, to our knowledge, this has not been specifically studied.

The use of supplemental oxygen during sleep is recommended because it may reduce morbidity and improve patient survival, especially regarding the pulmonary hypertension and cor pulmonale that develop in these patients (56,57,104).

Although patients with intrinsic lung disease often benefit from supplemental oxygen, those with neuromuscular and chest wall disorders often do not. Oxygen therapy alone is not only usually ineffective in relieving symptoms, but has also been shown to be dangerous and may lead to a marked acceleration of CO_2 retention (112,113).

Noninvasive Ventilation

As described above, the respiratory rate and drive to breathe are elevated in patients with intrinsic lung diseases such as IPF, as compared with patients with neuromuscular and chest wall diseases. The resulting dyspnea is severe, and $PaCO_2$ remains low, whereas in chest wall disorders it rises almost in proportion to the fall in the PaO_2 (116). Therefore, respiratory failure with an elevated $PaCO_2$ does not develop in patients with restrictive lung diseases, like IPF until the end stages of disease. It is then that the work of breathing, due to the reduced lung compliance, overcomes the ability of the respiratory muscles to ventilate the lungs adequately, and respiratory muscle fatigue develops (116). In IPF and other parenchymal lung diseases, the ventilatory device (preferably a bilevel device) needs to be set at a rapid respiratory rate, high inspiratory flow rate, small tidal volume (V_t), and short inspiratory and expiratory times, with a low-inspiratory sensitivity trigger setting. Positive end-expiratory pressure (PEEP) is of help in improving ventilation/perfusion abnormalities and thus oxygenation; however, supplemental oxygen is invariably required as the disease progresses (116). The rapid respiratory rate in these patients is due to hypoxemia and stimulation of pulmonary receptors, and NIV is often difficult to adapt to the patient until late in the course when PCO_2 rises. It is not recommended for patients with acute respiratory failure (53).

As alluded to earlier, the approach to NIV in patients with neuromuscular and chest wall disorders is different from that of interstitial disease, where oxygenation is a predominant abnormality. These disorders are fundamentally a hypoventilation derangement, and NIV is designed to decrease $PaCO_2$ (111,113). The polio epidemics during the last century heralded the development of negative pressure ventilation (iron lung) and the beginnings of modern

NIV. No randomized controlled trials are available, but reported outcomes were favorable. Spaingard (72,112) reported a 20-year experience in 40 patients with chronic respiratory failure caused by a variety of neuromuscular diseases, including muscular dystrophy (55%), spinal cord lesions (15%), spinal muscular atrophy (13%), and miscellaneous conditions (17%) (72,112). All patients could be discharged home with lowered $Paco_2$. Five- and 10-year survivals were 76% and 61%, respectively. Rocking beds developed to enhance the gravitational effects on the diaphragm, by raising and lowering the patients' heads, facilitated sleeping supine in patients with weakened or paralyzed diaphragms who often slept in reclining chairs. This improved sleep and decreased hypoventilation, particularly in polio patients (111). Pneumobelts were developed to optimize diaphragm function during the day, and cuirass (molded chest shell) ventilation enhanced negative pressure ventilation by freeing the extremities (previously confined in an iron lung) and allowed custom fitting for patients with chest wall abnormalities. These body ventilators have shown, in uncontrolled studies, to reverse hypoventilation, improve symptoms, and prolong life (72,111,112). These techniques have been supplanted by newer techniques of NIV positive pressure ventilation.

The exact mechanism for improved ventilation with noninvasive positive pressure ventilation (NPPV) is not known. The theories include the following: (a) respiratory muscle rest; (b) resetting the CO_2 sensitivity of the central ventilatory controller; and (c) improvement in pulmonary mechanics (112). Supportive evidence includes the improvement in daytime $Paco_2$, as well as a resetting of the central respiratory control set point for CO_2, with improved ventilatory response to hypoxia and hypercapnia (111,112). In 257 patients with neuromuscular diseases, Bach and associates (83) demonstrated that mouthpiece ventilation over an average of 9.6 years could allow 67 patients to be successfully switched from tracheostomy to NIV. Only 38 died over the monitoring period of 37 years. While randomized, controlled trials are not considered (111), withdrawal of NIV shows a deterioration of nocturnal oxygenation and ventilation, sleep quality, and symptoms (hypersomnolence and morning headache), which can be reversed promptly upon resumption of NIV (117).

Indications for beginning NIV start with an appropriate diagnosis. This may include patients with sequelae of polio, spinal cord injury, neuropathies, myopathies and dystrophies, ALS, chest wall deformities, and kyphoscoliosis. Treatment should begin at the time symptoms develop, as pre-emptive therapy has not been shown effective and may lead to later poor tolerance (111,112). Physiologic criteria include (one of the following): (a) $Paco_2$ >45 mm Hg; (b) nocturnal oximetry demonstrating oxygen saturation <88% for 5 consecutive minutes; and for neuromuscular disease, (c) maximal inspiratory pressures <60 cm H_2O or FVC <50% predicted (112). These are also the current Medicare requirements for reimbursement for NIV for restrictive/neuromuscular disease.

CPAP may be the preferred mode of ventilation in patients with minimal neuromuscular dysfunction, but significant OSA. Bilevel devices, which allow separate inspiratory and expiratory pressures, may be better tolerated and have similar outcomes in comparison to ventilators. In bilevel positive airway pressure, the amount of pressure support = inspiratory positive airway pressure (IPAP) – expiratory positive airway pressure (EPAP) is used to overcome hypoventilation and hypopneas (short decreases in airflow). Expiratory pressures should be kept just above the minimal level (in the 3- to 6-cm H_2O range) unless higher levels are needed to prevent obstructive apnea. Inspiratory pressure is gradually increased upward from low starting pressures (8 to 10 cm H_2O) (111), as tolerated by patient comfort. The IPAP can be adjusted to maintain an adequate tidal volume. Alternative protocols designed to enhance ventilatory assistance in order to stabilize gas exchange begin at high pressures (20 cm H_2O) and titrate downward, if the patient is unable to tolerate it (111). Pressure cycle ventilators are often used, as they are usually less expensive and have fewer alarms to disrupt sleep. Volume cycle ventilators may be preferred for patients with severe neuromuscular weakness who can be taught to "stack" breaths to achieve large tidal volumes, thus enhancing airflow during coughing and aiding in the expulsion of secretions (84,111). A back-up rate is available on ventilators and some bilevel devices. The role of the back-up rate is to prevent central apnea and to provide a minimum rate of assisted respiration. The respiratory efforts of some patients may be too feeble to trigger some devices to cycle between inspiration and expiration, thus requiring a fixed rate. The need for a back-up rate in all patients remains controversial. In the chronic setting, a back-up rate set sufficiently high to control breathing nocturnally (usually slightly below the awake spontaneous breathing rate) has been recommended in patients with neuromuscular disease in order to maximize respiratory muscle rest (111). Higher back-up rates of 23 per minute have more recently been shown by Parreira and colleagues (118) to improve nocturnal minute ventilation. Nasal masks may be better tolerated in patients for chronic respiratory failure. However, oronasal or full facemasks may be more efficient in lowering $Paco_2$. Nasal pillows may allow the claustrophobic patient to become tolerant of CPAP or NIV, and can be used to add heated humidity to prevent nasal mucosal irritation and obstruction from cold dry air exposure (111).

Many physicians across the United States and Canada are not well trained in the use of NIV in patients with pulmonary disease (119). As a result, many physicians (22.7%) were found to sometimes disclose this as a treatment option, whereas 2.3% never disclosed this information. Most patients should be told early about NIV, as when told later they often opt not to pursue this. Furthermore, they are more mentally and psychologically able to make an informed decision early on in treatment (119).

Prognosis

The mean length of survival in IPF from time of diagnosis varies between 3.2 and 5 years, with a median survival of 28.2 months from the onset of respiratory symptoms (56).

Patients with ILD are too short of breath to carry out activities of daily living and their quality of life is poor (116). Nocturnal hypoxemia has an effect on decreasing their perceived quality of life (54). Supplemental oxygen during sleep decreases heart and respiratory rate, but does not normalize the respiratory rate and has little impact on sleep efficiency and arousal index (103). Nocturnal oxygen has not been studied in large numbers of patients with IPF and no clear benefit is noted. Continuous oxygen therapy improves mortality in patients with lung diseases, in general (38).

The prognoses for patients with neuromuscular and chest wall diseases can be enhanced by specific interventions such as NIV. The outcomes of therapy are as described earlier for individual diseases. Long-term studies are in progress.

Future Directions

Research in this area of sleep and breathing disorders has expanded our ability to properly evaluate and treat patients with a broad range of pulmonary diseases and disorders. This has led to advances in such areas as NIV, with improvement in morbidity and mortality, especially acute exacerbations of COPD and chronic management of respiratory failure in neuromuscular and chest wall disorders. Long-term studies of outcomes are needed in other disorders to further define appropriate therapy and design measures to slow the progression of impairment.

Clinical Pearls

- PSG is not indicated in the routine evaluation of patients with pulmonary disease in the absence of symptoms or signs of a sleep disorder.
- Oximetry using the fastest recording settings (shorter averaging times) and on-line real time displayed data (high sampling rate) for analysis is preferred in sleep evaluations.
- Sleep-associated decreases in baseline SpO_2 (not oscillating) suggests alveolar hypoventilation requiring further evaluation.
- Control of nighttime symptoms in asthma may be a marker for adequate asthma therapy, in general.
- Lower end-expiratory pressures may be tolerated better early in initiation of NIV in patients with neuromuscular disorders.

- NIV should be preferred over supplemental oxygen in neuromuscular patients with early ventilatory impairment and hypoxemia.
- Patients with pulmonary diseases and disorders should be offered NIV early in the course of their illness in order to make informed decisions.

REFERENCES

1. McNicholas WT. Impact of sleep in COPD. *Chest.* 2000;117:48S–53S.
2. Block AJ, Boysen PG, Wynne JW, et al. Sleep apnea, hypopnea and oxygen desaturation in normal subjects. *N Engl J Med.* 1979;300:513–517.
3. DeMarco FJ, Wynne JW, Block AJ, et al. Oxygen desaturation during sleep as a determinant of the "blue and bloated" syndrome. *Chest.* 1981;79:621–625.
4. Coccagna G, Lugaresi E. Arterial blood gases and pulmonary and systemic pressure during sleep in chronic obstructive pulmonary disease. *Sleep.* 1978;1:117–124.
5. Boysen PG, Block AJ, Wynne JW, et al. Nocturnal pulmonary hypertension inpatients with chronic obstructive pulmonary pisease. *Chest.* 1979;76:536–542.
6. Petty TL. Definition, epidemiology, course, and prognosis of COPD. *Clin Cornerstone.* 2003;5:1–10.
7. Chaouat A, Weitzenblum E, Krieger J, et al. Association of chronic obstructive pulmonary disease and sleep apnea syndrome. *Amer J Respir Crit Care Med.* 1995;151:82–86.
8. Mulloy, E, Fitzpatrick M, Bourke S, et al. Oxygen desaturation during sleep and exercise in patients with severe chronic obstructive pulmonary disease. *Respir Med.* 1995;89:193–198.
9. NIH–Guidelines for the diagnosis and management of asthma. *NIH Publ* No. 97-4051A;1997:1–80.
10. Turner-Warwick M. Epidemiology of nocturnal asthma. *Amer J Med.* 1988;85(Suppl. 18):6–8.
11. Turner-Warwick, M. On observing patterns of airflow obstruction in chronic asthma. *Br J Dis Chest.* 1977;71:73–86.
12. Horn CR, Clark JH, Cochrane GM. Is there a circadian variation in respiratory morbidity? *Br J Dis Chest.* 1987;81:248–251.
13. Robertson CF, Rubinfield AR, Bowes G. Deaths from asthma in Victoria: a 12-month survey. *Med J Austr.* 1990;152:511–517.
14. British Thoracic Association. Death from asthma in two regions of England. *Br Med J.* 1982;285:1251–1255.
15. Ramsey BW. Management of pulmonary disease in patients with cystic fibrosis. *N Engl J Med.* 1996;355:179–188.
16. Douglas NJ, Flenley DC. Breathing during sleep in patients with obstructive lung disease. *Amer Rev Respir Dis.* 1990;141:1055–1070.
17. Bousquet J, Jeffery PK, Busse WW, et al. Asthma: from bronchoconstriction to airways inflammation and remodeling. *Amer J Respir Crit Care Med.* 2000;161:1720–1745.
18. Turki J, Pak J, Green SA, et al. Genetic polymorphisms of the beta 2-adrenergic receptor in nocturnal and non-nocturnal asthma: evidence that the gly-16 correlates with the nocturnal phenotype. *J Clin Invest.* 1995;95:1635–1641.
19. Catterall JR, Rhind GB, Whyte KF, et al. Is nocturnal asthma caused by changes in airway cholinergic activity? *Thorax.* 1988;43:720–724.
20. Morrison JF, Pearson SB, Dean HG. Parasympathetic nervous system in nocturnal asthma. *Br Med J.* 1988;296:1427–1429.
21. Selby C, Engleman HM, Fitzpatrick MF, et al. Inhaled salmeterol or oral theophylline in nocturnal asthma? *Amer J Respir Crit Care Med.* 1997;155:104–108.
22. Chen WY, Chai H. Airway cooling and nocturnal asthma. *Chest.* 1982;81:675–680.
23. Goodall RJR, Earnis JE, Cooper DN, et al. Relationship between asthma and gastroesophageal reflux. *Thorax.* 1981;36:116–121.
24. Kiljander TL, Salomar ED, Hietaven ER, et al. Gastroesophageal reflux in asthmatics: a double-blind, placebo-controlled crossover study with omeprazole. *Chest.* 1999;116:1257–1264.

25. Swillich CW, Neagley SR, Cicutto L, et al. Nocturnal asthma therapy: inhaled bitolterol versus sustained-released theophylline. *Amer Rev Respir Dis.* 1989;139:470–474.

26. Sanders C. The radiographic diagnosis of emphysema. *Radio Clin North Amer.* 1991;29:1019.

27. Harrigan RA, Jones K. ABC of clinical electrocardiography: conditions affecting the right side of the heart. *BMJ.* 2002;324:1201–1204.

28. Ferber R, Millman R, Coppola M, et al. Portable recording in the assessment of obstructive sleep apnea. *Sleep.* 1994;17:378–392.

29. Meyer RJ, Eveloff SE, Millman RP. One negative polysomnogram does not exclude obstructive sleep apnea. *Chest.* 1993;103:756–760.

30. Littner M. Polysomnography in the diagnosis of the obstructive sleep apnea–hypopnea syndrome. *Chest.* 2000;118:286–287.

31. Hanning CD, Alexander-Williams JM. Fortnightly review: Pulse oximetry. A practical review. *BMJ.* 1995;311:367–370.

32. Netzer N, Eliasson AH, Netzer C, et al. Overnight pulse oximetry for sleep-disordered breathing in adults. *Chest.* 2001;120:625–633.

33. Williams AY, Santiago S, Yu G, et al. Screening of sleep apnea using pulse oximetry and a clinical score. *Chest.* 1991;100:631–635.

34. Epstein LF, Dorlac GR. Cost-effectiveness analysis of nocturnal oximetry as a method of screening for sleep apnea–hypopnea syndrome. *Chest.* 1998;113:97–103.

35. Rauscher H, Popp W, Zwick H. Computerized detection of respiratory events during sleep from rapid increases in oxyhemoglobin saturation. *Lung.* 1991;169:335–342.

36. Davila DG, Richards KC, Marshall BL, et al. Oximeter performance: the influence of acquisition parameters. *Chest.* 2002;122:1654–1660.

37. Nocturnal Oxygen Therapy Trial Group. Continuous or nocturnal oxygen therapy in hypoxemic chronic obstructive lung disease: a clinical trial. *Ann Internal Med.* 1980;93:391–398.

38. The American Academy of Sleep Medicine Task Force. Sleep-related breathing disorders in adults: recommendations for syndrome definition and measurement techniques in clinical research. *Sleep.* 1999;22:667–689.

39. Dancey DR, Tullis ED, Heslegrave R, et al. Sleep quality and daytime function in adults with cystic fibrosis and severe lung disease. *Eur Respir J.* 2002;19:504–510.

40. Frangolias DD, Wilcox PG. Predictability of oxygen desaturation during sleep in patients with cystic fibrosis. *Chest.* 2001;119:434–441.

41. Milross MA, Piper AJ, Norman M, et al. Predicting sleep-disordered breathing in patients with cystic fibrosis. *Chest.* 2001;120:1239–1245.

42. Milross MA, Piper AJ, Normal M, et al. Low-flow oxygen and bilevel ventilatory support. *Amer J Respir Crit Care Med.* 2001;163:129–134.

43. Plywaczewski R, Sliwinski P, Nowinski A, et al. Incidence of nocturnal desaturation while breathing oxygen in COPD patients undergoing long-term oxygen therapy. *Chest.* 2000;117:679–683.

44. Berry RB, Desa MM, Branum JP, et al. Effect of theophylline on sleep and sleep-disordered breathing in patients with chronic obstructive pulmonary disease. *Amer Rev Respir Dis.* 1991;143:245–250.

45. Dolly FR, Block AJ. Medroxyprogesterone acetate and COPD: effect on breathing and oxygenation in sleeping and awake patients. *Chest.* 1983;84:394–398.

46. Fletcher EC, Schaaf JW, Miller J, et al. Long-term cardiopulmonary sequelae in patients with sleep apnea and chronic lung disease. *Amer. Rev Respir Dis.* 1987;135:525–533.

47. American College of Chest Physicians. Clinical indications for non-invasive positive pressure ventilation in chronic respiratory failure due to restrictive lung disease, COPD, and nocturnal hypoventilation—a consensus conference report. *Chest.* 1999;116:521–534.

48. de Miguel J, Cabello J, Sanzhez-Alarcos MJF. Long-term effects of treatment with nasal continuous positive airway pressure on lung function in patients with overlap syndrome. *Sleep Breathing.* 2002;6:3–10.

49. Meecham-Jones DJ, Paul EA. Nasal pressure support ventilation plus oxygen compared with oxygen therapy alone in hypercapneic COPD. *Amer J Respir Crit Care Med.* 1995;152:538–544.

50. Strollo PF. Practical aspects of CPAP therapy for sleep apnea. *Up To Date 2003;* Version 11.2:pp. 1–7.

51. Ficker JH, Wiest GH, Lehnert G. Evaluation of an auto-CPAP device for treatment of obstructive sleep apnea. *Thorax.* 1998;53:643–648.

52. Brochard L, Mencebo J, Wysocki M. Non-invasive ventilation for acute exacerbations of chronic obstructive pulmonary disease. *N Engl J Med.* 1995;333:817–822.

53. Mehta S, Hill N. Non-invasive ventilation. *Amer J Respir Crit Care Med.* 2001;163:540–577.

54. Clark M, Cooper B, Singh S, et al. A survey of nocturnal hypoxemia and health-related quality of life in patients with cryptogenic fibrosing alveolitis. *Thorax.* 2001;52:482–486.

55. McNicholas WT, Coffey M, Fitzgerald MX. Ventilation and gas exchange during sleep in patients with interstitial lung disease. *Thorax.* 1986;41:777–782.

56. American Thoracic Society. Idiopathic pulmonary fibrosis: diagnosis and treatment. *Amer J Respir Crit Care Med.* 2000;161:646–664.

57. Perez-Padilla R, West P, Lertzman M, et al. Breathing during sleep in patients with interstitial lung disease. *Amer Respir Dis.* 1985;132:224–229.

58. Turner GA, Lowe EE, Corsa BE, et al. Sleep apnea in sarcoidosis. *Sarcoidosis Vasc Diff Lung Dis.* 1997;14:61–64.

59. Blankfield RP, Hudgel DW, Tapolyai AA, et al. Bilateral leg edema, obesity, pulmonary hypertension and obstructive sleep apnea. *Arch Internal Med.* 2000;160:2357–2362.

60. Martin RJ, Sanders MH. Chronic alveolar hypoventilation: a review for the clinician. *Sleep.* 1995;18:617–634.

61. Zwillich CW, Sutton FD, Pierson DJ, et al. Decreased hypoxic ventilatory drive in the obesity-hypoventilation syndrome. *Amer J Med.* 1975;59:343–348.

62. Baydun A. Respiratory muscle strength and control of ventilation in patients with neuromuscular disease. *Chest.* 1991;89:330–338.

63. Lopes JM, Tabachnik E, Muller NL, et al. Total airway resistance and respiratory muscle activity during sleep. *J Appl Physiol.* 1983;54:773–777.

64. Teirstein AS, Lesser M. Worldwide distribution and epidemiology of sarcoidosis. In: Fenburg BL, ed. *Sarcoidosis and other granulomatous diseases of the lung.* Vol. 20. New York: Marcel Dekker, 1983;101–134.

65. Phillipson EA. Control of breathing during sleep. *Amer Rev Respir Dis.* 1978;118:909–939.

66. Leech J, Onal E, Aronson R, et al. Voluntary hyperventilation in obesity hypoventilation. *Chest.* 1991;100:1334–1338.

67. Ahmed Q, Chung-Park M, Tomaslefski JF. Cardiopulmonary pathology in patients with sleep apnea/obesity hypoventilation syndrome. *Human Pathol.* 1997;28:264–269.

68. White DP. Central sleep apnea. In: Kryger MN, Roth T, Clement CS, eds. *Principles and practice of sleep medicine.* 3rd edn. Philadelphia: W.B. Saunders, 2000;827–839.

69. Barbe F, Queva-Salva MA, McCann C, et al. Sleep-related respiratory disturbances in patients with Duchenne muscular dystrophy. *Eur Respir J.* 1994;7(E):1403–1408.

70. Hakins CA, Hillman DR. Daytime predictors of sleep hypoventilation in Duchenne muscular dystrophy. *Amer J Respir Crit Care Med.* 2000;161:166–170.

71. Phillips MF, Smith PEM, Carroll N, et al. Nocturnal oxygenation and prognosis in Duchenne muscular dystrophy. *Amer J Respir Crit Care Med.* 1999;160:198–202.

72. Splaingard ML, Peates RL Jr, Harrison GM, et al. Home-positive-pressure ventilation: twenty years' experience. *Chest.* 1983;84:376–384.

73. Simonds AK. Neuromuscular disease. In: Muir JF, Ambrosio N, Siminds AK, eds. *Noninvasive mechanical ventilation.* Vol. 6, Sheffield UK: European Respiratory Society, 2001:218–226.

74. Vianello A, Bevilacqua M, Salvador V, et al. Long-term nasal intermittent positive pressure ventilation in advanced Duchenne's muscular dystrophy. *Chest.* 1994;105:445–448.

75. Ptacek LJ, Johnson KJ, Griggs RL. Genetics and physiology of the myotonic muscle disorders. *N Engl J Med.* 1983;328:482–489.

76. Gilmartin JJ, Cooper BG, Griffiths CJ, et al. Breathing during sleep in patients with myotonic dystrophy and non-myotonic respiratory muscle weakness. *Quart J Med.* 1991;78:21–31.

77. Martinez-Rodriguez JE, Lin L, Iranzo A, et al. Decreased hypocretin-1 levels in the cerebrospinal fluid of patients with myotonic dystrophy and excessive daytime sleepiness. *Sleep.* 2003;26:287–290.

78. Damian MS, Gerlach A, Schmidt F, et al. Modafinil for excessive daytime sleepiness in myotonic dystrophy. *Neurology.* 2001;56:794–796.

79. Cochrane Database. Psychostimulants for hypersomnia in myotonic dystrophy. *Cochrane Database Systemic Rev.* 2002;4: CD003218.

80. Arnulf I, Similowski T, Salaches F, et al. Sleep disorders and diaphragm function in patients with amyotrophic lateral sclerosis. *Amer J Respir Crit Care Med.* 2000;161:849–856.

81. Aboussouan LS, Khan SU, Meeker DP, et al. Effect of noninvasive ventilation on survival in amyotrophic lateral sclerosis. *Ann Internal Med.* 1997;127:450–453.

82. Bach JR, Alba AS, Bohatiuk A, et al. Mouth intermittent positive pressure ventilation in the management of post-polio respiratory insufficiency. *Chest.* 1987;91:859–864.

83. Bach JR, Alba AS, Saporito LR. Intermittent positive pressure ventilation via the mouth as an alternative to tracheostomy for 257 ventilator users. *Chest.* 1993;103:174–182.

84. Bach JR. Update and perspective on noninvasive respiratory muscle aids–Part 2, The Expiratory Aids. *Chest.* 1994;105:1538–1544.

85. Steljes DG, Kryger MH, Kirk BW, et al. Sleep in post-polio syndrome. *Chest.* 1990;98:133–140.

86. Bruno RL. Abnormal movements in sleep as a post-polio sequelae. *Amer J Phys Med Rehab.* 1998;77:339–343.

87. Putman MT, Wife RA. Myasthenia gravis and upper airway obstruction. *Chest.* 1996;109:400–404.

88. Amino A, Shiozawa Z, Nagasaka T, et al. Sleep apnoea in well-controlled myasthenia gravis and the effect of thymrectomy. *J Neurol.* 1998;245:77–80.

89. McCool FD, Rochester DF. The lungs and chest wall diseases. In: Murry JF, Nadel JA, Mason RL, Boushey HA, eds. *Textbook of respiratory medicine.* 3rd edn. Philadelphia: W.B. Saunders, 2000:2357–2376.

90. Guilleurinault C, Kurland G, Winkle R, et al. Severe kyphoscoliosis, breathing and sleep. *Chest.* 1981;78:626–630.

91. Sawaicka EH, Branthwaite MA. Respiration during sleep and kyphoscoliosis. *Thorax.* 1987;42:801–803.

92. Swank S, Lonstein J, Mac J, et al. Surgical treatment of adult scoliosis. *J Bone J Surg.* 1981;63:268–287.

93. Anderson WM, Falestiny M. Women and sleep. *Primary Care Update Ob/GYN.* 2000;7:131–137.

94. National Sleep Foundation. In: Johnson ED, ed. *1998 Women and sleep poll.* Ann Arbor, MI, National Sleep Foundation, 1998: Datastat 199:1–122.

95. Santiago JR, Nolledo MS, Kinzler, et al. Sleep and sleep-disorders in pregnancy. *Ann Internal Med.* 2001;134:396–408.

96. Bourne T, Ogilvy AJ, Vickers R, et al. Nocturnal hypoxaemia in late pregnancy. *Br J Anaesth.* 1995;75:678–82.

97. Hacket PH, Roach RC. High altitude illness. *N Engl J Med.* 2001;345:107–114

98. Sutton JR, Houston CS, Mansell AR, et al. Effect of acetazolamide on hypoxemia during sleep at high altitude. *N Engl J Med.* 1979;301:1329–1331.

99. Beaumont M, Goldenberg F, Lejeune D, et al. Effect of zolpidem on sleep and ventilatory patterns at simulated altitudes of 4,000 meters. *Amer J Respir Crit Care Med.* 1996;153:1864–1869.

100. Yanovski SZ, Yanovski JA. Obesity. *N Engl J Med.* 2002;346:591–602.

101. Serafini FM, Anderson WM, Rosemurgy AS, et al. Clinical predictors of sleep apnea in patients undergoing bariatric surgery. *Obesity Surg.* 2001;11:26–31.

102. Burwell CS, Robin ED, Whaley RD, et al. Extreme obesity with alveolar hypoventilation: a Pickwickian syndrome. *Amer J Med.* 1956;21:811–818.

103. Vazquez JC and Perez-Padilla R. Effect of oxygen on sleep and breathing in patients with interstitial lung disease at moderate altitude. *Respiration.* 2001;68:584–589.

104. Bye PTP, Berthon-Jones M, Sullivan CE. Studies of oxygenation during sleep in patients with interstitial lung disease. *Amer Rev Respir Dis.* 1984;129:27–32.

105. Shea SA, Winning AJ, McKenzie E, et al. Does the abnormal pattern of breathing in patients with interstitial lung disease persist in deep, non-rapid eye movement sleep? *Amer Rev Respir Dis.* 1989;139:653–658.

106. Koichiro T, Kimura H, Kumitono F, et al. Arterial oxygen desaturation during sleep in interstitial pulmonary disease: correlation with clinical control of breathing during wakefulness. *Chest.* 1989;95:962–967.

107. Radu OA, Groth ML. Idiopathic pulmonary fibrosis: Is surgical lung biopsy really necessary? *Clin Pulmonary Med.* 2001;8:362–364.

108. Hunninghake GW, Zimmerman MB, Schwartz DA, et al. Utility of a lung biopsy for the diagnosis of idiopathic pulmonary fibrosis. *Amer J Respir Crit Care Med.* 2001;164:193–196.

109. Chapman JR, Charles PJ, Venables PJW, et al. Defginition and clinical relevance of antibodies to nuclear ribonucleoprotein and other nuclear antigens in patients with cryptogenic fibrosing alveolitis. *Amer Rev Respir Dis.* 1984;130:439–443.

110. Black LF, Hyatt RE. Maximal respiratory pressures: normal values and relationship to age and sex. *Amer Rev Respir Dis.* 1969;99:696–702.

111. Mehta S, Hill NS. Noninvasive ventilation. *Amer J Respir Crit Care Med.* 2001;163:540–577.

112. American College of Chest Physicians. Clinical indications for noninvasive positive pressure ventilation in chronic respiratory failure due to restrictive lung disease, COPD, and nocturnal hypoventilation—a consensus conference report. *Chest.* 1999;116:521–534.

113. Hening W, Allen R, Earley C, et al. The treatment of restless legs syndrome and periodic limb movement disorder. *Sleep.* 1999;22:970–999.

114. Chervin RD. Periodic leg movements and sleepiness in patients evaluated for sleep-disordered breathing. *Amer J Respir Crit Care Med.* 2001;164:1454–1458.

115. Zieschie R, Hofbauer E, Wittman K, et al. A preliminary study of long-term treatment with interferon gamma-1b and low-dose prednisone prednisolone in patients with idiopathic pulmonary fibrosis. *N Engl J Med.* 1999;341:1264–1269.

116. Shneerson JR. Noninvasive ventilation in chronic respiratory failure due to restrictive chest wall and parenchymal lung disease. In: Muir FF, Ambrosio N, Simonds AK, eds. Sheffield, UK: European Respiratory Society, 2001:204–217.

117. Caroll N, Branthwaite MA. Control of nocturnal hypoventilation by nasal intermittent positive pressure ventilation. *Thorax.* 1988;43:349–353.

118. Parreira VF, Jounieaux V, Delguste P, et al. Determinants of effective ventilation. *Eur Respir J.* 1997;10:1975–1982.

119. Rumbak MJ, Walker M. Should patients with neuromuscular disease be denied the choice of the treatment of mechanical ventilation? *Chest.* 2001;119:683–684.

Sleep and Internal Medicine

Susan M. Harding and Jeffrey W. Hawkins

INTRODUCTION

Sleep disturbances are common in many medical disorders. Medications utilized to treat these disorders may disrupt sleep. This chapter reviews the clinical aspects of how medical disorders including gastroesophageal reflux (GER), renal disease, infectious diseases, selected endocrine disorders, fibromyalgia syndrome, and chronic pain syndromes interfere with or alter sleep. Finally, sleep-associated medication side effects will be discussed.

SLEEP AND GASTROESOPHAGEAL REFLUX

Sleep's Influence on Esophageal Function

Sleep influences esophageal function. Physiologic changes occur from wake to sleep, from sleep to wake, and from

one sleep stage to another (1). The upper esophageal sphincter (UES) pressure decreases from 40 to 20 mm Hg with sleep onset and further decreases to 8 mm Hg during stable sleep, predisposing to aspiration (2). The lower esophageal sphincter (LES) is the primary antireflux barrier, and when the LES relaxes without a swallow, it is called a transient LES relaxation. Transient LES relaxations are the primary gastroesophageal reflux (GER) mechanism, accounting for 63% to 100% of GER episodes (3). Transient LES relaxations are confined to wake time and brief arousals, so GER events occur primarily during arousals (4). Sleep also affects esophageal acid clearance. Esophageal acid clearance is markedly prolonged during sleep and requires arousal (1,5). Furthermore, swallowing frequency is almost nonexistent during stable sleep, with swallowing occurring during brief arousals (2). Saliva production also ceases during sleep, impeding the ability to neutralize refluxate (6). Sleep facilitates proximal migration of acid in the esophagus if a GER event occurs (7). All these physiologic alterations during sleep can result in esophageal and extraesophageal GER manifestations.

Manifestations of Sleep-Related Gastroesophageal Reflux

Gastroesophageal reflux manifestations during sleep include sleep-related GER (ICD9-530.1), sleep-related asthma (493.0), and sleep-related laryngospasm (780.59-4). Furthermore, GER frequently occurs in patients with obstructive sleep apnea (OSA) (780.53-0).

Sleep-related Gastroesophageal Reflux

Sleep-related GER is a primary sleep disorder (8). GER occurring during sleep time is more injurious than in the diurnal condition, is associated with more severe esophagitis, and may play a role in the development of Barrett's esophagitis (9). Sleep-related GER is common, with 10% of respondents to a random sample telephone survey reporting nocturnal GER (10). It presents with multiple awakenings, substernal burning and/or chest discomfort, indigestion, and heartburn. Other symptoms include a sour or bitter taste in the mouth, regurgitation, water brash, coughing, and choking. Some patients may not have esophageal symptoms and present with excessive daytime sleepiness (EDS) without an obvious cause.

Diagnostic methods for detecting sleep-related GER include esophageal pH testing that has a sensitivity and specificity of approximately 90%. It can be integrated with polysomnography (PSG) for temporal correlation of sleep-related events. Esophageal pH testing is not required to make the diagnosis of sleep-related GER. Esophageal pH testing is performed by placing an esophageal pH probe 5 cm above the LES. Many laboratories include dual pH probes, in which a proximal pH probe is placed at the UES or in the pharynx. The pH probes are connected to a data recorder with an event marker for symptom correlation. Patients also record meal times, bedtime, and awakening times in a diary. A GER episode is defined by the presence of material that has a pH of less than 4.0 (11). Figure 30-1 shows a GER event associated with an arousal. Normative data is shown in Table 30-1 (12). Diagnostic accuracy is based on data recorded over a 24-hour period.

Sleep-Related Asthma

Gastroesophageal reflux is present in approximately 50% of asthmatics (13). Gastroesophageal reflux during sleep may alter airway activity (14). For instance, Cuttitta et al. (15) noted that GER episode duration correlated with increases in respiratory resistance. Furthermore, as part of the European Community Respiratory Health Survey, Gislason et al. (16) noted that 5% of randomly selected subjects had nocturnal GER more than once a week and that asthma was more frequent in those with nocturnal GER. Further research will delineate the association between sleep-related GER and airway reactivity.

Sleep-related Laryngospasm

Gastroesophageal reflux also has a role in sleep-related laryngospasm (780.59-4). Patients abruptly awaken with an intense feeling of suffocation often accompanied with stridor and choking sensations (8). Other features include

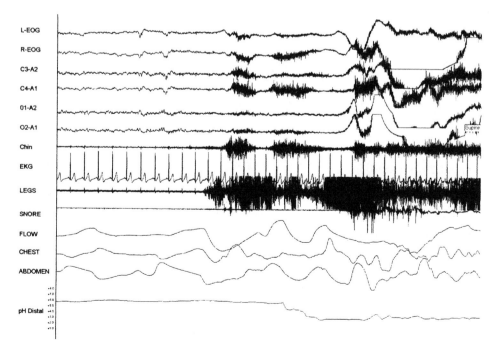

FIGURE 30-1. Thirty-second epoch showing esophageal pH integrated with PSG. The pH probe was placed 5 cm above the lower esophageal sphincter. Note the drop in esophageal pH to less than 4 during an arousal.

▶ **TABLE 30-1. Esophageal pH Normal Values**[a,b]

% Time pH < 4	Distal Probe (%) (5 cm above LES[b])	Proximal Probe (%) (1 cm below UES[c])
Total	<5.8	<1.1
Upright[d]	<8.2	<1.7
Supine[e]	<3.5	<0.6

[a] Based on 110 normal controls in our laboratory (12).
[b] LES, lower esophageal sphincter.
[c] UES, upper esophageal sphincter.
[d] Upright, refers to wake time.
[e] Supine, refers to bed time.

intense anxiety, rapid heart rate, sensation of impending death, and residual hoarseness. Differential diagnosis for sleep-related laryngospasm includes OSA, epilepsy, sleep-choking syndrome, sleep terrors, vocal cord dysfunction, and other upper-airway pathologies. Thunheer et al. (17) noted that nine of ten patients with sleep-related laryngospasm had GER documented by esophageal pH testing. Six patients responded to antireflux therapy, showing that GER may be associated with sleep-related laryngospasm.

Obstructive Sleep Apnea

Gastroesophageal reflux during sleep time is also associated with daytime sleepiness, snoring, and OSA. Janson et al. (18) noted that 16% of subjects with nocturnal GER symptoms snored nightly, compared with 5% of subjects without nocturnal GER. Nocturnal GER was also associated with daytime sleepiness and disruptive breathing during sleep. These findings demonstrate an epidemiologic link between nocturnal GER, sleep-disordered breathing (SDB), and snoring.

There is a temporal association between GER and apnea with both events occurring simultaneously 53% of the time (19). H_2 receptor antagonist therapy results in a reduction of both arousals and GER events. Senior et al. (20) reported that omeprazole reduced the apnea index from 41 events to 31 events an hour in patients with GER and OSA. OSA decreases sleep efficiency, which may trigger transient LES relaxations and promote GER. Gastroesophageal reflux may also contribute to the excessive daytime sleepiness (EDS) often found in OSA patients.

Continuous positive airway pressure (CPAP) resulted in improvement in sleep-related GER symptoms in a large cohort of OSA patients (21). In 331 OSA patients, sleep-related GER symptoms were present in 62%. There was a strong correlation between CPAP pressure and GER symptom improvement, with higher CPAP pressures resulting in fewer sleep-related GER symptoms.

Therapy of Sleep-related Gastroesophageal Reflux

All patients should be instructed about lifestyle modifications (13). Patients should not eat for at least 2 hours

before bedtime and avoid foods that promote GER, including high fat-containing foods, caffeine, chocolate, mint, alcohol, tomato products, citrus, and sodas. Medications that promote GER should be avoided, including calcium channel blockers, anticholinergic medications, theophylline, prostaglandins, and bisphosphonates. Smoking significantly decreases LES pressure, so all patients should be encouraged to stop smoking. Patients should lose weight if they are obese and sleep in loose-fitting clothing.

Positional therapy can also be useful. Sleeping with the head of the bed elevated 6 inches with a full-length wedge or placing blocks under the head of the bed reduces GER. Recently, Khoury et al. (22) noted that sleeping in the right lateral decubitus position was associated with higher esophageal acid contact times. The left lateral decubitus position resulted in significantly lower esophageal acid contact times and appears to be the best sleeping position for sleep-related GER.

Medical therapy includes antacids for acute symptom control, H_2 receptor antagonists, proton pump inhibitors, and prokinetic agents. H_2 receptor antagonists provide heartburn relief in 60% of patients and can be given prior to sleep onset. Proton pump inhibitors (PPI) provide superior gastric acid suppression. Dosing of PPIs should be 30 minutes before a meal, since these agents inhibit gastric acid secretion only in actively secreting parietal cells. When examining optimal dosing schedules of omeprazole, Kuo et al. (23) noted that giving 40 mg of omeprazole with dinner, or 20 mg before breakfast and dinner, resulted in better gastric acid suppression than giving 40 mg before breakfast only. Recent data show that there is nocturnal acid secretion in the stomach despite PPI therapy (24). Whether nocturnal gastric acid breakthrough is clinically important is not known.

Metoclopramide is the only prokinetic agent available for use in the United States, and it has a high prevalence rate (20% to 50%) of central nervous system (CNS) side effects. Prokinetic agents can be used concomitantly with gastric acid suppressive agents.

Antireflux surgery, primarily fundoplication (both open and laparoscopic methods), is successful in 80% to 90% of patients. However, long-term results show that 62% of surgically treated patients use antireflux medications regularly (25). This data implies that surgery does not always replace the need for antireflux medication.

Finally, nasal CPAP therapy reduces sleep-related GER symptoms (21). Kerr et al. (26) also noted that 8 cm of nasal CPAP resulted in marked reduction of esophageal acid contact times.

Clinical Pearls

■ Sleep-related GER occurs in 10% of people.
■ Symptoms include awakening with heartburn and/or regurgitation, but may be clinically silent, with patients presenting with EDS without an obvious cause.

- Esophageal pH testing integrated with PSG can be useful in diagnosing sleep-related GER.
- Sleep-related GER can also result in sleep-related laryngospasm, worsening airway reactivity in asthmatics, and is often seen in OSA patients.
- Therapy of sleep-related GER includes conservative therapy, positional therapy (head of bed raised or left lateral decubitus), and weight loss if obese.
- PPIs have superior gastric acid suppression compared with other medications and should be given before meals.
- Patients who have undergone fundoplication may still require antireflux medications postoperatively.
- Nasal CPAP improves sleep-related GER symptoms and esophageal acid contact times in OSA patients.

SLEEP DISTURBANCES IN PATIENTS WITH RENAL DISEASE

Sleep disturbances are also very common in renal disease patients. Most investigations examine patients with end-stage renal disease (ESRD) who are on chronic hemodialysis (HD) or continuous ambulatory peritoneal dialysis (CAPD). Sleep complaints occur in up to 80% of dialysis patients (27). Holly et al. (28) reported that the most common sleep complaints were: nighttime awakenings in 67%, early morning awakenings in 80%, restless legs in 72%, jerking legs in 83%, and daytime sleepiness in 28% of patients. Many patients napped more than 1 hour a day (28). Walker et al. (29) noted that 83% of patients had sleep-related complaints, with daytime sleepiness being the most commonly reported symptom (66%), followed by restless legs syndrome (RLS) (57%). Hays et al. (30) found that trouble sleeping and daytime sleepiness were in the the top 12 of most bothersome symptoms in patients with renal disease (30). Sleep-related symptoms can be very stressful to patients and impair their quality of life (QOL).

Not only do dialysis patients have a high prevalence of sleep complaints, they also have alterations in their sleep architecture. Numerous reports have examined PSG features of sleep in dialysis patients, including reduced total sleep times (TST) ranging between 260 and 360 minutes, poor sleep efficiencies as low as 66%, and large amounts of wake time (27). Minimal data evaluate whether improving sleep hygiene improves the patient's sleep architecture.

The prevalence of OSA is higher in renal disease patients compared with the general population. Kimmel et al. (31), performing PSG in 30 patients with chronic renal failure, found that 73% of patients had sleep apnea. Interestingly, CAPD patients had increased sleep fragmentation and lower oxygen saturations from apneas on nights when fluid was present in their abdomens (32). Several mechanisms have been proposed to explain the development of OSA in renal patients. The first proposal is that the accumulation of uremic toxins affects upper-airway muscle

tone through CNS regulation during sleep (27). Edema and volume overload may also predispose the upper airway to collapse. Furthermore, hypocapnia from metabolic acidosis may change the apnea threshold, predisposing to an unstable breathing pattern. Protein metabolism may also play a role, since a diet rich in branched-chain amino acids results in a lower apnea index (27). Confounding factors, including age, may be important since both sleep apnea and ESRD are more prevalent in older people. There is evidence showing that aggressive therapy of ESRD improves sleep apnea. For instance, case studies show that sleep apnea was no longer present after kidney transplantation (33). A decrease in apnea index was also noted with the use of a bicarbonate versus an acetate-based dialysate. Furthermore, Hanly et al. (34) reported that switching patients to slow nocturnal HD (8 to 10 hours a night) for up to seven nights compared to HD three times weekly for 4 hours resulted in a marked decrease in the number of respiratory events. Clinical implications from these investigations suggest that all patients with renal disease should be screened for sleep apnea/hypopnea syndrome, and if present, treated.

Patients with renal disease also have a high prevalence of RLS and periodic limb movement of sleep disorder (PLMS). Uremia is considered a secondary cause of RLS (35). Up to 80% of patients with RLS also have PLMS (36). RLS is extremely distressing and occurs in approximately 80% of dialysis patients. (Further discussion is found in Chapter 15.)

Patients with ESRD also have EDS. Stephanski et al. (37) noted that 77% of questioned CAPD patients reported taking daytime naps and 51% reported falling asleep unintentionally. A subset of their patient population underwent multiple sleep latency testing (MSLT) showing a mean sleep latency of 6.3 minutes, verifying pathologic daytime sleepiness. EDS is also found in HD patients. It is very difficult to address the underlying causes of this condition in these patients, especially with the high prevalence of OSA, PLMS, and RLS. Other potential causes of EDS include uremic encephalopathy, parathyroid hormone excess (which could have neurotoxic effects), and alterations in neurotransmitter levels (27). Dialysis may also release cytokines that have somnogenic properties, including interleukin-1 (IL-1) and tumor necrosis factor alpha (TNFα). Rapid changes in the acid–base balance and serum osmolality may also affect alertness. Furthermore, extrinsic factors may contribute to sleep disturbances. Dialysis schedules may interfere with sleep time and propagate an irregular sleep–wake schedule. For example, some patients report for dialysis as early as 0500 hours, 3 days a week. Patients also nap during dialysis sessions, thus interfering with normal circadian rhythm-timing processes. Peritoneal dialysis is also performed during sleep time, so that fluid shifts and noise from the machines may cause arousals and disrupt sleep. In patients with less severe renal disease, polyuria may also disrupt sleep.

Clinical Pearls

- Sleep complaints are present in approximately 80% of dialysis patients.
- PSG features of dialysis patients include poor sleep efficiency with significant wake time.
- OSA is prevalent in renal disease patients.
- Uremia is a secondary cause of RLS and PLM disorder.
- Renal patients often have EDS.
- Renal patients should be assessed for the presence of sleep disorders and if present, aggressively treated.

SLEEP IN INFECTIOUS DISEASE PATIENTS

Most of us have noticed an increased propensity to sleep when we have an infection. Bacterial cell wall products result in the release of somnogenic cytokines, including IL-1 (38). These immune responses are partially responsible for sleep alterations. Also, increasing core body temperature, as with an infection, results in increased amounts of delta sleep. With infection, sleep time requirements may need to be increased. Furthermore, infection may cause sleep disruption. This section will briefly discuss sleep alterations in HIV patients and will briefly discuss other infections. This section will not discuss CNS infections including African sleeping sickness (*Trypanosoma brucei*), meningeal encephalitis, and prion diseases.

Sleep in Patients with HIV Infection

Patients with HIV infection report many sleep-related symptoms including daytime sleepiness, difficulty in initiating and maintaining sleep, and multiple nocturnal arousals (39). HIV infection alters cytokines and other immune regulators that may impact sleep. Also, secondary infectious processes may disrupt sleep. Medications used to treat HIV infection may disrupt sleep. For instance, some patients report insomnia with the use of zidovudine (AZT). Vivid dreams have been reported in patients taking the non-nucleoside reverse transcriptase inhibitors nevirapine and efavirenz (40)

Many investigators have examined sleep architecture in HIV patients. Norman et al. (39) found an increase in delta sleep that was more prevalent during the later part of the sleep time. Furthermore, other investigators have noted that as HIV infection progresses, there is worsening of the sleep disturbance (41,42). During the early stages of asymptomic infection (CD_4 count greater than 400 per mm^3), there is mild difficulty in initiating and maintaining sleep, which is associated with mild and intermittent periods of daytime fatigue. PSG findings in these patients include an increase in total delta sleep percentage with more delta sleep occurring during the later sleep cycles. Alpha intrusion may also be noted along with mild alterations in the REM–NREM sleep cycles. In patients with mild symptoms of HIV (CD_4 count greater than 200 per mm^3 but less than 400 per mm^3), there is more difficulty in maintaining sleep, and patients note increasing fatigue. PSG findings include a decrease in sleep efficiency, with lesser amounts of delta sleep and more difficultly discriminating the NREM–REM sleep cycles. In the terminal stages of HIV infection (CD_4 counts less than 200 per mm^3), patients have more difficulty with daytime fatigue and severe difficulty in maintaining sleep. PSG findings include further decreases and sometimes even the absence of delta sleep, poor sleep efficiency, and difficulty in recognizing NREM–REM sleep cycles, with many spontaneous arousals. It has been postulated that the decrease in delta sleep as the disease progresses may be related to fluctuations in cytokines and neurologic involvement from the infection (43). Furthermore, HIV-positive individuals have many psychosocial stressors that may impact sleep quality (44).

Therapy of sleep disturbances in HIV-positive individuals includes good sleep hygiene practices, avoidance of alcohol, caffeine, and other sleep disruptive substances, screening for treatable sleep disorders. For example, and lipodystrophy may predispose patients to OSA development. Patients with HIV also have a high prevalence of depression, so this should be screened for and treated, if present. Some practitioners use intermittent sedatives–hypnotics for insomnia, which may be helpful in selected patients. As more aggressive therapeutic modalities are available to treat HIV infection, clinical outcome may be improved, and further attention to sleep disturbances may improve the patient's overall QOL.

Other Infectious Diseases

Patients with infectious mononucleosis experience malaise and fatigue during active infection. Some patients develop chronic sleepiness and fatigue and have prolonged sleep periods and nap throughout the day. Other chronic infections that may potentially cause fatigue include cytomegalovirus, hepatitis B and C, Lyme disease, and brucellosis (45).

Clinical Pearls

- Cytokines released during infections, including IL-1, have somnogenic properties.
- Increasing core body temperature increases delta sleep.
- With HIV infection, there are increased amounts of delta sleep early in the infection's natural history.

SLEEP IN ENDOCRINE DISORDERS

Sleep is also altered in patients with endocrine disorders including hypo- and hyperthyroidism, acromegaly, and Cushing's syndrome.

Hypothyroidism has been associated with sleep apnea (46). Potential mechanisms in which hypothyroidism could lead to sleep apnea include infiltration of tissues with myxedematous material leading to a smaller upper airway, impaired strength of the upper-airway muscles, and reduced central drive to the upper-airway muscles (46). No large cohort studies evaluate the prevalence of sleep apnea in hypothyroid subjects. Obesity may be a significant confounding factor. Pelttari et al. (47) examined 26 patients with hypothyroidism and 188 euthyroid control subjects finding that 50% of hypothyroid patients and 29% of control subjects had significant respiratory events. There are case reports of hypothyroid patients whose sleep apnea resolved after attaining normal thyroid function. Since rapid escalation of thyroid replacement therapy is associated with significant cardiovascular morbidity, sleep apnea should be diagnosed and treated prior to initiation of thyroid hormone replacement, if at all possible (48). Winkelman et al. (49) does not recommend performing screening thyroid function studies in all patients with suspected sleep apnea; however, screening may be appropriate in elderly women who have a higher risk of hypothyroidism. Hypothyroidism has other effects on sleep, including reduction in delta sleep percentage. EDS is also noted in these patients. On the other hand, hyperthyroidism has been associated with insomnia. There are conflicting data concerning the effect of hyperthyroidism on sleep architecture.

Growth hormone (GH) excesses resulting in acromegaly is also associated with sleep apnea. Grunstein et al. (50) noted that 60% of unselected acromegaly patients have sleep apnea. Potential pathophysiological mechanisms of this association include macroglossia and increased muscle mass of the upper airway. Since central sleep apnea is also noted in acromegalic patients, alterations in central ventilatory control may also play a role. In addition, acromegaly patients may also have EDS with an increase in REM sleep in the absence of other primary sleep disorders (51). There is limited data examining sleep characteristics with GH deficiency. One study showed a reduction in delta sleep, although more research is needed to make any conclusions.

Adrenocorticosteroid excess, as seen in Cushing's disease, is associated with sleep apnea in approximately 30% of patients (52). Other investigations have shown shortened REM latencies and poor sleep efficiencies, although more data are needed to draw further conclusions.

Clinical Pearls

- Hypothyroidism is associated with sleep apnea, although thyroid function screening is not recommended in all patients with suspected sleep apnea.
- Hyperthyroidism may be associated with insomnia.
- Growth hormone and adrenal corticosteroid excesses are also associated with sleep symptoms.

FIBROMYALGIA SYNDROME

Clinical Features

Fibromyalgia syndrome (FS) is defined by the American College of Rheumatology as the presence of widespread musculoskeletal pain for at least 3 months, which is bilateral above and below the waist, including axial pain and the presence of 11 of 18 tender points (53). Note that fibromyalgia is a syndrome and not a disease, and that the definition itself does not include a sleep disturbance. Investigators noted that adding a sleep disturbance to the definition did not improve the definition's operating characteristics. Fibromyalgia syndrome is very common, affecting between 6 and 10 million Americans. In population-based studies, FS is thought to affect 3% of the population and is most prevalent in people aged 30 to 50 years (54). Interestingly, 75% to 90% of people with FS are women. Furthermore, health-seeking behavior is related to psychiatric diagnoses and not to FS itself. Pain symptoms may be severe, but remain stable over years. Factors associated with symptom onset include infection in 55%, physical trauma in 14% to 23%, and emotional trauma and stress in 14% of FS patients. Twenty to 50% of FS patients also have depression and 53% to 65% of FS patients have a history of sexual abuse (55). Of FS patients, 23% have seasonal variations, with worse symptoms noted in December and January, and fewer symptoms in July. There are other modulating factors reported in FS patients. Poor sleep is an aggravating factor in 67% of patients, and rest is an ameliorating factor in 62% of patients (56).

Pathophysiology of Fibromyalgia Syndrome

The pathophysiology of FS is very complex. The main mechanism is thought to be central sensitization of nociceptive neurons in the dorsal horn of the spinal cord with activation of *N*-methyl-*D*-aspartate (NMDA) receptors (57). This central sensitization results in generalized heightened pain sensitivity due to pathological nociceptive processing within the CNS. There are changes in neurotransmitter systems, including substance P and serotonin, at spinal cord and higher centers. A threefold increase in substance P and a decrease in serotonin levels is present in cerebrospinal fluid (CSF) (58). There is evidence that FS patients have functional polymorphism of the 5-HT serotonin transporter gene. There are also alterations in endocrine function in FS patients, including decreases in growth hormone (GH), insulinlike growth factor 1 (IGF-1), free T_4, and prolactin levels (59). Korszun et al. (60) reported that melatonin levels in FS patients (compared to control subjects) are elevated between 2300 and 0650 hours (60)

There are also alterations in regional cerebral blood flow (rCBF) in FS patients, with lower rCBF to the thalamus and caudate nucleus (61). The thalamus plays a role in abnormal pain perception and processing, and the caudate nucleus is important for pain modulation. Gracely et al. (62) noted that pain is visible on functional MRI scans. With pain, FS patients had increased rCBG flow to 12 areas of the brain compared with 2 areas in the control subjects. These findings suggest that FS is characterized by both cortical and subcortical pain-processing augmentation. Psychosocial and health status factors also may be important. The role of nonrestorative sleep is also an issue in the idiopathogenesis of abnormal pain sensitivity in FS, which will be discussed below.

Sleep in Fibromyalgia Syndrome Patients

Sleep is altered in FS patients, with many patients having the alpha NREM sleep anomaly. Sleep complaints are very prevalent, with 76% of FS patients complaining of nonrestorative sleep, compared with 10% to 30% of control subjects (54). Patients report fragmented sleep and have sleep onset and sleep maintenance insomnia. They also associate pain with a prior nights' poor sleep.

There are also PSG findings. Based on seven controlled trials with 77 FS patients, FS patients had decreased TST, decreased delta sleep (adjusted for age), and decreased REM sleep percentages. There were more arousals, and long awakenings, and micro-arousals were three times more prevalent than in control subjects. The alpha NREM sleep anomaly was also noted (63).

Investigators examining the microstructure of sleep utilizing power spectral, frequency, and domain analysis in the EEG of FS patients found that sigma frequency (12 to 14 Hz) and delta frequency (<2 Hz) reflected a sleep-protective function associated with greater depth; beta frequency (14 to 38 Hz) reflected arousal and was associated with micro-arousals and lightening of sleep; and occipital alpha frequency (8 to 13 Hz) was arousal-associated (54). Interestingly, in normal control subjects, stage 4 sleep disruption by noise resulted in unrefreshing sleep, pain, and fatigue. Furthermore, in normal controls, deep joint pain stimulation reduced delta and sigma power and increased alpha and beta power on EEG spectral analysis.

The Alpha NREM Sleep Anomaly

The alpha frequency (8 to 13 Hz) during NREM sleep was first observed in 1973. In 1975, Moldofsky (63) identified it in FS patients, calling it "alpha intrusion," and noted that it was frequently seen during delta sleep. This alpha NREM sleep anomaly is not specific for FS and not all FS patients have it. Figure 30-2 shows a 10-second epoch of the alpha NREM sleep anomaly during delta sleep. Previous work has shown that the amount of alpha frequency correlates with overnight pain measures, mood, energy levels, and perceived shallow sleep. Branco et al. (64) noted that FS patients had more alpha in successive sleep cycles compared with control subjects. Furthermore, Drewes et al. (65) noted that the alpha frequency is more promi-

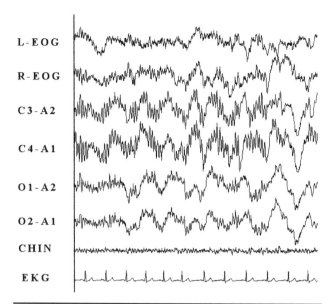

FIGURE 30-2. Alpha NREM sleep anomaly. This 10-second epoch shows alpha frequency (8 to 13 Hz) EEG wave forms superimposed on a background of delta frequency (<2 Hz) EEG. The alpha frequency is most evident in the central EEG leads ($C_3 - A_2$ and $C_4 - A_1$).

nent in the frontal area, so the alpha frequency may be more prominent on the central versus the occipital lead on routine PSG. In a recent review, Mahowald (66) stated that the alpha NREM sleep anomaly was not specific to fibromyalgia, was not a marker for fibromyalgia, was not associated with enhanced long-term or short-term memory during sleep, and was not associated with myalgic symptoms (66). He stated that this anomaly was found in 15% of 240 normal subjects and was found more frequently in people with undisturbed sleep (20%) than in those with disturbed sleep (8%). He raised the question whether the alpha frequency might actually be a sleep-maintaining process. To quote Mahowald, "Van Sweden's conclusion that 'alpha-delta or alpha sleep is still an atypical and aspecific sleep pattern with an unclear pathophysiology' is well stated."

Roizenblatt et al. (67) noted that FS patients have different alpha pattern characteristics and that these alpha pattern characteristics may identify FS patients into subcategories (67). Monitoring sleep microstructure using power spectral and frequency domain analyses in 40 FS patients (who were off their medications for more than 4 weeks) and 43 controls, they noted worsening of morning pain symptoms in 72% of FS patients compared with 12% of controls. Of FS patients, 93% also had an increase in the number of tender points after the sleep period and poor sleep quality was reported in 70% of FS patients compared to none in controls. Alpha rhythm was noted during NREM in 70% of FS patients and in 16% of controls. Furthermore, the investigators noted three distinct patterns of alpha activity: (a) *Phasic alpha* pattern activity in which alpha was episodic, occurring simultaneously with delta; this pattern was seen in 50% of FS patients and in 7% of controls; (b) the second pattern was *tonic alpha*, which was continuously present throughout NREM, independent of delta activity, and seen in 20% of FS patients and in 9% of controls; and (c) a *low alpha* pattern with minimal alpha, which was seen in 30% of FS patients and in 84% of controls. Furthermore, the phasic alpha pattern was associated with decreased sleep efficiency, decreased delta sleep, the subjective feeling of superficial sleep, and longer pain duration and morning stiffness. This phasic alpha pattern distinction may be useful in future research to identify patients for specific therapeutic modalities.

Therapy of Fibromyalgia Syndrome

Few randomized controlled trials evaluate sleep parameters with medication in FS patients, and no treatment has been shown to have long-lasting benefits. Trazadone increased delta sleep and decreased the alpha NREM sleep anomaly without altering wake time after sleep onset (WASU) or sleep latency (54). Amitriptyline improved sleep symptom scores. One-third of FS patients have a meaningful response with amitriptyline therapy at 1 month; however, by 6 months, the response declines (54). Fluoxetine helps sleep scores but not pain or tender point numbers. Goldenberg et al. (68) noted that combination therapy with amitriptyline and fluoxetine was more effective than single-agent therapy. Farber et al. (69), in a prospective multicenter, parallel, placebo-controlled trial of more than 400 FS patients, found that tropisteron, a 5-HT3-receptor antagonist, resulted in a 39% response rate, a 35% decrease in pain scores, and at a 5-mg dose, resulted in decreased symptom scores, decreased tender point number, and improvement in sleep and dizziness (69).

Exercise may also improve outcomes. In a Cochrane Review, Busch et al. (70) examined 16 randomized controlled trials that enrolled more than 700 FS patients. Exercise improved aerobic performance and tender point pressure threshold. Richards et al. (71) performed a parallel group, randomized, controlled trial examining more than 100 FS patients receiving either graded aerobic exercise, or relaxation and flexibility therapy. Exercise resulted in a reduction in tender point number, and improvement in the Fibromyalgia Impact Questionnaire score at 1 year follow-up.

Brief cognitive behavioral therapy may also be useful in FS patients. Williams et al. (72) performed a randomized controlled study of 145 FS patients evaluating brief cognitive–behavioral therapy, showing that cognitive therapy improved physical function; however, there was no improvement in the McGill Pain Registry score (72).

Many interventions do not improve outcomes. Sedatives and benzodiazepines do not provide any specific benefit; however, intermittent use may help insomnia symptoms. Non-benzodiazepine hypnotic medications, such as zaleplon and zolpidem, may improve subjective sleep and EDS, but do not alter the alpha NREM sleep anomaly or pain scores (73). Intermittent use of these agents may be helpful. Melatonin also did not provide any benefit, nor did 4 weeks of morning light therapy (63). There are many design faults in therapeutic trials, including small sample sizes, low statistical power, and heterogeneous subject groups and outcome measures. There is no consensus on optimal management for FS patients. Treatment success, unfortunately, is very limited, with less than 50% of patients having adequate symptom relief. At 3-year follow-up, only 3% of patients were pain-free, so that even though the pain remains stable, it does not go away.

Patient management is multidisciplinary and should be flexible and multimodal. Management includes education, pharmacologic interventions, including antidepressants, benzodiazepines, non-benzodiazepine sedatives, analgesic, and muscle relaxants, nonpharmacologic interventions including exercise, cognitive–behavioral therapy, biofeedback, hypnotherapy, and even acupuncture. Fibromyalgia patients commonly have OSA, PLMD, RLS and delayed-sleep phase, and should be screened and treated for these disorders. They should also be assessed and treated for maladaptive sleep behaviors, if present. Assessing for mental health needs and referring to appropriate mental health professionals also should not be overlooked. Develop a team approach. Take a patient-centered approach, since one standardized protocol will not be adequate for all patients. Include an inventory of social and family support systems and note any associated overlapping conditions including irritable bowel syndrome, chronic fatigue syndrome, and posttraumatic stress syndrome, all of which may impact upon their FS.

Sleep management includes sleep hygiene measures such as a regular sleep–wake schedule, a quiet bedroom environment, and the avoidance of alcohol and alerting substances, such as caffeine and nicotine. Relaxation techniques and an exercise program may be helpful. Review all over-the-counter medications, including herbal remedies, as these agents may interfere with sleep.

Potential therapies under development include human recombinant growth hormone (rGH) (74), sodium oxybate (75), and substance P inhibitors (76). Hopefully, future research will help improve our ability to manage FS patients.

Clinical Pearls

- Fibromyalgia syndrome affects 3% of the population and 75% to 90% are women.
- Pathophysiology of FS includes central sensitization resulting in generalized pain sensitivity.
- Fibromyalgia syndrome patients have nonrestorative, fragmented sleep and insomnia.

- PSG findings in FS patients include decreased TST, delta sleep, and REM sleep.
- The alpha NREM sleep anomaly is commonly seen in FS patients, but it is not specific for FS and is seen in 15% of normal people.
- The phasic alpha pattern characteristic is associated with the subjective feeling of superficial sleep, morning stiffness, and decreased sleep efficiency and delta sleep.
- Management of FS is multimodal and may require a team approach.

SLEEP AND CHRONIC PAIN (CP) SYNDROMES

Chronic pain also interferes with sleep. A 1996 Gallop Poll sponsored by the National Sleep Foundation found that 56 million Americans have nighttime pain that interferes with falling asleep or have early morning awakenings (77). Depression is present in more than 40% of patients and there is a synergistic effect of pain on depression (78). Of CP patients, 50% to 70% report sleep impairment with sleep disturbances correlating with higher pain intensity, depression, anxiety, and decreased activity levels.

There are also PSG findings in patients with CP syndromes. Harman et al. (79) reported polysomnographic findings in patients with chronic low back pain. In a study of 10 patients and 11 age-matched controls, there was no difference in sleep-onset, TST, or sleep-staging parameters. Low sigma power was noted in the chronic low back pain patients, which could potentially explain the poor sleep quality in these patients. Depressed patients with chronic low back pain had more occipital delta, more occipital and central alpha, and more beta activity than in the non-depressed chronic low back pain patients. These findings help support the idea that comorbid disorders, including depression, have a major impact on the ability to sleep.

Wilson et al. (80) noted that 45% of CP patients have major depression (of which 84% complained of insomnia) and that subjects without major depression have a lower incidence of insomnia (55%). Patients with major depression and insomnia have the highest level of pain-related impairment. Widerström–Noga et al. (81) examined chronic pain after spinal cord injury surgery in more than 200 subjects and noted that high pain intensity and the use of multiple pain descriptors are associated with sleep onset difficulty. Other factors predicting frequent sleep interruptions include high pain intensity, male gender, anxiety, and higher age at the time of injury. Management includes medications, and psychologic and behavior strategies (82). Medications used to treat chronic pain may also impact sleep and sleep architecture. For instance, opioids initially cause insomnia in naïve patients, with normalization over time. Nonsteroidal anti-inflammatory agents increase wake time and delay delta sleep onset (83). With the availability of oral long-acting opioids and implantable delivery systems

(epidural and intrathecal), we are finding that some patients have significant central sleep apnea (CSA) that is very resistant to therapy.

Clinical Pearls

- Chronic pain patients have sleep disruption.
- Depression is associated with more sleep complaints.
- Management includes medication, as well as psychologic and behavior strategies.

CHRONIC FATIGUE SYNDROME

Chronic fatigue syndrome (CFS) is a heterogeneous condition defined by: (a) fatigue for at least 6 months; and (b) finding no underlying cause for fatigue despite an exhaustive laboratory investigation (84). Sleep complaints are very common in CFS patients and include EPS, and difficulty in initiating and maintaining sleep. Fischler et al. (85) examined polysomnographic findings in 49 CFS patients and 20 controls and found less stage 4 sleep, more sleep fragmentation, lower sleep efficiency, and difficulty in sleep initiation in CFS patients. Watson et al. (86) reported subjective and objective measures of insomnia in monozygotic twins discordant for CFS. Interestingly, despite CFS patients reporting eight subjective measures of insomnia and poor sleep more commonly, objective PSG features of insomnia were very similar between groups. These data support the idea that CFS patients may suffer from sleep-state misperception. As in all other medical disorders previously described, all CFS patients should be screened for underlying sleep disorders and treated appropriately.

Clinical Pearls

- Screen for primary sleep disorders in patients with chronic fatigue syndrome.

DRUG EFFECTS ON SLEEP AND WAKEFULNESS

This section is a brief review of the more common prescriptive and over-the-counter medications used in internal medicine. Psychotropic and antiepileptic medications are covered in their respective chapters. This discussion should be considered as a general guide, as the specific drug effects in any individual may be influenced by age, sex, health, other drug interactions, and other unknown factors. Table 30-2 displays potential sleep effects on commonly used drugs.

Cardiovascular

The cardiovascular drugs discussed include antihypertensive, antiarrhythmic, and lipid-lowering drugs (87).

Antihypertensives

Beta-Adrenergic Receptor-blocking Agents

The frequency of side effects is dependent on dosage and patient age and health. Frequently reported symptoms include fatigue, insomnia, nightmares, vivid dreams, confusion, and depression (87,88). These effects are more common with the more lipophilic drugs (i.e., propanolol) than with the hydrophilic drugs (i.e., atenolol), and are more likely to occur in the older rather than younger patient (84). Other factors that may influence CNS effects include the drug's relative affinity for beta-2 or 5HT receptors, plasma catecholamine levels, and plasma concentration (89). Melatonin suppression has also been reported (90).

Alpha-2 Agonists

While sedation is the most common reported side effect of clonidine and methyldopa, insomnia and nightmares have also been reported (91). Methyldopa has also been associated with memory impairment (92).

Beta-Adrenergic Receptor Blockers with Alpha-1 Blocking Activity

Carvedilol and labetalol have been associated with somnolence and fatigue, with insomnia noted only occasionally (93).

Other Antihypertensives

Other antihypertensive medications have few reported detrimental effects on sleep or wakefulness. The alpha antagonists, prazosin and terazosin, have been occasionally associated with transient somnolence. Calcium-channel antagonists have minimal impact on sleep. The calcium-channel agents may, however, decrease the effectiveness of hypnotics and potentiate stimulant effects (94). Angiotensin-converting enzyme (ACE) inhibitors (captopril, etc.) have very few central side effects. The new angiotensin receptor antagonists (losartan) rarely is associated with insomnia (95). Vasodilators and diuretics do not appear to affect sleep, although micturition may cause more frequent awakenings.

Antiarrhythmics

Fatigue is the most common impairment with the use of these agents, with class II drugs (beta-adrenergic receptor-blocking agents) showing the highest rates. Insomnia and abnormal dreams have also been noted.

Lipid-lowering Agents

The effect of lipid-lowering agents on sleep and wake are somewhat variable, from no effect, to insomnia, to fatigue or drowsiness (96,97). These are generally uncommon occurrences.

Antihistamines

Histamine-1 Antagonists

First-generation histamine-1 antagonists are lipophilic and readily cross the blood–brain barrier. However, they antagonize muscarinic cholinergic and alpha-adrenergic receptors because of poor receptor selectivity. The second-generation H-1 antihistamines are large and hydrophilic and do not easily cross the blood–brain barrier. The major side effect of the first-generation H-1 antihistamines is sedation, while the second-generation H-1 antihistamines appear not to be as sedating. Cetirizine (Zyrtec) however, is a metabolite of hydroxyzine, and may be sedating at higher doses and potentiate the effects of alcohol (98,99). Performance impairment is slight with second-generation agents, whereas impairment with first-generation agents is substantially higher, with triprolidine presenting the highest risk (100). Although not certain, tolerance to the sedating effects may develop with chronic use.

Histamine-2 Antagonists

These drugs do not easily cross the blood–brain barrier and are unlikely to affect CNS function. However, in a small number of susceptible individuals, insomnia and somnolence may occur (101). Cimetidine has been most frequently associated with side effects and can slow benzodiazepine clearance and increase theophylline, carbamazepime, and beta-adrenergic receptor-blocking agent levels. In patients with renal failure, is present an increased frequency of lethary, sleepiness, and confusion (102).

Theophylline

Disturbed sleep is a common side effect in patients taking theophylline, which is chemically related to caffeine. Absorption is lower at night than in the daytime and is significantly affected by food (103). However, in patients whose respiratory function improves with theophylline, sleep may actually improve.

Corticosteroids

Although objective studies are inconsistent, corticosteroids have frequently been associated with disturbed sleep, most often a subjective increase in wakefulness (104). PSG data show a decrease in REM sleep, with a small increase in stage 2 sleep. Hydrocortisone may increase delta sleep, but dexamethasone does not (105).

Decongestants

Pseudoephedrine and phenylpropanolamine have similar pharmacologic properties similar to ephedrine, but are less potent CNS stimulants (102). These agents are associated with insomnia and are used extensively as nasal

TABLE 30-2. Medication Effects on Sleep

Drug Class	Comments	Sleep Continuity	Sleep Latency	TST[a]	STG[b] 1	STG[b] 2	Delta	REM
Anticholinergics Scopolamine		↓	↓			↑ Acute ↓ withdrawal		↓ Acute ↑ withdrawal
Antihypertensives Beta blockers Propranolol Atenolol	Insomnia, nightmares; effects more common with lipophilic drugs	↓			↑			↓
Alpha-2 agonists Clonidine	Sedation, ↓ concentration, nightmares			↑ Acute ↓ with chronic use ↑			↓	
Methyldopa	Sedation, insomnia, nightmares, memory impairment							↑
Beta antagonists with alpha-blocking activity Carvedilol Labetalol	Somnolence, fatigue, insomnia							
Catecholamine depleters Reserpine	Sedation, insomnia, nightmares	↓					↑	
Calcium antagonists Verapamil Nifedipine	Decrease effectiveness of hypnotics, potentiate stimulants							
ACE inhibitors Captopril	No negative effects on sleep							
ACE II inhibitors Losartan	Rare insomnia							
Alpha-1 antagonists Prazosin Doxazosin	Transiently sedating							
Vasodilators Hydralazine	Anxiety, insomnia							↑
Diuretics HCTZ	No impairment; ↑ micturition may lead to sleep disruption							

Drug	Sleep effects	Comments
Antiarrhythmics Disopyramide, Procainamide (IA) Mexiletine, Tocainide (IB) Flecainide; Propafenone (IC) III Amiodarone (II)	↑	Fatigue (IA); drowsiness, fatigue (IB); fatigue, insomnia (IC); fatigue, nightmares, insomnia (II)
Antihistamines		
H-1 antihistamines First generation Diphenhydramine Benadryl Second generation Loratadine Cetirizine	↑	Sedation Cetirizine classified as sedating by FDA (high doses) Insomnia/somnolence <2%; ↑ frequency, lethargy/somnolence in Renal insufficiency
H-2 antihistamines Cimetidine Ranitidine	↓ ←	Disturbed sleep
Xanthines Theophylline Caffeine	→ ← →	
Corticosteroids Hydrocortisone Dexamethasone	→ →	Increases delta (hydrocortisone) Does not increase delta (dexamethasone)
Decongestants Pseudoephedrine Phenylpropanolamine	→	Insomnia, ↑ plasma caffeine levels ↑ plasma caffeine levels
Nicotine	→ ← ↑ Withdrawal	Nonrestorative sleep
Opiates	↑ Withdrawal ↓ Attenuates ↑ Withdrawal[1]	Sedation

[a]TST, total sleep time; STG, sleep stage.

decongestants. While phenylpropanolamine is much less lipophilic, with less CNS effects, it has been reported to increase caffeine levels (106).

Nicotine

Nicotine is one of the most widely used drugs in the world. It is associated with sleep onset insomnia and nonrestorative sleep (107). PSG data show an increase in alpha activity with reduced delta sleep, and reduced sleep efficiency (108). Withdrawal is associated with worsened sleep continuity. Furthermore, acute smoking abstinence results in increased arousals during sleep and objective daytime sleepiness (109).

Opiates

Opiates produce analgesia as well as drowsiness, feelings of tranquility, and psychomotor retardation. They promote sleep in patients with pain and chronic pain syndromes, and may be useful in RLS therapy. Single and repeated doses of opiates in addicts and nonaddicts lead to more disturbed sleep. REM sleep is suppressed, although this may attenuate fairly quickly. Opiate withdrawal leads to disturbed sleep (110). Similar effects are seen with methadone, although this medication has less effect on arousal.

Clinical Pearls

- Medications affect sleep and sleep architecture, so a careful review of prescription and over-the-counter drugs and herbs should be done routinely.
- Beta-adrenergic receptor-blocking agents, especially lipophilic ones, are associated with fatigue, insomnia, nightmares, and vivid dreams.
- Use of first-generation histamine-1 antagonists often results in sedation.

ACKNOWLEDGMENT

Drs. Harding and Hawkins wish to acknowledge the kind editorial assistance of Arren M. Graf. Dr. Harding is a past recipient of the NIH-NHLBI Sleep Academic Award.

REFERENCES

1. Orr WC, Johnson LF, Robinson MG. The effect of sleep on swallowing, esophageal peristalsis, and acid clearance. *Gastroenterology.* 1984;86:814–819.
2. Kahrilas PJ, Dodds WJ, Dent J, et al. Effect of sleep, spontaneous gastroesophageal reflux, and a meal on upper esophageal sphincter pressure in normal human volunteers. *Gastroenterology.* 1987;92:466–471.
3. Mittal RK, Holloway, RH, Panagini R, et al. Transient lower esophageal sphincter relaxation. *Gastroenterology.* 1995;109:601–610.
4. Freidin N, Fisher MJ, Taylor W, et al. Sleep and nocturnal acid reflux in normal subjects and patients with reflux oesophagitis. *Gut.* 1991;32:1275–1279.
5. Orr WC, Johnson LF. Responses to different levels of esophageal acidification during waking and sleep. *Digest Dis Sci.* 1998;43:241–245.
6. Schneyer LH, Pigman W, Hanahan L, et al. Rate of flow of human parotid, sublingual, and submaxillary secretion during sleep. *J Dental Res.* 1956;35:109–114.
7. Orr WC, Elsenbruch S, Harnish MJ, et al. Proximal migration of esophageal acid perfusions during waking and sleep. *Amer J Gastroenterol.* 2000;95:37–42.
8. American Sleep Disorders Association. *The international classification of sleep disorders,* revised. Diagnostic and coding manual. Rochester, Minnesota: American Sleep Disorders Association, 1997.
9. Johnson LF, DeMeester TR. Twenty-four hour pH monitoring of distal esophagus. A quantitative measure of gastroesophageal reflux. *Amer J Gastroenterol.* 1974;62:325–332.
10. Farup C, Kleinman L, Sloan S, et al. The impact of nocturnal symptoms associated with gastroesophageal reflux disease on health-related quality of life. *Arch Internal Med.* 2001;161:45–52.
11. Richter JE, ed. *Ambulatory esophageal pH monitoring. Practical approach and clinical implications.* 2nd edn. Baltimore: Williams and Wilkins, 1997.
12. Harding SM, Richter JE, Guzzo MR, et al. Asthma and gastroesophageal reflux: acid suppressive therapy improves asthma outcome. *Amer J Med.* 1996;100:395–404.
13. Harding SM. Gastroesophageal reflux and asthma: insight into the association. *J Allergy Clin Immunol.* 1999;104:251–259.
14. Harding SM. Nocturnal asthma: role of nocturnal gastroesophageal reflux. *Chronobiol Intern.* 1999;16:641–662.
15. Cuttitta G, Cibella F, Visconti A. Spontaneous gastroesophageal reflux and airway patency during the night in adult asthmatics. *Amer J Respir Crit Care Med.* 2000;151:177–181.
16. Gislason T, Janson C, Vermeire P, et al. Respiratory symptoms and nocturnal gastroesophageal reflux. A population-based study of young adults in three European countries. *Chest.* 2002;121:158–163.
17. Thurnheer R, Henz S, Knoblauch A. Sleep-related laryngospasm. *Eur Respir J.* 1997;10:2084–2086.
18. Janson C, Gislason TR, De Backer W, et al. Daytime sleepiness, snoring and gastro-oesophageal reflux amongst young adults in three European countries. *J Internal Med.* 1995;237:277–285.
19. Ing AJ, Meng CN, Breslin ABX. Obstructive sleep apnea and gastroesophageal reflux. *Amer J Med.* 2000;108:120S–125S.
20. Senior BA, Khan M, Schwimmer C, et al. Gastroesophageal reflux and obstructive sleep apnea. *Laryngoscope.* 2001;111:2144–2146.
21. Green BT, Broughton WA, O'Connor JB. Marked improvement in nocturnal gastroesophageal reflux in a large cohort of patients with obstructive sleep apnea treated with continuous positive airway pressure. *Ann Internal Med.* 2003;163:41–45.
22. Khoury RM, Camacho-Lobato L, Katz PO, et al. Influence of spontaneous sleep positions on nighttime recumbent reflux in patients with gastroesophageal reflux disease. *Amer J Gastroenterol.* 1999;94:2069–2073.
23. Kuo B, Castell DO. Optimal dosing of omeprazole 40 mg daily: effects on gastric and esophageal pH and serum gastrin. *Amer J Gastroenterol.* 1996;91:1532–1538.
24. Peghini PL, Katz PO, Castell DO. Randitidine controls nocturnal gastric acid break through on omeprazole: a controlled study in normal subjects. *Gastroenterology.* 1998;115:1335–1339.
25. Spechler SJ, Lee E, Ahnen D, et al. Long-term outcome of medical and surgical therapies for gastroesophageal reflux disease: follow-up of a randomized controlled trial. *JAMA.* 2001;285:2331–2338.
26. Kerr J, Shoenut P, Steens RD, et al. Nasal continuous positive airway pressure. A new treatment for nocturnal gastro-esophageal reflux? *J Clin Gastroenterol.* 1993;17:276–278.
27. Parker KP. Sleep disturbances in dialysis patients. *Sleep Med Rev.* 2003;7:131–143.
28. Holley JL, Nespor S, Rault R. Characterizing sleep disorders in chronic hemodialysis patients. *ASAIO Trans.* 1991;37:M456–M457.

29. Walker S, Fine A, Kryger MH. Sleep complaints are common in the dialysis unit. *Amer J Kidney Dis.* 1995;26:751–756.
30. Hays RD, Kallich JD, Mapes DL, et al. Development of the Kidney Disease Quality of Life (KDQOL) instrument. *Qual Life Res.* 1994;3:329–338.
31. Kimmel PL, Miller G, Mendelson WB. Sleep apnea syndrome in chronic renal disease. *Amer J Med.* 1989;86:308–314.
32. Wadhwa NK, Seliger M, Greenberg HE, et al. Sleep related respiratory disorders in end-stage renal disease patients on peritoneal dialysis. *Peritoneal Dialysis Intern.* 1992;12:51–56.
33. Auckley DH, Schmidt-Nowara W, Brown LK. Reversal of sleep apnea hypopnea syndrome in end-stage renal disease after kidney transplantation. *Amer J Kidney Dis.* 1999;34:739–744.
34. Hanly PJ, Pierratos A. Improvement of sleep apnea in patients with chronic renal failure who undergo nocturnal hemodialysis. *N Engl J Med.* 2001;344:102–107.
35. Winkelman JW, Chertow GM, Lazarus JM. Restless legs syndrome in end-stage renal disease. *Amer J Kidney Dis.* 1996;28:372–378.
36. Wetter TC, Stiasny K, Kohnen R, et al. Polysomnographic sleep measures in patients with uremic and idiopathic restless legs syndrome. *Move Disorders.* 1998;13:820–824.
37. Stepanski E, Faber M, Zorick F, et al. Sleep disorders in patients on continuous ambulatory peritoneal dialysis. *J Amer Soc Nephrol.* 1995;6:192–197.
38. Krueger JM, Fang J, Hansen MK, et al. Humoral regulation of sleep. *News Physiol Sci.* 1998;13:189–194.
39. Norman SE, Chediak AD, Freeman C. et al. Sleep disturbances in HIV infected men. *AIDS.* 1996;4:775–781.
40. Morlese JF, Qazi NA, Gazzard BG, et al. Nevirapine-induced neuropsychiatric complications, a class effect of non-nucleoside reverse transcriptase inhibitors? *AIDS.* 2002;16:1840–1841.
41. Darko DF, McCutchan J, Kripke D, et al. Fatigue, sleep disturbances, disability and indices of progression in HIV infection. *Amer J Psych.* 1992;149:514–520.
42. Norman SE, Chediak AD, Freeman C, et al. Sleep disturbances in men with asymptomatic human immunodeficiency virus (HIV) infection. *Sleep.* 1992;15:150–155.
43. White JL, Darko DF, Brown SJ, et al. Early central nervous system response to HIV infection: sleep distortion and cognitive motor decrements. *AIDS.* 1995;9:1043–1050.
44. Cruess DG, Antoni MH, Gonzalez J, et al. Sleep disturbance mediates the association between psychological distress and immune status among HIV-positive men and women on combination antiretroviral therapy. *J Psychosom Res.* 2003;54:185–189.
45. Greenberg HE, Ney G, Scharf SM, et al. Sleep quality in Lyme disease. *Sleep.* 1995;18:912–916.
46. Grunstein RR, Sullivan CE. Sleep apnea and hypothyroidism: mechanisms and management. *Amer J Med.* 1988;85:775–779.
47. Pelttari L, Rauhala E, Polo O, et al. Upper airway obstruction in hypothyroidism. *J Internal Med.* 1994;236:177–181.
48. Abouganem D, Taylor AL, Donna E, et al. Extreme bradycardia during sleep apnea caused by myxedema. *Arch Internal Med.* 1987;147:1497–1499.
49. Winkelman JW, Goldman H, Piscatelli N, et al. Are thyroid function tests necessary in patients with suspected sleep apnea? *Sleep.* 1996;19:790–793.
50. Grunstein RR, Ho KY, Sullivan CE. Sleep apnea in acromegaly. *Ann Internal Med.* 1991;115:527–532.
51. Astrom C, Christensen L, Gjerris F, et al. Sleep in acromegaly before and after treatment with adenomectomy. *Neuroendocrinology.* 1991;53:328–331.
52. Shipley JE, Schteingart DE, Tandon R, et al. Sleep architecture and sleep apnea in patients with Cushing's disease. *Sleep.* 1992;15:514–518.
53. Wolfe F, Smythe HA, Yunus MB, et al. The American College of Rheumatology 1990 Criteria for the classification of fibromyalgia: Report of the multi-center criteria committee. *Arthritis Rheumatol.* 1990;33:160–172.
54. Harding SM. Sleep in fibromyalgia patients: subjective and objective findings. *Amer J Med Sci.* 1998;315:367–376.
55. Bradley LA, Alarcón GS. Sex-related influences in fibromyalgia. *Sex Gender Pain.* 2000;17:281–307.
56. Okifugi A, Turk DC. Stress and psychophysiological dysregulation in patients with fibromyalgia syndrome. *Appl Psychophysiol Biofeedback.* 2002;27:129–141.
57. Neeck G. Pathogenic mechanisms of fibromyalgia . [Review] *Ageing Res Rev.* 2002;1:243–255.
58. Pillemer SR, Bradley LA, Crofford LJ, et al. The neuroscience and endocrinology of fibromyalgia. *Arthritis Rheumatol.* 1997;40:1928–1939.
59. Neeck G, Crofford LJ. Neuroendocrine perturbations in fibromyalgia and chronic fatigue syndrome. *Rheum Dis Clin North Amer.* 2000;26:989–1002 .
60. Korszun A, Sackett-Lundeen L, Papadopoulos E, et al. Melatonin levels in women with fibromyalgia and chronic fatigue syndrome. *J Rheumatol.* 1999;26:2675–2680.
61. Mountz JM, Bradley LA, Modell JG, et al. Fibromyalgia in women. Abnormalities of regional cerebral blood flow in the thalamus and the caudate nucleus are associated with low pain threshold levels. *Arthritis Rheumatol.* 1995;38:926–938.
62. Gracely RN, Petzke F, Wolf JM, et al. Functional magnetic resonance imaging evidence of augmented pain processing in fibromyalgia. *Arthritis Rheumatol.* 2002;46:1333–1343.
63. Moldofsky H. Management of sleep disorders in fibromyalgia. *Rheumatol Dis Clin North Amer.* 2002;28:353–368.
64. Branco J, Atalaia A. Paiva T. Sleep cycles and alpha-delta sleep in fibromyalgia syndrome. *J Rheumatol.* 1994;21:1113–1117.
65. Drewes AM, Nielsen KD, Taagholt SJ, et al. Sleep intensity in fibromyalgia: focus on the microstructure of the sleep process. *Brit J Rheumatol.* 1995;34:629–635.
66. Mahowald ML, Mahowald MW. Nighttime sleep and daytime functioning (sleepiness and fatigue) in less well-defined chronic rheumatic diseases with particular reference to the "alpha-delta NREM sleep anomaly." *Sleep Med.* 2000;1:195–207.
67. Roizenblatt S, Moldofsky H, Benedito-Silva AA, et al. Alpha sleep characteristics in fibromyalgia. *Arthritis Rheumatol.* 2001;44:222–230.
68. Goldenberg D, Mayskiy M, Mossey C, et al. A randomized, double-blind crossover trial of fluoxetine and amitriptyline in the treatment of fibromyalgia. *Arthritis Rheumatol.* 1996;39:1852–1859.
69. Farber L, Stratz TH, Bruckle W, et al. Short-term treatment of primary fibromyalgia with the 5-HT3-receptor antagonist tropisetron. Results of a randomized, double-blind, placebo-controlled multicenter trial in 418 patients. *Intern J Clin Pharmacol Res.* 2001;21:1–13.
70. Busch A, Schachter CL, Peloso PM, et al. Exercise for treating fibromyalgia syndrome (Cochrane Review). *The Cochrane Library.* Issue 3. Oxford: Update Software, 2002.
71. Richards SCM, Scott DL. Prescribed exercise in people with fibromyalgia: parallel group randomized controlled trial. *BMJ.* 2002;325:185–187.
72. Williams DA, Cary MA, Groner KH, et al. Improving physical functional status in patients with fibromyalgia: a brief cognitive behavioral intervention. *J Rheumatol.* 2002;29:1280–1286.
73. Moldofsky H, Lue FA, Mously C, et al. The effect of zolpidem in patients with fibromyalgia: a dose ranging, double-blind, placebo controlled, modified crossover study. *J Rheumatol.* 1996;23:529–533.
74. Bennett RM, Clark SC, Walczyk J, et al. A randomized double-blind, placebo-controlled study of growth hormone in the treatment of fibromyalgia. *Amer J Med.* 1998;104:227–231.
75. Scharf MB, Baumann M, Berkowitz DV. The effects of sodium oxybate on clinical symptoms and sleep patterns in patients with fibromyalgia. *J Rheumatol.* 2003;30:1070–1074.
76. Russell IJ. The promise of substance P inhibitors in fibromyalgia. *Rheumatol Dis Clin North Amer.* 2002;28:329–342.
77. *National Sleep Foundation Gallop Poll on adult public's experiences with night-time pain.* Washington D.C., 1996.
78. Morin CM, Gibson D, Wade J. Self-reported sleep and mood disturbance in chronic pain patients. *Clin J Pain.* 1998;14:311–314.
79. Harman K, Pivik RT, D'Eon JL, et al. Sleep in depressed and non-depressed participants with chronic low back pain: electroencephalographic and behavior findings. *Sleep.* 2002;25:775–783.
80. Wilson KG, Eriksson MY, D'Eon JL, et al. Major depression and insomnia in chronic pain. *Clin J Pain.* 2002;18:77–83.
81. Widerström–Noga EG, Felipe-Cuervo E, Yezierski RP. Chronic pain

after spinal injury: interference with sleep and daily activity. *Arch Phys Med Rehabil.* 2001;82:1571–1577.

82. Moldofsky H. Sleep and pain. *Sleep Med Rev.* 2001;5:387–398.
83. Murphy PJ, Badia P, Myers BL, et al. Nonsteroidal anti-inflammatory drugs may affect normal sleep patterns in humans. *Physiol Behav.* 1994;55:1063–1066.
84. Komaroff AL, Fagioli LR, Geiger AM, et al. An examination of the working case definition of chronic fatigue syndrome. *Amer J Med.* 1996;100:56–54.
85. Fischler B, LeBon O, Hoffmann G, et al. Sleep anomalies in the chronic fatigue syndrome. A comorbidity study. *Neuropsychobiology.* 1997;35:115–122.
86. Watson NF, Kapur V, Arguelles LM, et al. Comparison of subjective and objective measures of insomnia in monozygotic twins discordant for chronic fatigue syndrome. *Sleep.* 2003;26:324–328.
87. McAinsh J, Cruickshank JM. Beta-blockers and central nervous system side effects. *Pharmacol Ther.* 1990;46:163–197.
88. Gleiter GH, Deckert J. Adverse CNS-effects of beta-adenoceptor blockers. *Pharmacopsychiatry.* 1996;29:201–211.
89. Yamada Y, Shibuya F, Hamada J, et al. Prediction of sleep disorders induced by β-adrenergic receptor blocking agents based on receptor occupancy. *J Pharmacokinet Biopharm.* 1995;23:131–145.
90. Brismar K, Hylander B, Eliasson K, et al. Melatonin secretion related to side effects of beta-blockers from the central nervous system. *Acta Med Scand.* 1988;223:525–530.
91. Paykel ES, Fleminger R, Watson JP. Psychiatric side effects of antihypertensive drugs other than reserpine. *J Clin Psychopharmacol.* 1982;2:14–39.
92. Solomon S, Hotchkiss E, Saravay SM, et al. Impairment of memory function by antihypertensive medication. *Arch Gen Psych.* 1983;40:1109–1112.
93. Pearce CJ, Wallin JD. Labetalol and other agents that block both alpha- and beta-adrenergic receptors. *Cleveland Clin J Med.* 1994;61:59–69.
94. Monti JM. Disturbances of sleep and wakefulness associated with the use of antihypertensive agents. *Life Sci.* 1987;41:1979–1988.
95. Reid JL. New therapeutic agents for hypertension. *Br J Clin Pharmacol.* 1996;42:37–41.
96. Rosenson RS, Goranson NL. Lovastatin-associated sleep and mood disturbances. *Amer J Med.* 1993;95:548–549.
97. Keech AC, Armitage JM, Wallendszus KR, et al. Absence of effects of prolonged simvastatin therapy on nocturnal sleep in a large randomized placebo-controlled study. Oxford Cholesterol Study Group. *Br J Clin Pharmacol.* 1996;42:483–490.
98. Nolen TM. Sedative effects of antihistamines: safety, performance, learning, and quality of life. *Clin Ther.* 1997;19:39–55.
99. Schweitzer DK, Muehlbach MJ, Walsh JK. Sleepiness and performance during three day administration of cetirizine or diphenhydramine. *J Allergy Clin Immunol.* 1994;94:716–724.
100. Hindmarch I. Psychometric aspects of antihistamines. *Allergy.* 1995;50(24 Suppl.):48–54.
101. Berlin RG. Effects of H_2-receptor antagonists on the central nervous system. *Drug Develop Res.* 1989;17:97–108.
102. Penston J, Wormsley KG. Adverse reactions and interactions with H_2-receptor antagonists. *Med Toxicol.* 1986;1:192–216.
103. Janson C, Gislason T, Boman G, et al. Sleep disturbances in patients with asthma. *Respir Med.* 1990;84:37–42.
104. Estrada de la Riva G. Psychic and somatic changes observed in allergic children after prolonged steroid therapy. *South Med J.* 1958;51:865–868.
105. Fehm HL Benkowitsch R, Kern W, et al. Influences of corticosteroids, dexamethasone and hydrocortisone on sleep in humans. *Neuropsychobiology.* 1986;16:198–204.
106. Lake CR, Rosenberg DB, Gallant S, et al. Phenylpropranolamine increases plasma caffeine levels. *Clin Pharmacol Ther.* 1990;47:675–685.
107. Wetter DW, Young TB. The relation between cigarette smoking and sleep disturbance. *Prev Med.* 1994;23:328–234.
108. Davila DG, Hunt RD, Offord KP, et al. Acute effects of transdermal nicotine on sleep architecture, snoring, and sleep-disordered breathing in nonsmokers. *Amer J Respir Crit Care Med.* 1994;150:469–474.
109. Prosise GL, Bonnet MH, Berry RB, et al. Effects of abstinence form smoking on sleep and daytime sleepiness. *Chest.* 1994;105:1136–1141.
110. Obermeyer WH, Benca RM. Effects of drugs on sleep. *Neurol Clin.* 1996;14:827–840.

Recording Artifacts and Solving Technical Problems with Polysomnography Technology

James Geyer and Jennifer Parr

ARTIFACTS IN POLYSOMNOGRAPHY RECORDINGS

Loose Electrode

Description: High-frequency noise superimposed on high-amplitude slow activity with possible superimposed electrode pops.

Method for reducing or eliminating the artifact: Reprep and repaste the electrode to decrease the impedance (Fig. A-1).

Muscle (EMG) Artifact

Description: Obscuration of the background EEG and occasionally EOG by myogenic (muscle) artifact.

Method for reducing or eliminating the artifact: Ask the patient to relax; opening the jaw slightly can dramatically reduced EMG artifact. Rereferencing electrodes can also decrease artifact (Fig. A-2).

EKG in the EEG Channel Artifact

Description: A representation of the EKG in the EEG channels secondary to volume conduction of the EKG waveform. The artifact in the EEG channels should be time locked to the EKG.

Method for reducing or eliminating the artifact: Re-reference the EEG channels to A1 + A2 (Fig. A-3).

Vibration Artifact

Description: The vibration caused by leg movements or snoring can result in high frequency artifacts in other channels. One can see a manifestation of the snore registering in the chin EMG channel.

Method for reducing or eliminating the artifact: This artifact is very difficult to reduce but should be recognized as a normal physiologic occurrence (Fig. A-4).

Electrode Pop Artifact

Description: Very sharp, spikelike deflection originating from a mechanically or electrically unstable electrode. The deflections should have no electrical field and should be isolated to a single electrode. The deflection may however be seen in multiple channels if that electrode is used as a component of a channel.

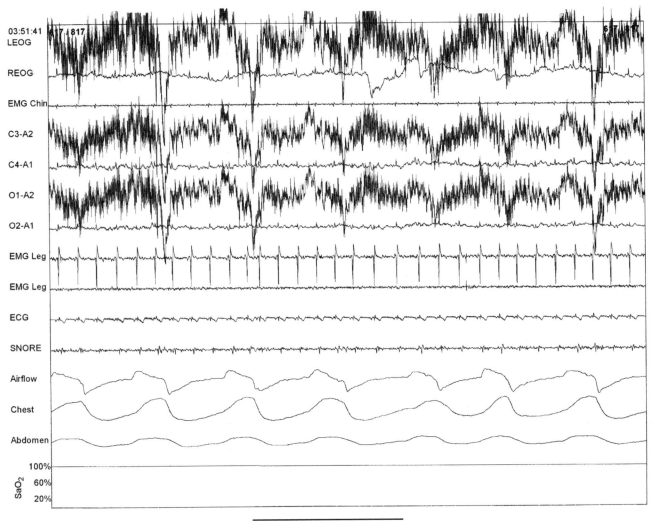

FIGURE A-1. Loose electrode.

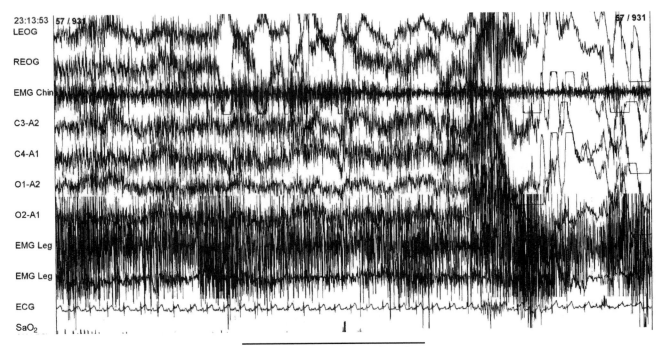

FIGURE A-2. Muscle (EMG) artifact.

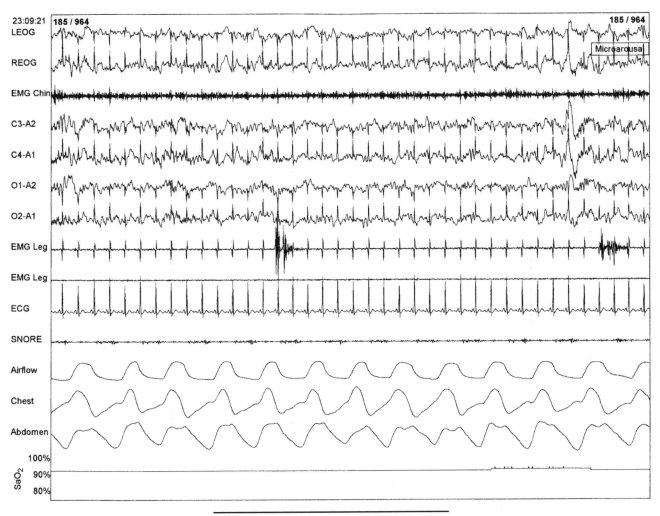

FIGURE A-3. EKG in the EEG channel artifact.

Method for reducing or eliminating the artifact: Reprep and repaste the electrode to decrease the impedance (Fig. A-5).

Cardio Ballistic Artifact

Description: A pulse wave may be seen in the chest belt or abdominal belt that has only a slight delay behind the EKG channel. A representation of the pulse wave may be seen in airflow channels, nasal pressure monitors, and in esophageal pressure-monitoring channels.

Method for reducing or eliminating the artifact: This artifact is very difficult to reduce but should be recognized as a normal physiologic occurrence (Fig. A-6).

Blink Artifact

Description: An electric dipole is created by the eye, with the cornea being electropositive and the retina being electronegative. Eyelid movement also creates an electrical potential. Eye and eyelid movement creates a frontally (with

variable amplitude and field depending upon the direction of gaze) predominate slow wave.

Method for reducing or eliminating the artifact: This artifact is very difficult to reduce but should be recognized as a normal physiologic occurrence (Fig. A-7).

Sweat Artifact

Description: Slow delta frequency rolling or swaying deflections are superimposed on the background EEG. One can see the sweat artifact most prominently in the O1-A2 channel.

Method for reducing or eliminating the artifact: Decrease the room temperature by lowering the air-conditioner temperature or by turning on a fan. Use of filtering to decrease in the artifact can result in alteration of physiologic waveforms (Fig. A-8).

Loose Belt Artifact

Description: Effort channels begin to flatten without any evident movement despite continued respiratory effort

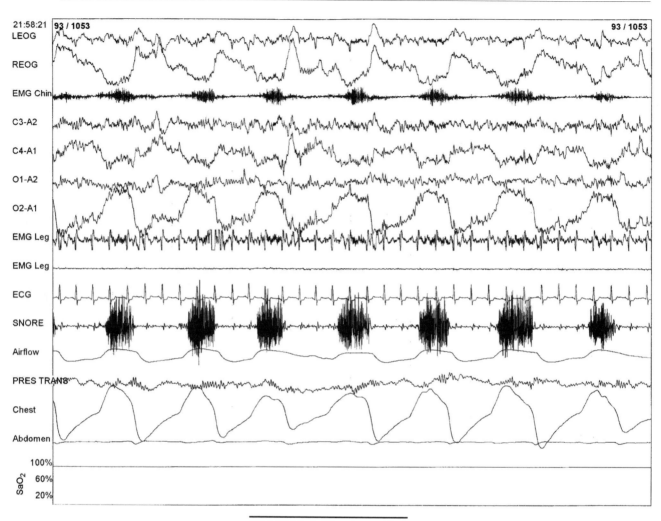

FIGURE A-4. Vibration artifact.

because the belt is no longer tight enough or in the appropriate location to accurately reflect movement.

Method for reducing or eliminating the artifact: Tighten the loose belt.

Swallow Artifact

Description: The glossokinetic potential occurs because the tip of the tongue is more electrically negative than the base of the tongue. Movement of the tongue may result in a slow wave, predominantly in the temporal regions. One can see the swallow occurring during the arousals.

Method for reducing or eliminating the artifact: This artifact is very difficult to reduce but should be recognized as a normal physiologic occurrence.

Misplaced Thermocouple Artifact

Description: The airflow-sensing thermocouple can move from its proper position. When the thermocouple moves, it

may no longer be able to monitor changes in temperature between inhalation and exhalation.

Method for reducing or eliminating the artifact: Place thermocouple in proper position.

Humidifier Condensation or Drainage in the Continuous Positive Air Pressure Tubing

Description: In the airflow channels, there may be an M-shaped waveform with each breath as the water moves backward and forward in the tubing.

Method for reducing or eliminating the artifact: Drain water from the tubing.

Rectus Spike Artifact

Description: The electric potential created by the rectus eye muscles can create a small spikelike discharge in the frontal and frontotemporal EEG derivations.

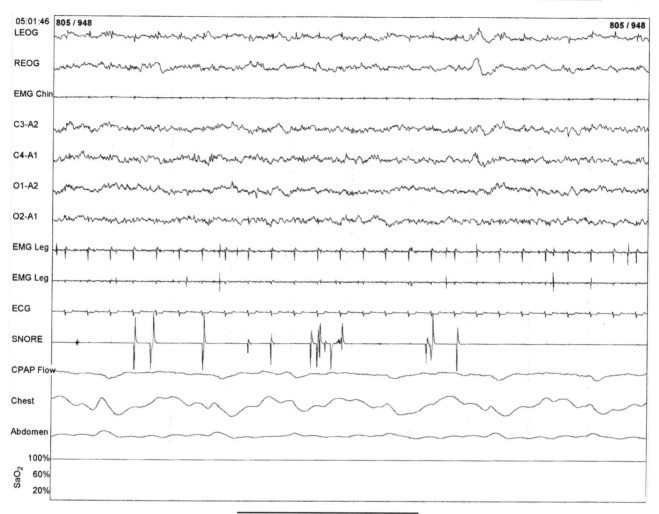

FIGURE A-5. Electrode pop artifact.

Method for reducing or eliminating the artifact: This artifact is very difficult to reduce but should be recognized as a normal physiologic occurrence.

Sixty-Hertz Artifact

Description: Lighting, electrical wiring, and machinery can produce electrical artifact, which occurs at approximately 60 Hz. This may be superimposed on baseline EEG, EKG, EOG, and EMG waveforms.

Method for reducing or eliminating the artifact: Reprep or reattach electrodes. Check ground lines. Turn off lighting and any unnecessary electrical equipment.

CONTINUOUS POSITIVE AIR PRESSURE COMPLICATIONS AND POTENTIAL RESPONSES

- Nasal drainage—treat with nasal saline spray, nasal steroid spray, or over-the-counter nasal decongestant sprays.

- Nasal congestion—increase heated humidity, nasal spine saline spray, nasal steroid spray, and when occurring on an infrequent basis, over-the-counter nasal decongestant sprays.
- Poor seal/mask leak—tighten headgear, refit mask, try a new style of mask.
- Sore nose—loosen headgear, if no improvement try a new mask style, topical antibiotic ointment.
- Nasal dryness—increase heated humidification, nasal saline spray.
- Nosebleeds—increase heated humidification, nasal saline spray.
- Allergy to mask material—change to a hypoallergenic mask.
- Patient reports pressure feels too high, but study shows that setting is correct—change to C-flex produced by Respironics.
- Difficulty exhaling—use lowest possible CPAP setting, change to a bilevel pressure system, change to C-flex by Respironics.
- Claustrophobia—educate patients on the possibility of

claustrophobia and that it will likely improve over time, select mask for patient comfort, meditation, CPAP adjustment periods during wakefulness, sedative medications, or anxiolytic medications at bedtime if necessary.

- Air swallowing (aerophagia) and gas—chin strap, bilevel pressure, educate patients on the possibility that this may occur.

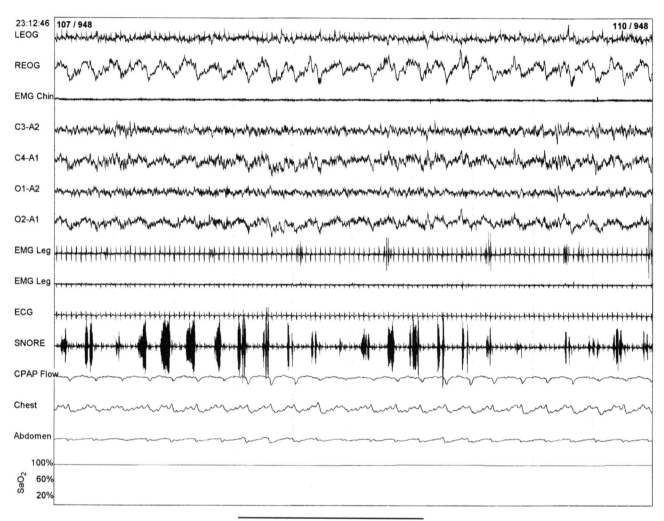

FIGURE A-6. Cardio ballistic artifact.

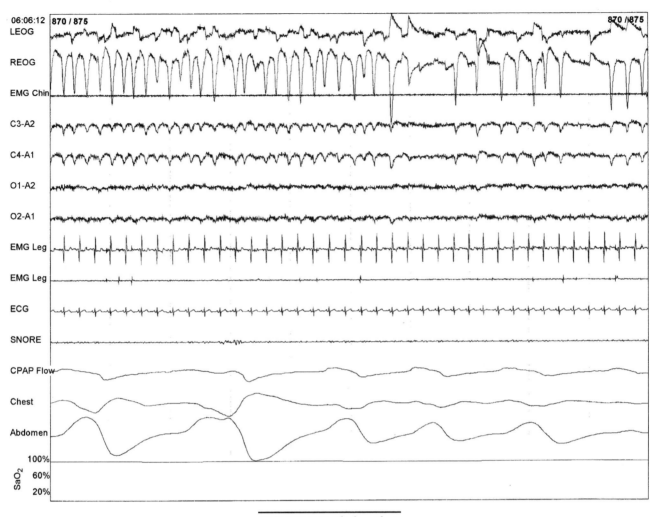

FIGURE A-7. Blink artifact.

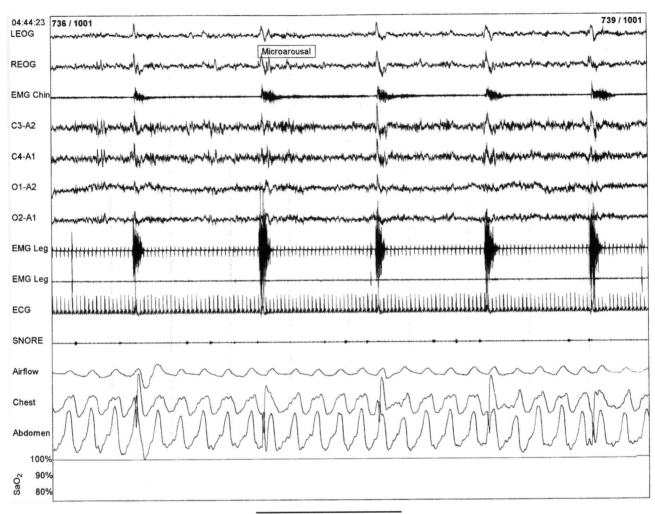

FIGURE A-8. Sweat artifact.

Sleep Questionnaires

Danielle A. Becker, Susan R. Bongiolatti, and Paul R. Carney

The following appendix provides a listing of several adult and pediatric sleep questionnaires and scales that may be of benefit to investigators. A variety of subjective measures are presented, including measures of sleep quality, daytime sleepiness, physicians' sleep knowledge, beliefs about sleep and insomnia, and the functional outcomes of sleep disturbance. This appendix is not exhaustive, but rather offers a selection of commonly referenced items found via literature review.

PEDIATRIC SLEEP QUESTIONNAIRES

Pediatric Daytime Sleepiness Scale (PDSS)

Drake C, Nickel C, Burduvali E, et al. The pediatric daytime sleepiness scale (PDSS): sleep habits and school outcomes in middle-school children. *Sleep*. 2003;26(4):455–458.

- Eight-item scale that assesses relationship between daytime sleepiness and school-rated outcomes
- Developed to measure daytime sleepiness in middle-school children

The Pediatric Sleep Survey

Owens JA. The practice of pediatric sleep medicine: Results of a community survey. *Pediatrics* 2001;108(3):E51.

- Forty-two-item questionnaire developed to assess pediatricians' familiarity with sleep in children
- Measures knowledge base, clinical screening, diagnostic, and treatment practices, and attitudes regarding impact of sleep disorders

Children's Sleep Habits Questionnaire (CSHQ)

Owens JA, Spirito A, McGuinn M. The Children's sleep habits questionnaire (CSHQ): psychometric properties of a survey instrument for school-aged children. *Sleep*. 2000;23(8):1043–1051.

- Forty-five-item parent report sleep-screening instrument designed for school-aged children
- Evaluates bedtime behavior and sleep onset, sleep duration, anxiety around sleep, sleep-disordered breathing, parasomnias, and morning waking–daytime sleepiness

OSA-18

Franco RA Jr, Rosenfeld RM, Rao M. First place – resident clinical science award 1999. Quality of life for children with obstructive sleep apnea. *Otolaryngol Head Neck Surg*. 2000;123:9–16.

- Eighteen-item health-related quality of life assessment for pediatric patients with obstructive sleep apnea
- Designed for caregivers to complete, covering sleep disturbance, physical symptoms, emotional symptoms, daytime functioning, and caregiver concerns

Pediatric Sleep Questionnaire (PSQ)

Chervin RD, Hedger K, Dillon JE, et al. Pediatric Sleep Questionnaire (PSQ): validity and reliability of scales for sleep-disordered breathing, snoring, sleepiness, and behavioral problems. *Sleep Med*. 2000;1:21–32.

- Seventy-item close-ended parent-report measure used to assess the presence of sleep-related breathing disorders
- Includes items on sleep-disordered breathing, daytime sleepiness, and sleep hygiene

OSA–QOL Questionnaire

Cohen SR, Suzman D, Simms C, et al. Sleep apnea surgery versus tracheostomy in children: an exploratory study of the comparative effects on quality of life. *Plastic Reconst Surg*. 1998;102(6):1855–1864.

- Seventy-six-item questionnaire on health and sleep related questions, medical visits and costs, and psychosocial functioning
- Developed to assess posttreatment quality of life in patients with obstructive sleep apnea

ADULT SLEEP QUESTIONNAIRES AND SCALES

Women's Health Initiative Insomnia Rating Scale (WHIIRS)

Levine DW, Kaplan RM, Kripke DF, et al. Factor structure and measurement invariance of the Women's Health Initiative Insomnia Rating Scale. *Psych Assess*. 2003;15(2):123–136.

- Five-item scale developed to assess insomnia symptoms
- Provides information on sleep latency, sleep maintenance, early morning awakening, and sleep quality

Sleep Timing Questionnaire (STQ)

Monk TH, Buysse DJ, Kennedy KS, et al. Measuring sleep habits without using a diary: the sleep timing questionnaire. *Sleep*. 2003;26(2):208–212.

- Eighteen-item single-administration instrument designed to assess the habitual timing of an individual's sleep (e.g., time one goes to bed and time one wakes up)
- Designed to yield measures of sleep equivalent to those obtained from a formal sleep diary

Berlin Sleep Questionnaire

Netzer NC, Stoohs RA, Netzer CM, et al. Using the Berlin Questionnaire to identify patients at risk for the sleep apnea syndrome. *Ann Internal Med*. 1999;131(7):485–491.

- Brief questionnaire developed to identify patients with sleep apnea
- Assesses risk factors for sleep apnea including snoring behavior, waketime sleepiness or fatigue, and the presence of obesity or hypertension

Functional Outcomes of Sleep Questionnaire (FOSQ)

Weaver TE, Laizner AM, Evans LK, et al. An instrument to measure functional status outcomes for disorders of excessive sleepiness. *Sleep*. 1997;20: 835–843.

- Thirty-item measure designed to assess the impact of disorders of excessive sleepiness on functional status
- Assesses five domains of everyday living and quality of life including: activity level, vigilance, intimacy, general productivity, and social outcome

Sleep Disorders Questionnaire (SDQ)

Douglass AB, Bornstein R, Nino-Murcia G, et al. The Sleep Disorders Questionnaire, I. Creation and multivariate structure of SDQ. *Sleep*. 1994;17(2):160–167.

- Questionnaire (175-item) developed from the Sleep Questionnaire and Assessment of Wakefulness (SQAW) that is designed to assess the presence of common sleep disorders
- Includes four main factors: sleep apnea, narcolepsy, psychiatric sleep disturbance, and periodic movement disorders

Sleep–Wake Activity Inventory (SWAI)

Rosenthal L, Roehers TA, Roth T. The sleep wake inventory: a self-report measure of daytime sleepiness. *Biol Psych*. 1993;34(11):810–820.

- Nineteen-item multidimensional self-report measure of sleepiness
- Includes six factors: excessive daytime sleepiness, psychic distress, social desirability, energy level, ability to relax, and nocturnal sleep

Dysfunctional Beliefs and Attitudes about Sleep (DBAS)

Morin, C. M. *Insomnia: psychological assessment and management*. New York: Guilford Press, 1993.

- Twenty-eight-item scale assessing beliefs, attitudes, expectations, and attributions about sleep and insomnia
- Questions reflect five themes: (a) misattributions or amplification of the consequences of insomnia, (b) diminished perception of control and predictability of sleep, (c) unrealistic sleep expectations, (d) misconceptions about the causes of insomnia, and (e) faulty beliefs about sleep-promoting practices

Epworth Sleepiness Scale (ESS)

Johns MW. A new method for measuring daytime sleepiness: The Epworth sleepiness scale. *Sleep*. 1991;14(6):540–545.

- Self-administered scale used to measure an individual's general level of daytime sleepiness
- Assesses likeliness to fall asleep in eight different situations (e.g., watching TV)

Karolinska Sleep Scale (KSS)

Akerstedt TR, Gillberg M. Subjective and objective sleepiness in the active individual. *Intern J Neurosci*. 1990;52:29–37.

- Nine-point verbally anchored self-rating scale of sleepiness

Pittsburgh Sleep Quality Index (PSQI)

Buysse DJ, Reynolds CF, Monk TH, et al. The Pittsburgh Sleep Quality Index: a new instrument for psychiatric practice and research. *Psych Res.*1989;28:193–213.

- Measure of sleep quality and disturbances during the previous month
- Yields a global sleep score and derived subscales including: (1) subjective sleep quality; (2) sleep-onset latency; (3) total amount of sleep; (4) sleep efficiency; (5) specific sleep disturbances; (6) use of sleep medication; and (7) daytime dysfunction

Verran and Snyder–Halpern (VSH) Sleep Scale

Snyder-Halpern R, Verran JA. Instrumentation to describe subjective sleep characteristics in healthy subjects. *Res Nursing Health*. 1987;10:155–163.

- Sixteen-item visual analog sleep scale
- Measures three dimensions of sleep: sleep disturbance, sleep effectiveness, and sleep supplementation (need for sleep after arousal)

St. Mary's Hospital Sleep Questionnaire (SMHSQ)

Ellis BW, Johns MW, Lancaster R, et al. The St. Mary's Hospital Sleep Questionnaire: a study of reliability. *Sleep*. 1981;4(1):93–97.

- Fourteen-item measure assessing an individual's previous night sleep, including sleep quantity, sleep quality, sleep latency, and early morning awakening
- Designed for repeated use with a particular focus on the needs of the hospital patient

Leeds Sleep Evaluation Questionnaire (LSEQ)

Parrott AC, Hindmarch I. Factor analysis of a sleep evaluation questionnaire. *Psychol Med*. 1978;8(2):325–329.

- Ten-item questionnaire providing subjective ratings of medication effects on aspects of sleep and early morning behavior
- Scales grouped chronologically and include ease of falling asleep, quality of sleep, ease of waking, and integrity of early morning behavior after wakefulness

Stanford Sleepiness Scale (SSS)

Hoddes E, Zarcone V, Smythe H, Phillips R, Dement WC. Quantification of sleepiness: a new approach. *Psychophysiology*. 1973;10:431–436.

- Seven-point self-rating scale that is used to quantify level of sleepiness versus alertness.

Starting a Sleep-Disorders Facility

James D. Geyer and Betty J. Seals

Due to the overwhelming evidence that sleep disorders affect a significant portion of the population, a sleep facility is a vital component in a community's medical delivery system. A sleep-disorders facility can be freestanding or established as a hospital-based program. Hospital-based programs have many advantages including support with marketing, billing, equipment maintenance and emergency response, just to name a few. This document is written based on the needs of developing a hospital-based facility, and the terms program and facility will be used interchangeably. Three things are essential to the development of a program. A successful hospital-based program is dependent upon research, planning, and commitment. Program implementation can be an expensive endeavor, which requires adequately trained staff, costly equipment, and appropriate space. The program can, however, become a significant resource to your medical community as well as a revenue-generating service if you have researched your community needs, planned appropriately for the operations of the program, and secured commitment from the key players in your organization.

RESEARCHING COMMUNITY NEEDS

With help from the hospital's marketing department, a demographic assessment should be made of the communities served by the hospital. If an adequate percentage of the population falls between the ages of 30 to 60 years, then a sleep-disorders program is usually indicated. Generally speaking, one sleep bed per 10,000 adults in this age range will be needed. This need can vary considerably based on public and physician awareness of sleep disorders. Therefore, the marketing department will also be needed to assist with educational programs for the medical community and the public.

OPERATIONAL PLANNING

Many states require accreditation from the American Academy of Sleep Medicine (AASM) as a prerequisite to reimbursement for sleep studies. Major insurance carriers within the program's state should be contacted during the planning process to understand their reimbursement requirements. Even if accreditation is not required for reimbursement, it is strongly suggested that the Standards of Accreditation from the AASM be used as a template for program development and that accreditation be a goal of the program. This will ensure a quality program. Two levels of accreditation can be granted—accreditation as a *Sleep Center* or accreditation as a *Laboratory for Sleep-Related Breathing Disorders*. Although the services of an accredited *Laboratory for Sleep-Related Breathing Disorders* are limited in scope, this type laboratory must meet many of the same high standards as a full-service center (1).

The first step of the planning process should be the selection of a medical director. This physician must be licensed in the state in which the program resides. Each accredited program must have a Diplomat of the American Board of Sleep Medicine (ABSM) on staff. Therefore, it is suggested that the medical director hold these credentials. The medical director will be a key player in the training and development of the technical staff working in the facility. This individual will also be responsible for the safety and proper testing of patients and ensure that patients tested in the facility meet the Clinical Practice Parameters as defined by the AASM (2). The medical director should also be involved in the marketing of the program as well as the education of the medical community and public about sleep disorders. In addition to the medical director, the program should also have an administrative director who will be responsible for the general management and daily operations of the facility.

With input from the medical and administrative directors, appropriate space should be chosen for the program. This space must be in a location that affords privacy, comfort, and security for patients. The patient testing rooms should be a minimum of 140 square feet with bathrooms in each room. Handicap-accessible rooms must be available and rooms should be light- and sound-insulated. It is essential that the facility be rapidly accessible by emergency personnel. A separate control room located on the same floor must be available for the technical staff. (3). Many facilities begin with two sleep testing rooms, along with a control room, and expand as growth occurs through physician education and public awareness. It is suggested that adequate space be chosen initially, with growth in mind. Relocating equipment can be costly as well as interruptive to program operations.

Equipment must be capable of reliable and continuous recordings with 12-channel or greater capabilities. Each sleep room should have one dedicated machine for polysomnographic recording, and all data from an overnight study should be collected on a single recorder (1). Review stations will also be necessary for summarizing or scoring collected data prior to physician interpretation. Equipment from at least three different vendors should be evaluated prior to purchase. Many varieties of equipment exist and the equipment best suited to your needs should be chosen. Ambulatory equipment as well as in-home portable equipment is becoming increasingly available, although indications for its use are subject to debate among sleep clinicians (1). A variety of technical artifacts can occur with ambulatory and in-home studies, which could result in uninterpretable recordings.

Choosing the appropriate technical staff is critical to the operations of a successful sleep program. The recruitment and interviewing process is time consuming but will prove to be beneficial to the appropriate selection of staff. Individuals with backgrounds in sleep testing are preferred but they can be difficult to find. Even more difficult to find are Registered Polysomnographic Technologists (RPSGT). Technicians with backgrounds in respiratory therapy or electroneurodiagnostics can be trained to function as sleep technologists. The knowledge obtained in these two fields will be used extensively in the sleep program. A medical director, who is a board-certified sleep specialist, should be involved in the training process of the technical staff. Training periods last 6 months to 1 year (1). Following training, the sleep technical staff should become credentialed as Registered Polysomnographic Technologists through a written exam administered by the Board of Registered Polysomnographic Technologists (BRPT). Specifics on the credentialing process can be obtained through the BRPT management office. RPSGT credentials demonstrate competence in all technical aspects of polysomnography (PSG) (4) and will symbolize quality for a program. A chief sleep technologist should be appointed for the program. This individual will be responsible for coordinating staff training as well as nightly work schedules for the staff. Accreditation by the AASM requires that at least one Registered Polysomnographic Technologist be on staff in an accredited sleep program. AASM standards also require patient-to-sleep-technologist ratio of two to one (3). Each sleep technologist usually works three 12-hour night shifts per week. Therefore, operation of a four-bed facility six nights per week will require four sleep technologists. A daytime technologist will also be needed, in addition to nighttime technologists. This daytime technologist will be responsible for summarizing or scoring the data collected during all nighttime recordings. After scoring by the daytime technologist, the sleep study will be ready for interpretation by the appropriate physician. The daytime technologist must also be capable of conducting tests on patients, including sleep studies and other procedures such as multiple sleep latency testing (MSLT). Per diem staff should also be trained to fill in during times of absenteeism by full-time staff. This will eliminate the risk of costly service interruptions.

COMMITMENT

A sleep-disorders program should not be established with the idea that it will guarantee revenue, but with the intention that it will provide a needed clinical patient service (1). Therefore, commitment to the program should come from all levels of administration in the host institution. Most well-run and quality-oriented programs do, however, prove to be profitable.

REFERENCES

1. American Academy of Sleep Medicine (formerly American Sleep Disorders Association). *Starting a sleep disorders center.* Revised ed. Minnesota: American Sleep Disorders Association Accreditation Committee, 1989.
2. American Academy of Sleep Medicine Accreditation Committee. *Clinical practice parameters developed by the standards of practice committee.* Rochester, NY: American Academy of Sleep Medicine, 2002.
3. American Academy of Sleep Medicine. *Standards for accreditation of a sleep disorders center.* Revised ed. Illinois: American Academy of Sleep Medicine Accreditation Committee, 2002.
4. Board of Registered Polysomnographic Technologists. *BRPT candidate handbook,* 2003.

Pharmacological Treatments[a]

Deborah M. Ringdahl, Christie G. Snively, and Paul R. Carney

---

[a] Note: Antidepressants are not FDA approved as hypnotics; all hypnotics should be tapered to avoid rebound insomnia.

▶ TABLE D-1.

Generic Name	Trade Name	Drug Class	Dosage	Usual Doses	Half-life (h)	Side Effects
Acetaminophen, 500 mg/ diphenhydramine citrate, 38 mg	Excedrin PM	Analgesic/antihistamine	Tabs, cap	2 Caps	Acetaminophen 2–4; diphenhydramine citrate 2–8	Anticholinergic effects (diphenhydramine); morning sedation
Acetaminophen, 500 mg/ diphenhydramine hydrochloride 25 mg	Tylenol PM	Analgesic/antihistamine	Tabs, caps	1 Cap	Acetaminophen 2–4; diphenhydramine hydrochloride 2–8	Anticholinergic effects (diphenhydramine); morning sedation
Clonazepam Diphenhydramine hydrochloride 50 mg	Klonopin Unisom	Benzodiazepine Antihistamine	0.5 mg, 1 mg tabs Tabs, caps	0.5 mg; 0.25 for elderly	34 Diphenhydramine hydrochloride, 2–8	Morning sedation Anticholinergic side effects, (diphenhydramine)
Doxepin	Sinequan	Antidepressant	10 mg, 25 mg, 50 mg, 75 mg, 100 mg, 150 mg tabs	50 mg 25 mg for elderly; not recommended for children	8–25	Drowsiness, anticholinergic effects, CNS overstimulation, nausea, extrapyramidal symptoms, hypotension
Estazolam	Prosom	Benzodiazepine (hypnotic)	1 mg, 2 mg tabs	Adults 1–2 mg at bedtime; elderly, low weight, debilitated, 0.5 mg–1 mg; max for skilled nursing care resident 0.5 mg; children and adolescents, not established.	17	Sedation, dizziness, weakness
Flurazepam	Dalmane	Benzodiazepine (hypnotic)	15 mg, 30 mg caps	Usual dose 15–30 mg at bedtime; elderly or debilitated 15 mg	2 (active metabolite 30–200)	Dizziness and lightheadedness, daytime sedation
Lorazepam	Ativan	Benzodiazepine	1 mg tabs	1 mg; 0.5 mg for elderly	15	Rebound insomnia if abruptly discontinued
Melatonin	Melatonix melatonin CR	Hormone (secreted by pineal gland)	0.3 mg circadian (phase shifting) 1–4 mg (hypnotic) tabs	No systematic studies	45 minutes (mean elimination (h))	Potentiates CNS depression with alcohol, other CNS depression; drowsiness, dizziness, anticholinergic effects, gastritis, paradoxical excitement, blood dyscrasias, hypotension

(continued)

TABLE D-1. (*Continued*)

Generic name	Trade Name	Drug Class	Dosage	Usual Doses	Half-life (h)	Side Effects
Mirtazapine	Remeron	Antidepressant	15 mg, 30 mg, 45 mg tabs	Hypnotic: 15 mg; 7.5 mg for the elderly; maybe less sedating at higher doses 30–45 mg	20–40	Somnolence, increased appetite, weight gain dizziness, nausea, dry mouth, constipation, asthenia, flu syndrome
Nefazodone	Serzone	Antidepressant	50 mg, 100 mg, 150 mg, 200 mg, 250 mg tabs	100 mg; 50 mg for the elderly; not recommended for children	2–4	Headache, nausea, dizziness, insomnia, asthenia, agitation, dry mouth, constipation, blurred or abnormal vision; *Rare:* severe liver injury/failure
Quazepam	Doral	Benzodiazepine (hypnotic)	7.5 mg, 15 mg tabs	15 mg at bedtime; decrease to 7.5 mg at bedtime after 1–2 days; elderly, 7.5 mg at bedtime and increase to 15 mg after 1–2 days; children not established	Active metabolite 100	CNS depression, ataxia, headache, dry mouth, GI upset
Temazepam	Restoril	Benzodiazepine (hypnotic)	7.5 mg, 15 mg, 30 mg caps	Usual dose 15 mg 30 minutes before bedtime; half dose is recommended in the elderly; children not established.	11	Sedation, dizziness; rebound insomnia if abruptly discontinued
Trazodone hydrochloride	Desyrel	Antidepressant	50 mg, 100 mg, 150 mg, 300 mg tabs	50 mg; 25 mg for elderly	5–9	Drowsiness, dizziness, rare anticholinergic effects, cardiac arrhythmias, extrapyramidal symptoms, hypotension (alpha blockade), priapism, impotence seizures
Triazolam	Halcion	Benzodiazepine (hypnotic)	0.125 mg 0.25 mg tabs	Adults 0.25 mg; low body weight 0.125 mg; max dose 0.5 mg; elderly 0.125 max 0.25 mg; children and adolescents not established.	2	Dizziness and lightheadedness, drowsiness, poor coordination, memory loss; rebound insomnia if abruptly discontinued
Zaleplon	Sonata	Sedative (hypnotic)	5–10 mg caps	10 mg immediately before bedtime or after going to bed (at least 4 hours before becoming active again); max 20 mg; elderly or debilitated: initially 5 mg at bedtime	1	Daytime drowsiness, amnesia, paresthesia, abnormal vision, hyperacusis, anorexia, depersonalization
Zolpidem tartrate	Ambien	Sedative (hypnotic)	5–10 mg tabs	Elderly or debilitated: initially 5 mg at bedtime, max 10 mg; not recommended for children under 18 yrs; elderly, debilitated, pregnancy, category B, nursing mothers, not recommended.	2–3	Dizziness, daytime drowsiness, diarrhea, drugged feeling, amnesia

REFERENCES

1. Clinical Pharmacology Online, Gold Standard Multimedia, 2004.
2. Kaplan HI, Sadock MD. *Pocket handbook of clinical psychiatry.* Baltimore, MD: Williams and Wilkins, 1996.
3. Murphy J. *Nurse practitioners prescribing reference.* Prescribing refer RPh. Prescribing Reference, 2004.
4. www.ArthritisCentral.com

Introduction to Electroencephalograms

James Geyer and Richard B. Berry

The international 10–20 system for electrode placement is illustrated in Fig. E-1. The common electrode designations are Fp, frontopolar; F, frontal; P, parietal; O, occipital; T, temporal with numerical subscripts representing position. The odd subscripts are on the left and the even on the right.

A montage is created by combining electrodes into channels. These derivations represent the voltage difference between electrodes. For example Fp1–F3 is the voltage difference between electrodes Fp1 and F3. By convention, if Fp1 is more negative than F3; the deflection is up. Bipolar montages compare two standard in a sequential fashion. Referential montages refer recording electrodes to one or more reference electrodes. In modern digital EEG recording, usually all electrodes are recorded against a common reference. Any two electrodes may then be compared by subtracting the signals (F7-ref) – (P7-ref) = F7 – P7.

A spike is defined as a transient with a pointed peak and a duration of 20 to 70 milliseconds (Fig. E-1). At polysomnography (PSG) paper speed (30-second page) spikes look like a single vertical line. A sharp wave is a transient with a pointed peak and a deflection of 70 to 200 millseconds. Interictal epileptiform activity is an abnormal, sharply contoured EEG activity that occurs between seizures. Because seizures rarely appear during recording, the physician must recognize the interictal pattern of epilepsy.

Localized spikes will show *phase reversal* if the bipolar chains cross the area of the seizure focus, typically with a field (electric representation in the nearby electrodes). This may help differentiate them from artifact. For example, in Fig. E-1, negative spike activity is seen at electrode T7. This results in downgoing deflections in F7-T7. In this figure "s" stands for spike and "w" for wave.

If the spike focus is between two monitoring electrodes, the derivation connecting them may show little or no activity and the derivations on either side will show phase reversal.

Since both the central and ear electrodes typically used in PSG recordings are active, epileptiform activity may arise from either electrode, making localization very difficult. At the usual PSG compressed time, base (paper speed) spikes are difficult to recognize. Digital equipment with an adjustable time base allows for closer inspection of the EEG, but filter settings and sampling frequency must be considered (Table E-1).

BENIGN ELECTROENCEPHALOGRAPHIC PATTERNS

14 and 6-Hz positive spikes—are brief posterior temporal "spikes" that occur during drowsiness and light sleep in adolescents.

Benign epileptiform transients of sleep (BETS) or **small sharp spikes of sleep** (SSSS)—occur in one-fourth of adults during drowsiness and light sleep. They consist of monophasic or biphasic spikes often followed by a slow wave; may have horizontal dipole.

6-Hz spikes (phantom spike and wave)—are small "spikes" that occur in the drowsy 2.5% of adults.

Wicket spikes—are 6- to 12-Hz, temporally maximal, intermittent trains of sharp activity resembling Mu rhythm or sporadic single spikes that are surface negative and essentially monophasic. They are most common in drowsiness and light sleep.

Rhythmic mid-temporal bursts of drowsiness (RMTD)—most common in drowsiness or light sleep in young adults. The EEG consists of rhythmic, notched, sharpened theta waves with unilateral or bitemporal predominance, lasting up to 10 seconds.

Subclinical rhythmic electrographic discharges in adults (SCREDA)—occurs with bursts of rhythmic sharp

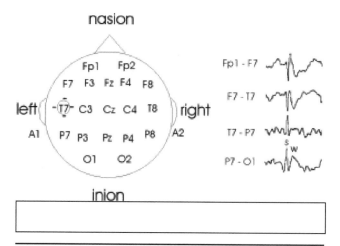

FIGURE E-1. Electrode position on the right and a spike on the left.

theta, with abrupt onset and offset in the parietal and temporal derivations. It can last for several seconds and look like a seizure, but the background may be visible and there is no postictal slowing.

ABNORMAL ELECTROENCEPHALOGRAMS

Delta activity (<4 Hz)—always abnormal in awake adults, except in elderly, if it represents less than 1% of the record.

Persistent polymorphic delta activity (PPDA) is seen in white matter lesions, postictal states, or ipsilateral thalamic lesions. Intermittent rhythmic delta activity (IRDA) may arise from dysfunction of subcortical centers influencing activation of cortex.

Epileptiform activity and epilepsy—occurs in 2% to 4% of nonepileptic patients. Patients with epilepsy have an abnormal first EEG 50% to 55% of the time. Sleep deprivation activates epileptiform activity in 34% to 41% of epileptic patients.

Seizures may occur with several different EEG patterns. Rhythmic sinusoidal discharges occur in two-thirds of clinical seizure onset and in one third of subclinical seizure onsets. Spike and wave and repetitive spike and beta activity are common ictal patterns. Interictal epileptiform activity may disappear immediately prior to seizure. Attenuation of background activity precedes 10% of partial seizures, 10% of tonic seizures, and 40% of infantile spasms. Increasing interictal activity is rare. The interictal epileptiform activity may be greater following the seizure. At PSG recording rates, seizure activity may mimic alpha activity.

Rolandic epilepsy—associated with centrotemporal spikes that have a horizontal dipole (positive centrally, negative centrotemporally). Spikes are unilateral in 60% of cases and increase during sleep.

Landau-Kleffner syndrome—an acquired childhood aphasia with a subacute or stuttering progression. There

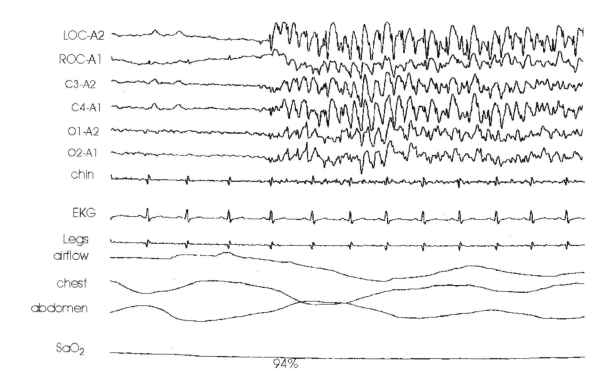

FIGURE E-2. Spike and wave activity present in all recording EEG electrodes.

▌**TABLE E-1.** **Typical Seizure Occurrence**

Seizure Type	Interictal Discharge		Ictal Discharge		
	NREM	REM	NREM	REM	After NREM[a]
Primary generalized	Common	Rare	Rare	Rare	Common
Focal	Common	Rare	Common	Rare	Possible

[a] After awakening from NREM sleep.

is continuous spike-and-wave activity in slow-wave sleep (SWS), with the seizures varying in type.

Absence epilepsy—classic EEG findings with a generalized, but frontally maximal 3-Hz spike-and-wave discharges. The frequency varies during a seizure. The background is normal between seizures.

Actigraphy: monitoring of body movement, especially for the study of insomnia, restless legs, and periodic limb movements.

Active sleep: the stage of sleep in infants that is considered to be most similar to REM sleep in adults.

Apnea hypopnea index AHI: the number of apneas and hypopneas per hour of sleep. (See also Respiratory Disturbance Index.)

Akathisia: restlessness and a strong urge to move.

Aliasing: distortion of a signal when sampled at or below the Nyquist frequency (twice the signal frequency).

Alpha rhythm: EEG activity, ranging between 8 and 13 Hz, which is typically most prominent in the parietooccipital region during wakefulness with eyes closed. The alpha rhythm is typically below 50 μV in adults; it slows by approximately 1 Hz during drowsiness.

Alpha delta sleep: alpha activity superimposed on delta activity during stage 3 and stage 4 sleep.

Alveolar hypoventilation: hypoventilation (increased arterial P_{CO_2}) typically associated with oxygen desaturations, despite the lack of apnea and hypopnea.

Apnea: cessation of airflow lasting at least 10 seconds (adults). Apneas may be obstructive, central, or mixed.

Arousal: an abrupt change from one stage of sleep to a lighter stage of sleep or from sleep to awakening.

Auto PAP (sometimes called auto CPAP): a positive airway pressure device with the ability to increase or decrease the level of CPAP in response to the presence or absence of respiratory variables that vary between devices. For example, the presence of apnea, hypopnea, snoring, or airflow limitation would trigger a slow increase in pressure depending on the algorithm used by the device.

Beta activity: EEG activity ranging between 13 and 35 Hz, usually associated with alert wakefulness or medications such as benzodiazepines and barbiturates.

Bilevel PAP: bilevel positive airway pressure with a higher pressure during inspiration and a lower pressure during expiration.

Bipolar recording: an electrode linked to a nearby electrode creates a bipolar montage.

Body mass index (BMI): weight in kilograms divided by square of height in meters squares.

Bruxism: tooth grinding or tooth gritting.

Capacitor: a device that stores separated charge. $I = C (dV/dT)$, where I = current, C = capacitance and dV/dT = the change in voltage in regard to time. $C = Q/V$, where C = capacitance, Q = charge, and V = voltage (potential difference).

Cataplexy: the sudden loss of muscle tone and deep tendon reflexes initiated with muscle weakness and paralysis. Cataplexy is typically precipitated by strong emotions, most commonly laughter, anger, or profound sadness. Cataplexy is one of the components of the classic tetrad of narcolepsy.

Central sleep apnea: cessation of airflow at the mouth and nose lasting at least 10 seconds, with no associated respiratory effort.

Cephalometry: measurement of the parameters of the upper airway and head.

Cheyne–Stokes respirations: a breathing pattern with a crescendo–decrescendo fluctuation in both respiratory rates and tidal volume. There is commonly an arousal at the maximum tidal volume.

Circadian rhythm: the fluctuation of physiologic and behavioral patterns including the sleep–wake cycle. The typical period of the circadian rhythm is between 23 and 25 hours. Recent studies have suggested that the average period in humans is just slightly longer than 24 hours.

CPAP: continuous positive airway pressure used primarily as a treatment for obstructive sleep apnea.

Delta activity: EEG activity ranging between 0 and 4 Hz. For sleep staging, delta activity is required to be <2 Hz with an amplitude greater than 75 μV peak to peak.

EEG (electroencephalogram): recording of the electrical activity of the brain.

EMG (electromyogram): recording of the electrical activity of the muscles.

Enuresis: bedwetting.

EOG (electro-oculogram): recording of the electrical activity of the eyes created by the dipole between the cornea and retina and by the electrical change created by eyelid motion.

First night effect: a change in the usual breathing and sleeping patterns of an individual caused by the foreign environment of the sleep laboratory and monitoring systems.

Fragmentary myoclonus: brief myoclonic jerks occurring at random in multiple muscle groups. This may occur as a normal component of phasic REM sleep.

Hypersomnolence: excessive sleepiness.

Hypnagogic: an event associated with the transition from wakefulness to sleep.

Hypnagogic hallucinations: vivid sensory images most commonly occurring with sleep onset REM periods.

Hypnic myoclonus: a "sleep start" or jerk occurring during the transition from drowsiness to sleep that may be associated with a sense of falling and possibly an awakening.

Hypnopompic: an event associated with the transition from sleep to wakefulness.

Hypopnea: a decrease in airflow lasting at least 10 seconds. Definitions of hypopnea vary. Two commonly used definitions are: (a) a 30% or greater reduction in flow from baseline associated with a 4% or greater drop in arterial oxygen saturation, or (b) either a 50% drop in airflow from baseline *or* any discernable drop in flow associated with an arousal or 3% or greater drop in the arterial oxygen saturation.

Impedance (Z): The effective resistance (voltage/current) of an AC current with frequency f depends on resistance (R), capacitance (C), and inductance (L). $Z = $ square root $[R^2 + (Xc^2 + X_L^2)]$. Here Xc is the capacitive reactance $= 1/\omega\, C$ and X_L is the inductive reactance $= \omega L$ and ω is $2\pi f$.

Insomnia: difficulty initiating or maintaining sleep.

K complex: a EEG waveform found in stage 2 sleep. The morphology consists of a sharp negative deflection followed by a higher voltage slow wave with a duration of at least 0.5 seconds. Sleep spindles frequently accompany the K complex.

Leakage current: currents caused by stray capacitance or stray inductance. Stray capacitance arises from the construction of the power cords and nearby electrical equipment or wiring separated by the insulators surrounding the wires. Stray inductance is created by the magnetic fields generated by current flowing through wires.

Microsleep: brief periods of sleep typically lasting up to 30 seconds, during which external stimuli are not fully recognized.

Montage: the arrangement of data displays from electrode combinations, oximetry data, and other monitoring systems.

Movement time: polysomnographic scoring term describing periods during which the EEG and EOG tracings are obscured by motion artifact for more than one-half of a scoring epoch. This term is used only when the preceding and following epochs are staged as sleep.

Mu rhythm: central alpha frequency activity typically occurring with archlike shapes that do not block with eye opening but do block with voluntary activity.

Nyquist theorem: the signal must be digitally sampled with a sampling rate of at least twice the maximum signal frequency in order to create a reliable digital representation of the signal.

Obstructive apnea: cessation of airflow at the mouth and nose lasting at least 10 seconds, with continued respiratory effort.

Parasomnia: episodic arousal or sleep stage-transition disorder, including disorders such as sleepwalking, and REM sleep behavior disorder.

Periodic limb movements: ankle dorsiflexion, great toe extension, possible knee flexion, and possible hip flexion occurring during sleep. The duration of the individual movements should be between 0.5 and 5 seconds. The movements should have a period of between 20 and 60 seconds.

Phasic events: events including motor activity or muscle twitches (leg EMG) and irregular respiratory activity, which occur during phasic REM sleep, often in association with REMs.

Polysomnogram: the recording of multiple physiologic variables during sleep.

Positive occipital sharp transients of sleep (POSTS): EEG waveforms consisting of surface-positive transient sharp activity, typically theta frequency, that may occur in small bursts of 4 to 5 Hz. POSTS are typically seen in light stage 1 and stage 2 sleep.

Quiet sleep: non-REM sleep in infants when the individual stages of non-REM sleep cannot be identified.

Referential recording: the recording electrodes are linked to one or several distant "reference" electrode(s).

Resistance: resistance dissipates the energy carried by currents, usually into heat. Extremely high resistance results in an insulator. Ohm's law states that $V = IR$, where $V = $ voltage, $I = $ current, and $R = $ resistance. In and AC circuit $V = IZ$, where Z is the impedance (see impedance).

Respiratory disturbance index (RDI): in some sleep centers this is equivalent to the AHI. In others the RDI $=$ AHI $+$ RERA index, where the RERA index is the number of respiratory effort-related arousals per hour of sleep.

Sawtooth waves: notched theta frequency activity occurring during REM sleep, with a duration of up to 10 seconds.

Sleep onset: the transition from wakefulness to sleep typically identified by slowing of the background EEG activity, vertex waves, and slow-rolling eye movements.

Sleep spindle: 11.5 to 15 Hz bursts of sine wave–shaped activity, typically lasting 0.5 to 1.5 seconds. The amplitude is typically highest over the central vertex region of the head, but is usually lower than 50 μV.

Stage 1 sleep: typically occurs at sleep onset or following arousal from other stages of sleep. The EEG should consist of lower voltage and slower activity than is seen during wakefulness. The alpha activity should consist of <50% of the scoring epoch. Vertex waves and POSTs are common. Sleep spindles and K complexes should be absent.

Stage 2 sleep: NREM sleep characterized by the presence of either sleep spindles or K complexes with a relatively low-voltage mixed-frequency background EEG. Delta activity meeting scoring criteria (less than 2 Hz in frequency and greater than 75 μV in amplitude peak-to-peak) should comprise less than 20% of a stage 2 sleep epoch.

Stage 3 sleep: NREM sleep characterized by an epoch containing between 20% and 50% delta activity, less than 2 Hz in frequency, and greater than 75 μV in amplitude.

Stage 4 sleep: NREM sleep characterized by an epoch containing greater than 50% delta activity, less than 2 Hz in frequency, and greater than 75 μV in amplitude.

Stage REM sleep: lowest resting muscle activity recorded during sleep, with intermittent bursts of rapid eye movements. The EEG consists of a low-voltage mixed-frequency activity and sawtooth waves. In patients with obstructive sleep apnea, the longest apneas and most severe arterial oxygen desaturation usually occur during REM sleep.

Theta rhythm: EEG activity ranging between 4 and 8 Hz.

Total recording time: the total amount of time from sleep onset to final awakening during a polysomnogram.

Total sleep time: the total amount of time spent sleeping during a polysomnogram.

Vertex wave: centrally predominant medium- to high-voltage, typically diphasic discharge beginning with an initial surface-negative deflection followed by a low-voltage surface-positive deflection. These occur primarily during stage 2 sleep.

Zeitgeber: a time cue serving to entrain the sleep–wake cycle. Daylight is a common cue to the time of day.

INDEX